Professional Nursing and Health Care Concepts

Concepts *for* Nursing Practice

SECOND EDITION

Jean Foret Giddens, PhD, RN, FAAN

Professor and Dean
Doris B. Yingling Endowed Chair
School of Nursing
Virginia Commonwealth University
Richmond, Virginia

ELSEVIER

ELSEVIER

3251 Riverport Lane
St. Louis, Missouri 63043

CONCEPTS FOR NURSING PRACTICE, SECOND EDITION

ISBN: 978-0-323-37473-6

Notices

Knowledge and best practice in this field are constantly changing. As new research and experience broaden our understanding, changes in research methods, professional practices, or medical treatment may become necessary.

Practitioners and researchers must always rely on their own experience and knowledge in evaluating and using any information, methods, compounds, or experiments described herein. In using such information or methods they should be mindful of their own safety and the safety of others, including parties for whom they have a professional responsibility.

With respect to any drug or pharmaceutical products identified, readers are advised to check the most current information provided (i) on procedures featured or (ii) by the manufacturer of each product to be administered, to verify the recommended dose or formula, the method and duration of administration, and contraindications. It is the responsibility of practitioners, relying on their own experience and knowledge of their patients, to make diagnoses, to determine dosages and the best treatment for each individual patient, and to take all appropriate safety precautions.

To the fullest extent of the law, neither the Publisher nor the authors, contributors, or editors, assume any liability for any injury and/or damage to persons or property as a matter of products liability, negligence or otherwise, or from any use or operation of any methods, products, instructions, or ideas contained in the material herein.

Previous edition copyrighted 2013.

Library of Congress Cataloging-in-Publication Data
Concepts for nursing practice / [edited by] Jean Foret Giddens.—Second edition.
   p. ; cm.
Includes bibliographical references and index.
ISBN 978-0-323-37473-6 (pbk. : alk. paper)
I. Giddens, Jean, editor.
[DNLM: 1. Nursing Process. 2. Nursing Care. 3. Nursing. WY 100.1]
RT42
610.73—dc23

2015026306

Content Strategist: Heidi Pohlman
Product Manager: Kristin Zurliene
Content Development Specialist: Heather Rippetoe
Publishing Services Manager: Jeff Patterson
Project Manager: Lisa A. P. Bushey
Designer: Renee Duenow

Working together
to grow libraries in
developing countries

Printed in China

Last digit is the print number: 9   8   7   6   5

www.elsevier.com • www.bookaid.org

Dr. Giddens earned a Bachelor of Science in Nursing from the University of Kansas, a Master of Science in Nursing from the University of Texas at El Paso, and a Doctor of Philosophy in Education and Human Resource Studies from Colorado State University. Dr. Giddens has 30 years' experience in nursing education spanning associate degree, baccalaureate degree, and graduate degree nursing programs in New Mexico, Texas, Colorado, and Virginia. She is an expert in concept-based curriculum development and evaluation, as well as innovative strategies for teaching and learning. Dr. Giddens is the author of multiple journal articles, nursing textbooks, and electronic media and serves as an education consultant to nursing programs throughout the country.

ACKNOWLEDGMENTS

Developing and writing *Concepts for Nursing Practice, Second Edition,* represents an amazing collaboration of educators and clinicians from multiple disciplines across the country. I extend my gratitude and appreciation to the contributors and reviewers for sharing their expertise and wisdom. I also am grateful to my colleagues at Elsevier for their expertise and guidance. Lastly, I extend deep appreciation to my husband Jay—without your friendship, love, and support, I could not accomplish such work.

CONTRIBUTORS

Alexander Anzardo, RN, BSN, PALS/BLS/ Trauma/Burn
PICU Nurse/Unit Leader
Kendall Regional Medical Center
Director of Nursing
Sweet Angels Health Services, Inc.
FNP/MSN Graduate Student
Florida International University
Miami, Florida

Gail E. Armstrong, DNP, PhD(c), ACNS-BC, CNE
Associate Professor
College of Nursing
University of Colorado
Aurora, Colorado

Nikki Austin, JD, MSN, RN
Of Counsel
Thorpe Shwer
Phoenix, Arizona

Kathleen M. Bell, MSN, RNC-OB, WHNP-BC
Director of Nursing
CrossOver Healthcare Ministry
Richmond, Virginia

Deb Bennett-Woods, EdD
Professor
Division of Health Services Education
Rueckert-Hartman College for Health Professions
Regis University
Denver, Colorado

Janet Prvu Bettger, ScD
Associate Professor
School of Nursing
Duke University
Durham, North Carolina

Janice Bissonnette, RN-NP, MScN, PhD
Advance Practice Nurse
Renal Transplantation/Nephrology
Clinician Investigator-Clinical Epidemiology Program/Ottawa Hospital Research Institute
The Ottawa Hospital
Ottawa, Ontario, Canada

Kevin Brigle, PhD, NP
Oncology Nurse Practitioner
Massey Cancer Center
Virginia Commonwealth University
Richmond, Virginia

Lorraine Buchanan, MSN, RN
Clinical Assistant Professor
School of Nursing
University of Kansas
Kansas City, Kansas

Lynne Buchanan, PhD, APRN-NP, BC
Associate Professor
College of Nursing
University of Nebraska Medical Center
Omaha, Nebraska

Lucy M. Caicedo, RN, BSN
Baptist Hospital Health System
Miami, Florida

Susan Caplan, PhD, MSN, APRN-BC
Assistant Professor
Rutgers, The State University of New Jersey
Newark, New Jersey

Barbara M. Carranti, MS, RN
Clinical Associate Professor
Department of Nursing
Le Moyne College
Syracuse, New York

Verna Benner Carson, BSN, MSN, PhD
President
C&V Senior Care Specialists, Inc
Fallston, Maryland

Helen Connors, RN, PhD, FAAN, ANEF
Professor
School of Nursing and Center for Health Informatics
University of Kansas
Kansas City, Kansas

Sean P. Convoy, BA, BSN, MSN, PMHNP-BC, DNP
Associate Professor
School of Nursing
Virginia Commonwealth University
Richmond, Virginia

Nancy Crigger, PhD, MA, APRN, BC, FAAN
Faculty Associate
Graceland University
Independence, Missouri

Robert M. Elgie, RN, MSN, BC
Clinical Instructor
College of Nursing
University of New Mexico
Albuquerque, New Mexico

Sylvia Escott-Stump, MA, RDN, LDN
Director
Dietetic Internship
East Carolina University
Greenville, North Carolina

Grethell Estrada, RN, BSN
Certified Brain Injury Specialist (CBIS)
FNP Graduate Student
Florida International University
Miami, Florida

Linda Felver, PhD, RN
Associate Professor
School of Nursing
Oregon Health & Science University
Portland, Oregon

Katherine A. Fletcher, PhD, RN, ACNS-BC, CNE
Clinical Professor
School of Nursing
University of Kansas
Kansas City, Kansas

Nelda Godfrey, PhD, ACNS-BC, FAAN
Associate Dean and Clinical Professor
School of Nursing
University of Kansas
Kansas City, Kansas

Sue K. Goebel, MS, RN, WHNP, SANE
Associate Professor of Nursing
Department of Health Sciences
Moss School of Nursing
Colorado Mesa University
Grand Junction, Colorado

Debra Hagler, PhD, RN, ACNS-BC, CNE, CHSE, ANEF, FAAN
Clinical Professor
College of Nursing and Health Innovation
Arizona State University
Phoenix, Arizona

Ingrid C. Hendrix, MILS, AHIP
Nursing Services Librarian
Health Sciences Library and Informatics Center
University of New Mexico
Albuquerque, New Mexico

Nancy Hoffart, PhD, RN
Founding Dean and Professor
Alice Ramez Chagoury School of Nursing
Lebanese American University
Byblos, Lebanon

Beth S. Hopkins, DNP, FNP
Clinical Assistant Professor
School of Nursing
Virginia Commonwealth University
Richmond, Virginia

Eun-Ok Im, PhD, MPH, RN, CNS, FAAN
Professor and Marjorie O. Rendell Endowed Professor
School of Nursing
University of Pennsylvania
Philadelphia, Pennsylvania

Nancy Jallo, PhD, FNP-BC, WHNP-BC, RNC-OB
Associate Professor
School of Nursing
Virginia Commonwealth University
Richmond, Virginia

Teresa Keller, PhD, RN
Associate Director and Assistant Dean
School of Nursing
New Mexico State University
Las Cruces, New Mexico

Sangmi Kim, RN, MPH
Doctoral Student
School of Nursing
University of Pennsylvania
Philadelphia, Pennsylvania

Kathie Lasater, EdD, RN, ANEF, FAAN
Professor
Oregon Health & Science University
Portland, Oregon

Judy Liesveld, PhD, PPCNP-BC
Associate Professor and Education Chair
College of Nursing
University of New Mexico
Albuquerque, New Mexico

Marieta Lima, RN, BSN, Vascular Access Certified
MSN/APRN Student
Florida International University
Miami, Florida

Carolyn McKenzie, RN, BSN, MSN, PhD, CNL
Associate Professor
University of North Carolina Chapel Hill
School of Nursing
Chapel Hill, North Carolina

Nicole Moore, RN, BSN
FNP Graduate Student
Duke University School of Nursing
Durham, North Carolina

Alissette Naveda, RN, BSN
ONS Member and MSN Graduate Student
Florida International University
Miami, Florida

Ann Nielsen, BS, MN, PhD, RN
Assistant Professor, Undergraduate Program Director
School of Nursing
Oregon Health & Science University
Portland, Oregon

Devon Noonan, PhD, MPH, FNP-BC
Assistant Professor
School of Nursing
Duke University
Durham, North Carolina

William Padron, RN, BSN, CPN, BLS, PALS, TRAUMA
PICU Staff Nurse and MCH Way Facilitator
Miami Children's Hospital
Miami, Florida

Iliana M. Pena, RN-BSN, Cardiac-Vascular BC
FNP Graduate Student
Florida International University
Miami, Florida

Katherine Pereira, DNP, RN, FNP-BC, ADM-BC, FAANP, FAAN
Associate Professor
School of Nursing
Duke University
Family Nurse Practitioner
Department of Medicine/Endocrinology
Duke University Medical Center
Durham, North Carolina

Shannon E. Perry, RN, PhD, FAAN
Professor Emerita
School of Nursing
San Francisco State University
San Francisco, California

Nancy Ridenour, PhD, APRN, BC, FAAN
Dean and Professor
College of Nursing
University of New Mexico
Albuquerque, New Mexico

Beth Rodgers, PhD, RN, FAAN
Professor and Research Chair
College of Nursing
University of New Mexico
Albuquerque, New Mexico

L. Jane Rosati, EdD, MSN, RN-BC
Professor
School of Nursing
Daytona State College
Daytona Beach, Florida

Carolyn E. Sabo, RN, EdD
Professor and DNP Program Coordinator
School of Nursing
University of Nevada, Las Vegas
Las Vegas, Nevada

Lana Sargent, MSN, BSN, FNP-BC, GNP-C
Assistant Professor
School of Nursing
Virginia Commonwealth University
Richmond, Virginia

Pamela Schultz, RN, BS, MS, PhD
Associate Dean and Director
School of Nursing
New Mexico State University
Las Cruces, New Mexico

Deborah Witt Sherman, PhD, ARNP, ANP-BC, ACHPN, FAAN
Professor
Nicole Wertheim College of Nursing and Health Sciences
Florida International University
Miami, Florida

Gwen Sherwood, PhD, RN, FAAN
Professor and Associate Dean for Academic Affairs
School of Nursing
University of North Carolina
Chapel Hill, North Carolina

Leigh Ann Simmons, PhD, MFT
Associate Professor
School of Nursing
Duke University
Durham, North Carolina

Diane J. Skiba, PhD, FAAN, FACMI, ANEF
Professor and Informatics Specialty Director
College of Nursing
University of Colorado
Aurora, Colorado

Leigh Small, PhD, RN, CPNP-PC, FNAP, FAANP, FAAN
Associate Professor and Department Chair
Family and Community Health Nursing
School of Nursing
Virginia Commonwealth University
Richmond, Virginia

Debra J. Smith, MSN, RN, CNE
Principal Lecturer
College of Nursing
University of New Mexico
Albuquerque, New Mexico

Angela Starkweather, PhD, ACNP-BC, CNRN, FAAN
Professor and Director
Center for Advancements in Managing Pain
University of Connecticut School of Nursing
Storrs, Connecticut

Amy Szoka, MSN, CNE, RN
Assistant Professor
Daytona State College
Daytona Beach, Florida

Susan F. Wilson, PhD, RN, CNE
Emeritus Associate Professor
Harris College of Nursing and Health Sciences
Texas Christian University
Fort Worth, Texas

P.J. Woods, PhD, MBA, RN
Associate Professor and DNP Program Director
College of Nursing
University of New Mexico
Albuquerque, New Mexico

REVIEWERS

Deb Bennett-Woods, EdD
Professor
Division of Health Services Education
Rueckert-Hartman College for Health
   Professions
Regis University
Denver, Colorado

Janice Bissonnette, RN-NP, MScN, PhD
Advance Practice Nurse
Renal Transplantation/Nephrology
Clinician Investigator-Clinical Epidemiology
   Program/Ottawa Hospital Research
Institute
The Ottawa Hospital
Ottawa, Ontario, Canada

Lorraine Buchanan, MSN, RN
Clinical Assistant Professor
School of Nursing
University of Kansas
Kansas City, Kansas

Barbara M. Carranti, MS, RN
Clinical Associate Professor
Department of Nursing
Le Moyne College
Syracuse, New York

**Annette M. Conklin, DNP, PhD, CNE,
   OCN**
Assistant Professor of Nursing
Math, Science, and Health Professions
Mercer County Community College
West Windsor, New Jersey

Shirlee Proctor Davidson, MSN, RN
Independent Practitioner and Consultant,
   Psychiatric-Mental Health Nursing
Liaison Consultation and Education
Santa Fe, New Mexico

Kelly Duffy, EdD, MSN, RN
Professor
RN-BSN Program
College of Nursing
Daytona State College
Daytona Beach, Florida

Sylvia Escott-Stump, MA, RDN, LDN
Director
Dietetic Internship
East Carolina University
Greenville, North Carolina

**Debra Hagler, PhD, RN, ACNS-BC, CNE,
   CHSE, ANEF, FAAN**
Clinical Professor
College of Nursing and Health Innovation
Arizona State University
Phoenix, Arizona

**Kathy Hammond, MS, RN, BSN, BSHE,
   RDN, LD**
Director of Education and Professional
   Development
Visiting Nurse Health System
Atlanta, Georgia;
Adjunct Assistant Professor
Department of Foods and Nutrition
University of Georgia
Athens, Georgia

Robbyn Harry-Ieremie, MSN, RN
Nursing Faculty
Indiana Wesleyan University
Marion, Indiana

Teresa Keller, PhD, RN
Associate Director and Assistant Dean
School of Nursing
New Mexico State University
Las Cruces, New Mexico

Kim K. Kuebler, DNP, ARNP, ANP-BC
Director
Multiple Chronic Conditions Resource
   Center
Savannah, Georgia

**Barbara J. Lutz, PhD, RN, CRRN,
   APHN-BC, FAHA, FNAP, FAAN**
McNeill Distinguished Professor
School of Nursing
College of Health and Human Services
University of North Carolina–Wilmington
Wilmington, North Carolina

**Claranne Mathiesen, MSN, RN, CNRN,
   SCRN**
Assistant Professor, Nursing
East Stroudsburg University
East Stroudsburg, Pennsylvania

Mary Courtney Moore, RN, RD, PhD
Research Professor
Molecular Physiology & Biophysics
Vanderbilt University School of Medicine
Nashville, Tennessee

Shannon E. Perry, RN, PhD, FAAN
Professor Emerita
School of Nursing
San Francisco State University
San Francisco, California

Carole Peterson, MSN, RN
Associate Professor, Nursing
Daytona State College
Daytona Beach, Florida

Christina J. Phillips, DNP, APRN, FNP-C
Clinical Assistant Professor
School of Nursing
University of Kansas
Kansas City, Kansas

L. Jane Rosati, EdD, MSN, RN-BC
Professor
School of Nursing
Daytona State College
Daytona Beach, Florida

**Lisa Ruth-Sahd, RN, DEd, MSN, CEN,
   CCRN**
Associate Professor, Nursing
York College of Pennsylvania
York, Pennsylvania

Carolyn E. Sabo, RN, EdD
Professor and DNP Program Coordinator
School of Nursing
University of Nevada, Las Vegas
Las Vegas, Nevada

**Angela Starkweather, PhD, ACNP-BC,
   CNRN, FAAN**
Professor and Director
Center for Advancements in Managing Pain
University of Connecticut School of
   Nursing
Storrs, Connecticut

Amy Szoka, MSN, CNE, RN
Assistant Professor
Daytona State College
Daytona Beach, Florida

Karen Gahan Tarnow, PhD, RN
Clinical Associate Professor
School of Nursing
University of Kansas
Kansas City, Kansas

For many educators, a concept-based approach to teaching and learning seems like a new, earth-shaking idea. Undoubtedly it seems that way because this approach essentially stands the more familiar content-driven modes of teaching and learning on their heads in the quest to construct more effective educational processes that surpass goals associated with content acquisition. But for all the differences, a concept-based approach is not an unorthodox view of learning at all. It is based on how a child learns to recognize, categorize, and talk about a dog or a flower; how a newcomer learns to thrive in a foreign environment; and how adults, including nurses, develop the skills necessary to become the life-long learners that are essential for evidence-based practice and for progress in the discipline and practice of nursing. Concepts are a central feature of all knowledge. They enable the joining together of otherwise isolated facts along with the ability to share what is in our own minds. Concepts also enable movement from one situation to the next without each instance seeming completely new and foreign. Learning concepts moves the education process beyond specific facts and seemingly isolated detail to a broader level that invites a dynamic approach to both learning and application of knowledge, one that is flexible, open to change, and accommodating of new discoveries. Concept-based learning provides the tools to make adjustments in knowledge as new information arises. It is the key to the critical thinking that nurses have espoused for decades as essential to effective nursing practice and to the growth of the discipline.

The future for nursing calls for graduates who have the ability to adapt to change on all levels, to be responsive to new evidence, and to resist complacency in their knowledge and their actions. Faculty who use this text to focus on the broader ideas that underpin nursing practice and to promote concept acquisition rather than memorization have in their hands an important tool to help students develop the thinking skills needed to be the lifelong, critical learners who are needed in the discipline. Nurses tend to be very skilled at describing what they "do." With this text, a big step forward is made in educating nurses who can describe what they "know" and in connecting the tasks of nursing with the conceptual knowledge that underlies all action.

Beth Rodgers, PhD, RN, FAAN
Professor and Research Chair
College of Nursing
University of New Mexico
Albuquerque, New Mexico

Wisdom means keeping a sense of the fallibility of our views and opinions, and of the uncertainty and instability of the things we most count on.

Gerard Brown

INTRODUCTION TO CONCEPTUAL LEARNING

Conceptual learning is increasingly viewed as a major trend for the future of education—not in nursing alone, but across numerous disciplines. This belief is based on the premise that *concepts* can be used effectively as unifying classifications or principles for framing learning while knowledge increases exponentially.

So, what is a *concept*? Simply stated, a concept is an organizing principle or a classification of information. A concept can be limited or complex in scope and can be useful as a basis for education from preschool through doctoral education. In advanced applications, concepts are considered building blocks or the foundation for theory.

By gaining a deeper understanding of a core set of concepts, a student can recognize and understand similarities and recurring characteristics, which can be applied more effectively than memorized facts. Teaching conceptually turns traditional learning upside down, focusing on generalities (concepts) and then applying this understanding to specifics (exemplars), instead of the traditional educational approach that focuses more heavily on content and facts.

HOW THIS BOOK IS ORGANIZED

The conceptual approach in nursing involves an examination of concepts that link to the delivery of patient care. There are multiple concepts applicable to nursing practice. This book does not attempt to present all nursing concepts, nor does it suggest that the featured concepts chosen are the most important. However, the 58 concepts featured in this book are commonly seen in nursing literature or are representative of important practice phenomena; they are the concepts that apply to the broadest group of patients of various ages and across various health care settings. A simplified concept analysis format using consistent headings is intentionally used for the presentation of concepts in this book so that students will find the approach intuitive; at the same time, an understanding of more formalized conceptual analyses will be fostered. Three overarching groups of concepts, or *units*, are featured:

- **Health Care Recipient Concepts (Unit 1)**—concepts that help us understand the individuals for whom we care
- **Health and Illness Concepts (Unit 2)**—concepts that help us make sense of the multiple health conditions experienced by our patients across the lifespan
- **Professional Nursing and Health Care Concepts (Unit 3)**—concepts that guide our professional practice in the context of health care

These three overarching units are further categorized into *themes*, into which concepts are organized to provide a structured framework. This structured approach promotes a thorough understanding of individual concepts and their important context within related health care concepts.

Each concept provides a full spectrum of information, with separate subheadings for concept definition, risk factors, health assessment, context of the concept to nursing and health care, interrelated concepts, case studies, and examples (exemplars) of concepts in practice. Each piece helps build an understanding of the concept as a whole, which in turn will promote the development of clinical judgment, a key outcome if nursing students are to practice effectively in today's complex health care environment.

FEATURES

Concept discussions include holistic concept diagrams that help visualize conceptual processes, along with *interrelated concepts* diagrams. These illustrations encourage students to build important associations among interrelated concepts. *Case Studies* provide an example of the concept applied in the context of patient care or practice setting.

An extensive list of *exemplars* (boxes at the end of every concept chapter) is based on incidence and prevalence across the lifespan and clinical settings. The new *Featured Exemplars* section provides a brief explanation of some of the most important exemplars. Using a custom technology, direct links to selected exemplars have been embedded into a core collection of Elsevier eBooks. This option of linking directly to a curated list of exemplars in a set collection of titles allows for a seamless user experience by uniting concepts to priority exemplars. Although instructors have complete flexibility to choose those concepts and exemplars best suited to their particular institution, these direct links are provided to allow quick access to those exemplars likely to be used in the majority of cases.

Interactive review questions incorporated into a self-assessment student testing engine are provided as an additional feature of this book's Evolve website (http:/evolve.elsevier.com/Giddens/concepts). These 250 student questions include multiple-choice and multi-select questions to simulate the NCLEX™ Examination testing experience, along with correct answer options and rationales.

Additional material to support faculty is included on the *Evolve Instructor Resources* site. A number of resources are provided to offer assistance in developing and teaching in a concept-based curriculum. Additionally, TEACH Lesson Plans, PowerPoints, and test banks have all been developed at both the RN and PN level to accommodate all learning needs.

CONCLUSION

Why use a conceptual approach? An exponential generation of new knowledge and information in all areas of our world (including health care and nursing) has made it literally impossible for anyone to know all information within the discipline of nursing. The study of nursing concepts provides the learner with an understanding of essential components associated with nursing practice without becoming saturated and lost in the details for each area of clinical specialty. If concepts are understood deeply, links can be made when these are applied in various areas of nursing practice.

The conceptual approach also fosters future advancement of the nursing discipline. This book serves as a guide to learning about concepts and their application in clinical nursing practice. The conceptual approach provides the foundation for learning, clinical practice, and research efforts needed to continue to build substantive knowledge to the discipline of nursing. The conceptual approach represents a journey that embraces change. Let the journey begin!

Jean Foret Giddens

CONTENTS

Health Care Recipient Concepts

ATTRIBUTES AND RESOURCES

1 *Development*
2 *Functional Ability*
3 *Family Dynamics*

PERSONAL PREFERENCES

4 *Culture*
5 *Spirituality*
6 *Adherence*
7 *Self-Management*

I n the not too distant past, health care was delivered in a disease-centered model whereby health care providers controlled and directed care with little input from patients regarding their desires or their concerns about the impact of the treatment plan on their lives. Patients were apprised of the plan as opposed to discussing options for disease management.

Health care has been actively moving toward a patient-centered model of health care in which patients and their families are active participants in their care.[1] Health care services are designed to meet the needs and wishes of the individual. Health care professionals counsel and provide advice related to health care decisions, based on their clinical expertise and evidence.[1] Fundamental to this is the ability to understand the unique attributes of each and every patient. For the successful delivery of patient-centered care, nurses should understand the concepts presented in this unit. The two themes within this unit are Attributes and Resources and Personal Preferences.

Attributes and Resources includes concepts associated with unique characteristics of the patient: Development, Functional Ability, and Family Dynamics. *Personal Preferences* includes concepts that influence an individual's attitudes and preferences regarding health care: Culture, Spirituality, Adherence, and Self-Management. These concepts are necessary to understand the decision making and behavior of patients, and they inform providers of strategies necessary to reach decisions that are mutually acceptable and agreeable to patients and providers.

REFERENCE

1. Institute of Medicine: *Crossing the quality chasm: A new health system for the 21st century*, Washington, DC, 2001, National Academies Press.

CONCEPT
1

Development

Leigh Small

A basic characteristic of all human life is change. Development is a complex process that involves the integration of an expansive variety of gradual changes that occur across multiple domains and result in an individual's functional abilities. These changes usually increase in complexity according to a dynamic, somewhat predictable sequence that begins at conception and continues over the lifespan until older age and/or death.[1-3] The individual's state of health, environmental context, and/or life experiences may alter an aspect of an individual's development causing it to stagnate or regress to an earlier stage. The ability to provide patient-centered, quality care requires nurses to understand and assess the different aspects of an individual's development and appropriately adjust the care they provide. It is also important for nurses to recognize when expected developmental progression in any area is not occurring so that collaborative interventions can be initiated.

DEFINITION

Development refers to *the sequence of physical, psychosocial, and cognitive developmental changes that take place over the human lifespan.*[3] Development does not occur as an isolated phenomenon. Rather, it represents the dynamic integration of three aspects of change: growth, differentiation, and maturation. *Physical growth* is a quantitative change in which an increase in cell number and size results in an increase in overall size or weight of the body or any of its parts. *Differentiation* is the process by which initially formed cells and structures become specialized. This is both a quantitative and a qualitative change from simple to complex in which broad global function becomes refined and specific. *Maturation* is the emergence of personal, behavioral, or adult-like physical characteristics or a "ripening." Maturation enables an individual to function in a fully developed and optimal way. Thus, maturation increases adaptability and competence in new situations.[3] Development, as well as the interrelated processes of growth, differentiation, and adaptation, is significantly impacted by genetics, environmental factors, culture, family values, and personal experiences.[3-5] Therefore, the overall concept of development, as defined in this context, affects all aspects of every individual and directs all aspects of nursing care. Times during which development is rapidly occurring (i.e., childhood and older adulthood) deserve special attention and in-depth knowledge as nursing

care will need to responsively adjust and nurses will need to adapt to the developmental changes of the patient more frequently and on an individual basis.

Unique sets of skills and competencies to be mastered at each developmental stage across the lifespan in order for the individual to cope with the environment are called *developmental tasks.*[6] Developmental tasks are broad in scope and are, to a significant degree, determined by culture.[7] They may relate to the individual or to the family. Examples of developmental tasks are stepping up steps unassisted and coping with the loss of a spouse.[8]

The order of developmental task attainment is more important than the chronological age at which each occurs because although development is ongoing, its speed varies across individuals. Furthermore, each individual has a unique developmental pace moderated by one's state of health, environment, and social/family context. Rate and level of development are also related to the physiological maturity of all systems—particularly the neurologic, muscular, and skeletal systems.

SCOPE

The scope of the concept, or extent to which development influences an individual (i.e., expected, delayed, or advanced development; Figure 1-1), spans the entire life course—from birth to death (Table 1-1). Normal human development is organized and progressive and usually occurs in a predictable sequence. Based on this expected sequence, stages of development have been identified. The traditional stages of development have been identified by general age groups and include embryologic, infant, toddler, preschool, school age, adolescent (teen), young adult, adult, middle age, and older adult. These stages identify characteristics found in the majority of individuals within a stated age range. Although individuals vary in the time of onset of each stage and in the length of time spent in each stage, the sequence itself rarely varies.

Types of Development

Development is a complex and interconnected concept that has been distilled into six overarching categories or domains: physical/physiological, motoric, social/emotional, cognitive, communication, and adaptive (Figure 1-2). The accelerated and decelerated paces of

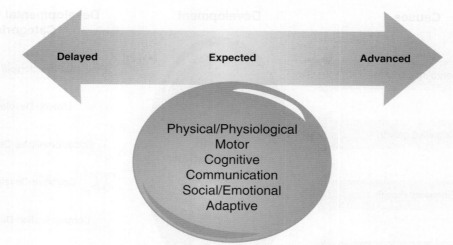

FIGURE 1-1 Scope of Development

TABLE 1-1 Identified Developmental Age Compared with Chronological Age

Developmental Age	Chronological Age
Birth	Conception through birth
Infant	Birth through 12 months
Toddler	12 months through 36 months
Preschooler	36 months through 5 years
Schoolager	5 years through 12 years
Adolescent	12 years through 18 years
Young adult	18–35 years
Middle adult	35–65 years
Older adult	
Young-old	65–75 years
Middle-old	75–85 years
Old-old	Over 85 years

development occur somewhat independently within each domain (e.g., physical/physiological, motor, social, cognitive, and communication). For example, while gross motor skills are changing (i.e., infant walking), language skills may not be developing as quickly. Similarly, an older school-aged child may be demonstrating advanced physical maturation but has not achieved advanced states of emotional maturation. Thus, age-related developmental expectancies or norms are always based on an age range—never an exact point in time when specific skills will be achieved.[1,3,9] While the pace of development within each of these domains occurs independently, the progression of skills in the subcategories is also interconnected and reliant on the development in the other domains.

Physical/Physiological Development

Physical/physiological development refers to the growth and changes in body tissues and organ systems and the resultant changes in body functions and proportions. Physiological development includes cellular proliferation, differentiation, and maturation that occurs in each organ and system that allows integrated human functioning necessary for life and health (i.e., infant hematopoietic maturity and secondary sexual characteristic development leading to sexual function). Overall physical growth and development occur in a bilateral and symmetrical way, progressing in a cephalocaudal (head-to-toe) direction (i.e., infants have a disproportionately larger head-to-body ratio compared with that of an adult) and proximodistally (from midline to periphery).

Motoric Development

Motoric development is frequently separated into two major categories: gross and fine motor. Very generally, motoric development progresses from achievement of gross motor to fine motor skills—a process referred to as refinement.[10,11] Gross motor skills involve the use of large muscles to move about in the environment. Examples of gross motor development include the sequential skills of sitting, standing, maintaining balance, cruising, walking, running, walking up stairs without assistance, and more complex physical tasks such as playing soccer. Fine motor skills involve the use of small muscles in an increasingly coordinated and precise manner. Examples of fine motor development include the achievement of the successive skills of batting at an object, reaching and holding an object, transferring an object from hand to hand, holding a pencil in a refined grasp, making marks with a pencil, writing letters, writing words, and the complex skill of creating masterful artwork. Other fine motor skills using the hands and fingers to eat, draw, dress, and play are all required to achieve optimal functioning.[12,13] Fine motor development is contingent upon cognitive and neurologic development.

Social/Emotional Development

Social and emotional development includes the development of self-understanding, understanding others, and understanding social interactions.[1,2,10,11] These different elements of social/emotional development usually occur in this order (e.g., self, others, and social interaction). Knowledge of social/emotional skills is critical because it directs effective communication with an individual(s) and may impact suggested environmental strategies for an individual to attain optimal functioning. For example, young preschool children cannot distinguish between their effort and their ability and are likely to overestimate their competence and abilities. Thus, caution should be used regarding self-reported ability(ies), and nurses should seek confirmation (e.g., "Johnnie says that he can swallow pills. Have you seen Johnnie take

FIGURE 1-2 Development Concept Categories

pills before or is Johnnie better able to swallow liquid medicine?"). Development of an understanding of others (perspective taking) includes a growing comprehension that other people have emotions and intentions and that objects do not. This understanding is foundational to the development of trust, moral development, and the ability to interact with others. These aspects of development underlie the ability of children to discern the difference between a truth and a lie. A complicating aspect of social/emotional development is emotional regulation, which directly impacts relational interactions (i.e., play, work, and social interactions).[14] This complex aspect of development declines during the aging process in an indeterminable rate, underscoring the need to consider and assess areas of social/emotional development across the lifespan.

Cognitive Development

The cognitive dimension of development relates to working memory capacity, cognitive self-regulation, and the processing and use of information about the environment and objects in the environment, as well as understanding the relationships between self and this information. These processes underlie the development of critical thinking skills and executive functioning, which includes learning, forming concepts, understanding, problem solving, reasoning, remembering, and thinking abstractly. Ultimately, these complex aspects of cognitive development, in combination with advanced social/emotional developmental stages, enable moral and spiritual development.[1]

Some have suggested that there are different aspects of intelligence that include analytical, creative, and practical components,[10,11] whereas others have conceptualized intelligence to include many different types of intelligence.[15] Because the brain has reached 90% of its adult weight and has completed a majority of synaptogenesis and myelination by 6 years of age, the individual is deemed to be at an optimal ready state for formal education—a process thought to stimulate cognitive development. In late adulthood, maintenance of cognitive abilities is affected by a decline in the speed of processing, decrements in executive functioning (e.g., attention and memory), and potentially by reduced or limited cognitive stimulation, which leads to continued synaptic pruning and decreased synaptogenesis. Lifespan cognitive development and "brain science," including the impact of the

environment and trauma, has become a primary focus of research recently.

Communication Development

Speech is the spoken expression of language. The three components of speech are (1) articulation, which refers to the pronunciation of sounds; (2) voice, which refers to the production of sound by the vocal cords; and (3) fluency, which refers to the rhythm of speech. Language involves a set of rules shared by a group of people that allows the communication of thoughts, ideas, and emotions. Communication is a process that requires both receptive and expressive skills. Receptive language function is the ability to hear and understand what others say. Expressive language function is the ability to develop and express one's own thoughts, ideas, and emotions.[16] Speech and language development synergistically occurs with cognitive, neurologic, and fine motor development and requires optimal sensory function (e.g., hearing), sensory integration, and interactional relationships to develop and refine.

Simple speech begins with utterances of consonants, increases to include vowels ("ba-ba" and "da-da"), then single words are formed ("no" and "me"), and two- and three-word combinations arise ("me do" and "you up"), leading to the development of meaningful phrases and sentences. This language explosion or "period of exuberance" is an outward demonstration of frontal lobe development and typically occurs in children 18 months to 3 years of age. This is a specific example of a critical developmental time point, meaning that if significant speech and language gains are not made during this time, the delay may have resultant sequelae (i.e., a variety of learning disorders). Speech and language continues to increase in complexity during the lifespan until older adulthood, a time during which communication and speech may decline or become impaired as a result of health impairment or disease (e.g., expressive aphasia that results from a stroke).

Adaptive Development

Adaptive development refers to the acquisition of a range of skills that enable independence at home and in the community. Adaptive skills are learned and include self-care activities such as dressing/undressing, eating/feeding, toileting, and grooming; management of one's immediate environment; and functional behaviors within the community, such as crossing the street safely, going to the store, and following rules of politeness when interacting with others.[17] Demonstration of skills in this developmental domain requires advanced and complex skills in each of the other developmental domains previously discussed and efficient sensory integration processes. Examples of adaptive development include cooperation; a level of moral and ethical decision making; and abilities to follow social and cultural folkways, mores, taboos, rules, and laws.

ATTRIBUTES AND CRITERIA

Expected Development

A person who is considered to have *normal* development is one who is demonstrating the expected developmental and physical maturation, physiological function, and/or expected tasks within or across the developmental domains (e.g., physical/physiological, motor, social, cognitive, and language) that are associated with the individual's chronological age.

Developmental level refers to an individual's stage of development (e.g., stage of epiphyseal closure in long bone development, Tanner stage of pubertal development, and stage of cognitive development) or ability to independently achieve an outcome (e.g., perspective taking and abstract reasoning).

A *developmental milestone* is an ability or specific skill that most individuals can accomplish in a certain age range.[1,9] The categories of age ranges typically include those individuals who are experiencing rapid developmental change such as infants, toddlers, preschoolers, school-aged children, and adolescents (teens), with emphasis on the growing child. However, milestone attainment and loss is appreciated across the lifespan. Common use of the term "developmental milestones" typically refers to changes that involve *motor, social, emotional, cognitive,* and *communication* skills. In the context of this concept presentation, development also includes *physical/physiological milestones* (Box 1-1). For example, every aspect of physical and physiological growth and maturation has been carefully mapped and normed to the general population and to several subpopulations (e.g., weight for age, body mass index for age and gender, and kidney and liver growth

---

BOX 1-1　Attributes of Development

- Physical/Physiological development
  - Growth
  - Physical characteristic development
  - Organ system maturation
- Motoric development
  - Fine motor development
  - Gross motor development
- Cognitive development
- Communication development
  - Speech
  - Language
- Social/emotional development
  - Social skills
  - Emotional control
- Adaptive development

---

and development). Classically defined, developmental milestones occur when a confluence of critical changes (i.e., neurologic, cognitive, motional, and physical) occur, marking a significant or critical point of maturation. As a result, these milestones provide a basis for developmental assessment and serve as major markers in tracking development.

Abnormal Development

If an individual does not accomplish milestones within a specified age range, or a critical period, he or she may be identified as being *developmentally delayed*, signifying that an essential element of neurologic and/or cognitive maturation has not occurred within an age range and should be investigated. The definition of developmental delay varies, but it usually involves a delay of at least 2.5 standard deviations in one or more areas or subcategories of development. In other words, a developmental delay would be identified if a developmental change was not found in an individual that can be found in 95% of others of the same chronological age range. Certain individuals may demonstrate advanced development in one or more developmental domains/categories (see Figure 1-1). The developmental changes assessed would include physiological and physical development, motor, cognitive, communication, social/emotional, and adaptive development.[18] Individual delays within a developmental domain may be demonstrated in subtle ways and may not affect overall functioning unless the delays are pronounced and developmental progress continues to lag over time.

An individual who has accomplished a developmental milestone rarely loses this ability unless the individual encounters a significant stressor (e.g., hospitalization or a new disease diagnosis). For example, once a child learns to sit or stand or becomes toilet trained, it is unusual for such skills to be lost without cause. The loss of developmental milestones, or *developmental regression*, is very subtle, and parents often miss this occurring in their own children. Recognizing the loss of a previously attained developmental milestone is as important of an assessment finding as the identification of achieving milestones. When developmental regression has occurred, the underlying cause must be identified with the goal of ameliorating the situation, addressing underlying health conditions impacting development, and restoring developmental gains as soon as possible.

Developmental arrest is the plateau of developmental change in some category and is noted when chronological age continues to progress but developmental change does not. Developmental arrest can be differentiated from lagging or slowed development because of its significant effects on an individual's functioning. Physical or growth arrest can be the result of underlying health abnormalities or social conditions (e.g., abuse, neglect, or social isolation) that may or may not have been diagnosed. Cessation in physiological development (organ or system maturation) frequently results in significant functional limitations or chronic health conditions. For example, some believe that developmental arrest that occurs *in utero* results in a congenital anomaly.[12]

It is estimated that at least 8% of all children from birth to age 6 years have developmental problems and/or delays in one or more areas of neurocognitive development. A *global delay* refers to lag in multiple neurocognitive developmental areas—speech and language, gross and fine motor skills, and personal and social development.[19] Some individuals are identified as having a *pervasive developmental disorder* (PDD), which means that they have a significant developmental delay in many basic milestones and skills that often cross developmental domains. PDD is usually identified by 3 years of age, which is a critical time in an individual's development. Frequently, children with PDD have delays that affect the ability to socialize with others, to communicate, and to use imagination—all skills that usually emerge during this age. Thus, children with these conditions often demonstrate confusion in their thinking and generally have problems understanding the world around them—challenges that continue throughout their life. Specific types of developmental delays are presented in the Clinical Exemplars section later in this chapter.

There are periods within each of the domains of development that are characterized not only by critical periods (mentioned previously) but also by susceptible or sensitive periods. These are points in the lifespan when there is greater susceptibility to positive or negative influences (e.g., genetic, environment, culture, family values, and personal experiences), with resulting beneficial or detrimental effects.[6] One example of the latter is the finding that young children with rapidly occurring frontal lobe development, the "period of exuberance," are particularly vulnerable to environmental toxins (e.g., lead intoxication) and exhibit marked detrimental effects from such exposures (e.g., stunted cognitive abilities or learning disabilities).[20]

THEORETICAL LINKS

Several theories have been developed throughout the years to understand different domains of neurocognitive development and define different developmental levels and/or stages within each domain. Four of the classic theories are presented: Freud's theory of psychosexual development (1930s and 1940s), Erikson's eight stages of psychosocial development (1940s), Piaget's theory of cognitive development (1960s), and Kohlberg's theory of moral development (1980s). Caution should be taken when considering each of these theories because controversy exists regarding their accuracy and applicability.

Freud's Theory of Psychosexual Development

The term *psychosexual*, as used by Freud, refers to any sensual pleasure. Freud believed that at different ages, particular areas of the body provide the chief source of sensual pleasure and that experiences with these pleasure centers significantly impact the development of personality. He outlined five stages of development: oral (birth–1 year), anal (1–3 years), phallic (3–6 years), latency (6–12 years), and genital (puberty–adulthood). He identified conflicts associated with each stage that must be resolved for development to occur. Under stress, individuals were thought to regress temporarily to an earlier stage. If resolution was not satisfactorily achieved, an individual may become fixated in the stage and personality development would be arrested.[21,22]

The validity and applicability of Freud's theory and associated underlying assumptions are frequently contested because his work was based on adults with mental health diagnoses and their reflections of past life experiences (retrospective data). However, the conceptual view that an individual matures and develops over time in a stagewise process and the environment impacts those changes (i.e., relationships) was novel at the time and proved to be a critical step for the field of psychology. It resulted in other theorists developing and testing hypotheses regarding specific aspects of cognitive and psychological development over the lifespan (i.e., psychosocial and moral development).

Erikson's Theory of Psychosocial Development

Erikson's theory of development focused on the psychosocial development of an individual across the lifespan. Erikson was a protégé of Freud, and the theory he developed was an expansion and refinement of Freud's theory specific to psychosocial development. Erikson identified eight stages of psychosocial development thought to occur between birth and death. These stages were identified by the conflict confronting the individual and included trust versus mistrust (birth–1 year), autonomy versus shame and doubt (1–3 years), initiative versus guilt (3–6 years), industry versus inferiority (6–11 years), identify versus role confusion (11–18 years), intimacy versus isolation (18–25 years), generativity versus self-absorption and stagnation (25–65 years), and integrity versus despair (65 years–death). He also had a stagewise philosophy (every individual moves only in a forward sequential way through each stage or development ceases), in which each stage had a particular task, identified in the form of a conflict, that must be resolved to progress to the next developmental level.[21,23]

Piaget's Theory of Cognitive Development

Piaget's theory of cognitive development sought to explain how children innately organize their world and learn to think.[24] In this theory, cognitive development is viewed as progressing from illogical to logical, from concrete to abstract, and from simple to complex. Underlying assumptions of this theory are that cognitive development is a product of inborn intellectual capacity, nervous system maturation, and perceptual ability, and exposure to new experiences serves as a stimulus for cognitive development. The theory posits that there are four general periods: sensory motor (birth–2 years), preoperational (2–7 years), concrete operational (7–11 years), and formal operations (11 years–adulthood). Each period is composed of a number of stages that are age-related, sequential, and stepwise forward.[14,25] These pioneering theories resulted in years of debate regarding the influence of nature versus nurture during a person's development; however, more contemporary theories allege that both play an important role.

Kohlberg's Theory of Moral Development

Kohlberg developed a theory that expands on Piaget's cognitive theory to address the development of an individual's moral reasoning across his or her lifespan.[26] According to Kohlberg, when a conflict in universal values occurs, a moral choice must be made. This choice is based on moral reasoning, which is postulated to develop progressively over three levels: preconventional (18 months–5 years), conventional (6–12 years), and postconventional (12–19 years). Each level is composed of two stages. In this theory, development of moral reasoning is dependent on cognitive skills and neurologic maturation, but it is not definitively linked to specific developmental stages.[26] This theory furthered thought regarding other areas that undergo change and development during one's life.

Contemporary Theories

More contemporary scientists and students who study development appraise theories with regard to three main aspects: Does the theory suggest that development is continuous (uninterrupted change over time) or discontinuous (stepwise progression)? Does the theory suggest that there is only one path of development for all children? and What is the relative influence of nature and nurture according to the theory being discussed? A careful review and appraisal of those early developmental theories has given rise to many current theories, such as the ecological systems theory, Vygotsky's sociocultural theory, and theories of multiple intelligences.

CONTEXT TO NURSING AND HEALTH CARE

Because of the frequency and intimacy of their patient contact, nurses are uniquely positioned to gain information about (assess) their patients and holistically intervene to improve patient health and functioning. Assessment of all six domains of development is well within a nurse's scope of practice and significantly impacts the care that nurses and other health care providers offer. Care modified or directed by a person's development will be most appropriate and more likely to bring patients to optimal well-being and functioning. Therefore, it is important to recognize risk factors and age-sensitive time periods during which developmental progress may be threatened.

Risk Recognition

Developmental progress, delay, arrest, advance, or decline occur in all social classes, ethnic groups, and across ages. Most frequently, these concepts are discussed in terms of pediatric populations (infancy through adolescence) because change in all categories of development is occurring rapidly.[27,28] Because development in all areas is interdependent, a delay, arrest, or decline during a time period of rapid developmental change may place an individual at risk. Several types of risk exist, including the following:

- **Prenatal:** Genetic conditions, congenital infections, and prenatal exposure to environmental toxins, illicit drugs and/or alcohol, or cigarette smoking
- **Birth risk:** Prematurity, low birth weight, birth trauma, and maternal infection
- **Individual risk:** Ill health, malnutrition, physical or mental disabilities, and cognitive impairments
- **Family risk:** Low parental education, poor health of family members, and large family size
- **Situational risk:** Acute life stress, acute mental or physical health crises, acute school/social problems, bullying, interpersonal violence, sexual abuse, and acute conflictual or violent family relationships
- **Social determinants of health:** Poverty, environmental toxins, adverse living conditions, rural or urban living, areas with high prevalence of disease, community with low cohesion, limited access to health-promoting foods and safe physical environments that facilitate healthy activity, and limited access to health care
- **Toxic stress:** Strict or authoritative parenting, child abuse or neglect, exposure to domestic violence, chronic social isolation, and chronic everyday stressors
- **Health status:** Chronic illness (e.g., congenital heart disease, cancer, brain injury, and cystic fibrosis), traumatic or severe injuries, and conditions requiring prolonged bed rest and/or multiple/prolonged hospitalizations[13]

Stressors, as perceived by children, may differ greatly from the stressors that caregivers may sense exist for a child. For example, loss of a pet, a move, integration into a new school, alterations in household members, and/or illness of sibling, family member, teacher, or friend may be extremely stressful for a child. In some cases in which children spend time with different adults in different contexts (e.g., child care and split time with a divorced parent), caregivers may be unaware that their child has experienced these stressors.

Developmental Assessment

Development, as a concept, has implications for all aspects of nursing practice across all populations and health care settings. A thorough developmental assessment of all domains and recognition of risk factors that may impact development are essential for early identification of developmental problems. These assessments are also necessary

to determine goals for rehabilitation and strategies to compensate and thus optimize function and overall health when limited progression is identified and/or following illness or injury.

Assessment of development should independently occur for every domain of development. These critical assessments require focused attention and intervention, particularly when working with preverbal or young children and older adults with limited abilities to articulate accurate information, in situations with an absent primary caregiver, or in chaotic living situations in which limited historical data are available.

Infants and Children

Gross screening for developmental risks and lags or delays primarily occurs as a part of well-child health visits.[27] These assessments should be completed by health care providers with specialized training in child development and require direct observation with planned developmental challenges and parent report of development task accomplishment. Valid and reliable screening instruments are used and frequently involve documentation of specific skills, parent and/or teacher reports, and child reports. A classic tool used to measure developmental status is the Denver Developmental Screening Test II (DDST II). The DDST II is designed for use with children from 1 month to 6 years of age and has been standardized for minority populations. It assesses gross motor, fine motor, language, and personal–social skills and milestones. The two primary limitations to the use of the DDST II involve the limited sensitivity (83%) and specificity (43%) of the tool,[29] leading to a number of referrals for further evaluation of children suspected of being developmentally delayed but who are not truly developmentally delayed. In addition, the use of this tool does not identify children who have other diagnoses (e.g., cerebral palsy) that may affect the developmental changes anticipated in a child's early years.[3,8,30] Thus, the DDST II is recognized as a gross screening tool with inherent error and not a diagnostic tool.

When delay is suspected in any specific area of development, a more in-depth assessment with a valid, reliable, and highly sensitive and specific tool for that particular area is needed for diagnostic purposes. For example, an in-depth language assessment may be needed after a gross screening by the DDST II. Given this situation, a tool such as the Early Language Milestones Scale (ELM Scale-2)[31] may be used to assess auditory visual, auditory receptive, and expressive language in children between the ages of 1 month and 3 years. Assessment of social/emotional development may include the Modified Checklist for Autism in Toddlers–Revised (M-CHAT-R). This tool has been found to be valid and reliable and to have strong sensitivity and specificity.[32] Other examples of developmental screening tools that include parental report are the Ages and Stages Questionnaire (ASQ),[8] the Parents' Evaluation of Developmental Status (PEDS), and the Learn the Signs/Act Early Interactive Milestones Checklist program sponsored by the Centers for Disease Control and Prevention's (CDC) National Center on Birth Defects and Developmental Disabilities.[33]

Detailed information and several assessment tools focused on child development are available from pediatric and developmental textbooks and from reliable websites such as that of the CDC.[33] The Bright Futures website, developed by the American Academy of Pediatrics, includes specific information for health care providers.[34] Many Internet resources are appropriate for parents and interested care providers (e.g., child care providers) but it should be emphasized that screening tools do not provide a diagnosis. A diagnosis requires a thorough neurodevelopmental history, physical examination, advanced testing and assessment for specific delay, and assessment for potential underlying associated health disturbance.[19]

Adolescents

Routine physical examinations monitor continued development in all areas into the adolescent years. During the adolescent years, teens' major developmental milestones include advanced cognitive thinking and risk-taking behaviors that accompany psychosocial, moral, and sexual development. To assess these areas of development, a HEADSS Adolescent Risk Profile may be used.[35] HEADSS is a screening tool that assesses the teen's *home, education, activities, drugs, sex*, and potential for *suicide* for the purpose of identifying high-risk adolescents and the need for more in-depth assessment, counseling, and/or anticipatory guidance. Other general adolescent screening tools can be used, including CRAFFT (*Car, Relax, Alone Forget, Friends, Trouble*), which is a behavioral health screening tool for use with children younger than age 21 years to assess for behavior health risk, and RAAPS (*Rapid Assessment for Adolescent Preventive Services*; https://www.raaps.org)[36] or GAPS (*Guidelines for Adolescent Preventive Services*) developed by the American Academy of Pediatrics.[37] It is important to note that teens often develop mental health issues. Some may be the result of the tumultuous social and emotional changes encountered during adolescence, as well as many chronic mental health conditions first manifest during prepubescence or adolescence (e.g., schizophrenia, substance dependence, and bipolar disorder). There are a multitude of specific, high-quality (valid and reliable) assessment tools that can be used with older school-aged children and adolescents to detect the presence and acuity of depression, anxiety, attention deficit with/without hyperactivity disorder, and other mental health and developmentally associated issues.

Adults

In adulthood, physical examinations and assessments should continue to monitor normal developmental patterns. However, the focus of these interactions frequently involves minor acute or chronic health disturbances. Physical/physiological, psychological, and cognitive characteristics of individuals are assessed relative to age. For example, older females' reproductive organs are monitored for the normal decline in function. This physiological change may result in associated symptoms that are disruptive to the individual (e.g., "hot flashes"). In addition, mental health is an aspect of health and wellness that should be assessed in all individuals (e.g., depression). Screening tools designed for use with adults include the Recent Life Changes Questionnaire, the Life Experiences Survey,[14] and the Stress Audit, all of which aim to identify adults in need of supportive interventions and/or services relative to stress and coping.[30]

Older Adults

When adulthood is reached, often there is limited focus on developmental assessment until individuals reach the older adult stage, unless an adult has a serious mental or physical illness or injury or suffers a traumatic event. When this is the case, frequently the focus is on functional assessment (or functional ability)—that is, an assessment of an individual's ability to carry out basic activities of daily living (BADLs) and instrumental activities of daily living (IADLs).[38] BADLs include skills such as hygiene, toileting, eating, and ambulating. IADLs are skills that are needed to function independently and include preparing meals, shopping, taking medications, traveling within the community, and maintaining finances. Functional assessment is described in greater detail in Concept 2 Functional Ability.

Care Delivery

Knowledge of the individual's development in all areas (i.e., physical/physiological, motoric, social/emotional, cognitive, communication, and adaptive) is critical to nursing care even when no developmental problems exist. It determines appropriate communication strategies, teaching levels and techniques, safety provisions, assistance with activities of daily living, and approaches to therapeutic interventions. An individual's developmental level also determines need for anticipatory guidance, health promotion, and accident or illness prevention interventions. To provide appropriate information on recommended health screenings, immunizations, and chemoprophylaxis as well as counseling on health topics such as injury prevention, cigarette smoking, alcohol and drug abuse, diet, exercise, and sexual behavior, the developmental level of all areas must be known.

Early identification and intervention are among the most important points when developmental delay(s) is present. In general, regardless of the type of developmental delay, the earlier that intervention occurs, the better the outcome. Management of neurocognitive developmental delay truly requires intradisciplinary collaboration. Early intervention services can include one or more of the following services: nursing, medicine, physical therapy, occupational therapy, psychological intervention, individual and/or family counseling, nutritional consulting, speech and language services, play therapists, audiology services, and assistive technologies. All of these services have as their interprofessional goal to maximally develop a specified area and develop other areas to compensate for an identified disability to optimize future development and functioning (e.g., readiness to learn in a preschool-aged child).

Physical/physiological developmental limitations and/or challenges are not addressed in this chapter, although the effects of such problems have been suggested and will affect each of the health and illness concepts and thus impact nursing care. For example, glucose regulation of a newborn is affected differently from that of an adult because of the inability of the newborn to feed itself, the limited amount of brown fat for calorie stores, and the differential caloric loss due to temperature instability.[13] Similarly, tissue integrity in an infant is significantly different than that of a teen, middle-aged adult, or older adult. Premature and young infants have a greater degree of skin barrier dysfunction resulting in a higher transepidermal water loss, increased percutaneous absorption of chemicals, and higher risk for injury and/or bacterial invasion/infection.[13] Therefore, the effect of physical/physiological development should be considered with review of each of the health and illness concepts contained in this text.

INTERRELATED CONCEPTS

Concepts used to describe the human person do not represent isolated phenomena but, rather, phenomena that interrelate with one another. The strength and direction of the impact of one conceptual phenomenon on another vary, given the central concept under consideration. The interrelated concepts are presented in Figure 1-3. Concepts representing major influencing factors and hence determinants of development include Functional Ability, Nutrition, and Culture with its unique variations in practices and expectations. These appear in green at the top of the diagram, and their influence on development is indicated by the arrow pointing in the direction of the concept. Family Dynamics and the concepts associated with Mood and Cognition have a reciprocal relationship with development, represented by the red ovals with double-headed arrows. The concepts below the influencers (identified in purple at the bottom of the diagram) are the health and illness concepts significantly impacted by development. Note that there are only a few concepts not affected by development. The relationships are indicated by an arrow pointing from development to each of the concepts.

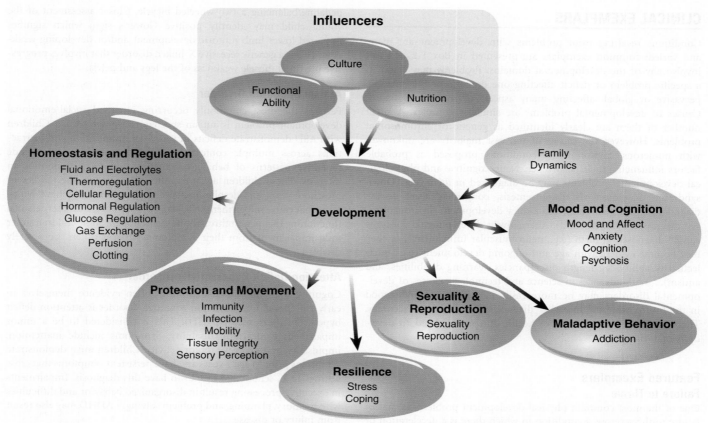

FIGURE 1-3 Development and Interrelated Concepts

The following text appears within the figure:

Influencers
- Culture
- Functional Ability
- Nutrition

Homeostasis and Regulation
- Fluid and Electrolytes
- Thermoregulation
- Cellular Regulation
- Hormonal Regulation
- Glucose Regulation
- Gas Exchange
- Perfusion
- Clotting

Development

Family Dynamics

Mood and Cognition
- Mood and Affect
- Anxiety
- Cognition
- Psychosis

Protection and Movement
- Immunity
- Infection
- Mobility
- Tissue Integrity
- Sensory Perception

Sexuality & Reproduction
- Sexuality
- Reproduction

Maladaptive Behavior
- Addiction

Resilience
- Stress
- Coping

BOX 1-2   EXEMPLARS OF DEVELOPMENTAL DELAY/DISORDERS

Physical/Physiological Developmental Delay/Disorder
- Angelman's syndrome
- Bladder exstrophy
- Hydronephrotic kidney disease
- Cleft lip/palate
- Congenital heart disease
- Cystic fibrosis
- Developmental hip dysplasia
- Down syndrome
- Failure to thrive
- Fragile X syndrome
- Hydrocephaly
- Klinefelter's syndrome
- Prader–Willi syndrome
- Spina bifida and other neural tube defects
- Turner's syndrome

Motoric Developmental Delay/Disorder
- Cerebral palsy
- Developmental dyspraxia
- Duchene's muscular dystrophy
- Hypertonia
- Hypotonia

Social/Emotional Developmental Delay/Disorder
- Autism spectrum disorder
- Asperger's syndrome

- Childhood (pediatric) disintegrative disorder not otherwise specified (PDD-NOS)
- Failure to thrive
- Aggressive/bullying/violent behaviors
- Dysfunctional attachments
- Generalized anxiety disorder
- Obsessive–compulsive disorder
- Reactive attachment disorder
- Separation anxiety disorder

Cognitive Developmental Delay/Disorder
- Attention deficit disorder
- Attention deficit hyperactivity disorder
- Fetal alcohol syndrome
- Rett syndrome

Speech and Communication Developmental Delay/Disorder
- Central auditory processing disorder
- Deafness/conductive hearing loss
- Expressive language disorder
- Receptive language disorder

Adaptive Developmental Delay
- Blindness
- Oppositional defiant disorder
- Traumatic brain injury

CLINICAL EXEMPLARS

Conditions resulting from problems with development are many and varied; common exemplars are presented in Box 1-2 and can involve any of the developmental domains. Problems may result in a specific problem or deficit affecting one domain, or they may be pervasive or global, affecting many aspects of multiple domains. Causes of developmental problems are similarly complex. A small number of them are clearly identified as genetic or chromosomal problems. However, the causes of the vast majority are unknown, with numerous environmental conditions proposed as probable factors influencing their occurrence. Neurocognitive and physiological developmental problems may be diagnosed *in utero* (e.g., Down syndrome diagnosed via amniocentesis, congenital heart disease diagnosed with a sonogram, and kidney development (hydronephrosis) diagnosed by ultrasound). Alternatively, developmental concerns can be diagnosed at birth (e.g., neuromuscular immaturity), or they may become evident with age and ongoing development (e.g., intellectual disability, leg length discrepancies, learning disabilities, and autism).[12] With advances in science and technology, causes of developmental disorders may be more easily identified and understood in the future, resulting in earlier diagnosis with increased accuracy. These advances should improve health outcomes related to developmental disruptions.

Featured Exemplars
Failure to Thrive

One of the most common physical development problems is that of failure to thrive/grow, a condition in which there is a deceleration or loss in weight and subsequent loss of linear growth (height/length). This has many etiologies categorized into three types: endogenous or organic (e.g., diagnosed/undiagnosed disease process, condition of the gastrointestinal tract, and inadequate nutrition), exogenous or nonorganic (e.g., inappropriate or dysfunctional feeding practices), or mixed type.[13] Weight/height loss or deceleration may be the result of emotional stress related to social isolation (e.g., neglect) or mental health difficulties (e.g., depression).

Cleft Lip and Palate

Physiological developmental problems often have their origins in intrauterine development or embryologic formation and/or cellular division. There may be subtle or overt manifestations that are detected by thorough assessments. One exemplar would be a soft palate abnormality identified through physical examination of the oropharynx. This represents a midline deformity with its beginning in embryologic development. This defect can be demonstrated subtly (e.g., soft palate deformities) or overtly (e.g., cleft lip). It may result in significant functional impairment (inability to suckle from a breast or bottle) and emotional distress (facial deformity), or it may cause little effect on an individual's functioning.

Duchene's Muscular Dystrophy

A classic example of problems with gross and fine motor development identifiable by impaired motoric developmental milestone achievement is Duchene's muscular dystrophy. In this example, a preschool-aged boy may be identified as having difficulty climbing stairs or pedaling/balancing a two-wheeled bicycle. Closer assessment of the young child may identify positive Gower's sign, which signifies impaired lower limb motoric development and/or developing weakness. This is a genetic recessive X-linked disorder that involves progressive proximal muscle weakness of the legs and pelvis.

Autism Spectrum Disorder

Perhaps the most commonly occurring impaired social/emotional development problem is autism spectrum disorder (ASD). Children with ASD demonstrate deficits in social communication and interactions across multiple contexts. Associated manifestations include repetitive patterns of behavior, activities, and focused nonhuman interests. These children are most often identified in the toddler or preschool years, and despite intensive interventions, they have symptoms that cause impairment in social, occupational, and interpersonal functioning that persist throughout their lifespan. Some children suffer mild impairment from their symptoms, whereas others are severely disabled.

Attention Deficit Hyperactivity Disorder

Cognitive and intellectual disabilities often evidence themselves in early childhood. One common cognitive disorder is attention deficit hyperactivity disorder (ADHD). This is considered to be a minor impairment or learning disability. Symptoms include inattention, impulsivity, and excessive motor activity. Children must demonstrate symptoms prior to age 7 years and have persistent symptoms that cross settings (e.g., school and home) to have this diagnosis. Impairments in executive processing result in disorganized behavior and difficulties with memory, planning, and problem solving.[11] ADHD may also result from injury or disease.

Central Auditory Processing Disorder

Impairments of speech and language are often recognized as learning disabilities. The diagnosis of central auditory processing disorder (CAPD) has become more commonly applied. This disorder affects how the brain receives and processes what is heard. This, like other learning disabilities, is a lifelong problem and often affects an individual's social interactions. Children demonstrate symptoms of this disorder differently based on their age and level of cognitive development. For example, young children may appear to have a speech delay, whereas school-aged children often have difficulty following spoken instructions, do not understand people who speak quickly, and cannot find the right words to say in conversation.

Traumatic Brain Injury

Adaptive development is the result of a complex integration of the multiple skills and abilities easily impacted by injury, illness, substance use, exposure to trauma, or an accumulation of toxic chronic stressors. Traumatic brain injury (TBI) is an example of an adaptive developmental disability defined as an external mechanical force resulting in permanent or temporary brain injury and associated cognitive, physical, or psychosocial dysfunction. Immediate symptoms associated with TBI include deficits in motor coordination, confusion, and irritation. However, persistent symptoms include deficiencies identifying, understanding, processing, and describing emotions; impulsivity; and mood swings. These chronic problems can result in lifelong cognitive and social deficits.

CASE STUDY

Source: AndreyPopov/iStock/Thinkstock

Case Presentation

A first-time mother and father bring their 3-month-old daughter to a clinic appointment. When the nurse asks the parents if they have any concerns about the baby, the mother responds, "I'm worried because she is still so small and she lifts her head up when she is on her stomach but she doesn't turn over from stomach to side. My neighbor says her grandchild was starting to turn over when she was about 4 months old and my friend's baby who is just about the same age weighs a pound and a half more than mine."

As part of the assessment, the nurse gathers the following information:

- Length at birth: 46 cm (18.4 in.)
- Current length: 57 cm (22.4 in.; increase of 11 cm in 90 days)
- Birth weight: 2786 g (6 lb., 2 oz.)
- Current weight: 5100 g (11.2 lb.; increase of 2314 g in 90 days, or 25.7 g/day)
- Motor (gross and fine): Kicks when placed on back; holds head up 90 degrees and chest off floor when prone; bears weight on legs when feet placed on solid surface; rudimentary reach/swipe toward objects; pulls objects toward midline
- Reflexes: Moro, tonic neck and stepping reflexes readily elicited
- Social/emotional behavior: Child attends to faces within 8–10 in. away and appears expressive with eye and mouth movements at site of mother or positive expressions of others

- Neuro/cognitive: Follows a moving object past midline180 degrees
- Speech and communication: Turns head toward sound; babbles

Based on knowledge of the different areas of development, the nurse assesses the infant's physical growth by comparing the birth weight and length with the current weight and length. The infant is between the 10th and 25th percentiles for weight and at the 25th percentile for length. The infant was born at 40 weeks of gestation; therefore, the physical growth is determined to be slightly less than the average height and weight for a female infant but with consistent growth acceleration from birth. The major 3-month gross motor, fine motor, social/emotional, neurocognitive, and speech and communication milestones are met according to this assessment, and the primitive reflexes found are supposed to be present. Follow up is needed to review the mother's prenatal and birth history inclusive of intrauterine ultrasound tests, α-fetoprotein test, screens for prenatal infections and immunization titers, and the hospital newborn hearing screening result and newborn screening for inborn errors of metabolism and congenital diseases.

The nurse reviews the assessment findings with the mother and explains that the infant's development falls within the normal ranges at this point. The nurse also explains the different elements of development and the individualized nature of developmental milestones achievement, emphasizing that children normally differ in size, growth, and speed of development. Realizing the importance of providing anticipatory guidance to parents as a way of outlining expected developmental gains over time to decrease unusual expectations and anxiety, and to educate parents regarding abnormal or concerning changes, the nurse provides the parents with a list of developmental milestones for reference and tracking and a list of primitive and postural reflexes with their onset and extinction times. The nurse goes on to explain that even though biologically related, children in the same family normally differ in growth and speed of development.

Case Analysis

This case exemplifies the concept of development in several ways, including the collection of assessment data for all aspects of development, the use of standardized tools and instruments, the analysis of findings, and the use of that information to have a conversation with the parents about variations in attainment of milestones.

ACCESS EXEMPLAR LINKS IN YOUR GIDDENS EBOOK

REFERENCES

1. Santrock JW: *Life-span development*, ed 14, New York, 2013, McGraw-Hill.
2. Feldman RS: *Child development*, ed 6, Englewood Cliffs, NJ, 2012, Pearson.
3. Hesselgrave J: Developmental influences on child health promotion. In Hockenberry JJ, Wilson D, editors: *Wong's nursing care of infants and children*, ed 9, St Louis, 2011, Mosby.
4. Seidel HM, Ball JW, Dains JE, et al: *Mosby's guide to physical examination*, ed 7, St Louis, 2010, Mosby.
5. Haith M, Benson J: *Encyclopedia of infant and early childhood development*, St Louis, 2008, Elsevier.
6. Perry SE, Hockenberry MJ, Lowdermilk DL, et al: *Maternal–child nursing care*, ed 5, St Louis, 2014, Elsevier.
7. Trawick-Smith J: *Early childhood development: A multicultural perspective*, ed 6, Upper Saddle River, NJ, 2003, Pearson.
8. Wilson SF, Giddens JF: *Health assessment for nursing practice*, ed 5, St Louis, 2012, Elsevier.
9. Sigelman CK, Rider EA: *Lifespan human development*, ed 6, Belmont, CA, 2008, Wadsworth.
10. Berk LE: *Exploring lifespan development*, ed 3, New York, 2014, Pearson.
11. Berk LE: *Development through the lifespan*, ed 6, New York, 2014, Pearson.
12. Chamley CA, Carson P, Randall D, et al: *Developmental anatomy & physiology of children: A practical approach*, New York, 2005, Churchill Livingstone.
13. Kliegman R, Stanton BF, Geme JW, et al: *Nelson's textbook of pediatrics*, ed 19, New York, 2011, Elsevier.
14. Sarason JG, Johnson JH, Siegal JM: Assessing the impact of life changes: Development of life experiences survey. *J Consult Clin Psychol* 46:932–946, 1978.
15. Gardener H: *Frames of mind: The theory of multiple intelligences*, ed 3, Philadelphia, 2011, Basic Books.
16. American Speech–Language–Hearing Association: Communication for a lifetime, (n.d.). Retrieved from <http://www.asha.org/public>.
17. LaBerge M, Gale T: *Adaptive behavior scales for infants and early childhood. Gale encyclopedia of public health*, Farmington Hills, MI, 2006, The Gale Group. Retrieved from <http://www.encyclopedia.com/doc/1G2-3447200017.html>.

18. Developmental Disabilities Resource Center: *What is a developmental disability?*, Lakewood, CO, 2010, Developmental Disabilities Resource Center. Retrieved from <http://www.ddrcco.com/resources-and-training/definition-of-developmental-disability.php>.

19. Tervo R: Identifying patterns of developmental delays can help diagnose neurodevelopmental disorders. *Clin Pediatrics* 45(6):509–517, 2006.

20. Etzel RA: Developmental milestones in children's environmental health. *Environ Health Perspect* A420–A421, 2010.

21. Crain W: *Theories of development: Concepts and applications*, ed 6, Englewood Cliffs, NJ, 2010, Pearson.

22. Freud S: *The ego and the id and other works* (vol 19), Strachy J, translator, London, 1966, Hogarth Press and the Institute of Psychoanalysis.

23. Erikson EH: *Childhood and society*, ed 2, New York, 1963, Norton.

24. Piaget J: *The theory of stages in cognitive development*, New York, 1969, McGraw-Hill.

25. Singer DG, Revenson TA: *A Piaget primer: How a child thinks*, New York, 1996, Penguin Books.

26. Kohlberg L: *The philosophy of moral development: Moral stages and the idea of justice*, San Francisco, 1981, Harper & Row.

27. Leifer G: *Introduction to maternity & pediatric nursing*, ed 6, St Louis, 2010, Saunders.

28. Whitley PP: Developmental, behavioural and somatic factors in pervasive developmental disorders: Preliminary analysis. *Child Care Health Dev* 30(1):5–11, 2004.

29. Glascoe FP1, Byrne KE, Ashford LG, et al: Accuracy of the Denver-II in developmental screening. *Pediatrics* 89(6 Pt 2):1221–1225, 1992.

30. Estes MEZ: *Health assessment & physical examination*, ed 5, Farmington Hills, MI, 2010, U.S. Delmar Cengage Learning.

31. Caplan J, Gleason JR: Test–retest and interobserver reliability of the Early Language Milestone Scale, ed 2 (ELM Scale-2). *J Pediatr Health Care* 7:212–219, 2006.

32. Robins DL, Casagrande K, Barton M, et al: Validation of the Modified Checklist for Autism in Toddlers, Revised with Follow-up (M-CHAT-R/F). *Pediatrics* 133(1):37–45, 2014.

33. Centers for Disease Control and Prevention, National Center on Birth Defects and Developmental Disabilities, Division of Birth Defects and Developmental Disabilities: Parent information, 2014. Retrieved from <http://www.cdc.gov/parents/index.html>.

34. Hagan JF, Shaw JS, Duncan P: *Bright futures: Guidelines/health supervision of infants, children, & adolescence*, ed 3, Elk Grove Village, IL, 2007, American Academy of Pediatrics.

35. Neinstein LS, Gordon CM, Katzman DK, et al: *Adolescent health care: A practical guide*, ed 5, New York, 2007, Lippincott Williams & Wilkins.

36. The Regents of the University of Michigan: Rapid assessment for adolescent services, 2014. Retrieved from <https://www.raaps.org>.

37. Klein JD, Allan MJ, Elster AB, et al: Improving adolescent health care in community health centers. *Pediatrics* 107(2):318–327, 2001.

38. Berman A, Snyder SJ: *Kozier & Erb's fundamentals of nursing concepts, process, and practice*, ed 9, Upper Saddle River, NJ, 2011, Pearson.

Functional Ability

Lana Sargent

Health is seen as the level of functional ability for an individual's mind and body. Historically, to be considered in "good health" meant that an individual was free from injury, disability, illness, or pain. A challenge to this view occurred when the World Health Organization (WHO) broadened the definition of health as a "state of complete physical, mental, and social well-being, not merely the absence of disease or infirmity."[1,p100] Expanding and refining the definition of what is considered "good health" or "healthy" is a paradigm shift that is inclusive and more representative of the human population, especially those individuals with disabilities or chronic health conditions. The expanded view of health as it relates to functional ability is supported by one of the four overarching goals of *Healthy People 2020*—to promote quality of life, healthy development, and healthy behaviors across all life stages.[2] A key factor in quality of life, and therefore in health, is an individual's ability to function. This view is further supported by the Institute of Medicine report *Crossing the Quality Chasm: A New Health System for the 21st Century*, which emphasizes that a goal of the U.S. health care system is "to improve the health and functioning of the people of the United States."[3,p39] Thus, the concept of functional ability has implications for collaborative health care across all populations and settings.

DEFINITION

Functional ability refers to the individual's ability to perform the normal daily activities required to meet basic needs; fulfill usual roles in the family, workplace, and community; and maintain health and well-being.[4] Specifically, it reflects the adaptive dimension of development, which is concerned with the acquisition of a range of skills that enable independence in the home and in the community. For the purposes of this concept analysis, functional ability is defined as the *cognitive, social, physical, and emotional ability to carry on the normal activities of life*.[5] Functional ability may differ from functional performance, which refers to the actual daily activities carried out by an individual. Functional impairment and disability refers to varying degrees of an individual's inability to perform the tasks required to complete normal life activities without assistance.

SCOPE

On the broadest and simplest level, the scope of functional ability represents a continuum from full function to disability (Figure 2-1). This simple linear perspective is useful to acknowledge that a functional ability is a continuum that varies from person to person and within the same person at different points in time. However, the interaction between the health of an individual and disability is a complex process that is influenced by developmental and biological factors, including current state of health, as well as by psychological, sociocultural, environmental, and politicoeconomic factors. Within the conceptual framework known as the disablement process, the term *function* refers to the positive or neutral interaction between a person's health condition and ability to perform social or physical activities.[6,7] At the other end of the spectrum, *disability* refers to the negative aspects to a person's health condition and social or physical limitation. *Impairment* refers to the physical abnormality that underlies these limitations and is caused by some type of disease process.[7] The scope of conceptualizing function as a complex process that changes based on lifespan, health, and environment is essential to nursing care and assessment across the entire life course from birth to death.

Lifespan Considerations

Functional ability changes across the lifespan as a function of development (occurring predominantly during the infant, toddler, preschool, school age, adolescent, and young adult developmental stages), although changes in environment, lifestyle, and technology require some continued development of functional skills across the entire lifespan. In infants and young children, expected development of functional ability is indicated by achievement of developmental milestones. Specialized age-appropriate tests of development are used when indicated to determine developmental delays (see Concept 1 Development). During young and middle adulthood, identification of problems with functional ability requires careful assessment of each developmental milestone. For older adults, functional status ordinarily refers to the safe, effective performance of activities of daily living (ADLs) essential for independent living.[8] For this age group, intentional

FIGURE 2-1 **Scope of Concept** Functional ability ranges from full function to disability.

screening focused on factors known to contribute to a decline in functional ability is essential. A comprehensive, interprofessional assessment, focused on observed functional, social, or cognition changes, should be performed for all individuals not exclusive of environment (institutionalized or community dwelling) or disease state.

ATTRIBUTES AND CRITERIA

Functional ability has two dimensions: attributes and antecedents. Attributes are defining characteristics of functional ability, and antecedents are events that must happen before functional ability can exist.

Attributes of functional capacity include the following:
- The capacity to perform specific functional abilities
- The actual or required performance of functional abilities

Antecedents of functional capacity include the following:
- Development of physiologic process: neural, endocrine, musculoskeletal, and metabolic
- Acquisition of developmental milestones and skills

At any given time, an individual with the capacity to perform a self-care activity may not complete that activity because of developmental, cultural, environmental, or social factors. Functional ability is further characterized by gradations of capacity or performance. It is not simply a matter of whether the individual *can* or *does* perform the activity but, instead, under what circumstances, with what type and amount of assistance, and in what length of time and with what degree of effort the person *can* or *does* perform the activity. All aspects of this concept presentation are based on these attribute and antecedent principals.

THEORETICAL LINKS

Functional ability is important across the life course because it is a major contributing factor to quality of life. It allows independence and participation in activities that are fulfilling to human nature. Functional ability is also important to health care providers and health care financers because it can indicate the existence and severity of disease, signal the need for services, monitor success of treatment/disease progression, and facilitate cost-effectiveness in the provision of care.[9] Several theories can be used to translate the complex interaction and dynamic process of functional ability across the life course.

A model of nursing with the concept of functional ability as a cornerstone is the *Roper–Logan–Tierney model of nursing*. According to this model, 12 activities of daily living are central to human life; these are presented in Box 2-1. This model was developed in Edinburgh and is used throughout Europe as well as in many other areas of the world to guide nursing education and practice by providing a framework to organize and individualize care. It has a focus on health rather than illness and promotes care directed toward health promotion and wellness. Ongoing patient assessment and facilitation of independence in the patient's normal activities of living are central to the model.[10,11]

The International Classification of Functioning, Disability and Health (ICF) is a framework created by WHO to describe this dynamic

---

BOX 2-1 **The 12 Activities of Daily Living According to the Roper–Logan–Tierney Model of Nursing**

Maintaining a safe environment	Personal cleansing and dressing
Breathing	Maintaining body temperature
Communication	Working and playing
Mobilizing	Sleeping
Eating and drinking	Expressing sexuality
Eliminating	Dying

Source: Data from Roper N, Logan WW: *The Roger–Logan–Tierney model of nursing: Based on activities of living*, London, 2004, Elsevier/Churchill-Livingstone.

(rather than linear) process that occurs between functional ability and disability (Figure 2-2). The ICF focuses on the changes in functional level; these may be temporary (e.g., recovering from an illness or injury) or long term (e.g., spinal cord injury). The ICF highlights the complex interactions of environment and personal factors and the effect they have on the domains of body function, activity, and the person's ability to participate in hobbies, sports, work, shopping, and driving. This criteria is used in the featured exemplars discussed later to illustrate the complex dynamic process of impairment or limitation in functional ability for certain health conditions.[12]

CONTEXT TO NURSING AND HEALTH CARE

Nursing practice has three major dimensions of concern relative to an individual's functional ability: (1) risk recognition, (2) functional assessment, and (3) planning and delivery of individualized care appropriate to level of functional ability. Functional ability is a complex concept that represents the interaction of the physical, psychological, cognitive, and social domains of the human person. Alterations in functional ability occur as primary or secondary problems. Primary problems are those in which the ability to perform a particular function never developed. Secondary problems, on the other hand, occur after functional ability has been attained. Thus, secondary problems represent a loss of functional ability.

Two examples of functional ability are the basic activities of daily living (BADLs or ADLs) and the instrumental activities of daily living (IADLs). The BADLs relate to personal care and mobility and include eating as well as hygienic and grooming activities such as bathing, mouth care, dressing, and toileting. IADLs are more complex skills that are essential to living in the community. Examples of IADLs are managing money, grocery shopping, cooking, house cleaning, doing laundry, taking medication, using the telephone, and accessing transportation. BADLs and IADLs are essential to independent living.[13]

Functional ability is a critical consideration in virtually all areas of health care and to all members of the health care team representing

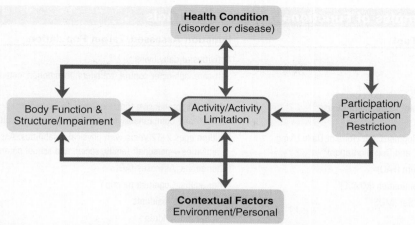

FIGURE 2-2 The International Classification of Functioning, Disability, and Health Model (ICF)
(Source: Redrawn from World Health Organization (WHO): *Towards a common language for functioning, disability and health,* Geneva, 2002, WHO. Retrieved from http://www.who.int/classifications/icf/training/icfbeginnersguide.pdf.)

interprofessional interest. It is a critical element in discharge planning from health care facilities. Successful transition is dependent on the functional level in combination with supportive services such as home care services, inpatient or outpatient rehabilitation services, or placement in a long-term care facility. In the rehabilitation setting, the focus is on restoring functional ability and evaluating the functional outcomes of treatment by means of a functional assessment. For long-term care services, functional impairment—defined as needing assistance with a minimum of two or three ADLs—is a common eligibility criterion.[14]

Risk Recognition

Risk recognition is essential to the early identification of factors that affect function. Actual functional deficiencies lead to subsequent mobilization of resources and support to enhance functional ability. The early identification is critical to the health status of individuals because research has shown that functional deficits are associated with poor health outcomes, whereas good functional ability is associated with positive outcomes. For example, a study of stroke patients revealed that major predictors of independence 5 months after stroke were independent living status and independent in ADLs.[15]

There are multiple risk factors for impaired functional ability because of the multiple variables that impact function, including developmental abnormalities, physical or psychological trauma or disease, social and cultural factors including beliefs and perceptions of health, and physical environment. Research has repeatedly documented age,[15] cognitive function,[16] and level of depression[17] as risk factors for and predictors of functional impairment. Comorbidities and socioeconomic factors have also been implicated. Preclinical disability, defined as task modification without report of difficulty in performing a specific activity, has also been found to be an important predictor of future functional decline and disability in the elderly. In a study of postpartum women, those with postpartum depression (PPD) were 12 times less likely to achieve prepregnancy functional levels than those without PPD. Postpartum depression predicted lower personal, household, and social functioning, but without deficit in infant care.[18] Sudden onset of functional decline is often indicative of acute illness or worsening of a chronic disease.

Risk reduction should be the focus of care for patients with identified risks. Teaching patient and family about factors associated with

maintenance of high-level functional ability is required. These factors include well-balanced nutrition, physical activity, routine health checkups, stress management, regular participation in meaningful activity, and avoidance of tobacco and other substances associated with abuse.[8] In addition, patients need teaching and guidance to develop effective action plans designed to decrease their specific risks. Finally, ongoing assessment of an individual's functional ability can provide continual adjustment of recourses in order to maximize independence rather than dependence.

Functional Assessment

Comprehensive functional assessment is a time-intensive, interprofessional effort requiring use of multiple assessment tools. Comprehensive functional assessment is indicated under specific circumstances. As discussed for Concept 1 Development, children who are delayed in meeting developmental milestones and accomplishing developmental tasks are referred for assessment across domains of development including that of adaptive behavior, which is analogous to functional ability. Comprehensive assessment of functional ability in older adults is indicated when the individual has demonstrated a loss of functional ability, has experienced a change in mental status, has multiple health conditions, or is a frail elderly person living in the community. Screening for functional deficits in older adults should be a part of routine care[19] just as screening for meeting developmental milestones is for children.

An individual's performance of ADLs is basic to functional assessment. ADLs as indicators of functional ability evolved in the late 1950s with the identification of a group of basic physical activities, the performance of which was to be used to evaluate the success of rehabilitation programs. A decade later, IADLs were identified as indicators of ability to live independently in the community. This led to the use of ADLs as a measure of need and eligibility for long-term care and other support services and to the development of an array of assessment tools.

Assessment Tools

The two basic types of assessment tools are self-report and performance-based. Self-report tools provide information about the patient's perception of functional ability, whereas performance-based tools involve actual observation of a standardized task, completion of which is judged by objective criteria. Performance-based assessments are

TABLE 2-1   Examples of Functional Assessment Tools

Functional Assessment Tool	Function Assessed/Target Population
Barthel Index[36]	Activities of daily living
FIMTM Instrument Functional Independence Measure[37]	Self-care, sphincter control, transfers, locomotion, communication, and social cognition
Dartmouth COOP Functional Health Assessment Charts[38]	Adults: Comprehensive functional and social health Adolescents: Comprehensive functional and social health
NGAGED (Now, Growth & Development, Activities of Daily Living, General Health, Environment, and Documentation)[39]	Children ages 2–12 years with physical disabilities: Assesses engagement in life activities—personal, family, social, and school parameters
Functional Activities Questionnaire (FAQ)[40]	Older adults: Assesses IADLs
Folstein Mini-Mental Status Examination (MMSE)[41]	Older adults: Cognitive function
Long Term Care Minimum Data Set (MDS)[42]	Nursing home residents
Functional Status Scale (FSS)[26]	Hospitalized children
The Edmonton Functional Assessment Tool[43]	Cancer patients: Functional performance
24-Hour Functional Ability Questionnaire (24hFAQ)[20]	Outpatient postoperative patients: Functional ability
Geriatric Depression Scale[44]	Older adults: Depression
Inventory of Functional Status after Childbirth[18]	Postpartum women: Functional status

preferred because they avoid potential for inaccurate measurement inherent in self-report. They also can measure functional ability with repetition and with consideration of time on task. Potential problems with self-report measures of functional activity stem from the effect of an individual's personal characteristics and preferences as well as environmental factors. Interpretation of what is meant by the question can vary from person to person. Even when vocabulary is correctly understood, the phrasing of the question can lead to an ambiguous response. For example, if a person is asked, "Can you …?" the answer is based on the person's perception of his or her ability to perform the task, not necessarily on actual ability. Thus, overstatements of ability may occur because of a lack of awareness that gradual changes in ability have occurred. Understatements of ability are possible when an individual has not attempted to perform the activity in question because of culture or preference or mistakenly believes that he or she is unable to perform the task. Ability can also be overreported or underreported by individuals based on personal reasons. Pride and the desire to be seen as self-sufficient, fear of losing independence, and fear of long-term care placement are common reasons for overstatement of ability, especially among elders.

Meaningful measurement of functional ability also has to address the areas of dependency and difficulty. Dependency refers to the amount of assistance needed to function, whether it involves the assistance of an adaptive device or another person. *No assistance*, *partial assistance*, or *total assistance* are examples of common options related to dependency used when scoring functional assessment tools. Common scoring options related to difficulty are *some, a lot*, or *unable to perform*. In addition to functional assessment tools that focus on complex, multidimensional abilities such as ADLs, there are tools designed to assess a specific area of function such as mental status, mobility status, or hand function. There are also tools designed for use with specific populations[20–23] and age groups.[24–27] Table 2-1 presents examples of the wide variety of functional assessment tools. Table 2-2 presents questions and observations associated with functional assessment.

Care Delivery

Knowledge of an individual's functional level in the physical, social/emotional, cognitive, and communication dimensions is essential to planning and implementing effective patient care. Functional level determines the patient's need for assistance as well as the type and amount of assistance required. It guides the nurse in helping with activities while ensuring use of adaptive equipment and maximizing the patient's independent function. This goal of optimal independent function along with the prevention of functional decline is essential to the improvement of health-related quality of life, which as an outcome of care is an objective for individuals of all ages with chronic illness or disability.[28]

Management of functional activity impairment involves a multidisciplinary effort. Early intervention can include one or more of the following services: nursing, medicine, physical therapy, occupational therapy, psychological intervention, individual and/or family counseling, nutritional consulting, speech and language services, audiology services, home health or homemaker assistance, community services (e.g., day care), support groups, and assistive technologies. When functional activity is impaired, early intervention is critical because, in general, the earlier the intervention, the better the outcome.[29]

INTERRELATED CONCEPTS

The human person is a complex integrated whole that is greater than the sum of its parts. It follows, therefore, that concepts used to describe aspects of the human person represent interrelated rather than isolated phenomena. The strength and direction of the impact of one conceptual phenomenon on another vary with the central concept under consideration. Because functional activity depends on the interplay of multiple elements within the physical, psychological, social, and cognitive dimensions, and because it allows for purposeful interaction with the environment, a multitude of concepts can be identified as influencing and/or being influenced by it. Figure 2-3 depicts the most prominent of these interrelationships. Concepts representing major influencing factors and hence determinants of functional ability are Development, Cognition, and Culture, with its unique variations in practices and expectations. These appear at the top of the diagram, and their influence on functional ability is indicated by the arrow pointing in the direction of this concept. Family Dynamics and Coping, as well as the physiologically focused concepts of Mobility, Nutrition, Sensory

TABLE 2-2 Guide to Functional Assessment Screening[13,42,45,46]

Functional Assessment Component	Sample Questions	Observations/Examinations
Vision	Do you have any difficulty seeing? Do you wear glasses or contact lens? Do you use any special equipment to help you see, such as a high-intensity light or magnifying glass? When was your last eye exam?	Observe for signs of impaired vision during interaction with patient: turning head to one side in an effort to see better; nonapplicable comments about room seeming dark; feeling for items. Have patient hold a magazine or newspaper and read a line of print. Have patient read a wall clock or sign at a distance.
Hearing	Do you have difficulty hearing? Does anyone tell you that you are hard of hearing? Do you have to ask people to repeat what they say? Can you hear well in crowds? Can you hear when the area is noisy?	Note patient's apparent hearing during your interaction with him or her. Rub your thumb and forefinger together in front of each of patient's ears; patient should easily hear the sound.
Mobility	Do you have any trouble moving? Do you feel steady when you walk? Do you use anything to help you walk? Do you have trouble getting out of bed? Do you have difficulty sitting down or standing up?	Observe patient's general movements; look for obvious limitation of movement in any body part. Have patient put hands together behind neck and then behind waist to assess external and internal rotation of shoulder. Assess lower extremity function, balance, and gait by asking patient to arise from a straight back chair, stand still, walk across room (approximately 10 feet), turn, walk back, and sit down. Note ability to stand up and sit down; balance when sitting, standing, and walking; gait; and ability to turn.
Fall history	Have you had any falls? Have you had any near falls? Do you take any precautions against falling?	
Continence	Do you ever lose control of your bowels? Do you ever lose control of your urine and wet yourself? Do you wear any type of protective pad or underclothes in case of an accident with urine or bowels?	
Nutrition	Have you gained or lost 10 pounds in the past 6 months without trying? What do you typically eat in a day? Do you have difficulty chewing or swallowing? When was your last dental visit?	Note general appearance as related to nutritional status: well nourished, undernourished, emaciated. Obtain weight and determine body mass index
Cognition	Do you have any trouble with your memory?	Note patient's ability to respond appropriately to questions and directions. Three-item recall at 1 minute; if patient fails this test, follow with MMSE.
Affect	Do you often feel anxious or overstressed? Do you often feel sad or down?	Note patient's expression and if this matches mood.
Home environment	Who do you live with? What type of house do you have: single home, multiple family, apartment? How many floors does the home have? Are there stairs you must use?	
Social participation	What keeps you busy all day? How often do you go out? How often do you have company?	
ADLs (basic and instrumental)	Use a reliable, valid assessment tool to assess function related to grooming, toileting, dressing, eating, walking, shopping, meal preparation, housekeeping, travel/driving, money management.	

Perception, Gas Exchange, and Perfusion, have a clearly reciprocal relationship with functional ability. These concepts surround either side of the concept with double-headed arrows because of their mutual interaction with it. The concepts of Elimination and Sexuality are shown at the bottom of the figure with arrows pointing from functional ability to them because of the primarily unidirectional relationship of these concepts.

CLINICAL EXEMPLARS

Alterations in functional ability may affect one very specific area of function or may be global and affect widespread function. Impaired functional ability is often complex and may involve an array of environmental as well as individual factors. Furthermore, similar alterations in function can be the result of very different causes.

FIGURE 2-3 Functional Ability and Interrelated Concepts

There are multiple exemplars of situations that change an individual's functional ability. Examples of specific exemplars are presented in Box 2-2 using two major categories of problems for distinction: primary and secondary. Causes of primary problems of functional ability may be genetic in origin (i.e., the result of a congenital defect) or may be a result of trauma, disease, or negative environmental factors occurring during the early years of development. Often, however, as with many developmental problems, the cause is unclear.

Secondary problems of functional activity are more commonly identifiable as the result of aging, disease, trauma, or negative environmental factors. Sudden onset of functional decline is a sign of acute disease such as pneumonia, urinary tract infection, or fluid and electrolyte imbalance. Alternatively, it can be a sign of worsening chronic disease such as diabetes, chronic obstructive pulmonary disease, or heart failure.[30] Depending on the extent of alteration in functional ability, the problem may be termed an impairment, a disability, or a handicap.

Featured Exemplars
Cerebral Palsy

Cerebral palsy (CP) refers to a group of neurologic disorders that affect body movement, posture, and muscle coordination. It is caused by abnormal development or injury to the developing brain in the area responsible for muscle control. This disorder occurs before birth, during the birth process, or within the first years of childhood, and it represents the most common motor disability in childhood. There are four main types of CP (spastic CP, dyskinesic CP, ataxic CP, and mixed CP); thus, the severity of symptoms is highly variable. Prevalence estimates of CP range from 1 to 4.5 per 1000 births.[31]

BOX 2-2 EXEMPLARS OF IMPAIRED FUNCTIONAL ABILITY

Causes of Primary Problems
- Angelman's syndrome
- Autism spectrum disorder
- Cerebral palsy
- Down syndrome
- Duchenne's muscular dystrophy
- Fetal alcohol syndrome
- Hypoplastic limb
- Malnutrition
- Receptive or expressive language disorder

Causes of Secondary Problems
- Alzheimer's disease
- Blindness
- Brain injury
- Cardiovascular disease
- Chronic pain
- Chronic fatigue
- Chronic obstructive pulmonary disease
- Deafness
- Malnutrition
- Multiple sclerosis
- Osteoarthritis
- Parkinson's disease
- Rheumatoid arthritis
- Schizophrenia
- Spinal cord injury
- Skeletal fracture
- Stroke

Autism Spectrum Disorder

Autism spectrum disorder (ASD) refers to a broad category of conditions with a wide range of impairments and disabilities affecting children in early childhood that lasts throughout life. Two general areas of dysfunction are social impairment and repetitive behaviors. Although the cause is not well understood, it is suspected that genetic and environmental factors may be involved. ASD represents a primary problem in functional ability because affected individuals have difficulties meeting BADLs or IADLs. The CDC estimates that 1 in 68 children have ASD; the rate in males is four or five times higher than in females.[32]

Alzheimer's Disease

Alzheimer's disease, an irreversible progressive brain disease, is the most common cause of dementia among older adults, affecting an estimated 5 million in the United States.[33] This disorder is characterized by the loss of cognitive functioning (memory, thinking, reasoning, and problem solving) and behavioral changes resulting in a decline of functional ability. The degree of symptoms and functional limitations is directly related to the progression of the disease. Because this occurs in older adults, it is considered a secondary problem in functional ability.

Rheumatoid Arthritis

Rheumatoid arthritis (RA) is a systemic autoimmune condition with genetic predisposition that creates an inflammatory process in the synovial membrane of the joints and other body tissues. Over time, the joint inflammation leads to erosion of the membrane cartilage, causing pain, swelling, and joint deformity; significant impairment in functional ability and mobility results. Affecting less than 1% of the general population, RA is most common among women and individuals older than age 60 years.[34] This is considered a secondary problem in functional ability.

Parkinson's Disease

Parkinson's disease (PD) is a neurologic disorder caused by a loss of dopamine-producing cells in the brain and resulting in motor disability. Four primary symptoms are tremors, rigidity, bradykinesia, and impaired balance and coordination. This condition most commonly occurs in adults older than age 50 years, with a higher incidence among men than women. Although symptoms are subtle and mild initially, these become more pronounced as the disease progresses and interfere with functional ability.[35] An estimated 1 million Americans have PD, with an estimated 50,000–60,000 new cases of PD diagnosed each year.

CASE STUDY

Source: kirstyokeeffe/iStock/ Thinkstock

Case Presentation

Mrs. Rose Finney is an 85-year-old woman with ovarian cancer. She presented at the oncology clinic for a scheduled appointment 6 weeks after surgical removal of her ovaries, uterus, a section of large bowel, and as much tumor mass as possible from other areas of her abdomen. The purpose of the visit was a postoperative checkup and planning for chemotherapy. Mrs. Finney was accompanied by a niece with whom she had stayed while recovering from the surgery. The niece lives out of state and the patient will be returning to her own home after this follow-up appointment. At this visit, the nurse interviewed the patient to obtain detailed self-report information related to functional ability. The following information was gathered:

- Alert, well-groomed, well-spoken, fiercely independent elderly woman recuperating remarkably well from extensive surgery
- Uncontrolled glaucoma with limited vision in one eye; 20/80 vision with glasses in other eye
- Slightly hard of hearing
- Arthritis in fingers along with lack of strength makes some tasks difficult (e.g., opening jars, using telephone)

- Uncertain walking outdoors, particularly in unfamiliar areas and when ground uneven; no assistive devices
- Medication: Synthroid every morning for 47 years
- Never married, no children
- Lives alone in a single home; bedroom on first floor but laundry facilities and garage are on basement level
- Does not drive
- Only living relatives in addition to the niece are two nephews: One lives out of state and other lives ½ hour away
- Telephone contact with closer nephew daily, occasional visits and trips for shopping and other errands
- Three friends in neighborhood, each of whom calls or visits on average every 2 weeks

Case Analysis

Mrs. Finney is at risk for falls as a result of unsteadiness, poor vision, and stair use in her home. In the event of an accident, she is at risk for inability to call for help as a result of living alone and having limited strength, poor eyesight, and arthritis, which makes telephone dialing difficult. Mrs. Finney needs reliable transportation for care appointments and for grocery shopping. Her poor eyesight also makes her at risk for problems with medication compliance during the chemotherapy treatment regimen. Additional monitoring will also be needed because of the risk of associated side effects as a result of chemotherapy.

ACCESS EXEMPLAR LINKS IN YOUR GIDDENS EBOOK

REFERENCES

1. World Health Organization: The constitution of the World Health Organization. *WHO Chron* 1:6–24, 1947.
2. U.S. Department of Health and Human Services: *Healthy People 2020*, 2015. Retrieved from <http://www.healthypeople.gov/>.
3. Institute of Medicine, Committee on Quality of Health Care in America: *Crossing the quality chasm: A new health system for the 21st century*, Washington, DC, 2001, National Academies Press.
4. American Thoracic Society: Quality of life resource, 2007. Retrieved from <http://qol.thoracic.org/sections/key-concepts/functional-status .html>.
5. Tappen RM: *Advanced nursing research: From theory to practice*, Sudbury, MA, 2011, Jones & Bartlett Learning.

6. Granger CV: A conceptual model for functional assessment. In Granger CV, Gresham GE, editors: *Functional assessment in rehabilitation medicine,* Baltimore, 1984, Williams & Wilkins, pp 14–25.

7. Verbrugge LM, Gates DM, Ike RW: Risk factors for disability among US adults with arthritis. *J Clin Epidemiol* 44(2):167–182, 1991.

8. Potter PA, Perry AG: *Fundamentals of nursing,* ed 7, St Louis, 2009, Mosby.

9. Min LC, Wenger NS, Reuben DB, et al: A short functional survey is responsive to changes in functional status in vulnerable older people. *J Am Geriatr Soc* 56(10):1932–1936, 2008.

10. Roper N, Logan WW: *The Roger–Logan–Tierney model of nursing: Based on activities of living,* London, 2004, Elsevier/Churchill-Livingstone.

11. Allegoode M, Tomey AM: *Nursing theorists and their work,* ed 7, St Louis, 2010, Mosby.

12. World Health Organization (WHO): *International Classification of Functioning, Disability, and Health,* Geneva, 2001, WHO.

13. Goldman L, Ausiello D, editors: *Cecil medicine,* ed 23, Philadelphia, 2008, Saunders.

14. Geron SM: Functional ability. In *Encyclopedia of aging,* 2002. Retrieved from <http://www.encyclopedia.com>.

15. Hankey GJ: *Stroke,* ed 2, London, 2007, Churchill Livingstone.

16. Royall DR, Lauterbach EC, Kaufer D, the Committee on Research of the American Neuropsychiatric Association: The cognitive correlates of functional status: A review from the Committee on Research of the American Neuropsychiatric Association. *J Am Geriatr Soc* 55:1705–1711, 2007.

17. Van der Weele GM, Gussekloo J, De Waal MM, et al: Co-occurrence of depression and anxiety in elderly subjects aged 90 years and its relationship with functional status, quality of life and mortality. *Int J Geriatr Psychiatr* 24(6):595–601, 2009.

18. Posmontier B: Functional status outcomes in mothers with and without postpartum depression. *J Midwifery Women's Health* 53(4):310–318, 2008.

19. Bierman AS: Functional status: The sixth vital sign. *J Gen Intern Med* 16(11):785–786, 2001.

20. Hogue SL, Reese PR, Colopy M, et al: Assessing a tool to measure patient functional ability after outpatient surgery. *Anesth Analgesia* 91(1):97–106, 2000.

21. Hudak PL, Amadio PC, Bombardier C: Development of an upper extremity outcome measure: The DASH (disabilities of the arm, shoulder and hand) [corrected]. The Upper Extremity Collaborative Group (UECG). *Am J Ind Med* 29(6):602–608, 1996. erratum in *Am J Ind Med* 30(3):372, 1996.

22. Leidy NK: Functional status and the forward progress of merry-go-rounds: Toward a coherent analytical framework. *Nurs Res* 43:196–202, 1994.

23. Pfeffer RI, Kurosaki TT, Harrah CH, Jr, et al: Measurement of functional activities in older adults in the community. *J Gerontol* 37(3):323–329, 1982. Reprinted with permission of The Gerontological Society of America, 1030 15th St NW, Suite 250, Washington, DC 20005, via Copyright Clearance. Retrieved from <http://www.ncbi.nlm.nih.gov/pubmed/7069156>.

24. Center for Functional Assessment Research at SUNY Buffalo: *Guide for the uniform data set for medical rehabilitation for children (WeeFIM), Version 4.0,* Buffalo, NY, 1993, State University of New York at Buffalo.

25. Odetola F: Assessing the functional status of children. *Pediatrics* 124(1):e163–e165, 2009.

26. Pollack MM, Holubkov R, Glass P, et al; Eunice Kennedy Shriver National Institute of Child Health and Human Development Collaborative Pediatric Critical Care Research Network: Functional status scale: A new pediatric outcome measure. *Pediatrics* 124(1):e18–e28, 2009.

27. Wasson JH, Kairys SW, Nelson EC, et al: A short survey for assessing health and social problems of adolescents. *J Fam Pract* 38:489–494, 1994.

28. Wilson IB, Cleary PD: Linking clinical variables with health-related quality of life. *JAMA* 59-65:1995, 1995.

29. Lubkin IM, Larsen PD: *Chronic illness impact and intervention,* ed 6, Boston, 2006, Jones & Bartlett.

30. Krevesic DM, Mezey M: Assessment of function. In Mezey M, Fulmer T, Abraham I, editors: *Geriatric nursing protocols for best practice,* ed 2, New York, 2003, Springer.

31. Centers for Disease Control and Prevention: Cerebral palsy, 2015. Retrieved from <http://www.cdc.gov/ncbddd/cp/facts.html>.

32. National Institute of Mental Health: Autism spectrum disorder, (n.d.). Retrieved from <http://www.nimh.nih.gov/health/topics/autism-spectrum-disorders-asd/index.shtml#part4>.

33. National Institute on Aging: Alzheimer's disease fact sheet, 2015. Retrieved from <http://www.nia.nih.gov/alzheimers/publication/alzheimers-disease-fact-sheet>.

34. Centers for Disease Control and Prevention: *Arthritis* 2014. Retrieved from <http://www.cdc.gov/arthritis/index.htm>.

35. National Institute of Neurologic Disorders and Stroke: NINDS Parkinson's disease information page, 2015. Retrieved from <http://www.ninds.nih.gov/disorders/parkinsons_disease/parkinsons_disease.htm>.

36. Neal LJ: Current functional assessment tools. *Home Healthc Nurse* 16(11):762–772, 1996.

37. Turner-Stokes T, et al: The UK FIM+FAM: Development and evaluation. *Clin Rehabil* 13:277–287, 1999.

38. Nelson E, Wasson J, Kirk J, et al: Assessment of function in routine clinical practice: Description of the COOP chart method and preliminary findings. *J Chron Dis* 40(Suppl 1):55S–63S, 1987.

39. Guillet SE: Assessing the child with disabilities. *Home Health Nurse* 16:402–409, 1998.

40. McDowell I, Newell C: *Functional disability and handicap. Measuring health: A guide to rating scales and questionnaires,* ed 2, New York, 1996, Oxford University Press.

41. Kurlowicz L, Wallace M: The mini mental status examination (MMSE). *J Gerontol Nurs* 25(5):8–9, 1999.

42. Centers for Medicare and Medicaid Services: *Long Term Care Minimum Data Set,* 2012. Retrieved from <http://www.cms.gov/Research-Statistics-Data-and-Systems/Files-for-Order/IdentifiableDataFiles/LongTermCareMinimumDataSetMDS.html>.

43. Kaasa T, Loomis J, Gillis K, et al: The Edmonton Functional Assessment Tool: preliminary development and evaluation for use in palliative care. *J Pain Symptom Manage* 13(1):10–19, 1997.

44. Sheikh JI, Yesavage JA: *Geriatric Depression Scale (GDS): Recent evidence and development of a shorter version. Clinical Gerontology: A Guide to Assessment and Intervention 165-173,* NY, 1986, The Haworth Press.

45. Nelson E, Landgraf JM, Hays RD, et al: The functional status of patients: How can it be measured in physicians' offices? *Med Care* 28:1111–1126, 1990.

46. Lachs MS, Feinsttein AR, Cooney LM, et al: A simple procedure for general screening for functional disability in elderly patients. *Ann Intern Med* 12(9):699–706, 1990.

Family Dynamics

Shannon E. Perry

The *family* has been viewed traditionally as the primary unit of socialization, the basic structural unit within a community. A family is a group of people who are related by heredity, marriage, or living in the same household. Thus, a family consists of (1) parents and their children; (2) those related by blood, such as ancestors and descendants; or, in a less restricted definition, (3) any group living together as if they were related by blood. A family is who they say they are.

There are a variety of family configurations: the nuclear family, married-parent families, extended families, married-blended families, cohabiting-parent families, single-parent families, no-parent families, and same-sex families.

Because families are the foundation of social context and family members act either as a support system or demonstrate a lack of support for members of the family, nurses must have an understanding of and appreciation for the ways in which family dynamics influence the delivery of health care to individuals. This concept presents family dynamics and includes definitions and exemplars of the application of this concept to professional nursing practice.

DEFINITION

For the purposes of this concept presentation, the term family dynamics is defined as *interrelationships between and among individual family members or "the forces at work within a family that produce particular behaviors or symptoms."*[1,p675] The dynamic is created by the way in which a family lives and interacts with one another. That dynamic—whether positive or negative, supportive or destructive, nurturing or damaging—changes who people are and influences how they view and interact with the world outside of the family. Influences on family dynamics are many and varied. These include such factors as the family configuration, relationship between the parents, number of children in the family, parental presence or absence, other people living in the home, chronic illness, disability, substance abuse, physical abuse, death, culture, socioeconomic status, unemployment, family values, and parenting practices.

When examining family dynamics, ages within the family should be considered. Young people often have ideas at variance with their parents. Grandparents will likely have views different from those of their grandchildren. The history of the people in the family is important. When a couple marry, they bring with them the culture and norms of their family of origin. This will influence the family

dynamics. The role each member plays in the family is significant; it may be important to exchange roles to increase understanding among family members and decrease resentment.

SCOPE

One emphasis in nursing today is providing wellness-oriented family centered care and empowering families to achieve control over their lives. Wherever nurses practice, they will work with families and observe family dynamics across the lifespan. Family dynamics occur between couples, with parents and children, and with extended family members. As implied by the word "dynamic," the interactions between family members are fluid and change with growth and development, time, and circumstances. Thus, the scope of family dynamics ranges from positive/healthy to negative/dysfunctional (Figure 3-1) and is shown on a continuum because these dynamics evolve and change over time and are influenced by multiple variables.

Quality of Relationships

Positive, healthy family dynamics are characterized by relationships that are loving and respectful. Family members support each other, provide nurturance and assistance, and form a unit within society. Family interactions and communications can become negative and dysfunctional as a result of social isolation, perceptions that are inaccurate, and faulty personal interpretations of information.[1] A husband may berate his wife for perceived shortcomings or denigrate a child for having difficulty with school. Siblings may squabble and place blame for incidents. In some instances, a parent and siblings may abuse one child. Observing dysfunctional interactions and communications of parents can lead children to imitate those negative behaviors.

Roles of Family Members

Within the family, individuals assume or are assigned roles: spouse, parent, child, sibling, grandchild, disciplinarian, leader, scapegoat, nurturer, enabler, hero, and so on. Healthy families are able to adapt and adjust to roles that may change over time. For example, as children grow and develop, crises are encountered, illnesses develop, or family members leave home. It may be difficult for family members, especially children, to understand roles, changes in roles, the way changes affect the balance of relationships within the family, and the effects of one family member's actions on the remainder of the family.

FIGURE 3-1 Scope of Concept on a Continuum from Negative/Dysfunctional to Positive/Healthy

Evolving Complexity of the Family

The dynamics change between a married couple when their first child is born. This is because the dynamics in a triad are more complex than those in a dyad (Figure 3-2); further increases in complexity occur when additional children are born. Extended family relationships add to the complexity, as do divorce, remarriage, and stepchildren. Same-sex families may not be accepted by, or may be estranged from, their families of origin, which precludes receiving support from them. In times of illness and stress, family interactions may change—sometimes for the better and sometimes for the worse. Family members can express concern for the ill member; extended family may gather and provide assistance and support. Old quarrels can be resolved, hurts can be forgiven, love can be expressed, and memories can be shared. At other times, quarrels can arise over past slights, the perceived or real burdens of caregiving, and the strain on family finances. Ill family members can become more demanding, believing they deserve special treatment and care. Death must be faced, burial details settled, and assets divided.

ATTRIBUTES AND CRITERIA

Defining attributes of family dynamics include the following:
- Family, however that is defined, is involved.
- The group of people, the family, have relational obligations.
- Communication, verbal or nonverbal, among family members occurs.
- Interactions among family members are fluid, flexible, and changeable (dynamic).

The family, whether a couple or a multigenerational group, communicates and interacts. The more members involved, the greater the complexity of interaction and communication. Communication and interaction are dynamic and changing and can be positive or negative. Positive interactions and communications are growth-producing and produce cohesion. Negative interactions and communications are divisive and disruptive and lead to dysfunction and alienation.

THEORETICAL LINKS

Family Systems Theory

Wright and Leahy describe systems theory as allowing nurses to "view the family as a unit and thus focus on observing the interaction among family members, and between the family and the illness or problem rather than studying family members individually."[2,p22] The following are key characteristics of family systems theory: (1) A family system is part of a larger suprasystem and is composed of many subsystems, (2) the family as a whole is greater than the sum of its individual members, (3) a change in one family member affects all family members, (4) the family is able to create a balance between change and stability, and (5) family members' behaviors are best understood from a view of circular rather than linear causality.[2]

Because a change in one family member affects all family members, a change in family dynamics occurs. For example, when Tama, a mother of three children, gives birth to her fourth child, the father and the siblings of the baby experience change, and the relationships among the members of the family change. The father, Peter, has to assume additional responsibilities for care of the family while the mother recuperates from the birth. He can prepare meals and do laundry; he can assume some care of the newborn. Siblings must share their mother's love and time with this new member; sibling rivalry may occur. The family attempts to balance this change and restore stability. As the newborn is incorporated into the family, the siblings resume their previous activities.

Because one family member changes, the family changes, and in turn this change affects the member who changed (circular causality). The mother is now the mother of four children with the additional responsibilities of caring for a newborn and three other children while maintaining her relationship with her partner.

Structural–Functional Theory

The origins of structural–functional theory are in social anthropology.[3,4] In this theory, the family is a social system. Family members have specific roles, such as the father role, mother role, and daughter or son role. Maintaining equilibrium between complementary roles is accomplished through family dynamics. This permits the family to function within the family unit and in society. Some families establish rigid boundaries and outsiders are kept at a distance. Some families may be isolated and may find that in times of crisis their resources are inadequate. Other families maintain open boundaries and give and accept assistance when needed. Some reciprocal relationships within the family can be detrimental, such as designating one member as the family scapegoat or viewing another family member as weak or dependent. Another family member may be identified as the strong or responsible one, and undue expectations may be placed on that member.

Family Stress Theory

The focus of the family stress theory is on the way families react to stress.[5] Stress of families can be studied in the contexts in which the family is living, both internal and external. Events that the family can change or control (e.g., family structure, psychological defenses, and philosophical values and beliefs) comprise the internal context. The external context is composed of the time and place in which a family finds itself and over which the family has no control (e.g., culture of the larger society, time in history, economic state of society, maturity of the individuals involved, success of the family in coping with stressors, and genetic inheritance).

Tama and Peter have a strong sense of family, are supportive of each other, and value family (internal context). They were prepared to cope with the stress on family finances incurred by the addition of the fourth child. However, at 6 weeks of age, the baby was diagnosed with pyloric stenosis and required hospitalization and surgery. This created additional stress on the family, including concern about the health of the

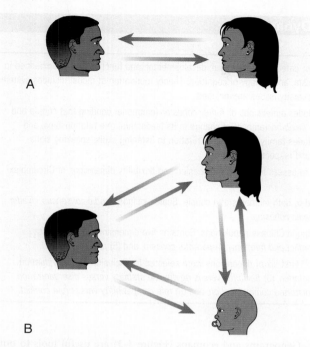

FIGURE 3-2 Complexity of Relationships within the Family **A**, Dyad. **B**, Triad.

baby, separation of the mother and infant from the family during the hospitalization, and increased strain on finances. The maternal grandmother assisted with the care of the children while the infant was hospitalized, introducing a different level of relationship and increasing the number of interactions within the family. Peter and his mother-in-law do not always agree on childrearing activities, meal preparation, or discipline, which creates additional stress.

Family Life Cycle (Developmental) Theory

Families pass through stages. Relationships among family members move through transitions. Although families have roles and functions, a family's main value is in relationships that are irreplaceable. Developmental stresses can disrupt the life cycle process.[6]

The family of Tama and Peter went through stages of dating and marriage to being a couple, to becoming parents of one child, and now as parents of four children. Tama and Peter's exclusive relationship expanded to include their firstborn. When the second child was born, the firstborn had to relinquish his role as an only child and develop a relationship with his sibling. The complexity of relationships increased exponentially as the size of the family increased.

Children grow and develop within the family and expand the cycle of their relationships through play groups, school, church, and social club activities. As they mature and change, family relationships will change.

As time goes on, Tama and Peter will progress to being grandparents, growing older, and relinquishing their places as primary in the lives of their children. Role reversals may occur as they age; their children as adults may need to care for them and, eventually, deal with their deaths.

CONTEXT TO NURSING AND HEALTH CARE

The family influences and is influenced by other people and institutions. This plays a pivotal role in health care. There are many situations in which the nurse interacts with the family while providing care. Understanding family dynamics and how these dynamics relate to

health is important to nurses for the provision of quality nursing care.[7] The family, whether present or absent, influences the patient, either positively or negatively. For nurses to be effective in their care of the family, they must recognize risks, assess situations, and plan and deliver care appropriate to the situation.

Risk Recognition

During interactions with patients and families, nurses must recognize family dynamics that promote health and family dynamics that place families at risk for dysfunction. Examples of situations that place stress on families follow.

Expanding Family

When a family is expanding through childbirth, adoption, or blending families, the dynamics among family members change. The birth of a baby is usually a joyous event while at the same time creating stress within the family. The infant may be born prematurely, with congenital defects, or die. Home arrangements, finances, and work obligations may change. The complexity of family interactions increases and provides opportunities for growth or misunderstanding. Family interactions can vary depending on the age of a child at adoption. A baby may be easily assimilated, whereas an older child brings additional challenges to becoming part of a family. Children of different ages with differing backgrounds must learn to live together when families are blended. Whether through death or divorce, a parent will be missed, and the stepparent must be acknowledged. Each of these situations brings challenges to families, and the ways they interact will be affected.

Cancer Diagnosis/Life-Threatening Illness

Breast cancer can be a devastating diagnosis. The woman who receives this news must face her own mortality, make decisions about treatment, and share her concerns with her family. In some instances, the family will provide the necessary understanding, support, and comfort throughout the treatment. In other instances, the family is the one needing support. Family members may have difficulty envisioning life without this wife/mother/daughter on whom they rely. While she is in need of support, she finds herself comforting her family and without the comfort and support she needs.

Intimate Partner Violence

Nurses may encounter women (or men) in emergency departments or other settings who have experienced intimate partner violence. Although the interaction of the perpetrator with the victim can appear loving and concerned, the behavior may conceal the actual dynamics of the couple. Parents may abuse one or more children. Adult children may abuse their parents.

Substance Abuse/Addiction

People abusing various substances may live in a dysfunctional family that provides little assistance in coping with their problems and addictions. Nurses working in mental health and psychiatric settings, as well as in all health care settings, may encounter such codependent individuals and families. The families may demonstrate enabling behaviors and try to "rescue" the person abusing substances instead of encouraging him or her to seek treatment.

Death and Dying

In hospitals, long-term care, and hospice settings, nurses care for individuals who are dying and their families. Whether the death is of a newborn with congenital anomalies or is premature, an elderly person of natural causes, or is a sudden death of a younger person as the result of an accident or illness, families react in various ways.

TABLE 3-1   Models and Tools to Assess Family Dynamics

Model	Purpose/Description
Calgary Family Assessment Model[2]	A multidimensional framework with three major categories: structural, developmental, and functional. It is embedded in larger worldviews of postmodernism, feminism, and biology of cognition. Theory foundation of model includes systems, cybernetics, communication, and change. Diversity issues are included.
Circumplex Model of Marital & Family Systems[14]	Family model grounded in systems theory. Includes dimensions of *family cohesion* (emotional bonding that couple and family members have toward one another), *flexibility* (amount of change in its leadership, role relationships, and relationship rules), and *communication* (includes family as a group in relation to listening skills, speaking skills, self-disclosure, clarity, continuity tracking, and respect and regard).
Family Adaptability and Cohesion Evaluation Scales (FACES IV)[15]	Updated version of self-report scale designed to assess full range of cohesion and flexibility dimensions of Circumplex Model.
Dyadic Adjustment Scale[16]	Self-report 32-item questionnaire administered to both members of a couple. Scales include *dyadic consensus, dyadic satisfaction, affectional expression,* and *dyadic cohesion.*
Chinese Family Assessment Instrument (C-FAI)[17]	Self-report measure to assess family functioning in Chinese populations. Contains five dimensions: (1) *mutuality,* (2) *communication and cohesiveness,* (3) *conflict and harmony,* (4) *parental concern,* and (5) *parental control.*
Family Dynamics Measure II (FDM II)[18]	Based on eight bipolar dimensions of Barnhill.[19] First six of dimensions were selected for inclusion: (1) *individuation versus enmeshment,* (2) *mutuality versus isolation,* (3) *flexibility versus rigidity,* (4) *stability versus disorganization,* (5) *clear communication versus unclear or distorted communication,* and (6) *role compatibility versus role conflict.*

Grieving takes many forms, and nurses should be cognizant of various manifestations of grief and ways to assist the family. Nurses provide supportive care and information; request spiritual advisors as desired by the family; and answer questions about postmortem examinations, organ donation, and disposition of the body.

Conducting a Family Assessment

A number of culturally sensitive tools have been developed to assess or measure family dynamics (Table 3-1). These and other models are often used in studies of family dynamics. The following example uses the Calgary Family Assessment Model to illustrate a system of family assessment.

The Calgary Family Assessment Model (CFAM)[2] is widely used by nurses to assess families. Wright and Leahy caution that the nurse must recognize that such an assessment is based on the perspective of the nurse (based on personal and professional life experiences) and interactions with interviewees.[2] The assessment is not "the truth" about the family but is just one perspective at one point in time.

The model is used to ask family members questions about themselves in order to gain understanding of the structure, development, and function at a point in time. Not all questions within the subcategories are asked at the first interview, and not all questions are appropriate for all families. Although individuals are interviewed, the focus of a family assessment is on the interaction among the individuals in the family.

The three major categories of the CFAM are structural, developmental, and functional.[2] There are several subcategories for each category. In this brief explanation of the model, only the major categories are addressed. Sample questions used in an assessment are included. Consult the Wright and Leahy text for a full explanation of the model.

Structural Assessment

Assessment of the structure of the family includes determining the members of the family, the relationship among family members in contrast to relationships with those outside the family, and the context of the family. Questions to assess the structure include the following:
- Who is in your family?
- Does anyone else live with you?
- Has anyone moved out recently?
- Is there anyone you think of as family who does not live with you?[2]

Genograms and ecomaps (Figure 3-3) are useful tools to outline the family's internal and external structures. These tools can be hand drawn. In addition, some computer programs are available to construct genograms.

Developmental Assessment

Most nurses are knowledgeable about the stages of child development and adult development, and there is increasing literature about development during senior years. However, family development is more than concurrent development of individuals in a family. Family development is different from family life cycle. Family development considers the vicissitudes of living with both predictable and unpredictable events. Family life cycle describes the typical trajectory followed by most families. The CFAM uses family life cycle to organize the assessment of family development.[2]

The following are sample questions for families in later life:
- When you review your life, what aspects did you enjoy the most?
- What aspects generate the most regret?
- As your health is declining, what plans have you made for your care or that of others in your family who are in ill health?

Functional Assessment of Family Relationships

Functional assessment addresses how individuals actually behave in relation to one another.[2] The two basic aspects of family functioning are instrumental and expressive. Instrumental aspects include routine activities of daily living, such as preparing meals, eating, sleeping, doing laundry, and changing dressings. Expressive aspects include communication (emotional, verbal, nonverbal, and circular), problem solving, roles, influence and power, beliefs, and alliances and coalitions.[2] The categories are not used to define a family's emotional health; it is the family's judgment of whether they are functioning well that is important.

Questions such as the following can be asked:
- Whose role is it to see that Granddad takes his medicine?
- Whose turn is it to bathe Granddad?
- Why is Jimmy not helping to take care of Granddad?
- How can we get Jimmy to help with the caretaking?

If the family is having trouble coping with instrumental issues, often expressive issues exist. However, the family can cope with

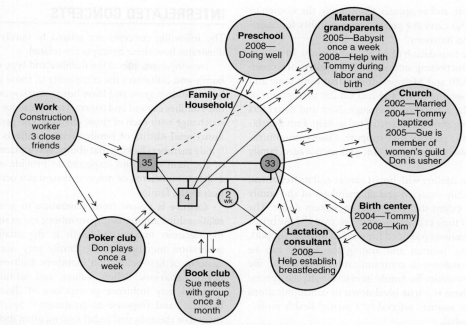

FIGURE 3-3 Example of Ecomap Describing Social Relationships and Depicting Available Supports (Source: From Lowdermilk DL, Perry SE, Cashion K, Alden KR: *Maternity and women's health care,* ed 11, St Louis, 2016, Elsevier.)

instrumental issues and still have expressive issues. Thus, assessment of both is essential.

Planning Care When Family Dynamics Are Dysfunctional

Knowledge of the quality and appropriateness of family dynamics enables nurses to set goals, create a plan of care, and provide that care while continuing to assess the family. Evaluation of the plan provides the opportunity to make any changes necessary based on changes observed in the dynamics of communication and interactions of the family.

Breast Cancer Diagnosis

When Alyssa was diagnosed with breast cancer and a radical mastectomy was performed, she spent much of her time before and after surgery comforting her husband and father, who had great difficulty accepting the diagnosis and facing the possibility of mortality associated with a diagnosis of cancer. The nurse observed no family member or friend providing encouragement or support for Alyssa.

The nurse could spend time listening to Alyssa, expressing empathy and answering Alyssa's questions. The nurse could volunteer to contact any friends or family members who would be supportive of Alyssa. A member of a cancer survivor group such as Reach to Recovery is often helpful because members have an understanding of exactly what Alyssa is experiencing.

Intimate Partner Violence

April arrived at the emergency department with significant bruising on her arms and legs, a black eye, and a forearm that is obviously broken. She is moaning and crying with pain. She is accompanied by her husband, Ronnie. He informed the nurse that April is clumsy and fell down the stairs. He hovers over her solicitously and refuses to leave her side when requested by the nurse. When the nurse tries to take a history, Ronnie interrupts and answers all the questions for April.

The nurse should suspect intimate partner violence (IPV) and endeavor to speak to April alone. For example, she can accompany April to the women's restroom, where Ronnie would not be present. She could ask April about IPV and assure her that no one deserves to be abused. She can provide April with phone numbers of organizations or persons who assist women experiencing IPV. The nurse may support April developing a plan to leave the abusive situation and in contacting the police.

Death and Dying

While Herman was dying of renal failure, his children argued loudly outside his room about who would be responsible for the hospital bills and burial costs.

After suggesting that the family move further away from Herman's room, the nurse can recommend that the family consult a social worker to deal with the financial implications of the hospitalization and the death of their father. In the meantime, spending time with their father and assuring him of their love and support are more therapeutic for both the family and the father. A hospice worker may be useful in helping the family deal with the death of their father.

Planning Care When Family Dynamics Are Positive
Expanding Family

A nurse caring for Tama during her labor and birth assists Peter to coach and support Tama. She ascertains how the children have been prepared for the birth of the baby, and she encourages Peter to bring the children to the birth center to visit their mother and meet the new baby. She provides teaching about sibling rivalry, breast-feeding, and postpartum recovery; encourages rest and good nutrition; offers exercises that will assist in recovery; and includes Peter and the siblings in appropriate teaching. She observes interactions among the family, identifies any obvious difficulties, and makes recommendations and referrals as appropriate.

Breast Cancer Diagnosis

A diagnosis of breast cancer can change family dynamics. The family must make decisions and strive to cope with the changes engendered by the diagnosis, treatment, and prognosis. Commonly, the women in the family are the ones who carry the greatest responsibility for maintaining family balance and harmony.[2]

Communication is the foundation of good relationships. In a study of perception of family functioning among family members of women who had breast cancer, Biffi and Mamede[8] found that both male and female family members became closer and had similar perceptions of the family identity and the adaptation to change. Sons and daughters assumed a problem-coping stance and attempted to help. Female relatives were important in the provision of support. Clear communication among family members relieved tension and encouraged family interactions.[9]

To support the woman dealing with breast cancer and its treatment, nursing care must be family centered and all members of the family must be included to the extent that they and the woman desire. The family can be informed of their crucial role in the recovery of the breast cancer survivor and suggestions provided for ways to provide support. Communication with the woman and among the family can be encouraged. When a breakdown in communication is observed, the nurse can facilitate opportunities for family interactions to clarify misunderstandings. When there is a true breakdown in communications that negatively affects the woman, referral to a mental health professional may be recommended.

Substance Abuse/Addiction

Complex family issues often occur in conjunction with treatment or hospitalization for substance abuse or addiction. Often, there is significant codependency, and treatment must include the family as part of therapy. High levels of collaboration among the referring provider, the patient, and the family contribute to the success of therapy. Family therapy can help patients and their families make systemic changes that will reduce the likelihood of rehospitalization.[9] Nurses working in psychiatric settings participate in individual and group therapy sessions. They may also participate in family therapy. Inclusion of the family in the plan of care is crucial for increasing the possibility of integrating the patient back into the family upon discharge from treatment or a psychiatric facility.

INTERRELATED CONCEPTS

The following concepts are related to family dynamics. Figure 3-4 illustrates how these concepts are related.

Development affects the number and type of interactions within a family and influences the complexity of those interactions. Infants are born; children grow and leave home; marriages occur; parents age and die. Families expand and contract as a consequence, and family dynamics change with each of those changes. The presence or absence of the **Functional Ability** of family members affects the self-concept of the family members lacking that ability, and it places stress on the members of the family who are expected to provide assistance. Whether the assistance is offered or not, resentment can occur and lead to dysfunction in the family.

Culture is passed from generation to generation and can affect relationships among family members; for example, the male is always the decision maker; childbirth is the affair of women. Second-generation members of the family may not share the values and customs of first-generation members. Culture has a direct effect on health behaviors. Beliefs, values, and attitudes that are culturally acquired may influence perceptions of illness, health care-seeking behavior, and response to treatment.[10] **Spirituality** encompasses a mental or metaphysical belief system, often including belief in a higher being and participation in organized religion. Families often share similar beliefs, but when beliefs diverge, conflicts can occur. Spirituality can bring great comfort in times of stress, illness, and hardship. It can also cause distress when expectations for assistance are not met.

A fundamental purpose of a family is **Reproduction**. The addition of children, whether by birth, adoption, or blending of families, increases the complexity of interactions in a family, introduces stress, and provides the potential for growth and maturation. Infertility creates different stresses through inability to have desired children, through the many tests and procedures undergone to ascertain the cause of the infertility, or through the procedures to try to achieve pregnancy. Physiological or psychological **Stress** can create challenges for individuals and families. Stress may be from disease onset or sequelae of addictions or substance abuse. It may exist over a period

FIGURE 3-4 Family Dynamics and Interrelated Concepts

of time such as from an acute infection or for a lifetime, as with a diagnosis of diabetes. The family can be a source of support for the one experiencing stress or, conversely, add to the stress by the family's lack of support.

CLINICAL EXEMPLARS

Positive and negative exemplars of family dynamics provide opportunity to see the great variety of situations in which family dynamics can be observed (Box 3-1). The importance of understanding family dynamics when caring for families should lead the nurse to study the factors involved, practice observation of families, and learn appropriate intervention techniques. A detailed discussion of each of these is beyond the scope of this text, but several important exemplars are briefly presented here. Refer to other references for further information about these exemplars and specific interventions for each.

Featured Exemplars
Expanding Family
The family expands by the birth or adoption of a child or by blending families with children through marriage or cohabitation. The family

---

BOX 3-1   EXEMPLARS OF FAMILY DYNAMICS

Changes to Family Dynamics
- Expanding family (birth or adoption of an infant; blended family)
- Caregiver role for family member
- Change in socioeconomic status of family
- Chronic illness of family member
- Marriage, divorce/remarriage
- Traumatic injury of family member
- Disability of family member
- Aging of family members
- End-of-life care
- Death of family member

Positive Family Dynamics
- Assistance with child care after birth of new infant
- Respite care for a caregiver
- Support after injury or death of a spouse
- Presence during surgery
- Family reunions
- Celebrations of birthdays and other significant events
- Praying together
- Supportive in-laws
- Sharing care of a dependent family member

Negative/Dysfunctional Family Dynamics
- Child abuse
- Codependency (related to substance abuse by a family member)
- Interfering in-laws
- Intimate partner violence
- Marital infidelity
- Placing blame for birth of a preterm infant or for death of a young child by SIDS
- Sibling rivalry
- Adolescent pregnancy

SIDS, sudden infant death syndrome.

---

can also expand by incorporating parents or other extended family members. The complexity of communication and interaction is increased in these instances in proportion to the number of individuals involved.

Sibling Rivalry
Sibling rivalry is competition or animosity between and among siblings. It is common with the birth of an infant when the older child competes with the infant for the time and attention of a parent but is usually quickly outgrown. As children grow, the rivalry may be heightened, resulting in arguing and fighting. Sibling rivalry may persist into adulthood. At times, the rivalry is healthy, encouraging the siblings to excel. At other times, lifelong animosity may persist.

Intimate Partner Violence
Intimate partner violence is physical, sexual, emotional, or psychological abuse, threatened or actual, by a current or ex-spouse, current or ex-boyfriend or girlfriend, cohabiting partner, or date. Both women and men can be victims. It involves social isolation, emotional distress, and personal safety.[11]

Child Abuse
Child abuse is intentional physical or emotional abuse or neglect, including sexual abuse, of a child, usually by an adult. It is a significant social problem affecting children and can result in disability or death. Child abuse is significantly underreported, so actual incidence is unknown.

Codependency
Codependency is characterized by a relationship in which a person is controlled or manipulated by another who has an illness or addiction. It is a dysfunctional pattern of living and problem solving. It occurs in a setting in which there is addiction, physical or emotional abuse, neglect, or a dysfunction that causes pain and stress.[12,13]

Absent Extended Family
The mobility of today's society means that many children move away from their family of origin or retired parents move to a retirement area, often hundreds of miles away. Extended family members often provide child care; help with cooking or cleaning in the event of illness or disability; provide transportation; and, by their presence, have the opportunity to pass on family stories and traditions. When they are absent, there is a void in support and limited opportunity for young children to know their grandparents, aunts and uncles, and other family members.

Aging of Family Members
For many people, healthy aging occurs with retention of their mental and physical capacities. For others, as they age, their capacities and roles may change. Disability and the need for care often come with aging. Hearing and sight may become impaired; mobility may decrease. The aged person may no longer be able to drive. Mental capacity and memory may decline. Adult children may have to provide care for their aging parents.

Death of a Family Member
As part of the cycle of life, family members will die. The death of an infant, child, young parent, middle-aged or older adult, or the aged will have different effects on the family. Tradition, culture, and spiritual beliefs will influence the response to death. Grief may be manifested in a variety of ways and may last a significant length of time.

CASE STUDY

Case Presentation

Source: Jupiterimages/Photos.com/ Thinkstock

Marge is a single parent who dropped out of high school to marry Andrew when she was 17 years old and pregnant. After 6 years of marriage and two children (Stacy, age 5 years, and Monica, age 2 years), Marge divorced Andrew because of his drinking, affairs, and lack of support of her and the children.

Andrew has a job delivering newspapers and spends free time drinking beer with friends. He only sporadically provides monetary support. Marge and the girls live in a small apartment. Because she has only a minimum wage job, Marge relies on food stamps and other types of assistance. Babysitters and rent are major expenses, and Marge continually worries about being able to pay rent. She would like to earn her GED to get a better job, but she lacks the time and resources to make that happen. Andrew sees the girls only occasionally—usually when Marge asks him to keep the girls so she can work extra shifts. He dislikes spending his time babysitting the girls and openly verbalizes his frustration with the "whiny girls."

Marge's parents live close by but believe that Marge deserves her situation. They were very against her leaving school to get married, and they consider Andrew a "deadbeat." They decline to help Marge financially, citing concerns for their own retirement. They also do not help with babysitting, and they accuse Marge of "spoiling the girls." Marge has always believed that her parents liked her older brother, Dominic, better. He is married and has three children who spend a great deal of time with Marge's and Dominic's parents. Dominic rarely interacts with Marge because they "don't have anything in common."

Recently, after the girls spent time with their father, Marge noticed bruises on the arms and the buttocks of Monica. When she asked the girls what happened, Stacey said, "Daddy got mad when Monica wet her pants and spanked her." A week later, while at a health clinic getting Stacy immunized for school, Marge shared with the nurse practitioner details of her life and situation: lack of money and support, working too many hours, fear of losing her apartment, and now—Andrew hurting Monica. She said she does not know what to do and began crying.

Case Analysis

Marge and Andrew, while married, were in the stage of "families with young children" in the "family life cycle," whereas their parents are in the stage of "families in later life." However, since the divorce, Marge and the children form the family unit. Both Marge and Andrew are in the young adult developmental stage.

The interactions among all the family members are dysfunctional. Marge's parents appear to favor her brother and his children while giving little support or encouragement to Marge. Exploration of the origins of this situation is necessary before any practical suggestions for resolution of differences can be offered. Family therapy involving Marge, Dominic, and their parents would be ideal but is unlikely to occur.

The nurse practitioner must be cognizant of the laws of the state in which he or she practices and must report the alleged abuse. Marge may need to consult with legal aid to change visitation rights for Andrew so that she can keep the children safe. Referral of Marge to a counseling center where she could obtain assistance with planning to obtain a GED, prepare for a higher-paying job, and obtain financial assistance would be a short-term solution. Marge must also plan for child care; she might be able to find a day-care center for low-income families for Monica.

This is a family with serious problems with interrelationships. There are many long-term problems with few or no short-term solutions. Counseling individually and as a family is necessary to attain more healthy interactions but may be unlikely to occur. It will take great resolve and work on Marge's part to achieve her goal of a healthy relationship with her parents and brother.

ACCESS EXEMPLAR LINKS IN YOUR GIDDENS EBOOK

REFERENCES

1. Mosby: *Mosby's dictionary of medicine, nursing & health professions*, ed 9, St Louis, 2013, Elsevier.
2. Wright LM, Leahy M: *Nurses and families: A guide to family assessment and intervention*, ed 5, Philadelphia, 2009, Davis.
3. Malinowski F: *The dynamics of cultural change*, New Haven, CT, 1945, Yale University Press.
4. Radcliffe-Brown A: *Structure and function in a primitive society*, New York, 1952, Free Press.
5. Boss P: *Family stress management*, ed 2, Thousand Oaks, CA, 2002, Sage.
6. McGoldrick M, Carter B, Garcia-Preto N: *The expanded family life cycle: Individual, family and social perspectives*, ed 4, Englewood Cliffs, NJ, 2010, Prentice-Hall.
7. White MA, Elder JH, Paavilainen E, et al: Family dynamics in the United States, Finland and Iceland. *Scand J Caring Sci* 24(1):84–93, 2010.
8. Biffi RG, Mamede MV: Perception of family functioning among relatives of women who survived breast cancer: Gender differences. *Rev Latino-American Enfermagem* 18(2):269–277, 2010.
9. Anderson RJ, Huff NL, Hodgson JL: Medical family therapy in an inpatient psychiatric setting: A qualitative study. *Families Systems Health* 26(2):164–180, 2008.
10. Martinez-Campos R: Community care: The family and culture. In Lowdermilk DL, Perry SE, Cashion K, et al, editors: *Maternity and women's health care*, ed 11, St Louis, 2016, Elsevier.
11. Esposito N: Violence against women. In Lowdermilk DL, Perry SE, Cashion K, et al, editors: *Maternity and women's health care*, ed 11, St Louis, 2016, Elsevier.
12. All About Counseling: Codependency, n.d. Retrieved from <http://www.allaboutcounseling.com/codependency.htm>.
13. Johnson RS: Codependency and codependent relationships, 2014. Retrieved from <http://bpdfamily.com/content/codependency-codependent-relationships>.
14. Olson DH, Gorall DM: Circumplex model of marital and family systems. In Walsh F, editor: *Normal family processes*, ed 3, New York, 2003, Guilford.
15. Olson DH: Circumplex model of family systems. *J Family Therapy* 22(2):144–167, 2000.
16. Spanier G: Measuring dyadic adjustment: New scales for assessing the quality of marriage and similar dyads. *J Marriage Family* 38(1):15–28, 1976.
17. Shek DTL: Assessment of family functioning in Chinese adolescents: The Chinese Family Assessment Instrument. In Singh NN, Ollendick T, Singh AN, editors: *International perspectives on child and adolescent mental health*, Amsterdam, 2002, Elsevier, pp 297–316.
18. Lasky P, Buckwalter KC, Whall A, et al: Developing an instrument for the assessment of family dynamics. *Western J Nursing Res* 7(1):40–57, 1985.
19. Barnhill LR: Healthy family systems. *Family Coordinator* 28:94–100, 1979.

Culture

Susan Caplan

Human beings need to construct meaning from their experiences, and this construction or created reality is known as culture.[1] Culture forms a person's worldview, which in turn shapes his or her beliefs about health and illness. The concept of culture is an important aspect of understanding human behavior[2] and, in particular, is a critical part of understanding how to provide person-centered nursing care.

DEFINITION

For the purpose of this concept presentation, culture is defined as *a pattern of shared attitudes, beliefs, self-definitions, norms, roles, and values that can occur among those who speak a particular language or live in a defined geographical region.*[3] These dimensions guide such areas as social relationships; expression of thoughts, emotions, and morality; religious beliefs and rituals; and use of technology.

A discussion of culture includes the subconcepts of enculturation, acculturation, assimilation, biculturalism, ethnicity, and ethnic identity. *Enculturation* is the process by which a person learns the norms, values, and behaviors of a culture, similar to socialization. *Acculturation* is the process of acquiring new attitudes, roles, customs, or behaviors as a result of contact with another culture. Both the host culture and the culture of origin are changed as a result of reciprocal influences. Unlike acculturation, *assimilation* is a process by which a person gives up his or her original identity and develops a new cultural identity by becoming absorbed into the more dominant cultural group.[4] Usually, when a minority group or individual assimilates, they do not have a choice about what aspects of the dominant culture they will adopt; rather, the dominant culture's values and practices are imposed upon the less dominant group. In contrast, in the case of *biculturalism*, the individual has a dual pattern of identification and chooses which aspects of the new culture he or she wishes to adopt and which aspects of the individual's original culture he or she wishes to retain.

Ethnicity refers to a common ancestry that leads to shared values and beliefs. It is transmitted over generations by the family and community. Ethnicity is a powerful determinant of one's identity, known as *ethnic identity*. Race is sometimes thought of in biological terms (for some people, it has a biological meaning) based on the erroneous belief in the existence of hereditary physical differences among people that define membership in a particular group.[5] However, there are no genetic characteristics that distinguish one group of people from

another and, in fact, there are more genetic differences among people who are labeled "black" than there are differences between "blacks" and people labeled "white."[5] As stated by Haney Lopez in 1994, "It is clear that even though race does not have a biological meaning, it does have a social meaning which has been legally constructed."[5,pp6–7]

SCOPE

The concept of culture is very broad and influences the shared beliefs, values, and behaviors of a group. Cultural norms impact all aspects of life, including everything from interpersonal relationships, family dynamics, and childrearing practices to gender roles, dietary preferences, communication, dress, and religious practices. Cultural norms also significantly influence how people make decisions about treatment preferences, medication adherence, self-care, and perceptions of illness, which in turn affects nursing care and health care delivery. The scope of these influences, in the context of health and illness, is illustrated in Figure 4-1. Kleinman makes the distinction between the Western biomedical model of disease and traditional models of illness.[6] Disease is a response to physiological causes explained by pathophysiology and manifested by symptoms and signs.[7] In contrast, traditional health beliefs define illness in terms of mind, body, and spiritual and social connections.[8] Therefore, all illnesses reflect the influence of the environment, including an individual's cultural experiences.

Causal Beliefs about Illness

Cultural differences can result in different explanations for illness.[9,10] In non-Western cultures, explanatory models of illness might include natural causes (e.g., bacteria, viruses, climate, and environmental irritants), the social world (e.g., punishment for individual behaviors or negative social interactions), or the supernatural world (e.g., ancestral spirits and deities). Western cultures are more likely to endorse solely biomedical causation theories, whereas many non-Western cultures have theories of disease causation that can be characterized as an imbalance with natural, social, or spiritual realms in addition to biomedical causes.[10,11]

Symptoms and Expression of Illness

The manifestation and symptoms of illness can be unique for different cultures. These "culture-bound syndromes or cultural idioms of distress"[12] occur in specific societies and have a constellation of symptoms

FIGURE 4-1 Scope of Culture Related to Health Care

that are recognized in that culture as a disease entity. For example, *ataque de nervios* is a Latino–Caribbean culture-bound syndrome that usually occurs in response to a specific stressor and is characterized by disassociation or trance-like states, crying, uncontrollable spasms, trembling, or shouting.[13,14] *Shenjing shuairuo* or "weakness of nerves" in Chinese culture is described in the *Chinese Classification of Mental Disorders* as a condition caused by a decrease in vital energy that reduces the function of the internal organ systems and lowers resistance to disease.[15] Its symptoms include fatigue, weakness, dizziness, and memory loss.[16] Also known as neurasthenia throughout Asia, the *International Classification of Diseases and Related Disorders* defines this disorder as characterized primarily by extreme fatigue after mental effort and bodily weakness of persistent duration.[17] Neurasthenia is a more socially acceptable illness label in Asia than depression, which might be considered a mental illness or illness label that is very stigmatizing.[18] Although many Americans would not consider anorexia nervosa or bulimia to be culture-bound syndromes, they conform to the definition of a culture-bound syndrome[19] because major risk factors for these illnesses are social pressure to be thin and media messages equating beauty and thinness that are more prevalent in Westernized, developed countries.[20,21]

Taboos

In many cultures, certain illnesses or behaviors that may be characteristic of illnesses are highly stigmatized and are often not revealed to health care providers. A patient may deny the existence of socially disapproved symptoms and/or decide not to seek treatment. This is particularly true for mental illnesses (e.g., schizophrenia and depression), behavioral disorders in children (e.g., attention deficit hyperactivity disorder (ADHD) and autism spectrum disorders), sexually transmitted infections (e.g., herpes or syphilis), and potentially fatal illnesses (e.g., Ebola and AIDS).

ATTRIBUTES AND CRITERIA

The following attributes are related to the concept of culture—that is, conditions common to all cultures: *Culture is learned* through families and other group members; *culture is changeable* and adaptive to new conditions; and cultural values, beliefs, and behaviors are *shared* by all within a group.

Culture Is Learned

Culture may be transmitted to individuals during childhood and adolescence by the process of socialization or enculturation. However, a culture is not limited to members who share the same country of origin or ethnicity and may not be determined solely in childhood; rather, it may encompass any group whose members share certain roles and values, norms, and attitudes—sometimes referred to as subcultures. Subcultures can include members of racial and ethnic minorities;

people of indigenous or aboriginal heritage; professions, such as nursing; people of different socioeconomic levels, such as the "culture of poverty";[22,23] individuals who are bisexual, gay, or lesbian or transgender; individuals affiliated with particular religious or spiritual groups; age groups, such as teenagers or the elderly; and persons with disabilities. Culture is determined by self-identification, and most people identify with a mix of cultures.

Changing and Adapting

Since the beginning of human history, culture has been constantly changing as people adapt to environmental and technical innovations and in response to globalization and influences of diverse cultural groups.[19,24] Population migration occurs as a result of regional overpopulation, changes in economic circumstances, the occurrence of catastrophic events (e.g., earthquakes, floods, and famines), and the existence of religious or ethnic conflicts. These migration processes result in ongoing encounters between individuals of different cultures, with subsequent changes and acculturation in both groups.[25]

Shared Beliefs, Values, and Behaviors

Language, rituals, customs (e.g., holiday celebrations), dietary practices, and manner of dress are among the most overt attributes of culture that are readily apparent to non-group members. Some of the more subtle attributes of culture, such as values, relationship to authority, social interactions, gender roles, and orientation toward the present or future, are probably the attributes of culture that are most relevant to health care and communication. These kinds of cultural attributes were examined in several landmark studies by Hofstede[26,27] that yielded five dimensions of these attributes. Four of the five dimensions, in addition to religiosity, have particular significance for health care and are presented in the following sections.

Individualism Versus Collectivism

This attribute places value on the degree of closeness and the structure of social relationships, as well as whether loyalties belong to immediate families or to the extended family or clan. The differences in these interpersonal interactions can be thought of as interdependent versus independent and are reflected in the concept of self. Western Europe and the United States are characteristic of individualist societies. Childrearing practices and a "family model of independence" produce a separated or independent sense of self.[28,pp20,29] The concept of self is distinct and separate from the "non-self," which includes the environment and social worlds.[30] Collectivistic cultures foster development of an interdependent self-concept. People who have an interdependent sense of self consider their social worth in relation to others. The value of collectivism or interdependence in self-concept is most clearly exemplified by Asian cultures, but it also applies to African, Latin American, and some southern European cultures and also some minority cultures within the United States.[28,31] Cultural differences in social practices are apparent in the differences in colloquialisms heard in the United States and Japan. For example, in the United States, "the squeaky wheel gets the grease," whereas in Japan, "the nail that stands out gets pounded down."[31,p224]

Power Distance

Power distance is the acceptance of an unequal distribution of power as legitimate or fair versus illegitimate from the point of view of the less powerful. In cultures that value a more equal distribution of power, people have the expectation that their opinions will be heard and equally valued. People who are less powerful have the right to criticize those in power. In contrast, in cultures in which a greater power distance is observed, people are unlikely to overtly challenge or disagree with people in positions of authority because such power is the result of longstanding formal and hierarchical arrangements.

Masculinity Versus Femininity

Masculinity versus femininity describes how gender roles are conceived and how greatly male and female roles differ. Some societies place greater value on masculine attributes (as defined by Western culture), such as achievement, material success, and recognition, versus more feminine attributes, such as harmonious relationships, modesty, and taking care of others. In some cultures, only men can enact masculine roles, whereas in other cultures gender roles are more flexible. In cultures with more fixed gender roles, women are usually given the role of caretaker for aging relatives and may suffer the stresses of caregiver strain.

Long-Term Versus Short-Term Orientation

Long- versus short-term orientation is the degree to which a culture is oriented to the future and long-term rewards versus the degree to which a culture is oriented to the past or present.[32,33] Long-term-oriented cultures favor thrift, perseverance, and adapting to changing circumstances. Short-term-oriented cultures are oriented to the present or past and emphasize quick results; they favor respect for tradition and fulfillment of social obligations, although status is not a major issue in relationships and leisure time is important. Among the most long-term-oriented countries are China, Hong Kong, Taiwan, and Japan, whereas the United States, Great Britain, Canada, and the Philippines are among the most short-term-oriented countries.[34]

In a health care context, a long-term orientation would be evidenced by the patient who comes in for preventive care visits, receives all of the recommended screening tests and immunizations, and is an active partner in his or her care. A short-term orientation might be evidenced by the individual who seeks treatment for health care problems only when the symptoms of an illness become unbearable.

Religiosity

Another cultural dimension is religiosity, which varies according to how much religion permeates one's day-to-day existence and to what degree religious practices can be separated from nonreligious practices.[35] Religion differs from spirituality in that religiosity is an organized and institutionalized practice associated with particular beliefs, whereas spirituality is an individualistic connection to a higher power, which may or may not entail belonging to a organized religion. The majority of people in the United States believe in God (74%), miracles (72%), and heaven (68%), although this has been diminishing over time and with each succeeding generation.[34] Thus, religious beliefs are in a state of flux in the United States.

THEORETICAL LINKS

The importance of culture and its influence on human behavior has not always been an accepted theoretical premise. Theories of human behavior have been dominated by the underlying premise of the "psychic unity" of humankind, a theory that states that all human social behavior is derived from evolution.[36] Scientists who believe in these concepts claim that through evolution and natural selection, certain genes in the species that enhance survival are most likely to be passed down from one generation to the next, and these genes specify cognitive functioning and the manner in which people perceive the world.[37] Therefore, thoughts, behaviors, and emotions develop universally and account for such diverse behaviors as favoring relatives (i.e., altruism), creating and following rules, or adopting specific beliefs about religion and warfare.[38] Language, culture, and religion

are incidental to or an outgrowth of these genetically determined behavioral processes. Karasz and McKinley[39] refer to "the 'culture-free' approach of traditional health psychology." Relatively recently, behavioral geneticists have shown us how the social environment has a major influence on how genes are expressed. Although there might be inherent biological factors that produce emotions and behavior, genes interact with the environment to produce differences in emotional responses.[40]

Leininger's Theory of Culture Care Diversity and Universality

Berry and Leininger emphasized the importance of understanding human behavior in the context of culture.[41-43] They applied the concepts of "emic" and "etic," which referred to an approach to understanding behaviors. The term *emic* refers to an approach to understanding culture from within (i.e., the insider's viewpoint), whereas *etic* refers to the application of constructs external to a culture to discover universal characteristics common to all cultures. The assumption of universality can also imply an imposition of an outsider's values, rules, and understanding to another culture or subculture. The concepts of emic and etic are essential aspects of Leininger's theory of culture care diversity and universality.[44]

The central tenet of this theory is that both etic and emic approaches could lead to more responsive approaches to caring, the most important focus of nursing. To provide meaningful and holistic care, social structure factors, such as religion, economics, education, technology, ethnic background, and history, have to be taken into account because these factors have major influences on health, well-being, and illness.[45] This comprehensive approach to nursing formed the basis of Leininger's development of transcultural nursing, the "formal area of humanistic and scientific knowledge and practices focused on holistic culture care ... to assist individuals or groups to maintain or regain their health (or well-being)."[45,p84]

Interprofessional Theory of Social Suffering

The interprofessional theory of social suffering states that relationships and social interactions shape our illness experiences and beliefs about the meaning of suffering. Memories of trauma and suffering exist collectively within a group or culture and are transmitted through shared experiences and learning. All illnesses are a form of social suffering, mediated by cultural and political institutions. Technological advances can treat an individual's disease, but they do not address the root causes of illness including poverty and the global political economy. Tuberculosis, depression, sexually transmitted infections, substance abuse, domestic violence, post-traumatic stress disorders, and AIDS are not individual problems but, rather, a reflection of social structure and health care and political inequities. It is also important to understand the individual's cultural interpretation of illness and suffering. These cultural representations of suffering and the response to it comprise the diversity of human responses to illness and pain. In some cultures, silent endurance is valued, whereas other cultures rail against unjust Gods.[46,ppix-xiv] Some cultures place a high priority on the well-being and health of their members, whereas other societies are characterized by greater inequities in the health status of their populations.

CONTEXT TO NURSING AND HEALTH CARE

Many nursing students have asked, "Why is there such an emphasis on culture in health care? That's all we keep hearing about." Culture is an essential aspect of health care because of the increasing diversity of the United States. In 2008, the U.S. population was estimated at 304 million. In that year, the non-Hispanic white population of the United States represented 67% of the total population.[47] By 2050, the non-Hispanic white population is expected to decrease to 50%. Half of the population will be composed of people who identify themselves as belonging to a racial or ethnic minority population, including black, Asian, and Pacific Islander; American Indian, Eskimo, and Aleut; and Hispanic. In 2008, approximately 12% of the U.S. population, or 36 million people, had a disability.[48] Persons with disabilities identify themselves as part of a culture based on shared life experiences; this identification has led to music, publications, and media products unique to that culture, as well as to the disability rights movement to address discrimination in housing, employment, and health care. An estimated 4% of the U.S. population ages 18–44 years identified themselves as lesbian, gay, bisexual, or transgender.[49] Persons who are lesbian, gay, bisexual, or transgender experience societal discrimination, societal stigma, and human rights abuses that have led to higher rates of mental illness in addition to higher rates of HIV and sexually transmitted infections.[50,51]

Health Disparities

The increasing cultural diversity in the United States has resulted in the national health objective proposed in *Healthy People 2020:* achieving the highest level of health for all people by addressing societal inequalities and "historical and contemporary injustices."[52] One of the major goals of *Healthy People 2020* is the elimination of health care disparities[53] and is closely allied with nursing's basic tenet of social justice, which is the belief that all people deserve quality health care and access to care is a basic human right.[54] *Healthy People 2020* emphasizes the need to provide culturally competent health care services and to improve health literacy and health education among non-English-speaking populations. This is presented in greater detail as Concept 54 Health Disparities.

Cultural Competency in Nursing

Cultural competence is an expected component of nursing education and professional nursing practice. Culturally competent care means conveying acceptance of the patient's health beliefs while sharing information, encouraging self-efficacy, and strengthening the patient's coping resources. The scope and standards of nursing practice specifically identify cultural competency as it relates to assessment, outcomes identification, planning, and implementation.[54] Cultural competency is more of an imperative now as we begin to understand that health care providers' unconscious biases contribute to disparities in treatment,[55] even though nurses and physicians continue to deny that their own behavior is a factor in health care inequalities.[56]

As a nursing student, you might be thinking, "Yes, but we are taught how to communicate with our patients and if I treat everyone with respect and understanding, isn't that sufficient?" Well, no. By treating everyone the same, we are not providing quality care because we are ignoring societal factors that contribute to worse health outcomes among vulnerable populations. It is true that communicating respectfully is an essential aspect of communication and every patient is an individual with unique needs. However, failure to recognize the fact that people identify themselves as members of certain groups who have shared experiences of social injustice and who are currently treated differently in health care will result in an inability to understand some of the most essential human experiences of our patients.[57]

Now, you may be saying to yourself, "Yes, I understand cultural competency is important, but really, there are so many other things that we need to learn as nurses."

Rubin defines expert nursing as the ability to recognize qualitative distinctions between patients.[58] The ability to make qualitative distinctions, or to be able to understand differences in the patient's life experiences, requires empathy. Empathy is necessary to understand the individual's self-perceptions of how he or she came to feel that way. Nurses who lack empathy are not practicing evidenced-based care, defined as comprising research-based information, clinical expertise, and patient preferences.[59]

In a cultural sense, this could be illustrated by the description of one nursing student's health assessment and history taking. She writes, "His parents are from India and he practices Hinduism. He goes to Mosques regularly and is a lot like my patient from Sudan, who is also very religious and celebrates Ramadan." This assumption of similarity between Muslim and Hindu practices and the confusion between the two evidences an inability to make qualitative distinctions in a person's history or to really attempt to understand that person's experience of religion. Individualized care or "patient-centered" care is facilitated by cultural competence that respects and acknowledges the patient's values, needs, and preferences.[60]

Developing Cultural Competence

The process of developing cultural competence consists of four interrelated constructs—cultural desire, self-awareness, cultural knowledge, and cultural skill—thus forming the broad components of cultural competency.[61-63]

Cultural Desire

A pivotal construct is *cultural desire*. Cultural desire refers to an interest and intent to understand people who are different from oneself. Cultural desire is a personal choice; this interest is foundational to cultural competence and provides the means for overcoming one's biases and their effect on care. Cultural desire leads to patient-centered care as the nurse becomes more attuned to differences between individuals. Like any other effort to master new skills and knowledge, motivation or cultural desire is a prerequisite.

Self-Awareness

Self-awareness involves identifying and understanding one's own cultural identity. You might think about some aspects of your own cultural identity. Did you grow up with people of the same ethnic background as yourself? Did you gather with extended family and engage in traditional activities? Do members of your family make frequent visits to their country of origin or old neighborhood? Do you participate in ethnic cultural events? Do you speak another language? Do you have pride in your cultural background?

Perhaps you are saying to yourself, "But I grew up in an area where everyone is the same as I am, and we don't have traditions from the countries where my great grandparents came from and we just eat normal American food and celebrate the same holidays as everyone else. *I don't have any cultural identification.*" If you feel that way, ask yourself, "What about the place I grew up? Is it like every other place in the United States? What about the meals I prepare? Does everyone in America celebrate the same holidays? Are all Americans the same? What are my own values and beliefs?"

Perhaps you are saying to yourself, "But I grew up in an area where everyone is from a different culture and I'm very comfortable interacting with other cultures." If you feel that way, ask yourself, "How would I feel living next door to a family with two parents of the same sex, or a halfway house for people with chronic severe mental illness? How comfortable do I feel interacting with homeless people? How would I feel if my son or daughter married someone from a religion that I know nothing about? What are my own biases?"

Biases not only are negative stereotypes but also can be any tendency to act, think, or feel in a certain way toward other people. For example, you may believe that Vietnamese people are hardworking, they want their children to do well in school, they expect that their children show respect to their parents, and they stick together. Many nurses believe, "But that really doesn't apply to me, because I know that even if I personally don't like someone or something they've done, I will treat everyone in a professional manner and will treat everyone the same." Nurses grow up with the values and beliefs of their cultures and the society around them. Perhaps you believe that abortion is wrong, that it is immoral to have same-sex relationships, that people with depression could really snap out of it if they wanted to, that people with substance abuse do not have a mental illness—they make choices. Perhaps you feel angry that some people receive health benefits that are "free" and are paid for by your tax dollars. After all, you work hard to earn money, "Why can't they?" "Why do all of those refugees who have moved into my community get Medicaid and can get medications that I can barely afford?" Is it possible to separate all of these feelings from our practice? Many studies in many fields indicate that those feelings carry over into the care we provide.

Even when one's own values and beliefs are directed against a particular group of people, they may still reflect the biases of the dominant cultural group. For example, nurses from independent cultures will develop nursing objectives based on the cultural value of autonomy— developing one's own potential and maintaining one's independence— and equate "more" of such traits with better health. A patient from a more interdependent, collectivist culture might not share such values. For this patient, it might be expected that he or she is dependent on other family members in times of ill health. Moreover, the family's needs and desires might be valued more highly than obtaining one's own personal goals. The use of the concept of "self-esteem" as part of a nursing diagnosis may reflect the bias that the self is construed similarly in all cultures. As Markus and Kitayama[31] explain, in interdependent cultures, the essence of self is defined by one's relationships to others rather than the inner self. Internal attributes such as desires, abilities, and personality traits are viewed as situation dependent and, therefore, unreliable. Self is not a constant but, rather, is fluid and changes according to the situation or the relationship. It is important for the nurse to assess the patient's own values and definition of health and to develop mutually agreed upon nursing care plans.

Knowledge

Knowledge as a domain of cultural competency does not imply learning facts about every culture but, rather, exposing one's self to other cultures and being motivated to learn. Knowledge can be acquired by reading journals that represent different groups; visiting ethnic neighborhoods and sampling different foods; learning a foreign language; attending a community meeting in a different neighborhood; speaking with someone from another culture; walking into botánicas, ethnic grocery stores, or herb shops; attending a service at a mosque or synagogue; speaking with a hospital translator; going to a gay pride march or Puerto Rican day parade; or reading a novel about someone growing up in another culture.

Skill

Skills are acquired over time by careful attention to the nurse–patient relationship. One element of cultural skill is communication. There are many resources available to learn basic medical terminology on the Web, including Internet and smartphone applications that serve as translators. There are also assessment questions designed to understand the sociocultural contexts of people's health care needs. The RESPECT model of cultural assessment, based on a series of eight questions developed by Kleinman,[64] provides a blueprint to develop skills needed to become culturally competent[65] (Box 4-1).

BOX 4-1 Eight Questions Associated with the RESPECT Model

1. What do you call the problem?
2. What do you think has caused the problem?
3. Why do you think it started when it did?
4. What do you think the sickness does? How does it work?
5. How severe is the sickness? Will it have a long or short course?
6. What kind of treatment do you think you should receive?
7. What are the chief problems the sickness has caused?
8. What do you fear most about the sickness?

Source: From Kleinman A: *Patients and healers in the context of culture*, Berkeley, CA, 1980, University of California Press.

RESPECT is an acronym for *r*espect, *e*xplanatory model, *s*ociocultural context, *p*ower, *e*mpathy, *c*oncerns and fears, and *t*herapeutic alliance/ trust.

Respect and *empathy* are attitudes that demonstrate to the patient that his or her concerns are valued and he or she is understood. The nurse can further assess for the patient's *explanatory model*, or understanding of what is the cause of his or her illness, and the *sociocultural context*, which comprises factors in a person's life that may contribute to the current state of health and expectations for treatment, such as poverty, stress, and social support. *Power* refers to the importance of acknowledging that the patient is in a vulnerable position and that there is a difference between patients and health care providers in terms of access to resources, knowledge level, and control over outcomes. The loss of power and control that a patient faces can contribute to *concerns and fears* about treatment, illness outcomes, and the future. Bearing in mind the meaning of these concepts in the nursing relationship enhances communication and assessment skills between patient and nurse and creates a *therapeutic alliance and trust*.

Conducting a Cultural Assessment

Assessment has long been recognized as the foundation for competent, patient-centered nursing care. It should be no surprise that cultural assessment is an expected component of nursing care. A cultural assessment helps nurses gain an understanding of the meaning of the illness to the patient, expectations the patient has regarding treatment and care, and the patient's perception about the process. The patient history includes many questions that link to a patient's cultural perspectives and preference. It is most important to apply elements previously described into the history and assessment so these critical data are recognized and understood. Data gained from an interview as it relates to cultural assessment are included in Box 4-2. In addition to data collected as part of an interview, the nurse should observe the patient's behavior (e.g., personal space and eye contact), clothing, and presence of articles as cues for additional or clarifying questions.

INTERRELATED CONCEPTS

Several concepts within this textbook are closely related to the concept of culture and are shown in Figure 4-2.

Health Disparities adversely affect groups of people who have systematically experienced greater obstacles to health based on their racial, ethnic, or cultural group; religion; socioeconomic status; gender; age; mental health; cognitive, sensory, or physical disability; sexual orientation or gender identity; geographic location; or other characteristics historically linked to discrimination or exclusion.[52] Culture affects Family Dynamics in many ways including the manner in which sick family members receive care, beliefs about sharing information with outsiders about a family member's illness, gender roles, and beliefs about appropriate childrearing practices. As one example the dominant practice in America of letting an infant cry him- or herself to sleep to learn how to self-soothe may be construed as a form of

---

BOX 4-2   Data Collected as Part of Cultural Assessment

Origins and Family
- Where born; if in other country, length of time in United States and circumstances
- Decision making within family
- Cultural group(s) identify with; presence of social network
- Important cultural practices

Communication
- Language spoken at home; skill in speaking, reading, and writing in English
- Preferred methods to communication with patient and/or family member (how to be addressed, to whom questions are directed, etc.)
- Ways respect is shown to others
- Eye contact, interpersonal space

Personal Beliefs about Health, Illness
- Meaning and belief about cause of illness
- Perception of control over health
- Practices or rituals used to improve health
- Perception of severity of illness
- Expectations for treatment; use of folk remedies, alternative medicine
- Practices that violate beliefs (taboos)
- Concerns or fears about illness or process of treatment

Daily Practices
- Dietary preferences and practices; forbidden foods
- Beliefs about food that pertain to health and illness
- Spiritual beliefs; religious practices
- Special rituals

---

neglect, particularly for people of cultures that believe in sharing a bed with an infant. Another cultural dimension is Spirituality, which varies according to how much spirituality permeates one's day-to-day existence, and the importance placed on spiritual practices.[34] Spirituality is an individualistic subjective experience of transformation or connection to a higher power, which may or may not entail belonging to a organized religion. Spirituality is closely interrelated with culture because many spiritual beliefs are embedded within cultural groups.

The concept Communication is closely related to culture because communication patterns, both verbal and nonverbal, are determined by cultural norms. Degree of eye contact, personal space, and the acceptability of touch all vary by cultures. Culture dictates the nature of relationships and the degree of hierarchy and structure in relationships. In some cultures, a high degree of formality and reserve is expected when addressing people of greater social status, whereas in other cultures there is less stratification by age or social standing and it is acceptable to be direct and open with everyone. Similarly, in some cultures, personal revelations or discussion of family problems are taboo, whereas in other cultures there are no such restrictions on communication.

Coping and dealing with life's difficulties are, to a large extent, culturally determined. Cultural belief systems form the basis of a coping strategy by creating a redefinition of negative circumstances.[66] These belief systems may encompass religious beliefs and religiosity, which may have a beneficial effect on health by fostering positive emotions such as hope, gratitude, and reverence.[67] Religiosity may result in decreased symptoms of distress and may help with coping by decreasing loneliness and fostering cultural identity.[68]

The expression and meaning of some symptoms such as Fatigue are influenced by culture. Some cultures seek a biomedical explanations for the medically unexplained symptom of fatigue (such as chronic fatigue syndrome and depression) or a lack of fulfillment whereas other cultures view fatigue as an imbalance of essential energies.[39] Likewise, Mood and Affect has a strong interrelationship to culture. Depression is the leading cause of non-fatal disease burden and years of life lived with disability worldwide.[69] Rates of depression are highest among the most vulnerable populations—people living in poverty, immigrants, and refugees.[70-72] Experiences of immigration may also contribute to mood disorders because immigrants experience depression from the stress of adjusting to a new culture, loss of family

FIGURE 4-2 Culture and Interrelated Concepts

BOX 4-3 EXEMPLARS OF CULTURE

Health Care Practices/Beliefs
- Symptoms of illness
- Treatment preferences
- Meaning of illness
- Control over health and illness
- Consequences of illness/preventive care
- Dietary practices
- Religious healing practices
- Complimentary alternative or integrative medicine

Family Roles
- Birthrights
- Childrearing practices
- Gender roles
- Family structure
- Decision making
- Death and dying
- Caregiver roles

Patient–Provider Communication
- Language preference
- Nonverbal communication (eye contact, personal space, touch, body posture)
- Power distance
- Taboos
- Revealing personal information
- Expression of emotion

and traditions, loss of social status, and memories of severe deprivation or political violence in their countries of origin.[73] Racial and ethnic minorities are less likely to receive treatment for mood disorders, and when they do receive treatment, it often does not meet the standard of care.[74] Patients have better outcomes when they are culturally and linguistically matched with their mental health provider.[75] Cultural values and beliefs, including the reluctance to share personal problems outside of the family, disclose personal problems, a value on self-sufficiency, recognition of mental health problems, and stigma about mental illness, also create barriers to treatment engagement.[76–79]

CLINICAL EXEMPLARS

There are multiple exemplars of culture in the context of health care delivery. These are best presented using the framework of health care practices and beliefs, family roles, and patient–provider communication. The most common exemplars of culture as it relates to health care and nursing practice are presented in Box 4-3.

Featured Exemplars
Language Preference
An estimated 57 million Americans speak a language other than English in the home.[80] Patients with limited English proficiency (LEP) face many health care barriers in terms of understanding health care information, adherence to treatment plans, and follow-up care due to impaired patient–provider communication. Health care providers must ensure that health care is delivered in a manner that takes into account the needs of patients with LEP, often through the use of interpreters. The Agency for Healthcare Research and Quality has a number of tools and guidelines available to help nurses provide quality care to LEP patients.[81]

Decision Making
The values of individualism versus collectivism form cultural differences in the role of the family in determining how people decide to obtain treatments and medical care. For independent cultures, an individual will put him- or herself first in the case of a life-threatening illness, whereas even in such dire situations, members of collectivist cultures may still consult other family members for the best course of action.

Taboo
A taboo is a prohibited or forbidden action or behavior based on moral judgment and/or religious beliefs in the context of one's culture. Taboos are present in all cultures, and what is considered taboo in one culture may not be considered taboo in another. Health care providers must maintain awareness that some procedures and treatment practices considered standard of practice may be considered taboo in some cultures. Examples include physical touch of a female patient for an examination without the consent of the husband and administration of blood products.

Power Distance
People from cultures with greater inequality of power distance may be unwilling to disagree with or question the authority of a health care provider, whereas people from cultures in which there is an expectation of equality of relationships may not be hesitant in expressing their wishes and needs for their own health care. Therefore, when a nurse provides education to the patient who is from a culture that values greater power distance, it might appear that the patient is willing to accept all the nurse's suggestions, when further prompting might elicit additional questions or concerns of the patient.

Symptoms of Illness
The symptoms of an illness may vary depending on how a culture understands and perceives the illness. Thus, health care providers must consider the possibility that their view of "expected symptoms" associated with certain disorders may be different from that of people from other cultures. For example, in some cultures, it is acceptable to verbalize that one is in pain, whereas in other cultures, the verbalization of pain is seen as a sign of weakness or control. As another example, mental health illnesses are described in bodily terms such as backaches, headaches, and fatigue rather than disturbances in mood and affect.[82,83]

Beliefs about Illness Control
Beliefs about control one has over health and illness are highly variable depending on one's culture and can impact decisions about health promotion practices or care during times of illness. Individuals who hold a belief that they have control over the course of an illness may "appear" to be more engaged in and actively pursue health screening and treatment options. In some cultures, the predominant belief is that what happens is out of one's control, sometimes referred to as fatalism or an external locus of control. In some contexts, an external locus of control can be a culturally protective mechanism and serves to preserve a sense of peace and well-being in situations that are out of one's control, such as a terminal illness.

CASE STUDY

Source: Tomwang112/iStock/Thinkstock

Case Presentation

Mr. Wong is a 78-year-old male from mainland China who has been admitted for rehabilitation following total hip replacement surgery. He has a poor appetite, has experienced weight loss, and has been unable to participate in physical therapy. Thus, he is not meeting his goals for rehabilitation. No evidence exists to suggest an underlying disease process.

Ms. Faye, the nurse assigned to care for Mr. Wong, is interested in learning what might be going on with Mr. Wong to better meet his treatment outcomes. Ms. Faye considers the possibility that he does not have adequate pain relief, which could affect his appetite and cause poor participation in physical therapy. She reviews his history to learn more about him. According the health history, Mr. Wong is a widower of 3 years; he has a son and daughter who live in distant cities. Mr. Wong emigrated from China at the age of 38 years and only speaks Cantonese. He has lived in an ethic neighborhood with other Chinese Americans and has worked as a short-order cook in a Chinese restaurant since arriving in the United States 40 years ago.

Ms. Faye arranges for Mr. Lee, a Cantonese translator who is also Chinese, to help her ask Mr. Wong a few questions. She first asks Mr. Wong if he is in pain. When he responds no, she follows with another question, asking him if he is depressed or anxious. Again, Mr. Wong responds no, that he is fine. During the interaction, Ms. Faye observes that Mr. Wong does not look at her or Mr. Lee, the translator.

After leaving the room, Ms. Faye expresses her frustration to Mr. Lee, mentioning how difficult it will be to help Mr. Wong when he will not communicate. Mr. Lee responds, "Elderly Chinese people believe that they must be stoic about pain and there is a stigma about talking about any mental health problems." This explanation had not occurred to Ms. Faye, who then recognizes her approach may have been offensive, and that she had failed to consider the underlying cultural differences beyond language.

Ms. Faye asks Mr. Lee to share more about traditional Chinese beliefs. She then asks Mr. Lee to help her ask Mr. Wong additional questions using a cultural assessment form as a guide. After gathering additional information from Mr. Wong and gaining additional insight from Mr. Lee, Ms. Faye incorporates strategies that include changes to how his food is prepared and served, changes in approaches to pain management, and involving Mr. Wong's son and daughter in his care.

Case Analysis

This case exemplifies culture in the context of health care delivery in several ways. First, it illustrated how some cultural information in a medical record may provide initial clues but does not substitute for conducting a thorough cultural assessment. Second, language can be a barrier to understanding, even if a translator is available. Third, the nurse exhibited cultural bias and an initial lack of self-awareness of personal biases.

ACCESS EXEMPLAR LINKS IN YOUR GIDDENS EBOOK

REFERENCES

1. Shweder RA: Cultural psychology—What is it? In Stigler JW, Shweder RA, Herdt G, editors: *Cultural psychology*, Cambridge, 1990, Cambridge University Press, pp 1–43.
2. Geertz C: *The interpretation of cultures*, New York, 1973, Basic Books.
3. Triandis HC: The psychological measurement of cultural syndromes. *Am Psychol* 51(4):407–415, 1996. Retrieved from: <http://dx.doi.org/10.1037/0003-066X.51.4.407>.
4. Cengage G: Acculturation. In Breslow L, editor: *Encyclopedia of public health, 2002*, eNotes.com, 2006. Retrieved January 2011 from: <http://www.enotes.com/public-health-encyclopedia/acculturation>.
5. Haney Lopez IF: The social construction of race: Some observations on illusion, fabrication, and choice, 29 *Harvard Civil Rights–Civil Liberties Law Review* 1–62, 6–7, 11–17, Winter 1994.
6. Kleinman A: *Rethinking psychiatry: From cultural category to personal experience*, New York, 1988, Free Press.
7. Huff RM: Cross-cultural concepts of health and disease. In Huff RM, Kline MV, editors: *Promoting health in multicultural populations*, Thousand Oaks, CA, 1999, Sage, pp 23–39.
8. Baer RD, Clark L, Pederson C: Folk illnesses. In Loue S, editor: *Handbook of immigrant health*, New York, 1998, Plenum, pp 183–202.
9. Huff RM, Kline MV: Health promotion in the context of culture. In Huff RM, Kline MV, editors: *Promoting health in multicultural populations*, Thousand Oaks, CA, 1999, Sage, pp 3–21.
10. Rivera SV: Latino cultural beliefs of the causes of a medical and a psychological illness. *Dissert Abstr Int Sect B Sci Eng* 62(2–B):1096, 2001.
11. Klonoff EA, Landrine H: Culture and gender diversity in commonsense beliefs about the causes of six illnesses. *J Behav Med* 17(4):407–418, 1994.
12. American Psychiatric Association: *Diagnostic and statistical manual of mental disorders*, ed 5, Washington, DC, 2013, Author.
13. Guarnaccia PJ, Lewis-Fernandez R, Marano MR: Toward a Puerto Rican popular nosology: Nervios and ataque de nervios. *Cult Med Psychiatr* 27(3):339–366, 2003.
14. Guarnaccia PJ, Lewis-Fernandez R, Martinez Pincay I, et al: Ataque de nervios as a marker of social and psychiatric vulnerability: Results from the NLAAS. *Int J Soc Psychiatr* 56:298–309, 2010.
15. Chinese Medical Association and Nanjing Medical University: *Chinese classification of mental disorders, Second Edition, Revised (CCMD-2-R)*, Nanjing, 1995, Dong Nan University Press.
16. Schwartz PY: Why is neurasthenia important in Asian cultures? *West J Med* 176(4):257–258, 2002.
17. World Health Organization: *International classification of diseases and related disorders (ICD-10)*, Geneva, 1992, Author.
18. U.S. Department of Health and Human Services: *Mental health: Culture, race and ethnicity—A supplement to mental health: A report of the Surgeon General*, Rockville, MD, 2001, Substance Abuse and Mental Health Services Administration. U.S. Public Health Service No. 01–3613.
19. Lopez SR, Guarnaccia PJ: Cultural psychopathology: Uncovering the social world of mental illness. *Annu Rev Psychol* 51:571–598, 2000.
20. Jacobi C, Hayward C, de Zwaan M, et al: Coming to terms with risk factors for eating disorders: Application of risk terminology and suggestions for a general taxonomy. *Psychol Bull* 130:19–65, 2004.

21. Taylor CB, Bryson SW, Altman TM, et al: Risk factors for the onset of eating disorders in adolescent girls: Results of the McKnight longitudinal risk factor study. *Am J Psychiatr* 160:248–254, 2003.

22. Lewis O: *The children of Sanchez: Autobiography of a Mexican family*, New York, 1961, Random House.

23. Moynihan DP: *The Negro family: The case for national action*, Washington, DC, 1965, Office of Policy Planning and Research, U.S. Department of Labor. Retrieved from: <http://www.dol.gov/oasam/programs/history/webid-meynihan.htm>.

24. Committee on Cultural Psychiatry Group for the Advancement of Psychiatry: *Cultural assessment in clinical psychiatry*, Washington, DC, 2002, American Psychiatric Publishing.

25. Redfield R, Linton R, Herskovits MJ: Memorandum for the study of acculturation. *Am Anthropol* 38:149–152, 1936.

26. Hofstede G: *Culture's consequences: International differences in work-related values*, Beverly Hills, CA, 1980, Sage.

27. Hofstede G: Empirical models of cultural differences. In Bleichrodt N, Drenth P, editors: *Contemporary issues in cross-cultural psychology*, Lisse, The Netherlands, 1991, Swets & Zeitlinger, pp 4–20.

28. Kagitcibasi C: Individualism and collectivism. In Berry JW, Segall MH, Kagitcibasi C, editors: *Handbook of cross-cultural psychology. Volume 3: Social behavior and applications*, ed 2, Needham Heights, MA, 1997, Allyn & Bacon.

29. Mesquita B: Emotions in collectivist and individualist contexts. *J Personality Soc Psychol* 80(1):68–74, 2001.

30. Landrine H, Klonoff EA: Culture and health-related schemas: A review and proposal for interdisciplinary integration. *Health Psychol* 11(4):267–276, 1992.

31. Markus HR, Kitayama S: Culture and the self: Implications for cognition, emotion, and motivation. *Psychol Rev* 98:224–253, 1991.

32. Hofstede G: *Culture and organizations: Software of the mind*, New York, 1997, McGraw-Hill.

33. Hofstede G, Bond MH: The Confucius connection: From cultural roots to economic growth. *Organiz Dyn* 16:5–21, 1988.

34. Shannon-Missal L: Americans' belief in God, miracles and heaven declines. *The Harris Poll* 2013. Retrieved from: <http://www.harrisinteractive.com/vault/Harris%20Poll%2097%20-%20Beliefs_12.16.2013.pdf>.

35. Matsumoto D, Yoo SH: Toward a new generation of cross-cultural research. *Perspect Psychol Sci* 1(3):234–250, 2006.

36. Tooby J, Cosmides L: Evolutionary psychology and the generation of culture. Part I: theoretical considerations. *Ethnol Sociobiol* 10:29–49, 1989.

37. Wilson EO: *Sociobiology: The new synthesis*, Cambridge, MA, 1975, Harvard University Press.

38. Fukuyama F: *The origins of political order: From prehuman times to the French Revolution*, New York, 2011, Farrar, Straus & Giroux.

39. Karasz A, McKinley PS: Cultural differences in conceptual models of everyday fatigue: A vignette study. *J Health Psychol* 12(4):613–626, 2007.

40. Caspi A, Moffitt TE, Morgan J, et al: Maternal expressed emotion predicts children's antisocial behavior problems: Using monozygotic-twin differences to identify environmental effects on behavioral development. *Dev Psychol* 40(2):149–161, 2004.

41. Berry JW: On cross-cultural comparability. *Int J Psychol* 4:119–128, 1969.

42. Berry JW: Imposed etics–emics–derived etics: The operationalization of a compelling idea. *Int J Psychol* 24:721–735, 1989.

43. Leininger MM: Leininger's theory of nursing: Culture care diversity and universality. *Nurs Sci Q* 1:152–160, 1988.

44. Leininger MM: *Culture care diversity and universality, a theory of nursing*, New York, 1991, National League for Nursing Press.

45. Leininger M, McFarland MR: *Transcultural nursing: Concepts, theories, research and practices*, ed 3, New York, 2002, McGraw-Hill.

46. Kleinman A, Das V, Locke M: Introduction. In *Social suffering*, Oakland, CA, 1997, University of California Press.

47. U.S. Census Bureau: American FactFinder, United States: American Community Survey. American Community Survey 1-year estimates, ACS demographic and housing estimates, 2008. Retrieved from <http://factfinder.census.gov>.

48. U.S. Census Bureau: American FactFinder, United States: American Community Survey. American Community Survey 1-year estimates, Selected social characteristics in the United States, 2008. Retrieved from <http://factfinder.census.gov>.

49. Mayer KH, Bradford JB, Makadon HJ, et al: Sexual and gender minority health: What we know and what needs to be done. *Am J Public Health* 98:989–995, 2008.

50. McLaughlin KA, Hatzenbuehler ML, Keyes KM: Responses to discrimination and psychiatric disorders among black, Hispanic, female, and lesbian, gay, and bisexual individuals. *Am J Public Health* 100:1477–1484, 2010.

51. Centers for Disease Control and Prevention: *HIV and AIDS among gay and bisexual men*, Atlanta, 2010, Author. Retrieved from: <http://www.cdc.gov/hiv/risk/gender/msm/facts/index.html>.

52. U.S. Department of Health and Human Services: *HHS Action Plan to Reduce Racial and Ethnic Disparities: A Nation Free of Disparities in Health and Health Care*, Washington, D.C., 2011, U.S. Department of Health and Human Services. <http://minorityhealth.hhs.gov/npa/files/Plans/HHS/HHS_Plan_complete.pdf>.

53. Healthy. People 2020. About Healthy People. 2015. Retrieved from <http://www.healthypeople.gov/2020/About-Healthy-People>.

54. American Nurses Association: *Nursing scope and standards of practice*, ed 2, Silver Spring, MD, 2010, Author.

55. Van Ryn M, Fu SS: Paved with good intentions: Do public health and human service providers contribute to racial/ethnic disparities in health? *Am J Public Health* 93(2):248–255, 2003.

56. Clark-Hitt R, Malat J, Burgess D, et al: Doctors' and nurses' explanations for racial disparities in medical treatment. *J Health Care Poor Underserved* 21(1):386–400, 2010.

57. Brown CR, Mazza GJ: *Healing into action*, Washington, DC, 1997, National Coalition Building Institute.

58. Rubin J: Impediments to the development of clinical knowledge and ethical judgment in critical care nursing. In Benner P, Tanner C, Cheslan C, editors: *Expertise in nursing practice: Caring, clinical judgment, and ethics*, ed 2, New York, 2009, Springer, pp 171–198.

59. Brown SJ: *Evidenced-based nursing: The research–practice connection*, ed 3, Burlington, MA, 2014, Jones & Bartlett, p 6.

60. Institute of Medicine: *Health professions education: A bridge to quality*, Washington, DC, 2003, National Academies Press.

61. Betancourt JR: Cross-cultural medical education: Conceptual approaches and frameworks for evaluation. *Acad Med* 78(6):560–569, 2003.

62. Campinha-Bacote J: A culturally conscious approach to holistic nursing. Program and abstracts of the American Holistic Nurses Association 2005 Conference, King of Prussia, PA, June 16–19, 2005.

63. Cavillo E, Clark L, Ballantyne JE, et al: Cultural competency in baccalaureate nursing education. *J Transcult Nurs* 20:137–145, 2009.

64. Kleinman A: *Patients and healers in the context of culture*, Berkeley, CA, 1980, University of California Press.

65. Mostow C, Crosson J, Gordon S, et al: Treating and precepting with RESPECT: A relational model addressing race, ethnicity, and culture in medical training. *J Gen Intern Med* 25(Suppl 2):146–154, 2010.

66. Folkman S, Lazarus RS: The relationship between coping and emotion: Implications for theory and research. *Soc Sci Med* 26:309–317, 1988.

67. Emmons RA: Emotion and religion. In Paloutzian RF, Park CL, editors: *Handbook of the psychology of religion and spirituality*, New York, 2005, Guilford, pp 235–252.

68. Rosmarin DH, Krumrei E, Andersson G: Religion as a predictor of psychological distress in two religious communities. *Cognitive Behav Ther* 38:54–64, 2009.

69. Lopez A, Mathers D, Ezzati CD, et al: *Global and regional burden of disease and risk factors, 2001: Systematic analysis of population health data*, London, 2006, Onwhyn.

70. Hiott A, Grzywacz JG, Arcury TA, et al: Gender differences in anxiety and depression among immigrant Latinos. *Families Systems Health* 24:137–146, 2006.

71. Huang FY, Chung H, Kroenke K, et al: Racial and ethnic differences in the relationship between depression severity and functional status. *Psychiatric Services* 57:498–503, 2006.

72. Kessler RC, Berglund P, Demler O, et al: The epidemiology of major depressive disorder: Results from the National Comorbidity Survey Replication (NCS-R). *JAMA* 289:3095–3105, 2003.

73. Caplan S: Latinos, acculturation, and acculturative stress: A dimensional concept analysis. *Policy Politics Nursing Practice* 8(2):93–106, 2007.

74. Institute of Medicine: *Unequal treatment: Confronting racial and ethnic disparities in health care*, Washington, DC, 2003, National Academy Press.

75. Sue S: Psychotherapeutic services for ethnic minorities: Two decades of research findings. *Am Psychologist* 43:301–308, 1988.

76. Corrigan PW, Morris S, Larson JE, et al: Self-stigma and coming out about one's mental illness. *J Community Psychol* 38:1–17, 2010.

77. Wang J, Lai D: The relationship between mental health literacy, personal contacts and personal stigma against depression. *J Affective Disorders* 110(1):191–196, 2008.

78. Nadeem E, Lange HM, Edge D, et al: Does stigma keep poor young immigrant and U.S.-born black and Latina women from seeking mental health care? *Psychiatric Services* 58:1547–1554, 2007.

79. Caplan S, Whittemore R: Barriers to treatment engagement for depression among Latinas. *Issues Mental Health Nurs* 34:412–424, 2013.

80. U.S. Census Bureau: American FactFinder, United States: American Community Survey. American Community Survey 1-year estimates, Languages spoken at home: 2009. Retrieved from <http://www.census.gov/compendia/statab/2012/tables/12s0053.pdf>.

81. Agency for Healthcare Research and Quality: *Improving patient safety systems for patients with limited English proficiency: A guide for hospitals*, Rockville, MD, 2012, Author. Retrieved from: <http://www.ahrq.gov/professionals/systems/hospital/lepguide/index.html>.

82. Escobar JI, Hoyos Nervi C, Gara MA: Immigration and mental health: Mexican Americans in the United States. *Harvard Rev Psychiatr* 8(2):64–72, 2000.

83. Kleinman A: Depression, somatization and the "new cross-cultural psychiatry." *Soc Sci Med* 11:3–10, 1977.

Spirituality

Verna Benner Carson

Spirituality is a concept in nursing that has probably always been present in practice—even in ancient times there was awareness that people were more than their bodies and that "more," although difficult to describe or to quantify, was just as real as the body that could be touched and ministered to. In ancient cultures, there was a sense that people had good and/or bad spirits residing in their bodies, and these spirits influenced the individual's behavior for good or evil. In early Judaism, the care of the sick was a religious obligation, and this obligation continued as Christianity grew and expanded throughout the world. The earliest hospitals were run by religious orders, and nurses were trained by the Catholic Sisters who ran many of these hospitals. These early "health professionals" did not describe what they did in "spiritual terms," but they believed that the care they provided honored God.

In the 1970s and 1980s, spirituality was virtually removed from nursing curricula as the education of nurses moved increasingly into colleges and universities. With a growing emphasis on "evidence-based" interventions, spirituality was nearly lost as a part of nursing education. However, spirituality and its significance were not totally removed from nursing. In the late 1970s, Jean Stallwood and Dr. Ruth Stoll were co-contributors to a chapter titled "Spiritual Dimensions of Nursing Practice" in the third edition of *Clinical Nursing* by Beland and Passos.[1] Following this, Stoll published a sentinel article on spiritual assessment in a 1979 edition of the *American Journal of Nursing*. Margaret Colliton wrote a chapter titled "The Spiritual Dimension of Nursing" in the fourth edition of *Clinical Nursing* by Beland and Passos.[2] In 1989, *Spiritual Dimensions of Nursing Practice,* written by Verna Benner Carson was released.[3] Nursing became a profession—developing its own theories and educational methods, and professors of nursing began to examine the "more of nursing"—in other words, what made nursing unique and effective. These nurses recognized that nursing was more than making beds, bathing patients, administering medications, and performing the myriad other tasks that the nurses of today still perform. What was that "other" that nurses provided? Nurses arrived at multiple answers to this question, but one of the concepts identified was the nurse's ability to assess and address the spiritual needs of patients.

DEFINITION

The concept of *spirituality* is an elusive concept to define. Authors that write about spirituality in nursing advocate the position that a patient's quality of life, health, and sense of wholeness are affected by spirituality, yet still the profession of nursing struggles to define it. Why? There are a number of explanations for this. One explanation is that spirituality represents "heart" not "head" knowledge, and "heart" knowledge is difficult to encapsulate into words. A second explanation is that spirituality is unique to each person, so a precise definition is somewhat elusive.

The definitions of spirituality encompass the following: a principle, an experience, attitudes and belief regarding God, a sense of God, and the inner person. According to Mary Elizabeth O'Brien, "Spirituality, as a personal concept, is generally understood in terms of an individual's attitudes and belief related to transcendence (God) or to the nonmaterial forces of life and of nature."[4,p4] O'Brien concluded that most descriptions of spirituality include not only transcendence but also the connection of mind, body, and spirit, in addition to love, caring, and compassion and a relationship with the Divine.[4]

Ruth Stoll defined spirituality in 1989 when she wrote,

It is who I am—unique, and personally connected to God. That relationship with God is expressed through my body, my thinking, my feelings, my judgments, and my creativity. My spirituality motivates me to choose meaningful relationships and pursuits. Through my spirituality I give and receive love; I respond to and appreciate God, other people, a sunset, a symphony, and spring. I am driven forward, sometimes because of pain, sometimes in spite of pain. Spirituality allows me to reflect on myself. I am a person because of my spirituality—motivated and enabled to value, to worship, and to communicate with the holy, the transcendent.[5,p6]

Stoll's definition is clearly related to a belief in God and derives from a Christian theistic worldview. It is important to note that individuals can view themselves as being very spiritual—believing that there is a transcendent being—and yet have no association with organized religion.

Because there is such a wide deviation in the ways that spirituality is defined, for the purposes of this concept presentation, we use the following definition of spirituality, suggested by Dr. Harold Koenig, a major author and researcher on topics related to spirituality and who credits this definition to Dr. Kenneth Pargament: "Spirituality represents a search for the sacred or transcendent (God, Jesus, Muhammad, the Buddha, Brahman, Ultimate Truth of Reality)."[6,pp74-75]

There are a few similar and related terms to spirituality worth mentioning to provide distinction and clarification. *Faith*, as defined by Dyess, refers to an "evolving pattern of believing, that grounds and guides authentic living and gives meaning in the present moment of inter-relating."[7,p2728] *Religiosity*, another similar term, is an external expression (public or private) in the form of practicing a belief or faith, whereas spirituality is an internalized spiritual identity (or experiential). Specifically, religiosity is defined as "the adherence to religious dogma or creed, the expression of moral beliefs, and/or the participation in organized or individual worship, or sacred practices."[8,p200]

SCOPE

The scope of spirituality is quite broad and encompasses life itself and its meaning as perceived by each individual. Spirituality may be based on religious convictions, teachings, and experiences that provide moral direction and a sense that individuals are part of a larger plan and that each of us belongs to a Higher Being. However, spirituality might have no connection at all to religion and the transcendent but be experienced in the "highs" and "lows" of life with a view that these experiences are viewed as a normal part of living.

What is true is that everyone has a spiritual nature, a sense that there is more than what is experienced day to day, month to month, year to year until death. Spirituality encompasses the mundane activities of life that keep us grounded as well as those magnificent times and experiences when our innermost spirit soars with any number of emotional responses, including exquisite joy, dark and deep sorrow, laughter and fun, and all emotions in between (Figure 5-1). When we desire with all our might to hold onto a particular event along with the feelings and thoughts that accompany that event, our desire is linked to awareness at some level that convinces us that the event has forever changed us in a profound manner—this is a spiritual response. Births, deaths, marriages, separations, divorces, terrible diagnoses, joy, and sorrow all possess this ability to touch our spirits in a profound manner. The person is not the same as he or she was before this event occurred. The meaning and significance of the event might only be experienced by one individual; others who might be participants in the event might be left virtually untouched and unchanged. These life-changing spiritual events include just about any occurrence that has intense and personal relevance to those involved in the event. Examples of spiritually life-changing events include births, deaths, weddings, divorces, illnesses, diagnoses, and loss of abilities, loss of independence, and death. These events, having the power to change individuals and families, also have the power to draw people toward the transcendent.

ATTRIBUTES AND CRITERIA

The attributes of the concept of spirituality in the context of nursing care are presented in Box 5-1 and described further here:

> ### BOX 5-1 Attributes of Spirituality
>
> - Spirituality is universal.
> - Illness impacts spirituality.
> - Patient and/or family must be willing to share and act on spiritual beliefs.
> - Spiritual beliefs and practices are impacted by family and culture.
> - Nurse must be willing to assess and integrate patient beliefs into care.
> - Nurse must be willing to consult with/refer to appropriate spiritual expert.
> - Community-based religious organization can provide support/resources.

- Spirituality is universal. All individuals, even those who profess no religious belief, are driven to derive meaning and purpose from life.
- Illness impacts spirituality in a variety of ways. Some patients and families will draw closer to God or however they conceive that Higher Power to be in an effort to seek support, healing, and comfort. Others may blame and feel anger toward that Higher Power for any illness and misfortune that may have befallen a loved one or their entire family. Still others will be neutral in their spiritual reactions.
- There has to be willingness on the part of the patient and/or family to share and/or act on spiritual beliefs and practices.
- The nurse needs to be aware that specific spiritual beliefs and practices are impacted by family and culture.
- The nurse needs to be willing to assess the concept of spirituality in patients and families and, based on this ongoing assessment, to integrate the spiritual beliefs of patients and families into care.
- The nurse needs to be willing to refer the patient or family to a spiritual expert—that is, a minister, priest, rabbi, or imam.
- Community-based religious organizations can provide supportive care to families and patients, and nurses need to be aware of these resources.

THEORETICAL LINKS

A theoretical model that closely aligns with spirituality is Atchley's continuity theory of the spiritual self.[9] According to this theory, there is recognition that individuals develop preferences as part of their personalities that influence their spiritual self as they age. The continuity theory of the spiritual self is based on the assumption that spirituality sensitizes and guides individuals through a variety of human experiences throughout life. Several key constructs include (1) deep inner silence, (2) insight, (3) compassion, (4) connection with the ground of being, (5) transcendence of personal self, (6) wonder, and (7) transformation. Furthermore, the continuity theory of the spiritual self proposes a significant role for spiritual beliefs and practices in coping with problems later in life, particularly the experiences of illness, death, and dying. This closely illustrates the notion that spirituality is a lifelong journey.

Boswell and Boswell-Ford[8] conducted a study using the continuity theory to analyze religious concepts and spirituality. The researchers found that older adults adapt spiritual beliefs and practices through an awareness of their spiritual experiences and that private religiosity is more highly correlated with experiential spirituality than is public religiosity.

FIGURE 5-1 Scope of Spirituality

CONTEXT TO NURSING AND HEALTH CARE

Many health care providers recognize assessment and meeting of spiritual needs as forms of caring. When spirituality is left out of care, nursing and indeed all of health care is incomplete. The quality of health care is impacted by spirituality.

Spirituality is the driving force when health professionals feel "called" to do what they do. Spirituality is the reason for inquiring about the stories of patients and families because we know that only in the stories do we capture the meaning of health and illness to the persons in our care. Spirituality is what motivates us to go the extra mile and keeps us going because we see that the needs are so great! Spirituality infuses the work we do with love, compassion, and a sense of gratitude for being participants in God's healing work.[10,pviii]

Professional Mandates to Provide Spiritual Care

As a profession, nursing prides itself on being holistic in its approach to patient care. Nurses tout their ability to conduct thorough assessments of patients' needs, planning nursing strategies to meet these needs and providing the necessary care that patients require. However, nurses shy away from providing spiritual care. The neglect of the spiritual is a serious deficit in nursing. Every professional document that focuses on standards of nursing practice includes a statement regarding nursing's responsibility to address spiritual concerns. In *Nursing Intervention Classification*,[11] two standard nursing interventions are identified that directly relate to spiritual care: Spiritual Support (No. 540) and Spiritual Growth Facilitation (No. 5426). Also, in the *Nursing Outcome Classification*,[12] two spiritual outcomes are identified: Spiritual Health (2001) and Personal Health Status (2006). In addition, the North American Nursing Diagnosis Association International (NANDA-I) includes three standard nursing diagnoses: "spiritual distress," "spiritual distress, risk for," and "spiritual well-being, readiness for enhanced."[13] In the guidelines for professional nursing, "spiritual" or "spirituality" is mentioned 18 times with specific instructions that spiritual beliefs need to be integrated into care, that nurses need to collaborate with other nurses as well as patients to provide spiritually and culturally appropriate interventions; and that the Bachelor of Science in Nursing graduate needs to be able to conduct comprehensive assessments including the spiritual realm.[14]

The emphasis on spirituality in major nursing documents, including statements on ethics, standards of nursing diagnosis, and classification, makes it clear that assessing for and addressing spiritual issues is not an option for nurses but, rather, a mandate.

Assessment of Spirituality

Providing spiritual care starts with an assessment of a patient's spirituality. The very act of engaging in a conversation about spirituality conveys to the patient and family that we are willing to discuss spiritual/

religious beliefs and issues. This initial spiritual conversation may very well lead to other opportunities to talk about the impact of spiritual matters on the patient's current health-situation issues, such as how the patient will cope, what impact this health crisis will have on the patient's sense of purpose and meaning in life, what adaptations or changes need to be made to accommodate the current health problem, and what difficult choices face the patient/family. Every one of these issues is spiritual in nature. We may not have the answers, nor is it necessary to have the answers; it is usually best to encourage the patient and family to talk openly about these issues until they are able to arrive at their own answers.

Conducting a spiritual assessment is a powerful way to open up the topic of spirituality with a patient and/or the patient's family. There are a number of spiritual assessment tools that are easy to use. One that was developed by Dr. Harold Koenig includes the following five questions:

1. Do religious/spiritual beliefs provide comfort to you or cause you stress?
2. How might your religious/spiritual beliefs influence your health care decisions?
3. Are there any religious/spiritual beliefs that might interfere with or conflict with your medical treatment?
4. Ar4.e you a member of a religious/spiritual community and, if so, is it supportive?
5. Are there any other spiritual needs that someone should address?[15]

Another spiritual assessment tool, developed by Puchalski and Romer (2000), uses the acronym tool FICA.[16] The four questions for this tool are presented in Box 5-2.

Nursing Interventions for Spiritual Care

Spiritual care involves recognizing and honoring the religious beliefs and practices of those in our care, but it can also be shared laughter or tears or remembering a patient's birthday. Spiritual care can be

---

> ## BOX 5-2 FICA Tool for Spiritual Assessment
>
> - **F**aith or beliefs: What are your spiritual beliefs? Do you consider yourself spiritual? What things do you believe in that give meaning to life?
> - **I**mportance and influence: Is faith/spirituality important to you? How has your illness and/or hospitalization affected your personal practices/beliefs?
> - **C**ommunity: Are you connected with a faith center in the community? Does it provide support/comfort for you during times of stress? Is there a person/group/leader that supports/assists you in your spirituality?
> - **A**ddress: What can I do for you? What support/guidance can health care provide to support your spiritual beliefs/practices?

Source: Adapted from Puchalski C, Romer AL: Taking a spiritual history allows clinicians to understand patients more fully, *J Palliative Med* 3(1):129–137, 2000.

keeping vigil with a family as a loved one struggles to recover. It can be crying with that same family when their loved one dies. It can be supporting a chronically ill individual who is struggling to redefine his worth and personal meaning in light of the illness and its demands. It can be a gentle backrub coupled with soothing words that allows a worried patient to sleep. It can be a shared prayer or religious reading that has special meaning to the patient. Spiritual care cannot be boxed in and narrowly defined. Spiritual care is not limited to those who believe a certain way or who define God according to a specific doctrine. Spiritual care is for everyone. People may express their spirituality in unique ways, but everyone has a spiritual nature that can be touched through the kindness, compassion and ministrations of another.

The provision of spiritual care can be thought about in three distinct approaches that include *communication*, *action*, and *presence*.

Communication

Excellent communication is a learned skill that involves hearing, not just the words being spoken but also those that are not spoken. The ability to listen is both an art and a learned skill. It requires that the nurse completely attends to the patient with open ears, eyes, and mind. Listening is an active process that requires the nurse's concentration. Nurses must attend to both the auditory and the visual stimuli that they receive from the patient, and then they must analyze these stimuli to ascertain the patient's intent. Several barriers may interfere with the nurses' ability to listen actively. Nurses must develop sensitivity to their own internal barriers to active listening as well as to demonstrate great sensitivity to the patient's belief system.

Frequently, patients hint at their real concerns and openly reveal them only when we go beyond their words to their feelings and the deeper meaning behind their communication. Likewise, people often do not reveal their most intimate personal thoughts and feelings in a direct manner but, rather, cloak them in obscure language. This masking of what represents the true self is a protective measure—fearing that the listener may react in a hurtful way. Thus, rather than expose oneself to the possibility of being hurt, the patient may hide what he or she really feels and may only allude to it in a roundabout way. This places a burden on the nurse to pick up and pursue clues that the patient or family member gives.

Several barriers may result in the nurse's inability to be totally present and communicate effectively with the patient. First, the nurse may be distracted by other things and may not pay attention to the patient. Second, the nurse may miss the meaning of the patient's message because of failure to clarify the meaning of a word, a phrase, or a facial expression. Third, the nurse may interject personal feelings and reactions into the patient's situation rather than allow the patient to explore and discuss his or her own feelings and reactions. The last barrier occurs when the nurse is busy formulating a response while the patient is still talking. In this instance, the nurse does not hear the patient's message.

Action

The second spiritual intervention, that of taking action, refers to how the nurse carries out nursing activities, including the following:

- Giving verbal support and encouragement of spiritual beliefs
- Making a referral to a chaplain or pastoral care professional
- Using religious literature that is meaningful to the patient and/or the patient's family
- Using prayer with the patient's or family's consent

Underlying these actions is the need for the nurse to convey a powerful message of love and concern. The following example from a nurse demonstrates this:

There was a nun at the far end of our unit; I didn't usually take care of her. No one wanted to take care of her. Everyone thought she was going to die, and she wasn't the easiest person—kind of crotchety and grouchy. Anyway, one day we were short-staffed, and I was asked to take Sister's medicine to her. I was told to take along applesauce to make it easier for her to take her pills. I did that, and when I was done, I offered her a glass of cold water, for which she seemed grateful. I never took care of her again. Two years later, I saw this very tiny nun walking toward our nurse's station—it was Sister. She said, "I know that voice! Where is she?" (I have a slight Boston accent, or so I am told.) Sister came up to me and hugged me. She said, "You gave me the glass of cold water. That was the kindest thing anyone did for me, and I have never forgotten it." Can you believe that a glass of water could be that powerful?[17,p108]

Presence

Probably the greatest tool available to nurses for meeting spiritual needs is their own presence and ability to touch another person both physically and spiritually. Presence requires more than just showing up when someone is sick or standing by the bedside, although these actions are important. To fully demonstrate presence, the nurse needs to be an active listener and to be able to demonstrate empathy, humility, vulnerability, and commitment.

A nurse demonstrates presence through the personal relationship that is developed with the patient and the patient's family. This relationship allows the nurse and patient to mutually experience the uniqueness of the other. It is in this relationship that the nurse is able to learn about the patient's spiritual and/or religious needs, wants, hurts, joys, and ambitions. It is through this relationship that the nurse communicates personal spiritual strength and willingness to care, listen, and be available to the patient. The presence of the nurse touches the patient's distressed spirit, just as a cool hand might soothe a fevered brow.[17]

Why Some Nurses Neglect Spiritual Care

Although spirituality should be incorporated into the care of all patients, this is unfortunately not the case. There are a number of explanations for this lack of response to spiritual needs. First, often the nurse fails to recognize spiritual needs of the patient and/or family. If a specific spiritual assessment is not done, the failure to recognize the need is understandable. There are times when the nurse recognizes spiritual needs but feels inadequate to meet these needs. This may be linked to a lack of understanding, skill, or confidence to effectively implement appropriate interventions. An insufficient focus on spirituality in nursing education often leaves nurses feeling inadequate and ill prepared in this area. Furthermore, some nurses believe that they must be personally "religious" to address and meet the spiritual needs of patients. Finally, another common reason nurses often fail to incorporate spirituality into nursing care relates to personal discomfort experienced by the nurse when discussing an area that does not have concrete answers.[6]

All of these reasons lead nurses to either avoid this area of inquiry or, if they recognize a spiritual need, immediately make a referral to the hospital chaplain. Certainly making a referral to the hospital chaplain and/or a representative from the patient's faith tradition such as a priest, minister, rabbi, or an imam is a better response than ignoring the patient's spiritual needs. However, such a response means that the nurse has cut her- or himself off from being present to a patient and/or family at the time when a spiritual need is expressed.[6] In addition, when patients express a spiritual need, there is generally

FIGURE 5-2 Spirituality and Interrelated Concepts

immediacy about that need that warrants a response from the nurse—even if the response is just to encourage the patient to elaborate on his or her concerns. The freedom to be able to speak about spiritual issues to a willing listener is probably enough for many patients. However, nursing should be able to provide more than just a listening ear.

INTERRELATED CONCEPTS

Several concepts in this book are closely interrelated with the concept of spirituality and have previously been mentioned. One could make that case that spirituality is interrelated with all concepts presented in this book. Although this may be the case, it is useful to examine those that have the closest links to better understand this concept (Figure 5-2). One of the closest interrelated concepts is Culture. Culture refers to a pattern of shared attitudes, beliefs, and values. Spirituality is deeply embedded in an individual's personal belief system and is strongly influenced by the context of that individual's culture. Likewise, spirituality, in itself, can influence culture. When large numbers of individuals share specific spiritual beliefs and/or practices, this can be identified as a religious group with cultural norms. Figure 5-2 shows the relationship between spirituality and culture as a bidirectional arrow for these reasons. Family Dynamics are also closely aligned with spirituality. A person's belief system is strongly influenced within the family unit from early in life. Specific religious practices within a family shape one's view of religiosity, which closely links with an individual's spirituality. It is also possible that disagreements or changes in one's spiritual beliefs, if different from those held by family members, can lead to changes in relationships. Figure 5-2 shows the relationship between spirituality and family dynamics as a bidirectional arrow for these reasons. A bidirectional arrow is also shown between family dynamics and culture to show that these concepts form a concept cluster. The concept of Development is interrelated because an individual's spirituality is, in part, dependent on the developmental stage of the individual. Spirituality changes during one's life, partly based on life experiences and emotional maturity. Another concept closely linked to spirituality is Cognition. Spirituality is an abstract concept involving deep-seated beliefs and values—the individual's cognitive status impacts thought, awareness, and ability for purposeful actions

> **BOX 5-3** **EXEMPLARS OF SPIRITUALTY**
>
> - Faith
> - Hope
> - Prayer
> - Compassion
> - Meditation
> - Dietary traditions
> - Ceremonies
> - Sacraments
> - Religious articles (e.g., candles, oils, and rosaries)
> - Religious texts (e.g., the Bible, Toran, and Qur'an)
> - Practice of organized religion
>   - Christian-based faiths
>   - Judaism
>   - Islamic
>   - Buddhism
>   - Hinduism

related to spirituality. Finally, the concept of Communication closely aligns with spirituality. Communication is one of three distinct approaches involved with spiritual care previously discussed. The nurse must be able and willing to actively listen to the patient and notice nonverbal cues as a foundation for understanding the patient's needs, beliefs, and values. Because this is a professional nursing concept, this is shown as a different color in Figure 5-2.

CLINICAL EXEMPLARS

There are many exemplars of the concept spirituality in the context of health care. It is not expected that nurses will develop expertise in each exemplar. However, nurses should be willing to assess the patient's need and to confidently and competently discuss and support the patient's spiritual preferences. Common exemplars are presented in Box 5-3.

Featured Exemplars
Faith

The term *faith* can refer to a specific religious tradition or belief in something that cannot be touched or seen. Members of an organized religious tradition speak about beliefs and traditions they not only hold dear but also believe are historically trustworthy even though they cannot touch, see, reproduce, or feel the experience. In the context of health care, faith represents a measure of confidence that a force is at work that will lead to a positive outcome (i.e., "God will help me recover"). Faith may also be expressed by patients as confidence in the skill and knowledge of their physicians and nurses.

Hope

Hope refers to beliefs, wishes, or actions taken in situations of uncertainty. Hope is linked to faith but tends to have an emphasis on the fear of the unknown. Hope is based more on facts of a situation but links to the future belief in things unseen. For instance, patients hope for relief from pain even in the face of relentless pain. Hope is a concept that nurses need to foster. When hope for a cure is not possible, nurses can direct patients to reconfigure what they are hopeful about—for example, relief from pain, comfort when needed, and a peaceful death.

Prayer

Prayer is conversation with God or a Higher Power, however that Higher Power is conceived. The conversation may take many forms. Sometimes prayer is supplication, or asking God for something such as healing for self or others or removal of pain. At other times, prayer can serve as a way to get to know God better and to be in God's presence. At even other times, prayer may be thanksgiving to God for His goodness.

Sacraments

The term *sacrament* is derived from the Latin *sacramentum,* which means "a sign of the sacred." Sacraments, recognized by Christian faiths, represent special occasions for experiencing God's saving presence. There are variations in the number and meaning of sacraments among the Christian faiths. For example, the Catholic Church recognizes seven sacraments (Baptism, Holy Communion, Reconciliation, Confirmation, Marriage, Holy Orders, and Anointing of the Sick), whereas most protestant denominations recognize two sacraments (Baptism and Holy Communion). In the health care setting, patients are most likely to request Holy Communion or Reconciliation, although Baptism may be requested for an infant in an emergency situation.

CASE STUDY

Source: Juanmonino/iStock/Thinkstock

Case Presentation

Robert Klein, a 16-year-old with bilateral amputation below the knee, was assigned to Mrs. Carlton, a registered nurse on a rehabilitation unit. Mrs. Carlton, who had two teenage sons, found it very difficult to work with Robert. When she was in his room, she felt tearful and was unable to carry on a conversation with him and experienced difficulty engaging him in rehabilitation for fear of causing him pain. Her thoughts were on how awful this must be for Robert and what it would be like if this happened to one of her sons. Mrs. Carlton was sympathetic to Robert, but she was ineffective because her close identification with his feelings interfered with her ability to focus on his needs.

One morning, Mrs. Carlton walked into Robert's room and found him crying. Her first response was to leave the room as she thought, "I can't handle this today." But she was able to stop herself, and she went over to Robert and touched his shoulder. He continued to sob and said, "What am I going to do? I wish I were dead. My whole life is sports. I would have qualified for an athletic scholarship if this hadn't happened. I feel like my life is over."

Mrs. Carlton recognized the feelings of despair that Robert was expressing and said to him, "It seems to you like your life is over. You are feeling that this is such an unfair thing to have happened to you. I agree with you, it is, but let's talk about it." Mrs. Carlton responded to Robert in an empathetic manner. She communicated to him that she was present for him, that she understood his feelings, and that she would be with him if he wanted to talk about his situation at greater length. Mrs. Carlton's response did not change Robert's present or his future—her understanding did not change the reality that Robert had experienced a bilateral below the knee amputation. However, her commitment to be present to Robert, her ability to really listen attentively to what he had to say, her encouragement of him, and her ability to put into words for him the deep spiritual issue he was facing helped him to open up and draw from his inner spiritual strength.

Case Analysis

Mrs. Carlton's initial response to Robert was not therapeutic, nor did it represent spiritual care. She responded by overidentifying with Robert's situation and instead of focusing on his needs, she focused on the "what if's" and put herself and her own sons in the same situation, thus removing herself from being present to Robert. When she found him despondent and in deep spiritual distress, she was able to remain in his room—to be present to him and to listen and validate his spiritual pain—life as he knew it would be forever changed. He would need to discover other avenues to find meaning, purpose, and direction. However, in this moment with Mrs. Carlton's presence, he could feel validated, loved, and perhaps even a bit hopeful.

ACCESS EXEMPLAR LINKS IN YOUR GIDDENS EBOOK

REFERENCES

1. Stallwood J, Stoll R: Spiritual dimensions of nursing practice. In Beland IL, Passos JY, editors: *Clinical nursing: Pathophysiological and psychosocial approaches*, ed 3, New York, 1975, Macmillan, pp 1086–1098.
2. Colliton MA: The spiritual dimension of nursing. In Beland IL, Passos JY, editors: *Clinical nursing: Pathophysiological and psychosocial approaches*, ed 4, New York, 1981, Macmillan, pp 492–501.
3. Carson VB, editor: *Spiritual dimensions of nursing practice*, Philadelphia, 1989, Saunders, pp 150–180.
4. O'Brien ME: The need for spiritual integrity. In Yura H, Walsh MB, editors: *Human needs and the nursing process*, East Norwalk, CT, 1982, Appleton & Lange.
5. Stoll R: The essence of spirituality. In Carson VB, editor: *Spiritual dimensions of nursing practice*, Philadelphia, 1989, Saunders.
6. Koenig H: Why include spirituality? In *Spirituality in patient care: Why, how, when and what*, ed 3, West Conshohocken, PA, 2013, Templeton Press, pp 6–7.
7. Dyess SM: Faith: A concept analysis. *J Adv Nurs* 67(12):2723–2731, 2011.
8. Boswell GE, Boswell-Ford KC: Testing a SEM model of two religious concepts and experiential spirituality. *J Relig Health* 49:200–211, 2010.
9. Atchley R: *Spirituality and aging*, Baltimore, MD, 2009, Johns Hopkins University Press.
10. Carson VB, Koenig H: *Spiritual dimensions of nursing practice*, rev ed, West Conshohocken, PA, 2008, Templeton Press.
11. Bulechek G, Butcher H, Dochterman J, et al, editors: *Nursing interventions classification (NIC)*, ed 6, St Louis, 2013, Elsevier.
12. Moorhead S, Johnson M, Maas M, et al, editors: *Nursing outcomes classification (NOC)*, ed 5, St Louis, 2013, Elsevier.
13. NANDA International: *Nursing diagnoses: Definitions and classifications 2012–2014*, ed 9, Des Moines, IA, 2014, Wiley–Blackwell.
14. Stoll R: Guidelines for spiritual assessment. *Am J Nurs* 79:1574–1577, 1979.
15. Koenig HG: Spiritual history. *JAMA* 288(4):2002.
16. Puchalski C, Romer AL: Taking a spiritual history allows clinicians to understand patients more fully. *J Palliat Med* 3(1):129–137, 2000.
17. Carson VB, Koenig HG: *Spiritual caregiving: Healthcare as a ministry*, Philadelphia, 2004, Templeton Foundation Press, pp 15–17.

Adherence

Janice Bissonnette

As a health care recipient concept representing patient preferences, adherence has numerous definitions across health care, which has led to contradictory meanings.[1–11] In nursing, the concept of adherence is closely associated with patient-centered care and the expertise required by nurses to support a patient's long-term adherence to treatment.[10,11] Nursing plays a major role in supporting patients' acceptance and adjustment to the impact of illness on their lives. Adherence from a patient-centered approach supports the goal of nursing by advocating for what is best in the context of each patient's life. This concept presentation serves as a preliminary step to broadening nurses' appreciation for the complexity of adherence as a patient behavior and represents an integration of what we know about adherence.

DEFINITION

The North American Nursing Diagnosis Association International (NANDA-I) defines "adherence behavior" as a "self-initiated action taken to promote wellness, recovery, and rehabilitation."[12,p458] Haynes et al. defined adherence as the extent to which patients follow the instructions they are given for prescribed treatments.[13] Christensen offered an alternative definition, in keeping with a less paternalistic approach.[14] Adherence in this setting is patient focused and is the extent to which a person's actions or behavior coincide with advice or instruction from a health care provider intended to prevent, monitor, or ameliorate a disorder.

Cohen, in a concept analysis of adherence related to the nursing practice of patients with cardiovascular disease, defined adherence as "persistence in the practice and maintenance of desired health behaviors and is the result of active participation and agreement."[15,27] Adherence is also associated with terms such as compliance, concordance, obedience, observance, conformity, acceptance, cooperation, mutuality, persistence, and therapeutic alliance.[16–19]

Before the late 1990s, compliance was the more commonly used term to describe a patient's behavior related to following a recommended treatment.[20,21] The definition of compliance behavior, as an outcome for nursing diagnostic categories, is distinctly different from that for adherence behavior. In this context, compliance behavior is "the action taken on the basis of professional advice to promote wellness, recovery, and rehabilitation."[12,p458] The term compliance was the primary descriptor for a patient's obedience to prescribed treatments.[22] Variation and debate exist on how to define adherence; how it differs from compliance or concordance; and how the behavior of adherence relates to patients, health care professionals, and system factors.[2,8,9,23–26] The historical transition and change in terminology from compliance to adherence, and concordance, requires a standardization of the taxonomy for "adherence" as a concept for nursing practice.[9,10,27–29] In nursing practice, it is important to determine if adherence, as a profile of the patient's behavior, provides an effective way of characterizing the behavior that individuals demonstrate in response to a prescribed treatment regimen.

SCOPE

The scope of adherence essentially ranges from a total lack of adherence to complete adherence (Figure 6-1). The degree of adherence within this range includes the patient's intentional or rationale decision to stop the medication or change the dose or frequency of the medication.[17,30] Also included in this range is the patient's unintentional change in medication-taking behavior, which represents a nonpurposeful overlooking of taking the medication.[29,31]

The same applies for health-promotion activities—for example, reducing the amount of recommended exercise, increasing the amount of recommended salt in the diet on weekends, or not attending physician's appointments. Despite the potential for any degree of nonadherence to influence a patient's disease control or health, it is unclear where, within this range, patients become most at risk for negative outcomes.[27]

The primary situation preceding the evaluation of a patient's adherence behavior is the recommendation or prescription of a treatment by a health care professional. Often, the focus is on the patient's adherence to long-term medications or treatments and health-promotion activities in the face of chronic disease.[26] The theme underlying the patient's total or positive adherent behavior suggests the patient views/believes the professional to be a trusted and knowledgeable source concerning recommended treatment for the disease or health state in question. The action or behavior of adherence assumes some degree of willingness and motivation on the part of the patient to accept all or part of the prescription or recommendation. What is not clear with the behavior of adherence is the degree to which the patient agreed with or was involved in the prescription or recommendation.

Within health care, the consequences of nonadherence fall into three areas: patient related, health professional related, and health care system related.[26,29] Patient-related consequences include increased

Non-adherence	Partial adherence:	Partial adherence:	Total adherence
Complete omission	**Intentional**	**Non-intentional**	
	Adjusting dose/frequency	Non-purposefully	
	(increase or decrease)	forgets/misses/neglects	

FIGURE 6-1 Scope of Adherence

mortality and morbidity, conflict, attributional uncertainty, embarrassment, and changes in quality of life.[27] Health professional-related consequences include ambivalence, misinterpretation, avoidance, decisional conflict, and empathy.[31–34] Health care system-related consequences include increased cost and health care service use.[26,27] Nurses are present in the majority of health care settings in which patients receive treatment recommendations. This provides an opportunity to assess motivation and integrate and reinforce treatment adherence strategies with patients.

ATTRIBUTES AND CRITERIA

The attributes of a concept support identification of situations or behaviors that are best characterized by using the concept of interest. The cluster of attributes comprises the real-life definition of a concept, as opposed to the dictionary definition.[35] A number of attributes are associated with adherence (Box 6-1).

In the context of a number of nursing diagnoses, adherence behavior is the anticipated outcome. For the diagnosis of *Health-Seeking Behaviors*, defined as "the state in which an individual in stable health is actively seeking ways to alter personal health habits, and/or the environment in order to move toward a higher level of health,"[12,p162] adherence behavior is the outcome. The nursing diagnosis of *Individual Management of Therapeutic Regimen, Effective*, defined as "a pattern of regulating and integrating into daily living a program for treatment of illness and its sequelae that are satisfactory for meeting specific health goals,"[12,p179] adherence behavior is the outcome.

A variable that has significant influence on adherence is motivation. Adherence does not occur if an individual is not motivated to do so.[36] Moreover, the degree or source of motivation may influence the extent of adherence. One of the oldest definitions of motivation stems from the psychological use of the term in 1904, which suggests the term represents an inner or social stimulus for action.[37] Motivation, as with adherence, also runs along a continuum. Ryan and Deci stated that people "vary not only in the *level* of motivation (i.e., how much motivation), but also in the *orientation* of that motivation (i.e., what type of motivation)."[38,p54] Two major types of motivation are based on the goals that inspire people to act. Intrinsic motivation refers to "doing something because it is inherently interesting or enjoyable," and extrinsic motivation refers to "doing something because it leads to a separable outcome."[38,p55]

THEORETICAL LINKS

Social psychologists have developed a number of behavioral approaches to guide the assessment of a patient's medication-taking behavior and the overall enhancement of adherence behavior. The social cognition models are the most common theories supporting the behavior change associated with adherence or nonadherence.[14,39–45] Common psychological theories include the theory of planned

behavior[43] and the health belief model.[44] The primary outcome in each of these models is a specific health behavior based on a deliberate process of decision making. Preexisting intentions, beliefs, or degree of confidence in his or her success influences the patient's decision-making process.

Theory of Planned Behavior

The theory of planned behavior (TPB) proposes a model about how human action is guided.[42,43] It predicts the occurrence of a specific behavior if that behavior is intentional. As depicted in Figure 6-2, the model integrates the variables of attitude (e.g., behavioral beliefs), subjective norms (e.g., normative beliefs and motivation), and perceived behavioral control (e.g., confidence and influence on control beliefs), which predict the intention to perform the behavior. In this model, intentions and motivation precede the actual behavior.

The key assumptions of TPB relate to the prediction of whether a person *intends* to do something. The predicators are the patient's attitude or motivation (i.e., if the patient is in agreement with completing the treatment), the subjective norm (i.e., the amount of social pressure the patient feels to proceed with the treatment), and the perceived behavioral control (i.e., the level of control the patient feels he or she has over the treatment or choice of treatment). By influencing or enhancing these three "predictors," nurses can increase the chance that the individual will intend to proceed with a recommended or prescribed treatment and then actually do it.[42,43]

For example, a patient presents to a nurse clinician in a diabetes clinic with elevated fasting glucose and hemoglobin A_{1c} (HbA$_{1c}$) measurements. Will the patient tell the nurse that the elevated measurements are attributable to the fact that he has not been taking his insulin regularly or following his diet? The answer to this question depends on whether the patient *intends* and is motivated to do so. In other words, it is not an automatic, habitual, or thoughtless action. The intention, in turn, depends on the following considerations:

- Whether the patient has a positive or negative *attitude* about revealing his nonadherent behavior.

FIGURE 6-2 The Theory of Planned Behavior

- To what extent the patient perceives that he experiences social pressure to adhere to healthy lifestyle practices for control of his diabetes and associated health risks, including whether the patient believes the following:
  - The nurse wants to know how he manages his diabetes.
  - Family/friends/significant others would approve of him telling the nurse (normative beliefs).
  - These people's opinions are important to the patient.
  - Whether the patient finds it difficult to discuss his diabetes self-management and adherence with the nurse, resulting in an appropriate treatment plan.

The final behavior is predicted by the degree to which each of the previously mentioned components influences the patient's intention to act.

The Health Belief Model

The health belief model (HBM) first conceptualized beliefs as predictors of preventive health behavior to help explain the failure of some individuals to use these behaviors.[44] The theory hypothesizes that people are likely to initiate a health-related behavior to the extent that they (1) perceive they could become ill or be susceptible to the problem (e.g., perceived susceptibility), (2) believe that the illness has serious outcomes or will disrupt their daily functioning (e.g., perceived severity), (3) believe that the required recommendation will be effective in reducing symptoms (e.g., perceived benefits), and (4) believe that there are few barriers to initiating the recommendation (e.g., perceived barriers).[44]

For example, using the same scenario previously described, a patient presents to a nurse clinician with elevated fasting glucose and HbA$_{1c}$ measurements. Will the patient tell the nurse the elevation is because he has not been taking his insulin regularly or following his diet? The answer to this question depends on the patient's perceptions of susceptibility, risk, benefits, and barriers. Engaging in a conversation of insulin adherence, in turn, depends on the following factors:

- Whether the patient perceives his diabetes as severe and his perceptions of susceptibility to the health risks associated with diabetes
- The extent to which the patient perceives that insulin therapy and diet control are beneficial in the control of his diabetes and reduction of risk factors
- Whether the patient perceives barriers exist with the use of insulin therapy and diet control

The extent or degree of these perceptions influences the patient's engagement and persistence in the behavior—in this case, whether

the patient participates in a conversation about his insulin-taking behavior.

CONTEXT TO NURSING AND HEALTH CARE

Dimensions of Adherence

Interactions between patient variables and health care provider systems can influence the degree to which a patient follows a prescribed regimen. Some suggest patients are more likely to adhere when the treatment recommended fits with their expectations.[14] Adherence as a behavior is currently thought to be composed of distinct elements representing adherence to medication, management of adherence, and adherence-related science.[36] Adherence represents three dimensions of thought and attitudes regarding patient behavior associated with recommended treatment and therapies: compliance, persistence, and concordance (Figure 6-3).

Compliance

Compliance or "obedience" with a prescribed treatment promotes an undertone of blame toward the patient when the patient's behavior does not meet health professionals' expectations.[4,46] The definition for medication compliance, developed by the International Society for Pharmacoeconomics and Outcomes Research group, is "the extent to which a patient acts in accordance with the prescribed interval and dose of a dosing regimen."[46,p46] In this context, compliance is the *behavior of conforming* to treatment for a recommended length of time. The World Health Organization (WHO) attempted to change this by introducing adherence as an alternative to the more paternalistic concept of compliance.[26] Adherence suggests the patient's agreement to prescribed recommendations rather than passive cooperation in obedience to them.[26] Some authors describe the main function of such terms as compliance and adherence as ideological, in that these terms serve as a framework from which health care professionals convey their ideas concerning how patients should behave.[28,47–50]

David Sackett, one of the original and major researchers in medical compliance, published randomized clinical trial results of strategies for improving medication compliance in patients with hypertension.[22] The majority of compliance research published from the 1970s to the 1980s was by physicians or behavioral scientists, containing no input from nursing.[22,23] The concept of adherence became more prominent in nursing literature in the late 1990s through the works of Marston.[51]

FIGURE 6-3 Dimensions of Adherence

Persistence

Another dimension of adherence behavior associated with health care therapies is persistence. Persistence appears primarily within the context of chronic disease management therapies.[48] In contrast to compliance, medication persistence is the time from initiation to discontinuation of a recommended or prescribed treatment and is a *measure of continuation*.[48] In nursing practice, the patient's degree of persistence is of most value when assessing his or her adherence behavior. Confirming how often a patient renews or refills his or her prescriptions is a measurement of the patient's persistence with continuation of the treatment.

Concordance

Concordance is the most recent term added in an attempt to more accurately reflect the behavior of adherence and suggests that patients and health care professionals come to a *mutual agreement* on regimen through a process of negotiation and shared decision making.[24,49] The behavior of concordance reflects development of an alliance with patients based on realistic expectations.[49]

Interdisciplinary Lens of Adherence

In moving beyond the ideological and semantic debate, the practical reality of not following a recommended course of treatment, particularly in chronic illness, remains a major cause of poor health outcomes and increased health care costs.[22,23] In 2003, WHO launched a global initiative to improve worldwide rates of adherence to therapies commonly used in treating chronic conditions. Adherence rates with prescribed regimens in chronic illness average 50%, ranging from 0% to 100% depending on the method of measurement.[22]

Evangelista reviewed the literature on adherence and compliance from all health disciplines in an attempt to distinguish between the everyday health care practice use and that associated with scientific use.[7] Adherence is a dynamic concept, influenced in part by the social context of its use. The social or disciplinary context for the purpose of this section is nursing practice, with identification of interrelations between and with other health disciplines. Similar inductive approaches have been applied by nurse researchers for the analysis of such concepts as chronic pain, symptom clusters, conflict in nursing work environments, and adaptive systems.[52–54] Understanding the perspective and use of adherence from each discipline is fundamental for clarification of the concept and for identification of contextual variations.[54–56] The following sections present the major characteristics of adherence emerging from the disciplines of nursing, mental health, general medicine, and pharmacy.

Nursing

Before the introduction of the concept of adherence, Marston, as one of the first nursing authors to enter the compliance debate, raised

concerns about medicine's multiple definitions of compliance in addition to the lack of objective compliance measures.[51] Marston encouraged nurses to participate in the debates related to compliance to improve the nursing knowledge of compliance from a more holistic nurse–patient perspective.[51] In 1973, NANDA accepted noncompliance as a nursing diagnosis. The new diagnostic category reflected little recognition of the impact on nursing practice but resulted more in response to the medically based literature.[57]

Kim suggested that the diagnostic taxonomies for nursing appeared to unify communication and documentation between nurses but did not add to the development of nursing science because of the lack of association with an explanatory framework.[56] From 1973 to the present, members of NANDA-I, supported by additional nursing authors, pursued the removal of noncompliance from this diagnostic nomenclature because the term emphasized a paternalistic obligation to follow orders.[51–57] Interestingly, as discussed previously, the nursing diagnosis of noncompliance remains in use, with adherence behavior as the expected outcome.

Mental Health

Adherence to therapies is a key component of care in mental health settings.[33,34,39,40,58,59] Estimates of medication nonadherence for patients with mental disease are 24–90%.[39,40] One in four patients experiencing psychosis demonstrates nonadherence.[39,40] Adherence and compliance continue to be described as interchangeable concepts in the mental health literature.[39,40] An important theme identified from the mental health literature was the association between the patient's nonadherence and the patient's feelings of embarrassment when questioned about the nonadherence.[60–62] Hui et al. reported an underrecognition by mental health clinicians of both the patient's nonadherent behavior and the patient's associated feelings of embarrassment.[34] Nonadherence became a symptom of mental illness as opposed to a distinct entity. In more recent publications, various psychosocial interventions have been presented and studied. The key elements of these interventions include psychoeducational strategies, cognitive–behavioral therapy, and motivational interviewing. Results are inconclusive, but authors suggest adherence interventions with an intensive approach and a combination of strategies show results that are more favorable.[58]

Medicine

In the general medicine literature, adherence and compliance are synonymous. Adherence is most frequently associated with efforts to develop a statistically based measurement to predict the presence or risk of adherence and correlation to a health outcome or disease-specific outcomes.[13,15] The chronic disease states most commonly studied for nonadherence rates include asthma, diabetes, HIV/AIDS, transplantation, cardiovascular disease, hypertension, epilepsy, and cancer.[1,5,6,8,15,16,32] Research within these disease states attempts to provide answers to the questions of how to predict, measure, or intervene with nonadherent patient behavior.[13]

Pharmacy

The pharmacy literature mirrors the general medicine literature in the area of nonadherence. Pharmacology research focuses on the development of measurement tools for nonadherence, with reference to pharmacist-led interventions to improve patient adherence as a means of achieving therapeutic goals.[25,46,47,58] The most common formal definition was from Haynes and colleagues.[13] Some authors describe the general intent of using the term adherence to reflect a more active, voluntary, and collaborative relationship between the patient and the health care provider but continue to use compliance and adherence interchangeably.[49,50]

FIGURE 6-4 Adherence and Interrelated Concepts

Power Structure in Health Care

The historical and present-day use of compliance, adherence, and concordance continues to reflect the power structure within the social system of health care. In its ongoing attempt to develop and maintain a power hold, nursing has confronted this power structure without having a clear understanding of its impact on nursing practice. Very few researchers to date have explored the health care professional's perceptions and understanding of adherence, and none has focused on the causal relationship between motivation and adherence as distinct concepts. The question that now comes to mind is the following: Do we need to rethink how we see or explore the phenomena and concern with patients' "obedience" with treatment recommendations?

If asked, patients would not label themselves as nonadherent, noncompliant, nonconcordant, or disobedient. When confronted with questions of nonadherent behavior, patients admit to feeling blamed and accused, stating very few attempts were being made by nurses or physicians to understand the motivations or basis of decisions to "nonadhere."[4,14] As with the notion of informed consent, if patients understand the consequences of nonadherence, do we have the right to make a judgment on that individual's choice? After 40 years of studying compliance and adherence, with no clear development of guidance on how to best intervene, perhaps now is the time to accept this as a phenomenon of human nature with no one solution or one investigational approach.[11,63,64]

Research attempting to provide an objective measure of adherence reveals variability in identifying a gold standard measure as well as limited success in interventional efficacy directed at improving adherence rates.[13,14] There remains an inconsistent definition of adherence as it relates to health care recommendations, which has led to the ongoing labeling of patients as nonadherent and unmotivated. Despite the possible replacement of adherence with the new language of persistence or concordance, Russell et al. noted that the understanding of what is best for patients' lives is seldom addressed in the literature.[10]

INTERRELATED CONCEPTS

Several concepts featured in this textbook influence the degree of adherence; those with greatest influence are presented in Figure 6-4. Understanding how each concept influences nonadherence is a critical part of understanding why the problem occurs and which patients are at highest risk for nonadherence. Sociodemographic characteristics such as Culture, Spirituality, and stage of Development have been shown to have varying degrees of influence on adherence. Younger patients have consistently demonstrated poorer adherence to prescribed treatment, with adherence again declining in patients older than age 65 years[14] particularly those with impaired Cognition and those with limited Functional Ability. Similar results have suggested that those with less than 12 years of education and lower household income demonstrate poorer rates of adherence.[14] The quality of Family Dynamics and perceived family support also play a role in patient adherence, particularly among those with chronic disease.[14]

CLINICAL EXEMPLARS

There are countless clinical exemplars of adherence—so many, in fact, that it would be impossible to explain every situation on the spectrum of nonadherence to adherence. Box 6-2 presents the most common situations whereby adherence behavior is most commonly discussed or most important. The three primary categories are medication management, dietary modification, and preventative health activities.

Featured Exemplars
Medication-Taking Behavior

The most common exemplar for adherence is medication-taking behavior. Medication-taking behavior is associated with short- and long-term medication regimens. According to WHO, nonadherence

BOX 6-2 EXEMPLARS OF ADHERENCE BEHAVIOR

Medication Management

Short-Term Medication Treatment
- Antibiotics
- Anticoagulants

Long-Term Medication Treatment
- Antihypertensive agents
- Antirejection medications
- Birth control
- Cholesterol-lowering agents
- Insulin

Diet
- Diabetic diet
- Low-cholesterol diet
- Renal diet
- Sodium restrictions

Preventative Health Activities
- Annual influenza vaccination
- Regular exercise
- Smoking cessation
- Use of sunscreen

with long-term medications is an ongoing problem that results in serious health risks.[26] The total cost of nonadherence is estimated to be $100 billion annually for the health care system in the United States.[64] Results of a systematic review by Cramer et al. found that adherence and persistence with cardiovascular and glucose-lowering medications are poor.[16] In this review, only 59% of patients took medication for greater than 80% of the expected therapy days.[16]

Dietary Modification

Another common exemplar of adherence behavior is following a diet—either for weight loss or as a specific treatment measure for a medical condition. In the context of chronic illness such as chronic kidney disease, patients face a long-term commitment to dietary restrictions (e.g., fluid, sodium, and protein) and challenges with ongoing exercise. Nonadherence rates are estimated between 50% and 80% for chronic disease management and lifestyle changes.[26]

Exercise

Exercise is the cornerstone of health-promotion behavior and is a common treatment measure for chronic conditions. If patients do not perceive any benefit to the exercise, or if they do not like the activity, sustaining and maintaining the motivation for the change becomes very difficult. Health care professionals, such as nurses, can influence adherence behavior through motivational interviewing, supporting patients' knowledge development, and using negotiation for realistic and mutually agreed upon goal setting.[65,66]

CASE STUDY

Source: diego cervo/iStock/Thinkstock

Case Presentation

Martin Herrera is a 65-year-old male admitted to the cardiology unit for a non-ST-elevated myocardial infarction (non-STEMI). Mr. Herrera is now 3 days post stent insertion and is preparing for discharge the next day. Prior medical history for Mr. Herrera includes known coronary artery disease, anterior wall MI 2 years ago, hyperlipidemia, hypertension, and metabolic syndrome. In addition, Mr. Herrera continues to smoke, although he has reduced his smoking to 20 cigarettes per day. In preparing Mr. Herrera for discharge, the nurse reviews his discharge medications, medication-taking behavior before admission, and specific cardiovascular disease (CVD) risk reduction strategies (e.g., weight control, exercise, and smoking cessation). Mr. Herrera admitted to not taking his medications on a regular basis, often missing them 2 or 3 days a week. The most common reason given by Mr. Herrera was forgetfulness and "it won't make a difference anyways."

To begin the assessment of adherence, it is first important to clarify with the patient (1) his beliefs and perceptions about his health risk status, (2) his existing knowledge about CVD risk reduction, (3) any prior experience with health care professionals, and (4) his degree of confidence in controlling the disease. Clarification of these areas reveals the following: (1) Mr. Herrera believes that because he has a very strong family history of CVD, noting his father died at age 66 years and his brother at age 60 years, nothing he does will change the final outcome; (2) Mr. Herrera states that he saw a video while in the hospital and was given a bunch of pamphlets, but he does not really remember any specifics; in addition, he has never participated in a smoking cessation program; (3) he is seen by a cardiologist every 12 months, but he did not attend his last appointment because he was told if he did not quit smoking the cardiologist was transferring him for follow-up by his family physician; and (4) Mr. Herrera states that he tried to quit smoking but was only able to reduce to 10 cigarettes a day and believes he is unlikely to smoke any less.

Case Analysis

This case study illustrates the concept of adherence in the context of a nursing assessment for CVD risk reduction. According to the TPB model, Mr. Herrera's attitude, beliefs, and perceptions influence his intention or motivation to adhere to his recommended medications and treatment plan. The comments made by Mr. Herrera suggest a negative attitude toward his ability to control the disease outcomes or benefits of recommended treatments and a lack of confidence with lifestyle changes (e.g., smoking cessation). The nurse can focus on these particular assumptions and work with Mr. Herrera to help him develop a better understanding of his disease severity and progression as well as the benefits of recommended treatments. To improve Mr. Herrera's motivation and adherence to treatment, it will be important to help him develop reminder strategies that fit into his lifestyle and support long-term adherence (e.g., persistence and agreement) and to address Mr. Herrera's misperceptions of the benefits of medications and lifestyle change to control CVD progression (e.g., decisional conflict and knowledge alignment).

ACCESS EXEMPLAR LINKS IN YOUR GIDDENS EBOOK

REFERENCES

1. Akerblad A, Bengtsson F, Ekselius L, et al: Effects of an educational compliance enhancement programme and therapeutic drug monitoring on treatment adherence in depressed patients managed by general practitioners. *Int Clin Psychopharmacol* 18(6):347–354, 2004.
2. Bissonnette J: A concept analysis: Adherence. *J Adv Nurs* 63(6):634–643, 2008.
3. Buchmann W: Adherence: A matter of self-efficacy and power. *J Adv Nurs* 26:132–137, 1997.
4. Carpenter R: Perceived threat in compliance and adherence research. *Nurs Inquiry* 12(3):192–199, 2005.
5. Dunbar-Jacob J, Mortimer-Stephens MK: Treatment adherence in chronic disease. *J Clin Epidemiol* 54:S57–S60, 2001.
6. De Geest S, Dobbels R, Fluri C, et al: Adherence to the therapeutic regimen in heart, lung and heart–lung transplant recipients. *J Cardiovasc Nurs* 20(55):S85–S95, 2005.
7. Evangelista LS: Compliance: A concept analysis. *Nurs Forum* 34(1):5–11, 1999.
8. Gray R, Wykes T, Cournay K: From compliance to concordance: A review of the literature on interventions to enhance compliance with antipsychotic medication. *J Psychiatr Ment Health Nurs* 9:277–284, 2002.
9. Murphy N, Canales M: A critical analysis of compliance. *Nurs Inquiry* 8(3):173–181, 2001.
10. Russell S, Daly J, Hughes E, et al: Nurses and "difficult" patients: Negotiating non-compliance. *J Adv Nurs* 43(3):281–287, 2003.
11. Lehane E, McCarthy G: Medication non-adherence—Exploring the conceptual mire. *Int J Nurs Pract* 15:25–31, 2009.
12. Johnson M, Bulechek G, McCloskey-Dochterman J, et al: *Nursing diagnoses, outcomes, & interventions: NANDA, NOC, and NIC linkages*, St Louis, 2001, Mosby.
13. Haynes RB, Yoa X, Degani A, et al: Interventions to enhance medication adherence [review]. *Cochrane Database Systemat Rev* (issue 4), 2005.
14. Christensen AJ: *Patient adherence to medical treatment regimens: Bridging the gap between behavioral science and biomedicine*, New Haven, CT, 2004, Yale University Press.
15. Cohen SM: Concept analysis of adherence in the context of cardiovascular risk reduction. *Nurs Forum* 44(1):25–36, 2009.
16. Cramer JA, Benedict A, Muszbek N, et al: The significance of compliance and persistence in the treatment of diabetes, hypertension and dyslipidaemia: A review. *Int J Clin Pract* 62:76–87, 2008.
17. Donovan JL, Blake DR: Patient non-compliance, deviance or reasoned decision making? *Soc Sci Med* 34:507–513, 1992.
18. Kontz M: Compliance redefined and implications for home care. *Holistic Nurs Pract* 3:54–56, 1989.
19. Kyngäs H, Duffy M, Kroll T: Concept analysis of compliance. *J Clin Nurs* 9:5–12, 2000.
20. Playle JF, Keeley P: Non-compliance and professional power. *J Adv Nurs* 27:304–311, 1998.
21. Dracup A, Meleis AJ: Compliance: An interactional approach. *Nurs Res* 31:31–36, 1982.
22. Sackett DL, Haynes RB: *Compliance with therapeutic regimens*, Baltimore, MD, 1976, Johns Hopkins University Press.
23. Sackett DL, Haynes RB, Gibson ES, et al: Randomized clinical trial of strategies for improving medication compliance in primary hypertension. *Lancet* 1:1205–1207, 1975.
24. Bissell P, May C, Noyce P: From compliance to concordance: Barriers to accomplishing a re-framed model of health care interactions. *Soc Sci Med* 58:851–862, 2004.
25. Farmer K: Methods for measuring and monitoring mediations regimen adherence in clinical trials and clinical practice. *Clin Ther* 21(6):1074–1090, 1999.
26. Sabaté E: *Adherence to long-term therapies: Evidence for action*, Geneva, 2003, World Health Organization.
27. Simpson S, Eurich D, Majumdar S, et al: A meta-analysis of the association between adherence to drug therapy and mortality. *BMJ* 2006. doi: 10.1136/bmj.38875.675486.55.
28. Stevenson F, Cox K, Britten N, et al: A systematic review of the research on communication between patients and health care professionals about medicines: The consequences for concordance. *Health Expect* 7:235–245, 2004.
29. Vermeire E, Hearnshaw H, Van Royen P, et al: Patient adherence to treatment: Three decades of research—A comprehensive review. *J Clin Pharm Ther* 26:331–342, 2001.
30. Crow J: Intentional non-adherence. *Pract Nurse* 26(6):12–17, 2003.
31. Lehane E, McCarthy G: Intentional and unintentional medication non-adherence: A comprehensive framework for clinical research and practice? A discussion paper. *Int J Nurs Stud* 44:1468–1477, 2007.
32. Wilson HS, Hutchinson SA, Holzemer WL: Reconciling incompatibilities: A grounded theory of HIV medication adherence and symptom management. *Qual Health Res* 12(10):1309–1322, 2002.
33. Hui C, Chen E, Kan C, et al: Anti-psychotics adherence among out-patients with schizophrenia in Hong Kong. *Keio J Med* 55(1):9–14, 2006.
34. Hui C, Chen E, Kan C, et al: Detection of non-adherent behaviour in early psychosis. *Austral N Z J Psychiatr* 40(5):446–451, 2006.
35. Rodgers BL: Concept analysis: An evolutionary view. In Rogers BL, Knafl KA, editors: *Concept development in nursing: Foundations, techniques and applications*, ed 2, Philadelphia, 2000, Saunders, pp 77–102.
36. Vrijens B, De Geest S, Hughes DA, et al: A new taxonomy for describing and defining adherence to medications. *Br J Clin Pharmacol* 73:691–705, 2012.
37. American Psychological Association: motivation (n.d.), *Online etymology dictionary*. Retrieved from <http://dictionary.reference.com/browse/motivation>.
38. Ryan RM, Deci EL: Intrinsic and extrinsic motivations: Classic definitions and new directions. *Contemp Educ Psychol* 25:54–67, 2000.
39. Kamali M, Kelly B, Clarke M, et al: A prospective evaluation of adherence to medication in first episode schizophrenia. *Eur Psychiatr J Assoc Eur Psychiatr* 21(1):29–33, 2006.
40. Pratt S, Mueser K, Driscoll M, et al: Medication nonadherence in older people with serious mental illness: Prevalence and correlates. *Psychiatr Rehabil J* 29(4):299–310, 2006.
41. Dunbar-Jacob J: Models for changing patient behavior. *Am J Nurs* 107(6):20–25, 2007.
42. Ajzen I, Fishbein M: *Understanding attitudes and predicting social behavior*, Englewood Cliffs, NJ, 1980, Prentice-Hall.
43. Ajzen I: The theory of planned behavior. *Organiz Behav Hum Decision Processes* 50:179–211, 1991.
44. Rosenstock IM: Historical origins of the health belief model. In Becker MH, editor: *The health belief model and personal health behavior*, Thorofare, NJ, 1974, Charles B. Slack, pp 1–8.
45. Bandura A: Social cognitive theory: An agentic perspective. *Annu Rev Psychol* 52:1–26, 2001. Breen J: Transitions in the concept of chronic pain. *Adv Nurs Sci* 24(4):48–59, 2002.
46. Raynor DK, Nicolson M, Nunney J, et al: The development and evaluation of an extended adherence support programme by community pharmacists for elderly patients at home. *Int J Pharm Pract* 8(3):157–164, 2000.
47. Chisholm MA: Enhancing transplant patients' adherence to medication therapy. *Clin Transplant* 16(1):30–38, 2000.
48. Cramer JA, Burrell A, Fairchild CJ, et al: Medication compliance and persistence: Terminology and definitions. *Value Health* 11(1):44–47, 2008.
49. Fraser S: Concordance, compliance, preference or adherence. *Patient Pref Adher* 4:95–96, 2010.
50. Lutfey K, Wishner W: Beyond "compliance" is "adherence": Improving the prospect of diabetes care. *Diabetes Care* 22:635–639, 1999.
51. Marston MV: Compliance with medical regimens: A review of the literature. *Nurs Res* 19(4):312–333, 1970.

52. Kim HS, McGuire D, Tulman L, et al: Symptom clusters: Concept analysis and clinical implications for cancer nursing. *Cancer Nurs* 28(4):270–282, 2005.

53. Almost J: Conflict within nursing work environments: Concept analysis. *J Adv Nurs* 53(4):444–453, 2006.

54. Holden L: Complex adaptive systems: Concept analysis. *J Adv Nurs* 52(6):651–657, 2005.

55. Rodgers BL: Concepts, analysis and the development of nursing knowledge: The evolutionary cycle. *J Adv Nurs* 14(4):330–335, 1989.

56. Kim HS: Structuring the nursing knowledge system: A typology of four domains. *Schol Inquiry Nurs Pract* 1(2):99–110, 1987.

57. Bakker RH, Kasterman MC, Dassen TW: Non-compliance and ineffective management of therapeutic regimen: Use in practice and theoretical implications. In Rant MJ, LeMone P, editors: *Classification of nursing diagnoses: Proceedings of the twelfth conference/North American Nursing Diagnoses Associations*, Glendale, CA, 1997, CINHAL Information Systems, pp 196–201.

58. Kane JM, Kishimoto T, Correll CU: Non-adherence to medication in patients with psychotic disorders: Epidemiology, contributing factors and management strategies. *World Psychiatry* 12(3):216–226, 2013.

59. Sajatovic M, Valenstein M, Blow FC, et al: Treatment adherence with antipsychotic medications in bipolar disorder. *Bipolar Disord* 8(3):232–241, 2006.

60. Nose M, Barbui C, Tansella M: How often do patients with psychosis fail to adhere to treatment programmes? A systematic review. *Psychol Med* 33(7):1149–1160, 2003.

61. Akerblad A, Bengtsson F, Von Knorring L, et al: Response, remission and relapse in relation to adherence in primary care treatment of depression: A 2-year outcome study. *Int Clin Psychopharmacol* 21(2):117–124, 2006.

62. Pope M, Scott J: Do clinicians understand why individuals stop taking lithium? *J Affective Disord* 74(3):287–291, 2003.

63. Trostle JA: Medical compliance as an ideology. *Soc Sci Med* 27:1299–1308, 1988.

64. Jones G: Prescribing and taking medicines: Concordance is a fine theory but is mostly not being practiced. *Br Med J* 327:819, 2003.

65. Salamon KS, Brouwer AM, Fox MM, et al: Experiencing type 2 diabetes mellitus: Qualitative analysis of adolescents' concept of illness, adjustment and motivation to engage in self-care behaviors. *Diabetes Educ* 38:543–551, 2012.

66. Copeland L, McNamara R, Kelson M, et al: Mechanisms of change within motivational interviewing in relation to health behaviors outcomes: A systematic review. *Patient Educ Couns* 98:401–411, 2015.

Self-Management

Leigh Ann Simmons and Devon Noonan

Improvements in public health and medical care during the past century have increased the population's life expectancy, and now a larger proportion of individuals live with one or more chronic diseases. As a consequence, the current major focus of health care services is the ongoing prevention and treatment of chronic diseases that have no cure as opposed to primarily treating acute disease.[1] In fact, data show that by 2020, approximately 80% of all health care expenditures will be for the prevention and treatment of chronic disease.[2] This shift toward chronic disease care has required health care systems to revamp their approaches to medical treatment. The paternalistic approach, which views the provider as "expert" and the patient as "passive recipient" of medical advice, works well for acute illness but is largely ineffective at treating chronic diseases that require daily management by patients and their caregivers.[2] Rather, evidence suggests that patient-centered approaches, which emphasize patient–provider partnerships in which patients are active participants in their care, are most effective for addressing chronic disease.[2,3]

Self-management is the primary means by which patients and their caregivers play active roles in their health and medical care. Chronic diseases have significant consequences for patients, including persistent symptoms, daily medication use, changes in health behaviors (e.g., exercise and diet), effects on social and work circumstances, and emotional distress.[1] Patients with chronic disease must continuously and over time engage in health care practices and make decisions about health behaviors that influence the course and progression of their disease.[1] These self-management practices reduce risk for complications and comorbid illness and improve long-term prognosis and quality of life.[4] Thus, self-management is an essential component of chronic disease care, and providers must teach patients to develop their self-management skills.[1] However, self-management is not limited to controlling chronic disease. Health maintenance also requires individuals to engage in daily health-promoting behaviors that support long-term well-being and reduce chronic disease risk and onset. This chapter describes the concept of self-management within nursing practice.

DEFINITION

There are a number of definitions for self-management in the literature. Clark and colleagues defined self-management as "the day-to-day tasks an individual must undertake to control or reduce the impact of disease on physical health status."[5,p5] Barlow et al. defined self-management as "the individual's ability to manage the symptoms, treatment, physical and psychosocial consequences, and lifestyle changes inherent in living with a chronic condition."[3,p178] For pediatric patients, Modi et al. defined self-management as "the interaction of health behaviors and related processes that patients and families engage in to care for a chronic condition."[6,p475] Although the definitions of self-management vary slightly, there are some core expectations and skills consistent across these definitions.[7] First, patients and their caregivers must have sufficient knowledge of the chronic condition and its treatment. Second, they must monitor the condition and respond to information about the current disease state with appropriate cognitive or behavioral responses (e.g., a patient with diabetes may need to adjust the timing of insulin based on home blood sugar monitoring). Third, they must be able to accurately convey important information about their condition and its management to health care providers so that providers can impart the information necessary for patients to develop an effective self-management plan.[1] However, as noted previously, self-management of key health behaviors (e.g., diet, physical activity, sleep, and stress) is also critical for maintaining good health. Given the previously mentioned definitions in concert with the skills necessary to manage both health and chronic disease, the following definition is proposed for purposes of this concept presentation:

> *Self-management is the ability of individuals and/or their caregivers to engage in the daily tasks required to maintain health and well-being or to manage the physical, psychological, behavioral, and emotional sequelae of a chronic disease based on their knowledge of the condition, its consequences, and the plan of care co-developed with their health care team.*

SCOPE

From a very broad perspective, the scope of self-management as a concept ranges from optimal self-management to a complete absence of self-management. The level or degree of self-care varies from person to person and in different situations. Thus, self-management is not a continuous state but, rather, can be conceptualized on a continuum that can change and is influenced by a number of variables (Figure 7-1).

Self-management exists within a broad system of collaborative care that includes a partnership among patients, their caregivers, their

FIGURE 7-1 Scope of Self-Management

health care providers, and the health care system.[8,9] Within this system, each member has an essential role in the partnership.[1] Patients and their families become the principal caregivers responsible for day-to-day management and accurate reporting of how their health or chronic condition is progressing. Providers become teachers and advisors who are responsible for helping patients and their caregivers to understand health-promoting behaviors. In the case of chronic disease, providers also must help patients and caregivers to understand the condition, acquire necessary management skills, and develop an effective management plan. The health care system becomes the care coordinator that organizes and finances the collection of services available to patients for health enhancement and chronic disease prevention and management to ensure continuity.[10] Optimal self-management is the by-product of the effective partnership among these members such that health is maximized and the negative consequences of chronic disease, including greater symptomatology, poor disease-related outcomes, reduced quality of life, morbidity, mortality, and excessive health care expenditures, are limited.[4]

The scope of self-management also can be characterized in terms of approaches to enhancing the knowledge and skills of patients and their caregivers. Self-management education can be provided one-to-one, in groups, or a combination of both. Information may be relayed in person, telephonically, or using self-instruction via mailers, manuals, books, audio- or videotapes, web-based applications, and mobile applications.[3,4] The content of self-management education may include information on guidelines for optimal health-promoting behaviors, the causes and consequences of common chronic diseases, medication management, symptom management, lifestyle behaviors, managing psychosocial effects, social support, and communicating with providers.[3] A variety of entities and individuals may disseminate self-management information and education.[3,4] These include, but are not limited to, voluntary health care agencies (e.g., the American Heart Association and the American Diabetes Association), state and federal public health systems (e.g., local public health departments and the Centers for Disease Control and Prevention), educational and community-based settings (e.g., schools, worksites, and the YMCA), inpatient institutions (e.g., hospitals and long-term care facilities), ambulatory clinics (e.g., primary and specialty clinics and also ambulatory surgical centers), diverse health care providers (e.g., nurses, pharmacists, and physicians), and peers (e.g., others with the same diagnosis who have successfully managed their disease). Most self-management education programs are run separately from clinical patient care but in collaboration with health care professionals.[11]

Finally, self-management is essential across the lifespan.[4,11] During the infant, toddler, and school-age years, parents or other caregivers take primary responsibility for self-management skills on behalf of their children. During adolescence, parents and children often share responsibility for these tasks until early adulthood, when now-grown children assume full responsibility from their parents for managing their health or condition. As adults, individuals continue to self-manage their health or chronic condition unless they develop significant disability (e.g., age-associated cognitive decline and accident) that

prevents them from handling some or all of the required tasks. In this case, partners, children, or other caregivers assist with or assume management as needed. The provider's role in assisting patients with self-management depends on the life stage and requires the provider to facilitate patients and caregivers to effectively transition roles and responsibilities in self-management strategies.

ATTRIBUTES AND CRITERIA

Five key attributes characterize self-management: self-efficacy, patient engagement, health education, patient–provider partnership, and disease management.

Self-Efficacy

Self-efficacy is having the confidence in one's knowledge and abilities to reach a desired outcome.[12] Patients increase self-efficacy through (1) educational experiences that improve knowledge about their health or their chronic condition and its management, (2) ongoing successful performance of the daily tasks required to enhance health or manage their disease and minimize symptoms, (3) engaging in shared decision making and collaborative problem solving with providers and caregivers about their health or disease, and (4) linkages to individual and community-based support services.[4]

Patient Engagement

Patient engagement is linked to self-efficacy and refers to having the knowledge, skills, ability, and willingness to be an active participant in one's health and health care.[13,14] Patients with greater self-efficacy are more likely to be engaged in the process of their care and to develop the necessary partnerships with their health care team that enable them to optimize their health or manage their chronic disease.

Health Education

Health education refers to any combination of learning experiences designed to help patients and their caregivers improve health (or a chronic condition) by enhancing their knowledge, skills, and confidence or influencing their attitudes.[15] As a central feature of chronic disease care, patients frequently need to be taught about the condition itself, as well as how to manage it. This self-management education complements traditional patient education, and it includes core features such as problem-solving skills, decision making, utilizing resources, forming a strong patient–provider team relationship, taking action, and self-tailoring.[16]

Patient–Provider Relationship

The *patient–provider relationship*, in which patients take responsibility for their health (or chronic condition) and the "provider," which represents members of the health care team as well as the health system in which care is being provided, serves as the vehicle through which optimal self-management occurs. A strong patient–provider relationship is essential to patient-centered care in which patients' needs, concerns, problems, and values remain at the center of care, and self-management approaches are responsive to patients' unique needs and preferences.[10,16]

Disease Management

Disease management is a system of coordinated health care interventions and communications for patients with chronic conditions that require significant self-management efforts.[17] The primary goal of disease management programs is to improve population health and reduce health care costs by mitigating the future complications of chronic conditions through effective self-care.

THEORETICAL LINKS

Two key theories within the field of psychology underpin self-management and its attributes: social cognitive theory and cognitive–behavioral theory.

Social Cognitive Theory

Social cognitive theory is based on the idea that individuals' expectations influence their behaviors.[18,19] Thus, individuals with high self-efficacy, or those who believe they can organize and execute a course of action necessary to produce a desired outcome, are more likely to view difficult tasks as things to be mastered versus avoided. Individuals in good health remain confident they can maintain their health by practicing positive health behaviors. Among individuals with chronic disease, those with greater self-efficacy—or those who believe they can perform well—will be more likely to successfully manage their condition. Self-management education that helps patients increase self-efficacy by improving their knowledge of the disease and the tasks essential to managing the disease and its symptoms frequently results in better health behaviors and outcomes.

Cognitive–Behavioral Theory

Cognitive–behavioral theory is similar to social cognitive theory in that the theoretical foundation is the notion that thoughts affect behavior. Thus, helping people to change the way they think about (1) their health or illness and (2) themselves in relation to their health or illness is necessary to help them self-manage effectively (Figure 7-2).[20,21] Several features of cognitive–behavioral theory are evident in self-management education and practices. Specifically, cognitive–behavioral theory assumes an active, involved patient who is responsible for engaging in specific actions as part of a plan the patient develops with his or her provider that is responsive to the patient's individual needs and preferences.

CONTEXT TO NURSING AND HEALTH CARE

Nurses help patients and their caregivers with self-management throughout the lifespan in diverse clinical and community-based settings and across the continuum of care from health enhancement/wellness to chronic disease prevention, management of ongoing disease, and recovery from an acute event. The following sections describe the role of self-management in nursing care for each of these areas.

Health Enhancement and Wellness

Across the lifespan, nurses help patients and their caregivers engage in positive behaviors that optimize health and promote well-being. A critical component of patient self-management for health enhancement and wellness is that patients must schedule and attend wellness visits and screening appointments determined necessary. They also must engage in the lifestyle behaviors that promote good health, including maintaining a normal body mass index (BMI), eating a

FIGURE 7-2 Cognitive Behavior Theory (Source: Redrawn from Stangor C: Introduction to psychology, v. 1.0, Washington, DC, 2015, Flat World Education. Retrieved from http://catalog.flatworldknowledge.com/bookhub/127?e=stangor-ch13_s01.)

healthy diet, getting regular physical activity, getting sufficient sleep, managing stress, and reducing unintentional injuries through safety measures such as wearing a seat belt or helmet and using age-appropriate car seats for children. Nurses may impart some of this information to patients during one-to-one clinical visits; however, community-based and public health initiatives also serve as a source of information on how individuals can self-manage their daily decisions to maximize health.

Predisease/Disease Prevention

Predisease is a state in which individuals do not meet full diagnostic criteria for a diagnosis, but they have one or more clinical markers that indicate they are not completely healthy either.[22] Some common predisease states include prediabetes, prehypertension, and precancerous lesions, and these are most often diagnosed as a result of age-, sex-, and risk-based screening. For many predisease states, there are some important self-management tasks for patients to begin, such as changes in diet or physical activity, quitting smoking, using sunscreen, or even starting a low-dose medication. Nurses play an important role in helping patients to understand both the predisease state and the ultimate disease, including family, lifestyle, and environmental factors that contribute to the disease, their risk of developing the disease based on their current health status and risks, and the potential benefit of making changes to reduce the risk of developing full disease. A core component of this education is assessing patients' capacity for making changes. That is, nurses need to understand the social and environmental contexts in which patients are trying to self-manage in order to partner with them to help them decide how to approach the necessary changes. For example, if a patient needs to exercise but lives in an unsafe neighborhood, the nurse and patient will need to work collaboratively to identify a safe means for exercising, such as walking in place at home while watching television.

Disease/New Diagnosis

When patients receive a new disease diagnosis, frequently they must make significant lifestyle changes. Helping patients to self-manage new disease requires nurses to provide education in both the disease and its management. Education about the causes and consequences of the disease helps patients to understand the importance of self-management in general and the specific self-management tasks in which they will need to engage. Much of the chronic disease education nurses provide occurs individually or in groups in ambulatory clinical settings and community-based settings. However, broader public health initiatives from voluntary health care entities, such as the American Heart Association or the American Diabetes Association, also serve as a source of important information for individuals with chronic disease, and nurses can leverage these sources when working with patients and their caregivers. As with predisease states, considering patients with chronic disease holistically and understanding their capacity for making changes is critical to successful management over time.

Acute Event Management

An acute event, such as a stroke, myocardial infarction (MI), asthma exacerbation, or hip fracture, is frequently a life-changing occurrence, especially for individuals who were unaware of or did not understand their risk for the event. Self-management after an event is critical to the patient making a full recovery, including achieving the most optimal health possible given his or her disease state and preventing recurrence of the event, comorbidity, or even mortality. As with a new diagnosis, recovery from an acute event requires the patient to self-manage new medications; changes in lifestyle behaviors; and greater health care utilization due to increased monitoring, specialty care, and ancillary health services (e.g., dietician and exercise physiologist). If the patient was already managing a chronic disease, these changes may not be as significant as they might be for a patient who was unaware of his or her risk for the event. Thus, nursing interventions will involve tailoring self-management education to the patients' pre-event state. For example, a patient with diagnosed coronary artery disease (CAD) who was already taking lipid-lowering drugs and daily low-dose aspirin and has an MI will need different self-management education than a patient who did not have diagnosed CAD prior to the MI.

INTERRELATED CONCEPTS

A number of concepts within nursing care are interrelated with self-management and are presented in Figure 7-3. Adherence to treatment recommendations and self-management tasks is necessary in order to sustain optimal management as evidenced by few or no symptoms and limited interferences with quality of life or activities of daily living. As previously discussed, Patient Education is a central feature of self-management. Health care professionals must provide patients with education that helps them to understand the causes and consequences of their disease and the strategies for managing their condition long term. Self-management education does not replace general health education but, rather, complements it with a specific focus on building capacity for ongoing self-care practices that promote optimal health for the individual. Health Promotion is related to self-management in that the focus of health promotion is on helping individuals and communities to take control over and ultimately improve their health.[9] Whereas some health-promotion efforts focus primarily on individuals and how they might manage their behaviors and choices, many approaches move beyond the individual to address a broad range of community, social, and environmental determinants of health that also require management at various levels.[9] Collaboration between patients and providers also was identified previously in the chapter as a central feature of self-management. Optimal self-management of chronic conditions depends on patients and providers working together to identify priorities, goals, and specific plans of action to achieve those goals.[4] Care Coordination is also essential for patients with chronic disease to self-manage effectively. Frequently, patients need additional information about their disease from specialists and/or more knowledge and skills regarding diet, physical activity, smoking cessation, medication adherence, and other lifestyle behaviors that affect their condition. Thus, chronic disease care becomes a team-based approach wherein multiple providers work together to support patients in their ongoing self-management. These providers can range from specialty physicians and nurse practitioners to registered nurses and other allied health professionals such as nutritionists, exercise physiologists, and health behavior specialists. Coordination among these providers regarding services and recommendations is essential for patients to effectively self-manage their conditions without becoming overwhelmed by the amount of information they receive. Finally, Health Disparities populations have been shown to have higher rates of chronic disease and poorer self-management practices, leading to worse health outcomes.[23] Self-management education for these patients must consider how a lack of resources or education may be exacerbating poor self-management, and strategies should be tailored to specific needs of these populations.

FIGURE 7-3 Self-Management and Interrelated Concepts

CLINICAL EXEMPLARS

Self-management cuts across all areas of health care and populations served—from wellness and health promotion to chronic disease management. For this reason, there are far more exemplars of self-management than could possibly be presented in this text. Box 7-1 presents a list of the most common exemplars by age group and context that represent the concept. Next, six of these exemplars are featured with a short description.

Featured Exemplars
Prenatal Care
Regular prenatal care helps to inform women about the steps they can take to ensure a healthy pregnancy. These include consuming a safe and healthy diet, taking a prenatal vitamin with minimum daily folic acid requirements, getting regular exercise, avoiding exposure to harmful environmental substances, avoiding alcohol and drugs, and managing preexisting conditions. Ongoing monitoring of the mother's weight, blood pressure, and urine along with results from evidence-

based screenings serve as the basis for recommended changes in self-management practices to reduce risk for maternal and infant complications.[24] Women who develop complications of pregnancy, such as gestational diabetes, gestational hypertension, or preeclampsia, will need to receive education about their condition and learn how to manage it through changes in diet, physical activity levels, stress, and medication.

Pediatric Asthma
Asthma is one of the most common and costly chronic disorders in children, affecting nearly 10% of all youth younger than age 18 years and accounting for nearly $56 billion in health care expenditures.[25,26] It is also one of the leading causes of school absenteeism. If not managed properly, asthma can be life-threatening. Proper self-management includes helping patients and their parents/caregivers to adhere to daily medications, understand triggers, know how to self-monitor and assess symptoms for rescue treatment, and make changes to the environment (reduce/eliminate secondhand smoke exposure, dust mite covers on bedding, etc.).

BOX 7-1 EXEMPLARS OF SELF-MANAGEMENT

Health Enhancement/Wellness
- Pediatric well child visit
- Prenatal care
- Adult/older adult annual wellness visit

Predisease/Disease Prevention
Pediatric
- Prediabetes
- Overweight
- Prehypertension

Prenatal
- Prehypertension
- Preeclampsia
- Excess gestational weight gain early in pregnancy

Adults
- Prehypertension
- Prediabetes
- Overweight
- Precancerous lesions
- Osteopenia
- Vision impairment
- HIV infection

Disease/New Diagnosis
Pediatric
- Asthma
- Overweight/obesity
- Diabetes
- Malnutrition
- Developmental disabilities
- Behavioral/mental health

Prenatal/Maternal
- Pregnancy-induced hypertension
- Eclampsia
- Gestational diabetes
- Depression

Adult/Older Adult
- Coronary artery disease
- Type 2 diabetes
- Obesity
- Coronary obstructive pulmonary disease
- Osteoporosis
- Arthritis
- Glaucoma
- Dementia
- Depression
- AIDS

Acute Medical Events
Pediatric
- Orthopedic (sprains, ligament tears, broken bones)
- Accidental ingestion (e.g., poison substance, medication)
- Trauma
- Burns
- Sports-related head injuries (concussions)

Prenatal Care
- Premature labor
- Premature rupture of the membranes
- Trauma

Adult/Older Adult
- Congestive heart failure
- Myocardial infarction
- Stroke
- Falls (hip fracture)
- Pneumonia
- Acute renal failure
- Infection/sepsis
- Trauma
- Suicide attempt

Type 2 Diabetes

Type 2 diabetes is one of the most prevalent preventable chronic diseases among adults in the United States and worldwide. In addition, the number of children being diagnosed with type 2 diabetes is increasing with higher prevalence of pediatric overweight and obesity.[27] Self-management of weight through regular physical activity and a healthy diet is the most cost-effective means to prevent or delay onset of type 2 diabetes. Once diagnosed, self-management is equally critical to prevent complications, morbidities, and mortality. Self-management tasks include regular visits to a provider, medication adherence, and health-promoting lifestyle behaviors (e.g., physical activity and balanced diet).

HIV/AIDS

More than 1.1 million people ages 13 years or older in the United States have HIV infection, and approximately 16% of these individuals do not know they are infected. Every year, nearly 50,000 people are newly diagnosed with HIV, and another 32,000 are diagnosed with AIDS. Risk for HIV/AIDS is highest among men who have sex with men, injection drug users, blacks/African Americans, and Latinos. Regular health care visits to monitor viral load, opportunistic infections, cardiovascular health, medication adherence, and safe sex practices are among the critical self-management practices individuals with HIV/AIDS must undertake to minimize risk for morbidity and mortality.[28]

Congestive Heart Failure

Congestive heart failure (CHF) is one of the most common complications of CAD. Approximately 5 million U.S. adults live with CHF, and it is the most common diagnosis for hospital patients ages 65 years or older.[29] Sudden death is common among heart failure patients; more than half of individuals with CHF die within 5 years of diagnosis, and it contributes to nearly 275,000 deaths annually. As with most chronic conditions, patients with CHF benefit from education about their disease and self-managing diet, physical activity, weight, and medication adherence.

Depression

Depression is a common mental health disorder affecting approximately 1 in 10 U.S. adults. Individuals most affected by depression are midlife adults ages 45–64 years, women, minorities, individuals without a high school education, and individuals without health insurance. Treatment for depression includes the use of medication and psychological therapy. In addition, patients must learn to manage moods including suicidal thoughts, recognize triggers and relapse, and set goals for behavioral management of their disease.[30]

CASE STUDY

Case Presentation

Source: goce risteski/iStock/Thinkstock

Margaret is a 5-year-old female with a past medical history at age 3 years of an acute asthma exacerbation requiring five total inpatient days, two of which were in the pediatric intensive care unit. Her parents made an appointment with the nurse practitioner to get advice on how to better manage Margaret's asthma. In the past year, they have taken Margaret to the emergency department three times and to urgent care twice. She has been on oral steroids (prednisolone) four times in the past 12 months, and she uses her rescue inhaler (albuterol) at least twice weekly when she is well. In the first 4 months of the school year, Margaret has missed 12 days of kindergarten due to asthma.

The nurse practitioner (NP) evaluates Margaret. Her vital signs and BMI are within normal rage. Her parents report that Margaret receives her maintenance medications most days, missing on average 1 or 2 days per week. The NP inquires about the family's living situation and learns that Margaret lives with her biological parents and a 7-year-old Labrador retriever, which is an indoor dog. Her paternal grandmother, a smoker, also lives with the family during the winter months. The family's house is 76 years old with carpeted living and sleeping areas and a basement. The parents do not have Margaret's bedding encased with dust mite protectors. The parents deny any mold, mice, or cockroaches in the home. The parents report that Margaret occasionally wheezes during exercise, but she does not pretreat with her rescue inhaler.

The NP discusses with Margaret's parents the importance of daily medication adherence as the first line of defense. When she investigates further, she learns that the nebulizer administration sometimes gets in the way of her parents adhering to the daily schedule. The NP discusses with them increasing the daily dose and changing the administration route to the metered dose inhaler with spacer, which they already use for the rescue medications. The parents agree this would make daily adherence easier. The NP also educates the family on asthma triggers and the role of smoking. She asks the parents to discuss with the grandmother smoking outdoors when she is visiting. The parents agree they will discuss with each other how to approach the conversation. The NP educates the parents about bedding encasements for mattresses and pillows and provides a flyer with online stores to purchase them. The parents agree to purchase these encasements. Due to the parents' report of coughing with physical activity, the NP recommends pretreating Margaret with two puffs of the rescue inhaler before exercise, and the parents agree. Finally, the NP discusses the importance of keeping track of medication administration and symptoms using an application on a phone or paper-based recording tool in order to determine triggers and patterns in symptoms. The mother downloads a tool in the office to begin tracking. Based on the conversation, the parents and NP together update the asthma action plan and agree on a follow-up plan. The NP asks the family to follow-up in 3 months or sooner if Margaret needs to go to the emergency department or urgent care.

Case Analysis

Margaret has several risk factors for having subsequent acute asthma acerbations, including past hospitalizations, exposure to triggers, and inconsistent use of her maintenance medications. Important factors in the successful self-management of Margaret's asthma include helping her parents adhere to Margaret's daily medication schedule, understanding Margaret's triggers (i.e., exercise/activity), managing these triggers effectively to avoid exacerbations, and making changes to the environment (reduce/eliminate secondhand smoke exposure, dust mite covers on bedding, etc.). The NP sets realistic goals with the parents for the self-management of Margaret's asthma, including changing the administration route of her maintenance medications to the metered dose inhaler with spacer, which is easier to use and may increase the parents' self-efficacy in remaining adherent. The NP also recommends a plan to help Margaret's parents eliminate common environmental asthma triggers in their home, including secondhand smoke and dust mites. Margaret's parents demonstrate motivation by initiating self-management strategies suggested by the nurse, such as downloading a medication tracker to ensure maintenance medication compliance and agreeing on a follow-up plan with the NP for continued evaluation of Margaret's asthma self-management plan.

ACCESS EXEMPLAR LINKS IN YOUR GIDDENS EBOOK

REFERENCES

1. Holman H, Lorig K: Patient self-management: A key to effectiveness and efficiency in care of chronic disease. *Public Health Rep* 119(3):239–243, 2004.

2. Lawn S, Schoo A: Supporting self-management of chronic health conditions: Common approaches. *Patient Educ Couns* 80(2):205–211, 2010.

3. Barlow J, Wright C, Sheasby J, et al: Self-management approaches for people with chronic conditions: A review. *Patient Educ Couns* 48(2):177–187, 2002.

4. Battersby M, Von Korff M, Schaefer J, et al: Twelve evidence-based principles for implementing self-management support in primary care. *Joint Commission J Quality Patient Saf* 36(12):561–570, 2010.

5. Clark NM, Becker MH, Janz NK, et al: Self-management of chronic disease by older adults: A review and questions for research. *J Aging Health* 3(1):3–27, 1991.

6. Modi AC, Pai AL, Hommel KA, et al: Pediatric self-management: A framework for research, practice, and policy. *Pediatrics* 129(2):e473–e485, 2012.

7. Barlow J: How to use education as an intervention in osteoarthritis. *Best Pract Res Clin Rheumatol* 15(4):545–558, 2001.

8. Wagner EH, Austin BT, Von Korff M: Organizing care for patients with chronic illness. *Milbank Q* 74:511–544, 1996.

9. World Health Organization: *Innovative care for chronic conditions: Building blocks for actions: Global report*, Geneva, 2002, Author.

10. Lawn S, McMillan J, Pulvirenti M: Chronic condition self-management: Expectations of responsibility. *Patient Educ Couns* 84(2):e5–e8, 2011.

11. Warsi A, Wang PS, LaValley MP, et al: Self-management education programs in chronic disease: A systematic review and methodological critique of the literature. *Arch Intern Med* 164(15):1641–1649, 2004.

12. Bodenheimer T, Lorig K, Holman H, et al: Patient self-management of chronic disease in primary care. *JAMA* 288(19):2469, 2002.

13. Hibbard JH, Stockard J, Mahoney ER, et al: Development of the patient activation measure (PAM): Conceptualizing and measuring activation in patients and consumers. *Health Serv Res* 39(4 Pt 1):1005, 2004.

14. Hibbard JH, Mahoney ER, Stock R, et al: Do increases in patient activation result in improved self-management behaviors? *Health Serv Res* 42(4):1443–1463, 2007.

15. World Health Organization: Health education. 2014. Retrieved from: <http://www.who.int/topics/health_education/en>.

16. Lorig KR, Holman HR: Self-management education: History, definition, outcomes, and mechanisms. *Ann Behav Med* 26(1):1–7, 2003.

17. Population Health Alliance: Disease management. 2010. Retrieved from: <http://www.populationhealthalliance.org/research/phm-glossary/d.html>.

18. Bandura A: Self-efficacy: Toward a unifying theory of behavioral change. *Psychol Rev* 84(2):191, 1977.

19. Bandura A: The explanatory and predictive scope of self-efficacy theory. *J Soc Clin Psychol* 4(3):359–373, 1986.

20. Hupp SD, Reitman D, Jewell JD: Cognitive–behavioral theory. *Handbook Clin Psychol Children Adolescents* 2:263–288, 2008.

21. Schwarzer R: Social–cognitive factors in changing health-related behaviors. *Curr Directions Psychological Sci* 10(2):47–51, 2001.

22. Viera AJ: Predisease: When does it make sense? *Epidemiol Rev* 33(1):122–134, 2011.

23. National Center for Health Statistics: *Health, United States, 2007*, With chartbook on trends in the health of Americans, Hyattsville, MD, 2007, Author.

24. NICHD/NIH: What is prenatal care and why is it important? Pregnancy: Condition information. 2013. Retrieved from: <http://www.nichd.nih.gov/health/topics/pregnancy/conditioninfo/Pages/prenatal-care.aspx>.

25. American Lung Association: Asthma & children fact sheet. 2014. Retrieved from: <http://www.lung.org/lung-disease/asthma/resources/facts-and-figures/asthma-children-fact-sheet.html>.

26. Barnett SBL, Nurmagambetov TA: Costs of asthma in the United States: 2002–2007. *J Allergy Clin Immunol* 127(1):145–152, 2011.

27. Centers for Disease Control and Prevention: *National diabetes statistics report: Estimates of diabetes and its burden in the United States*, Atlanta, GA, 2014, Author.

28. Centers for Disease Control and Prevention: Monitoring selected national HIV prevention and care objectives by using HIV surveillance data—United States and 6 U.S. dependent areas—2011. *HIV Surveillance Rep* 18(5):2013.

29. Emory Healthcare: Heart failure statistics. 2014. Retrieved from: <http://www.emoryhealthcare.org/heart-failure/learn-about-heart-failure/statistics.html>.

30. Centers for Disease Control and Prevention: Depression in the United States. 2012. Retrieved from: <http://www.cdc.gov/features/dsdepression>.

Health and Illness Concepts

The provision of health care is geared toward three general goals: to promote health, to prevent disease, and to treat illness when it arises. These do not represent three separate and competing goals; rather, these goals characterize the health and illness continuum and apply to all people across the lifespan. The concepts presented in Unit 2 are related to these goals within the context of the patients who receive our care.

Health and illness concepts are complex and represent a multitude of health-related conditions. These concepts are presented similarly and include concept definition, scope of concept, risk factors, physiological processes and consequences, assessment, collaborative management, a model case, interrelated concepts, and clinical exemplars. Presented from a lifespan and health-continuum perspective, these concepts focus on the commonalities of conditions represented as opposed to specific disease conditions. For each concept, nurses should understand the concept and notice situations that place an individual at risk for less than optimal function; furthermore, nurses should know how to recognize alterations when they occur, and they should have a general understanding of interventions both to promote optimal health and to restore health if an alteration occurs.

The following six themes are used to organize 31 concepts in this unit:
- Homeostasis and Regulation
- Sexuality and Reproduction
- Protection and Movement
- Resilience
- Mood and Cognition
- Maladaptive Behavior

CONCEPT
8

Fluid and Electrolytes

Linda Felver

Fluid in the body circulates in the blood and lymph vessels, surrounds the cells, and provides the environment inside cells in which they perform their cellular chemistry. The amount, concentration, and composition of the fluid in the body influence function at all levels from the cell to the whole person. The body continuously adjusts the characteristics and location of its fluid through specific physiological processes that nurses must understand in order to assist individuals to maintain or restore their fluid and electrolyte balance and function optimally. This concept presents a conceptual analysis of fluid and electrolytes including the process of maintaining balance and the recognition and management of imbalances when they occur.

DEFINITION

The concept fluid and electrolytes refers to the *process of regulating the extracellular fluid volume, body fluid osmolality, and plasma concentrations of electrolytes*. Fluid is water plus the substances dissolved and suspended in it. Important characteristics of fluid are its volume (amount) and its degree of concentration (osmolality). Electrolytes are substances that are charged particles (ions) when they are placed in water. Examples of electrolytes are sodium ions (Na^+), potassium ions (K^+), calcium ions (Ca^{2+}), and magnesium ions (Mg^{2+}). In health care settings, people often omit the word "ion" when discussing electrolytes, referring to potassium ions as "potassium," for example. All body fluids contain electrolytes; body fluids in different locations normally contain different concentrations of electrolytes that are necessary for optimal function.

Maintaining physiological balance of body fluid and electrolytes is a dynamic interplay between three processes: intake and absorption, distribution, and output. *Intake and absorption* refers to the addition of fluid and electrolytes to the body (intake) and their movement into the blood (absorption). *Distribution* is the process of moving fluid and electrolytes between the various body fluid compartments. These fluid compartments include inside the cells (*intracellular*) and outside the cells (*extracellular*). The extracellular fluid (ECF) compartment includes fluid between the cells (*interstitial*) and fluid inside blood vessels (*vascular*).[1] *Output* is removal of fluid and electrolytes from the body, through normal or abnormal routes.

Fluid and electrolyte balance is a dynamic interplay because fluid and electrolyte output occurs continuously. Intake of fluid and electrolytes influences output to some degree, but intake can easily become less than or more than output. Fluid and electrolyte distribution can

shift rapidly when conditions change. Optimal fluid and electrolyte balance keeps the volume, osmolality, and electrolyte concentrations of fluid in the various body fluid compartments within their normal physiological ranges.

SCOPE

From the most abstract perspective, the concept of fluid and electrolytes is quite simple: One either has optimal balance or an imbalance. Fluid and electrolyte imbalances can be too little, too much, or misplaced. Conceptually, *fluid balance* has two aspects: extracellular volume and osmolality. *Electrolyte balance* requires separate consideration. Extracellular fluid volume, body fluid osmolality, and plasma electrolyte concentrations each can be visualized as a continuum with three categories: optimal balance and two types of imbalances (Figure 8-1).

NORMAL PHYSIOLOGICAL PROCESS

Understanding the physiological processes of fluid and electrolyte balance provides the foundation for understanding the consequences of imbalances or disruptions. The three physiological processes whose interplay creates fluid and electrolyte balance were defined previously: intake and absorption, distribution, and output. This discussion describes these processes in more detail. Optimal balance occurs when both of the following characteristics are present:
- Intake and absorption of fluid and electrolytes match the output of fluid and electrolytes.
- Volume, osmolality, and electrolyte concentrations of fluid in the various body fluid compartments are within their normal ranges.

To maintain optimal fluid and electrolyte balance, output must be matched by appropriate intake, and the intake must be absorbed (Figure 8-2).

Intake and Absorption

The most common route of fluid and electrolyte intake is oral. Other routes include intravenous (IV) administration and less common avenues such as insertion into the rectum, introduction through nasogastric or other tubes into the gastrointestinal (GI) tract, instillation into body cavities, and infusion into subcutaneous tissues (hypodermoclysis)[2] or bone marrow (intraosseous).[3] The amount and type of intake can be manipulated deliberately to maintain fluid and

FIGURE 8-1 Scope of Fluid and Electrolyte Balance **A,** Scope of extracellular fluid volume (ECV) balance. **B,** Scope of body fluid osmolality balance. **C,** Scope of electrolyte balance. Potassium (K^+) is used as an example.

FIGURE 8-2 Optimal Balance of Fluid and Electrolytes Optimal balance with fluid and electrolyte output balanced by intake.

electrolyte balance. Habit and thirst are strong influences on oral fluid intake.[4] The most important stimulus to thirst is increased osmolality of body fluids, although dry oral mucous membranes, angiotensin II, angiotensin III, and arterial baroreceptor stimulation during severe hypovolemia also trigger thirst.[5]

Fluid and electrolytes that enter the body by all routes except IV must be absorbed into the bloodstream. IV fluid and electrolytes do not need absorption because they enter the bloodstream directly. Absorption is especially important to consider for oral intake of the electrolytes Ca^{2+} and Mg^{2+}, which have specialized absorption mechanisms in the intestines. Ca^{2+} absorption in the duodenum, its most important absorptive site, is dependent on adequate availability of vitamin D.[1] A healthy intestinal epithelium in the terminal section of the ileum is necessary for Mg^{2+} absorption. If fluid and electrolytes are not absorbed, they remain in the GI tract and leave the body in the feces.

Distribution

After fluid and electrolytes enter the blood, they are distributed to various body compartments. Normal fluid and electrolyte distribution is necessary for optimal function. The process of filtration distributes the ECF between the two major extracellular compartments: vascular and interstitial. The process of osmosis distributes water between ECF and cells because of osmotic forces. Numerous factors distribute electrolytes between the ECF and electrolyte pools.[6]

Fluid Distribution between Vascular and Interstitial Compartments

Fluid distribution between the vascular and interstitial compartments occurs by *filtration*, the net result of simultaneous opposing forces at the capillary level. Two forces tend to move fluid out of capillaries and two other forces tend to move fluid into capillaries.[1] The forces that are stronger at any particular time determine which way the fluid moves. *Hydrostatic pressure* pushes fluid out of its compartment. Capillary blood hydrostatic pressure (a relatively strong force) pushes fluid out of the capillaries; interstitial fluid hydrostatic pressure (a relatively weak force) pushes fluid out of the interstitial compartment back into capillaries. *Colloid osmotic pressure*, caused by large protein particles in the fluid, pulls fluid into its compartment. Thus, capillary blood colloid osmotic pressure (normally a relatively strong force) pulls fluid into the capillaries; interstitial fluid colloid osmotic pressure (normally a very weak force) pulls fluid out of the capillaries into the interstitial compartment. With normal fluid distribution, the net result of these opposing forces filters some of the ECF from capillaries into the interstitial compartment at the arterial end of capillaries, bringing oxygen and nutrients to cells. At the venous end of the capillary, some interstitial fluid filters back into the capillary, carrying waste products to be excreted.

Water Distribution between ECF and Intracellular Fluid

The structure of cell membranes allows water to cross the membrane readily but Na^+ enters with difficulty. This is the reason why cell membranes are called *semipermeable*. The process of *osmosis* is movement of water across a semipermeable membrane that separates compartments with different concentrations of particles. As noted previously, the osmolality of a fluid is its degree of concentration. Technically, it is the number of particles per kilogram of water.[7] Osmosis occurs almost instantaneously when the osmolality changes on one side of the semipermeable cell membrane. This rapid equilibration keeps the ECF and intracellular fluid at the same osmolality.

Electrolyte Distribution

With the exception of Na^+, which has a high ECF concentration that reflects osmolality, electrolytes have low concentrations in the ECF compared to their concentrations in electrolyte pools.[6] The K^+ pool is inside cells, which contain almost 98% of total body potassium.[8] Bone is an important Ca^{2+} pool. Mg^{2+} pools include inside cells and bones. Physiologically inactive forms of Ca^{2+} and Mg^{2+} bound to albumin or organic anions such as citrate also can be considered electrolyte pools.

Numerous opposing factors influence distribution of electrolytes between the ECF and the electrolyte pools. For example, two hormones influence Ca^{2+} distribution: parathyroid hormone (PTH) from the parathyroid glands and calcitonin from the thyroid.[1] Calcitonin moves Ca^{2+} into bone; PTH shifts Ca^{2+} from bone into the ECF.[9] Unusual amounts of factors that shift electrolytes can alter their distribution and cause plasma electrolyte deficits or excesses, which are discussed later in this chapter.

Output

The normal excretory routes of fluid and electrolytes are renal (urine), gastrointestinal (feces), through the skin (insensible perspiration and sweat), and the lungs (water vapor). Some of these routes (urine, sweat, and, to some degree, feces) are regulated physiologically to maintain optimal balance, but the regulatory mechanisms can be overwhelmed. Other excretory routes, including insensible water exiting through skin and lungs, are mandatory, regardless of fluid balance.[7] Abnormal routes of fluid and electrolyte output include emesis, hemorrhage, drainage through tubes or fistulas, and other routes of fluid and electrolyte loss often seen in clinical situations.[6] These abnormal output routes do not have physiological regulatory mechanisms.

Renal excretion provides the largest output of fluid and electrolytes in normal circumstances. The hormone aldosterone (along with natriuretic peptides not discussed in this concept presentation) regulates renal excretion of Na^+ and water (isotonic fluid), whereas antidiuretic hormone (ADH) regulates excretion of water.[1] Aldosterone increases renal excretion of K^+ directly and probably Mg^{2+} indirectly.[8,9]

Aldosterone

The adrenal cortex secretes aldosterone in response to angiotensin II, one of the components of the renin–angiotensin system. When the ECV is low, the resulting decreased blood flow through the renal arteries increases release of renin, formation of angiotensin I, and then formation of angiotensin II, thus increasing secretion of aldosterone. Aldosterone acts on the kidneys to remove Na^+ and water from the renal tubules and return them to the blood, which restores or even expands the ECV.[1] The liver cells normally metabolize aldosterone, which stops its action. Decreased renin release or damage to the adrenal cortex will decrease aldosterone secretion, thus increasing renal Na^+ and water excretion. Aldosterone is the major hormonal regulator of ECV.[1] Conditions involving excessive or insufficient secretion of aldosterone cause ECV imbalances.

Aldosterone also facilitates renal excretion of K^+. Increased concentration of plasma K^+ stimulates aldosterone secretion, which causes the kidneys to excrete more K^+ and helps return plasma K^+ concentration to normal. If plasma K^+ concentration decreases, aldosterone secretion is suppressed and the kidneys excrete less potassium. Another influence on renal excretion of K^+ is the amount of flow in the distal nephrons where K^+ is secreted into renal tubular fluid. More flow in the distal nephrons increases K^+ output in urine.[8,10] This situation is clinically important with osmotic diuresis and with use of potassium-wasting diuretics, both of which cause excessive K^+ output. Cortisol and other glucocorticoids have some aldosterone-like action on the kidneys.

Antidiuretic Hormone

ADH regulates renal excretion of water but not Na^+. Its name describes its action on the kidneys; the antidiuretic effect removes water from the renal distal tubules and collecting ducts and returns it to the blood, which dilutes the ECV and other body fluids. The posterior pituitary normally releases ADH at a level that maintains osmolality (degree of concentration) within normal limits. When body fluids become too concentrated (osmolality too high), osmosensitive cells in the hypothalamus trigger more release of ADH from the posterior pituitary. Increased renal action of ADH retains more water and dilutes body fluids back to their normal osmolality.[1,11] On the other hand, when body fluids become too dilute (osmolality too low), the osmosensitive cells in the hypothalamus suppress release of ADH from the posterior pituitary. Less ADH action on the kidneys allows more water excretion in the urine and concentrates body fluids back to their normal osmolality. The serum Na^+ concentration usually reflects the osmolality of body fluids. Conditions that cause excessive or deficient ADH release cause plasma Na^+ concentration imbalances.

Age-Related Differences
Infants and Children

Neonates and infants are not able to communicate thirst except by crying, which can affect their fluid intake if their caregivers are not vigilant. They also have a high percentage of body weight as water and more extracellular fluid than intracellular fluid. As infants grow, creating more cells, the percentage of weight as water decreases and the amount of intracellular fluid exceeds the amount of extracellular fluid. Those conditions persist throughout the rest of the age span. Because neonates and infants have a large body and lung surface area compared to their body mass, they have a higher fluid exchange ratio than any other age group. In addition, neonates and infants have immature kidneys that have little reserve capacity, reaching maturation during childhood.[12]

Older Adults

The thirst sensation is blunted in older adults.[13] Thus, the osmolality of their body fluids can rise higher before older adults become thirsty, so they may have a decreased fluid intake. Older adults also have decreased lean body mass, which decreases the percentage of their body weight that is water compared to that of young and middle-aged adults. Although older adults who do not have renal disease have functioning kidneys, they have decreased renal reserve due to a decreased number of nephrons that occurs with normal aging.

VARIATIONS AND CONTEXT

As mentioned previously, the primary problems seen are imbalance of fluids and imbalance of electrolytes (Figure 8-1). The term *imbalance* often is used to indicate disrupted fluid or electrolyte balance. Fluid imbalances can reflect imbalance of fluid volume or imbalance of fluid concentration. Any electrolyte can be out of balance, but for the purposes of this concept presentation, the two electrolytes that have greatest importance are sodium and potassium. This section explains the categories of imbalances and the common causes that lead to imbalances.

Categories of Fluid and Electrolyte Imbalances

Extracellular Fluid Volume Imbalances

As their name indicates, extracellular fluid volume (ECV) imbalances are abnormal amounts of fluid in the extracellular compartment (vascular plus interstitial). Fluid that has the same effective concentration as normal body fluid is called isotonic fluid.[11] Normal ECF is isotonic Na^+-containing fluid. The Na^+ is necessary to hold the water in the extracellular compartment.

There are two types of ECV imbalances. ECV deficit is too little Na^+-containing isotonic fluid in the extracellular compartment; ECV excess is too much Na^+-containing isotonic ECF. With ECV imbalances, the amount of isotonic fluid changes, but its concentration remains the same unless an osmolality imbalance is present at the same time.

Osmolality Imbalances

Osmolality imbalances are changes in the degree of concentration of body fluid. If osmolality changes, it equilibrates rapidly between ECF and intracellular fluid as a result of osmotic shifts of water across cell membranes. Although osmolality can be measured directly, in many clinical settings it is tracked using the serum Na^+ concentration, which usually rises or falls in parallel with osmolality.[11] Na^+ stays in the ECF when water moves into or out of cells, which is why the serum Na^+ concentration changes when the osmolality changes.

There are two types of osmolality imbalances. Hypernatremia (increased serum Na^+ concentration) indicates that body fluids are too concentrated (osmolality is too high). Hyponatremia (decreased serum Na^+ concentration) indicates that body fluids are too dilute (osmolality is too low). Osmolality imbalances can occur alone or with ECV imbalances. The combination of ECV deficit and hypernatremia is known as clinical dehydration.[6]

Electrolyte Imbalances

Electrolyte imbalances are abnormal plasma concentrations of electrolytes such as K^+, Ca^{2+}, and Mg^{2+}. Although Na^+ also is an electrolyte, its concentration reflects the osmolality, as discussed previously. Electrolyte concentrations are measured from blood samples and do not necessarily correlate with the concentrations inside cells.

There are two types of electrolyte imbalances: plasma concentration deficits and excesses. Names of electrolyte imbalances are constructed from a prefix that indicates whether the concentration is too low (*hypo-*) or too high (*hyper-*), a combining form that indicates the specific electrolyte involved (e.g., *-kal-* for K^+, *-calc-* for Ca^{2+}, and *-magnes-* for Mg^{2+}), and the suffix *-emia* that signifies "in the blood." Electrolyte imbalances can occur alone or with ECV and/or osmolality imbalances.

Causes of Fluid and Electrolyte Disturbances

Practically speaking, there are only three overarching causes leading to fluid and electrolyte imbalances. All of these imbalances involve at least one of the following conditions:

- Fluid and electrolyte output is *greater than* intake and absorption
- Fluid and electrolyte output is *less than* intake and absorption
- Altered fluid and electrolyte distribution

Output Greater Than Intake and Absorption

When fluid and electrolyte output is greater than intake and absorption, ECV deficit, increased osmolality (hypernatremia), and various plasma electrolyte deficits can occur (Figure 8-3). Two situations cause output to exceed intake and absorption (Figure 8-3A):

- Normal output but deficient intake or absorption
- Increased output not balanced by increased intake

Normal output but deficient intake or absorption. Body fluid output through the combination of urine, feces, skin, and respirations is dilute Na^+-containing fluid. Therefore, daily intake of some Na^+ and considerable water is necessary to maintain optimal fluid balance. Although the kidneys are able to reduce their fluid output to some degree in response to decreased fluid intake, some renal output is obligatory, as is water output through the skin and respiration.[7,14] When intake is less than normal output, the fluid imbalance a person develops depends on the type of fluid that is deficient. For example, people who do not drink enough water to match their water output can make their body fluids too concentrated (osmolality too high; hypernatremia). See hypernatremia in Box 8-1 for examples.

Deficient electrolyte intake and absorption with normal output can cause plasma electrolyte deficits such as hypokalemia or hypomagnesemia. Box 8-2 lists specific causes of electrolyte deficits due to normal output but decreased intake or absorption.

Increased output not balanced by increased intake. Another situation in which fluid and electrolyte output becomes greater than intake arises when output increases but intake does not increase enough to balance it. For example, diarrhea increases output of Na^+, water, and K^+. During diarrhea, an intake of Na^+, water, and K^+ that does not balance the increased output creates a high risk for ECV deficit, increased osmolality (hypernatremia), and hypokalemia.[11,14] Boxes 8-1 and 8-2 show other examples of imbalances due to increased output not balanced by increased intake. To prevent these imbalances, fluid and electrolyte intake must increase to balance increased output.

Output Less Than Intake and Absorption

When fluid and electrolyte output is less than intake and absorption, ECV excess, decreased osmolality (hyponatremia), and plasma electrolyte excesses can occur. Two situations cause intake to be greater than output (Figure 8-3B):

- Output less than excessive or too rapid intake
- Decreased output not balanced by decreased intake

Output less than excessive or too rapid intake. Individuals with normal renal function may overwhelm their output capacity by excessive or very rapid intake of fluid and electrolytes. This situation most commonly occurs with IV infusions. Any person receiving IV fluid is

ECV deficit
Osmolality too high
Plasma electrolyte deficits

ECV deficit
Osmolality too high
Plasma electrolyte deficits

A   Normal output but deficient intake or absorption

Increased output not balanced by increased intake

ECV excess
Osmolality too low
Plasma electrolyte excesses

ECV excess
Osmolality too low
Plasma electrolyte excesses

B   Output less than excessive or too rapid intake

Decreased output not balanced by decreased intake

FIGURE 8-3 Disrupted Balance of Fluid and Electrolytes **A,** Imbalance from fluid and electrolyte output greater than intake and absorption. **B,** Imbalance from fluid and electrolyte output less than intake and absorption.

at risk for developing fluid and electrolyte imbalances from excessive or too rapid infusion of the solution, even if the infusion is intended to replace a fluid or electrolyte deficit. The specific imbalance that develops depends on the type of IV solution being administered.[15] Nurses need to be especially alert when infusing IV solutions that contain K[+] because hyperkalemia caused by too rapid infusion can cause dangerous cardiac dysrhythmias.[7,14]

Excessive oral intake that overwhelms normal output mechanisms also is possible. The most common example is mild ECV excess that occurs when people eat salty foods and drink water. They may notice tight rings or shoes and overnight weight gain, which resolve in a day or two as the kidneys excrete the excess Na[+] and water. People who have conditions that cause chronic ECV excess, such as compensated heart failure, often are prescribed Na[+]-restricted diets to avoid exacerbating their ECV excess.[16,17]

When people drink a lot of water without salt, they normally produce less antidiuretic hormone and their kidneys excrete the extra water. However, massive rapid oral intake of water can overwhelm renal water excretion capacity and make body fluids too dilute (osmolality too low; hyponatremia).[18,19] See hyponatremia in Box 8-1 for examples. Oral intake of electrolyte-rich foods by people who have normal renal function usually is not a problem because the kidneys excrete any excess.

Decreased output not balanced by decreased intake. People who have oliguria from any cause have decreased output of fluid and electrolytes, and their intake must be decreased as well to prevent imbalances. For example, people who have oliguric renal disease develop ECV excess, hyperkalemia, and hypermagnesemia unless their intake is decreased appropriately.[7] See other examples in Boxes 8-1 and 8-2.

Combining excessive or too rapid intake of fluid and electrolytes with decreased output creates a potentially dangerous situation in which imbalances can develop rapidly. An IV solution that infuses in excess amounts or too rapidly into an individual who is oliguric can cause life-threatening ECV excess (Na[+]-containing fluid) or hyperkalemia (K[+]-containing fluid).[6,7,14]

Altered Fluid and Electrolyte Distribution

Alterations of distribution, the process of moving fluid and electrolytes between their various compartments, can create fluid or electrolyte imbalances (Figure 8-4):

- Shift of vascular fluid into the interstitial space causes edema.
- Rapid shift of ECF into a "third space" can create ECV deficit.
- Electrolyte shift from ECF into its electrolyte pool causes plasma electrolyte deficits.
- Electrolyte shift from its electrolyte pool into ECF causes plasma electrolyte excesses.

Shift of vascular fluid into interstitial space. As explained previously, fluid distribution between the vascular and interstitial compartments occurs by filtration, the net result of simultaneous opposing forces at the capillary level. Altered filtration can allow too much fluid to accumulate in the interstitial compartment, which is called edema. For example, ECV excess causes edema by increasing the capillary blood hydrostatic pressure. Inflammation causes edema because it involves local vasodilation (increases capillary blood hydrostatic pressure) and increased microvascular permeability (protein leakage increases the interstitial fluid colloid osmotic pressure). The edema of hypoalbuminemia is caused by decreased blood colloid osmotic pressure.

BOX 8-1 Causes of Disrupted Fluid Balance

ECV Deficit (Too Little Extracellular Volume)
Normal Output but Deficient Intake of Na⁺ and Water
- Lack of access to Na^+ and water

Increased Output Not Balanced by Increased Intake of Na⁺ and Water
- Vomiting
- Acute or chronic diarrhea from any cause, including laxative abuse
- Draining GI fistula, gastric suction, or intestinal decompression
- Hemorrhage or burns
- Overuse of diuretics
- Lack of aldosterone (adrenal insufficiency, Addison's disease)

Rapid Fluid Shift from ECV into a Third Space
- Acute intestinal obstruction
- Ascites that develops rapidly

ECV Excess (Too Much Extracellular Volume)
Output Less Than Excessive or Too Rapid Intake of Na⁺ and Water
- Excessive IV infusion of Na^+-containing isotonic solution (0.9% NaCl, Ringer's)
- High oral intake of salty foods and water with renal retention of Na^+ and water

Decreased Output Not Balanced by Decreased Intake of Na⁺ and Water
- Oliguria (e.g., acute kidney injury, acute glomerulonephritis, end-stage renal disease)

- Aldosterone excess (e.g., cirrhosis, chronic heart failure, primary hyperaldosteronism)
- High levels of glucocorticoids (e.g., corticosteroid therapy, Cushing's disease)

Hypernatremia (Body Fluids Concentrated; Osmolality Too High)
Normal Output but Deficient Intake of Water
- No access to water or inability to respond to or communicate thirst (e.g., aphasia, coma, infancy)
- Tube feeding without additional water intake

Increased Output Not Balanced by Increased Intake of Water
- Vomiting or diarrhea with replacement of Na^+ but not enough water
- Diabetes insipidus (lack of antidiuretic hormone)

Hyponatremia (Body Fluids Dilute; Osmolality Too Low)
Output Less Than Excessive or Too Rapid Intake of Water
- IV 5% dextrose in water (D_5W) infusion with excess rate or amount
- Rapid oral ingestion of massive amounts of water (e.g., child abuse, club initiation, psychiatric disorders)
- Overuse of tap water enemas or hypotonic irrigating solutions
- Massive replacement of water without Na^+ during vomiting or diarrhea

Decreased Output Not Balanced by Decreased Intake of Water
- Excessive antidiuretic hormone

Shift of vascular fluid into the interstitial space

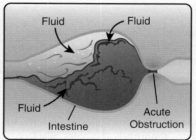

Rapid ECF shift into "third space"

Electrolyte shift from ECF into its electrolyte pool

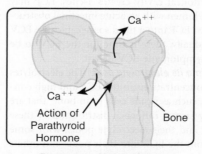

Electrolyte shift from its electrolyte pool into ECF

FIGURE 8-4 Imbalance from altered fluid and electrolyte distribution

BOX 8-2 Causes of Disrupted Electrolyte Balance

Hypokalemia (Plasma K⁺ Deficit)
Normal Output but Deficient K⁺ Intake
- Prolonged anorexia or diet lacking K⁺-rich foods
- No oral intake plus IV solutions not containing K⁺

Increased Output Not Balanced by Increased K⁺ Intake
- Vomiting
- Acute or chronic diarrhea from any cause, including laxative abuse
- Use of K⁺-wasting diuretics or other drugs that increase renal K⁺ excretion
- Excessive aldosterone effect (e.g., large amounts of black licorice, cirrhosis, chronic heart failure, primary hyperaldosteronism)
- High levels of glucocorticoids (e.g., corticosteroid therapy, Cushing's disease)

Rapid K⁺ Shift from ECF into Cells
- Alkalosis, excessive β-adrenergic stimulation, or excessive insulin

Hyperkalemia (Plasma K⁺ Excess)
Output Less Than Excessive or Too Rapid K⁺ Intake
- IV K⁺ infusion with excess rate or amount
- Massive transfusion (>8 units for adults) of stored blood

Decreased Output Not Balanced by Decreased K⁺ Intake
- Oliguria (e.g., severe hypovolemia, circulatory shock, acute kidney injury, end-stage renal disease)
- Use of K⁺-sparing diuretics, angiotensin-converting enzyme inhibitors, or other drugs that decrease renal K⁺ excretion
- Lack of aldosterone (e.g., adrenal insufficiency, Addison's disease)

Rapid K⁺ Shift from Cells into ECF
- Lack of insulin or acidosis due to mineral acids
- Massive sudden cell death (e.g., crushing injuries, tumor lysis syndrome)

Hypocalcemia (Plasma Ca²⁺ Deficit)
Normal Output but Deficient Ca²⁺ Intake or Absorption
- Diet lacking Ca²⁺-rich foods
- Poor Ca²⁺ absorption (e.g., chronic diarrhea, lack of vitamin D)

Increased Output Not Balanced by Increased Ca²⁺ Intake and Absorption
- Steatorrhea (binds Ca²⁺ in GI secretions as well as dietary Ca²⁺)

Ca²⁺ Shift from ECF into Bone or Physiologically Unavailable Form
- Hypoparathyroidism
- Large load of citrate from massive blood transfusion (binds Ca²⁺)
- Alkalosis (more Ca²⁺ binds albumin) or elevated plasma phosphate level
- Acute pancreatitis (Ca²⁺ binds necrotic fat in abdomen)

Hypercalcemia (Plasma Ca²⁺ Excess)
Output Less Than Excessive Ca²⁺ Intake and Absorption
- Vitamin D or Ca²⁺ overdose (includes shark cartilage supplements)

Decreased Output Not Balanced by Decreased Ca²⁺ Intake
- Use of thiazide diuretics

Ca²⁺ Shift from Bone into ECF
- Hyperparathyroidism
- Cancers that secrete bone-resorbing factors

Hypomagnesemia (Plasma Mg²⁺ Deficit)
Normal Output but Deficient Mg²⁺ Intake or Absorption
- Diet lacking Mg²⁺-rich foods
- Poor Mg²⁺ absorption (e.g., chronic diarrhea, ileal resection, chronic alcoholism)

Increased Output Not Balanced by Increased Mg²⁺ Intake and Absorption
- Prolonged vomiting, gastric suction, or draining GI fistula
- Steatorrhea (binds Mg²⁺ in GI secretions as well as dietary Mg²⁺)
- Use of diuretics or other drugs that increase urinary Mg²⁺

Mg²⁺ Shift into Physiologically Unavailable Form
- Large load of citrate from massive blood transfusion (binds Mg²⁺)
- Alkalosis (more Mg²⁺ binds albumin)

Hypermagnesemia (Plasma Mg²⁺ Excess)
Output Less Than Excessive Mg²⁺ Intake and Absorption
- Overuse of Mg²⁺-containing laxatives or antacids

Decreased Output Not Balanced by Decreased Mg²⁺ Intake
- Chronic oliguric renal disease

Rapid ECF shift into "third space." The term "third space" refers to a location where ECF accumulates abnormally (becomes misplaced) that is neither the vascular nor the interstitial compartment. The peritoneal cavity and the intestinal lumen are examples of third spaces. ECF accumulating in the peritoneal cavity creates ascites. ECF may shift rapidly into the intestinal lumen with an acute intestinal obstruction (Figure 8-4). Rapid shift of ECF into a third space can cause ECV deficit. If the shift occurs gradually, there is time for the ECV to be replenished without causing symptomatic ECV deficit.

Electrolyte shift from ECF into its electrolyte pool. The electrolytes K⁺, Ca²⁺, and Mg²⁺ have low concentrations in the ECF and high concentrations in other locations, such as inside cells or in bone, that are called electrolyte pools. Many factors influence distribution of these electrolytes between the ECF and their electrolyte pools, with some factors moving electrolytes from the ECF into their pools and others moving them in the opposite direction. Abnormal concentrations of these factors that shift electrolytes into their pools can cause plasma electrolyte deficits (Figure 8-4).[6] Although these distribution shifts may not change whole body electrolyte concentration, they cause signs and symptoms by changing the ratio of electrolytes inside and outside cells or the amount of physiologically active electrolyte. See hypokalemia, hypocalcemia, and hypomagnesemia in Box 8-2 for examples.

Electrolyte shift from its electrolyte pool into ECF. The factors that distribute electrolytes between the ECF and electrolyte pools can be altered in a way that shifts electrolytes from their pools into the ECF, causing plasma electrolyte excesses (Figure 8-4).[6] These distribution shifts may not change whole body electrolyte concentration but cause signs and symptoms by changing the ratio of electrolytes inside and outside cells. See hyperkalemia and hypercalcemia in Box 8-2 for examples.

CONSEQUENCES

Disruptions of fluid and electrolyte balance have different physiological consequences, depending on the type of imbalance. ECV and K⁺,

Mg^{2+}, and Ca^{2+} concentration imbalances can interfere with perfusion and oxygenation. Osmolality imbalances impair cerebral function.[11] K^+, Mg^{2+}, and Ca^{2+} concentration imbalances impair neuromuscular function.[6]

Impaired Perfusion and Oxygenation

A normal volume of ECF is necessary to provide tissue perfusion and oxygenate cells. Moderate or severe ECV deficit reduces tissue perfusion by decreasing arterial blood pressure (BP). Very severe ECV deficit leads to hypovolemic shock, a condition that severely impairs perfusion and oxygenation.[20] ECV excess also can impair oxygenation. Edema fluid from ECV excess pushes cells farther from capillaries, creating a larger distance for oxygen to diffuse before it reaches cells. This subtle change is part of the reason for delayed healing of injuries to edematous tissue. A more dramatic example of impaired oxygenation from ECV excess is pulmonary edema that arises from sudden or very severe ECV excess. Fluid in the alveoli interferes with gas exchange and thus oxygenation.

K^+, Mg^{2+}, and Ca^{2+} concentration imbalances can cause cardiac dysrhythmias, some of which can impair perfusion by reducing cardiac output.[8,9,21] Severe hyperkalemia causes cardiac arrest.

Impaired Cerebral Function

Osmolality imbalances cause shriveling (hypernatremia) or swelling (hyponatremia) of cells. Impaired cerebral function occurs with either condition.[7] The usual cerebral impairment with osmolality imbalances is decreased level of consciousness (LOC), which occurs on a continuum from drowsiness to coma. Seizures may occur if the osmolality changes very rapidly, rises very high, or falls very low.[18,22] The brain cell dysfunction caused by osmolality imbalances is reversible with well-managed return of osmolality to normal, avoiding rapid changes that can injure fragile brain structures.[23,24]

Impaired Neuromuscular Function

Plasma concentration imbalances of K^+, Ca^{2+}, and Mg^{2+} impair neuromuscular function, although they impair it in different ways. The ratio of K^+ inside to outside cells is a major determinant of resting membrane potential of muscle cells.[8] Plasma K^+ deficit and excess change the resting membrane potential of skeletal muscle by altering that ratio. Although the state of the resting potential is different in hypokalemia and hyperkalemia, the effect on skeletal muscles is similar: flaccid muscle weakness.[7,8]

Extracellular Ca^{2+} concentration is a major determinant of the speed of ion fluxes through the membranes of nerve and muscle cells. Mg^{2+} suppresses release of the neurotransmitter acetylcholine at neuromuscular junctions. Plasma concentration imbalances of Ca^{2+} and Mg^{2+} impair neuromuscular function by altering these processes. Plasma deficits of Ca^{2+} and Mg^{2+} increase neuromuscular excitability, which is why hypocalcemia and hypomagnesemia have similar signs and symptoms: muscle twitching and cramping, hyperactive reflexes, and seizures if very severe. In contrast, plasma excesses of Ca^{2+} and Mg^{2+} decrease neuromuscular excitability, causing similar manifestations of muscle weakness, depressed reflexes, and lethargy.[7,9]

RISK FACTORS

Populations at Risk

Optimal fluid and electrolyte balance is necessary for physiological function for all individuals, regardless of race, culture, age, or socioeconomic status. Populations at greatest risk for imbalance are the very young and the very old. Preterm infants are at great risk for fluid and electrolyte disturbances due to very immature kidneys and large surface area of skin and lungs; the degree of risk is related to weight and gestational age at the time of birth. Term infants and young children also are more at risk than adults due to immature kidneys, high metabolic rate, and large fluid exchange ratio.[12] Older adults have a blunted thirst sensation and decreased renal reserve due to a normal gradual loss of nephrons, which make them more susceptible to fluid and electrolyte disturbances.[13]

Individual Risk Factors

The greatest individual risk factors are associated with serious injury or significant health conditions. Because so many different disease processes and behaviors can disrupt fluid and electrolyte balance, it is more useful to think about risk factors in terms of what the disease or behavior is causing rather than focus on the disease itself. Nurses can deduce logically the individual risk factors for fluid and electrolyte imbalances by considering the dynamic interplay of the processes involved in fluid and electrolyte balance. Box 8-3 lists common situations and conditions that place an individual at risk for fluid and electrolyte imbalances.

BOX 8-3 Common Risk Factors for Fluid and Electrolyte Disturbances

Conditions
- Vomiting
- Diarrhea
- Malabsorption
- Fever
- Inadequate or excessive intake of fluid or electrolytes
- Inadequate or excessive water intake

Adverse Effects from Medications
- Diuretics
- Laxatives
- Antacids
- Corticosteroids
- Infusion of IV fluids
- Blood transfusions

Acute Medical Conditions, Injury, and Trauma
- Hemorrhage
- Burns
- Crush injuries
- Head injuries
- Acute pancreatitis
- Acute kidney injury

Chronic Medical Conditions
- Heart failure
- Diabetes mellitus
- Cancer
- Chronic oliguric kidney disease
- Chronic liver disease
- Chronic alcoholism
- Eating disorders (anorexia nervosa, bulimia)

TABLE 8-1 Clinical Manifestations of Disrupted Fluid Balance

EXTRACELLULAR VOLUME IMBALANCES		OSMOLALITY IMBALANCES	
Too Little Volume (ECV Deficit)	**Too Much Volume (ECV Excess)**	**Too Dilute (Hyponatremia)**	**Too Concentrated (Hypernatremia)**
Sudden weight loss, skin tenting, dry mucous membranes, vascular underload: rapid thready pulse, postural BP drop, lightheadedness, flat neck veins when supine, oliguria, syncope, shock if severe	Sudden weight gain, dependent edema, vascular overload: bounding pulse, distended neck veins when upright, dyspnea, pulmonary edema if severe	Impaired cerebral function: decreased LOC, nausea, seizures if severe; serum Na^+ <130 mEq/L	Impaired cerebral function: decreased LOC, thirst (not older adults), seizures if severe; serum Na^+ >145 mEq/L

BP, blood pressure; LOC, level of consciousness.

TABLE 8-2 Clinical Manifestations of Disrupted Electrolyte Balance

PLASMA K^+ IMBALANCES		PLASMA Ca^{2+} IMBALANCES		PLASMA Mg^{2+} IMBALANCES	
Hypokalemia	**Hyperkalemia**	**Hypocalcemia**	**Hypercalcemia**	**Hypomagnesemia**	**Hypermagnesemia**
Bilateral ascending flaccid muscle weakness, abdominal distention, constipation, postural hypotension, polyuria, cardiac dysrhythmias; serum K^+ <3.5 mEq/L	Bilateral ascending flaccid muscle weakness, cardiac dysrhythmias, cardiac arrest if severe; serum K^+ >5.0 mEq/L	Increased neuromuscular excitability: positive Chvostek's and Trousseau's signs, muscle cramps, twitching, hyperactive reflexes, carpal and pedal spasms, tetany, seizures, laryngospasm, cardiac dysrhythmias; serum total Ca^{2+} <9 mg/dL (4.5 mEq/L)	Decreased neuromuscular excitability: anorexia, nausea, constipation, muscle weakness, diminished reflexes, decreased LOC, cardiac dysrhythmias; serum total Ca^{2+} >11 mg/dL (5.5 mEq/L)	Increased neuromuscular excitability: positive Chvostek's and Trousseau's signs, insomnia, hyperactive reflexes, muscle cramps and twitching, nystagmus, tetany, seizures, cardiac dysrhythmias; serum Mg^{2+} <1.5 mEq/L	Decreased neuromuscular excitability: flushing, diaphoresis, diminished reflexes, hypotension, decreased LOC, muscle weakness, respiratory depression, bradycardia, cardiac dysrhythmias; serum Mg^{2+} >2.5 mEq/L

LOC, level of consciousness.

ASSESSMENT

Assessments for fluid and electrolyte imbalances often occur in the context of other conditions that cause such imbalances. Nurses can use the risk factors for these imbalances to guide their assessment.

History

Because many of the presenting signs and symptoms of fluid and electrolyte imbalances have other causes, taking a careful history is important. The standard questions for history taking are not repeated here, but they are expected. In addition to focusing on the renal, endocrine, or other conditions that may cause the fluid or electrolyte imbalance, the history must include questions regarding fluid and electrolyte intake and output. Recent vomiting or diarrhea should be explored as to frequency and quantity, as well as the type and quantity of water, Na^+, and K^+ replacement. Medication history, including dietary supplements, is an important focus because numerous medications influence fluid and electrolyte balance.[6,7,14]

Examination Findings

Clinical manifestations of fluid and electrolyte imbalances often are part of a larger clinical picture of the underlying disease process that caused the imbalance. For example, the ankle edema, bounding pulse, and distended neck veins caused by ECV excess in individuals who have left-sided heart failure will be noted as part of the wider cardiac, respiratory, and functional examination.[25] However, the quadriceps muscle weakness and constipation of hypokalemia may escape detection until the manifestations become severe, unless they are assessed specifically.

Astute clinicians incorporate assessment for the individual's most likely fluid and electrolyte imbalances into every physical assessment rather than waiting until the signs and symptoms become severe. For example, a person who has chronic diarrhea needs assessment for ECV deficit, hypernatremia, hypokalemia, hypocalcemia, and hypomagnesemia in addition to assessments related to the cause of the diarrhea and its consequences on skin integrity.[6]

Tables 8-1 and 8-2 present signs and symptoms of fluid and electrolyte imbalances. These manifestations arise from the physiological consequences described previously in this concept presentation. Interpretation of assessment findings may be complicated by the presence of acid–base imbalances (see Concept 9 Acid–Base Balance).

Diagnostic Tests

Diagnosis of ECV deficit and excess usually is made on the basis of history and clinical examination. Laboratory tests performed on blood samples provide the definitive diagnosis for osmolality and electrolyte imbalances. Normal ranges are provided in Tables 8-1 and 8-2.

CLINICAL MANAGEMENT

Primary and secondary prevention strategies as well as interventions for people who have fluid and electrolyte imbalances are useful in all clinical settings.

Primary Prevention

Primary prevention of fluid and electrolyte imbalances is based on the principle that intake must balance output to maintain optimal fluid and electrolyte balance. For example, teaching people to replace body fluid output from vomiting or diarrhea with Na^+-containing fluid can prevent ECV deficit. Similarly, teaching individuals who take potassium-wasting diuretics how to increase their dietary K^+ intake and the importance of taking prescribed K^+ supplements helps prevent hypokalemia. Teaching for people who have oliguric renal disease focuses on decreasing their intake of Na^+, K^+, and Mg^{2+} because their output is decreased.[14]

In addition to teaching people how to maintain optimal fluid and electrolyte balance, nurses engage in primary prevention in clinical settings when they see risk factors for various imbalances and intervene to modify intake or output appropriately. For example, nurses provide accessible fluids at a patient's preferred temperature as an independent nursing intervention; they request an order for an antiemetic or antidiarrheal medication as a collaborative intervention.

Secondary Prevention (Screening)

Screening to detect disrupted fluid and electrolyte balance is not performed in the general population except as part of a routine physical exam that would include assessment for physical signs of ECV excess or deficit and standard laboratory tests including measurement of serum Na^+, K^+, and Ca^{2+} levels.

Collaborative Interventions

Because fluid and electrolyte intake is easier to modify than output, interventions to restore optimal fluid and electrolyte balance often focus on intake.

Fluid and Electrolyte Support

ECV deficit, hypernatremia, and plasma electrolyte deficits are treated by fluid or electrolyte replacement and by treatment of any underlying cause. ECV deficit requires isotonic Na^+-containing fluid, hypernatremia requires water, and electrolyte deficit usually requires replacement of the deficient electrolyte.[14,26] A person who has clinical dehydration will need both isotonic Na^+-containing fluid and extra water. These fluids and electrolytes can be administered orally, by IV infusion, or through other routes, depending on patient status and the resources of the setting. Nursing responsibilities during fluid and electrolyte replacement include safely administering the replacement, measuring fluid intake and output, monitoring for complications of therapy, and teaching patients and families regarding the therapy.[27]

Treatments for ECV excess, hyponatremia, and plasma electrolyte excesses usually involve some type of restriction: Na^+ restriction for ECV excess, water restriction for hyponatremia, and decreased intake of the electrolyte that is excessive.[8,17,19] Nurses need to be sure that people know the reason for the restriction and receive culturally appropriate teaching regarding how to change their diet or fluid intake.[28] In addition to the appropriate restrictions, medications may be used to treat ECV excess, hyponatremia, and plasma electrolyte excesses.

Medication Management

In addition to the fluid and electrolyte replacements mentioned previously, people who have disrupted fluid and electrolyte balance may receive other medications. Depending on the situation, these medications are directed toward various goals: treat the underlying cause (e.g., antiemetic for imbalances due to vomiting or vasopressin for ADH deficiency), increase the output of fluid or electrolytes (e.g., diuretics for ECV excess or severe hyperkalemia), shift electrolytes into their pools to decrease plasma concentration (e.g., insulin and glucose for acute hyperkalemia or calcitonin for acute hypercalcemia),[29,30] or counteract life-threatening effects of the imbalance (e.g., calcium salts to counteract the effect of hyperkalemia on cardiac function).[29] In addition, medications that can contribute to the individual's fluid and electrolyte imbalances must be discontinued or their dosage should be modified.

Independent Nursing Interventions

Independent nursing interventions to provide safety and comfort are foundational for people who have fluid and electrolyte imbalances. For example, safety is high priority for patients with decreased level of consciousness from osmolality imbalances or substantial muscle weakness from severe hypokalemia. Comfort measures are especially important for people who need to restrict fluid or Na^+. People who have fluid restrictions frequently are uncomfortable from thirst. Interventions such as performing frequent oral hygiene, lubricating the lips, keeping fluids out of sight, providing the allowed liquids in insulated containers, and instructing people to swish fluids in their mouths before swallowing promote comfort during fluid restriction. Individuals who need to restrict Na^+ intake because of chronic ECV excess can be comforted with the knowledge that salt taste often changes after a few weeks of salt restriction so that the food that seems tasteless at first probably will have more enjoyable flavor in a few weeks.[16] Learning about herbs and spices also is useful for individuals restricting sodium.

Nurses use many different interventions to facilitate oral intake of Na^+-containing fluid for people who have mild ECV deficit or oral water intake for people with mild hypernatremia. For example, they can make fluids available frequently, provide them at the individual's preferred temperature, and assist individuals to keep their own intake records. Increased fluid intake also is important for individuals with hypercalcemia to prevent renal damage. Teaching people how to prevent fluid and electrolyte imbalances by balancing output with appropriate intake is extremely important. Box 8-4 summarizes nursing interventions for people with disrupted fluid and electrolyte balance.

INTERRELATED CONCEPTS

The concept of fluid and electrolytes has many interrelationships with other concepts discussed in this book. Fluid and electrolytes and Acid–Base Balance are closely related; changes in one can cause changes in the other, and situations such as vomiting and diarrhea can lead to both. Hormonal Regulation has a powerful influence on fluid and electrolytes because of the significant role hormones play in maintaining balance. Nutrition greatly influences fluid and electrolyte intake. Elimination creates fluid and electrolyte output; elimination alterations such as oliguria and diarrhea can disrupt fluid and electrolyte balance. Fluid and electrolyte imbalances can influence Perfusion and

---

BOX 8-4 Nursing Interventions for People with Disrupted Fluid and Electrolyte Balance

Provide safety and comfort.
Facilitate oral intake if appropriate.
Administer collaborative interventions:
    Adjustment of fluid intake or output
    Treatment of the underlying cause
Monitor for complications of therapy.
Teach how to prevent imbalances or when to seek help (if chronic imbalance).

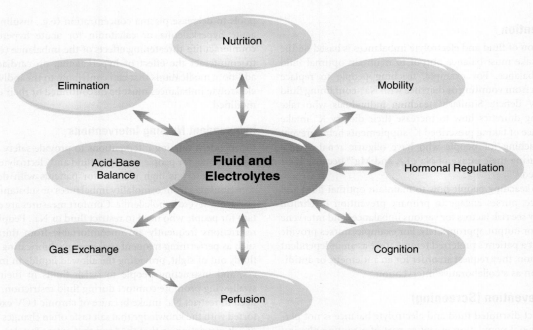

FIGURE 8-5 Fluid and Electrolytes and Interrelated Concepts

BOX 8-5   EXEMPLARS OF FLUID AND ELECTROLYTE IMBALANCE

Fluid Imbalances
- ECV deficit
- ECV excess
- Hypernatremia (increased osmolality)
- Hyponatremia (decreased osmolality, water intoxication)
- Dehydration (ECV deficit plus hypernatremia)

Electrolyte Imbalances
- Hypokalemia
- Hyperkalemia
- Hypocalcemia
- Hypercalcemia
- Hypomagnesemia
- Hypermagnesemia

Gas Exchange (ECV imbalances), Cognition (osmolality imbalances), and Mobility (electrolyte imbalances that cause muscle weakness). These interrelationships are illustrated in Figure 8-5.

CLINICAL EXEMPLARS

An exemplar of optimal fluid and electrolyte balance is a person of any age whose fluid and electrolyte output is balanced by appropriate type and amount of intake and whose fluid and electrolyte distributions are normal. This person has ECV, osmolality, and plasma electrolyte values within the normal range.

Box 8-5 lists exemplars of disrupted fluid and electrolyte balance. Using the general individual risk factors presented previously in this concept, nurses can understand the risk factors for each exemplar. For example, hypokalemia can occur from normal output but deficient K+ intake, increased output not balanced by increased K+ intake, or rapid K+ shift from ECF into cells. Specific causes of each exemplar are organized in Boxes 8-1 and 8-2 under these general individual risk factors.

Featured Exemplars

ECV Excess

ECV excess is too much fluid volume in the vascular and interstitial compartments. Signs and symptoms of ECV excess include distended neck veins when upright (vascular fluid overload) and dependent edema (interstitial fluid overload). People at high risk of ECV excess often have decreased excretion of Na+ and water because they have oliguria or excessive amounts of aldosterone. For example, chronic heart failure decreases cardiac output, which stimulates excessive renin release, which then increases aldosterone secretion, causing ECV excess.[17,25] People who receive IV isotonic Na+-containing solutions also develop ECV excess if the infusion is excessive.

Dehydration

Dehydration is the clinical combination of ECV deficit and hypernatremia, although the term sometimes is used loosely in clinical settings to indicate ECV deficit alone. ECV deficit is not enough fluid volume in the vascular and interstitial compartments; hypernatremia is abnormally increased serum Na+ concentration, denoting increased body fluid osmolality (too concentrated). Clinical dehydration causes signs and symptoms of both conditions: rapid thready pulse, postural hypotension, and flat neck veins when supine (vascular fluid underload); skin tenting (interstitial fluid underload); and decreased level of consciousness caused by osmotic shift of water out of brain cells. Although dehydration may occur in people of any age, those at highest risk of clinical dehydration are infants, children, and older adults who have gastroenteritis (vomiting and diarrhea) and whose fluid and salt output is not replaced sufficiently.

Hyponatremia

Hyponatremia is abnormally decreased serum Na+ concentration; body fluids have decreased osmolality (are too dilute). Water moves into cells by osmosis, causing them to swell. Swollen brain cells impair cerebral function, the basis of the signs and symptoms of hyponatremia.[7] People at high risk of hyponatremia usually have rapid intake of large amounts of water that overwhelms their ability to excrete it renally. For example, they may receive too much IV 5% dextrose in water (D5W) or drink massive amounts of water in a few hours.[15,18,19] People who secrete excessive ADH also develop hyponatremia because ADH causes renal retention of water that dilutes the blood.[23]

Hypokalemia

Hypokalemia is abnormally decreased plasma K^+ concentration. Intracellular K^+ may be low, normal, or even high. Skeletal muscle weakness, constipation, and cardiac dysrhythmias occur from the abnormal K^+ distribution. People at high risk for hypokalemia usually have increased K^+ output that they have not balanced with increased K^+ intake. For example, diarrhea increases fecal K^+ output; aldosterone excess, K^+-wasting diuretics, and cortisol excess all increase renal K^+ output.[8,24] Other people at high risk of hypokalemia have chronically low K^+ intake or rapid shift of K^+ from the ECF into cells.

Hypercalcemia

Hypercalcemia is abnormally increased plasma Ca^{2+} concentration. Signs and symptoms include constipation and decreased level of consciousness. People at high risk for hypercalcemia usually have shift of Ca^{2+} from their bones into the ECF. The two most common examples are hyperparathyroidism and cancer that secretes circulating substances that act like PTH and remove Ca^{2+} from bones.[30] People who overdose on vitamin D also have high risk for hypercalcemia due to absorption of more Ca^{2+} than they can excrete.[31]

Hypomagnesemia

Hypomagnesemia is abnormally decreased plasma Mg^{2+} concentration. It increases neuromuscular excitability, causing muscle cramps, hyperactive reflexes, cardiac dysrhythmias, and even seizures, depending on its severity. The people most at risk for hypomagnesemia have low Mg^{2+} intake or absorption or have increased Mg^{2+} output that is not balanced by increased Mg^{2+} intake. For example, people who abuse alcohol on a chronic basis have very high risk for hypomagnesemia from a combination of decreased Mg^{2+} intake, Mg^{2+} malabsorption, and increased Mg^{2+} output through vomiting and increased renal excretion.[32] People who receive massive citrated blood transfusions also have high risk for hypomagnesemia because the citrate binds Mg^{2+}, making it physiologically unavailable.

CASE STUDY

Source: Barbara Penoyar/ Photodisc/Thinkstock

Case Presentation

Mrs. Malone, age 83 years, lives in an apartment with her cat. She has hypertension, hyperlipidemia, and chronic left-sided heart failure, which are managed with the diuretic furosemide, KCl, several other medications, and dietary Na^+ restriction. Mrs. Malone volunteers at a nearby elementary school, where earlier in the week several students were sent home sick after vomiting. Mrs. Malone developed vomiting and diarrhea. Although the vomiting stopped, the diarrhea persisted. She drank more water than usual, ate rice and dry toast, and stopped taking her KCl to avoid upsetting her stomach. After 2 days of diarrhea, Mrs. Malone became lightheaded when she got out of bed and had difficulty standing up after using the toilet because her legs were so weak. She telephoned her nurse practitioner (NP), who advised her to drink some broth with salt in it as well as some orange juice. Mrs. Malone needed considerable teaching regarding the importance of Na^+ intake to replace her increased Na^+ output in diarrhea, but eventually she did agree to try the rehydration schedule her NP advised. After checking back by telephone later in the day and learning that Mrs. Malone was no longer lightheaded but still had "weak legs," the NP advised Mrs. Malone to restart her KCl, continue drinking orange juice, and make an appointment to have her plasma K^+ concentration checked.

Case Analysis

Mrs. Malone had chronic heart failure. Her reduced cardiac output and other mechanisms of heart failure increased activation of her renin–angiotensin–aldosterone system, causing more renal retention of Na^+ and water and creating chronic ECV excess. To counteract her decreased Na^+ and water output, she used the prescribed furosemide, a K^+-wasting diuretic that increases Na^+ and water output. Because this diuretic also increases K^+ output, Mrs. Malone also took KCl to increase her K^+ intake. She adhered to her Na^+-restricted diet because she had learned that Na^+ kept water in her body and "made her ankles swell more" (her understanding of ECV excess). When Mrs. Malone developed increased Na^+, water, and K^+ output from vomiting and diarrhea, her intake did not increase appropriately, so she developed ECV deficit (lightheaded upon standing) and hypokalemia (bilateral quadriceps weakness). Learning about the vomiting and diarrhea, her NP asked appropriate assessment questions over the telephone to elicit these symptoms and planned appropriate fluid and electrolyte replacement therapy. The NP taught Mrs. Malone the reason for the temporarily increased Na^+ intake, even though she usually followed a Na^+-restricted diet, and asked Mrs. Malone to make a follow-up appointment.

ACCESS EXEMPLAR LINKS IN YOUR GIDDENS EBOOK

REFERENCES

1. Hall JE: *Guyton and Hall textbook of medical physiology*, ed 13, Philadelphia, 2016, Saunders.
2. Gabriel J: Subcutaneous fluid administration and the hydration of older people. *Brit J Nurs* 23(14):S10, 2014.
3. Cheung WJ, Rosenberg H, Vaillancourt C: Barriers and facilitators to intraosseous access in adult resuscitations when peripheral intravenous access is not achievable. *Acad Emer Med* 21(3):250, 2014.
4. Arai S, Stotts N, Puntillo N: Thirst in critically ill patients: From physiology to sensation. *Am J Crit Care* 22(4):328, 2013.
5. Yugandhar VG, Clark MA: Angiotensin III: A physiological relevant peptide of the renin angiotensin system. *Peptides* 46:26, 2013.
6. Felver L: Fluid and electrolyte homeostasis and imbalances. In Copstead LC, Banasik JL, editors: *Pathophysiology*, ed 5, St Louis, 2013, Saunders.
7. Halperin ML, Goldstein MB, Kamel KS: *Fluid, electrolyte and acid–base physiology*, ed 4, Philadelphia, 2010, Saunders.
8. Medford-Davis L, Rafique Z: Derangements of potassium. *Emer Med Clin N Am* 32(2):329, 2014.

9. Chang W-T, Radin B, McCurdy MT: Calcium, magnesium, and phosphate abnormalities in the emergency department. *Emer Med Clin N Am* 32(2):349, 2014.

10. Khow KS, Lau SY, Li JY, et al: Diuretic-associated electrolyte disorders in the elderly: Risk factors, impact, management and prevention. *Curr Drug Safety* 9(1):2, 2014.

11. Harring TR, Deal NS, Kuo DC: Disorders of sodium and water balance. *Emer Med Clin N Am* 32(2):379, 2014.

12. Sulemanji M, Vakili K: Neonatal renal physiology. *Sem Pediatr Surg* 22(4):195, 2013.

13. El-Sharkawy AM, Sahota O, Maughan RJ, et al: The pathophysiology of fluid and electrolyte balance in the older adult surgical patient. *Clin Nutr* 33(1):6, 2014.

14. Hale A, Hovey MJ: *Fluid, electrolyte, and acid–base imbalances,* Philadelphia, 2013, Davis.

15. Wang J, Xu E, Xiao Y: Isotonic versus hypotonic maintenance IV fluids in hospitalized children: A meta-analysis. *Pediatrics* 133(1):105, 2014.

16. Wessler JD, Hummel SL, Maurer MS: Dietary interventions for heart failure in older adults: Re-emergence of the hedonic shift. *Prog Cardiovascular Dis* 57(2):160, 2014.

17. Philipson H, Ekman I, Forslund HB, et al: Salt and fluid restriction is effective in patients with chronic heart failure. *Eur J Heart Failure* 15(11):1304, 2013.

18. Cicognani C, Vezzadini C, Zoni R, et al: An overlooked cause of acute symptomatic seizures: Psychogenic polydipsia. *Am J Med* 126(5):e1, 2013.

19. Sterns R: Disorders of plasma sodium—Causes, consequences, and correction. *N Engl J Med* 372(1):55, 2015.

20. Richards JB, Wilcox SR: Diagnosis and management of shock in the emergency department. *Emer Med Pract* 16(3):1, 2014.

21. Maxwell AP, Linden K, O'Donnell S, et al: Management of hyperkalemia. *J Royal Coll Physicians Edinburgh* 43(3):246, 2013.

22. Williams CN, Belzer JS, Riva-Cambrin J, et al: The incidence of postoperative hyponatremia and associated neurological sequelae in children with intracranial neoplasms. *J Neurosurg Pediatr* 13(3):283, 2014.

23. Spasovski G, Vanholder R, Allolio B, et al: Clinical practice guidelines on diagnosis and treatment of hyponatremia. *Nephrol Dialysis Transplant* 29(Suppl 2):i1, 2014.

24. Bataille S, Baralla C, Torro D, et al: Undercorrection of hypernatremia is frequent and associated with mortality. *BMC Nephrol* 15:37, 2014.

25. Kasper DK, Fauci A, Hauser SL, et al, editors: *Harrison's Principles of Internal Medicine,* ed 19, New York, 2015, McGraw-Hill.

26. Wunderlich R: Principles in the selection of intravenous solutions replacement: Sodium and water. *J Infus Nurs* 36(2):126, 2013.

27. Infusion Nurses Society: Infusion nursing standards of practice. *J Infus Nurs* 34(1S):S1, 2011.

28. Giger JN: *Transcultural nursing: Assessment and intervention,* ed 6, St Louis, 2013, Mosby.

29. McCullough PA, Beaver TM, Bennett-Guerrero E, et al: Acute and chronic cardiovascular effects of hyperkalemia: New insights into prevention and clinical management. *Rev Cardiovasc Med* 15(1):11, 2014.

30. Fallah-Rad N, Morton AR: Managing hypercalcaemia and hypocalcaemia in cancer patients. *Curr Opin Support Palliative Care* 7(3):265, 2013.

31. Vogiatzi MG, Jacobson-Dickman E, DeBoer MD, et al: Vitamin D supplementation and risk of toxicity in pediatrics: A review of current literature. *J Clin Endocrinol Metab* 99(4):1132, 2014.

32. Weglicki WB: Hypomagnesemia and inflammation: Clinical and basic aspects. *Annu Rev Nutr* 32:55, 2012.

Acid–Base Balance

Linda Felver

The human body requires precise control of multiple physiological processes for optimal function. The concentration of hydrogen ions in body fluids influences cellular function and thus organ, system, and whole person function. An abnormal hydrogen ion concentration impairs cellular and organ function and can be fatal. The body maintains the hydrogen ion concentration within the normal range by continuously making adjustments through specific processes. Nurses providing care to acutely and chronically ill patients must understand these processes in order to optimize their function. This concept presents an analysis of acid–base balance, including the recognition and management of acid–base imbalances when they occur.

DEFINITION

For the purposes of this concept analysis, acid–base balance is defined as *the process of regulating the pH, bicarbonate concentration, and partial pressure of carbon dioxide of body fluids*. The definitions of acid and base are the foundation for the concept of acid–base balance. An *acid* is a substance that releases hydrogen ions (H^+), and a *base* is a substance that takes up H^+. The most important base in the body is bicarbonate (HCO_3^-). The pH of a solution, technically defined later in this concept analysis, is a measure of its degree of acidity. A low pH means the solution is acidic; a high pH means it is basic (alkaline).

Acid–base balance is a dynamic interplay between three processes: acid production or intake, acid buffering, and acid excretion. *Acid production* is generation of acid through cellular metabolism. Our cells continuously generate two kinds of acid during metabolism: carbonic acid (H_2CO_3) and metabolic acids. Although the chemical structures of metabolic acids vary, both normal and abnormal types of cellular metabolism generate metabolic acids. Occasionally, *acid intake* occurs, which involves entry into the body of acids or substances that the body converts to acids (acid precursors). *Acid buffering* is a process by which body fluids resist large changes in pH when acids or bases are added or removed. Body fluids normally have buffers, which are pairs of chemicals that take up H^+ or release it to keep pH in the normal range. *Acid excretion* is removal of acid from the body. These concepts are described in greater detail later in this concept analysis.

Acid–base balance is described as a dynamic interplay because acid production is occurring constantly, the body fluids constantly have cellular acids added to them that must be buffered to preserve function,

and the acid excretion mechanisms must function continuously to keep acids from accumulating in the body. Optimal acid–base balance keeps the pH of the blood and body fluids within the normal physiological range (7.35–7.45).

SCOPE

Considered conceptually, the scope of acid–base balance is on a continuum from acidotic (low pH) on one end to optimal balance (normal pH and other parameters) in the middle and alkalotic (high pH) on the other end (Figure 9-1). These link to three categories associated with this concept: optimal acid–base balance and two types of disrupted acid–base balance—acidosis (too much acid) and alkalosis (too little acid). The term acid–base imbalance often is used to indicate disrupted acid–base balance.

NORMAL PHYSIOLOGICAL PROCESS

The processes whose dynamic interplay is involved in acid–base balance are acid production, acid buffering, and acid excretion. When optimal acid–base balance is occurring, the buffers are not overwhelmed by the amount of acid that is generated and acid excretion keeps pace with acid production. The blood pH and other measures of acid–base status are in the normal range (7.35–7.45 for adults; a wider range for infants). This section explains these functions in detail. The process is illustrated in Figure 9-2.

Acid Production

Cellular metabolism continuously generates carbonic acid and metabolic acids. Increased cellular metabolism produces more of these acids.

Carbonic Acid Production

Cellular metabolism generates carbonic acid (H_2CO_3) in the form of carbon dioxide (CO_2) and water (H_2O). The enzyme carbonic anhydrase in erythrocytes and other cells facilitates the conversion in either direction, depending on the location in the body. In the tissues, in which CO_2 is abundant because it is being produced, the excess CO_2 in the blood drives the equilibrium toward making H_2CO_3. H_2CO_3 is a weak acid, which means that it dissociates (separates into H^+ and HCO_3^-) only partially in solution:

FIGURE 9-1 Scope of Concept Acid–base balance ranges from optimal balance to acidotic and alkalotic imbalances.

$$CO_2 + H_2O \approx H_2CO_3 \approx H^+ + HCO_3^-$$

Bicarbonate in the blood is transported to the lung capillaries, where the CO_2 level is low because CO_2 diffuses into the alveoli and is exhaled. Carbonic anhydrase in the lungs converts H_2CO_3 back to CO_2 and H_2O, the form in which it is excreted through exhalation.

Metabolic Acid Production

Metabolic acid, the other type of acid produced by cellular metabolism, is a general term that includes all acids except carbonic acid. Examples of metabolic acid are citric acid, pyruvic acid, and lactic acid. Cells can produce abnormal metabolic acids, such as the ketoacid β-hydroxybutyric acid, when cellular metabolism is disrupted or

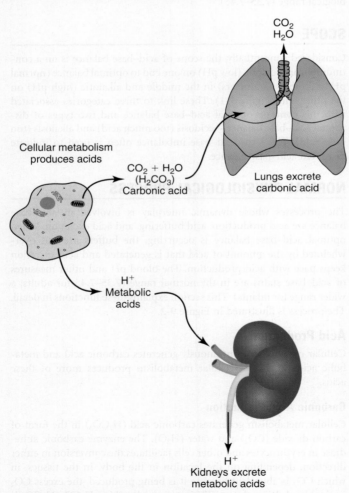

FIGURE 9-2 Acid Production and Excretion (Source: From Potter PA, Perry AG, Stockert P, Hall A: *Fundamentals of nursing*, ed 8, St Louis, 2013, Mosby.)

incomplete. The symbol that represents all metabolic acids is **HA**. The A indicates anion, which means negatively charged particle. Some, but not all, of these molecules dissociate into H^+ and A^- because they are weak acids. Metabolic acid moves from the cells that produce it into the body fluids, where it is buffered before it reaches the kidneys, where it is excreted.

Acid Buffering

Buffers help keep the pH of the blood and other body fluids in the normal range despite the metabolic acid continuously produced by the cells. A buffer is a pair of chemicals (a weak acid and its base) that are in equilibrium in a solution. These two parts of a buffer system must be present in a specific ratio to keep the pH normal. The most important buffer in the extracellular fluid is the bicarbonate buffer system, which consists of carbonic acid (the weak acid) and bicarbonate (its base).[1] When the bicarbonate-to-carbonic acid ratio is 20:1, the blood pH is in the normal range. If the ratio changes significantly, the blood pH becomes abnormal.

The bicarbonate buffer system buffers metabolic acid that is produced by cells or ingested. The bicarbonate portion of the buffer combines with the H^+ from the metabolic acid to make carbonic acid:

$$H^+ + HCO_3^- \approx H_2CO_3$$

This process could decrease the available bicarbonate and increase the concentration of carbonic acid, but normally the 20:1 ratio of bicarbonate to carbonic acid is restored immediately because the lungs excrete the carbonic acid as carbon dioxide and water. Most of the function of bicarbonate buffers in normal physiology is buffering metabolic acid. Bicarbonate buffers cannot buffer carbonic acid because carbonic acid is part of the buffer. If too much metabolic acid is present, the plasma bicarbonate concentration will decrease below its normal range because so much bicarbonate was used in buffering.

In abnormal circumstances in which there is too little metabolic acid present, the carbonic acid portion of the bicarbonate buffer system will release H^+. This process simultaneously raises the bicarbonate concentration and may restore the pH. However, if entirely too little metabolic acid is present, the plasma bicarbonate concentration will increase above its normal range. Thus, the plasma bicarbonate concentration is an indicator of the metabolic acid status in the blood.

Acid Excretion

The two types of acid produced by cellular metabolism differ in that carbonic acid is converted to gases and metabolic acid is not. The lungs excrete the gaseous form of carbonic acid, and the kidneys excrete metabolic acid.

Carbonic Acid Excretion

The lungs serve as the excretory organ for carbonic acid. The lungs are not able to excrete metabolic acid because it cannot be converted into a gaseous form. Changes in rate and depth alter the amount of carbonic acid that is excreted. Hyperventilation (increased rate and depth of respiration) excretes more carbonic acid; hypoventilation (decreased rate and depth of respiration) excretes less carbonic acid. The chemoreceptors influence respiratory rate and depth in response to blood levels of CO_2 and H^+ and, in some situations, oxygen. When the amount of CO_2 increases in the blood, the chemoreceptors increase the respiratory rate and depth,[2] which excretes more CO_2 and H_2O (carbonic acid) and helps restore the CO_2 level to its normal range. If the blood has too little CO_2, the chemoreceptors decrease the respiratory rate and depth, which enables CO_2 level to rise to its normal range because the cells constantly are producing it. These are examples of *correction*: fixing the problem and returning the blood values to their normal range.

Because chemoreceptors respond to H^+ concentration as well as to blood levels of CO_2, they modify respiratory rate and depth in response to the level of metabolic acid as well as carbonic acid. If too much metabolic acid accumulates, the chemoreceptors trigger hyperventilation (increased respiratory rate and depth). This does not correct the problem because the lungs cannot excrete metabolic acid, but hyperventilation removes more carbonic acid from the body, thus making the blood less acidic. The result is too little carbonic acid to help balance too much metabolic acid. The technical term for this process is *compensation*: moving the pH toward its normal range while making other blood values abnormal. If too little metabolic acid is present, the chemoreceptors cause hypoventilation.[3] This compensatory process moves the pH down toward its normal range by allowing too much carbonic acid to help balance the too little metabolic acid.

Metabolic Acid Excretion

The kidneys excrete metabolic acid but are unable to excrete carbonic acid. They have several mechanisms for excreting metabolic acid. Glomerular filtrate that enters the renal tubules contains HCO_3^- from blood. Cells that line the renal proximal tubules perform chemical processes that essentially take H^+ from the blood and secrete it into renal tubular fluid while moving HCO_3^- the opposite direction, from the renal tubules into blood. The A^- portion of metabolic acids enters renal tubular fluid in the proximal tubules as well. Infants and older adults have reduced ability to excrete large amounts of metabolic acids.[4]

Secretion of metabolic acid into the renal tubules adds free H^+ to the fluid, which potentially could damage renal cells. However, many of these H^+ combine with other molecules in the renal tubular fluid, and they no longer influence the pH. For example, renal tubular fluid contains buffers, especially phosphate buffers that were filtered at the glomerulus. Many of the secreted H^+ are buffered; buffered H^+ in urine are called *titratable acid*.[5] Additional free H^+ bind to ammonia (NH_3) that renal tubular cells produce when additional metabolic acid needs to be excreted. The H^+ no longer are free but are part of ammonium ions (NH_4^+), which do not contribute to the pH. NH_4^+ ions do not return to the cells but remain in the renal tubular fluid and are excreted in the urine:

$$H^+ + NH_3 \approx NH_4^+$$

By adjusting their H^+ secretion rate and the amount of ammonia they make, the kidneys are able to excrete more or less metabolic acid, which assists in maintaining optimal acid–base balance. If too much metabolic acid is present in the blood, the kidneys increase their secretion of H^+ and make more NH_3. These mechanisms correct the problem by removing more HA from the blood and simultaneously increasing blood HCO_3^- concentration (moves the opposite direction from the H^+). Similarly, if too little metabolic acid is present, the kidneys decrease their secretion of H^+ and make less NH_3 so that more metabolic acid remains in the blood and more HCO_3^- is excreted in the

urine. These corrective mechanisms normalize the pH by fixing the problem.

If too much carbonic acid accumulates, the kidneys cannot excrete it, but they can excrete more metabolic acid than usual.[6] This renal response to decreased pH compensates for the problem by causing too little metabolic acid in the blood, which somewhat balances the too much carbonic acid. Similarly, if the pH increases because there is too little carbonic acid, the renal compensatory response is less secretion of H^+ and less generation of NH_3. The resulting increase of metabolic acid is an attempt to balance the lack of carbonic acid, normalizing the pH by making other blood values abnormal.

Age-Related Differences
Infants and Children

Infants have several physiological differences worth noting. An infant has a much greater percentage of total body weight attributed to fluid (75%) compared to an adult (58%), more extracellular fluid than intracellular fluid, and an immature renal system that is inefficient in excreting a sudden acid load. In addition, an infant's metabolic rate is twice that of an adult, and the fluid exchange ratio is far greater than that of an adult. These differences place infants more at risk for acidosis as well as fluid and electrolyte imbalances compared to older children and adults.

Older Adults

A normal physiological change associated with aging is reduced size and function of the kidneys, which play a critical role in maintaining acid–base balance. Despite this age-related gradual loss of nephrons, the kidneys of the older adult typically are able to manage their role in fluid, electrolyte, and acid–base balance under normal circumstances. However, older adults have reduced renal reserve. They are less able to excrete a large acid load renally, and their ability to compensate may be less effective. This makes older adults more susceptible to acid–base disturbances as well as to fluid and electrolyte imbalances.

VARIATIONS AND CONTEXT

Conceptually, variations in acid–base balance are referred to as acid–base imbalance, of which there are two major categories: acidosis and alkalosis. Each of these categories has two underlying subtypes: respiratory and metabolic (Figure 9-3). When these conditions are developing, the body attempts to manage the changing acid–base balance through the corrective and compensatory responses described previously. Table 9-1 summarizes the corrective and compensatory responses to disrupted acid–base balance.

FIGURE 9-3 Categories of Acid–Base Imbalances

TABLE 9-1 Respiratory and Renal Responses to Disrupted Acid–Base Balance

Stimulus	Respiratory Response	Renal Response
Too much carbonic acid (respiratory acidosis)	Cause Hypoventilation Correction Hyperventilation	Compensation Increased secretion of H+ More NH₃ production
Too little carbonic acid (respiratory alkalosis)	Cause Hyperventilation Correction Hypoventilation	Compensation Decreased secretion of H+ Less NH₃ production
Too much metabolic acid (metabolic acidosis)	Compensation Hyperventilation	Cause More metabolic acid than kidneys can excrete Correction Increased secretion of H+ More NH₃ production
Too little metabolic acid (metabolic alkalosis)	Compensation Hypoventilation	Cause More bicarbonate than kidneys can excrete (too little metabolic acid) Correction Decreased secretion of H+ Less NH₃ production

Acidosis (Too Much Acid)

In a situation of too much acid, the buffers have been overwhelmed and body fluids have too much acid. Acid excretion is not able to keep up with acid production or intake. Conditions of too much acid are called *acidosis* and are given an additional descriptor that explains whether there is too much carbonic acid or too much metabolic acid. Because the lungs excrete carbonic acid, the condition of too much carbonic acid is called *respiratory acidosis*.[6] Similarly, because the kidneys excrete metabolic acid, the condition of too much metabolic acid is called *metabolic acidosis*. In some cases of metabolic acidosis, the base bicarbonate has been lost from the body, which causes relatively too much metabolic acid. In situations of too much acid, the pH is below the normal range (or in the low part of the normal range), and some other measures of acid–base status are abnormal. These laboratory values are explained in the Assessment section.

Alkalosis (Too Little Acid)

In situations of too little acid, the buffers also are not able to keep the pH in the normal range and body fluids do not have enough acid. Too much of the base HCO_3^- has been added to the buffer system or acid excretion is greater than acid production. Conditions of too little acid are called *alkalosis*—either *respiratory alkalosis* when there is too little carbonic acid or *metabolic alkalosis* when there is too little metabolic acid. In these situations of too little acid, the pH is above the normal range (or in the high part of the normal range) and some other mea-

sures of acid–base status are abnormal. The Assessment section explains these measures.

CONSEQUENCES

A firm grasp of the physiological processes that comprise acid–base balance makes it possible to understand the consequences when these processes are disrupted. Acid–base imbalances trigger compensatory mechanisms, as described previously. The time course of those mechanisms has important clinical implications. In addition to triggering compensatory mechanisms, pH changes impair cellular and organ function.

Time Course of Compensatory Mechanisms

Disruptions of acid–base balance cause the blood pH to move outside its normal range. In these situations, the buffers have been overwhelmed and the acid excretion mechanisms must work to keep pH from reaching the fatal limits. If the pH falls abnormally low from too much acid, both the lungs and the kidneys will excrete more acid, even though only one of these organs will be excreting the type of acid that is excessive. The other organ is compensating. Depending on the time course and the severity of the problem, the disruption may be uncompensated, partially compensated, or fully compensated.[6]

As explained in the previous section, if a problem with the respiratory system disrupts acid–base balance and the lungs are unable to correct it, renal compensatory mechanisms adjust the pH toward normal. It takes several days for renal compensatory mechanisms to become clinically significant;[6] therefore, a short-lived respiratory acidosis or alkalosis will not become compensated. Rapid treatment of an acute respiratory acidosis will correct the problem before renal compensation can occur. On the other hand, people who have chronic respiratory acidosis or an acute episode that lasts several days do develop some degree of renal compensation, either partial or full. Episodes of respiratory alkalosis occur from hyperventilation and usually do not last long enough for renal compensation to occur.

Analogously, if a problem with the kidneys disrupts acid–base balance and the kidneys are unable to correct it, respiratory compensatory mechanisms adjust the pH toward normal.[6] Respiratory compensation begins a few minutes after the pH becomes abnormal, so it is common to have some degree of compensation for a disruption of acid–base balance that involves too much or too little metabolic acid. When the disruption is severe, it will be only partially compensated.[1] In cases of metabolic alkalosis (too little metabolic acid), compensatory hypoventilation is limited by the respiratory drive for oxygen so that full compensation usually does not occur.[3] It is important to realize that even if compensatory mechanisms do not return pH to the normal range, they do prevent pH from becoming more abnormal.

Impaired Cellular and Organ Function

Disruptions of acid–base balance alter cell function, especially in the brain. The disorders involving carbonic acid (respiratory acidosis and alkalosis) generally cause more neurologic signs and symptoms than those involving metabolic acid (metabolic acidosis and alkalosis).[7] This difference occurs because CO_2 from carbonic acid crosses the blood–brain barrier easily and changes the pH of cerebrospinal fluid rapidly. Metabolic acid and HCO_3^- cross the blood–brain barrier with difficulty and produce fewer neurologic manifestations or cause them more slowly.

The enzymes inside cells work most effectively when pH is normal. Abnormal extracellular pH can cause intracellular pH to change, especially with respiratory acidosis and alkalosis. The resulting change in enzyme activity contributes to cell dysfunction. Acidosis decreases the level of consciousness (LOC). With alkalosis, initial excitation may occur, followed by decreased LOC if the pH increase becomes more severe.[7] In addition to brain cell dysfunction that causes altered LOC and other neurologic manifestations, cardiac cell dysfunction from acid–base imbalances can cause dysrhythmias.[8,9] Concurrent potassium imbalances caused by acid–base imbalances also cause cardiac dysrhythmias.[10]

RISK FACTORS

Populations at Risk

All individuals, regardless of race, culture, age, or socioeconomic status, need optimal acid–base balance for physiological function. From a population perspective, those at greatest risk for acid–base disturbances are the very young and the very old. Preterm infants are at great risk for acid–base disturbances due to immature lungs, kidneys, thermoregulation, and metabolic processes; the degree of risk is largely related to the weight and gestational age at the time of birth. Term infants are also more at risk than adults due to immature kidneys, elevated metabolic rate, and large fluid exchange ratio.

Older adults have decreased renal reserve due to a normal gradual loss of nephrons, making their ability to correct and to compensate for imbalances less effective Thus, they are more susceptible to acid–base disturbances.

Individual Risk Factors

Acid–base imbalances usually occur as a consequence of another underlying condition. The most common underlying conditions associated with acid–base disturbances are presented in Box 9-1. These are organized under general causes that provide a framework for remembering the conditions. For example, respiratory acidosis (too much carbonic acid) can arise from alveolar hypoventilation, ineffective neuromuscular action of the chest respiratory pump, or suppression of the neural drive from the brain stem that triggers respirations. Nurses can use these categories to understand specifically how the exemplars cause respiratory acidosis and generalize their knowledge to other conditions that cause respiratory acidosis by similar mechanisms. Nurses can also deduce logically the risk factors for acid–base imbalance by considering the processes whose dynamic interplay creates acid–base balance. Those at greatest risk for acid–base imbalances are individuals who have at least one of the following risk factors:[11]

- Excessive production or intake of metabolic acid
- Altered acid buffering due to loss or gain of bicarbonate
- Altered acid excretion
- Abnormal shift of H^+ into cells

Excessive Production or Intake of Metabolic Acid

The cells are capable of making excessive amounts of metabolic acid that overwhelm the acid buffering and excretory capacities. A common clinical example of too much metabolic acid due to acid production is diabetic ketoacidosis, in which abnormal cellular metabolism caused by lack of insulin produces ketoacids faster than the kidneys are able to excrete them.[1,12] Diabetic ketoacidosis is a type of metabolic acidosis. Other high-risk populations for ketoacidosis are people who do not have enough carbohydrate intake and people who abuse alcohol.[13] In addition to production of excessive metabolic acid within the body, excessive intake of acid or acid precursors also causes

metabolic acidosis. Although metabolic acidosis from intake of acid or acid precursors is less common, it is significant clinically in populations such as small children who accidentally ingest boric acid (intended for ant poisoning), individuals who overdose on aspirin (acetylsalicylic acid), or people who drink methanol or antifreeze (acid precursor).[14]

In summary, risk factors for excessive production or intake of metabolic acid include the risk factors for ketoacidosis or poisoning with acids or substances the body converts to acid. All of these

---

BOX 9-1   Common Underlying Conditions Leading to Acid–Base Imbalance

Respiratory Acidosis (Too Much Carbonic Acid)
Alveolar Hypoventilation
- Type B COPD (chronic bronchitis)
- End-stage type A COPD (emphysema)
- Severe asthma episode
- Bacterial pneumonia
- Pulmonary edema

Ineffective Respiratory Pump
- Guillain–Barré syndrome

Central Suppression of Respiration
- Opioid overdose

Metabolic Acidosis (Too Much Metabolic Acid)
Excessive Production or Intake of Metabolic Acid
- Diabetic ketoacidosis
- Starvation ketoacidosis
- Alcoholic ketoacidosis
- Lactic acidosis (from tissue anoxia)
- Thyroid storm
- Aspirin overdose

Decreased Excretion of Metabolic Acid
- Oliguria from any cause

Loss of Bicarbonate
- Prolonged diarrhea
- Draining intestinal or pancreatic fistula

Respiratory Alkalosis (Too Little Carbonic Acid)
Hyperventilation
- Acute hypoxia
- Acute pain
- Acute anxiety or emotional distress
- Central stimulation of respirations by inflammation from head injury or meningitis

Metabolic Alkalosis (Too Little Metabolic Acid)
Gain of Base (Bicarbonate)
- Excessive ingestion or infusion of $NaHCO_3$
- Massive blood transfusion (citrate metabolized to HCO_3^-)
- Diuretic therapy (contraction alkalosis)

Excessive Excretion of Metabolic Acid
- Repeated vomiting
- Mineralocorticoid excess

situations place people at risk for metabolic acidosis. The cells cannot stop producing metabolic acid, so decreased acid production is not a risk factor.

Altered Acid Buffering Due to Loss or Gain of Bicarbonate

The base bicarbonate is a component of the major buffer system that buffers metabolic acids. It is possible to lose or gain bicarbonate and thus alter the buffering capacity. People who lose a significant amount of bicarbonate, such as through prolonged diarrhea, lose buffering capacity and have relatively too much metabolic acid. Thus, bicarbonate loss causes metabolic acidosis.[15] Conversely, gaining a significant amount of bicarbonate, such as by ingesting baking soda (sodium bicarbonate) as an antacid or by receiving excessive intravenous (IV) sodium bicarbonate, alters the normal balance of buffer chemicals, which creates too little metabolic acid. Thus, bicarbonate gain causes metabolic alkalosis.[8,16] In summary, risk factors for altered acid buffering include prolonged diarrhea and excessive sodium bicarbonate intake in people of any age.[11] These conditions place them at risk for metabolic acidosis or metabolic alkalosis.

Altered Acid Excretion

Cellular metabolism generates two types of acid that are excreted by two different organ systems. For this reason, altered acid excretion occurs in many disease processes that affect lung and kidney function. Carbonic acid excretion occurs by gas exchange in the lung alveoli followed by exhalation; thus, it is possible to decrease or increase carbonic acid excretion. People at high risk for decreased carbonic acid excretion have acute or chronic respiratory diseases or other conditions that interfere with alveolar ventilation.[11] The cells continue producing carbonic acid, but the respiratory system is unable to excrete enough of it. The result is respiratory acidosis—too much carbonic acid. For example, people who have type B chronic obstructive pulmonary disease (COPD) (chronic bronchitis) have decreased carbonic acid excretion due to structural changes in their lungs and excessive mucus production that obstructs airflow.[17] They develop chronic respiratory acidosis. So do people of any age who have severe acute respiratory conditions such as asthma or bacterial pneumonia. Infants and small children have increased risk of respiratory acidosis with acute conditions because their airways have such small diameters.

Although decreased carbonic acid secretion is the most common problem with carbonic acid secretion, it is possible to excrete excessive carbonic acid through hyperventilation.[18] This situation causes too little carbonic acid, creating respiratory alkalosis. High-risk populations for too little carbonic acid due to hyperventilation include people who are hypoxic, are experiencing acute pain, or are upset and anxious. These conditions that cause respiratory alkalosis tend to be more short term than many causes of respiratory acidosis.

Excretion of metabolic acid also may be altered, either decreased or increased. People who have prolonged oliguria for any reason cannot excrete enough of the metabolic acid that their cells continue to produce. Thus, they develop metabolic acidosis. These high-risk populations include people of any age with acute or chronic oliguric renal disease and those with circulatory shock.[9,19] Infants have immature kidneys that are not yet fully effective in excreting metabolic acid; older adults often have reduced ability to excrete a metabolic acid load. These difficulties in excreting metabolic acid make them vulnerable to metabolic acidosis, especially in conjunction with increased acid production or intake.

Increased excretion of metabolic acid through the kidneys can occur in people with excessive aldosterone; however, the most common condition involving excessive removal of metabolic acid from the body is vomiting,[20] which removes hydrochloric acid. Vomiting also triggers bicarbonate retention by the kidneys, which alters buffering capacity and contributes to the resulting metabolic alkalosis.

In summary, risk factors for altered acid excretion include respiratory or other conditions that interfere with the ability to excrete enough carbonic acid, conditions causing hyperventilation that excretes too much carbonic acid, kidneys that are unable to excrete enough metabolic acid, and situations in which the kidneys or repeated episodes of vomiting remove too much metabolic acid from the body.[11]

Abnormal Shift of H⁺ into Cells

Factors that shift substantial numbers of H^+ into cells can cause too little acid to be in the blood. The most common example in this category of risk factors is hypokalemia (abnormally low plasma potassium concentration).[10] When hypokalemia is present, some potassium ions (K^+) leave cells and hydrogen ions (H^+) enter cells to maintain a balance of electrical charge. The result is too little metabolic acid in the blood, known as metabolic alkalosis. The primary risk factor for abnormal shift of H^+ into cells is hypokalemia. Risk factors for hypokalemia are discussed in Concept 8 Fluid and Electrolytes.

ASSESSMENT

Disruptions of acid–base balance almost always result from other conditions. For this reason, assessments of acid–base status usually are performed in the context of other conditions.

History

Clinical manifestations associated with disrupted acid–base balance often are due to an underlying condition and associated fluid and electrolyte imbalances. Acid–base imbalances cause nonspecific signs such as decreased LOC that have many possible causes. It is critical that nurses consider presenting symptoms in the context of other current health conditions. The history focuses on the respiratory, renal, or other conditions that could cause the acid–base problem. The standard questions for any history apply and are not repeated here. Other areas to explore in the history include the following: a recent history of vomiting or diarrhea (repeated vomiting causes metabolic alkalosis; prolonged diarrhea causes metabolic acidosis); use of heartburn or indigestion medications (a few days of baking soda/sodium bicarbonate ingestion can cause metabolic alkalosis); recent attempts to lose weight and methods employed (high-fat, low-carbohydrate diet or fasting predispose to starvation ketoacidosis); and use of medications, dietary supplements, and alcohol.[15,16,21]

Examination Findings

Unless the acid–base imbalance is severe, specific signs and symptoms of disrupted acid–base balance often are overshadowed by the clinical manifestations of the underlying cause. For example, in a person who has type B COPD (chronic bronchitis), the dyspnea and excessive mucus production usually are more obvious than the mild drowsiness from partially compensated respiratory acidosis. With severe acute asthma, the chest tightness, coughing, wheezing, use of accessory respiratory muscles, and poor oxygenation typically overshadow the manifestations of acute respiratory acidosis.[17] People who have end-stage renal disease experience many clinical manifestations from this chronic oliguric condition that predominate over lethargy from the metabolic acidosis that may occur between dialysis sessions, unless it becomes severe.

With substantial rapid changes of pH, such as with ketoacidosis, dramatic changes in LOC can overshadow the signs and symptoms of the underlying condition. For example, a person who develops diabetic

TABLE 9-2 Clinical Manifestations of Disrupted Acid–Base Balance

Type of Problem	TOO MUCH ACID		TOO LITTLE ACID	
	Too Much Carbonic Acid (Respiratory Acidosis)	Too Much Metabolic Acid (Metabolic Acidosis)	Too Little Carbonic Acid (Respiratory Alkalosis)	Too Little Metabolic Acid (Metabolic Alkalosis)
Common clinical findings	Headache Decreased LOC Hypoventilation (cause of problem) Cardiac dysrhythmias If severe: hypotension	Decreased LOC) Hyperventilation (compensatory mechanism) Abdominal pain Nausea and vomiting Cardiac dysrhythmias	Excitation and belligerence, lightheadedness, unusual behaviors; followed by decreased LOC if severe Perioral and digital paresthesias, carpopedal spasm, tetany Diaphoresis Hyperventilation (cause of problem) Cardiac dysrhythmias	Excitation followed by decreased LOC if severe Perioral and digital paresthesias, carpopedal spasm Hypoventilation (compensatory mechanism) Signs of volume depletion and hypokalemia if present
Blood gas findings	Blood gases: pH decreased (or low normal if fully compensated); $PaCO_2$ increased; HCO_3^- increased from compensation	Blood gases: pH decreased (or low normal if fully compensated); $PaCO_2$ decreased from compensation; HCO_3^- decreased	Blood gases: pH increased; $PaCO_2$ decreased; HCO_3^- decreased if compensation	Blood gases: pH increased; $PaCO_2$ increased from compensation; HCO_3^- increased

LOC, level of consciousness.

ketoacidosis typically will have been experiencing the polyuria, polydipsia, polyphagia, and weight loss of hyperglycemia before the onset of ketoacidosis. These manifestations often are realized only in retrospect, after abdominal pain and decreased LOC from the ketoacidosis have become the focus of attention and the metabolic acidosis is resolved.

Table 9-2 presents signs and symptoms of the various disruptions of acid–base balance. These manifestations arise from the impaired cellular and organ function described previously in this concept analysis. Decreased level of consciousness occurs on a continuum from decreased attention span and drowsiness on one end to stupor and coma on the other. Interpretation of assessment findings may be complicated by the presence of fluid and electrolyte imbalances (see Concept 8 Fluid and Electrolytes).

Diagnostic Tests

Arterial blood gas measurement is the definitive test for acid–base balance.[6,21,22] This section provides the conceptual basis for interpreting these diagnostic tests. The commonly used values are pH, $PaCO_2$, HCO_3^- concentration, and base excess. The partial pressure of oxygen in arterial blood (PaO_2) and the saturation of oxygen in arterial blood (SaO_2), which are measures of oxygenation, are not discussed here.

pH

The pH is defined technically as the negative logarithm of the H^+ concentration. H^+ ions arise from dissociation of acids, both carbonic acid and metabolic acid. The H^+ concentration is very small and awkward to write[2]; for that reason, the pH is calculated. The pH scale ranges from 1 to 14, with a pH of 7 being neutral. Because pH is a negative logarithm, a low pH indicates a solution that is acidic (has a high H^+ concentration). A high pH indicates a solution that is alkaline (has a low H^+ concentration). The pH of the blood has a normal range of 7.35–7.45 in adults, which is slightly alkaline. The normal range is lower in neonates and infants. In clinical settings, the term *acidemia* is used when the pH declines below the lower limit of normal (becomes *acidotic*). Even though the blood still may be

slightly alkaline (>7.0), it is more acidic than the normal range. The term *alkalemia* denotes a blood pH that is above the normal range (becomes *alkalotic*).

$PaCO_2$

$PaCO_2$ is the partial pressure of CO_2 in the arterial blood. It indicates how well the lungs are excreting carbonic acid (CO_2 and H_2O).[11] The normal range of $PaCO_2$ is 35–45 mm Hg (4.7–6.0 kilopascals (kPa)) for adults (lower in infants). Increased $PaCO_2$ level indicates CO_2 accumulation in the blood (too much carbonic acid) caused by primary or compensatory hypoventilation; decreased $PaCO_2$ level indicates excessive CO_2 excretion (too little carbonic acid) caused by primary or compensatory hyperventilation.

HCO_3^- Concentration

The serum HCO_3^- concentration indicates how well the kidneys are excreting metabolic acid.[11] The normal adult range is 22–26 mEq/L (22–26 mmol/L); the range is lower in infants. Increased HCO_3^- concentration indicates that the blood has too little metabolic acid; decreased HCO_3^- concentration indicates that the blood has too much metabolic acid.

Base Excess

Base excess, which normally ranges from −2 to +2 mmol/L, is an indicator of how well the buffers are managing metabolic acid.[6,23] Values less than −2 mmol/L (negative base excess) indicate too much metabolic acid; values greater than +2 mmol/L indicate too little metabolic acid. When people develop metabolic acidosis, clinicians may calculate other values, such as the anion gap and the Stewart strong ion difference, to assist in diagnosing the specific cause.[6,24,25]

CLINICAL MANAGEMENT

Clinical management of acid–base balance encompasses all clinical settings with primary and secondary prevention as well as interventions for people with acid–base imbalances.

Primary Prevention

The primary prevention for disrupted acid–base balance focuses on prevention of the major risk factors previously discussed rather than on prevention of disrupted acid–base balance itself. For example, prevention of respiratory diseases helps to prevent risk factors for accumulating too much carbonic acid. Thus, efforts to convince people not to begin smoking or to assist them to stop smoking, although targeted directly at prevention of respiratory disease, also indirectly prevent disruption of acid–base balance. Similarly, careful diabetes teaching and management help prevent ketoacidosis as well as other potential complications of diabetes. Teaching people how to lose weight safely without totally eliminating carbohydrates can help prevent starvation ketoacidosis as well as achieve weight management goals. Poison prevention efforts can help prevent excessive ingestion of acids or acid precursors. Instruction regarding hand hygiene and safe food storage helps prevent diarrhea and vomiting, two common risk factors for disrupted acid–base balance. In summary, most of the primary prevention strategies aimed at specific disease processes and behaviors detrimental to health in general also help prevent disrupted acid–base balance that can arise from these risk factors.

Secondary Prevention (Screening)

Screening measures to detect disrupted acid–base balance are not performed in the general population.

Collaborative Interventions

Patients experiencing acid–base imbalance require aggressive collaborative management aimed at treating the underlying condition. If left untreated, acid–base imbalances can be fatal.

Most medical and nursing management is directed at the disease process that disrupts acid–base balance. In general, collaborative interventions to manage acid–base imbalances caused by an underlying respiratory condition include respiratory support. Likewise, collaborative interventions to manage acid–base imbalances caused by an underlying metabolic condition usually include fluid and electrolyte support.

Respiratory Support

People who have too much or too little carbonic acid usually receive some type of respiratory support, such as airway management and oxygen therapy. For example, with primary respiratory acidosis (too much carbonic acid), the focus of collaborative interventions is treatment of the disease process that is impairing alveolar ventilation. By treating the underlying cause of the disruption, acid–base balance may return to normal, or at least to a more stable state. People who are hyperventilating develop respiratory alkalosis (too little carbonic acid). Collaborative interventions for these people focus on treating the underlying factor (e.g., hypoxia, acute pain, or acute anxiety) that drives the hyperventilation. Hyperventilation that is a compensatory response to metabolic acidosis (too many metabolic acids) should be allowed to continue while the metabolic acidosis is treated.

Fluid and Electrolyte Support

People whose acid–base balance is disrupted by too much or too little metabolic acid usually receive fluid and electrolyte support as part of collaborative interventions to treat the underlying problem. For example, providing insulin and fluids to treat diabetic ketoacidosis removes the original problem and normalizes acid–base balance. Dialysis for a person who accumulates too much metabolic acid from

> **BOX 9-2 Nursing Interventions for People with Disrupted Acid–Base Balance**
>
> - Ongoing assessment
> - Implement safety measures
> - Implement comfort measures
> - Support compensatory mechanisms
> - Implement collaborative interventions focused on
>   - Treatment of the underlying cause
>   - Adjustment of the pH (controversial)
> - Monitor for complications of therapy
> - Patient teaching
>   - Management of chronic underlying conditions
>   - Recognition of early problems; when to seek help

> **BOX 9-3 EXEMPLARS OF ACID–BASE IMBALANCE**
>
> - Respiratory acidosis
> - Metabolic acidosis
> - Respiratory alkalosis
> - Metabolic alkalosis

oliguric renal disease treats multiple aspects of the condition, including the disrupted acid–base balance.

Very low pH can be fatal; therefore, in situations of very severe metabolic acidosis in which pH is dangerously low, the collaborative focus occasionally expands to adjusting the pH itself. The most common agent used for pH adjustment is IV sodium bicarbonate, but its use is controversial.[9,15] Administration of IV sodium bicarbonate may cause extracellular fluid volume (ECV) excess or hypernatremia, delay renal excretion of ketoacids, or even lead to metabolic alkalosis from excessive administration. Monitoring for signs and symptoms of these complications, in addition to monitoring the patient's acid–base balance, is crucial.

Independent Nursing Interventions

Independent nursing interventions provide safety and comfort for people who have disrupted acid–base balance. Safety is high priority for patients with decreased LOC. In addition, interventions can promote compensatory mechanisms. For example, patients who are hyperventilating in compensation for metabolic acidosis need careful positioning to facilitate chest expansion and frequent oral care to prevent drying and cracking of their lips and oral mucous membranes. Another important type of intervention is teaching culturally appropriate[26] ways to prevent disruptions of acid–base balance or when to seek help if they have chronic problems. Box 9-2 summarizes nursing interventions for people with disrupted acid–base balance.

INTERRELATED CONCEPTS

Numerous concepts discussed in this book have interrelationships with acid–base balance. For example, **Fluid and Electrolytes** and acid–base balance are closely related because changes in one of them can cause changes in the other. **Gas Exchange**, **Perfusion**, and **Nutrition** facilitate optimal acid–base balance by allowing normal acid production, whereas alterations such as ischemia, hypoxia, starvation, and high-fat, low-carbohydrate diets can disrupt that process. Similarly, **Elimination**

FIGURE 9-4 Acid–Base Balance and Interrelated Concepts

facilitates optimal acid–base balance through acid excretion, whereas changes such as oliguria and diarrhea can disrupt acid–base balance. An individual who has disrupted acid–base balance can experience altered Cognition. These interrelationships are illustrated in Figure 9-4.

CLINICAL EXEMPLARS

An exemplar of optimal acid–base balance is a healthy person of any age. This person's acid production is balanced by acid excretion with adequate buffering. Optimal acid–base balance also can occur in a person with acute or chronic illness (e.g., osteoporosis) that does not seriously impair respiratory, gastrointestinal, endocrine, or renal function. The four exemplars representing acid–base disturbances are presented in Box 9-3 and are summarized briefly in the following Featured Exemplars section.

Featured Exemplars
Respiratory Acidosis

Respiratory acidosis is excess carbonic acid (measured as elevated $PaCO_2$) in the blood. Cellular metabolism continually produces carbonic acid, which must be excreted by the lungs or it accumulates in the blood. People at high risk of primary respiratory acidosis have acute or chronic respiratory diseases or other conditions that interfere with alveolar ventilation. These conditions arise from problems in the alveoli or airways (e.g., type B COPD and severe acute asthma), problems with respiratory muscle function (e.g., Guillain–Barré syndrome), or problems with the brain stem control of respirations (e.g., overdose of opioids or other central nervous system depressants). People develop mild compensatory respiratory acidosis if they have primary metabolic alkalosis.[3]

Respiratory Alkalosis

Respiratory alkalosis is too little carbonic acid (measured as decreased $PaCO_2$) in the blood. People at high risk for primary respiratory alkalosis are hyperventilating, which excretes carbonic acid faster than it is produced by cellular metabolism. Common causes of hyperventilation are acute hypoxia, acute pain, and emotional distress.[11] People develop compensatory respiratory alkalosis if they have primary metabolic acidosis.

Metabolic Acidosis

Metabolic acidosis is excess metabolic acid (measured as decreased HCO_3^-) in the blood. Cellular metabolism continually produces metabolic acid, which must be buffered in the blood by the HCO_3^- buffer system and excreted by the kidneys or the acid accumulates in the blood. People at high risk of primary metabolic acidosis have excessive production or intake of metabolic acid (e.g., ketoacidosis and salicylate overdose), decreased renal excretion (e.g., acute or chronic oliguria), or lose HCO_3^- buffers from the body (e.g., prolonged diarrhea).[14] These high-risk people include those with undiagnosed or inadequately treated type 1 diabetes, chronic alcohol abuse with malnutrition, untreated hyperthyroidism, circulatory shock, acute kidney injury, and oliguric chronic kidney disease.[9,12,13,19] People develop compensatory metabolic acidosis if they have a primary respiratory alkalosis that lasts for at least several days.

Metabolic Alkalosis

Metabolic acidosis is too little metabolic acid (measured as increased HCO_3^-) in the blood. People at high risk of primary metabolic alkalosis most frequently have excessive intake of HCO_3^- through use of baking soda as antacid, receiving IV $NaHCO_3$, or from metabolizing the citrate in massive blood transfusions.[8] Mild metabolic alkalosis is common with diuretic therapy.[4,27] People who have prolonged vomiting excrete metabolic acid more rapidly than it is produced while also retaining HCO_3^- renally.[20] People develop compensatory metabolic alkalosis if they have a primary respiratory acidosis that lasts for at least several days.

CASE STUDY

Source: samer chand/iStock/
Thinkstock

Case Presentation

Kevin Harney, age 14 years, did not appear for breakfast when his mother called him. "That's unusual," she thought, "He has been so hungry lately. And he is so skinny, he really needs the food!" She found Kevin lying on his bed, breathing rapidly and deeply. He responded slowly with one or two words at a time to her increasingly frantic questions. Some of his answers did not make sense. Kevin's parents took him to the nearest emergency department, where his laboratory tests showed arterial blood pH 7.20, $PaCO_2$ 21 mm Hg (2.8 kPa), serum HCO_3^- concentration 8 mEq/L (8 mmol/L), and glucose concentration 450 mg/dL (25 mmol/L). Kevin was diagnosed with diabetic ketoacidosis

(DKA) arising from previously undiagnosed type 1 diabetes. During Kevin's hospitalization, interventions focused initially on intensive collaborative management of his disrupted acid–base balance with insulin and IV fluid to treat the diabetes. As a safety intervention, Kevin was positioned on his side to prevent aspiration if he vomited. During this phase of management, attention also was given to supporting his parents, explaining that Kevin's unusual breathing pattern actually was beneficial to him and letting his mother assume the task

of protecting Kevin's lips by keeping them lubricated. Careful monitoring of blood values and physical assessment parameters was used to follow his progress and modify therapy when his condition changed. As Kevin began to be more responsive and stable, the focus of nursing interventions expanded to teaching Kevin and his parents about type 1 diabetes, how to manage it, and how to recognize the signs of hyperglycemia. Although not directed specifically at acid–base balance, this teaching helped prevent future episodes of DKA through disease management.

Case Analysis

Kevin developed DKA, a type of metabolic acidosis (too much metabolic acid), from a combination of excessive production and decreased excretion of metabolic acid. Because of his type 1 diabetes, Kevin's pancreas no longer was able to secrete insulin. The resulting metabolic problems included hyperglycemia and incomplete metabolism of fat that generated large amounts of ketoacids (increased acid production). Although Kevin did not have kidney disease, his kidneys were unable to excrete enough ketoacids to prevent their accumulation. An initial osmotic diuresis from hyperglycemia often decreases the ECV and decreases glomerular filtration rate, causing oliguria when the ECV becomes low. Oliguria decreased the excretion of the ketoacids, contributing to their accumulation. As his blood pH decreased, Kevin's chemoreceptors triggered compensatory hyperventilation. Kevin's arterial blood gas values demonstrate his disrupted acid–base balance: decreased pH (acidosis from too much acid), decreased $PaCO_2$ (carbonic acid removed by compensatory hyperventilation), and decreased HCO_3^- concentration (used in buffering the excess metabolic acids). Interventions directed at treating Kevin's diabetes and promoting safety, comfort, and teaching provided effective care.

ACCESS EXEMPLAR LINKS IN YOUR GIDDENS EBOOK

REFERENCES

1. Halperin ML, Goldstein MB, Kamel KS: *Fluid, electrolyte and acid–base physiology*, ed 4, Philadelphia, 2010, Saunders.
2. Hall JE: *Guyton and Hall textbook of medical physiology*, ed 12, Philadelphia, 2011, Saunders.
3. Feldman M, Alvarez NM, Trevino M, et al: Respiratory compensation to a primary metabolic alkalosis in humans. *Clin Nephrol* 78(5):365, 2012.
4. Khow KS, Lau SY, Li JY, et al: Diuretic-associated electrolyte disorders in the elderly: Risk factors, impact, management and prevention. *Curr Drug Saf* 9(1):2, 2014.
5. Ayers P, Dixon C: Simple acid–base tutorial. *J Parenteral Enteral Nutr* 36(1):18, 2012.
6. Berend K, de Vries AP, Gans RO: Physiological approach to assessment of acid–base disturbances. *N Engl J Med* 371(15):1434, 2014.
7. Espay AJ: Neurological complications of electrolyte disturbances and acid–base balance. *Handb Clin Neurol* 119:365, 2014.
8. Al-Abri SA, Olson KR: Baking soda can settle the stomach but upset the heart: Case files of the Medical Toxicology Fellowship at the University of California, San Francisco. *J Med Toxicol* 9(3):255–258, 2013.
9. Kraut JA, Madias NE: Lactic acidosis. *N Engl J Med* 371(24):2309, 2014.
10. Lee Hamm L, Hering-Smith KS, Nakhoul NL: Acid–base and potassium homeostasis. *Semin Nephrol* 33(3):257, 2013.
11. Felver L: Acid–base homeostasis and imbalances. In Copstead LC, Banasik JL, editors: *Pathophysiology*, ed 5, St. Louis, 2013, Saunders.
12. Kamel SK, Halperin ML: Acid–base problems in diabetic ketoacidosis. *N Engl J Med* 372(6):546, 2015.
13. Allison MG, McCurdy MT: Alcoholic metabolic emergencies. *Emerg Med Clin North Am* 32(2):293, 2014.
14. Klig JE, Sharma A, Skolnik AB: Case 26-2014: A 21-month-old boy with lethargy, respiratory distress, and abdominal distention. *N Engl J Med* 371(8):767, 2014.
15. Rice M, Ismail B, Pillow MT: Approach to metabolic acidosis in the emergency department. *Emerg Med Clin North Am* 32(2):403, 2014.
16. Soifer JT, Kim HT: Approach to metabolic alkalosis. *Emerg Med Clin North Am* 32(2):453, 2014.
17. Kasper DL, Fauci AS, Hauser SL, et al, editors: *Harrison's principles of internal medicine*, ed 19, New York, 2015, McGraw-Hill.
18. Hale A, Hovey MJ: *Fluid, electrolyte, and acid–base imbalances*, Philadelphia, 2013, Davis.
19. Chen W, Abramowitz MK: Treatment of metabolic acidosis in patients with CKD. *Am J Kidney Dis* 63(2):311, 2014.
20. Tutay GJ, Capraro G, Spirko B, et al: Electrolyte profiles of pediatric patients with hypertrophic pyloric stenosis. *Pediatr Emerg Care* 29(4):465, 2013.
21. Wiener SW: Toxicologic acid–base disorders. *Emerg Med Clin North Am* 32(1):149, 2014.
22. Lian JX: Using ABGs to optimize mechanical ventilation. *Nursing* 43(6):46, 2013.
23. Levi Y, Jeroukhimov I, Peleg K, et al: Base excess as a predictor for injury severity in pediatric trauma patients. *J Emerg Med* 45(4):496, 2013.
24. Kraut JA, Nagami GT: The serum anion gap in the evaluation of acid–base disorders: What are its limitations and can its effectiveness be improved? *Clin J Am Soc Nephrol* 8(11):2018, 2013.
25. Moviat M, van den Boogaard M, Intven F, et al: Stewart analysis of apparently normal acid–base state in the critically ill. *J Crit Care* 28(6):1048, 2013.
26. Giger JN: *Transcultural nursing: Assessment and intervention*, ed 6, St Louis, 2013, Mosby.
27. Peixoto AJ, Alpern RJ: Treatment of severe metabolic alkalosis in a patient with congestive heart failure. *Am J Kidney Dis* 61(5):822, 2013.

Thermoregulation

L. Jane Rosati and Amy Szoka

The human body has the capability of regulating body temperature at a near constant value, a process known as thermoregulation. Temperature regulation is critical for optimal physiological function. Thermoregulation is a foundational nursing concept; thus, it is essential that nurses apply this concept in nursing practice.

DEFINITION

Optimal physiological function of the human body occurs when a near-constant core temperature is maintained. Normal body temperature ranges from 36.2° to 37.6°C (97.0°–100°F), or an average of 37°C (98.6°F).[1] Fluctuation outside this range is an indication of a disease process, strenuous or unusual activity, or extreme environmental exposure. Thermoregulation is defined as *the process of maintaining core body temperature at a near constant value.*[1] The term *normothermia* refers to the state in which body temperature is within the "normal" range. The term *hypothermia* refers to a body temperature below normal range (<36.2°C), and *hyperthermia* refers to a body temperature above normal range (>37.6°C). An extremely high body temperature is referred to as *hyperpyrexia.*

SCOPE

Thermoregulation is an aspect of homeostasis that balances heat gain and heat loss. Body temperatures can range from above normal to below normal; thus, the scope of this concept is considered in this way (Figure 10-1). Physiological adjustments to body temperature are controlled by the hypothalamus—often considered the thermostat center of the body. The nurse uses the average target temperature of 37°C (98.6°F) to assess this state.

NORMAL PHYSIOLOGICAL PROCESS

Thermoregulation occurs through a dynamic and complex physiological process controlled by the hypothalamus that balances heat loss and gain. The hypothalamus establishes a "set point"—meaning the temperature level for optimal physiological functioning. The hypothalamic set point for core body temperature is 37°C (98.6°F). Compensatory and regulatory actions maintain a steady core temperature. When a person sits or stands, walks or runs, digests food, or even changes his or her respiratory rate, regulation of body functions takes place as the body compensates. A basic review of heat production, heat conservation, and heat loss is foundational to an understanding of thermoregulation.

Heat Production and Conservation

Body heat is continually produced through metabolic activity by chemical reactions occurring in the cells. The greatest amount of heat is produced by muscles and through metabolic activity in the liver. Metabolic activity involves the ingestion and metabolism of food and the basal metabolic rate—or the energy required to maintain the body at rest. Basal metabolic rate tends to be higher among younger individuals and decreases as the body ages. Food consumption, physical activity, and hormone levels affect the amount of heat produced. The contraction of muscles produces heat through muscle tone and shivering. Chemical thermogenesis occurs as a result of epinephrine release, which increases metabolic rate. In addition to heat production, the body conserves heat through peripheral vasoconstriction. This process shunts warm blood away from the superficial body tissues and skin surfaces and increases muscle activity to minimize heat loss.

Heat Loss

Not only does the body continually produce heat through metabolic activity but also it continuously loses heat. Heat loss occurs as a result of multiple mechanisms, including radiation, conduction, convection, vasodilation, evaporation, reduced muscle activity, and increased respiration.

Heat loss to *radiation* occurs through a process of electromagnetic waves that emit heat from skin surfaces to the air. The degree of heat loss through radiation is directly related to the difference between ambient air temperature, skin temperature, and exposure. *Conduction* is a transfer of heat through direct contact of one surface to another; warmer surfaces lose heat to cooler surfaces. A loss of heat by air currents (caused by wind or a fan) moving across the body surface is referred to as *convection.*[2] Warmer air at the body surface is replaced by the cooler air, resulting in cooling of the skin surface. Wet skin or clothing accelerates this process.

In addition to radiation, conduction, and convection, heat loss can occur through other physiological compensatory mechanisms. Heat loss can be increased through peripheral *vasodilation*, which brings a greater volume of blood to the body surface. Increased heat loss occurs by conduction (explained previously). This process is not

FIGURE 10-1 Scope of thermoregulation ranges from hypothermia to normothermia, hyperthermia, and hyperpyrexia.

effective, however, if ambient air temperature is greater than body temperature. A reduction in muscle tone and muscle activity occurs as another mechanism to minimize heat production. This process explains the fatigue or "washed out" feeling experienced in hot weather or after sitting in a hot tub for a period of time.[3] Perspiration is yet another mechanism involved with heat loss; this process is explained by evaporation of moisture from the skin surface. This provides a significant source of heat reduction and normally accounts for 600 mL of water loss per day. In extreme heat, an individual can lose as much as 4 L of fluids in an hour; for this reason, replacement of fluids and electrolytes is essential to prevent dehydration. Heat is also lost during the process of respiration. Cool ambient air is inhaled and warmed in the respiratory tract and by the microcirculation within the alveoli. The warmed air is then exhaled. For this reason, elevated respiratory rates are seen among individuals with elevated temperature, and lower respiratory rates are seen in individuals with hypothermia.

Temperature Control

Temperature control is mediated by the hypothalamus through hormonal control. The hypothalamus is located below the thalamus in an area of the brain called the diencephalon. This is a small but important part of the brain located between the midbrain and the cerebrum (Figure 10-2).

Thermoregulation involves a negative feedback system, which reverses or opposes a change in a controlled condition.[3] Multiple thermoreceptors are located throughout the body. Peripheral thermoreceptors (located in the skin) and central thermoreceptors (located in the spinal cord, abdominal organs, and hypothalamus) provide skin and core temperature information to the hypothalamus. The hypothalamus activates a series of responses to lower or raise body temperature based on information received by the thermoreceptors.

When the thermoreceptors signal a drop in body temperature, the hypothalamus initiates a series of heat-producing and heat-conserving mechanisms through endocrine and sympathetic nervous system connections. Thyrotropin (or thyroxine)-stimulating hormone–releasing hormone (TSH-RH) is secreted by the hypothalamus, which in turn stimulates the anterior pituitary to release thyroid-stimulating hormone. Thyroid-stimulating hormone acts on the thyroid gland to release thyroxine (T_4), which activates the adrenal medulla to cause the release of epinephrine into the blood. Epinephrine increases heat production by increasing the metabolic rate, stimulating glycolysis, and causing vasoconstriction (see Figure 10-2). The hypothalamus also stimulates the sympathetic nervous system, which triggers the adrenal cortex to increase muscle tone and initiate a shivering and vasoconstriction response.

When the thermoreceptors signal an increase in body temperature, the same mechanisms are reversed (the classic feature of a negative feedback system). The release of TSH-RH is discontinued (thus stopping the T_4 and epinephrine responses), and the sympathetic nervous system is signaled to induce vasodilation, decrease muscle tone, and

initiate sweat production (see Figure 10-2). Sweat glands rapidly produce and release increased levels of perspiration; heat dissipates from the body as sweat evaporates from its surface.

Age-Related Differences

Ineffective thermoregulation occurs at both ends of the age spectrum. Infants and elderly have less efficient physiological mechanisms for heat production and conservation.

Infants

Several important physiological differences among infants exist related to thermoregulation. Newborns do not have heat-conserving capacity; thus, thermoregulation is linked closely with metabolism and oxygen consumption. The newborn infant has a unique source of heat from brown adipose tissue (or brown fat). This tissue is associated with intensified metabolic activity, thus creating greater heat production capacity compared to normal adipose tissue. Brown fat provides an important mechanism for heat production. Because newborn infants generally do not shiver, a process referred to as *nonshivering thermogenesis* (involving increased metabolism and oxygen consumption) helps to offset heat loss.[4] Although newborn infants produce sufficient body heat, they have a propensity for heat loss due to a greater body surface area to weight ratio. The flexed posture of newborns moderates heat loss somewhat by reducing surface area exposure. Another physiological difference leading to newborn heat loss is limited insulation due to a thin layer of subcutaneous fat. Blood vessels are closer to the skin, further contributing to heat loss tendencies.

Thermoregulation becomes more efficient as the infant becomes older. Advanced physiological responses to temperature variations emerge that include the ability of muscles to contract, shivering response, vasoconstriction and vasodilation of the capillaries, and increased adipose tissue.

Older Adults

Several physiological changes associated with aging affect thermoregulation among older adults. Slower circulation, including decreased vasoconstrictor responses, reduced function of thermoregulatory capacity of the skin (including decreased or absent sweating), and reduced heat production (associated with slower metabolic and physical activity), decreased shivering response, and reduced perception of environmental temperature are seen among older adults.[3]

VARIATIONS AND CONTEXT

Variations in body temperature are represented by higher or lower body temperature from normal and are classified into three major categories: fever, hyperthermia, and hypothermia.

Fever

Fever represents a complex pathophysiological reaction involving the immune system in response to *pyrogens* (fever-producing agents) that

Thermostat

HYPOTHALAMUS

INCREASED TEMPERATURE:
Blood vessels dilate, giving flushed appearance.
Sweat glands become more active.

DECREASED TEMPERATURE:
Blood vessels constrict, heat is trapped in deeper tissues.
Sweat glands become less active.
Skeletal muscles contract, causing shivering.

Bus Stop

FIGURE 10-2 Temperature Regulation The hypothalamus controls body temperature and signals for mechanisms to increase heat production or to facilitate heat loss. (Source: From Herlihy B: *The human body in health and illness,* ed 5, St Louis, 2014, Elsevier.)

trigger the hypothalamus in the brain to adjust heat production, heat conservation, and heat loss mechanisms to maintain a higher core temperature, representing an increased hypothalamic set point. (Recall that *set point* is the established value determined by the hypothalamus for optimal physiological function.) There are two kinds of pyrogens. *Exogenous pyrogens* (those of external origin) include bacterial endotoxins, viruses, antigen–antibody complexes, etc. *Endogenous pyrogens* are produced by phagocytic white blood cells as part of the immune response and include interleukin-1, interleukin-6, tumor necrosis factor, and interferon. When exogenous pyrogens invade the body, endogenous pyrogens are released that trigger the production of prostaglandin E_2, which in turn elevates the thermal set point and increases core body temperature.[2]

Hyperthermia

Although elevated body temperature occurs in both hyperthermia and fever, the underlying processes are quite different. Hyperthermia occurs when the body temperature rises above 37.6°C with an unchanged hypothalamic set point. The three physiological mechanisms that coordinate body temperature are also the three mechanisms that can lead to hyperthermia: excessive heat production, inadequate ability to cool, or hypothalamic regulator dysfunction. When heat-related conditions occur, the body's natural ability to dissipate heat is interrupted, resulting in an increase in body temperature that exceeds heat loss. This can occur as a result of several factors, including environment (temperature, humidity, and lack of air movement),

excessive physical exertion (particularly in hot, humid environments without sufficient water replacement), genetic abnormality, metabolic diseases, injury to the hypothalamus, and as a result of pharmacologic agents.

Hypothermia

Hypothermia occurs when the core body temperature declines below 36.2°C and is further classified as mild (34–36°C or 93.2–96.8° F), moderate (30–34°C or 86–93°F), or severe (<30°C or <86°F). Three physiological factors can lead to hypothermia: excessive heat loss, insufficient production of heat, or dysfunction of hypothalamic regulatory mechanisms. Hypothermia may be either accidental or therapeutic. Accidental hypothermia results from environmental exposure (including staying out in the cold too long, wearing insufficient clothing for weather conditions, wet clothing, and cold water submersion) or as a complication from serious systemic disorders. Therapeutic hypothermia is intentionally induced to reduce metabolism and thereby preserve tissue by preventing tissue ischemia.

CONSEQUENCES

Although the body tolerates some variation in body temperature, physiological consequences can occur as a result of elevated or lowered temperature. The two variables that affect the extent of consequences for hypothermia and hypothermia are (1) the extent of temperature change and (2) the duration of temperature variation.

Consequences of Hyperthermia

A significant increase in body temperature leads to many physiological changes that can be fatal as a result of cardiovascular collapse and damage to the nervous system. Mentioned previously, one compensatory response to elevation in body temperature is sweating—a measure that helps to cool the body. Excessive and prolonged sweating coupled with a sustained high body temperature can result in sodium loss and dehydration if fluid replacement does not occur. Over time, excessive body temperature can lead to hypotension, tachycardia, and decreased cardiac output, progressing to reduced perfusion and coagulation within the microcirculation and cardiovascular collapse. Sustained high core body temperature coupled with reduced perfusion leads to cerebral edema, central nervous system degeneration, and renal necrosis.

Consequences of Hypothermia

The physiological consequences of hypothermia are dependent on the severity and duration of exposure. As core body temperature decreases, compensatory mechanisms including shivering (muscle contraction to simulate warmth) and vasoconstriction (to reduce heat loss) occur. However, because prolonged vasoconstriction would lead to peripheral tissue ischemia, intermittent reperfusion of peripheral tissues occurs. Prolonged hypothermia eventually leads to reduced perfusion in the microcirculation attributable to increased viscosity of the blood and reduced blood flow and coagulation. Also, the vasoconstrictive efforts controlled by the hypothalamus eventually fail, causing vasodilation and thus accelerating the loss of body heat. Individuals experiencing significant hypothermia have been known to remove clothing because of reduced cognition and because the vasodilation can create a false warming sensation.

RISK FACTORS

Risk factors can be described in terms of both populations at risk and individual risk factors. Recognition of risk factors is essential so that appropriate preventive measures can be initiated. Risk factors that affect thermoregulation include age, environment, and physiological condition of the individual.

Populations at Risk

Although all humans are at risk for alterations in thermoregulation, certain population groups have significantly greater risk—particularly the very young and the very old.

Infants and Young Children

Infants (particularly premature infants) have undeveloped temperature regulation capacity. Infants usually produce sufficient body heat, but they lack the ability to conserve heat produced; a large surface area relative to body mass makes them susceptible to excessive temperature loss.[4] Infants and young children are also at risk because they are unable to independently take measures to correct changes in temperature. They are completely dependent on the appropriate actions of caregivers for maintenance of a normothermic temperature range. Unfortunately a number of heat-related deaths among children result from being left in vehicles, in which life-threatening temperatures develop quickly.[5]

Older Adults

The elderly experience fluctuations in temperature because of a diminished ability to regulate body temperature due to a less effective thermoregulatory response (described previously).[2] The elderly also have a reduced perception of heat and cold; thus, they may not recognize when to take appropriate action in a timely manner. Elderly who lack resources to stay warm or cool in temperature extremes are also at risk for thermodysregulation. According to the Centers for Disease Control and Prevention (CDC), heat- and cold-related deaths drastically rise among adults older than age 75 years.[6]

Other Population Groups

The risk for heat- and cold-related deaths is twice as high for males compared to females, and non-Hispanic Blacks have higher rates of heat-related and cold-related deaths than any other race and ethnic group. The CDC reported that non-Hispanic Blacks had a heat-related mortality rate 2.5 times that of non-Hispanic Whites; likewise, non-Hispanic Blacks had a cold-related mortality rate 2.0 times that of non-Hispanic Whites.[6] People of low socioeconomic status may lack resources for adequate clothing, heating, and cooling. The homeless population (because of their frequent exposure to the elements and lack of adequate shelter) is particularly at high risk for hyperthermia or hypothermia. Populations living in certain geographical areas in the United States that have hot or cold climates are also at increased risk. Most heat-related deaths occur in the southern and western states; western states also have the highest cold-related death rates.[6]

Individual Risk Factors

Impaired Cognition

Individuals with impairments in cognition (either acute or chronic) are at risk for imbalanced temperature because of the potential inability to recognize dangerous environmental exposures or the inability to react appropriately. Persons under the influence of drugs or alcohol are at risk because sensory alterations affect judgment or there may be a loss of consciousness, thus increasing the risk for environmental exposure. Because alcohol acts as a vasodilator (dilation of surface blood vessels leads to loss of body heat), it is a common underlying factor in hypothermic deaths.[6]

Underlying Health Conditions

A number of medical conditions are associated with altered thermoregulation (Box 10-1). Individuals with preexisting medical conditions (e.g., congestive heart failure, diabetes, or gait disturbance) are at increased risk for hypothermia because their bodies have a reduced

---

BOX 10-1 Medical Conditions as Risk Factors for Altered Thermoregulation

- Autoimmune conditions
- Burns
- Chronic medical conditions
- Hypothalamic injury
  - Traumatic brain injury
  - Stroke
  - Brain neoplasm
- Infection
- Inflammation
- Long surgical procedures
- Metabolic conditions
  - Hyperthyroidism
  - Hypothyroidism
- Prematurity/preterm birth
- Protein calorie malnutrition
- Traumatic injury

ability to generate heat. Individuals who undergo surgical procedures are also at risk for hypothermia, particularly if the procedure is long.[7,8] Poor nutritional status also places an individual at increased risk for hypothermia.

Several medical conditions (infections, autoimmune disorders, trauma, and thyroid disturbances) place individuals at risk for elevated body temperature. Dehydration may also be associated with elevated body temperature because of the need for fluids to cool the body. Individuals who have experienced traumatic brain injury are at risk for problems with thermoregulation, particularly if the area of the brain damaged leads to hypothalamic dysfunction.[1]

Genetics

A less common risk factor for impaired thermoregulation is genetic predisposition. The classic example of this is malignant hyperthermia, a condition associated with an inherited autosomal dominant pattern. Malignant hyperthermia is often considered a surgical complication because it is actually a biochemical chain reaction triggered by commonly used general anesthetics and succinylcholine.

Recreational or Occupational Exposures

Individuals may suffer impairments in thermoregulation as a consequence of participating in recreational activities or working in conditions associated with temperature extremes. Strenuous activity in high ambient temperatures, particularly with high humidity, can lead to hyperthermia. Winter recreational activities such as hiking, snowmobiling, and skiing can lead to hypothermia if an individual has inadequate clothing for the activity or if the individual becomes lost or injured. Cold water exposure also quickly leads to hypothermia, particularly if the air temperature is also cold.[9]

ASSESSMENT

Body temperature is included in nearly all assessments because this provides baseline information about homeostasis and general health. When problems associated with thermoregulation present, a history and examination are warranted.

History

Typically, a history does not include specific questions related to normal body temperature or thermoregulation. However, in the event of thermoregulation imbalance, a history provides valuable information needed to understand the problem. The age, health history, family history (for malignant hyperthermia), and social history provide necessary information to establish risk factors. Additional questions include presence of recent injury, illnesses, or environmental exposure. If there has been recent environmental exposure, the type, severity, and length of exposure should be determined.

Symptoms associated with hyperthermia vary depending on degree of elevated temperature and underlying conditions. Reported symptoms may include "feeling feverish" or "feeling hot," chills, general malaise, lethargy, weakness, dizziness, loss of appetite, or muscle cramps. The primary symptom most commonly associated with hypothermia is feeling cold.

Examination Findings
Vital Signs

Nursing assessment for alterations in thermoregulation begins with a set of vital signs. Body temperature is measured using a thermometer. The most common routes to measure temperature include oral, rectal, auxiliary, temporal artery, and tympanic.[10] However, when an individual has hyperthermia or hypothermia, the most reliable means

available for assessing core temperature is a rectal temperature. A lubricated probe is inserted into the rectal canal at a depth of 1–1.5 in. in the adult and 0.5–1 in. in the child. In the critical care setting, the pulmonary artery catheter may be used to measure core temperature. Additional core temperature sites include the esophagus and urinary bladder.[11]

Temperature measurement among infants and children can be accomplished with tympanic thermometer, oral thermometer (a pacifier thermometer), axillary, or temporal artery, although the temporal artery method may not be as reliable in children younger than age 2 years.

Hyperthermia

Although the general appearance of an individual experiencing hyperthermia varies (depending on the underlying cause and the degree of temperature elevation), several common clinical findings are observed. Vasodilation occurs, causing the skin to appear flushed and warm or hot to touch. If the sweat mechanism has been activated, the individual will be diaphoretic, although this finding may be absent. Patients will often present with dry skin and mucous membranes, decreased urinary output, and other signs of dehydration and electrolyte imbalance. Because of the effects of high body temperature on the brain and central nervous system, seizures may occur and the patient's cognitive status may range from slightly confused or delirious to coma.

Hypothermia

The clinical presentation of hypothermic patients also varies, depending on the severity of the condition. Peripheral vasoconstriction causes the skin to feel cool and have slow capillary refill; skin color is pale and becomes cyanotic. Muscle rigidity and shivering is typically present in an effort to generate heat. The shivering response diminishes or ceases when the core temperature decreases to 30°C. Cognition is affected because of a gradual reduction in cerebral blood flow. A person may experience poor coordination and sluggish thought processes at 34°C; this progresses to confusion and eventually stupor and coma by the time the temperature decreases to 30°C. Dysrhythmias (e.g., atrial and ventricular fibrillation) may occur due to myocardial irritability. As hypothermia progresses, the metabolic rate declines and perfusion of blood is significantly reduced, leading to diminished urinary function, coma, and cardiovascular collapse.[12]

CLINICAL MANAGEMENT
Primary Prevention

Most cases of hyperthermia and hypothermia are preventable by reducing risk. The nurse's role in primary prevention is through patient education. Avoidance of exposure to temperature extremes is an obvious way to prevent problems associated with thermoregulation. When this is unavoidable, planning is essential to ensure adequate resources are available. Primary prevention measures include environmental control and shelter, appropriate clothing for different conditions, and physical activity.

Environmental Control and Shelter

Maintaining optimal ambient temperature in the home or having adequate shelter during temperature extremes is essential. If a home does not have air conditioning in the summer months, opening windows and using fans are encouraged. If home heating is inadequate during cold weather, patients should be advised to wear adequate and/ or additional clothing and use blankets for additional warmth. Wind drafts should be blocked and curtains hung at windows to improve insulation.

Community resources, including homeless shelters, can be used to assist those who are unable to stay cool during warm months and warm during the cold months. Individuals can also be encouraged to go to public buildings such as indoor shopping malls or libraries, where ambient temperatures are usually adequately regulated. For those exposed to the elements, seeking adequate shelter can be life-saving. Shelter includes finding shade and ideally a breeze when temperatures are high and avoiding the wind and precipitation when temperatures are low.

Appropriate Clothing

The selection of appropriate clothing is another primary prevention strategy. Although this applies for both types of temperature extremes, adequate clothing is essential to prevent hypothermia with cold temperatures. Evaporative heat loss is five times greater when clothing is wet; thus, dry clothing is essential. A newborn is susceptible to rapid heat loss directly after birth, and hypothermia may result. Immediately after delivery, the infant should be dried quickly, wrapped in blankets, and moved to a heated environment. Care should be taken to limit the time the infant's skin is wet (e.g., bathing and wet diapers or clothing).

Patients should be advised to dress in layers and cover the head. New parents should be instructed about heat loss in newborns and young children; dressing the infant and child appropriately for the weather and adequate regulation of temperature in the home are essential. When environmental temperature is low, infants should be provided with a hat to guard against heat loss, just as the elderly patient may need a sweater or clothing with long sleeves for comfort. The elderly (or their caregivers) may need to be reminded to dress in clothing appropriate for the weather.

Physical Activity

Physical activity increases body temperature. Increasing physical activity helps to warm the body when exposed to low temperatures and can prevent hypothermia. Physical exertion in hot conditions increases risk for hyperthermia because the heat gains may exceed heat loss. Resting, maintaining adequate hydration, wearing appropriate clothing, and seeking shelter will help to reduce risk under such conditions.

Secondary Prevention (Screening)

The goal of secondary prevention refers to the detection of a disease or condition. The only screening mechanism that applies to the concept of thermoregulation is screening for malignant hyperthermia (MH). Because susceptibility to MH is inherited (autosomal dominant disorder), genetic screening is available and recommended for individuals who have relatives with genetic mutations.

Collaborative Interventions

Management of the patient with altered thermoregulation is dependent on the core body temperature and the overall physical condition of the individual. Generally, infants and young children, the elderly, and individuals in poor health not only have greater risk factors but also have less physical capacity for physiological compensation when changes in core body temperature occur.

Elevated Body Temperature

The underlying cause of the elevated body temperature should be identified (e.g., a fever associated with an inflammatory process or hyperthermia associated with exposure). Regardless of the cause, the goal is to minimize cardiovascular and neurologic complications associated with excessive body temperature. Care of the individual whose temperature has exceeded 37°C should include removal of excess blanketing and clothing while observing for continued signs of hyperthermia (increased respiration, increased or decreased perspiration, high fever, and seizures). Signs and symptoms that persist beyond 1 hour require further intervention. Hydration, nutritional support, and other palliative measures to reduce core temperature should be implemented. Cool packs may be placed in the axillary and groin areas; a cooling blanket or lukewarm bath may also facilitate temperature reduction. Care should be taken to not induce shivering. More aggressive cooling efforts include gastric or colonic lavage with cool fluids.

The presence of fever is considered an expected finding with a systemic inflammatory response. Mild to moderate fever generally does little harm and may actually have beneficial effects to counteract the inflammation. However, complications such as dehydration and increased metabolic demand can occur.[13] Symptomatic relief of persistent or intermittent fevers can be treated with antipyretics such as nonsteroidal anti-inflammatory drugs (e.g., naproxen or ibuprofen and aspirin) and acetaminophen. Aspirin is also useful for reducing fever but should be used with caution; aspirin is not recommended for children because of the risk of Reye's syndrome. The use of a drug called dantrolene sodium can reverse the effects of malignant hyperthermia. Intracellular calcium levels are elevated in malignant hyperthermia; dantrolene counteracts this abnormality by reducing muscle tone and metabolism. Administration of dantrolene intravenously has dramatically reduced the mortality rate of malignant hyperthermia.[14]

Hypothermia

The goal of managing hypothermic patients is to increase the body temperature to the normal range. An initial step is to remove the individual from the cold. If hypothermia is mild, passive and active external rewarming measures are indicated. Passive measures include dry and warm clothing, warm drinks, and exercise, and these may be sufficient. However, active rewarming measures may be necessary and include providing warm blankets or heating pads, drawing a warm water bath, and placing the patient in a heated environment.

CLINICAL NURSING SKILLS FOR THERMOREGULATION

- Assessment
- Monitoring vital signs
  - Temperature measurement
  - Heart rate
  - Respiratory rate
  - Blood pressure
- External warming devices
  - Warm blankets
  - Administer warm oral fluids
- Active core warming
  - Warm intravenous fluids
  - Heated humidified oxygen
  - Warm fluid lavage
- Cooling measures
  - Cool water bath
  - Cool intravenous fluids
  - Cool fluid lavage
  - Cooling blankets

FIGURE 10-3 Thermoregulation and Interrelated Concepts

When core body temperature falls below 30°C, active core rewarming measures are indicated—meaning there is an application of heat directly to the core. Core rewarming should be done slowly and carefully to minimize the risk of triggering dysrhythmias; thus, continuous cardiac monitoring and core body temperature observation are necessary. Active core rewarming strategies include infusion of warm intravenous solutions, gastric lavage with warm fluid, peritoneal lavage with warm fluid, and inhalation of warmed oxygen. If hypothermia is severe, cardiopulmonary bypass or arteriovenous rewarming may be indicated.[9]

INTERRELATED CONCEPTS

A large number of concepts are clearly interrelated to thermoregulation. Those that have greatest importance are presented in Figure 10-3.

Infection is defined as the invasion and multiplication of microorganisms in body tissues, which may be clinically unapparent or result in local cellular injury due to competitive metabolism, toxins, intracellular replication, or antigen–antibody response. When infection is present, physical symptoms often include fever and chills. Because the hypothalamus regulates body temperature, Intracranial Regulation is closely associated with thermoregulation. Traumatic brain injury, with its associated cerebral edema, ischemia, energy failure, oxidative stress, and neuronal death, may directly affect the temperature control center.[15] Often, when injury occurs to the brain or spinal cord, there is interruption of the sympathetic nervous system that prevents peripheral temperature sensations from reaching the hypothalamus. Perfusion is impacted by body temperature. Measures to minimize or maximize heat loss include vasodilation and vasoconstriction within the blood vessels; severe extremes in body temperature can result in cardiovascular collapse. The skin plays an important role in body temperature regulation. The skin acts as a protective layer to reduce heat loss. In addition, thermoreceptors in the skin alert all individuals to extremes in temperatures, thus preventing injury. These mechanisms require intact skin and Tissue Integrity. Metabolism of nutrients provides the body with fuel needed for the generation of heat and body activities. Malnutrition increases risk for hypothermia because of an inability to generate adequate heat. For this reason,

BOX 10-2 EXEMPLARS OF ALTERED THERMOREGULATION

- Fever
- Hyperthermia
- Heat cramps
- Heat exhaustion
- Heatstroke
- Malignant hyperthermia
- Hypothermia
- Frostbite
- Therapeutic hypothermia

Nutrition is interrelated with thermoregulation. Fluid and Electrolytes are affected by thermoregulation. Efficient perspiration requires adequate fluid balances. Fluid and electrolyte imbalances can occur when excessive body temperature exhausts available fluids for perspiration.

CLINICAL EXEMPLARS

Although there are many situations and conditions that can cause altered thermoregulation, the distinct exemplars are fairly straightforward (Box 10-2). It is beyond the scope of this book to describe all possible causative factors and exemplars in detail, although brief descriptions of featured exemplars are presented next. Refer to medical surgical, pediatric, geriatric, critical care, and other textbooks for detailed information about exemplars.

Featured Exemplars
Fever

The most common exemplar of thermoregulation is fever. Fever is a temporary elevation in body temperature caused by the immune system's release of endogenous pyrogens (a protein produced by leukocytes) in response to an invasion of bacteria, viruses, fungi, toxins, or drugs. Specifically, pyrogens trigger the hypothalamus to increase the thermostatic set point. The elevated body temperature is thought to increase the production of white blood cells, thus enhancing the immune system response. Fever can also occur due to an exaggerated immune response such as autoimmune disorders or allergic reaction.

Malignant Hyperthermia

Malignant hyperthermia (MH) is a hypermetabolic disorder of skeletal muscle triggered by the induction of anesthetic agents and leads to severe hyperthermia. Susceptibility to MH is inherited as an autosomal dominant disorder; several forms of genetic mutations increase susceptibility. Many of these gene mutations are linked to inherited muscle diseases such as central core disease and multi-minicore disease. Epidemiologic studies reveal that malignant hyperthermia complicates 1 in approximately 100,000 surgeries in adults and 1 in approximately 30,000 surgical procedures in children.[14]

Heatstroke

Heatstroke occurs as a result of exposure to excessively high temperatures in the environment. The condition often occurs when performing physical exertion in a hot environment without proper ventilation. Hyperthermia results because the body cannot adequately cool itself and keep the temperature at the correct level. The central nervous system may not be functioning properly due to disease or injury. The condition is characterized by alterations in mental status, an increase in body temperature, with hot dry skin; severe conditions can be fatal.

Preterm and Newborn Hypothermia

Preterm and newborn hypothermia occurs with heat loss by radiation, evaporation, and conduction. Mechanisms of heat loss cause the newborn to be dependent on environmental temperature to keep warm. It is recommended that a newborn's axillary temperature be regulated at 36.5°C or 97.8°F. A subnormal temperature requires a radiant warmer for additional heat. Preterm infants are often kept under a radiant warmer or in an incubator with protection from draft air. Swaddling, a cap for the head, and/or skin-to-skin contact are additional ways to keep the infant warm.

Environmental Exposure Hypothermia

Environmental exposure hypothermia occurs from exposure to cold temperature or immersion in cold water; it is exacerbated by weather elements such as precipitation, humidity, and wind. Without proper clothing or shelter, environmental exposure presents a challenge to thermoregulatory systems of the body. The body compensates by initiating thermoregulatory mechanisms such as shivering and vasoconstriction, but eventually a hypothermic state occurs if the exposure is extensive in time and/or severity. Hypothermia due to environmental exposure can occur at any age, although very young and older adults are at greatest risk.[6]

CASE STUDY

Source: shironosov/iStock/Thinkstock

Case Presentation

Tom Anderson is an 86-year-old white male who lives with his 82-year-old wife in their home in upstate New York. During the past few years, Mrs. Anderson has noticed a decline in her husband's mental status. Early on a January morning, Mrs. Anderson was awaked at 4 AM by the doorbell. When she opened the door, a neighbor was standing with her husband, who was wearing nothing but his pajamas. The neighbor explained that he saw Mr. Anderson wandering outside on the snowy street. Tom was shivering uncontrollably and confused; the outdoor temperature was only 19°F. Mrs. Anderson immediately called 911 and had her husband transported to the hospital.

Upon arrival to the emergency department, the nurse noted the following assessment findings:

- Mental status: Confused; not oriented to person, place, or time
- Vital signs: Temperature, 33.1°C rectally; pulse, 62 beats/min; respirations, 12 breaths/min; blood pressure, 100/62 mm Hg
- Skin: Pale, cyanosis around lips and extremities
- Uncontrollable shivering

The nurse immediately placed Mr. Anderson in a dry gown, covered him with warming blankets, and placed him in a warm room. The findings were immediately reported to the physician, and the following measures were implemented:

- Stat electrocardiogram followed by continuous cardiac monitoring
- Continuous vital sign and pulse oximeter monitoring
- Intravenous infusion of 1000 mL of 0.9% normal saline to run over 8 hours; solution to be warmed to 98.6°F
- Cover patient with warming blanket set at 98.6°F
- Apply warm oxygen at 3 L/min via nasal cannula
- Blood draw for hemoglobin and hematocrit, electrolytes, blood gases, blood urea nitrogen and creatinine, blood glucose, and toxicology screen

After several hours in the emergency department, Mr. Anderson's core body temperature slowly increased to 35.4°C; he stabilized but remained confused. He was admitted to the medical unit for further evaluation.

Case Analysis

The case illustrates several aspects of this concept. Risk factors include age, altered cognition, and environmental exposure. The clinical findings were consistent with hypothermia. The treatment measures center on passive and active rewarming interventions.

REFERENCES

1. Braine M: The role of the hypothalamus. Part 1: The regulation of temperature and hunger. *Br J Neurosci Nurs* 5(2):66–72, 2009.
2. McCance K, Huether S: *Pathophysiology*, ed 6, St Louis, 2010, Mosby.
3. Thibodeau G, Patton K: *Structure and function of the body*, ed 14, St Louis, 2011, Elsevier.
4. Hockenberry M, Wilson D: *Wong's nursing care of infants and children*, ed 9, St Louis, 2011, Mosby.
5. San Jose State University, Department of Geosciences: Hyperthermia deaths of children in vehicles, 2011. Retrieved from <http://ggweather.com/heat>.
6. Centers for Disease Control and Prevention: Deaths attributed to heat, cold, and other weather events in the United States, 2006–2010, *National Health Statistics Reports*, 76, July 2014, <http://www.cdc.gov/nchs/data/nhsr/nhsr076.pdf>.
7. Uzoigwe CE, Khan A, Smith RP, et al: Hypothermia and low body temperature are common and associated with high mortality in hip fracture patients. *Hip Int* 24(3):237–242, 2014.
8. Kiekkas P, Theodorakopoulou G, Stefanopoulos N, et al: Post-operative hypothermia and mortality in critically ill adults: Review and meta-analysis. *Aust J Adv Nurs* 28(4):60–67, 2011.
9. Lewis S, Dirksen S, Heitkemper M, et al: *Medical–surgical nursing: Assessment and management of clinical problems*, St Louis, 2011, Mosby.
10. Ball JW, Dains JE, Flynn JA, et al: *Seidel's guide to physical examination*, ed 8, St Louis, 2015, Elsevier.
11. Lawson L, Bridges EJ, Ballou I, et al: Accuracy and precision of noninvasive temperature measurement in adult intensive care patients. *Am J Crit Care* 16(5):485–496, 2007.
12. Miller CA: *Nursing for wellness in older adults*, ed 6, Philadelphia, 2011, Lippincott Williams & Wilkins, pp 530–538.
13. Mayo Clinic. Fever, 2014. Retrieved from <http://www.mayoclinic.org/diseases-conditions/fever/basics/complications/con-20019229>.
14. Malignant Hyperthermia Association of the United States (MHAUS): Current concepts in the understanding of malignant hyperthermia, 2014. Retrieved from <http://www.anesthesiologynews.com/download/MalignantHyperthermia_ANO214_WM.pdf>.
15. Tran LV: Understanding the pathophysiology of traumatic brain injury and the mechanisms of action of neuro-protective interventions. *J Trauma Nurs* 21(1):30–35, 2014.

CONCEPT
11

Sleep

Beth Rodgers

Sleep is an essential component of life. The adequacy of sleep affects physiological, psychological, and social functioning. Sufficient quality sleep is crucial to metabolic regulation, cognitive functioning, quality of life, mood, and nearly every other aspect of existence. Sufficient quality of sleep is required to decrease risks for devastating chronic conditions that affect the respiratory, cardiovascular, metabolic, and endocrine systems. Despite the critical nature of sleep, a large percentage of people report that their sleep is inadequate either in quantity or in quality.[1] This widespread problem with sleep deprivation constitutes a significant public health concern because people are at greater risk for chronic illness, decreased quality of life, and accidents and injuries due to what often are very treatable problems with sleep.[2-9] Nurses in all settings have an important role in identifying sleep problems, instituting effective strategies to improve sleep, and promoting healthy sleep as part of an overall program of wellness and disease management.

DEFINITION

People tend to think they have a good understanding of sleep, especially because everyone does it and, in fact, every living mammal engages in sleep. It does not seem very complicated to close your eyes and drift into a state detached from the busy day of wakefulness. Sleep really is quite complex, however, even more so because the activities and events associated with sleep take place completely outside of the individual awareness. The very nature of sleep means that the person who is sleeping is not aware of the process. Historically, sleep was considered to be merely a period of inactivity. With the development of the ability to monitor brain activity, however, it became apparent that sleep really is a period of considerable action. In more recent years, researchers have discovered that a large number of physiological processes take place during sleep, including neurologic, metabolic, and endocrine activity.

Sleep is a relatively new field of study, and specialization and dictionary definitions often do not match the prevailing state of science. The *Oxford Dictionary of English*, for example, presents a definition of sleep as "a condition of body and mind such as that which typically recurs for several hours every night, in which the nervous system is relatively inactive, the eyes closed, the postural muscles relaxed, and consciousness practically suspended."[10] This definition is partially accurate, but it fails to acknowledge the essential processes that take place during sleep. Merriam–Webster presents a similar approach,

with the definition of sleep as "the natural periodic suspension of consciousness during which the powers of the body are restored."[11] All definitions have in common a change in consciousness that includes loss of awareness of the surrounding environment. More detailed definitions can be very specific about what is happening in the brain or in differentiating specific stages of sleep. For general purposes, the most important idea is that sleep is *natural, necessary, involves a shift in physiological and neurologic activity, and is intended to be restorative.*

SCOPE

Sleep occurs in a cyclic pattern following intermittent periods of wakefulness for the majority of humans. The time spent in sleep varies across individuals, as does the time of day during which sleep occurs. Despite such natural variation, there is a recurring need in all humans for a period of physical inactivity and a change in level of consciousness that allows for restoration and for specific physiological mechanisms to take place. Ideally, after a quality period of sleep, the individual returns to an alert state feeling refreshed and restored.

For a variety of reasons, some people may not feel restored and refreshed after a period of sleep. This may be due to lifestyle or behavior patterns that prevent the individual from receiving the needed volume and quality of sleep. Lack of restorative sleep also may be indicative of a "sleep disorder," which is a diagnosis of a specific pattern of sleep that is not compatible with the health needs of the individual.

Thus, from a broad perspective, the scope of sleep ranges from restorative sleep that results in an individual feeling rested to impaired sleep leaving the individual not feeling rested or refreshed. Impaired sleep can be intermittent or chronic, with chronic sleep being associated with physical, cognitive, and social challenges (Figure 11-1).

NORMAL PHYSIOLOGICAL PROCESS

Following a period of wakefulness, humans need to enter a period of rest and sleep that enables them to experience physiological restoration. Sleep occurs in stages and, under normal circumstances, in a fairly consistent pattern of movement through the stages. In general, the stages of sleep can be divided into two major categories: non-rapid eye movement (NREM) and rapid eye movement (REM) sleep. In normal sleep, the individual proceeds through four stages of NREM sleep and

FIGURE 11-1 Scope of Sleep

then to the REM stage (Figure 11-2). Movement must be through all four stages before reaching REM. Each stage lasts generally from 5 to 15 minutes, and the entire cycle through all four stages plus REM typically takes 90–110 minutes. The duration of REM sleep gets progressively longer during the night, producing more deep sleep consistent with this state.

Non-Rapid Eye Movement Sleep

In stage 1 (N1 or NREM stage 1), referred to as light sleep, the individual can be awakened easily. In this stage, brain waves slow and, on EEG, the slower wave pattern known as alpha waves appears. The individual at this point is likely to drift in and out of sleep and can be awakened easily. Sensations known as hypnagogic hallucinations can occur during this stage. A common sensation of this type is the feeling of falling. Uncontrolled muscle jerks sometimes occur at this stage along with sudden movements that can startle the individual and restore wakefulness.

In stage 2 (N2), eye movement ceases; brain waves become even slower, with the exception of an occasional burst or more rapid brain waves. Pulse rate and respirations slow, and body temperature decreases as the individual moves toward deeper stages of sleep. Stage 3 (N3) and stage 4 (N4) are the periods of deep sleep. N3 is characterized by very slow brain waves called delta waves interspersed with smaller, faster waves. In N4, the EEG shows almost exclusively delta waves. In this type of sleep, it is difficult to awaken the individual and muscle activity is very limited or may be completely absent. A person awakened from stage 3 or 4 of sleep could be disoriented for a brief period of time before regaining awareness.

Presleep sleepiness

FIGURE 11-2 Stages of Adult Sleep Cycle (Source: From Potter PA, Perry AG: *Fundamentals of nursing*, ed 8, St Louis, 2013, Mosby.)

Rapid Eye Movement Sleep

REM sleep commonly begins approximately 90 minutes after the onset of sleep. The first REM period may be rather short, sometimes lasting only 10 minutes. Periods of REM become progressively longer as the individual completes successive sleep cycles, and the final period of REM may last as long as 1 hour. EEGs of REM sleep show patterns of brain activity that are very similar to those produced when an individual is awake. In individuals who have normal sleep patterns (i.e., no sleep disorder), cardiac and respiratory rates increase and become uneven, and the rapid eye movement for which this stage is named takes place. This also is the stage of active dreaming related to the increase in brain activity. Although the brain is more active, there is a form of muscular paralysis that prevents the individual, in normal circumstances, from engaging in movement or other action that could be very dangerous given the activity of the brain during this time.

Restorative Processes of Sleep

Deep sleep is essential for the body to accomplish important restorative processes. Not only does such restoration contribute to wakefulness and alertness during non-sleeping hours but also the body undertakes a number of important physical processes, including tissue regeneration, muscle and bone development, and immune enhancement. Regulation of body metabolism and fat deposition also are affected by the depth and duration of deep sleep. Other hormones associated with sleep and essential for health include cortisol, human growth hormone, and leptin and ghrelin—the hormones that regulate appetite and body fat deposition. Sex and reproductive hormones also are affected by sleep and include secretion of testosterone and hormones associated with fertility—follicle-stimulating hormone and luteinizing hormone. An increase in the hormone melatonin at the onset of sleep helps to promote and maintain sleep, and a decrease in levels leads to eventual awakening. The immune system is enhanced as well during sleep as proteins associated with fighting illness are produced. The circadian rhythm, or the typical 24-hour (more or less) cycle through which the body passes, including both awake and sleep cycles, is responsible for regulating all of the physiological processes in the body. An adequate amount and quality of sleep, therefore, is essential to all of the regulatory mechanisms that take place in the body.

Age-Related Differences

Sleep is quite consistent throughout the lifespan in regard to physiological processes and the need for restoration and renewal. There also is general consistency in the circadian rhythm. Normal variations that occur with aging pertain primarily to the amount of total sleep needed and the amount of time spent in the various stages of sleep. Individual variation does occur and, in many cases, can be considered within normal limits. Such variation is discussed later. The most noticeable changes associated with age include the amount of sleep and the sleep architecture (the constitution of the sleep pattern). The amount of sleep typically needed by people in each age group is as follows:[12-15]

- Infants: 14–16 hours each day
- Toddlers: 9 or 10 hours at night in addition to 2 or 3 hours of daytime naps
- School-age children: 9–11 hours
- Teenagers: 9 hours
- Adults: 7–9 hours

It is important to remember that these are general recommendations and some variation will occur. Infants tend to sleep in shorter periods but with multiple episodes of sleep throughout the day. Sleep time gradually decreases during the first several months of life so that by approximate age 6 months, the infant can sleep throughout the night with at least one nap during the day. Infants spend as much as 50% of their sleep time in REM compared to approximately 20% in adults. EEG differences have been documented to show changes in brain activity that occur in sleep at different stages of life.[15]

Older adults may have more difficulty falling asleep, an occurrence referred to as increased sleep latency. They also may experience more awakenings during the night, which leads to a fragmented sleep pattern. Older adults often will awaken more quickly when aroused from sleep. The amount of time spent in deep sleep may decrease, with a corresponding increase in the time spent in N2. These are not necessarily age-related changes; it is likely that medical conditions, such as pain, discomfort, and medication side effects, interfere with the quality of sleep in older adults. Nonetheless, this pattern of changes in latency and time spent in various stages of sleep is very common as adults age.

VARIATIONS AND CONTEXT

The National Sleep Foundation conducts periodic studies of sleep habits and outcomes in the United States. In its 2008 study, 49% of people reported not feeling well rested at least several nights per week in the prior month, 65% reported experiencing some type of sleep problem several nights or more per week in the prior month, and 28% reported sleepiness interfering with their daily functioning at least a couple of days per week. This survey has shown consistently that sufficient quality and quantity of sleep are ongoing problems for adults in the United States.

Poor Sleep Patterns

Although the amount of sleep needed by each individual varies, research has shown that those who claim they function well on minimal sleep actually respond to tests in a manner consistent with someone who is sleep-deprived. In addition, they are at greater risk of physical problems consistent with inadequate sleep regardless of their subjective assessment of functioning and sleep quality.[1]

Many variations in sleep are the result of controllable phenomena: personal choices about bedtime; dietary habits, ingestion of alcohol or stimulants, frequent napping, and so on. The environment in which someone sleeps can lead to poor sleep quality as well—for example, noise or disruptive light, a television left on, a bed partner who moves frequently or snores, or a lack of safety in the home environment. Caregiving responsibilities, such as ill or elderly housemates or infants and children with interrupted sleep patterns, can affect the sleep of others in the vicinity. Work and job responsibilities may result in poor sleep due to fragmentation as a result of working more than one job or problems associated with shift work. Any of these can result in a substantial disturbance in sleep. Situational challenges such as worry or stress also can contribute to periodic episodes of ineffective sleep. In such situations, it is common for an individual to have difficulty falling asleep or remaining asleep. Waking several times during the night to deal with worries or stress easily can lead to ineffective sleep. Most people experience ineffective sleep at some, or multiple, points in their lives. When the problem is recurrent or ongoing, the individual may be said to have a sleep disorder.

Sleep Disorders

Many individuals have a sleep disorder defined in accordance with existing diagnostic standards such as those set by the American Academy of Sleep Medicine. Variations in sleep can occur along several different dimensions. There may be insufficient time spent sleeping, poor quality of sleep despite adequate time, problems falling or staying asleep, intermittent or situational disturbances in sleep, and any number of situations that result in a lack of feeling rested and refreshed

on awakening. Problems with sleep become a "sleep disorder" when the difficulty is recurring or chronic. Sleep disorders are fairly common and similar regardless of age. Disorders in children are similar to those of adults, although enuresis (bed-wetting) is more a factor in children, as are sleep-onset anxiety, night terrors, and behavioral problems around bedtime. Obstructive sleep apnea occurs in an estimated 1–3% of children, although the causative factors may differ, with tonsillar enlargement being a significant component in children.[16]

Primary Sleep Disorders

Primary sleep disorders are those that exist as an independent condition. The most common categories of primary disorders include insomnia, sleep-related breathing disorders, sleep-related movement disorders, parasomnias, circadian rhythm sleep disorders, and hypersomnia:

- Insomnia exists when there is difficulty falling asleep or staying asleep.
- Sleep-related breathing disorders involve either a problem with the airway, as seen in obstructive sleep apnea, or a problem with the neurologic drive to breathe during sleep (central sleep apnea).
- Sleep-related movement disorders include restless leg syndrome and periodic limb movement disorder.
- Parasomnias include a variety of behaviors, such as sleepwalking, sleep terror, and REM behavior disorder.
- Circadian rhythm sleep disorders occur when the drive to sleep does not occur according to what would be considered a normal sleep–wake pattern, such as someone who stays awake until early morning and does not have the drive to fall asleep as nighttime progresses.
- Hypersomnia is characterized by excessive sleepiness or falling asleep at inappropriate times. Narcolepsy is an example of hypersomnia as a primary sleep disorder.

Secondary Sleep Disorders

Secondary sleep disorders occur as the result of some other situation, and correcting that situation should resolve the problem with sleep. Secondary disorders are often caused by medical conditions, mental health conditions, and side effects of medical treatments. Box 11-1 presents medical conditions that are commonly known to interfere with sleep. A secondary sleep disorder may also be associated with use of any medication that has either a sedative or a stimulating effect because either of these actions can interfere with restorative sleep (Box 11-2). Prematurity in infants also may lead to problems with sleep secondary to the state of neurologic or cardiovascular development.

CONSEQUENCES

Excessive daytime sleepiness is a very distressing side effect of insufficient or poor quality sleep. In addition to the psychological and emotional challenges of sleepiness, the physiological consequences of poor sleep are widespread and can be serious. When sleep is inadequate, a large number of basic regulatory mechanisms of the body do not function effectively. Commonly occurring physiological consequences of poor sleep include hypertension, heart disease and heart failure, stroke, obesity, and developmental disorders that may be related to physiological factors such as alternations in growth hormone. Reproductive disorders can occur due to disruption in hormonal regulation. Mortality is increased significantly for people who report less than 6 or 7 hours of sleep per night, and studies have shown that sleep is a greater risk factor for mortality than smoking, high blood pressure, and heart disease.[2-6] Sleep apnea particularly increases the risk for

- Alzheimer's disease
- Anxiety
- Arthritis
- Asthma
- Cancer
- Chronic obstructive pulmonary disease
- Chronic kidney disease
- Depression
- Diabetes
- Epilepsy
- Febrile conditions
- Fibromyalgia
- Gastroesophageal reflux disease
- Heart failure
- Hyperthyroidism
- Menopause
- Pain
- Parkinson's disease
- Stroke

BOX 11-2 Common Pharmaceutical Categories That Impair Sleep

- Antiarrhythmics
- Antihistamines
- Beta-blockers
- Corticosteroids
- Diuretics
- Nicotine products
- Selective serotonin reuptake inhibitors
- Theophylline
- Thyroid hormone

metabolic syndrome, diabetes, hypertension, and heart disease, and it has been identified as a potential causative factor for these conditions. Research has revealed that the common stereotype of individuals having sleep apnea because of obesity is not accurate and that the obesity may actually be the outcome. Sleep, therefore, is essential to effective weight management, and anything that diminishes the amount or quality of sleep can have significant consequences. Immune function also is diminished in cases of inadequate sleep. Sleep is essential for all of the body's physiological mechanisms, so results of poor sleep are widespread and significant. It is quite common clinically to see individuals with multiple health problems, including diabetes, heart disease, and hypertension, who have a concomitant sleep disorder as a potential causative or aggravating factor in the physical problems. In children, poor sleep quality or insufficient sleep may be manifested primarily by developmental and behavioral abnormalities that may have physiological components as well.[2–6]

RISK FACTORS

Every human being is at risk for sleep problems. Wherever sleep exists as a part of the life pattern, there is the potential for challenges with

sleep or diagnosable sleep disorders. Although the risk for sleep problems is widespread, several known factors place an individual or groups at greater risk; also, risk factors are not easily generalizable because some risk factors are unique for specific sleep problems. Assessment of sleep can be made easier by recognizing common risk factors associated with various conditions.

Populations at Risk

As a population, middle-aged and older individuals are at greater risk for nearly all adult sleep disorders. Hormonal changes, changes in routine and lifestyle with advancing age, and the development of medical conditions (and subsequent symptoms and treatments) are all common among people as they age.[17–19] Women tend to be at greater risk for some sleep disorders, including insomnia and restless leg syndrome. Pregnant and perimenopausal women often experience sleep disturbances as a result of hormone fluctuations that can disrupt sleep through night sweats or lead to symptoms of insomnia. Pregnant women have the additional challenge of changes in body shape that create discomfort and difficulty breathing when lying down, along with pressure on the bladder that can lead to frequent awakenings. Men are at higher risk for obstructive sleep apnea (OSA) than women until menopause, at which point the risk for women increases to near that of men. African Americans, Hispanics, and Pacific Islanders are at greater risk for OSA than Caucasian populations. Children also have a greater risk for OSA than the general population, primarily as a result of tonsillar enlargement. Obesity can increase the risk for OSA in children as well.[16,17,20]

Individual Risk Factors

The most notable individual risk factors are related to family history, individual behaviors, and underlying conditions.

Family History

Family history is a significant factor in the occurrence of most sleep disorders, including OSA, narcolepsy, and insomnia. The nurse is not likely to have this information, however, unless a thorough history is obtained. The completion of a thorough history is complicated by the fact that it is quite common for people to not know that a family member did, in fact, have a sleep disorder.

Individual Behavior

Individuals who work variable shifts, particularly involving night shifts (e.g., emergency medical technicians and firefighters), are at risk for ineffective sleep and sleep disorders, especially if they try to maintain a typical daytime period of wakefulness on days they are not working. Also at risk for sleep disorders are those who work very long hours and monotonous routines such as truck drivers.

Individuals who have undergone recent life change or are experiencing increased stress are at high risk for sleep problems, particularly insomnia. Those who have irregular daily routines often experience problems with inadequate sleep or poor sleep quality, and the idea that it is possible to "catch up" is believed by many; research shows, however, that such attempts to catch up are not effective and do not compensate for poor sleep at other times. Drug and alcohol use along with dietary behaviors such as consumption of stimulants also interfere greatly with sleep. Other dietary habits, television watching in bed, disturbance from light, or a bed partner who is restless or has different sleep times all can interfere with the quality of sleep an individual receives. Child care and other responsibilities can disrupt sleep as well. Many people live in environments in which they do not feel safe either for domestic reasons or because of the environment surrounding their residence. An overwhelming number of people who report poor "sleep hygiene" experience insufficient and poor quality sleep.[1,19]

Underlying Medical Conditions

A significant risk factor for ineffective sleep is having one or more underlying medical conditions and pharmaceutical agents used to treat medical conditions that interfere with sleep, or the treatments for those conditions interfere with sleep (see Boxes 11-1 and 11-2). Symptoms that commonly interfere with sleep include pain, problems breathing, and anxiety.

Persons with retrognathia (receding jaw) and micrognathia (small jaw structure) or with craniofacial abnormalities are at greater risk for OSA, as are children with tonsillar enlargement. Obesity commonly is reported as a risk factor for OSA as well, although it is important to note that the obesity may occur as a consequence of OSA and not necessarily as a cause. The association of OSA and obesity means that OSA should be considered as a possibility in anyone who is obese, particularly as the obesity advances to more severe levels. Sleep disorders also are commonly associated with heart disease and respiratory conditions as both an outcome and a risk factor. Therefore, individuals with heart and respiratory problems should be evaluated for sleep quality. In women, polycystic ovarian syndrome has been found to be highly associated with sleep disorders, including OSA.[17-19,21,22]

ASSESSMENT

Although assessment of sleep is a component of health assessment, this is not addressed consistently by health care personnel. Practitioners do not always ask patients about sleep, and when concerns are discussed, clinicians may have difficulty differentiating fatigue or tiredness from sleepiness. In view of the importance of sleep to overall health, nurses should incorporate sleep assessment with all patients with whom they interact to determine if individuals are getting sufficient restorative sleep.

Assessment of sleep is complicated by the fact that individuals cannot subjectively determine the quality of their sleep. Individuals with OSA, for example, might say they "sleep" 10 hours each night and do not understand why they are so "tired." However, during that 10 hours, they have no way of knowing what is happening to their bodies. People also quite commonly report feeling "tired," but "tired" may be the result of many different conditions or factors. Tired, fatigued, and sleepy are very different in origin. Someone who has difficulty falling asleep or awakens frequently might complain of "insomnia," but awareness of what actually happens during sleep is usually limited. In terms of assessment, then, it is important to recognize that time spent in bed is not a good indicator of amount or quality of sleep. Problems with sleep result in "sleepiness," which can be differentiated from tiredness or fatigue. There are instruments that, with a few questions, can determine someone's sleepiness or likelihood of falling asleep under certain circumstances. These are not typically applied outside of specialty centers, but they are a good example of how attention to "sleepiness" can help to identify sleep problems.[23-28]

History

Start by asking the individual how he or she feels upon awakening. Ideally, the person awakens feeling rested and refreshed. Any response to the contrary indicates less than ideal sleep. The individual may not feel rested and refreshed on awakening, lack energy to do the things he or she enjoys, or feel less productive at work. Statements indicating weakness, malaise, lack of appetite, and so on may accompany reports of fatigue.

A description of what happened while trying to sleep should come next. If the individual reports difficulty falling asleep, assessment should include a discussion of what happens when the individual tries to sleep. Are thoughts racing? Is there discomfort that prevents sleep? Does the individual feel safe while sleeping? Does the individual awaken during the night or awaken early in the morning? What awakens him or her? What happens around any awakening? Inquire about the sleeping environment, including the bedroom and comfort factors such as light and temperature. Specific inquiry regarding physical symptoms, including discomfort or need to urinate that might lead to awakening, can be helpful, along with any other symptoms such as headache, dry mouth, or nasal stuffiness. Inquire about the thoughts, worries, or concerns the individual might be aware of when awakening. Can the person return to sleep quickly after being awakened? What position is the individual in when awakening? Is the bed in disarray, indicating the person has been very active while sleeping? If there is a bed partner, any observations made about the person's behavior while asleep can be very informative.

A detailed history of behavior prior to sleep is key to determining whether or not a sleep problem exists and what the nature of that problem might be. Fatigue is an extremely common symptom of impaired sleep, and, in many cases, the cause is behavioral in origin. The individual stays up late during the week, perhaps to watch television or have some quiet time after tasks are completed, and then arises early the next morning. The use of medications, recreational drugs, stimulants, alcohol, sedentary or active lifestyle, and dietary habits can be associated with sleep problems. Daytime napping may contribute to poor sleep at night, as may other possible factors, such as stress, dietary habits, or lack of exercise.

A thorough review of systems is important to identify problems that might indicate an underlying sleep disorder, such as pins and needles feelings in the legs or pain or nocturnal urination that disrupt the pattern of sleep. Headache, respiratory problems, dry mouth or sore throat, heartburn or reflux, a feeling of the heart beating either very fast or irregularly, a pins and needles feelings, or pain in any part of the body are all possible findings on the history and review that may be indicative of a sleep disorder. Also, family history is significant because there is a strong familial predisposition for most of the sleep disorders.

Examination Findings

Relatively few physical exam findings directly indicate a sleep disorder. However, sleep disorders are more common in people with upper airway or craniofacial construction that can lead to a more easily obstructed upper airway. Micrognathia, retrognathia, enlarged tonsils, somewhat thicker tongue, and a generally smaller upper airway are common in people with OSA. A measurement known as the Mallampati score is a determination of the difficulty of inserting an oral airway and reflects the openness of the upper airway. This measurement is used in assessment of sleep disorders. A Mallampati score of 3 or 4 is common in individuals with OSA. Neck circumference of 16 or greater in women and 17 or greater in men also is associated with OSA. Although obesity may be a result of sleep problems and not a cause, there is a higher incidence of OSA in people with higher body mass index (BMI). Therefore, a BMI of 30 or greater may indicate a possibility of OSA. OSA also can occur in people who with normal or lower BMI, so it should not be relied on as an exclusive screening tool for OSA. People who are obese often have OSA, but not everyone with OSA is obese.[29,30]

Physical examination of respiratory and cardiac function is helpful because such conditions often are associated with sleep disorders either as sequelae or by raising problems with circulation and oxygenation that then interfere with sleep. Cardiac function and coloration can indicate oxygenation status and thus can alert the nurse to possible sleep problems. Neurologic changes also tend to have an impact on sleep quality; therefore, abnormalities detected on examination of this system might point to the existence of challenges to sleep.

Diagnostic Tests

A variety of tests can be conducted that might identity conditions that have occurred as a result of sleep problems. The only definitive tests for sleep problems are those that measure activity and events related to sleep and wakefulness. These are most often done after referral to a sleep medicine specialist who can determine the most likely cause of the sleep problem and order appropriate tests. There are tests that are focused on determining ability to stay awake, time needed to fall asleep, actigraphy that monitors time spent in awake and sleeping states, and an array of other related tests. An actigraph is a device that is worn on the wrist to record movement. Analysis of the recording using special software can provide an estimate of sleep patterns and may be a helpful adjunct to subjective reports and sleep diaries. Actigraphy has been found to be a valid measure in a variety of populations, although it is not a definitive diagnostic tool.[31]

Polysomnogram

One of the most important tests to identify sleep disorders is the polysomnogram (PSG). A PSG is conducted while an individual sleeps and include monitoring of an array of physical parameters. PSGs can be used to evaluate a variety of sleep disorders, including difficulty falling asleep, difficulty staying awake, and sleep-related breathing disorders. PSGs are conducted using an array of electrodes and monitoring devices that can vary depending on the specific reason for conducting the study. Generally, however, a PSG will involve EEG-type electrodes to monitor sleep patterns and stages, stretching belts to measure respiratory effort, leads to monitor muscle activity (typically on the limbs but also for chin/jaw and eye movement), nasal and oral airflow, pulse oximetry. Monitors to document body position also may be indicated, and the entire experience often is recorded on videotape. Registered PSG technicians conduct these studies in clinical facilities designed specifically for overnight sleep studies and that also include video monitoring and, if indicated, the capability for initiating and titrating positive airway pressure (PAP) therapy for people found to have OSA during the PSG. Individuals who work at night and sleep during the day should have their studies done during the daytime to match their usual routine. A limited version of an overnight sleep study can be done outside of a sleep lab, typically in the home setting. Although home studies typically lack some of the monitoring capability of lab studies, they are effective in documenting sleep-related breathing problems and are used in some settings as an alternative to more costly studies or in cases of long waits for an overnight study.

Sleep Journals

Other means of data collection to help in the diagnosis of sleep problems are subjective in nature, particularly the maintenance of a sleep journal. Individuals may be asked to record a summary of their daily activities, dietary intake, bedtime, discussion of what happened during the night, and time of awakening. Subjective assessment on awakening, such as whether or not the individual feels refreshed and restored on awakening, can be an important adjunct to other means of measuring and assessing sleep. As noted previously, subjective assessment of sleep is fraught with difficulties because an individual who is sleeping is not aware of what is happening during sleep.

CLINICAL MANAGEMENT

Clinical management of sleep problems varies with the nature and type of problem or disorder. Regardless of more specific interventions that might be indicated, improvement in sleep begins with understanding and implementing behaviors that are conducive to quality sleep, an approach that is referred to generally as sleep hygiene. The major components of sleep hygiene are the sleeping environment and personal behavior. Proper sleep hygiene often is enough to remedy problems with sleep and is the foundation for quality sleep. It also is something that nurses can work with independently and make a significant difference in the lives of people with whom they work (and their own as well).

Primary Prevention

Sleep hygiene includes attention to the environment for sleep and to personal behavior. The sleeping environment should be comfortable, well ventilated, quiet, and as dark as possible. The optimal temperature for sleep usually is a bit cool; either cold or too warm a temperature can interfere with sleep quality. The bed should be used only for sleep and sexual activity. Bedding and blankets should be evaluated along with other factors of the environment to determine if something in the bed or environment overall is detracting from the quality of sleep.

Personal behaviors and habits are widespread causes of sleep problems. A lack of time spent in sleep often contributes to daytime sleepiness. A large number of sleep complaints and problems stem from not spending enough time sleeping. The healthiest pattern is to have a consistent bedtime and awakening time and to adhere to that pattern at all times. Napping generally is discouraged except in cases in which the naptime is short (30 minutes or so) and the individual has no problem falling asleep at bedtime. Dietary habits, particularly alcohol and stimulants, should be avoided as bedtime approaches, generally 4–6 hours before bed. Alcohol, stimulants, eating a heavy meal, spicy food, or sugary foods should be avoided 4–6 hours before bedtime. Regular exercise is very conducive to healthy sleep, although many people find that it is not beneficial to exercise close to bedtime.

Use of over-the-counter sleep products can interfere significantly with quality sleep patterns, and it is easy for an individual to feel dependent on the product for sleep. Older adults, particularly, may consume products that contain antihistamines and other sedating drugs without being aware that these actually can contribute to persistent sleep problems. Many products marketed for nighttime pain relief contain other drugs that may disrupt sleep. Primary prevention, therefore, focuses on good sleep hygiene and the elimination, when possible, of factors that may interfere with or limit the quality of sleep.[32–36]

Secondary Prevention (Screening)

A number of instruments can be used for more focused screening of sleep problems. The American Academy of Sleep Medicine has a screening tool that addresses a variety of sleep problems. Selected aspects of this tool can be adapted and used for screening as appropriate to the population and as screening reveals aspects of sleep that warrant more specific focus.[36]

Other organizations focused on sleep, along with a number of clinical agencies, have developed their own screening tools for use in assessing sleep quality and the presence of sleep problems specific to the populations with which they work. Nurses will not have difficulty finding age and developmentally appropriate screening tools. Because of the subjective nature of sleep quality, considerable screening can be accomplished with some fairly simple questions that determine whether the individual awakens rested and refreshed and whether some lifestyle or behavioral factors might be responsible for any problems in this area.

Collaborative Interventions
Sleep Hygiene

Sleep hygiene, as noted previously, is the foundation of any approach to improving sleep and thus is applicable as a prevention strategy and an intervention for sleep disturbances. Without a good foundation of appropriate lifestyle and behavioral approaches to sleep, other interventions will fall short of the desired outcome of quality and restorative sleep. Despite the importance of a solid foundation of sleep hygiene, that alone is not always sufficient to resolve existing sleep problems. Collaboration with individuals capable of prescribing other interventions, then, becomes necessary. In most cases, referral should be made to a sleep specialty center for more thorough assessment and diagnosis.

Pharmacologic Agents

Pharmaceutical preparations also may be needed in some situations related to poor sleep quality. In general, sleep aids and other medications designed to address sleep problems should be used only after a thorough assessment and measures related to improved "sleep hygiene" have been implemented. Common pharmacologic agents used to treat sleep disorders are presented in Box 11-3. These should be used with caution, and the patient should be monitored for effectiveness. For some conditions, such as restless leg syndrome, specific agents targeting the nervous system are used. These would require referral to a neurologist or sleep specialist for assessment and determination of an appropriate treatment regimen. Melatonin can be used in cases of circadian rhythm problems and difficulties associated with maintaining a functional sleep–wake pattern. Pharmaceutical-grade (standardized) melatonin should be used to ensure quality and consistency in strength.

Invasive Procedures

For individuals with upper respiratory system obstructions such as upper airway resistance syndrome or OSA, dentists and oral surgeons with additional and specialized education in sleep disorders can perform surgical procedures to provide more openness to the airway or construct oral appliances that aid in keeping the airway open during sleep.[37–48]

INTERRELATED CONCEPTS

A number of concepts are related to sleep through their essential role in healthy sleep patterns. The number of concepts that are related to sleep is quite extensive. The concepts of greatest concern in discussing sleep directly are presented in Figure 11-3.

Perfusion and gas exchange are shown with bidirectional arrows in Figure 11-3 because poor perfusion can cause problems sleeping and poor sleep exacerbates many cardiac and respiratory conditions, such as coronary artery disease, chronic obstructive pulmonary disease, and

---

BOX 11-3   Common Pharmacologic Agents Used to Treat Sleep Disorders

- Anticonvulsants
  - Gabapentin (Neurontin)
- Antidepressants
  - Amitriptyline (Elavil)
  - Bupropion (Wellbutrin)
  - Doxepin (Sinequan)
  - Fluoxetine (Proxac)
- Antihistamines
  - Diphenhydramine (Benadryl)
- Benzodiazepines
  - Diazepam (Valium)
  - Flurazepam (Dalmane)
  - Lorazepam (Ativan)
  - Trazolam (Halcion)
- Benzodiazepine receptor-like agents
  - Zolpidem (Ambien)
  - Zaleplon (Sonata)
  - Eszopiclone (Lunesta)
- Melatonin-receptor agonists
  - Ramelteon (Rozerem)

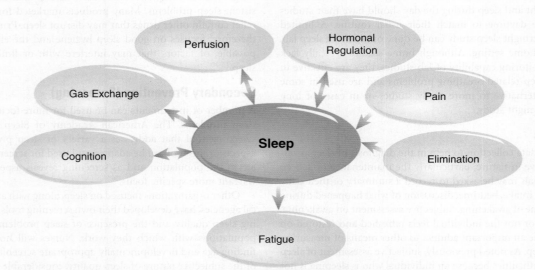

FIGURE 11-3 Sleep and Interrelated Concepts

- Circadian rhythm sleep disorders
  - Jet lag/shift work sleep disruptions
  - Advanced sleep phase disorder
  - Delayed sleep phase disorder
- Insomnia
- Narcolepsy
- Parasomnias
  - Sleep walking
  - Night terrors
  - Enuresis
- Sleep disordered breathing
  - Central sleep apnea
  - Obstructive sleep apnea
  - Obesity hypoventilation syndrome
- Sleep-related movement disorders
  - Restless leg syndrome
  - Periodic limb movement disorder

asthma. Cognition is also shown with a bidirectional arrow because many individuals with impaired cognition experience sleep disturbances and impaired sleep can affect cognitive function. Individuals experiencing pain often have problems sleeping—unless the pain can be adequately managed. Changes in hormonal regulation, such as increased thyroid secretion, can alter stages of sleep, and altered sleep can affect hormone regulation. Problems with elimination are known to be disruptive to sleep, particularly in adults; enuresis (bed-wetting) is an example of a childhood sleep dysfunction. Fatigue is an extremely common outcome complaint associated with impaired sleep.

CLINICAL EXEMPLARS

There are many types of sleep disorders that serve as exemplars of this concept. Exemplars are presented in Box 11-4, organized by the disorder category as appropriate. Although a detailed discussion of each of these exemplars is beyond the scope of this text, several are briefly described next. Refer to pediatric, medical, surgical, and geriatric references for additional information.

Featured Exemplars

The most common conditions encountered in regard to sleep are complaints of insomnia, obstructive sleep apnea, and general "tiredness."

Insomnia

The term insomnia refers to the inability to fall asleep or stay asleep and can last a few days (transient) or can occur over time. Insomnia can be associated with an number of conditions, including acute stress, pain, depression, and underlying medical conditions, and it can occur as a result of drug or alcohol use. A common scenario involves an individual who is stressed by work or life events, lies in bed with thoughts racing, cannot stop thinking about the events of the day or concerns, and consequently cannot fall asleep or cannot maintain sleep, waking up in the middle of the night only to have the disturbing thoughts gathering attention again.

Jet Lag/Shift Work Sleeping Disorders

The most common circadian rhythm sleep disorder occurs among individuals who work variable shifts (particularly night shifts) and

those who do extensive travel. This condition is characterized by disruptions in the sleep–wake cycle, thus affecting the individual's ability to sleep. For those who travel across time zones, the term jet lag is often used because the individual's body time is not synchronized with the environmental time, thus affecting the sleep–wake cycle. There is a direct correlation between the severity of symptoms and the number of time zones crossed.

Narcolepsy

Narcolepsy is a poorly understood chronic neurologic disorder caused by a deficiency of a neuropeptide (hypocretin) that results in the inability of the brain to properly regulate sleep–wake cycles. This condition is most common among adults and is characterized by overwhelming daytime sleepiness; individuals with this condition often find it difficult to stay awake for long periods of time, and they may experience brief periods of falling asleep throughout the day. This condition can lead to poor school and work performance, creating significant challenges including reduction in functional ability.

Obstructive Sleep Apnea

OSA is a condition characterized by interruption of sleep due to temporary airway obstruction by the soft palate, base of the tongue, or both. These structures collapse against the pharyngeal walls due to reduced muscle tome during sleep. The episodes, lasting up to 30 seconds, result in decreased oxygen saturation and fragmented sleep. A person with OSA typically will describe being extremely tired despite having spent sufficient time in bed. Other symptoms include heavy snoring, chronic daytime sleepiness, and fatigue; a sore throat or headache on awakening may also be reported.

Obesity Hypoventilation Syndrome

Obesity hypoventilation syndrome (OHS), one of the most severe forms of sleep-disordered breathing, is characterized by poor gas exchange (resulting in reduced oxygen and increased carbon dioxide levels in the blood) during sleep. Although the exact cause is unknown, OHS is thought to be caused by impaired respiratory mechanics (due to excessive weight against the chest wall) and depressed respiratory control during sleep. Most individuals with OHS are overweight or obese and often have a short, thick neck. Common symptoms include reports of poor sleep quality, daytime sleepiness, fatigue, and headaches.

Somnambulism

The common term for somnambulism is sleep walking. This condition occurs most frequently among children (especially school-aged children) but can occur among adults as well. Somnambulism is characterized by getting out of bed and doing an activity in a partial-wakefulness state during NREM sleep. The activity is often goal-directed and can range from sitting up in bed to walking around the house, moving objects, and even driving a car with no recall of the event on awakening.

Sleep Terrors

Sleep terrors (also known as night terrors) are a parasomnia characterized by sudden episodes of intense fear, screaming, panic, and confusion while still asleep. The episode can last from just a few seconds to several minutes. There is usually increased respiratory rate, heart rate, dilated pupils, and diaphoresis. Night terrors are not associated with dreams during REM sleep, and there is usually no recall of the awakening. Night terrors occur most often during early to middle childhood, although they can occur among adults, particularly those under significant stress or associated with substance use.

CASE STUDY

Source: Michael Greenberg/Digital Vision/Thinkstock

Case Presentation

Jim Wyatt is a 42-year-old Caucasian male, 5 ft. 11 in. and 200 pounds, with a BMI) of 27.9 (considered overweight according to BMI tables). He reports being tired "all the time." Other health problems include hypertension that is poorly controlled with three prescription medications and an HgbA1C level that has been rising, with the most recent measure at 6.2. On a typical day, he awakens at 6:30 AM, often with a significant headache and feeling like he has not gotten a good night's sleep. He adds that on most mornings, he has a dry mouth as well. He is worried that his work performance is suffering, and he has trouble staying awake at meetings. He had one minor traffic accident recently when his car went off the road after he fell asleep at the wheel. He often will nap when he gets home from work, and he falls asleep watching television after dinner. He attempts to go to bed at approximately 9:30 or 10 PM each night with the hope of getting enough sleep so he will not be so tired the next day. He has stopped going to social events in the evening due to the difficulty he has staying awake. On a recent camping trip, his companions teased him about his loud snoring. He explains that his father "was the same way." On physical exam, the nurse notes that he is having difficulty staying awake while he is talking and he has a neck circumference of 17 ½ in. On examination of his oropharynx, the nurse cannot visualize the uvula or tonsils.

Case Analysis

Mr. Wyatt has many common symptoms of OSA. Physically, the neck circumference of greater than 17 in. is highly correlated with OSA. He also reveals a positive family history indicative of OSA. No matter how much he sleeps, he never feels rested. This situation has been getting worse, as evidenced by his laboratory values showing possible metabolic problems and also what may be treatment-resistant hypertension. His quality of life is suffering, as is his work performance. Naps and sleeping longer at night do not help because the apnea continues. No matter how much time he spends thinking he is "sleeping," he is not getting the restorative sleep that he needs to be healthy, productive, and energetic. He has many of the characteristics of someone with significant OSA. It is important to remember, however, that people who do not fit the typical physical pattern may also have OSA. They are likely to have many of the signs, however, such as snoring and feeling tired regardless of the amount of sleep they get.

ACCESS EXEMPLAR LINKS IN YOUR GIDDENS EBOOK

REFERENCES

1. National Sleep Foundation: Sleep in America Poll: Sleep in the modern family. Summary of findings. 2014. Retrieved from: <http://sleepfoundation.org/sites/default/files/2014-NSF-Sleep-in-America-poll-summary-of-findings—FINAL-Updated-3-26-14-.pdf>.

2. Taveras EM, Rifas-Shiman SL, Oken E, et al: Short sleep duration in infancy and risk of childhood overweight. *Arch Pediatr Adolesc Med* 162(4):305–311, 2008.

3. Knutson KL, Ryden AM, Mander BA, et al: Role of sleep duration and quality in the risk and severity of type 2 diabetes mellitus. *Arch Intern Med* 166(16):1768–1774, 2006.

4. Nilsson PM, Rööst M, Engström G, et al: Incidence of diabetes in middle-aged men is related to sleep disturbances. *Diabetes Care* 27(10):2464–2469, 2004.

5. Kasasbeh E, Krishnaswamy G: Inflammatory aspects of sleep apnea and their cardiovascular consequences. *South Med J* 99(1):58–67, 2006.

6. Colten HR, Altevogt BM, editors: *Sleep disorders and sleep deprivation: An unmet public health problem*, Washington, DC, 2006, Committee on Sleep Medicine and Research, Board on Health Sciences Policy, National Academies Press.

7. Bin YS, Marshall NS, Glozier N: Secular trends in adult sleep duration: A systematic review. *Sleep Med Rev* 16:223–230, 2012.

8. Sigurdson K, Ayas N: The public health and safety consequences of sleep disorders. *Can J Physiol Pharmacol* 85:179–183, 2007.

9. Hublin C, Partinen M, Koskenvuo M, et al: Sleep and mortality: A population-based 22-year follow-up study. *Sleep* 30(10):1245–1253, 2007.

10. Oxford University Press: Sleep. In *Oxford Dictionary of English*, Oxford, 2005, Oxford University Press.

11. Merriam–Webster: Sleep. n.d. Retrieved from: <http://www.merriam-webster.com/dictionary/sleep>.

12. Acebo C, Sadeh A, Seifer R, et al: Sleep/wake patterns derived from activity monitoring and maternal report for healthy 1- to 5-year-old children. *Sleep* 28(12):1568–1577, 2005.

13. Floyd JA, Janisse JJ, Jenuwine ES, et al: Changes in REM-sleep percentage over the adult lifespan. *Sleep* 30(7):829–836, 2007.

14. Iglowstein I, Jenni OG, Molinari L, et al: Sleep duration from infancy to adolescence: Reference values and generational trends. *Pediatrics* 111(2):302–307, 2003.

15. Redeker NS: Developmental aspects of normal sleep. In Redeker NS, McEnany GP, editors: *Sleep disorders and sleep promotion in nursing practice*, New York, 2011, Springer, pp 19–32.

16. Baweja R, Calhoun S, Baweja R, et al: Sleep problems in children. *Minerva Pediatr* 65(5):457–472, 2013.

17. Hiestand DM, Britz P, Goldman M, et al: Prevalence of symptoms and risk of sleep apnea in the US population: Results from the National Sleep Foundation Sleep in America 2005 Poll. *Chest* 130(3):780–786, 2006.

18. Chen X, Wang R, Zee P, et al: Racial/ethnic differences in sleep disturbances: The Multi-Ethnic Study of Atherosclerosis (MESA). *Sleep* 38(6):877–888, 2015.

19. Ralls FM, Grigg-Damberger M: Roles of gender, age, race/ethnicity, and residential socioeconomics in obstructive sleep apnea syndromes. *Curr Opin Pulm Med* 18(6):568–573, 2012.

20. Allen RP, Picchietti D, Hening WA, et al: Restless legs syndrome: Diagnostic criteria, special considerations, and epidemiology— A report from the Restless Legs Syndrome Diagnosis and Epidemiology Workshop at the National Institutes of Health. *Sleep Med* 4(2):101–119, 2003.

21. Moran LJ, March WA, Whitrow MJ, et al: Sleep disturbances in a community-based sample of women with polycystic ovary syndrome. *Hum Reprod* 30(2):466–472, 2015.

22. Ye L, Pien GW, Ratcliffe SJ, et al: Gender differences in obstructive sleep apnea and treatment response to continuous positive airway pressure. *J Clin Sleep Med* 5(6):512–518, 2009.

23. Bloom HG, Ahmed I, Alessi CA, et al: Evidence-based recommendations for the assessment and management of sleep disorders in older persons. *J Am Geriatr Soc* 57:761–789, 2009.

24. Lee KA, Ward TM: Critical components of a sleep assessment for clinical practice settings. *Issues Mental Health Nurs* 26:739–759, 2005.

25. Damiani MF, Quaranta VN, Falcone VA, et al: The Epworth Sleepiness Scale: Conventional self vs physician administration. *Chest* 143(6):1569–1575, 2013.

26. Ulasli SS, Gunay E, Koyuncu T, et al: Predictive value of Berlin Questionnaire and Epworth Sleepiness Scale for obstructive sleep apnea in a sleep clinic population. *Clin Respir J* 8(3):292–296, 2014.

27. Billings ME, Rosen CL, Auckley D, et al: Psychometric performance and responsiveness of the Functional Outcomes of Sleep Questionnaire and Sleep Apnea Quality of Life Index in a randomized trial: The HomePAP study. *Sleep* 37(12):2017–2024, 2014.

28. Farney RJ: The STOP-Bang equivalent model and prediction of severity of obstructive sleep apnea: Relation to polysomnographic measurements of the apnea/hypopnea index. *J Clin Sleep Med* 7(5):459–465, 2011.

29. Karakoc O, Akcam T, Gerek M, et al: The upper airway evaluation of habitual snorers and obstructive sleep apnea patients. *ORL* 74(3):136–140, 2012.

30. Zonato AI, Bittencourt LR, Martinho FL, et al: Association of systematic head and neck physical examination with severity of obstructive sleep apnea–hypopnea syndrome. *Laryngoscope* 13(6):973–980, 2003.

31. Kawada T: Sleep parameters from actigraphy and sleep diary: Is the agreement important for sleep study? *Sleep Med* 14(3):298–299, 2013.

32. Irish LA, Kline CE, Gunn HE, et al: The role of sleep hygiene in promoting public health: A review of empirical evidence. *Sleep Med Rev* 2014. [Epub ahead of print]; pii, S1087-0792(14)00100-2.

33. Kline CE, Irish LA, Buysse DJ, et al: Sleep hygiene behaviors among midlife women with insomnia or sleep-disordered breathing: The SWAN Sleep Study. *J Women's Health* 23(11):894–903, 2014.

34. Hood HK, Rogojanski J, Moss TG: Cognitive–behavioral therapy for chronic insomnia. *Curr Treatment Options Neurol* 16(12):321, 2014.

35. Kloss JD, Nash CO, Walsh CM, et al: A "Sleep 101" program for college students improves sleep hygiene knowledge and reduces maladaptive beliefs about sleep. *Behav Med* 2014.

36. American Academy of Sleep Medicine: Screening questions–Sleep history & physical. n.d. Retrieved from: <http://www.aasmnet.org/Resources/MedSleep/%28Harding%29questions.pdf>.

37. Earley CJ: Latest guidelines and advances for treatment of restless legs syndrome. *J Clin Psychiatry* 75(4):e08, 2014.

38. Philip P, Chaufton C, Taillard J, et al: Modafinil improves real driving performance in patients with hypersomnia: A randomized double-blind placebo-controlled crossover clinical trial. *Sleep* 37(3):483–487, 2014.

39. Pergolizzi JV, Jr, Taylor R, Jr, Raffa RB, et al: Fast-acting sublingual zolpidem for middle-of-the-night wakefulness. *Sleep Disord* 2014:527109, 2014.

40. Idzikowski C: The pharmacology of human sleep, a work in progress? *Curr Opin Pharmacol* 14:90–96, 2014.

41. Victorri-Vigneau C, Gérardin M, Rousselet M, et al: An update on zolpidem abuse and dependence. *J Addict Dis* 33(1):15–23, 2014.

42. Schwartz TL, Goradia V: Managing insomnia: An overview of insomnia and pharmacologic treatment strategies in use and on the horizon. *Drugs Context* 2013:212257, 2013.

43. Vellante F, Cornelio M, Acciavatti T, et al: Treatment of resistant insomnia and major depression. *Clin Ter* 164(5):429–435, 2013.

44. Burke TM, Markwald RR, Chinoy ED, et al: Combination of light and melatonin time cues for phase advancing the human circadian clock. *Sleep* 36(11):1617–1624, 2013.

45. Shah C, Sharma TR, Kablinger A: Controversies in the use of second-generation antipsychotics as sleep agent. *Pharmacol Res* 79:1–8, 2014.

46. Schroeder AM, Colwell CS: How to fix a broken clock. *Trends Pharmacol Sci* 34(11):605–619, 2013.

47. Tamrat R, Huynh-Le MP, Goyal M: Non-pharmacologic interventions to improve the sleep of hospitalized patients: A systematic review. *J Gen Intern Med* 29(5):788–795, 2014.

48. FDA-approved drugs to treat sleep disorders. *J Psychosoc Nurs Ment Health Serv* 51(10):9–10, 2013.

Cellular Regulation

Kevin Brigle and Jean Giddens

The cell is always speaking—the secret is to learn its language.

—*Andrew S. Bajer, Cell Biologist*

Cells are the smallest form of life; they are the functional and structural units of all living things. The regulation of cellular activity is an intricate and tightly regulated process not only through the lifespan of an individual cell but also between cells. To maintain health and keep our bodies running smoothly, cells are constantly working, changing, sending and responding to chemical cues, and correcting mistakes whenever possible. When this is not possible, specific cellular pathways are activated to remove individual cells that are no longer functioning as they have been programmed to do. Although the complex interconnected circuits of cellular regulation have tremendous fidelity, irreparable errors can occur at many steps along these pathways, leading to permanent abnormal changes that can significantly impact biophysical and psychosocial health and functional status. Nurses should be familiar with the scope and process of cellular regulation, the consequences of altered cellular regulation, and the health care priorities to implement when conditions of altered cellular regulation develop.

DEFINITION

The term cellular regulation refers to *all functions carried out within a cell to maintain homeostasis, including its responses to extracellular signals (e.g., hormones, cytokines, and neurotransmitters) and the way each cell produces an intracellular response.*[1] Included within these functions is cellular *replication* and *growth*. Common terms used to describe detailed aspects of cellular reproduction and growth include *proliferation* and *differentiation*. Proliferation refers to the reproduction of new cells through cell growth and cell division. Differentiation refers to the acquisition of a specific cell function, a normal process by which a less specialized cell becomes a more specialized cell type. These terms are further described later. Another important term associated with this concept is *neoplasia*, an abnormal and progressive multiplication of cells, leading to the formation of a neoplasm (also known as a tumor). A *neoplasm* refers to new but abnormal tissue growth that is uncontrolled and progressive. Neoplasms are categorized as either *benign* or *malignant* (or cancerous).

SCOPE

The concept of cellular regulation is very broad and represents all aspects of cellular function. Some of the basic functions that cells have in common include creating fuel for the body, manufacturing a complex array of proteins, transporting materials, and disposing of wastes. Included in cellular regulation is cellular division and reproduction—processes that are strictly controlled for normal cells. The scope of this concept analysis focuses on the *cellular growth and reproduction* aspect of cellular regulation and the development of malignant neoplasms described previously. In this context, normal cellular growth is at one end of the spectrum, whereas malignant neoplasia is at the opposite end (Figure 12-1).

NORMAL PHYSIOLOGICAL PROCESS

Normal Cellular Reproduction and Growth

Cellular replication is an extraordinarily efficient process with millions of cells generated on a daily basis over the course of one's life. New cells are formed through a process of cell division referred to as proliferation. The rate of proliferation varies according to the needs of the tissue involved. For example, rapid proliferation occurs within epithelial cells, bone marrow, and the gastrointestinal tract, whereas slower proliferation occurs in muscles, cartilage, and bone.

There are two kinds of normal cell division: mitosis and meiosis. Mitosis is essentially a duplication process: Two genetically identical "daughter" cells are produced from a single "parent" cell. Mitosis may take place in cells in all parts of the body, keeping tissues and organs in optimal working order. Normal cells capable of mitosis divide for only one of two reasons: to develop normal tissues or to replace lost or damaged normal tissues. Meiosis generates "daughter" cells that are purposely distinct from one another and from the original "parent" cell. Essentially all cells are capable of mitosis, but only a few special cells are capable of meiosis—those that will become eggs in females and sperm in males. Basically, mitosis is necessary for growth and maintenance of normal tissues, whereas meiosis is utilized for sexual reproduction.

FIGURE 12-1 Scope of Cellular Regulation

Replication

Cellular replication is activated in the presence of cellular degeneration and death or on the basis of physiological need. That is, when replication is functioning normally, new cells are created at the same rate as older cells die. The determination and timing of cellular division are strictly controlled by molecular "stop" and "go" signals. For example, when a wound occurs, injured cells send "go" signals to the surrounding cells, which respond to the extracellular signals by activating intracellular proliferation pathways. This results in controlled cellular growth and division that, in time, seals the wound. Conversely, "stop" signals are sent by the newly formed tissue when the wound healing process nears completion and cell replacement is no longer required. However, in a pathologic process, these signals can function abnormally whereby a "go" signal can be produced when it should not be or a "stop" signal may be ignored by surrounding cells. Such errors could result in uncontrolled growth and the development of neoplasms. However, due to the redundancy of error-correcting mechanisms in cellular regulation, it takes more than one incorrect "stop" or "go" signal for neoplasia to develop. The human body is quite efficient at protecting its essential systems, and it generally requires multiple errors compounded over time for healthy cells to turn malignant.[2]

With normal reproduction, cells proceed through a cycle (known as the cell cycle) whereby the entire cellular contents of the parent cell are duplicated, after which it undergoes mitosis and splits into two identical daughter cells. This pathway follows an orderly progression whereby certain steps need to precede others in order for the process to continue. Initially, the cell must leave the resting state, G_0 (gap 0), in order to enter the cell cycle. The cell cycle is divided into four distinct phases: G_1 (gap 1), S (synthesis), G_2 (gap 2), and M (mitosis or cell division). Phases G_1 through G_2 are known as interphase, during which chromosomes (the genetic material) are copied and the cell typically doubles in size. During the M phase, mitosis (or cellular division) occurs, leading to the formation of two identical cells. Surveillance checkpoints exist at the junction of each phase to ensure that damaged or incomplete DNA is not passed on to daughter cells. Abnormal cells may be removed through error-correcting or cell death pathways. The initial entry into the cell cycle is an irreversible act, and it commits the cell to either mitosis or death. Cells cannot reverse the process and go backward to G_0; thus the most fundamental aspect of cell cycle control is the regulation of entry and exit. In neoplastic tumors, the duration of cell cycle is equal to or longer than that of normal cells. However, the proportion of cells that have committed to the cell cycle and are in active cell division (vs. cells in G_0 phase) is much higher than that in normal tissue. This results in a net increase in cell number and the formation of a tumor.

Differentiation

Most mature normal cells are functionally and morphologically differentiated into a specialized cell type. *Differentiation* means that a cell acquires functions that are *different* from those of the original cell from which it derived. Differentiation is a normal process by which a less specialized cell develops to possess a distinct form and specialized function. Differentiation dramatically changes a cell's size and shape (morphology) and its responsiveness to extracellular signals. These specialized changes are largely due to highly controlled modifications in gene expression specific to each differentiated cell type. Thus, different cells can have very different physical characteristics despite having the exact same complement of human genes. *Morphology* refers to the science of structure and form without regard to function. Each cell type has a specific morphology and at least one specific function.

Surveillance of Cellular Replication and Growth

Normal cellular replication and growth requires precise, error-free interpretation of both extra- and intracellular cell signals. Cell signaling is a complex communication system, requiring accurate communication pathways within the cell (intracellular coding) and among cells (extracellular coding). Intracellular signaling is a multistep pathway often initiated by an extracellular signal provided by a nearby or even distant cell. Many factors can cause dysregulated cellular signaling, including genetic mutations and aberrant protein expression. When a signaling mistake occurs in the cell cycle, a host of surveillance mechanisms are present to recognize the error and repair the mistake. If the error cannot be repaired, the cell can be actively destroyed through a process known as *apoptosis* or programmed cell death. These error-recognition processes help ensure accurate replication of daughter cells.

VARIATIONS AND CONTEXT

Despite the exquisite fidelity of cellular reproduction and growth, mistakes may occur at almost any point in the cell cycle. As stated previously, surveillance mechanisms usually recognize and correct these errors or, if unable to do so, destroy the cells to avoid passing the errors to subsequent daughter cells. However, when a mistake goes undetected or a repair is ineffective and the aberrant cell is not destroyed, cellular mutations can become fixed, leading to neoplasia and the formation of tumors. These tumors can be benign or malignant, and comparisons between these two categories of neoplasms are presented in Table 12-1.

Benign Neoplasm

Benign neoplastic cells tend to retain most of the morphologic and functional characteristics of the normal cells from which they were derived but represent groups of abnormal cells with excessive growth. Benign neoplastic cells are capable of replication and mitosis, but they are not capable of metastasis (the spread to locations outside their site of origin). Examples of common benign neoplastic tissues include endometriosis, nevi, and hypertrophic scars.

Benign tumors do not invade adjacent tissue or metastasize to distant organs. However, they can result in significant health consequences. A benign tumor can obstruct or mechanically press on other body structures, resulting in pain, physiological dysfunction, or even

TABLE 12-1 Comparison of Benign and Malignant Neoplasms

Characteristic	Benign	Malignant
Encapsulated	Usually	Rarely
Differentiated	Normally	Poorly
Metastasis	Absent	Capable
Recurrence	Rare	Possible
Vascularity	Slight	Moderate to marked
Mode of growth	Expansive	Infiltrative and expansive
Cell characteristics	Fairly normal; similar to parent cells	Cells abnormal, become more unlike parent cells

Source: From Lewis SL, Dirksen SR, Heitkemper MM, Bucher L: *Medical–surgical nursing: Assessment and management of clinical problems*, ed 9, St Louis, 2014, Mosby.

TABLE 12-2 Targeting the Hallmarks of Cancer and the Enabling Characteristics

Cancer Cell Phenotype[a]	Targeting Agent
Sustaining proliferative growth signaling	Cyclin-dependent kinase inhibitors[b]
Evading growth suppressors	Epidermal growth factor inhibitors[b]
Resisting cell death	Programmed death receptor blocking antibodies[b]
Avoiding immune destruction	Immune activators of cytotoxic T cells[b]
Enabling replicative immortality	Telomerase inhibitors
Inducing angiogenesis	Inhibitors of VEGF signaling[b]
Activating invasion and metastases	Inhibitors of HGF/c-Met[b]
Deregulating cellular energetics	Aerobic glycolysis inhibitors
Genome instability and mutation	Poly-ADP-ribose polymerase inhibitors[b]
Tumor-promoting inflammation	Selective anti-inflammatory drugs[b]

[a]The first eight phenotypes represent acquired functional capabilities of cancer cells that are necessary for tumor growth and progression. The last two phenotypes represent the enabling characteristics that help the cancer cell acquire these functional capabilities.
[b]A class of antineoplastic agents in which there is a drug with Food and Drug Administration approval.
Source: Data from Hanahan D, Weinberg RA: Hallmarks of cancer: The next generation, *Cell* 144(5):646–674, 2011.

death. For example, a benign brain tumor may compress brain structures, leading to various manifestations of neurologic symptoms and dysfunction. Other benign tumors, such as lipomas, may have more of a psychosocial impact because they may be outwardly visible and thus affect physical appearance of an individual.

Malignant Neoplasm

A malignant neoplasm (cancer) is characterized by cells having abnormal growth patterns, multiple abnormal functions, and the ability to disseminate to distant sites. These new abnormal characteristics give the malignant cell an advantage that allows it and its offspring to thrive and survive, even in unfavorable conditions. Malignant neoplastic cells arise from previously normal cells due to unrepaired errors in multiple cancer-causing genes. The identity of these genes varies from one cancer type to another, and in fact, they vary even within a given type of cancer. All cancers evolve to acquire a similar set of functional capabilities, referred to as the "eight hallmarks of cancer" aided by two "enabling characteristics" (Table 12-2).[3] Acquisition of these eight individual capabilities depends on a multistep succession of mutations, eventually resulting in a progressive expansion of subclones, one or more of which will evolve into a tumor of increasing growth dominance. Tumors are much more than insulated masses of identical proliferating tumor cells. Rather, they are very complex tissues composed of many distinct cell types (including nonmalignant "normal cells") that interact with one another and with the cancer cells. In this complex tumor microenvironment, cancer cells are able to recruit the associated "normal" cells to serve as contributors to support their proliferation, invasion, and metastases. In fact, an important part of modern cancer therapy has been the development of antineoplastic agents that target these normal "helper cells" rather than the cancer cells themselves.[4] Because cancer cells are often resistant to single-agent treatment modalities, new agents are being developed that would be used in combination to target each of these eight common capabilities of cancer cells and the associated enabling characteristics (see Table 12-2).

CONSEQUENCES

Malignant tumors acquire characteristics that allow them to spread, invade, and destroy normal tissue. Like any other tissue, cancer tumors require oxygen and nutrition to sustain their rapid growth. For this to happen, the tumor releases factors that encourage tumor neovascularization. This process, known as tumor angiogenesis, facilitates further growth and invasion capability. When neovascularization is not possible or is halted, cancer cells are able to reprogram their energy metabolism, allowing for sustained and rapid growth under anaerobic conditions as well.[5] Regardless of the energy source, as the tumor increases in size and metastasizes, it acts like a parasite, robbing normal body tissues of nutrients and oxygen and destroying invaded tissues. Unless treatment is successful, the result is fatigue, weight loss, pain, organ failure, and eventual death.

Despite the fact that many cancers are curable, people often associate the disease with inevitable pain and death. The most common psychosocial consequences associated with a cancer diagnosis are fear, stress, and anxiety. When a malignant tumor is first discovered, patients and their family members often experience tremendous stress for days to weeks during the diagnostic and staging process. Often, the fear of the unknown can be as anxiety provoking as the diagnosis itself. Some individuals cope with the stress through a mechanism of denial, whereas others become very proactive and are interested in every aspect of the diagnostic and treatment process. In instances in which a child is diagnosed with cancer, the entire family is impacted. Parents often exhibit depression, stress, and anxiety, whereas children commonly experience fear, anger, guilt, and grief, often expressed through behavioral changes.[6]

In addition to fear and anxiety, changes in family dynamics are common. Financial challenges often occur as a result of medical expenses and reduced income associated with lost time at work, both for the patient and the caregivers. Changes in self-image and self-identity may result if patients experience a significant change in their physical appearance or their family role due to the disease process. This, in turn, can lead to alterations in interpersonal relationships and the development of mood disorders. The psychosocial effects of cancer are particularly pronounced for cancer survivors and their families when cancer recurs.[7]

RISK FACTORS

As of January 2014, there were an estimated 14.5 million Americans living with a history of cancer. In 2015, an estimated 1,658,370 new cancer cases (excluding basal and squamous cell skin cancers) will be diagnosed, and an estimated 589,430 patients will die from their disease.[8] Cancer is the second most common cause of death in the United States, exceeded only by heart disease, and it accounts for nearly 25% of all deaths. Among men, the three most common new cancer diagnoses are prostate, lung/bronchus, and colon/rectum. For women, the three most common sites are breast, lung/bronchus, and colon/rectum. Lung cancer is the most common cause of death among both men and women, followed by breast cancer and colorectal cancer for women and prostate cancer and colorectal cancer for men. In contrast to the high number of cancer diagnoses in adults, only 10,380 children (ages 0–14 years) are expected to be diagnosed with cancer in 2015 (fewer than 1% of all cancer diagnoses). Although it is relatively uncommon, cancer remains the second leading cause of death in this age group, exceeded only by accidents. An estimated 1250 cancer deaths are expected to occur among children in 2015. Leukemia and cancers affecting the brain or central nervous system are the most common childhood cancers. Combined, they represent more than 50% of all new cases in children.

Populations at Risk

When cancer death rates were evaluated across populations, certain racial and ethnic minorities appeared to be at higher risk, and for years this was attributed to biologic differences. In recent years, it has been shown that these disparities in cancer burden largely reflect obstacles to receiving health care services related to cancer prevention, early detection, and high-quality treatment, with poverty as the overriding factor. In addition, racial and ethnic minorities tend to receive lower-quality health care than whites even when insurance status, age, severity of disease, and health status are comparable. In minority groups, communication barriers and provider assumptions can affect interactions between patients and physicians, which further contributes to miscommunication and the delivery of substandard care.

Individual Risk Factors
Age

Although it is not a modifiable risk factor, the risk for developing an invasive cancer increases significantly as a person ages. It is estimated that 78% of new cancer diagnoses occur among those ages 55 years or older. Between the ages 40 and 59 years, the probability of developing cancer (among those who were previously cancer free) is 8% for men and 9% for women, and the probability increases to 30% for men and 25% for women age 70 years or older.[8]

Smoking/Tobacco

Another known risk factor for cancer is smoking. At least 30% of all cancer-related deaths and 87% of all lung cancer deaths can be attributed to smoking. In addition, smoking is a known risk factor for 16 different types of cancers. Nonsmokers exposed to environmental tobacco smoke are also at increased risk of lung cancer, and second-hand smoke is estimated to cause 21,400 lung cancer deaths worldwide each year. Nontraditional tobacco products such as snuff, lozenges, and chewing tobacco are promoted as alternatives in smoke-free environments, but they are also associated with increased risk of cancer associated with the oral cavity, esophagus, and pancreas.[9]

Infectious Agents

Certain bacteria and viruses are known to cause cancer. Examples include the hepatitis B and hepatitis C viruses (liver cancer), human papillomavirus (cervical, oropharyngeal, and anal cancer), and *Helicobacter pylori* bacteria (gastric cancer). Vaccines are available to prevent infection by hepatitis B and the human papillomavirus and thus provide immediate opportunities for preventing cancers, especially in at-risk populations.[10]

Genetic Risk

Only approximately 5% of all cancers result from an inherited genetic alteration that is associated with an increased risk of developing certain types of cancer. In some cases, a specific gene mutation results in an extraordinarily high risk of cancer, such as women with a *BRCA1* gene mutation that confers a 70% lifetime risk of developing either breast or ovarian cancer. Fortunately, these types of mutations are rare in the population as a whole. Although approximately 20 other "cancer syndromes" are known (e.g., Lynch syndrome), more common are the generally unexplained genetic susceptibilities and familial tendencies that increase cancer risk in certain families. The development of breast cancer among first-degree relatives is an example.[11]

Radiation

There are two main types of radiation (ultraviolet and ionizing) exposure that are linked to an increased risk of developing certain types of cancer. Ionizing radiation includes medical radiation from tests used to both diagnose (x-rays and computed tomography scans) and treat (radiation therapy) disease, and it is responsible for an increased risk of developing leukemia and breast and thyroid cancer. An equally important source of ionizing radiation is from radon gas, which is a natural decay product of uranium in the earth. Exposure to radon gas dramatically increases risk for lung cancer. Ultraviolet radiation from the sun is the main cause of melanoma and the ubiquitous nonmelanoma skin cancers (basal and squamous). Although the latter of these is highly curable, the obvious intervention to decrease risk is to avoid the sun and use protective measures.[12]

Carcinogens

Environmental carcinogens have been associated with the development of many types of cancer. Exposure to these carcinogens is often due to lifestyle choices (e.g., smoking), but other carcinogens are present as environmental pollutants in the air, water, soil, or food. Although the risk level per person is thought to be quite low (accounting for only 6% of cancer deaths), the large number of people involuntarily exposed to these pollutants leads to a large population effect. Probably more significant are high levels of exposure to agents (e.g., asbestos, dioxins, tetrachloroethylene, and arsenic) that increase risk disproportionately in specific low-income occupations and in some poor and disenfranchised communities.[12]

Nutrition and Physical Activity

Diet, body weight, and activity levels are interrelated and seem to act in complex ways to either promote or reduce the risk of cancer. Combined, more than 30% of all cancers are attributed to poor nutrition, a sedentary lifestyle, and excessive weight. It is difficult to absolutely define the effects of diet on cancer because an individual's diet typically includes foods that may protect against cancer as well as foods that may increase the risk of cancer. However, a number of epidemiologic studies suggest that high intake of fresh fruits and vegetables is associated with lower cancer rates. Obesity is associated with increased risk for both developing new cancers and cancer recurrence. Weight loss has been shown to reduce cancer risk, although the exact mechanism is not well understood. In addition to these risk factors being significant for cancer, they are also responsible for significant disability and death from other causes, such as heart disease, hypertension and stroke, diabetes, and arthritis.[13]

ASSESSMENT

Assessment involves the collection of data from the health history, a physical examination, and diagnostic studies. It is not the intention of this text to describe the process of assessment or to describe the specific findings of all problems associated with cellular reproduction and growth because these are highly variable based on the involved tissue, organ, or body system. However, on initial diagnosis, several presenting symptoms and clinical findings often serve as "red flags" that are unusual and worthy of further investigation. The nurse should have an awareness of the significance of these symptoms and findings.

History

Individuals are usually asymptomatic when neoplasms are early in their development. As the tumor grows, an individual may become aware of its physical presence or may notice symptoms caused by the tumor. The most common presenting complaints include discovery of a lump, mass, or lesion; the onset of new symptoms (e.g., unusual or unexplained bleeding, pain, cough, or fatigue); changes in appearance of a body part; or signs associated with alterations in major body functions (e.g., appetite, weight, mental status, swallowing, or elimination). Often, the presenting symptoms are quite vague, and the nurse should conduct a symptom analysis to collect as much information as possible. This includes questions regarding the duration of the symptom, its location, characteristics, aggravating and relieving factors, and treatments undertaken, if any. In addition to documenting the symptoms, these questions also provide early information about the patient's coping skills or his or her potential denial of the problem. A medical history, a family history, and a psychosocial history will provide additional information that may later prove valuable (e.g., history of smoking or a family history of cancer).

Examination Findings

When a patient presents with a specific symptom that raises concern, the examination should be focused to learn more about the presenting problem. However, patients do not always experience symptoms and, thus, the nurse needs be aware of possible indicators of neoplastic growth when conducting the physical exam. Abnormal findings that may suggest the presence of a neoplasm include visible lesions, physical asymmetry, palpable masses, abnormal sounds, or the presence of blood such as on pelvic exam or in a guaiac test for occult blood.

Diagnostic Tests

A diagnostic workup is indicated when a symptom, examination finding, or screening test suggests the presence of a tumor. The tests discussed here are those most commonly used in the detection and diagnosis of tumors.

Radiographic Tests

Radiographic tests provide an image of tumors so that size, location(s), and activity can be assessed. The most common radiographic tests used for the diagnostic process related to cellular regulation include radiographs (x-rays), magnetic resonance imaging, computed tomography, or radioisotope scans, ultrasound, and diagnostic mammography.

Direct Visualization

Some tumors can be evaluated by insertion of a lighted scope into a lumen or body cavity (e.g., colonoscopy, endoscopy, or cystoscopy). These tests not only provide visualization of the tumor but also allow for biopsy to provide tissue samples for pathologic analysis.

Laboratory Tests

Several laboratory tests are useful in the diagnostic process. Perhaps the two most useful tests associated with the diagnostic process are the complete blood count and the chemistry panel. Although these tests are not diagnostic in themselves (except in the case of some hematologic malignancies), they may provide information about the overall health status of the patient or provide clues as to the presence of neoplasm. For example, an undiagnosed malignancy might first be detected in a patient having unexplained anemia or changes in his or her white blood cells. A limited number of tumor markers (e.g., carcioembyonic antigen and prostate-specific antigen) or cancer-specific genetic changes (e.g., Philadelphia chromosome) can be detected in the blood samples that may help provide a diagnosis. If a certain type of cancer is suspected, specific studies may be ordered that would be helpful in determining risk, such as genetic tests for the *BRCA1* and *BRCA2* genes that are linked to breast cancer.

Pathology

Pathology is the study of the origin and course of disease and is moreover the branch of medicine that deals with the laboratory examination of cells and tissues for diagnostic purposes. Pathologic evaluation of a tissue sample is the only definitive way to determine if a tumor is malignant or benign. It may also provide information such as the tissue type (histology), the degree of differentiation (grade), or the presence or absence of certain markers on the cell surface.

Cytology is the microscopic study of cells obtained either by aspiration (a fine-needle biopsy) or from a smear, a washing, or a scraping. A surgical biopsy involves removal of larger amounts of tissue for pathologic review. An incisional biopsy removes just part of the tumor or affected tissue, whereas excisional biopsy removes the entire tumor or tissue for evaluation. The type of biopsy done is based on the type of tissue to be removed, its location, and the amount of tissue required to make a diagnosis. Different biopsy approaches include going through the skin (percutaneous), through a scope (endoscopic), or directly during surgery. Percutaneous and endoscopic biopsy procedures are often facilitated with stereotactic approaches that allow for exact positioning of the biopsy instruments directly at the site of the tumor.

Classification: Grading and Staging

If a malignant tumor is identified, clinical staging is done as part of the diagnostic workup to define the extent or spread of the disease and to aid as a guide to treatment. Staging includes determining the size of the tumor, its location(s), and the presence or absence of metastasis. Grading of the tumor includes determining both the tissue origin of the malignancy and its histologic grade (i.e., the degree of differentiation).

Grading Cellular Differentiation

Grading is the measure of the degree of differentiation of a neoplasm. Some pathology grading systems apply only to malignant neoplasms, whereas others apply to benign neoplasms as well. The neoplastic grading system is a measure of a cell's *anaplasia* or how different it appears from its tissue of origin. A cancer cell that is well differentiated looks more like the normal cell from which it derived, whereas

TABLE 12-3 TNM Classification System

Primary Tumor (T)[a]	
TX	Tumor cannot be measured.
T0	No evidence of primary tumor (tumor cannot be found).
Tis	Tumor *in situ*, meaning malignant cells only within superficial layer of tissue; no extension into deeper tissue.
T1	Description of primary tumor based on size and/or
T2	invasion into nearby structures; the higher the T
T3	number, the larger the tumor and/or the more it
T4	has grown into nearby tissues.
Regional Lymph Nodes (N)[b]	
NX	Nearby lymph nodes cannot be evaluated.
N0	No evidence of cancer cells in regional lymph nodes.
N1	Description of size, location, and/or number of lymph
N2	nodes involved; the higher the N number, the
N3	more extensive the lymph node involvement.
Metastases (M)[c]	
MX	Metastases cannot be evaluated.
M0	No evidence of metastases can be found.
M1	Description of extent of metastasis; the higher the
M2	M number, the more extensive the metastasis.
M3	
M4	

[a]Describes the primary (original) tumor based on size (measured in centimeters).
[b]Describes whether or not the cancer has spread into regional (nearby) lymph nodes.
[c]Describes whether or not the cancer has metastasized (spread) to other parts of the body.
Source: Adapted from American Cancer Society: http://www.cancer.org.

a poorly differentiated cell has little resemblance to the original normal cell and typically represents a more advanced and aggressive cancer. Different grading systems are used to classify the appearance of malignant cells, although the most common is that recommended by the American Joint Committee on Cancer (Box 12-1).[14] Cancer-specific grading scales are also used for certain types of malignancies, such as the Gleason score[15] (prostate cancer), the Bloom–Richardson grading system[16] (breast cancer), and the Fuhrman system[17] (kidney cancer).

Clinical Staging

For all solid tumors, the TNM classification system is used to determine the stage of the disease.[14] This system assesses the growth and spread of the tumor based on three factors: *T*umor size and invasiveness, the presence or absence of spread to regional lymph *N*odes, and the presence or absence of *M*etastasis to distant organs (Table 12-3). Once the T, N, and M categories are determined, a stage (I–IV) is assigned, with stage I being early stage disease and stage IV being the most advanced disease. The actual assignment into these stages is specific to the cancer type. Hematologic cancers (i.e., liquid tumors) cannot be staged using the TNM classification system, and each of these malignancies has its own unique staging system. In recent years, unique genetic changes have been identified in certain tumor types (especially the hematologic malignancies), and this new information is being incorporated into the staging and prognostic systems specific to those cancers.

CLINICAL MANAGEMENT

Primary Prevention

Preventing cancer from occurring is the most definitive way to lessen the burden of cancer. Risk factors can be eliminated or reduced through behavior modification, modification of the environment, vaccination, or treatment of infections. Major risk reduction is possible through smoking cessation, avoiding excessive sun exposure, participating in regular physical activity, and eating a balanced diet.[12] Combined, these four risk factors account for nearly 60% of all cancers. Although it is not a common approach, another primary prevention strategy is prophylactic surgery for individuals at risk. For example, a woman with the *BRCA1* genetic marker has a 65% and 40% chance of developing breast and ovarian cancer, respectively. She might elect to have a bilateral mastectomy and oophorectomy to prevent the development of these two cancers.

Secondary Prevention (Screening)

The goal of secondary prevention is early disease detection so that prompt treatment can be initiated. Screening refers to the application of a test to a population that has no overt signs or symptoms of the disease in question in order to detect disease at a stage when treatment is more effective. Screening tests are used to identify people who require further investigation to determine the presence or absence of disease, but they are not primarily diagnostic tests. Whereas some screening tests may positively identify a malignancy (e.g., colonoscopy), others often only identify suspected problems (e.g., mammography). Individuals who a have positive screening test of any type need to be referred for a full diagnostic workup.

There are multiple types of cancer screening, and a discussion of each is beyond the scope of this text. Examples of common screening tests for cancer include mammography for breast cancer, prostate-specific antigen testing for prostate cancer, and colonoscopy and guaiac testing for occult blood in the stool for colon cancer. The U.S. Preventive Services Task Force establishes evidence-based screening recommendations for the general population.[18] Because the recommendations are based on the latest scientific evidence, screening recommendations will periodically change.

Collaborative Interventions

Interventions for neoplasia are addressed in terms of treatment goals, which include cure, control, and palliation. The interventions discussed here may be used in various sequences or combinations.

Surgery

Surgery is the oldest intervention for cancer treatment. In addition to primary treatment, surgical intervention is also used for diagnosis, staging, and cytoreduction (debulking). Surgery may also be used to prevent cancer, to relieve the symptoms of cancer, or to enhance functional and cosmetic outcomes. Primary surgical resection is rarely curative, and it is frequently combined with other treatment modalities to improve cure rates and increase disease-free intervals. Additional therapies that are done following surgery are called *adjuvant* therapy and may include chemotherapy or radiation. If these therapies occur prior to the surgical procedure, they are considered *neoadjuvant* therapy.

Nursing care associated with the patient undergoing surgical procedures for any aspect of cancer (prevention, cure, palliation, and reconstruction) includes patient education, pre- and postoperative care, infection prevention, pain management, and psychosocial care.[19]

Radiation Therapy

Radiation therapy is a local treatment for cancer and may be used anywhere in the disease trajectory. It can take the form of either palliative or potentially curative treatment. Radiation is essentially a small packet of energy in the form of photons (e.g., x-rays and ultraviolet light) or particles (e.g., protons, neutrons, alpha-particles, and electrons) that is delivered directly to the site of the neoplasm. When these packets of energy penetrate the tissue, ionization induces direct biologic damage to the cells. Because these packets often pass through healthy tissue on their way to the neoplasm, damage to unaffected cells is an unintended consequence.[20] Radiation therapy may be delivered in several ways, the most common of which is external beam therapy using a linear accelerator. Another delivery technique, known as brachytherapy, delivers a high dose of radiation to a limited volume of tissue. Using this technique, short-range radiation sources are enclosed in a protective capsule and placed directly at the site of the tumor. Thus, the radiation affects only a very localized area and limits exposure of radiation to healthy tissues. The nursing management of patients receiving either type of radiation therapy largely involves patient education and the management of symptoms associated with the therapies.[21]

Chemotherapy

The word *chemotherapy* means treatment with chemicals, but the term has evolved over time to mean the systemic treatment of cancer. The general goal of systemic chemotherapy is to prevent cancer cells from multiplying, invading, and metastasizing to distant sites. Unlike surgery or radiation therapies, which are local and regional treatments, systemic chemotherapy agents act at the site of the tumor as well as at distant sites where tumor cells may have already metastasized. The principle of chemotherapy is based on the phases of the cell cycle, and most chemotherapeutic drugs are classified according to the specific phase of the cell cycle in which they exert their cytotoxic effects.[22] The role of the nurse in cancer chemotherapy is vast, pivotal, and rewarding. Nurses are responsible for assessment and education of the patient, handling and administration of chemotherapeutic agents, management of side effects, and management of psychosocial issues. Before they can administer chemotherapy in the clinic, nurses must undergo special training and certification through the Oncology Nursing Society.[23]

Hormonal Therapy

Another effective form of cancer treatment involves the use of antihormonal agents to treat malignancies that are responsive to hormones, such as breast, prostate, and endometrial cancers. Current approaches use agents that are hormonal agonists or antagonists, depending on type of cancer and the nature of the disease process. Hormonal therapies were developed based on their ability to target and block specific receptors and their various associated feedback loops. Thus, these agents are considered the first form of targeted cancer therapy.[24]

Targeted Therapy

Targeted therapy is the most rapidly evolving and expanding class of anticancer agents due to their specificity at targeting cancer cells and their generally reduced side effect profile. These agents are designed to interfere with molecules that are necessary for tumor growth, progression, and metastases. This is in contrast to chemotherapy agents that act against all actively dividing cells. These agents take several forms but generally fall into the categories of antibodies, antibody–drug conjugates, or small molecule inhibitors, of which there are many different classes. Targeted therapies have been developed that prevent growth signaling, interfere with tumor blood vessel formation, stimulate the immune system to destroy cancer cells, or even deliver toxic drugs directly to cancer cells. In all, more than 30 of these agents have been approved by the U.S. Food and Drug Administration for use in the treatment of a wide variety of cancers. They are the cornerstone of the treatment arm of what is termed "precision medicine," a form of medicine that seeks to use information about a person's genes and proteins to prevent, diagnose, and treat disease.[25]

Biologic Therapy

Biotherapy (also known as immunotherapy) refers to modulation of the immune response for a therapeutic goal. Biotherapy is a global term used to describe the use of biologic agents to activate the immune system (biologic response modifiers) and more recently includes approaches that manipulate cells within immune system using techniques such as gene therapy. Within the scope of the biologic response modifiers is the broad class of drugs termed "biologic agents," which are substances that are extracted or produced from biologic material. Such agents include colony-stimulating factors, gene therapy, monoclonal antibodies, nonspecific immunomodulatory agents, angiogenesis inhibitors, vaccines, and cell-based systems. Note that many of these biologic response modifiers also fall into the category of targeted therapy because they have very specific targets within the immune system.[26] These agents often have unique side effects that are quite different from those of traditional chemotherapy agents. As with chemotherapy, nurses wishing to administer and manage the side effects of these novel agents must receive special training and certification through the Oncology Nursing Society.[23] Due to the unique nature of biotherapy, nurses play a significant role in patient education and psychosocial support. As with many of the targeted therapies, these agents can be quite expensive, and there are frequently economic issues for the patient receiving biotherapy.

Bone Marrow and Hematopoietic Stem Cell Transplantation

Hematopoietic (blood-forming) pluripotent stem cells are found in the bone marrow. When given the proper signals, these stem cells mature and give rise to fully formed erythrocytes, leukocytes, and platelets. Stem cells can be collected from the blood through a process called apheresis, or they may be harvested directly from multiple bone marrow biopsy samples. When these stem cells are infused into a patient, the procedure is called a "stem cell" or "bone marrow" transplant, with the nomenclature essentially reflecting the source of the stem cells. Regardless of the source, the principle of the procedure is to replace diseased hematopoietic cells with these highly specialized stem cells that will then give rise to the full spectrum of healthy hematopoietic cells. The transplant can be autologous (by harvesting and

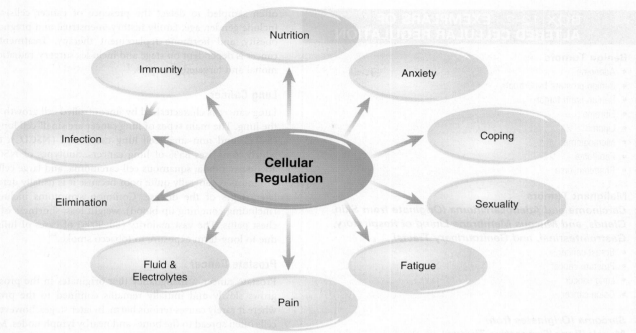

FIGURE 12-2 Cellular Regulation and Interrelated Concepts

using one's own stem cells) or allogeneic (whereby the stem cells come from a matched family donor or matched unrelated donor).[27] Stem cell transplantation is usually done for the purpose of cure or quality-of-life years gained. Patients undergoing transplantation can have many complex medical issues, and nurses working with these patients require very specialized training.

Symptom Management Resulting from Cancer and Cancer Treatment

Patients who undergo cancer treatment or who have an advanced cancer diagnosis experience multiple complications related to both the disease and its treatment. For these patients, nursing interventions are geared toward managing both the physical and the psychosocial aspects of these complications. Nurses can support the patient and family members by identifying coping mechanisms and resources. Although identifying all of the specific complications and adverse effects associated with the previously discussed treatment modalities is beyond the scope of this text, the most common and important complications and side effects are briefly presented in the following section.

INTERRELATED CONCEPTS

Cellular regulation is closely related to many of the concepts presented in this textbook. The interrelated concepts may be associated with the disease process, as consequence of treating the disease, or a combination of both. The most important interrelated concepts are presented in Figure 12-2, and they are briefly described here. **Nutrition** is an important interrelated concept because many patients with cancer experience calorie and especially protein malnutrition. Cancer cells divert nutrients from normal cells to sustain their cellular growth and expansion. In addition, many patients undergoing cancer treatment lose weight due to reduced or lost appetite (anorexia), nausea, vomiting, stomatitis, diarrhea, or physical inability to eat as part of the disease process.[28] Compromised **Immunity** is a concern especially among patients with a hematologic malignancy and is a common side effect of the myelosuppressive effects of chemotherapy or radiation.

Although this is typically transient, patients are vulnerable to many opportunistic infections. Disease- or treatment-related immunodeficiency puts cancer patients at significant risk for **Infection**. Moreover, due to their immunocompromised status, they may not present with the typical signs and symptoms of infection that are present in healthy patients. This can be fatal if it results in a delay in recognizing and treating an infection. In fact, infection is a very common cause of death for cancer patients undergoing treatment.[29] **Pain** is a common symptom associated with cancer and is among the most feared. It may result directly from cancer-caused tissue destruction, or it may be treatment related. It is a complex symptom to manage because of the wide variability in pain perception among patients. Unfortunately, pain is often underassessed and undertreated in cancer patients.[30] **Fatigue** is a common symptom associated with cancer and its treatment. Fatigue in patients with cancer, known as *cancer-related fatigue (CRF)*, is distinct and more debilitating than general fatigue. The unique and more debilitating symptoms associated with CRF are thought to be related to high levels of circulating inflammatory cytokines present in patients with cancer. A multitude of additional contributing factors may include side effects from medications, anemia, anorexia, weight loss, depression, and general organ dysfunction often associated with later-stage cancer.[31] Many cancer patients experience an altered pattern of **Elimination**—the most common of which is diarrhea. Conversely, some chemotherapy agents and most pain medications (opioids) cause significant issues with constipation. Also, bowel obstructions may occur as a result of the disease process, such as in the case of colorectal cancer, or an enlarged prostate may block urinary flow.

Fluid and Electrolyte imbalances can occur as a result of cancer or its treatment. Early in treatment when the disease burden is high, patients are at risk for tumor lysis syndrome manifested by elevated levels of uric acid, phosphate and potassium levels. Other imbalances such dehydration, hypercalcemia and third spacing of fluids are common in patients with more advanced disease. **Anxiety**, **Coping**, and **Sexuality** have important and interrelated impacts on patients with cancer due to the significant psychosocial issues that can be associated with their diagnosis and treatment.[32]

■■■ BOX 12-2 EXEMPLARS OF ALTERED CELLULAR REGULATION

Benign Tumors
- Adenoma
- Benign prostate hypertrophy
- Benign brain tumor
- Fibroma
- Lipoma
- Meningioma
- Papilloma
- Rhabdomyoma

Malignant Tumors
Carcinoma and Adenocarcinoma (Originate from Skin, Glands, and Mucous Membrane Lining of Respiratory, Gastrointestinal, and Genitourinary Tracts)
- Breast cancer
- Prostate cancer
- Lung cancer
- Colon cancer

Sarcoma (Originates from Muscle/Bone/Connective Tissues)
- Chondrosarcoma
- Ewing's sarcoma
- Fibrosarcoma
- Kaposi's sarcoma
- Rhabdomyosarcoma
- Osteosarcoma

Lymphomas (Originates from Lymph System)
- Hodgkin's lymphoma
- Non-Hodgkin's lymphoma

Leukemia (Originates from Hematopoietic System)
- Chronic lymphocytic leukemia (CLL)
- Chronic myeloid leukemia (CML)
- Acute lymphocytic leukemia (ALL)[a]
- Acute myeloid leukemia (AML)[a]

[a]Common among children.

CLINICAL EXEMPLARS

There are hundreds of examples of abnormal cellular reproduction and growth and, in fact, there are more than 200 different types of cancer. Although it is beyond the scope of this text to describe all types of abnormalities related to cellular regulation, some of the most common are presented in Box 12-2 and are featured here. Specific and detailed information related to each of these exemplars is readily available in nursing and medical textbooks, as well as on reputable websites, such as those of the American Cancer Society (http://www.cancer.org) and the National Cancer Institute (http://www.cancer.gov).

Featured Exemplars

Breast Cancer

Breast cancer originates in the tissues of the breast. The most common is ductal carcinoma, which begins in the lining of the milk ducts. Invasive breast cancer is one that has spread from where it began in the breast ducts to surrounding normal breast tissue. Lymphatic vessels in the breast drain to the axillary lymph nodes; thus, lymph nodes are often sampled to detect the presence of cancer cells. Risk factors include gender, age, family history, menstrual and pregnancy history, obesity, and hormone replacement therapy. Treatment for breast cancer is dependent on stage and includes surgery, radiation, and hormonal and targeted therapies.[33]

Lung Cancer

Lung cancer is characterized by uncontrolled cell growth of tissues of the lung. The main types of lung cancer are small-cell lung carcinoma (SCLC) and non-small-cell lung carcinoma (NSCLC), the latter of which comprises 85% of lung cancers. Subtypes of NSCLC include adenocarcinoma, squamous cell carcinoma, and large cell carcinoma. Prognosis is generally quite poor because it is usually detected only at later stages of the disease. Common symptoms include coughing (including coughing up blood), weight loss, shortness of breath, and chest pains. The vast majority (80–90%) of cases of lung cancer are due to long-term exposure to tobacco smoke.[34]

Prostate Cancer

Prostate cancer, a malignancy that originates in the prostate, usually grows slowly and initially remains confined to the prostate gland, where it rarely causes serious harm. In later stages, however, the cancer cells often spread to the bones and nearby lymph nodes. Most prostate cancer grows very slowly and may need minimal or no treatment. However, other types can be quite aggressive and will spread quickly if left unattended. Prostate cancer is the most common type of cancer in men; risk factors include older age, a family history of the disease, and race. Approximately 99% of all cases of prostate cancer occur in men older than age 50 years.[35]

Acute Lymphocytic Leukemia

Acute lymphocytic leukemia (ALL) is a malignancy of the white blood cells characterized by the overproduction and accumulation of cancerous white blood cells known as blasts. As blasts accumulate in the bone marrow, they inhibit the production of normal cells such as red and white blood cells and platelets, resulting in symptoms such as fever, infection, shortness of breath, tachycardia, bleeding, and bruising. The blasts are capable of leaving the blood and bone marrow and infiltrating other organs. ALL is the most common type of cancer in children, and treatment generally results in a cure. ALL was one of the first cancers for which an effective chemotherapeutic treatment was developed.[36]

Fibroma

A fibroma is a benign tumor mostly composed of fibrous or connective tissue that can form anywhere in the body and at any age, but fibromas are most often seen in adults. Common types of fibroma include angiofibromas, dermatofibromas, ovarian fibromas, and plantar fibromas. Most fibromas are harmless, and treatment is not required unless there are disturbing symptoms or cosmetic concerns. Depending on the site and size of the fibroma, removal may be accomplished by a simple surgical procedure or by cryotherapy. Neurofibromas, associated with an autosomal dominant mutation in the *NF1* gene, are associated with extensive lesion formation and can result in symptoms ranging from physical disfiguration to cognitive disability.[37]

Lipoma

A lipoma is a benign tumor composed of adipose or body fat and is the most common benign form of soft tissue tumor, occurring in approximately 1 in every 1000 people, usually in adults. They are generally slow growing, often arising over a period of months or years.

Most lipomas are small, soft to the touch, movable, and generally painless. They can occur almost anywhere in the body, including in muscles and internal organs. In most cases, lipomas do not need to be treated, although they may be surgically removed if there is concern about location, they are causing pain, or they are impacting physical appearance.[38]

CASE STUDY

Source: Jeremy Woodhouse/
Blend Images/Thinkstock

Case Presentation

Katrina Wells, a 54-year-old African American female, works a sedentary job in telecommunications. She has been overweight most of her life and has never engaged in physical activity on a regular basis. Because of limited finances and limited health care coverage, Katrina seeks health care only when she is ill.

Through a community outreach program, Katrina met Lydia Robinson, a nurse who helped her gain access to basic preventive health care services. Acting on the advice of Lydia, Katrina agreed to have a screening mammogram. The radiologist who reviewed the mammography films discovered a small mass in the upper outer quadrant of Katrina's left breast. She was contacted by the radiologist and told she had an abnormal mammography result and that she needed to return to the imaging center for further workup. Katrina, not knowing what this meant, asked if she had cancer. She was told that cancer was a possibility but that further testing was needed to determine if this was the case.

Katrina was upset by this information, and she was not sure she wanted any additional tests. Her mother had breast cancer, and Katrina watched her lose her breast and hair, in addition to becoming very sick from the medications. Lydia helped Katrina understand the need for the additional workup. During the next 4 weeks, Katrina underwent several tests as part of her diagnostic workup. Lydia helped Katrina by explaining the process and providing emotional support. The diagnostic mammogram and ultrasound examination of the breast revealed a 7.4-mm lesion, and a needle biopsy confirmed the diagnosis of breast cancer.

The pathology showed it to have low-risk features and that it would be responsive to hormonal therapy. Katrina was referred to a surgical and medical oncologist at the local cancer center for treatment.

An oncology clinical nurse specialist at the cancer center met with Katrina at her first oncology appointment to begin guiding her through the treatment process. Due to the small size of the lesion and the low-risk features, she was told she would not need chemotherapy. Her treatment would involve only surgery and radiation, followed by 5–10 years of hormonal therapy to decrease the risk of recurrence. She underwent a lumpectomy followed by 5 weeks of radiation to the left breast and axillary region. Following completion of radiation, she was started on an oral aromatase inhibitor, which she was to take daily for at least the next 5 years. She was to continue visiting the medical oncologist at the cancer center every 3–6 months during that time. At those visits, she would get a clinical breast exam and reinforcement about how to do a breast self-exam between visits. The staff at the cancer center also arranged for her to get yearly mammograms to screen for a new or recurrent breast cancer.

Case Analysis

This case exemplifies several aspects of cellular regulation gone awry. Katrina had several important risk factors for cancer: obesity, sedentary lifestyle, family history of cancer, and limited access to health care. Health policy initiatives for community outreach programs have been instituted to reduce cancer disparities, and without them, it is unlikely Katrina would have been screened. Her breast cancer was detected fairly early while it was still small and had not yet acquired aggressive features. Katrina did require multimodality treatment (surgery, radiation, and hormonal therapy) in an effort to effect a cure, but she was spared the need for aggressive chemotherapy. Katrina experienced the common fears and anxiety associated with a diagnostic workup for cancer, and Lydia helped her cope with these fears and assisted her throughout the diagnostic process. The caring atmosphere exemplified by Lydia and the health care providers at the cancer center was just as important as the physical care they provided.

ACCESS EXEMPLAR LINKS IN YOUR GIDDENS EBOOK

REFERENCES

1. Gomes AP, Blenis J: A nexus for cellular homeostasis: The interplay between metabolic and signal transduction pathways. *Curr Opin Biotechnol* 34:110–117, 2015.
2. Hanahan D, Weinberg RA: The hallmarks of cancer. *Cell* 100(1):57–70, 2000.
3. Hanahan D, Weinberg RA: Hallmarks of cancer: The next generation. *Cell* 144(5):646–674, 2011.
4. Hanahan D, Coussens LM: Accessories to the crime: Functions of cells recruited to the tumor microenvironment. *Cancer Cell* 21(3):309–322, 2012.
5. Cairns RA, Harris IS, Mak TW: Regulation of cancer cell metabolism. *Nat Rev Cancer* 11(2):85–95, 2011.
6. Peek G, Melnyk BM: Coping interventions for parents of children newly diagnosed with cancer: An evidence review with implications for clinical practice and future research. *Pediatr Nurs* 36(6):306–313, 2010.
7. Vivar CG, Canga N, Canga AD, et al: The psychosocial impact of recurrence on cancer survivors and family members: A narrative review. *J Adv Nurs* 65(4):724–736, 2009.
8. Siegel RL, Miller KD, Jemal A: Cancer statistics, 2015. *CA Cancer J Clin* 65(1):5–29, 2015.
9. World Health Organization: *WHO report on the global tobacco epidemic, 2008—The MPOWER package*, Geneva, 2008, World Health Organization.
10. de Martel C, Ferlay J, Franceschi S, et al: Global burden of cancers attributable to infections in 2008: A review and synthetic analysis. *Lancet Oncol* 13(6):607–615, 2012.
11. Garber JE, Offit K: Hereditary cancer predisposition syndromes. *J Clin Oncol* 23(2):276–292, 2005.
12. Anand P, Kunnumakkara AB, Sundaram C, et al: Cancer is a preventable disease that requires major lifestyle changes. *Pharm Res* 25(9):2097–2116, 2008.
13. Willett WC: Diet and cancer. *Oncologist* 5(5):393–404, 2000.
14. Edge SB, Byrd DR, Compton CC, et al: *AJCC cancer staging manual*, vol 649, New York, 2010, Springer.
15. Egevad L, Granfors T, Karlberg L, et al: Prognostic value of the Gleason score in prostate cancer. *BJU Int* 89(6):538–542, 2002.

16. Genestie C, Zafrani B, Asselain B, et al: Comparison of the prognostic value of Scarff–Bloom–Richardson and Nottingham histological grades in a series of 825 cases of breast cancer: Major importance of the mitotic count as a component of both grading systems. *Anticancer Res* 18(1B):571–576, 1998.

17. Ficarra V, Martignoni G, Maffei N, et al: Original and reviewed nuclear grading according to the Fuhrman system. *Cancer* 103(1):68–75, 2005.

18. U.S. Preventive Services Task Force: Recommendations. Retrieved from <http://www.uspreventiveservicestaskforce.org/Page/Name/recommendations>, 2015.

19. Lewis SL, Dirksen SR, Heitkemper MM, et al: *Medical–surgical nursing: Assessment and management of clinical problems*, ed 9, St Louis, 2014, Mosby.

20. Baskar R, Lee KA, Yeo R, et al: Cancer and radiation therapy: Current advances and future directions. *Int J Med Sci* 9(3):193–199, 2012.

21. Iwamoto RR, Haas M, Gosselin TK: *Manual for radiation oncology nursing practice and education*, Pittsburgh, PA, 2012, Oncology Nursing Society.

22. Fernando J, Jones R: The principles of cancer treatment by chemotherapy. *Surgery* 33(3):131–135, 2015.

23. Neuss MN, Polovich M, McNiff K, et al: 2013 updated American Society of Clinical Oncology/Oncology Nursing Society chemotherapy administration safety standards including standards for the safe administration and management of oral chemotherapy. *J Oncol Pract* 9:5s–13s, 2013.

24. Abraham J, Staffurth J: Hormonal therapy for cancer. *Medicine* 39(12):723–727, 2011.

25. Wujcik D: Science and mechanism of action of targeted therapies in cancer treatment. *Semin Oncol Nurs* 30(3):139–146, 2014.

26. Lizee G, Overwijk WW, Radvanyi L, et al: Harnessing the power of the immune system to target cancer. *Annu Rev Med* 64:71–90, 2013.

27. Copelan EA: Hematopoietic stem-cell transplantation. *N Engl J Med* 354(17):1813–1826, 2006.

28. Holder H: Nursing management of nutrition in cancer and palliative care. *Br J Nurs* 12(11):667–674, 2003.

29. Cameron D: Management of chemotherapy-associated febrile neutropenia. *Br J Cancer* 101:S18–S22, 2009.

30. Canivet D, Delvaux N, Gibon AS, et al: Improving communication in cancer pain management nursing: A randomized controlled study assessing the efficacy of a communication skills training program. *Support Care Cancer* 22(12):3311–3320, 2014.

31. Wang XS, Woodruff JF: Cancer-related and treatment-related fatigue. *Gynecol Oncol* 136(3):446–452, 2015.

32. Pedersen B, Koktved DP, Nielsen LL: Living with side effects from cancer treatment? A challenge to target information. *Scand J Caring Sci* 27(3):715–723, 2013.

33. National Cancer Institute: Breast cancer, (n.d.). Retrieved from <http://www.cancer.gov/cancertopics/types/breast>.

34. National Cancer Institute: Lung cancer, (n.d.). Retrieved from <http://www.cancer.gov/types/lung>.

35. National Cancer Institute: Prostate cancer, (n.d.). Retrieved from <http://www.cancer.gov/cancertopics/types/prostate>.

36. National Cancer Institute: Acute lymphocytic leukemia, (n.d.). Retrieved from <http://www.cancer.gov/cancertopics/types/leukemia>.

37. Cedars-Sinai: Fibroma, (n.d.). Retrieved from <http://www.cedars-sinai.edu/Patients/Health-Conditions/Soft-Tissue-Tumors—Benign.aspx>.

38. Cleveland Clinic: Lipomas. Retrieved from <http://my.clevelandclinic.org/health/diseases_conditions/hic_lipomas>, 2012.

Intracranial Regulation

Debra Smith

The brain is a highly complex organ that processes internal and external stimuli and controls body functions. As the largest component of the central nervous system (CNS), the brain lies within the cranium and is protected by the skull. The intracranial regulation (ICR) concept includes normal and abnormal processes of intracranial function. Nurses care for individuals experiencing a wide variety of ICR issues in both community and inpatient settings.

DEFINITION

The term *cranium* refers to the collective bone structure that encloses the brain—also known as the skull.[1] The prefix *intra-* refers to within. Thus, the term intracranial refers to those components that lie within the skull, which include the brain, circulatory system, and dura mater. *Regulation* is a term that refers to compliance and maintenance of balance. In the case of ICR, it is referring to maintaining a balance to promote an environment that is conducive to optimal brain functioning. The concept of ICR includes anything that affects the contents of the cranium and impacts the regulation of maintaining an optimally functioning brain. For the purpose of this concept presentation, ICR is defined as *mechanisms or conditions that impact intracranial processing and function.* Although the brain receives input from outside the cranium, specifically through the peripheral nervous system and the spinal cord component of the CNS, this concept does not include problems with the peripheral nervous system or spinal cord. ICR focuses on those conditions that specifically affect the contents of the cranium. As will be discussed further, there are many variables that can upset this balance with potentially devastating results.

SCOPE

The scope of this concept ranges from normal to impaired function (Figure 13-1). When functioning optimally, ICR allows individuals to function normally. Impairment can be caused by a number of factors including reduced blood flow to the brain, compromised neurotransmission, and damage to brain tissue. The resulting neurologic dysfunction can range from minimal to severe.

NORMAL PHYSIOLOGICAL PROCESS

The brain is the primary structure associated with intracranial regulation and is part of the CNS, serving as the primary control center for the body. Anatomically, the brain is divided into the following areas: the cerebrum, the diencephalon, the cerebellum, and the brain stem (Figure 13-2). Normal intracranial regulation involves interaction among these structures through a complex communication system. Table 13-1 presents general functions of these structures for reference. Neurons are cells within the nervous system designed for the transmission of information within the brain and throughout the body. Neurons direct signals from cell to cell through dendrites and axons. Optimal ICR is dependent on the transmission of nerve impulses across neuronal synapses by neurotransmitters.

Brain function depends on a consistent supply of blood delivering oxygen and nutrients. A sufficient volume of blood and cardiac function is required for adequate perfusion. The level of oxygen in the blood is dependent on gas exchange in the lungs and hemoglobin capacity. Likewise, because carbohydrates are the main source of fuel for the brain, optimal ICR is dependent on blood glucose levels. Several other unique physiological processes are in place to protect and preserve critical brain functions, and these are described next.

Cranial Vault/Skull

The skull is composed of multiple bones that act as a rigid, noncompliant protective covering of the brain. Within the skull are three components: brain tissue (80%), blood (10%), and cerebrospinal fluid (CSF) (10%).

Intracranial pressure (ICP) is the sum of the pressure exerted by these three volumes in the skull. In adults, ICP is normally ≤15 mm Hg; a sustained ICP of ≥20 mm Hg is considered intracranial hypertension. Because the total volume inside the skull cannot change, a change in one compartment necessitates a change in another. This interrelationship of volume and compliance of the three cranial components is known as the Monro–Kellie doctrine.[2]

Blood–Brain Barrier

Between the arterial and venous network of the brain is a unique capillary system called the blood–brain barrier (BBB), which consists of a tight layer of endothelial cells. This restrictive barrier makes it difficult for neurotoxic substances to pass into the brain.[3] This barrier may become compromised secondary to decreased perfusion.

Meninges

There are three layers of protective membranes that surround the brain and spinal cord: dura mater, arachnoid layer, and pia mater. The area

FIGURE 13-1 Scope of Intracranial Regulation

FIGURE 13-2 Structures of the Brain (Source: Modified from Lewis SL, et al, editors: *Medical–surgical nursing: Assessment and management of clinical problems*, ed 9, St Louis, 2014, Mosby.)

TABLE 13-1	Structures of the Brain and General Functions	
Brain Structure	**Description**	**Functions**
Cerebrum	Largest brain structure located at the top; divided into two hemispheres (right and left) and four lobes (frontal, parietal, temporal, occipital)	Thinking, consciousness, sensory perception, movement, emotions, memory
Cerebellum	Located under occipital lobe of the cerebrum	Balance, muscle coordination, posture
Diencephalon	Located between the cerebrum and the midbrain; consists of two structures—the thalamus and hypothalamus	Sensory relay, emotions, alerting mechanism (thalamus); regulation of body temperature, fluid balance, sleep, and appetite (hypothalamus)
Brain stem	Located at the base of the brain; consists of the medulla oblongata, pons, and midbrain	Conduction pathway between brain and spinal cord for movement, cardiac, respiratory, and vasomotor control; conduction pathway for visual and auditory impulses

between the arachnoid layer and the pia mater is referred to as the subarachnoid space, which contains CSF. ICR problems are frequently referred to in relation to the meningeal layer location—for example, subarachnoid hemorrhage, subdural hematoma, or epidural hematoma. Meningitis is an inflammatory condition of the meninges.

Autoregulation

Cerebral blood flow (CBF) is normally maintained at a relatively constant rate by intrinsic cerebral mechanisms referred to as autoregulation. Autoregulation adjusts regional CBF in response to the brain's metabolic demands by changing the diameter of cerebral blood vessels. Cerebral arterial walls are thinner than those in the systemic circulation because of a lack of smooth muscle and a decreased thickness of the tunica media. They also do not have the ability to develop collateral circulation in response to ischemia. Autoregulation allows the cerebral circulation to deliver a constant supply of blood despite wide fluctuations in systemic blood pressure.

Cerebral Spinal Fluid

CSF is produced at a rate of approximately 20 mL/hour, circulates within the subarachnoid space, and then is absorbed into the venous system. It acts to cushion and support the brain and other structures of the CNS and provides nutrients. CSF analysis provides useful diagnostic information related to certain nervous system conditions (see Diagnostic Tests).

Hyperventilation

Another protective mechanism in response to increasing cerebral volume is spontaneous hyperventilation. Carbon dioxide is a potent vasodilator. Hyperventilation is a compensatory mechanism that causes vasoconstriction, which reduces cerebral blood volume and ICP.

Age-Related Differences

The brain undergoes significant development during infancy and childhood. At birth, brain function is primarily limited to primitive reflexes and is sufficiently developed to sustain extrauterine life. Extensive development occurs thereafter during the first few years, not only in size but also in function. Throughout childhood, a child's growth and development is influenced by evolving cognitive, emotional, and motor functions within the brain. Cranial sutures are ossified by age 12 years, with no expansion of the skull after age 5 years.[4] Before the sutures are entirely closed, there is some room for expansion in the case of cerebral edema and increasing ICP.

Aging is associated with a reduction in brain size, weight, and number of neurons. Atrophy of neuronal dendrites causes a slowing of neurotransmission and neural processes. These changes, however, are not directly associated with mental function, and cognitive abilities remain intact in the absence of disease, although cognitive function is enhanced with continued stimulation.

VARIATIONS AND CONTEXT

There are several categories that describe impairment or dysfunction associated with ICR. These include problems associated with perfusion, neurotransmission, glucose regulation, and pathologic processes. These categories are briefly described next, and the pathologic consequences of these impairments are detailed in the sections that follow. All of these impairments can occur across the lifespan, although some are more prevalent in particular age groups.

Impaired Perfusion

For the brain to function optimally, there must be a consistent supply of blood delivering oxygen and nutrients. Impairment in blood flow, reduced oxygenation of the blood, or reduced blood glucose can lead to significant dysfunction. Intracerebral perfusion can be disrupted in a number of different conditions, such as internal blockage of a vessel, severe hypotension, or loss of vessel integrity attributable to damage or excessive external pressure on a vessel that exceeds perfusion pressure. For example, an ischemic stroke is the result of inadequate perfusion past the thrombus or embolus. Perfusion can also be disrupted as the result of an intracranial hemorrhage, such as a subdural hematoma or subarachnoid hemorrhage caused by a traumatic brain injury (TBI). A disruption of cerebral perfusion leads to a wide variety of ICR problems depending on the area of the brain that is affected and the length of time before perfusion is restored.

Compromised Neurotransmission

Optimal functioning of the brain is dependent on the transmission of nerve impulses across neuronal synapses by neurotransmitters. Normal transmission requires fully functioning neurons, nerves, and neurotransmitters. Presynaptic neurons release neurotransmitters that travel to postsynaptic neurons. Neurotransmitters can be either excitatory or inhibitory. Many components of this process can be disrupted. Degenerative diseases (see Pathology) disrupt brain functioning by the loss of neurons, which also disrupts neurotransmission. The concentration of the neurotransmitter acetylcholine is reduced in Alzheimer's disease secondary to the destruction of acetylcholine-secreting neurons. Neurotransmitters can be affected by drugs and toxins, which can modify their function or block their attachment to receptor sites on the postsynaptic membrane. For example, heroin binds to presynaptic endorphin receptors and reduces pain by blocking the release of the neurotransmitter that causes pain.[3] Seizures are aberrant neuronal activity that can manifest clinically as disrupted motor control, sensory perception, behavior, and/or autonomic function.

Glucose Regulation

Because the brain cannot store glucose, a constant supply is needed to maintain optimal functioning. Areas of the brain that are particularly sensitive to hypoglycemia are the cerebral cortex, hippocampus, and cerebellum. Prolonged hypoglycemia may cause widespread neuronal injury. Children, who have smaller glycogen stores, are particularly susceptible to hypoglycemia, which can adversely affect brain tissue.

Hyperglycemia (glucose level >126 mg/dL) can also cause problems by augmenting brain injury in acute stroke. Some of the deleterious effects of hyperglycemia are worsened ischemic damage, an increased infarction size, and increased BBB permeability. The optimal glucose range is being studied but is yet to be determined.[5]

Pathology

There are many pathologic states that disrupt intracranial functioning and regulation. Pathology of the brain can take many forms, such as brain tumors, degenerative diseases, and inflammatory conditions.

Many degenerative diseases of the brain are clinical exemplars of the ICR concept. Alzheimer's disease is a degenerative process that results in the loss of neurons primarily in the gray matter of the brain. Parkinson's disease is a result of damage to the basal ganglia, and Huntington's disease is a degeneration of striatal neurons. Although the degenerative process varies with each of these diseases, the result is the same—disruption of brain regulation and function.

The most common inflammatory conditions of the brain are abscesses, meningitis, and encephalitis. Although the etiology varies with each condition, the result is an inflammatory response that can result in disrupted cerebral function and regulation.

CONSEQUENCES

Regardless of the specific condition or cause, when there is impaired blood flow, compromised neurotransmission, and damage to brain tissue from trauma or other pathologic conditions, significant pathophysiological consequences can occur.

Cerebral Edema

Cerebral or brain parenchymal edema occurs for many reasons. Box 13-1 shows common causes of cerebral edema. It is a symptom

---

BOX 13-1   Causes of Cerebral Edema

Mass Lesions
- Brain abscess
- Brain tumor (primary or metastatic)
- Hematoma (intracerebral, subdural, epidural)
- Hemorrhage (intracerebral, cerebellar, brain stem)

Head Injuries and Brain Surgery
- Contusion
- Hemorrhage
- Post-traumatic brain swelling

Cerebral Infection
- Meningitis
- Encephalitis

Vascular Insult
- Anoxic and ischemic episodes
- Hemorrhagic stroke
- Ischemic stroke (thrombotic or embolic)
- Venous sinus thrombosis

Toxic or Metabolic Encephalopathic Conditions
- Lead or arsenic intoxication
- Hepatic encephalopathy
- Uremia

Source: From Lewis SL, et al, editors: *Medical–surgical nursing: Assessment and management of clinical problems*, ed 9, St Louis, 2014.

that is common to many ICR conditions. Cerebral edema may be classified as vasogenic, cytotoxic, or interstitial. Regardless of the classification or origin of cerebral edema, the result is an increase in brain size that will negatively affect perfusion and oxygenation to the brain. As discussed next, signs and symptoms will become evident to varying degrees based on the location and amount of cerebral edema.

Increased Intracranial Pressure

Elevated ICP is a potentially devastating complication of neurologic injury caused by many different conditions. Pathologic ICP is evident at sustained pressures ≥20 mm Hg. Several conditions may cause increased ICP, such as TBI, ruptured aneurysm, CNS infections, hydrocephalus, and brain tumors. Symptoms of increased ICP include headache, decreased level of consciousness, and vomiting. Signs may include cranial nerve VI palsies, papilledema, and periorbital bruising; a late sign is Cushing's triad (see increased intracranial pressure later in this concept presentation).[2] The untoward consequence of increased ICP is impaired perfusion (see Measurement of Cerebral Perfusion Pressure).

Brain Tumors

A tumor can occur in any part of the brain and spinal cord. Brain tumors are most commonly a result of metastasis from another primary site outside the brain. Clinical manifestations will depend on the size and location of the tumor.

RISK FACTORS

Populations at Risk

All populations are potentially at risk for problems with ICR because there are such a wide variety of conditions included in this concept. Depending on the condition, some populations are at a higher risk. ICR problems related to degenerative pathology have a higher incidence in the elderly population. Injury-related ICR problems are more commonly seen in the adolescent and young adult age groups. The leading causes of TBI are falls and motor vehicle accidents.[6] Falls are more of an issue with the very young and elderly populations. Because of risk-taking behavior, motor vehicle accidents are more prevalent in the young adult population.

Individual Risk Factors

Individual risk factors are dependent on the cause of injury or pathology. For example, the risk factors for stroke include age, hypertension, diabetes, smoking, obesity, and cardiovascular disease. Some of the degenerative pathologic conditions have a strong genetic component and put certain individuals at higher risk.

ASSESSMENT

History

A thorough history should be solicited from the patient or a family member if the patient is unable to provide information. Patient presentation will help direct the practitioner to the most relevant areas of inquiry. Information in a history that provides data about intracranial function can relate to multiple systems. Asking pertinent questions will provide clues to the examiner of ICR problems and will help to focus the physical examination. Potential ICR areas on which to focus include the following:

- Numbness, paralysis, tingling, neuralgia
- Loss of consciousness, dizziness, fainting, confusion
- Changes in recent or remote memory

- Changes in vision, hearing, balance, gait
- Speech problems (expressive and/or receptive)
- Chewing/swallowing problems
- Muscle weakness or loss of bowel or urinary control
- Onset of unexplained tremors or other motion disturbances
- Unexplained, severe headache
- Vomiting
- Symptom onset
- History of head injury

Examination Findings

Objective examination findings that convey neurologic status are found throughout a physical examination. Specific signs of dysfunction vary depending on the ICR problem. Many age-related degenerative changes occur in the CNS. When assessing an older adult, it is important to distinguish between the expected changes and changes potentially related to an ICR problem that could improve with appropriate treatment. Findings common to most conditions are a change in mental status and motor function. Some of the more common examination techniques and tools are discussed next, but these are not all-inclusive.

Mental Status

A complete mental status examination includes assessment of the individual's emotional responses, mood, cognitive functioning, and personality. Depending on the patient's presenting condition, the nurse will decide which components of the exam are relevant.[7] If it is not practical or necessary to do a complete mental status exam, the Mini-Mental Status Examination is an option, which is a simplified scored form of the cognitive portion of the mental status examination. It consists of 11 questions and takes only 5–10 minutes to administer.[8]

Cognitive functioning should be intact in the healthy elderly client, although some changes may occur as individuals grow older.[7] When assessing an elderly patient, it is essential to determine the patient's baseline neurologic functioning in order to establish if there are significant changes.

Glasgow Coma Scale

The Glasgow Coma Scale (GCS) is used to give a standardized numeric score of the neurologic patient assessment. This is a widely used measurement tool that consists of three components: eye opening, verbal response, and motor response. Although this is an objective measurement tool, there is room for subjective interpretation of assessment findings. To minimize subjectivity and facilitate consistency, when transferring care of a patient, nurses should complete the GCS together and agree on the values. Changes in the GCS will help to determine treatment methods and priorities. Table 13-2 describes the components of the GCS.

Cranial Nerves

As the name implies, the cranial nerves originate in the cranium; therefore, assessment of the cranial nerves should be included in a thorough neurologic assessment. Abnormal findings will help to locate the affected area of the brain. Assessment techniques can be found in nursing assessment textbooks.

Intracranial Pressure

The earliest sign of increased ICP is a change in level of consciousness. Another early sign is headache. Headache characteristics associated with increased ICP include nocturnal awakening, pain worsened by cough/defecation, recurrent and localized, and progressive increase in

TABLE 13-2 Glasgow Coma Scale

Appropriate Stimulus	Response	Score
Eyes Open • Approach to bedside • Verbal command • Pain	Spontaneous response	4
	Opening of eyes to name or command	3
	Lack of opening of eyes to previous stimuli but opening to pain	2
	Lack of opening of eyes to any stimulus	1
	Untestable[a]	U
Best Verbal Response • Verbal questioning with maximum arousal	Appropriate orientation, conversant; correct identification of self, place, year, and month	5
	Confusion; conversant, but disorientation in one or more spheres	4
	Inappropriate or disorganized use of words (e.g., cursing), lack of sustained conversation	3
	Incomprehensible words, sounds (e.g., moaning)	2
	Lack of sound, even with painful stimuli	1
	Untestable[a]	U
Best Motor Response • Verbal command (e.g., "raise your arm, hold up two fingers") • Pain (pressure on proximal nail bed)	Obedience of command	6
	Localization of pain, lack of obedience but presence of attempts to remove offending stimulus	5
	Flexion withdrawal,[a] flexion of arm in response to pain without abnormal flexion posture	4
	Abnormal flexion, flexing of arm at elbow and pronation, making a fist	3
	Abnormal extension, extension of arm at elbow usually with abduction and internal rotation of arm at shoulder	2
	Lack of response	1
	Untestable[a]	U

[a]Added to the original scale by some centers.
Source: Modified from Lewis SL, Dirksen SR, Heitkemper MM, Bucher L: *Medical–surgical nursing: Assessment and management of clinical problems*, ed 9, St Louis, 2014.

FIGURE 13-3 Coronal Section of Brain Showing Potential Sites for Placement of ICP Monitoring Devices (Source: Modified from Lewis SL, Dirksen SR, Heitkemper MM, Bucher L: *Medical–surgical nursing: Assessment and management of clinical problems*, ed 9, St Louis, 2014, Mosby.)

frequency or severity. Vomiting, usually not preceded by nausea, is often a nonspecific sign of increased ICP.[9]

Infants have less specific symptoms of increased ICP, such as irritability, bulging fontanel, lethargy, flat affect, and poor feeding. Retinal hemorrhage in children with increased ICP should raise suspicion of nonaccidental head trauma. Infants with elevated ICP may develop macrocephaly, split sutures, or a bulging fontanel.[10]

ICP is measured using a catheter placed in one of the following locations in the cranium: intraventricular, intraparenchymal, subarachnoid, or epidural (Figure 13-3). The most common placement is in the lateral ventricle. Patients must be in an intensive care environment for this type of monitoring. Most commonly, ICP monitoring is done in trauma patients with a closed head injury. Some other indications include stroke, intracerebral hemorrhage, hydrocephalus, and subarachnoid hemorrhage. Guidelines for management of severe head injury recommend that ICP monitoring is indicated in comatose head injury patients with a GCS score of 3–8 and with an abnormal computerized tomography (CT) scan. The goal of care is to keep ICP <20 mm Hg.[9] Catheters are available that monitor ICP, drain CSF, and

measure brain oxygenation. When the patient has increased ICP, the catheter may be used for therapeutic drainage of CSF in order to reduce ICP.

If hydrocephalus is present, a ventriculostomy may be used to remove CSF. In children, a "sun setting" appearance of the eyes is evident with increased ICP.[10] In some instances, a permanent catheter is placed to drain CSF, which is known as a ventriculoperitoneal shunt.

Cushing's triad is useful in explaining the late signs of increased ICP. It is an ominous late sign of increased ICP and an indication of impending herniation. The triad consists of hypertension (with widened pulse pressure), bradycardia, and changes in respiratory pattern in the presence of increased ICP. Pupil and vision changes may become apparent as edema impinges on cranial nerves II, III, IV, and/or VI.[7]

Measurement of Cerebral Perfusion Pressure

Cerebral blood flow increases with hypercapnia and hypoxia. Ischemia results from inadequate cerebral perfusion or increased cerebral oxygen consumption. To maintain adequate perfusion, it is necessary to optimize cerebral perfusion pressure (CPP), which is calculated by subtracting the ICP from the mean arterial pressure. When CPP is <60 mm Hg, cerebral blood flow is compromised and autoregulation is impaired.[2] CPP should be kept between 60 and 70 mm Hg in patients with elevated ICP to avoid ischemic injury. CPP >70 mm Hg should be avoided because of an increased risk for adult respiratory distress syndrome.[9]

Normal CPP range for children is not well established, but it is likely lower than that of adults because systolic blood pressure is lower in children. Appropriate CPP values are probably 40–60 mm Hg.[10]

The National Institutes of Health Stroke Scale

The National Institutes of Health Stroke Scale (NIHSS) is an example of one type of specific tool for nurses to use when assessing a patient following stroke. This scale, composed of 11 items, has been widely used and validated. The NIHSS score on admission has been correlated to stroke outcome and is recommended for all patients with suspected stroke.[11]

Diagnostic Tests

When an ICR problem is suspected, time is of the essence. Diagnostic tests that can quickly give the most pertinent information are recommended initially.

Neuroimaging Studies

Imaging studies are essential to obtain in patients presenting with sudden neurologic deterioration, and they may also be utilized with nonemergent conditions such as suspected brain tumor. A noncontrast CT or magnetic resonance imaging (MRI) scan should be performed as soon as possible to determine the origin of a neurologic injury. Current guidelines recommend a head CT for all TBI patients with a GCS of 14 or lower, which can detect skull fractures, intracranial bleeding, and cerebral edema.[9] Advanced CT and MRI technologies, such as magnetic resonance angiography and positron emission tomography, are available that can distinguish between brain tissue that is irreversibly infarcted and that which is potentially salvageable, which will help when deciding appropriate treatment.

Skull Radiograph

Depending on the mechanism of action and patient presentation, a skull x-ray may be ordered to detect fractures, bone erosion, calcification, and/or abnormal vasculature.

Electroencephalogram

An electroencephalogram (EEG) measures and records the brain's electrical activity through multiple electrodes placed on the scalp. Video EEG monitoring refers to continuous EEG monitoring over a prolonged period of time while simultaneously recording the patient's movements and activity. This monitoring combination is useful in diagnosing and localizing the area of seizure origin. The EEG is also helpful in identifying psychogenic nonepileptic seizures. The origin of these seizures may be associated with psychological conditions or other physical problems, but they are not caused by electrical activity in the brain.[12]

Brain Biopsy

To determine the type and stage of a brain tumor, a biopsy is performed, usually during a surgical procedure. Preliminary histologic type can usually be determined quickly in the operating room; then the tumor is sent to pathology for complete analysis and final determination.

Lumbar Puncture

The lumbar puncture (spinal tap) may be indicated when infection is suspected. A lumbar puncture should be deferred until after the head CT scan if intracranial hypertension is suspected because brain herniation may be precipitated by increasing the pressure gradient between the cranial vault and the spinal cord.

CLINICAL MANAGEMENT

Primary Prevention

Primary prevention strategies are intended to maintain optimal health and prevent injury or disease. This applies to intracranial regulation in many ways. Leading a healthy lifestyle, which includes smoking cessation, maintaining a healthy weight, controlling blood pressure, and exercising, can decrease the risk of vascular disease impacting the cerebral arteries. This is linked to risk reduction for stroke. Injury prevention measures such as proper use of seat belts and/or helmets, knowledge of firearm safety, and participation in violence prevention programs reduce the risk of TBI. *Healthy People 2020*[13] has identified the following three objectives specifically related to the prevention and reduction of brain injury:

- Reduce fatal traumatic brain injuries.
- Reduce hospitalization for nonfatal traumatic brain injuries.
- Reduce emergency department visits for nonfatal traumatic brain injuries.

Secondary Prevention (Screening)

There are no true screening tests available related to ICR. In the event of injury or the presence of clinical findings suggesting intracranial dysfunction, specific diagnostics tests are initiated to determine a cause.

Collaborative Interventions

There are many interventions related to caring for patients with ICR issues. A few of the most common examples are discussed. The overarching goal of caring for patients is to prevent secondary injury (damage to the vulnerable adjacent tissues) by improving cerebral perfusion; this is primarily achieved by decreasing cerebral edema and ICP, which will improve oxygenation to prevent cell death.

Pharmacotherapy

Because impairments in intracranial regulation represent a large number of conditions, there are many classes of pharmacologic agents associated with this concept. Table 13-3 presents these agents, and they are described further here.

Osmotic diuretics. Osmotic diuretics create an osmolar gradient that draws water across the BBB, leading to a decrease in interstitial volume and a subsequent decrease in ICP. Mannitol is the agent used

TABLE 13-3 Pharmacologic Agents Commonly Used to Treat Problems with ICR

Classification	Indications Specific for Intracranial Regulation	Most Common Agents Used
Osmotic diuretics	Reduction of ICP by reducing fluid	Mannitol
Sedatives	Reduction of metabolic demand to reduce ICP	Propofol, lorazepam
Analgesics	Pain control to reduce oxygen demand	Fentanyl, morphine
Antiepileptics	Seizure control	Phenytoin, valproic acid
Glucocorticoids	Cerebral edema associated with pathologies	Dexamethasone
Antipyretics	Fever control to reduce metabolic demand	Acetaminophen
Antihypertensives	Reduce blood pressure in hemorrhagic stroke	Labetalol, transdermal nitroglycerin paste, nicardipine
Antiparkinsonian agents	Restore balance of dopamine in brain	Levodopa, pramipexole, ropinirole, bromocriptine, selegiline
Cholinesterase inhibitors	Mild to moderate dementia	Doneprezil, rivastigmine, galantamine
	Moderate to severe dementia	Memantine

most commonly to achieve ICP control in a variety of conditions, and it has been shown to improve cerebral blood flow. Hypertonic saline is increasingly being used, but research has not clearly determined the volume, tonicity, or most effective method of administration.[14]

Sedatives. Sedatives can decrease ICP by reducing metabolic demand. Propofol (Diprivan) is frequently used in the intensive care unit setting because it has a short half-life and is easily titrated, permitting frequent neurologic assessment. Barbiturate coma is sometimes used as a final effort in the case of uncontrolled increased ICP, but there is little clinical evidence to support its use.[14] Benzodiazepines, such as lorazepam (Ativan), are another sedative option.

Analgesics. Pain increases oxygen demand; therefore, in addition to controlling pain for patient comfort, it should be controlled to avoid compromising sufficient oxygen delivery to ischemic neuronal cells. The use and choice of sedative agents should be individualized according to specific clinical circumstances and provider expertise. Short-acting narcotics, such as fentanyl or morphine, are generally preferable to allow for periodic neurologic assessments.

Antiepileptics. Seizures can exacerbate or cause increased ICP and increase oxygen demand. Antiepileptics may be used as a prophylactic or treatment measure. These medications act by stabilizing nerve cell membranes and preventing the distribution of the epileptic discharge. Initial seizure management of TBI patients includes phenytoin (Dilantin) or valproic acid (Depakote). Patient education is important because there are many serious side effects associated with antiepileptic medications. The U.S. Food and Drug Administration issued a warning in 2008 related to the risk of suicidal thoughts and behaviors associated with 11 antiepileptic medications.[15]

Glucocorticoids. Glucocorticoids may be indicated for use in some ICR problems and are contraindicated in others. Dexamethasone (Decadron) may be effective in reducing cerebral edema related to tumors, abscesses, and CNS infections. Glucocorticoids are associated with a poor outcome in treating moderate to severe head injury and should not be used in this patient population.[9]

Antipyretics. Fever may worsen the outcome after stroke and severe head injury by aggravating secondary brain injury caused by increased metabolic demand. Normothermia should be maintained through the use of antipyretic medications, such as acetaminophen, or by implementation of other treatment modalities such as mechanical cooling.

Antihypertensive medications. Depending on the ICR condition, antihypertensive medications may be detrimental or beneficial. Mean arterial pressure must be adequate to maintain sufficient CPP to limit secondary injury. Because of this, higher systemic blood pressures are tolerated in patients with ICR conditions that impair CPP. In these patients, antihypertensive medications are not recommended, and medications may be initiated in order to sufficiently raise the systemic pressure, particularly if the ICP is elevated. Several studies have shown that lowering the systemic blood pressure in patients with acute ischemic stroke has been associated with clinical deterioration. Conversely, reducing blood pressure in patients with a hemorrhagic stroke may be beneficial by minimizing further bleeding and continued vascular damage.[4]

Antiparkinsonian medications. Antiparkinsonian medications attempt to restore the balance of dopamine through one of several mechanisms, depending on drug type. The most effective drugs, called dopaminergic drugs, replace dopamine, or mimic its action in the brain. Another group of drugs delays the breakdown of dopamine, thus increasing the level in the brain.

Levodopa (Sinemet) is the most commonly used antiparkinsonian medication; it is converted to dopamine in the CNS, where it serves as a neurotransmitter. To minimize the side effects of dopamine in the periphery, another medication is administered with levodopa. In the United States, this drug is carbidopa, which prevents the conversion of levodopa to dopamine until it reaches the brain.

Dopamine agonists mimic the effect of dopamine by stimulating the same cells as dopamine. Monoamine oxidase B (MAO-B) is an enzyme that breaks down levodopa in the brain. MAO-B inhibitors prolong the effectiveness of dopamine and also levodopa.

Cholinesterase inhibitors. Cholinesterase inhibitors are prescribed to patients with mild to moderate dementia to make acetylcholine more available, improving cortical function. In moderate to severe dementia, an *N*-methyl-D-aspartate (NMDA) receptor antagonist may have a neuroprotective function as well as decrease dementia symptoms. However, it does not slow progression of the disease.[16]

Surgical Interventions

Many types of cranial surgery are available to address ICR problems. Some examples are craniotomy, craniectomy, and shunt and stereotactic procedures.

A *decompressive craniectomy* removes the rigid confines of the skull, allowing for expansion of the cranial contents and lowering the ICP. Potential complications of this surgery include herniation through the skull defect, spinal fluid leakage, wound infection, and epidural and subdural hematoma.

A *craniotomy* may be performed to remove a lesion or tumor; repair a damaged area; or relieve pressure and/or drain blood secondary to epidural, subdural, or intracerebral hematomas.

Frequently, the origin of seizures is either the hippocampus or the amygdala, which is located in the temporal lobe of the brain (see Diagnostic Tests, Electroencephalogram). If seizures are found to arise from these areas, a temporal lobectomy surgery is performed to resect the identified area. This surgery is becoming more common and has been successful in obtaining seizure control.

Stereotactic procedures allow precise localization of a specific area of the brain and may be utilized for dissection or to obtain a biopsy.

Shunt procedures place an artificial pathway for excessive CSF to be drained from an area of the brain to an extracranial location using a tube or implanted device. Accumulation of CSF may be due to overproduction, obstruction, or problems with normal reabsorption. Placement of a ventriculoperitoneal shunt is a common example of this type of procedure.

Ongoing Assessment

With prevention of secondary injury being the goal of patient care, it is of upmost importance to recognize changes in the patient's condition early. For this reason, thorough and frequent neurologic assessment is critical in the care of a patient with ICR problems. A complete neurologic assessment includes determination of level of consciousness and measurement of GCS score along with cognitive, motor, sensory, and reflex testing.

Vital signs should be monitored consistently on all patients with an ICR problem. The frequency will be dictated by the condition and acuity of the patient. Assessment should be frequent enough to detect significant changes early so that the appropriate interventions can be implemented to prevent patient deterioration (see the discussion of Cushing's triad in the Intracranial Pressure section).

ICP/CPP Monitoring

As discussed previously, it is imperative that the brain receive a constant, adequate blood supply to optimize brain functioning. Severely head-injured patients should receive continuous ICP and CPP monitoring. If these values are not optimal, several possible collaborative and nursing interventions are available. Most guidelines recommend that treatment for elevated ICP should be initiated when ICP is >20 mm Hg.

Interventions to Lower ICP

Positioning. The intracranial venous system consists of canals and sinuses, and unlike the peripheral venous system, it lacks valves. Interventions promoting venous outflow from the head decrease cerebral volume and help to lower ICP. Such interventions include head-of-bed elevation and proper alignment of the head and neck with the body. Head-of-bed elevation of 30 degrees is usually recommended to decrease ICP. It is also important to keep the head and neck midline (to prevent compression of jugular veins) and to limit hip flexion. Head-of-bed elevation potentially could decrease cerebral perfusion by increasing venous return. Therefore, head-of-bed elevation is recommended as long as the CPP remains at an appropriate level.

Activity management. Balance is needed between being efficient and not increasing oxygen demand when providing nursing care. Clustering of many nursing tasks at once will increase oxygen demand and may compromise cerebral perfusion. Distribution of care procedures over a longer time frame is preferable.

Airway management. Endotracheal suctioning stimulates coughing, which increases ICP. Patients with increased ICP should undergo endotracheal suctioning only when suctioning is indicated; in addition, these patients may need to be sedated before the procedure. Careful assessment is necessary to maintain an adequate airway and minimize complications of increased ICP.

Hyperventilation. Prophylactic hyperventilation ($PaCO_2$ ≤25 mm Hg) in TBI is not recommended because it decreases perfusion, which will negatively impact oxygen delivery. Hyperventilation is recommended only as a temporary measure to reduce elevated ICP.[9] A 1 mm Hg change in $PaCO_2$ is associated with a 3% change in cerebral blood flow.[2] Hyperventilation can also increase extracellular lactate and glutamate levels, which may contribute to secondary brain injury.[14]

Bowel management. Constipation increases intra-abdominal pressure and causes straining when defecating, thereby raising ICP. Stool softeners or laxatives may be necessary to minimize these untoward effects on ICP.

Nutrition Management

Nutrition management is a high priority when caring for patients with ICR conditions. The nurse should advocate for an early dietary consultation in order to ensure prompt and adequate nutrition to facilitate healing. Depending on the ICR impairment and patient condition, enteral or parenteral feeding may be appropriate. Swallowing function should be assessed before initiation of enteral feeding for certain patients, particularly following a stroke.

Patient Education

Patient education is always a primary nursing function, which is no exception when caring for patients with ICR conditions. Education should be focused on all levels of health promotion. Problems involving the brain can have devastating and long-lasting effects. Nurses are uniquely qualified and available to assist patients and their families throughout the course of their care.

Rehabilitation

Particularly after a stroke or head injury, rehabilitation is an important part of patient care. The focus is on returning the patient to optimal functioning. The composition of the rehabilitation team will depend on the patient's needs, which may include speech therapy, physical therapy, and occupational therapy along with medical and nursing care as needed. As soon as the patient is stabilized in the acute care setting, rehabilitation should begin. It may take months to years to determine how much function will be regained.

INTERRELATED CONCEPTS

Many concepts are closely related to ICR. Those considered most important are shown in Figure 13-4.

Cognition is dependent on an optimally functioning brain. If ICR is disrupted, depending on the area of the brain affected, cognitive function may be impaired either temporarily or permanently. The degree of cognitive function impairment is dependent on the number of neuronal cells affected.

The brain controls movement, coordination, and balance. Thus, optimal Mobility is dependent on an intact neurologic system and effective intracranial regulation. Individuals who have intracranial regulation problems may become immobile as a result of unsteadiness; imbalance; or the inability to initiate or execute purposeful movement to the arms, legs, or trunk.

Perfusion and Gas Exchange are intimately involved with ICR and have been discussed thoroughly in the Normal Physiological Process and Physiological Consequences sections. Without adequate perfusion of oxygen- and nutrient-rich blood, the neurons are unable to function. Hormonal Regulation is dependent on normal intracranial

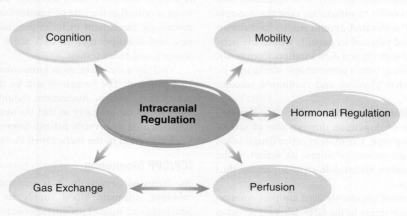

FIGURE 13-4 Intracranial Regulation and Interrelated Concepts

---

BOX 13-2 EXEMPLARS OF INTRACRANIAL REGULATION

Perfusion
Ischemic Stroke
- Embolic stroke
- Thrombotic stroke

Hemorrhagic Stroke
- Intracerebral hemorrhage
- Intraventricular hemorrhage
- Ruptured aneurysm
- Subarachnoid hemorrhage

Head Injury
- Epidural hematoma
- Skull fractures
- Subdural hematoma
- Traumatic brain injury

Neurologic Transmission
- Epilepsy
- Seizure

Pathology
Brain Neoplasm
- Benign brain tumor
- Malignant brain tumor

Degenerative Conditions
- Alzheimer's disease
- Dementia
- Huntington's disease
- Multiple sclerosis
- Parkinson's disease

Inflammatory Conditions
- Bacterial meningitis
- Brain abscess
- Encephalitis
- Viral meningitis

---

regulation because of the location of the hypothalamus and pituitary glands within the brain. Damage to these structures or surrounding brain tissue (from trauma or disease) can have disastrous effects on hormonal regulation.

CLINICAL EXEMPLARS

There are many clinical exemplars of intracranial regulation. Common exemplars are presented in Box 13-2. Although exemplars are listed under a specific category, there are instances in which an exemplar could fit under more than one category. For example, brain tumors can be considered *pathology* and can also cause problems with *neurotransmission*. Similarly, if a brain tumor is large enough and exerts enough pressure, it can also disrupt *perfusion*. The categories are not meant to be all-inclusive or exclusive but, rather, a suggested organization framework for ICR conditions. A brief discussion of common clinical exemplars follows. For detailed explanations and the nursing care for all the exemplars, see medical–surgical, pediatric, and gerontology textbooks.

Featured Exemplars
Stroke

A stroke occurs when there is a loss of blood flow to an area of the brain causing the neurons to die. Two major classifications of stroke are ischemic stroke and hemorrhagic stroke; ischemic stroke is the most common. Stroke is the third leading cause of death and serious long-term disability. Nearly three-fourths of all strokes occur in people older than age 65 years. The risk of having a stroke more than doubles each decade after age 55 years. In the United States, stroke death rates are higher for blacks than for whites, even at younger ages.[17] (See Case Study.)

Traumatic Brain Injury

TBI occurs when a blow to the head causes injury to the brain. The most common causes are motor vehicle accidents, falls, and violence.

Brain injury can range from mild to severe. With significant injury, the brain tissue swells, leading to cerebral edema and increased ICP; intracranial bleeding may also occur, further contributing to increased ICP. TBI is the leading cause of death and disability in children and adults ages 1–44 years.[9]

Epilepsy

Epilepsy, a brain disorder characterized by recurrent unprovoked seizures, is caused by inappropriate and excessive nerve impulses within clusters of neurons leading to uncontrolled and often violent muscle spasms and loss of consciousness. Epilepsy affects approximately 2 million people in the United States. More than one-third of people with epilepsy continue to have seizures despite treatment. Risk factors are more common in children younger than age 2 years and adults older than age 65 years. Approximately 10% of Americans will experience a seizure sometime during their lifetime.[18]

Alzheimer's Disease

Alzheimer's disease (AD) is one of many degenerative conditions that affect ICR. It is the most common form of dementia, affects more than 5 million Americans, and is the sixth leading cause of death in the United States. Almost two-thirds of those with AD are women. The most common form occurs in individuals older than age 65 years.[19] The exact cause of AD is unknown, but it is thought to be associated with abnormal plaque formation in the brain tissue and neuron tangles.

Meningitis

Meningitis is a pathologic condition affecting ICR; it is caused by inflammation of the meninges. The five types are viral, bacterial, fungal, parasitic, and noninfectious.[20] Viral meningitis is by far the most common type and less severe; bacterial meningitis is less common but is usually severe and associated with higher mortality. The populations at risk, transmission, and treatment vary widely, depending on the cause; however, more than 50% of cases occur in infants and children younger than age 5 years.

CASE STUDY

Source: JPC-PROD/iStock/ Thinkstock

Case Presentation

Mr. James Hobson is a 69-year-old male with a history of hypertension that is fairly well controlled on medication. He has been smoking one or two packs of cigarettes a day for the past 52 years and has a body mass index of 37.3. He awoke yesterday morning complaining of blurry vision and some weakness on the left side of his body. He thought he had just slept wrong, so he was not concerned. Later in the morning, he was having trouble walking and his wife convinced him to call his physician. The physician's office called 911, and Mr. Hobson was transported to the nearest hospital.

Upon arrival to the emergency department, the physical exam findings were as follows: heart rate, 112 beats/minute; blood pressure, 172/90 mm Hg; respiratory rate, 24 breaths/minute; O_2 saturation, 90%; arm and leg weakness (3/5); and somewhat decreased sensation. He was awake and responding to questions appropriately, although slowly. The following diagnostics tests were ordered: noncontrast CT (NCCT) of the head; electrocardiogram; complete blood count with platelets, cardiac enzymes, and troponin; electrolytes; blood urea nitrogen; creatinine; glucose; prothrombin time/international normalized ratio; and partial thromboplastin time. An NCCT will exclude or confirm the presence of hemorrhage. The sensitivity of an NCCT to show ischemia increases after 24 hours. This patient's CT scan did not show any signs of hemorrhage. Currently, thrombolytics are administered to treat an ischemic stroke within 3 hours of symptom onset. Studies are underway to evaluate the safety and efficacy of extending this window to $4\frac{1}{2}$ hours. Because it was unclear exactly when the symptoms began, the decision was made not to administer a thrombolytic.

Case Analysis

A stroke is an excellent exemplar of the ICR concept. The condition originates inside the cranium, which affects functioning within and outside the cranium. Sudden loss of focal brain function is the core feature of the onset of hemorrhagic and ischemic stroke.[4] When an ischemic stroke occurs because of a clot (thrombotic or embolic), perfusion is compromised to areas of the brain distal to the blockage. Clinical manifestations will vary depending on the ischemic area of the brain. Other conditions may mimic a stroke presentation (seizures, syncope, migraine, and hypoglycemia), so it is important to perform appropriate diagnostic testing early. A thorough history is imperative to determine onset of symptoms as early as possible because this will determine treatment and time is of the essence—particularly in the case of an ischemic stroke. A CT scan or MRI will determine if a stroke has occurred and its origin—hemorrhagic or ischemic.

ACCESS EXEMPLAR LINKS IN YOUR GIDDENS EBOOK

REFERENCES

1. Merriam–Webster: Cranium, (n.d.). Retrieved from: <http://www.merriam-webster.com/dictionary/cranium>.
2. Smith ER, Amin-Hanjani S: Evaluation and management of elevated intracranial pressure in adults, 2013. Retrieved from: <http://www.uptodate.com/contents/evaluation-and-management-of-elevated-intracranial-pressure-in-adults?source=search_result&search=elevated+icp&selectedTitle=1~150>.
3. Lewis SL, Dirksen SR, Heitkemper MM, Bucher L, editors: *Medical–surgical nursing: Assessment and management of clinical problems*, ed 8, St Louis, 2011, Mosby.
4. Perry S, Hockenberry M, Lowdermilk D, et al: *Maternal child nursing care*, ed 5, New York, 2014, Mosby.
5. Oliveira-Filho J, Koroshetz WJ: Initial assessment and management of acute stroke, 2015. Retrieved from: <http://www.uptodate.com/contents/initial-assessment-and-management-of-acute-stroke?source=search_result&search=acute+stroke&selectedTitle=1~120>.
6. Centers for Disease Control and Prevention: Traumatic brain injury in the United States: Fact sheet, 2015. Retrieved from: <http://www.cdc.gov/TraumaticBrainInjury/get_the_facts.html>.
7. Ball J, Dains J, Flynn J, et al: *Seidel's guide to physical examination*, ed 8, St. Louis, 2015, Elsevier.
8. Alzheimer's Society: Mini-Mental Status Examination (MMSE), (n.d.). Retrieved from: <http://www.alzheimers.org.uk/site/scripts/documents_info.php?documentID=121>.
9. Brain Trauma Foundation: TBI guidelines, (n.d.). Retrieved from: <https://www.braintrauma.org/coma-guidelines/searchable-guidelines>.
10. Brasher WK, Tasker RC: Elevated intracranial pressure (ICP) in children, 2013. Retrieved from: <http://www.uptodate.com/contents/elevated-intracranial-pressure-icp-in-children?source=search_result&search=elevated+ICP+children&selectedTitle=1~150>.
11. National Institute of Health: NIH stroke scale, 2003. Retrieved from: <http://www.ninds.nih.gov/doctors/nih_stroke_scale.pdf>.
12. Epilepsy Foundation: Types of seizures, 2013. Retrieved from: <http://www.epilepsy.com/learn/types-seizures/non-epilepsy-seizures>.
13. *Healthy People 2020*: Injury and violence prevention, 2015. Retrieved from: <https://www.healthypeople.gov/2020/topics-objectives/topic/injury-and-violence-prevention>.
14. Hemphill JC, Phan N: Management of acute severe traumatic brain injury, 2013. Retrieved from: <http://www.uptodate.com/contents/management-of-acute-severe-traumatic-brain-injury?source=search_result&search=management+of+acute+severe+traumatic+brain+injury&selectedTitle=1~150>.
15. U.S. Food & Drug Administration: Suicidal behavior and ideation and antiepileptic drugs, 2014. Retrieved from: <http://www.fda.gov/drugs/drugsafety/postmarketdrugsafetyinformationforpatientsandproviders/ucm100190.htm>.
16. Press D, Alexander M: Treatment of dementia, 2015. Retrieved from: <http://www.uptodate.com/contents/treatment-of-dementia?source=search_result&search=treatment+of+dementia&selectedTitle=1~150>.
17. Internet Stroke Center: U.S. stroke statistics, (n.d.). Retrieved from: <http://www.strokecenter.org/patients/about-stroke/stroke-statistics>.
18. Centers for Disease Control and Prevention: Chronic disease prevention & health promotion: Targeting epilepsy At a Glance, 2009. Retrieved from: <http://www.cdc.gov/nccdphp/publications/AAG/pdf/epilepsy.pdf>.
19. Alzheimer's Association: Alzheimer's facts and figures, (n.d.). Retrieved from: <http://alz.org/alzheimers_disease_facts_and_figures.asp#prevalence>.
20. Centers for Disease Control and Prevention: Meningitis, 2015. Retrieved from: <http://www.cdc.gov/meningitis/index.html>.

Hormonal Regulation

Jean Giddens

Hormonal regulation is a complex physiological process with integrated responses involving various glands, hormones (produced and secreted by the glands), and the action of hormones on the target tissues. Although each gland and hormone has a specific function, collectively hormonal regulation has five overarching functions: fetal differentiation of the reproductive and central nervous system, sequential growth and development during childhood and adolescence, reproduction, metabolic activity, and adaptive responses.[1] Imbalances of hormonal regulation can lead to significant health and social consequences. This concept presentation focuses on the normal process of hormonal regulation, hormonal imbalance, assessment, and interventions to optimize hormone balance.

DEFINITION

The term *hormonal regulation* is often used in the context of describing a specific group of hormones or metabolism. The focus of this concept presentation is broad, encompassing the general regulatory process including hormone production, secretion, and action. Clearly, the function and physiological action of each hormone are unique, and a presentation of details for each gland, each hormone, and conditions associated with imbalances is not intended; rather, a global perspective is proposed. Given this perspective, what is meant by hormonal regulation? For the purposes of this concept presentation, hormonal regulation is defined as *physiological mechanisms that regulate the secretion and action of hormones associated with the endocrine system.*

Several additional terms are important to fully understand this concept. An *endocrine gland* refers to a specialized cluster of cells, tissue, or an organ that produces and secretes hormones directly into the bloodstream. This distinction is important because there are also other types of glands (known as exocrine glands) that excrete other nonhormonal substances or fluids through ducts to body organs, cavities, or the skin. Examples include sweat glands, salivary glands, mammary glands, and bartholin glands. Exocrine glands are excluded from this concept presentation because they do not secrete hormones. A *hormone* is a chemical substance that stimulates cellular action in target tissues. *Target tissue* refers to the specific tissue that hormones can influence. A final term worth mentioning is *receptor site*, which refers to a location on the surface of a cell where hormones attach and gain access to the cell, allowing for physiological influence.

SCOPE

The scope of hormonal regulation ranges from the normal range of circulating hormone (based on physiological need) to abnormal secretion, in either excess or deficient amounts. This range, shown in Figure 14-1, is presented as a continuum because the secretion of hormones is variable, and it changes in response to physiological feedback. Typically, the prefix "hypo" before reference to the gland or hormone involved is used to describe deficient states, and the prefix "hyper" is used to describe states of excess. The scope of hormonal regulation can also be thought about from the perspective of the hormones and glands represented. Hormonal regulation represents the hormones produced and secreted from the hypothalamus, anterior pituitary, posterior pituitary, thyroid, parathyroid, adrenal cortex, ovary, testes, and pancreas.

NORMAL PHYSIOLOGICAL PROCESS

Hormones are produced by glands. The structural categories of hormones include protein and peptide hormones, steroid hormones, and monoamine hormones, with the majority being protein or peptides.[2] Figure 14-2 presents the locations of various adrenal glands, and Box 14-1 summarizes these glands, the hormones they produce, the target tissue, and the physiological effect.

Hormone Production, Secretion, and Transport

Many physiological functions are directed by hormones, which serve as chemical messengers that influence or control functions of other organs or body tissues. Hormones are produced and secreted by endocrine glands. The secretion of a hormone by the gland is in response to a certain level of a substance (e.g., sodium or glucose level) or in response to an alteration within the cellular environment. Once secreted from the gland, hormones are transported to their target tissue. In some cases, the target tissue is adjacent to the endocrine gland that produces the hormone, but more often the hormone is transported to one or more target tissues throughout the body by the circulatory system.[3] Water-soluble hormones circulate in the blood in free form, whereas most lipid-soluble hormones bind to a carrier (e.g., a protein) for transportation.

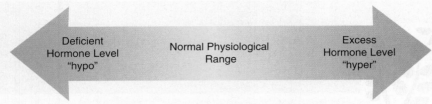

FIGURE 14-1 Scope of Hormonal Regulation

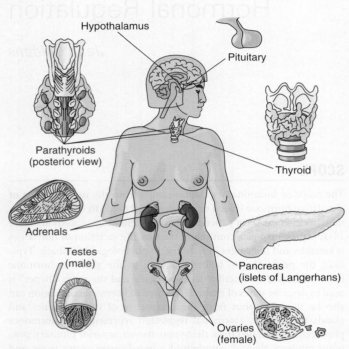

FIGURE 14-2 Location of Various Endocrine Glands (Source: From Ignatavicius DD, Workman ML, Medical-surgical nursing: patient-centered collaborative care, ed 7, St Louis, 2013, Elsevier.)

Hormone Action on Target Tissue

Hormones have very specific cellular effects but only on designated cells within the target tissue. Hormones depend on receptor sites to gain access and exert their specific physiological action within the cell.[4] Target cells have unique receptor sites for the designated hormone, much like a specific key is needed for a lock. For this reason, hormones are unable to influence cells unless they have the appropriate receptor site allowing a hormone to act on a cell. The more receptors on the cell, the higher affinity or sensitivity the cell has for that particular hormone. The cell has the ability to adjust the number of receptors (or sensitivity) based on the concentration of circulating hormone. When the circulating concentration of a hormone increases, fewer receptor sites are needed; when the concentration decreases, more receptor sites become available.

Control of Hormone Secretion

Maintaining hormone levels in normal physiological range is accomplished through feedback systems, although the specific mechanism varies depending on the gland or hormone involved. Four types of feedback control are negative feedback, positive feedback, biological rhythms, and central nervous system control.

Negative Feedback

Hormonal regulation occurs through negative and positive feedback mechanisms. The most common type of feedback system for hormonal regulation is the negative feedback system, whereby information regarding a hormone level or the effect of a hormone is communicated back to the gland that secrets the hormone which directs the need for hormone secretion or suppression.[1] One of the simplest examples is the secretion of insulin based on serum glucose levels. When serum glucose rises, the pancreas secretes insulin. Insulin has an effect on transporting glucose into the cell. As serum glucose levels drop, the pancreas inhibits insulin secretion. In this example, serum glucose levels trigger or inhibit the release of insulin.

Negative feedback is more complex when multiple glands and hormones are involved, but the same general process applies. For example, the secretion of thyroid hormones involves three glands (hypothalamus, anterior pituitary gland, and the thyroid gland). The hypothalamus secretes thyroid-releasing hormone, which triggers the release of thyrotropin, which in turn stimulates the secretion of triiodothyronine (T_3) and thyroxine (T_4) from the thyroid gland. As plasma levels of T_3 and T_4 rise, this information is communicated back to the hypothalamus and anterior pituitary gland to inhibit thyroid-releasing hormone and thyroid-stimulating hormone (TSH) secretion.

Positive Feedback

Positive feedback occurs when an increasing level of hormone triggers further elevation of hormone stimulation. The classic example of positive feedback is seen with the menstrual cycle, in which luteinizing hormone (LH) is secreted by the pituitary gland, which triggers the ovaries to secrete estradiol, which in turn stimulates the pituitary gland to secrete more LH.[2]

Biological Rhythms

The secretion of some hormones is controlled by biological rhythms. One example of this is the influence of the circadian rhythm on cortisol secretion. Cortisol secretion is highest in the morning and lowest in the late evening. Disruptions in biological rhythms and sleep deprivation can affect the normal secretion patterns of some hormones.[5]

Central Nervous System Stimulation

Another type of control mechanism for the secretion of hormones is through central nervous system stimulation.[1] For example, when an individual experiences a stressful situation, the sympathetic division of the autonomic nervous system is activated, triggering the release of epinephrine from the adrenal medulla (the fight-or-flight response). When the perceived stress is resolved, the adrenal medulla reduces the release of epinephrine.

Age-Related Differences

Glands and the action of hormones are influenced by the aging process, particularly during adolescence and among older adults.

BOX 14-1 Endocrine Glands, Hormones Secreted, and Physiological Effects

Hypothalamus
- Corticotropin-releasing hormone (CRH)/*anterior pituitary*/release of corticotropin hormone
- Thyrotropin-releasing hormone (TRH)/*anterior pituitary*/release of thyrotropin
- Gonadotropin-releasing hormone (GNHRH)/*anterior pituitary*/release of LH and FSH
- Growth hormone-releasing hormone (GHRH)/*anterior pituitary*/release of GH
- Growth hormone-inhibiting hormone (GHIH)/*anterior pituitary*/inhibition of GH
- Prolactin-inhibiting hormone (PIH)/*anterior pituitary*/inhibition of PRL
- Melanocyte-inhibiting hormone (MIH)/*anterior pituitary*/inhibition of MSH

Anterior Pituitary
- Thyrotropin/*thyroid*/stimulates synthesis and release of thyroid hormone
- Corticotropin/*adrenal cortex*/stimulates synthesis and release of corticosol
- Luteinizing hormone (LH)/*ovary and testis*/stimulates ovulation and progesterone secretion in females; testosterone secretion in males
- Follicle-stimulating hormone (FSH)/*ovary and testis*/stimulates estrogen secretion and follicle maturation in females; spermatogenesis in males
- Prolactin (PRL)/*mammary glands*/stimulates breast milk projection
- Growth hormone (GH) (also known as somatotropin)/*bone, muscle, and soft tissue*/promotion of growth and metabolism
- Melanocyte-stimulating hormone (MSH)/*skin*/pigmentation

Posterior Pituitary
- Antidiuretic hormone (AHD)/*kidney and blood vessels*/promotes water reabsorption
- Oxytocin/*uterus and mammary glands*/stimulates uterine contractions

Thyroid
- Triiodothyronine (T_3) and thyroxine (T_4)/*body-wide*/increased metabolism
- Calcitonin/*bones and kidneys*/lowers serum calcium and phosphate

Parathyroid
- Parathyroid hormone (PTH)/*bone, kidney, and gastrointestinal tract*/increases serum calcium and phosphate

Adrenal Cortex
- Glucocorticoids (cortisol)/*body-wide*/stress response, glucose regulation, immunity
- Mineralcorticoids (aldosterone)/*kidney*/retains water and Na^+, exertion of K^+

Adrenal Medulla
- Catecholamines (epinephrine and norepinephrine)/*heart, blood vessels, lung, kidney, liver, pancreas, and skin*/stress response: fight-or-flight reaction

Gonads
- Estrogen/*uterus, ovary, and breast*/reproduction
- Progesterone/*uterus, ovary, breast, and skin*/development of ova, female sex characteristics
- Testosterone/*sex organs, muscle, and skin*/development of sperm, male sex characteristics

Pancreas
- Insulin/*liver, muscles, and fat tissue*/regulates metabolism, lowers blood glucose
- Glucagon/*liver, muscles, and fat tissue*/elevates blood glucose

Adolescence

Reproductive glands and hormones lie mostly dormant during childhood and become active at the onset of adolescence.[6] During puberty, the anterior pituitary increases secretion of gonadotropins (LH and follicle-stimulating hormone). In the male, this stimulates the maturation of the testes, production of testosterone, and development of external genitalia. In the female, this stimulates estrogen production, the maturation of ovaries leading to ovulation, and development of external genitalia.

Older Adults

In response to advancing age, most glands become smaller with reduced hormone production.[1] This does not necessarily lead to hormonal regulation impairments, but the physiological activity of the hormone is reduced, which is linked to some common physiological changes associated with aging. For example, frailty has been shown to be associated with a pattern of hormonal changes in elderly men.[7] Also, menopause in women occurs as a normal response to aging and is associated with a reduction of estrogen produced by the ovaries. Reduced metabolism results in cold intolerance and reduced appetite. A reduction in the production of antidiuretic hormone also occurs, leading to a more dilute urine and thus leaving the older adult more at risk for dehydration.

VARIATIONS AND CONTEXT

Many problems can lead to hormone imbalance. Two general categories of hormonal imbalance can occur for each hormone secreted by endocrine glands: hormonal deficiency or excess. Problems with hormone deficiency or excess are usually associated with an issue in production/secretion or in the regulatory mechanisms directing the glands. Glands can be affected in a number of ways, including by trauma; congenital, genetic, and inflammatory conditions (including autoimmune conditions); and tumors. Damage to a gland can result in a reduction or loss of the ability of that gland to produce and secrete a hormone.

For example, damage to the thyroid gland can result in the inability to produce thyroid hormones. A number of other conditions can result in excessive production and secretion of a hormone. Signaling errors, caused by improper levels of other hormones or ineffective negative feedback mechanisms, can lead to excessive production or inhibition of hormone secretion. Other physiological triggers can result in undesired elevations or deficiencies in hormones. For example, excessive and sustained stress can result in chronic elevated circulating cortisol; interruption of the circadian cycle (e.g., from sleep deprivation) can result in reduced secretion of melanin.

Although hormonal deficiency or excess is often caused by a production/secretion problem, other variations can occur if the hormone loses its effect on the tissue or is unable to gain access to the cells due to a problem with receptor sites—often referred to as insensitivity.[8] A classic example of this is seen in type 2 diabetes, in which insulin insensitivity develops at the receptor sites.

CONSEQUENCES

Understanding the physiological consequences of hormone imbalance requires an understanding of the physiological effects of the hormones, presented in Box 14-1. Thus, an excess or deficiency of any hormone can create significant physiological challenges. The severity of such effects can vary widely—from the devastation a partnered couple experiences with infertility to life-threating states such as seen in thyroid storm or diabetes insipidus and diabetic ketoacidosis. Common consequences from impaired hormonal regulation can include alterations in growth and development, alterations in cognition, alterations in metabolism, alterations in reproduction, changes in growth, and altered adaptive responses. The disruption of any hormone production may result in potential complications associated with the underlying condition and the potential for lifetime hormonal replacement therapy.

RISK FACTORS

All individuals of all population groups have the potential for problems with hormonal regulation. Risk factors for hormonal imbalance are usually considered in the context of the specific gland and hormone involved. For example, the risk factors involving the anterior pituitary gland and the secretion of growth hormone differ significantly from risk factors associated with the hormonal imbalance involving the pancreas and secretion of insulin. Although risk factors are typically described at the level of each gland and hormone dysfunction, there are several risk factors that are shared by many hormonal imbalances (Box 14-2). One of the most obvious is hormone supplement therapy. Exogenous supplementation of any hormone places an individual at risk for excess or deficient hormone levels due to the variability in dosing needs and medication adherence. In response to advanced age, most glands become smaller with reduced hormone production, which increases the risk for certain hormonal deficiencies and reduced metabolism. Obesity and sedentary lifestyle are associated with many hormonal imbalances, such as diabetes and polycystic ovarian syndrome.[8] Genetics, chromosomal abnormalities, and family history, particularly a history of autoimmune responses, increase risk for several hormone deficiencies.

ASSESSMENT

Because hormonal regulation affects all body systems, and because each hormone has a specific role, there are not standard questions and examination procedures for all glands and hormones. Instead, hormonal function is considered adequate unless the patient, a parent, or other family members report a symptom or a clinical finding presents itself that suggests an abnormality. Such a situation triggers an in-depth history, examination, and diagnostic tests based on the presenting sign and/or symptom. For this reason, this section provides a very broad discussion regarding endocrine assessment.

History

The history provides the foundation for assessment. Baseline history always includes gender, age, marital status, past medical history (including age at menarche, last menstrual period, and reproductive history for females), current conditions, current medications, psychosocial history, and family history.[9] Often, these baseline data provide important clues if a hormonal imbalance is suspected. For example, some hormonal imbalances are more common in men than in women; some are more common among older adults than in children.

From a functional perspective, the symptoms or problems most likely reported by a parent of a child, an adolescent, or an adult patient are often associated with basic physiological functions. These include abnormal growth patterns, physical development, activity, energy level, sleep, nutrition, elimination, sexual response or reproductive problems, and unexplained changes in weight. Any of these types of symptoms warrants a symptom analysis of the presenting problem.

Examination Findings

Because of the anatomic location of the glands, most glands, with the exception of the thyroid gland and testes, are inaccessible to direct examination. Thus, most of the examination focuses on evidence of physiological or clinical effects of hormonal function.

Vital Signs, Height, and Weight

Physical examination begins with an assessment of vital signs, height, and weight. For children, the height and weight should be analyzed based on standardized growth charts. Many hormones can affect changes in weight and vital signs, especially those secreted by the thyroid, pancreatic, and adrenal glands. Abnormal growth patterns may be associated with growth hormone (or growth hormone-inhibiting or -releasing hormone).

Inspection

Many clues about hormonal balance (or imbalance) may be noted during a general inspection, particularly by a health care professional with a critical eye.[9] Note the overall skin color and texture, hair texture, body posture, facial characteristics, and affect. Findings associated with one or more hormonal imbalances include unusual dryness, pigmentation, wounds, or other lesions; malformation of the fingernails; unusual hair texture; and excessive hair growth in unexpected areas (e.g., on the face of women) or excessive hair loss. Note anxious or fidgety behavior, a flat affect or an overly animated affect, puffiness around the face, and protrusion of the eyes (exophthalmos). Notice the neck and determine if there is a thickening or enlargement that might be caused by an enlarged thyroid gland. Abnormal findings of the external genitalia (e.g., size, shape, color, and pubic hair distribution) for the patient's age/developmental level may also reveal important clues associated with hormonal imbalance.

Palpation and Auscultation

The thyroid gland and testes are anatomically positioned to allow for direct palpation; ovaries can be palpated through bimanual palpation. The thyroid gland, located on the anterior neck just below the cricoid cartilage, is not particularly easy to palpate unless it is abnormally large or has nodules. An enlargement of the thyroid (goiter) or the presence of nodules are abnormal findings. If the thyroid is enlarged, the area should be auscultated for bruits, which would indicate increased vascular flow. The testes are palpated through the scrotal sac. They should be firm, small, and smooth.[9] An irregular shape or texture are abnormal findings. Ovaries can be indirectly palpated through a bimanual examination as part of a pelvic examination. This examination is usually done by an advanced practice nurse (e.g., a nurse practitioner) or a physician.

Diagnostic Tests

Laboratory Tests

A number of laboratory tests are used to determine hormonal function.

Hormone level. One of the most common ways to assess hormonal function is a direct measure of the hormone level in the blood (or other body fluids such as urine). If a hormone is secreted at a consistent rate (e.g., thyroid hormone), then a single sample can be drawn at any time. However, some glands secrete hormones on a cyclic pattern; thus, the specific time the sample is drawn is critical for test analysis. For example, a cortisol level tests adrenal function. Secretion of cortisol is highest in the morning and lowest in the evening; thus, blood sample should be drawn at 8 AM and 4 PM.[10] When the test involves the collection of urine, this is often done as a 24-hour urine sample. This often requires specific handling of the sample during the collection period.

An indirect assessment of the hormone function involves evaluating the blood or urine for components affected by the hormone function. For example, blood glucose provides an indirect measure of the pancreatic cells that produce insulin or insulin usage.

Stimulation and suppression testing. These tests are done to evaluate the process for hormone secretion and inhibition. Stimulation testing involves giving the patient a stimulus substance or hormone to stimulate the targeted gland to trigger hormone release. A measure of the hormone level follows, with an elevation in hormone level as the normal (expected) finding. A suppression test involves giving the patient a suppression substance or hormone to suppress the targeted gland from producing hormone. A measure of the hormone level follows, with a decrease in hormone level as the normal (expected) finding.[10]

Imaging

In some cases, imaging of the gland is necessary for diagnostic purposes. Ultrasound imaging can be used for imaging the thyroid, parathyroid, ovaries, and testes. Magnetic resonance imaging or computed tomography scans are very effective to evaluate pituitary, adrenal glands, pancreas, and ovaries. These scans may involve the injection of a radioactive isotope that allows imaging of the substance in the target tissue.[11]

Biopsy

In some cases, pathology analysis of the gland tissue is needed. A biopsy may be performed to collect tissue sample of the gland involved. Because of the relative ease of accessibility, the thyroid gland is the most common gland for this analysis.

CLINICAL MANAGEMENT

Primary Prevention

Primary prevention refers to strategies aimed to optimize health and prevent disease. Primary prevention strategies typically include education, diet, exercise, weight control, injury avoidance, and avoidance of environmental hazards.[12] These basic primary prevention strategies affect hormonal regulation as well. Maintaining a healthy lifestyle optimizes overall health and thus provides an optimal physiological environment for hormonal regulation to occur. For example, diet, exercise, and weight control affect the production and function of some hormones, such as insulin, glucagon, and thyroid hormones.[13] Measures

to manage stress can prevent excess secretion of cortisol. Maintaining routine sleep–wake patterns optimizes the secretion of hormones dependent on a circadian cycle. Preventing head injury through the use of helmets reduces risk of injury to the hypothalamus and pituitary glands.

Secondary Prevention (Screening)

Secondary prevention refers to the early identification of a disease so that prompt treatment can be initiated. The two primary endocrine-related screening recommendations are for thyroid and diabetic conditions and include recommendations for infants and adults.

Infants

A routine congenital thyroid screening in infants is recommended as part of the uniform screening panel. This recommendation includes the screening of every newborn for 31 core conditions, including two endocrine disorders—congenital adrenal hyperplasia and congenital hypothyroidism.[14]

Adults

The two pertinent areas for screening include thyroid and diabetes. According to the U.S. Preventative Services Task Force (USPSTF), there is insufficient evidence to recommend routine screening for thyroid problems among asymptomatic adults.[15] Regarding gestational diabetes screening, the USPSTF found insufficient evidence to recommend routine screening before 24 weeks of gestation, but it does recommend routine screening in all asymptomatic women after 24 weeks of gestation.[16] In the draft update to the 2008 screening recommendations for type 2 diabetes, USPSTF recommended screening for abnormal blood glucose and type 2 diabetes mellitus in adults who are at risk for diabetes.[17]

Collaborative Interventions

The management of individuals with endocrine disturbances is complex, and a detailed discussion for each is beyond the scope of this concept. However, common underlying care principles include a combination of diet, fluid management, pharmacotherapy, surgical options, radiation, and psychosocial support. This section presents the common interventional categories associated with hormonal disturbances and is not intended to be comprehensive for any specific endocrine disorder.

Pharmacotherapy

Pharmacologic treatment for individuals with hormone imbalance typically involves hormone replacement (for deficiencies) or drugs that block production or use of hormones in states of excess hormone production. For this reason, the pharmacologic agents are presented with the underlying problem.

Hypopituitarism. Synthetic human growth hormone is used for growth hormone (GH) deficiencies caused by pituitary insufficiency, as well as other conditions such as Turner's syndrome, chronic kidney disease, and children small for gestation age. Testosterone is used as supplement for men with gonadotropin deficiency. Estrogen and progesterone supplements, also referred to as hormone replacement therapy, are indicated for women with gonadotropin deficiency and for the relief of postmenopausal symptoms.[18] Estrogen is also known to regulate secretion and action of GH in men and women.[19]

Hyperpituitarism. Dopamine agonists (bromocriptine mesylate, cabergoline, and pergolide) inhibit release of GH; octreotide (somatostatin) and pegvisomant (Somavert) block GH receptors.

Posterior pituitary antidiuretic hormone deficiency. Desmopressin (DDAVP) and avasopressin (Pitressin) represent replacement therapy for antidiuretic hormone (ADH). Chlorpropamie (Diabinese) has antidiuretic action and increases ADH production in the hypothalamus.

Posterior pituitary antidiuretic hormone excess. Tolvaptan (Samsca) and conivaptan (Vaprisol) are vasopressin antagonists that promote water excretion without loss of sodium.

Adrenal insufficiency (Addison's disease). Cortisone, hydrocortisone (Cortef), prednisone, and fludrocortisone (Florinef) are used for the treatment of adrenocorticoid deficiency.

Hypercortisolism (Cushing's disease). Aminoglutethimide (Elipten and Cytadren), metyrapone (Metopirone), and cyproheptadine (Periactin) interfere with adrenocorticotropic hormone (ACTH) production.

Hypothyroidism. Levothyroxine sodium (Synthroid) is a synthetic hormone preparation that represents the most common form of thyroid replacement therapy.

Hyperthyroidism. Propythiouracil (PTU) and methimazole (Tapazole) block thyroid hormone production.

Hypoparathyroidism. Because parathyroid regulates calcium, therapy involves calcium, vitamin D, and magnesium sulfate supplements.

Diabetes. A variety of insulin preparations are used for individuals with type 1 diabetes and represent hormone replacement. In type 2 diabetes, several agents are used to increase insulin secretion and/or improve insulin receptor sensitivity. These include sulfonylurea agents glipizide (Glucotrol) and glimepiride (Amaryl); meglitinide analogs repaglinide (Prandin) and nateglinide (Starlix); and insulin sensitizers, which include biguanides (metformin [Glucophage]) and thiazolidinediones (rosiglitazone [Avandia] and pioglitazone [Actos]).[3]

Nutrition Therapy

Nutrition management is the cornerstone of many endocrine disorders, with diabetes being the most obvious (and which is discussed in detail in Concept 15 Glucose Regulation).

Fluid and Electrolyte Management

Some hormone imbalances or associated treatments can lead to an actual or potential for fluid and electrolyte imbalances. This is particularly true with antidiuretic hormone imbalances, hypercortisolism, aldosterone imbalances, parathyroid hormone disturbances, and as a result of insulin deficiency (diabetic ketoacidosis).[8] Thus, monitoring fluid intake and output and monitoring serum electrolytes is a central component of care for many of these conditions.

Surgery

Hypophysectomy. A hypophysectomy is the surgical removal of the pituitary gland and often an associated tumor. The most common cause of hyperpituitarism is a benign tumor within the anterior pituitary gland (pituitary adenoma).[3] This procedure may also be done when there is hypersecretion of ACTH from the pituitary gland, leading to adrenocortical hypersecretion.

Adrenalectomy. Removal of one or both adrenal glands is a treatment option for three different types of hormonal regulation problems. Adrenocortical hypersecretion and hyperaldosteronism are often caused by a benign adrenal tumor affecting the adrenal cortex, although some cases are bilateral.[20] A pheochromocytoma is a catecholamine-producing tumor of the adrenal medulla and leads to excessive release of epinephrine and norepinephrine. Patients require lifelong glucocorticoid and mineralocorticoid replacement if both adrenal glands are removed. If only one gland is removed, replacement therapy is needed temporarily until the remaining adrenal gland can sufficiently increase hormone production.

Thyroidectomy. A complete removal or partial removal of the thyroid gland is indicated for individuals with an excessively large goiter (causing compression on the esophagus or trachea) or who do not have adequate response to pharmacotherapy with antithyroid agents or with radioactive iodine (RAI) therapy. The four types of procedures are lobectomy (removal of one lobe), bilateral subtotal thyroidectomy, near total thyroidectomy, and total thyroidectomy.[21] The patient must be monitored for serious complications (hemorrhage, respiratory distress, hypocalcaemia, tetany, thyroid storm, and laryngeal nerve damage) in the postoperative period.[22] Patients who undergo a total thyroidectomy require lifelong thyroid replacement therapy.

Parathyroidectomy. Hyperparathyroidism is often caused by a benign tumor in the parathyroid glands. Removal of one or more of the four parathyroid glands may be indicated for hyperparathyroidism. The minimally invasive radio-guided technique shows promise as a surgical option.[23] Because the parathyroids are located on the thyroid gland, similar concerns for postoperative monitoring apply. In addition, calcium levels are monitored to avoid hypocalcemic crisis.

Radiation

RAI is indicated for the treatment of hyperthyroidism. It is given as an oral preparation, usually as a single dose. RAI makes its way to the thyroid gland, where it destroys some of the cells that produce thyroid hormone. RAI is completely eliminated from the body after approximately 4 weeks. The extent of thyroid cell destruction is variable; thus, the patient has ongoing monitoring of thyroid function. If thyroid production remains too high, a second dose may be needed.[3]

Psychosocial Support

A hormonal imbalance often represents a change in an individual's lifestyle and can affect an individual's physical appearance, libido, sexual functioning, and mood. Combined, these changes can affect interpersonal relationships, self-confidence, and often requires an adjustment (particularly if it is a chronic condition). Patients may benefit from individual counseling and support groups as a means for effective coping.

Patient Education

The complexity of many hormonal imbalances requires significant patient education regarding diet, activity, and medications to achieve optimal disease management. Patients who undergo hormone replacement therapy must understand the need to take medications regularly, consistently, and within the dosing parameters established for their condition. Patients must also know the signs and symptoms of excessive or insufficient hormone supplements. Patients with conditions requiring specific dietary and/or fluid management must be taught how to incorporate dietary patterns into their culture and lifestyle.

INTERRELATED CONCEPTS

All body systems are affected by hormones; for this reason, all health and illness concepts are interrelated in some way. However, concepts with the closest interrelationships are presented in Figure 14-3. **Intracranial Regulation** has a significant role in hormonal regulation because of its influence on the function of the hypothalamus and pituitary glands. Many hormonal imbalances occur as a result of brain injury or damage to these glands located in the brain. Likewise, optimal intracranial regulation and cognitive function depend on normal regulation of hormones. Maintaining balance of **Fluid and Electrolytes** is highly dependent on the secretion and regulation of aldosterone and antidiuretic hormone. **Glucose Regulation** and **Nutrition** are highly dependent on the regulation of insulin and glucagon. **Stress** has a close relationship because of the role that glucocorticoids and catecholamines play in the stress response. The processes of **Development** and **Reproduction** are dependent on hormones such as growth hormone,

FIGURE 14-3 Hormonal Regulation and Interrelated Concepts

estrogen, progesterone, testosterone, LH, follicle-stimulating hormone, prolactin, and oxytocin.

CLINICAL EXEMPLARS

There are clearly many exemplars of hormonal regulation. The classic exemplars are presented in Box 14-3, organized by the glands producing hormones. It is beyond the scope of this text to discuss each endocrine condition, and this information is easily found in pathophysiology, adult health, and pediatric textbooks. A brief description of some of the most important or common exemplars is featured next.

Featured Exemplars

Hypothyroidism

Hypothyroidism refers to insufficient secretion of thyroid hormones. Typically, this is caused by reduced production of thyroid hormone by the thyroid gland, but it can also be a result of dietary intake of substances (e.g., iodide and tyrosine) enabling thyroid hormone production. Because thyroid hormones influence metabolic rate, thyroid insufficiency has a significant effect on systemic cellular metabolism, creating body-wide symptoms including fatigue, weight gain, depression, reduced cardiac and respiratory rates, as well as myxedema. This condition occurs most often among women between ages 30 and 60 years, with increased incidence with age.[24]

Type 1 Diabetes Mellitus

Type 1 diabetes mellitus is a metabolic condition resulting from the destruction of pancreatic beta cells, leading to a loss of insulin production. Insulin is a hormone that is necessary to facilitate movement of glucose into the cell for metabolic activity. Insulin deficiency is clinically associated with hyperglycemia, with significant systemic effects over time. The cause of type 1 diabetes is unknown, but it may be associated with an autoimmune response with genetic predisposition. Native Americans, non-Hispanic blacks, and Hispanics have significantly higher rates of diabetes compared to non-Hispanic whites and Asian Americans.[25]

Hypercortisolism (Cushing's Syndrome)

Cushing's syndrome affects an estimated 10–15 per 1 million people each year[26] and is characterized by chronic excess glucocorticoid (cortisol) secretion from the adrenal cortex. This is caused by the hypothalamus, the anterior pituitary gland, or the adrenal cortex. Cushing's syndrome can also be caused by taking corticosteroids in the form of medication (e.g., prednisone) over time—referred to as exogenous Cushing's syndrome. Regardless of the cause, excess secretion of cortisol has a systemic effect, affecting immunity, metabolism, and fat distribution (truncal obesity) and causing reduced muscle mass, loss of bone density, hypertension, fragility to microvasculature, as well as thinning of the skin.

Syndrome of Inappropriate Antidiuretic Hormone

Antidiuretic hormone is responsible for fluid balance and is normally secreted by the posterior pituitary gland in response to elevated plasma osmolarity. As the name suggests, the syndrome of inappropriate antidiuretic hormone (SIADH) is a condition in which ADH is secreted despite normal or low plasma osmolarity, resulting in water retention and dilutional hyponatremia. In response to increased plasma volume, aldosterone secretion increases and further contributes to sodium loss.[3] A large number of clinical conditions can cause SIADH, including malignancies, pulmonary disorders, injury to the brain, and certain pharmacologic agents.

Adrenal Insufficiency (Addison's Disease)

Adrenal insufficiency, also known as Addison's disease, occurs with an insufficient secretion of adrenocortical steroids (cortisol and aldosterone). Adrenal insufficiency can occur from dysfunction of the pituitary gland and insufficient secretion of ACTH, which signals adrenocortical steroid release from the adrenal glands, or from damage to the adrenal cortex, in which adrenocortical steroids are produced.[8] Adrenal insufficiency results in fluid and electrolyte imbalances, particularly hyponatremia, hyperkalemia, and hypovolemia. This condition can be life-threatening if the physiological requirement for cortisol and aldosterone exceeds supply—often association with severe physiological stress such as surgery, trauma, or sepsis.

CASE STUDY

Source: NADOFOTOS/iStock/Thinkstock

Case Presentation

Marci Myers, a 38-year-old female, presented to a community-based clinic with generalized complaint of feeling "odd" for the past few months. Michael, a nurse practitioner, evaluated her. Marci denied any previous medical conditions and takes no medications other than vitamin supplements. When Marci was asked to explain her symptoms further, she described a variety of sensations, including palpitations in her chest, shortness of breath, generalized weakness and fatigue, heat intolerance, and insomnia. She described often feeling restless and was told by her coworkers that she is irritable, but in her opinion she is not—she just does not feel herself. When asked about recent weight loss, Marci was unsure but admitted that her clothes might be a bit looser than they used to be, and she has not been dieting. During the interview, Marci appeared somewhat restless, and a slight trembling to her hands was noted. Her vital signs were as

follows: heart rate, 106 beats/minute; respiratory rate, 24 breaths/minute; blood pressure, 132/80 mm Hg; and temperature, 36.9°C. Marci's skin was very warm and slightly damp. The thyroid gland felt somewhat enlarged when palpated, and the rest of the examination was unremarkable. Laboratory tests for T_3, T_4, and free T_4 index were ordered to assess thyroid hormone regulation. All three of these tests were elevated. Because the nurse practitioner suspected Marci had hyperthyroidism, he referred her to an endocrinologist.

Further diagnostic testing done by the endocrinologist included thyrotropin-stimulating test (which was low), thyroid-releasing hormone stimulation test (showed no response), thyroid antibodies titer (was elevated), thyrotropin receptor antibodies (TSH-RAb) test (showed high titers), and a thyroid scan (showed an enlarged thyroid gland and increased radioactive iodine uptake). These tests confirmed a diagnosis of hyperthyroidism caused by Graves' disease.

Case Analysis

The thyroid gland secretes hormones that affect overall metabolism. Thyroid regulation occurs through a negative feedback loop involving the hypothalamus, anterior pituitary, and thyroid gland. Normally, thyroid hormone production is triggered by thyrotropin, which is stimulated by thyrotropin-releasing hormone (TRH); sufficient circulating plasma levels of T_3 and T_4 prevent further secretion of thyrotropin and TRH. In Graves' disease, these regulatory mechanisms are overridden by an autoimmune process associated with hyperfunction of the thyroid gland. An increase in the number and size of thyroid cells leads to thyroid enlargement (goiter) and an overproduction of thyroid hormone (thyrotoxicosis) with an associated suppression of thyrotropin and TRH. The excess secretion of thyroid hormone contributes to the classic symptoms associated accelerated metabolism, noted above. Infiltrative ophthalmopathy (exophthalmos) occurs in many, but not all cases of Graves' disease. The fact that Marci's symptoms began a few months ago suggests an initial mild disturbance with subtle symptoms that have become more pronounced over time.

ACCESS EXEMPLAR LINKS IN YOUR GIDDENS EBOOK

REFERENCES

1. McCance K, Huther S: *Pathophysoiology: The biologic basis for disease in adults and children*, ed 7, St Louis, 2013, Elsevier.
2. Wu J, McAndrews J: Introduction to the endocrine system. Part 1: Basic concepts and anatomy. *Am Medical Writers Assoc J* 27(4):153–156, 2012.
3. Ignatavicius D, Workman M: *Medical–surgical nursing: Patient-centered collaborative care*, ed 8, St Louis, 2015, Elsevier.
4. McAndrews J, Wu J: Introduction to the endocrine system. Part 2: Physiology. *Am Medical Writers Assoc J* 28(2):51–56, 2013.
5. Konishi M, Takahaski M, Naoya E, et al: Effects of sleep deprivation on autonomic and endocrine functions throughout the day and on exercise tolerance in the evening. *J Sports Sci* 31(3):248–255, 2013.
6. Hockenberry M, Wilson D: *Wong's essentials of pediatric nursing*, ed 9, St Louis, 2013, Elsevier.
7. Tajar A, O'Connell M, Mitnitski AB, et al: Frailty in relation to variations in hormonal levels of the hypothalamic–pituitary–testicular axis in older men: Results from the European Male Aging Study. *J Am Geriatr Soc* 59:814–821, 2011.
8. Lewis S, Dirkson S, Heitkemper M, et al: *Medical–surgical nursing: Assessment and management of clinical problems*, ed 9, St Louis, 2014, Elsevier.
9. Wilson S, Giddens J: *Health assessment for nursing practice*, ed 5, St Louis, 2013, Elsevier.

10. Fischbach F, Dunning MB: *A manual of laboratory and diagnostic tests,* ed 9, Philadelphia, 2014, Lippincott Williams & Wilkins.

11. Pagana K, Pagana T, Pagana T: *Mosby's diagnostic laboratory test reference,* ed 12, St Louis, 2015, Mosby.

12. Pender N, Murdaugh C, Parson MA: *Health promotion in nursing practice,* ed 7, Upper Saddle River, NJ, 2015, Pearson.

13. Schubert M, Sabapathy S: Acute exercise and hormones related to appetite regulation: A meta-analysis. *Sports Med* 44:387–403, 2014.

14. Advisory Committee on Heritable Disorders in Newborns and Children: Recommended uniform screening panel, 2015. Retrieved from <http://www.hrsa.gov/advisorycommittees/mchbadvisory/heritabledisorders/recommendedpanel/index.html>.

15. U.S. Preventative Services Task Force: Thyroid dysfunction: Screening, 2015. Retrieved from <http://www.uspreventiveservicestaskforce.org/Page/Topic/recommendation-summary/thyroid-dysfunction-screening>.

16. U.S. Preventative Services Task Force: Gestational diabetes mellitus, Screening, 2014. Retrieved from <http://www.uspreventiveservicestaskforce.org/Page/Topic/recommendation-summary/gestational-diabetes-mellitus-screening?ds=1&s=gestational%20diabetes>.

17. U.S. Preventative Services Task Force: Draft recommendation statement: Abnormal glucose and type 2 gestational diabetes mellitus in adults: Screening, 2014. Retrieved from <http://www.uspreventiveservicestaskforce.org/Page/Document/draft-recommendation-statement43/screening-for-abnormal-glucose-and-type-2-diabetes-mellitus>.

18. Archer D, Sturdee D, Baber R, et al: Menopausal hot flashes and night sweats: Where are we now? *Climacteric* 14:515–528, 2011.

19. Birzniece V, Sutanto S, Ho K: Gender difference in neuroendocrine regulation of growth hormone axis by selective estrogen receptor modulators. *J Clin Endocrinol Metab* 97(4):E521–E527, 2012.

20. Lacroix A: Heredity and cortisol regulation in bilateral macronodular adrenal hyperplasia. *N Engl J Med* 369(22):2147–2149, 2013.

21. March P, Schub T: *Thyroidectomy,* Glendale, CA, 2005, Cinahl Information Systems.

22. Massick D, Garrett M: Hypocalcemia after minimally invasive thyroidectomy. *ENT: Ear Nose Throat J* 93(9):414–417, 2014.

23. Rubello G: Minimally invasive parathyroidectomy. *J Postgrad Med* 59(1):1–3, 2013.

24. National Institute of Diabetes and Digestive and Kidney Diseases: Hypothyroidism, 2013. Retrieved from <http://www.niddk.nih.gov/health-information/health-topics/endocrine/hypothyroidism/Pages/fact-sheet.aspx>.

25. Centers for Disease Control and Prevention: National diabetes statistics report, 2014. Retrieved from <http://www.cdc.gov/diabetes/pubs/statsreport14/national-diabetes-report-web.pdf>.

26. Guaraldi F, Salvatori R: Cushing syndrome: Maybe not so uncommon of an endocrine disease. *J Am Board Fam Med* 25(2):199–208, 2012.

Glucose Regulation

Katherine Pereira

Glucose is fundamental to the process of human life. Glucose is the preferred energy source for most cells in the body, and the neurologic system is dependent on glucose for energy needs. When glucose metabolism becomes impaired, serious health consequences occur. Because this concept represents a foundational basis of health, the nurse must possess a solid understanding of energy and glucose regulation, including the ability to recognize and respond to situations in which this process is impaired.

DEFINITION

Glucose regulation is achieved through a delicate balance between nutrient intake, hormonal signaling, and glucose uptake by the cell. Once glucose enters the cell, it is oxidized through cellular respiration into adenosine triphosphate (ATP). The efficiency of glucose metabolism is reflected in circulating blood glucose levels. For the purposes of this concept presentation, glucose regulation is defined as *the process of maintaining optimal blood glucose levels.*

A few other key terms are important to mention. *Glycogen* is the major form of stored glucose, primarily in the liver and muscle cells. *Glycogenolysis* refers to the breakdown of glycogen to glucose. *Gluconeogenesis* refers to the process of producing glucose from non-carbohydrate sources (e.g., proteins and fats).

SCOPE

The scope of glucose regulation can conceptually be represented by the categories of normal/optimal regulation and impaired regulation throughout the lifespan. Normal blood glucose (BG) levels range between 70 and 99 mg/dL in the fasting state and 100 and 140 mg/dL in the 2-hour postprandial state, otherwise referred to as *euglycemia.* Impaired regulation can be further categorized by the etiology and is reflected in abnormally high or low BG levels. *Hyperglycemia* refers to a state of elevated BG levels, generally defined as greater than 100 mg/dL in the fasting state or greater than 140 mg/dL 2 hours postprandial. *Hypoglycemia* refers to a state of insufficient or low BG levels, defined as less than 70 mg/dL. Figure 15-1 shows the spectrum of glucose metabolism and regulation: hypoglycemia, euglycemia, and hyperglycemia.

NORMAL PHYSIOLOGICAL PROCESS

In the healthy individual, glucose regulation occurs with little awareness given to the process. To help maintain glucose homeostasis, a variety of hormones are required. Insulin is the only hormone produced that lowers elevated BG levels after carbohydrate intake. Several counterregulatory hormones (hormones that oppose the action of other hormones) are required to raise BG if levels begin to decrease or in anticipation of increased needs. When this system works efficiently, glucose levels remain normal, even in the setting of extreme stress.

After the consumption of food, insulin is released in response to rising glucose levels. Insulin facilitates glucose metabolism by binding to insulin receptors on the cell wall, *signaling* glucose transporter molecules that facilitate glucose entry into the cell. Insulin suppresses glucagon secretion and facilitates glycogen storage.

Glucagon is one of several counterregulatory hormones released in response to cellular deficiency of glucose. Glucagon suppresses insulin and stimulates hepatic glucose production (from glycogen), resulting in elevated glucose levels. Gluconeogenesis is required if blood glucose and glycogen stores are insufficient and can also occur with stress conditions, or from use of steroid medications, with resulting increased risk of loss of muscle mass. Other counterregulatory hormones released include cortisol, growth hormone, norepinephrine, and epinephrine. Counterregulatory hormones all lead to utilization of glycogen stores, and these hormones are also increased with stress-related conditions, both physical (e.g., pain, illness, and injury) and emotional, and are therefore often referred to as stress hormones.

VARIATIONS AND CONTEXT

Problems with glucose regulation arise when glucose-regulating hormones are either deficient or excessive, or when the timing of production is not balanced with blood glucose needs. An imbalance of glucose regulation results in either too much or insufficient glucose.

FIGURE 15-1 Scope of Glucose Regulation

Hyperglycemia

Hyperglycemia occurs as a result of insufficient insulin production or secretion, excessive counterregulatory hormones secretion, or from deficient hormone signaling. The word *diabetes* means "sweet urine," and the term *diabetes mellitus* is used to describe a group of disorders characterized by chronic hyperglycemia and disturbances in carbohydrate, protein, and fat metabolism.

Insufficient Insulin Production/Secretion

Insulin is produced, stored, and released by pancreatic β cells (located in pancreatic islets). Damage or destruction of the β cells results in insufficient or cessation of insulin secretion. Insufficient insulin secretion results in a hyperglycemic state because glucose is unable to enter the cells for cellular metabolism. Damage to the β cells is usually caused by an autoimmune response with genetic disposition or can occur secondarily from other diseases such as pancreatitis or pancreatic cancer.

Deficient Hormone Signaling

The term *insulin resistance* refers to a state in which the body cells respond abnormally to the signaling action of insulin; in other words, there is not a problem with insulin supply but, rather, with how the cell responds to insulin signaling due to a reduction of insulin receptors or glucose transporter molecules,[1] resulting in sluggish glucose uptake by the cell. The pancreas overproduces insulin to compensate for reduced cellular glucose update, resulting in hyperinsulinemia. When insulin resistance persists for long periods of time, the insulin producing capacity of the pancreas is exhausted and hyperglycemia ensues.[2]

Excessive Counterregulatory Hormone Secretion

Excessive secretion of any of the counterregulatory hormones can result in hyperglycemia. These include glucagon (previously described) and cortisol, a hormone that raises blood glucose through gluconeogenesis. Causes of increased cortisol secretion include chronic stress, pain, sleep deprivation, and acute injury or illness. It can also occur as

an adverse effect of medications (particularly with high doses of corticosteroids) or due to Cushing's disease. Elevated cortisol levels also exacerbate insulin resistance (described previously).

Hypoglycemia

Hypoglycemia is a state of low glucose levels and typically occurs as a result of insufficient nutritional intake, adverse reaction to medications, excessive exercise, and/or as a consequence of disease states. Often, hypoglycemia occurs due to a combination of these factors.

Insufficient Nutritional Intake

Malnutrition leads to depletion of glucose stores in the liver and adipose tissue and thus prevents hepatic mechanisms for maintenance of normal glucose levels. Free fatty acids are mobilized as substrates for glucose production and resulting production of ketone bodies. Prolonged starvation and malnutrition can eventually lead to life-threatening hypoglycemia.

Adverse Reaction to Medication

Hypoglycemia is generally attributed to inappropriate dosing of exogenous insulin or the sulfonylurea form of oral hypoglycemic agents, which increases endogenous insulin production. Once an individual requires insulin therapy to maintain glucose control, creating a physiological insulin replacement regimen while avoiding hypoglycemia can be difficult, and this is one of the great challenges of caring for patients with diabetes.

Excessive Exercise

The work of muscle contraction requires energy, and initially this energy is derived from glucose stored in muscle cells as glycogen. As an exercise interval lengthens, glucose stores are quickly depleted, and then glucose from the circulation and hepatic glucose stores is utilized for energy, lowering blood glucose levels. During post exercise recovery, muscle cells then replenish glycogen stores with additional glucose from the circulation also lowering glucose levels, and this is sometimes referred to as "lag effect."

CONSEQUENCES

A number of significant physiological consequences are associated with poor glucose regulation. Hyperglycemia and insulin resistance are known to be toxic and proinflammatory states, causing cellular changes, cell death, and contributing to the various long-term health problems. Likewise, hypoglycemia can result in impaired function of the neurological system and thus grave danger to the patient. The consequences of hyperglycemia and hypoglycemia are discussed separately.

Physiological Consequences of Hyperglycemia

Insulin resistance is understood to be a proinflammatory state, thus contributing to atherogenesis and plaque formation,[3] and is also thought to be associated with increased cancer risk, with hyperinsulinemia appearing to act as a cellular growth factor. Reduced cancer risk has been noted among persons taking the insulin-sensitizing agent metformin.[4] Hypertension is present in 50% of insulin-resistant individuals and 80% of those with type 2 diabetes, both sharing a common mechanism of high oxidative stress and inflammation.[5] Hyperinsulinemia causes hypertension through its role in reducing elasticity of blood vessels.[6] Reinforcing this influence on hypertension is the recognition that reducing carbohydrate intake can lower blood pressure levels.[7,8] Other conditions associated with insulin resistance and proinflammatory states are non-alcoholic steatohepatitis and sleep apnea.[9]

Angiopathy

Individuals with long-standing or chronic hyperglycemia are at risk for developing several significant physiological complications attributable to angiopathy (damage to blood vessels). Chronic elevations of blood glucose damage the basement membrane of small blood vessels and impair adequate oxygenation to the tissues. These are known microvascular effects and directly lead to end-organ disease, including damage to the eye (retinopathy and vision loss) and the kidney (chronic kidney disease that can lead to end-stage renal disease).

Chronic hyperglycemia further damages medium and larger blood vessels, leading to hypertension and cardiovascular and peripheral vascular disease. The risk for myocardial infarction and stroke is two to four times higher for those with type 2 diabetes compared to those without diabetes.[10] The vascular damage to small blood vessels in the lower extremities leads to impaired blood supply to the lower extremities and peripheral vascular disease, increasing the risk of foot ulcers and chronic wound infection (sometimes leading to amputation).

Peripheral Neuropathy

Hyperglycemia is toxic to nerves, resulting in nerve damage and leading to peripheral neuropathy causing symptoms such as burning and numbness in the lower extremities. Once protective sensation is lost in the feet, the risk for foot ulcers and foot lesions greatly increases. Peripheral neuropathy is seen with prediabetes and may be the presenting symptom of impaired glucose utilization.[11]

Fluid, Electrolyte, and Acid–Base Imbalances

A potential consequence of severe hyperglycemia is dehydration because of a water deficit resulting from osmotic diuresis. Hyperosmolar hyperglycemic state (HHS) usually presents as severe hyperglycemia (>600 mg/dL), dehydration and accompanied impaired mental status, and is more common in elders with type 2 diabetes.[12] There is also an increasing incidence of HHS in children with type 2 diabetes, in direct correlation with increasing type 2 diabetes rates in children.[13] An acid–base disturbance, diabetic ketoacidosis (DKA), is a hyperglycemic state

(associated type 1 diabetes) whereby an absolute insulin deficiency is accompanied by the use of fatty acids and subsequent excess of ketone bodies and metabolic acidosis.

Physiological Consequences of Hypoglycemia

To a large degree, the impact of the body's processes to contend with and overcome adverse effects of inadequate glucose availability is largely unknown. Because the brain depends on glucose as its only source of fuel, hypoglycemia can progress from mild symptoms of nervousness, irritability, diaphoresis, anxiety, and palpitations to neurological changes, seizures, loss of consciousness, and death.[14] Recurrent hypoglycemia can lower the glucose level that typically stimulates counterregulatory hormones; thus, symptoms of hypoglycemia do not occur until glucose levels are dangerously low, and frequent hypoglycemia is associated with a three- or fourfold increased risk of death[15] and a higher risk of chronic cognitive impairment and accelerated cognitive decline.[16]

Chronic hypoglycemia leads to the condition of hypoglycemia unawareness in which the counterregulatory hormonal response is blunted, describing a state of autonomic failure. This includes diabetes neuropathy and other symptoms of gastroparesis with associated symptoms of early satiety, poor food absorption, constipation, fecal incontinence, and diarrhea. The spectrum of autonomic neuropathy includes impaired pupil response to light, erectile dysfunction, loss of vaginal lubrication, painless cardiac ischemia, impaired exercise tolerance, orthostatic hypotension, resting tachycardia, dry skin, and impaired temperature regulation.[17] Hypoglycemia occurs two or three times more frequently in those with type 1 diabetes.[18]

RISK FACTORS

Impaired glucose regulation can potentially occur in any individual regardless of age, race, cultural identity, or gender. However, there are well-known risk factors for impaired glucose regulation.

Populations at Risk
Pregnant Women

Pregnancy and the associated hormonal changes (specifically hormones produced by the placenta) produce a state of insulin resistance and associated risk for hyperglycemia, especially postprandial hyperglycemia. All pregnant women are screened for gestational diabetes during the 24- to 28-week gestational mark, and women with known prediabetes or multiple risk factors for type 2 diabetes are screened at the first prenatal visit.[19]

Infants

The large for gestational age infant is at high risk for hypoglycemia after birth. The prevalence of neonatal hypoglycemia is also higher among infants whose mothers had diabetes during pregnancy.[20] Hypoglycemia is generally attributed to neonatal hyperinsulinemia that occurs in response to elevated glucose levels *in utero*. Small for gestational age and premature infants are at risk of hypoglycemic states because of increased energy needs and insufficient glycogen stores.

Older Adults

Older adults as a group are at greater risk for impaired glucose metabolism and hyperglycemia because of an increase in visceral fat and associated reduction in lean muscle mass, where most glucose is metabolized. This is often accompanied by age-related reduced insulin production and resulting reduced capacity to regulate and metabolize glucose concentration.[21]

Racial/Ethnic Groups

Certain racial and ethnic populations have greater genetic predisposition to insulin resistance, leading to a higher risk for type 2 diabetes especially American Indians/Alaska Natives (age-adjusted percentile of 15.9%), African Americans (13.2%), Hispanic/Latino (12.8%, with Puerto Ricans and Mexican Americans having the highest rate), and Asian Americans (9.0%) compared to 7.6% among whites.[10] There is a growing trend of increased diabetes prevalence seen in societies that become more modernized, affluent, and westernized and thus increasingly sedentary, as seen in China.[22] Other ethnic groups, particularly those of northern European descent, have a genetic tendency for the autoimmune form of diabetes.[23] Other autoimmune disorders are found in increased frequency among persons with type 1 diabetes, including celiac disease, adrenal insufficiency, pernicious anemia, vitiligo, and autoimmune thyroid disorders.[24]

Individual Risk Factors

Genetic Risk Factors

Research is rapidly expanding an understanding of the genetics of diabetes. Currently, there are at least 40 known genetic markers, including *HLA* genes, associated with the risk of diabetes.[25] Insulin resistance is the common feature associated with metabolic syndrome and type 2 diabetes.[26] Persons with a family history of type 2 diabetes, obesity, or factors associated with metabolic syndrome are at increased risk of insulin resistance and type 2 diabetes.[27,28]

Lifestyle Risk Factors

A number of lifestyle choices promote and worsen insulin resistance. One of these is a poor diet with a high intake of saturated and trans-fatty acids (with the excess caloric intake leading to obesity) and a low fiber intake. An inappropriately high intake of calories, particularly carbohydrates, will also adversely impact glucose metabolism, regardless of the presence of insulin resistance or type 2 diabetes. Obesity and a lack of physical activity also contribute to insulin resistance.

Chronic Conditions

Many medical conditions are associated with impaired glucose regulation—diabetes and metabolic syndrome are most notable. Many medical conditions interfere with oral intake, creating the need for enteral or parenteral nutrition that may impact glucose regulation. Malabsorption and resulting nutrient deficiencies required for cellular metabolism of glucose, including vitamin D deficiency, contribute to insulin resistance[29] and are further related to suppressed insulin production.[30] Glucose regulation is also affected by physiologic stress such as traumatic injury, cancer, and surgery.

Medications

Many medications used for treatment of health conditions are known to affect glucose regulation, which can place an individual at risk for hyperglycemia or hypoglycemia. Although there are too many to list, some of the most common include insulin, oral hypoglycemic agents, corticosteroids, estrogen, ACE inhibitors, β-blockers, potassium-depleting diuretics, bronchodilators, antipsychotics, and many antibiotics.

ASSESSMENT

History

The history includes personal medical history (including a list of current medications), social history, family history, and a review of

TABLE 15-1 Comparison of Clinical Presentation of Hypoglycemia and Hyperglycemia

	Hypoglycemia	Hyperglycemia
Symptoms	Symptoms related to degree of hypoglycemia and can include weakness, dizziness, headache, hunger, blurred vision, difficulty concentrating, feeling shaky, palpitations	No specific symptoms for elevated blood glucose, but symptoms may be associated with dehydration or acidosis and may include nausea, vomiting, abdominal cramps, fatigue, excessive hunger (polyphagia), excessive thirst (polydipsia)
Mental status	Anxious, irritability, confusion, seizures, unconsciousness, coma	Can range from alert to confused and coma, particularly if in untreated ketoacidosis
Skin	Diaphoresis, cool, clammy	Warm, moist
Respiratory/cardiovascular	Tachycardia; no change in respirations	Deep, rapid respirations; acetone odor to breath; tachycardia if dehydrated
Other	Muscle tremors, normal hydration, no ketones	Dehydration, polyuria, ketones

systems. In each area of the assessment, the nurse considers data consistent with actual or potential problems with glucose regulation. Central obesity and diabetes are two clear conditions to note in a personal or family history. Also, as previously mentioned, certain medications may place an individual at greater risk for impaired glucose regulation, so medication use should be noted.

The nurse should recognize common clinical manifestations of impaired glucose regulation (Table 15-1). Individuals may or may not have symptoms of hyperglycemia. Individuals in ketoacidosis may display *polyphagia* (excess hunger), which may occur due to cells not receiving adequate glucose, and *polydipsia* (excess thirst) and consequent *polyuria* (excess urination) due to an osmotic diuresis (when the renal glucose threshold of 180 mg/dL is exceeded, water is pulled along with it).

Other symptoms to ask about in a history include complications associated with long-standing hyperglycemia. Those with retinopathy might describe reduced vision. Those with peripheral neuropathy may report reduced sensation or pins-and-needles sensation in the lower extremities. Wounds that do not heal or generalized pain may be suggestive of poor peripheral perfusion. Insulin-resistant individuals and those with type 2 diabetes may experience sleep apnea, which can result in worsening glucose control and chronic fatigue.[31] It is also well established that individuals with diabetes are at higher risk for developing depression[32] and thus should be screened for depressive symptoms (lack of interest, feelings of sadness or worthlessness, difficulty with sleep, appetite or weight changes, suicidal thoughts, and difficulty concentrating).

FIGURE 15-2 Acanthosis nigricans is a physical exam finding frequently seen in individuals who are insulin resistant. (Source: Courtesy of Dr. Ann Brown, Duke University School of Medicine.)

Examination Findings

The examination should always include vital signs and anthropometric measurements such as height and weight to determine body mass index and waist/hip measurements (to determine waist-to-hip ratio). These measurements assess for hypertension and determine overweight or obesity as well as central obesity. Obesity and central obesity are both associated with insulin-resistant states.

Several physical findings are common among individuals with long-standing states of impaired glucose metabolism. Acanthosis nigricans, a velvety darkening of the skin that is sometimes seen on the posterior neck, axillae, and skin folds of the groin, is a cutaneous marker of insulin resistance and a "red flag" for diabetes risk (Figure 15-2). Skin tags are often seen with insulin resistance, commonly seen on the neck and axillae.

The lower extremities should be examined for evidence of peripheral vascular disease (poor perfusion and chronic wounds). A foot exam includes inspection of skin for blisters, ulcers, skin lesions, nail abnormalities, and excessive callusing. Sensation and motor strength of the extremities should be assessed to evaluate for neuropathy. Assessing visual acuity and inspection of intraocular structures may provide important information associated with retinopathy, although a dilated eye exam provides a more detailed retinal exam.

Diagnostic Tests

Diagnostic testing is an essential component associated with assessment for impairments in glucose regulation and metabolism. Laboratory tests can help reveal the etiology of impaired glucose metabolism, measure and assess blood glucose management, and evaluate consequences of impaired glucose metabolism on other disease conditions.

Blood Glucose Testing

Measurement of blood glucose is used widely for screening and monitoring glucose metabolism. A fasting glucose level greater than 100 and less than 126 mg/dL is indicative of prediabetes or impaired fasting glucose, a level of 126 mg/dL or greater on two separate occasions is indicative of diabetes, and a random blood glucose measurement greater than 200 mg/dL with signs and symptoms of diabetes is conclusive. The glucose tolerance test (GTT) is the most sensitive measure of glucose metabolism and can often detect early diabetes.

Glycosylated hemoglobin (also known as HgbA1C) is a laboratory measurement reflecting the average blood glucose reading and estimates glucose control for the prior 3 months. HgbA1C is used for diagnostic screening and monitoring disease management. A reading of 6.5% or greater is indicative of diabetes and can be obtained if the patient has not been fasting. Goals for HgbA1C is not as sensitive as GTT,[33] however, and it has been associated with significant variability related to ethnicity.[34]

Antibody Testing

Assessment of antibodies is used to confirm type 1 diabetes. The most common test is the glutamic acid decarboxylase antibody test. A C-peptide test (an indirect measure of insulin levels) and fasting insulin level may also be measured to help determine the quantity of residual insulin production.

Lipid Analysis

The most common lipid assessments include measurements of total cholesterol, high-density lipoprotein (HDL) cholesterol, and triglycerides. From these results, the low-density lipoprotein (LDL) cholesterol level is calculated, which is referred to as calculated LDL. Triglyceride levels are generally a reflection of glycemic control, meaning that when glucose levels are high, triglycerides will also be high. HDL levels indicate severity of insulin resistance, and low HDL cholesterol is seen frequently in insulin-resistant individuals.

Renal Function Tests

An early indication of renal disease associated with diabetes is microscopic protein loss in the urine, measured by the amount of albumin (microalbuminuria). Significant loss of albumin into the urine (>300 μg/dL) is associated with renal damage and the risk for development of end-stage renal disease. Two other standard laboratory tests to assess renal function are blood urea nitrogen and creatinine.

C-Reactive Protein

C-reactive protein (CRP) is made by the body during times of stress or infection. It is often elevated in those with diabetes, and it is associated with the inflammatory process of insulin resistance and cardiovascular disease risk. CRP can also be elevated in those with inflammatory processes such as rheumatoid arthritis.

CLINICAL MANAGEMENT

Primary Prevention

Primary prevention measures for optimal glucose regulation emphasize healthy lifestyle behaviors. The general measures include maintaining optimal body weight, regular physical activity, and eating a balanced diet. The Diabetes Prevention Program found that those with prediabetes could reduce the progression to type 2 diabetes by 58% through the combination of exercise for 30 minutes, 5 days a week, and a modest weight loss of 7% body weight. Metformin can also reduce progression to diabetes by 31%, and it is a recommended diabetes prevention strategy for those younger than age 60 years with prediabetes.[35]

Maintaining Optimal Body Weight

Obesity is directly linked to insulin resistance and the development of diabetes. In 2012, 12% of children ages 7–11 years were classified as obese, as were 21% of those ages 12–19 years;[36] in addition, 78.6 million adults (34.9% of the population) in the United States were classified as obese. The increase in diabetes prevalence in recent years correlates directly with the increase in overweight and obesity and the decline in regular physical activity during the past two decades.

Exercise

Exercise dramatically improves insulin resistance and cellular metabolism by increasing the number of GLUC4 transporter molecules within muscle cells,[37] thus facilitating glucose diffusion into the cell and lowering glucose levels. The American Diabetes Association recommends moderate-intensity aerobic exercise for at least 150 minutes per week and additional moderate resistive training 2 or 3 days per week for those with diabetes and for diabetes prevention. Resistive training works large muscle groups that often are not used during aerobic activities such as walking, but contraction of these muscles dramatically improves insulin resistance and insulin-mediated glucose uptake.[38]

Diet

Primary prevention further includes avoiding excess caloric intake, sweet drinks, and striving for a healthy weight. ChooseMyPlate.gov and the *2010 Dietary Guidelines* should be promoted; these emphasize consuming a diet high in whole grains, fruits and vegetables that are deep orange in color, leafy green vegetables, and legumes/beans along with low-fat milk and a variety of lean protein sources. These foods contribute to optimal cellular metabolism through provision of vitamin, minerals, fiber, and appropriate amounts of macronutrients and kilocalories needed for health. In addition, lower sodium guidelines can help lower blood pressure and reduce the risk of cardiovascular disease.

Secondary Prevention (Screening)

Secondary prevention refers to the early detection of disease through screening. Population-based screening recommendations vary across organizations, although blood glucose screening among adults with risk factors for diabetes and among all pregnant women after 24 weeks of gestation is widely recommended. There are no specific recommendations for population-based screening for hypoglycemia.

For individuals with diabetes, there are several regular screening measures for early detection of complications. *Healthy People 2020* and the American Diabetes Association recommend HgbA1$_C$ measurements at least twice per year (or every 3 months if not meeting glycemic targets); annual renal function tests; and annual dental, foot, and dilated eye examinations.[19,39] Individuals with type 1 diabetes are at higher risk for other autoimmune processes, and therefore thyroid function is monitored annually.

Collaborative Interventions

Management of conditions within the diabetes syndrome requires an interdisciplinary approach, with glycemic control as the goal to which all interventions are geared. The Diabetes Control and Complications Trial (DCCT) was the first randomized controlled trial to prove that improved glycemic control could lead to a significant reduction in diabetes-related complications in patients with type 1 diabetes.[40] The United Kingdom Prospective Diabetes Study (UKPDS) noted similar results in reducing complications for type 2 diabetes with good glycemic control.[41] These two landmark trials are the basis of diabetes treatment goals with the end aim to prevent complications and improve the quality of life for those with diabetes. Specific collaborative interventions include patient education for self-management, glucose monitoring, nutrition therapy, and pharmacologic agents.

Patient Education for Self-Management

Diabetes education is aimed at promoting self-care behaviors for those with diabetes. Health care professionals can provide insight into management decisions, but the diabetic patient is involved in daily decision making for disease management. Self-care behaviors as a component of diabetes management includes diet, exercise, weight control loss, medication management, getting adequate rest, and maintaining awareness of complications.

Monitoring and Managing Blood Glucose

Monitoring and managing blood glucose involves regular monitoring of BG level and using these data to determine medication or dietary action (if needed) to correct an imbalance. Two approaches to BG monitoring are incorporated in diabetic management: self-monitoring of blood glucose (SMBG) and HgbA1$_C$.

Self-monitoring of blood glucose. SMBG is done with a standard BG meter or a continuous glucose monitor that can reveal BG concentration changes that occur every 5 minutes. BG meters measure fingerstick capillary glucose levels and are calibrated to read equivalent to plasma glucose with a variance of approximately 10% from the laboratory setting. Because BG concentration fluctuates throughout the day, SMBG assists with decisions related to carbohydrate intake and medications. Patient or caregiver teaching is essential for accurate SMBG and is most helpful if the patient records readings regularly along with other details related to diet, activity, and stress. Many glucose monitors allow data to be downloaded at a clinic or office for viewing during a patient encounter. Glucose logs are helpful in identifying glucose trends that allow for provider medication adjustment.

Monitoring glycosylated hemoglobin. A person with prediabetes or diabetes can benefit from regular monitoring of HgbA1$_C$ levels to determine progression to overt diabetes. The goal HgbA1$_C$ for most patients is 7.0% or less, although higher glucose (~8.0%) may be appropriate for certain individuals to minimize the risk for episodes of hypoglycemia. Specifically, young children, elderly patients with impaired renal function, and patients taking β-blockers should have less stringent glycemic goals.[19]

Correcting hypoglycemia. One of the ongoing risks associated with glucose-lowering agents is hypoglycemia. The *15/15 rule* is recommended for correcting hypoglycemia: 15 g of quick-acting carbohydrate can raise blood glucose levels by approximately 50 mg/dL. Some examples of quick-acting, 15-g portions of carbohydrate are shown in Box 15-1. The blood glucose level should be checked after 15 minutes to determine effectiveness. If hypoglycemia is not corrected, the process is repeated until euglycemia is achieved (15 g of quick-acting carbohydrate followed by a repeat BG check after 15 minutes). Exceptions to the 15/15 rule include severe hypoglycemia, whereby 30 g of quick-acting carbohydrate is provided (for the conscious individual). If the patient is unconscious, either intravenous dextrose or glucagon is given. Patients receiving glucagon should be rolled onto their side or face down to reduce the risk of aspiration (nausea and vomiting are side effects of high-dosage glucagon).

BOX 15-1   Optimal 15 Gram Carbohydrates for Treatment of Hypoglycemia

- ½ cup regular soda or juice
- 1 cup milk
- ½ ampule of dextrose 50% (D50)
- 1 mg of glucagon
- 3–4 glucose tablets
- 1 tablespoon honey
- 4–6 pieces hard candy
- 15 jelly beans

It is not uncommon for patients to experience a "rebound" of blood sugar to very high levels after an episode of hypoglycemia (sometimes referred to as the Somogyi effect). During the stress of a hypoglycemic event, counterregulatory hormones (including growth hormone, cortisol, epinephrine, and norepinephrine) are released, all of which promote glycogenolysis and gluconeogenesis, resulting in elevated glucose levels after a hypoglycemic episode. For example, a patient can have a drop in glucose to 40–70 mg/dL and then experience a rebound high up to 300–400 mg/dL, creating a "roller coaster" of glucose levels.

Nutrition Therapy

Nutrition therapy is a cornerstone of diabetic management. Individualized dietary strategies should be developed in conjunction with the patient in accordance with his or her needs, readiness, and ability to alter lifestyle. For patients with type 2 diabetes, education often includes strategies to facilitate weight loss. Most individuals with insulin resistance, reactive hypoglycemia, or type 2 diabetes tolerate a range of up to 50–60 g of carbohydrate (three or four servings) per meal very well, especially if the meal is low in glycemic index. Nutrition education for those with type 1 diabetes is focused on knowledge of various nutrient components of each meal (carbohydrates, protein, and fats) to optimize nutrition as related to insulin therapy.

Pharmacologic Agents

The American Diabetes Association and the American Association of Clinical Endocrinologists emphasize an individualized approach to medication therapy for those with diabetes, in which factors such as life expectancy, support system, comorbidities, patient engagement and understanding of the disease process, risk for hypoglycemia, disease duration, and vascular complications are considered when creating a medication management plan.[42]

Oral hypoglycemic agents. Oral hypoglycemic agents are used in the treatment of type 2 diabetes and help to manage glycemic control by reducing insulin resistance and enhancing insulin secretion. These agents are as follows:

- Insulin sensitizers: The first-line oral agent for type 2 diabetes is the insulin sensitizer metformin in the biguanide class. Pioglitazone is in the thiazolidinedione class. Both metformin and pioglitazone help correct the defect of insulin resistance seen in type 2 diabetes.
- Insulin secretagogues: Sulfonylureas and the shorter acting non-sulfonylurea secretagogues enhance insulin secretion from the pancreas, but they are effective only for those who have effective insulin-secreting capacity in the pancreas. As the duration of diabetes diagnosis lengthens, these agents typically become increasingly less useful.
- Incretin agents: The incretin drugs (both the GLP-1 agonists and DPP-4 inhibitors) reduce postprandial glucose levels, and they are weight neutral or facilitate weight loss.
- SGLT-2 inhibitors: These agents increase the amount of glucose excreted by the kidneys and also are associated with some weight loss. They can also cause an osmotic diuresis and increase risk for dehydration and orthostatic hypotension.

Insulin. Patients who require insulin replacement need both basal (or long-acting) insulin and mealtime (or short-/fast-acting) insulin to achieve euglycemia. Normal insulin secretion patterns consist of a steady secretion of very small amounts of insulin throughout the day and night, with pulsations of insulin secretion at mealtimes. Insulin replacement therapy attempts to mimic this normal pattern by using basal and mealtime insulin. The following types of insulin replacement therapy are used:

TABLE 15-2   Characteristics of Various Insulin Preparations

Insulin	Onset of Action	Peak of Action	Duration of Action
NPH	1.5–4 hr	4–12 hr	Up to 24 hr
Glargine (Lantus)	45 min to 4 hr	Minimal	Up to 24 hr
Detimir (Levimir)	45 min to 4 hr	Minimal	Up to 24 hr
Regular Humulin R Novolin R	30–60 min	2–5 hr	Up to 12 hr
Aspart (Novolog)	10–30 min	0.5–3 hr	3–5 hr
Lispro (Humalog)	10–30 min	0.5–3 hr	3–5 hr
Glulisine (Epidra)	10–30 min	0.5–3 hr	3–5 hr
Premixed Preparations			
Humulin 50/50 50% NPH/50% regular			
Humulin 70/30 70% NPH/30% regular			
Novolin 70/30 70% NPH/30% regular			
Humalog mix 50/50 50% NPH/50% lispro			
Novolog mix 50/50 50% NPH/50% aspart			
Novolog mix 75/25 75% NPH/50% aspart			

Source: Beaser RS: *Joslin's diabetes deskbook: A guide for primary care providers*, ed 3, Boston, 2013, Joslin Diabetes Center.

- Basal insulin therapy: Basal insulin therapy can be provided with either neutral protamine hagedorn (NPH) insulin, glargine, or detimir insulin.
- Mealtime insulin therapy: Mealtime insulin therapy can be provided with regular insulin or rapid-acting analogs such as lispro, aspart, and glulisine insulin.
- Mixed preparations: Mixed insulin preparations combine long-acting basal insulin with mealtime insulin. Examples of mixed insulin include 70/30 NPH/lispro, 70/30 NPH/regular, and 75/25 NPH/aspart.

The onset of action, peak of action, and length of action of various insulin preparations are shown in Table 15-2.

Statin agents. Statin medications are used for the primary prevention of cardiovascular disease (CVD) in all individuals with diabetes ages 40–75 years and an LDL cholesterol of 70–189 mg/dL without any evidence of CVD. Evidence suggests statin agents reduce the rate of myocardial infarction, stroke, and death in those with diabetes.[43] It is thought that statin medications possess anti-inflammatory properties that confer additional CVD risk reduction beyond their LDL-lowering properties.[44]

Glucose Control

Glucose control in the hospitalized patient has taken on new importance due to landmark clinical trials that note significant reduction in mortality, wound infections, and length of stay when glucose levels are kept near glycemic goals of 140–180 mg/dL.[45,46]

In the outpatient setting, pattern management based on carbohydrate counting can be effective in stabilizing BG level with reduced frequency of hypo- and hyperglycemia, and it is now the recommended approach. In this approach, assessments of home glucose readings, grams of carbohydrate consumed, and the number of insulin units used help to verify the needed ratio of insulin to carbohydrate intake. Typically, most adults with type 1 diabetes require 1 unit per every 15 g of carbohydrate, or 1 carb serving. A very active adult or a young child may need as little as 1 unit for every 30 g of carbohydrate, whereas an obese, insulin-resistant individual with type 2 diabetes may need as much as 1 unit for every 2 or 3 g of carbohydrate intake. If there is a consistent pattern of hyper- or hypoglycemia by this time period, or by the next meal, the amount of insulin or carbohydrate can be adjusted up or down as needed. Once a ratio is determined, this will generally apply to other meals, although exceptions do occur. For example, the "dawn phenomenon" causes the early morning BG level to rise through increased production of cortisol and growth hormone, which are both counterregulatory hormones. With breakfast, as a consequence, there is often a decreased tolerance to carbohydrate intake with increased need for insulin (endogenous or exogenous).

An insulin correction factor can be used to correct hyperglycemia in addition to using the mealtime insulin-to-carbohydrate ratio. The *1800 rule* predicts the drop in BG level for each 1 unit of extra regular insulin beyond the bolus insulin needed to cover meal carbohydrate intake. The insulin correction factor is determined by dividing the total daily dose (TDD) of insulin units into the number 1800. For example, if a person is taking a usual TDD of 100 units, the predicted insulin correction factor is 18 (1800/100 = 18). In other words, each additional unit of insulin taken will decrease the BG level by 18 points. The higher the TDD, the lower the insulin correction factor, and thus the patient will require higher doses of correction insulin. Likewise, the lower the TDD, the less correction insulin required by the patient. Another person may be taking only 10 units of TDD insulin, which predicts that 1 extra unit of rapid-acting insulin would drop the BG 180 points (1800/10 = 180). The insulin correction factor is also referred to as the insulin sensitivity factor. The calculation factor for regular insulin in 1800/TDD, and for aspart/glulisine/lispro it is 1500/TDD.

INTERRELATED CONCEPTS

Glucose regulation affects and is affected by most, if not all, physiological processes. As the primary energy substrate, all life processes are dependent on normal glucose metabolism and regulation. Figure 15-3 shows some of the most important interrelated concepts.

Hormonal Regulation is shown as a close interrelated concept because of the significant influence that hormones have on the regulation of glucose. Proper Nutrition and regular physical activity (Mobility) are needed for optimal regulation of glucose concentration and management of conditions in which regulatory mechanisms are impaired. Long-term consequences of hyperglycemia lead to micro- and macrovascular changes (Perfusion), poor wound healing (Tissue Integrity), impaired immune function (Immunity), reduced renal function (Elimination), and changes in vision and peripheral sensation (Sensory Perception).

The concepts Family Dynamics, Adherence, and Culture influence the behavioral changes needed for optimal health promotion or disease management. Family relationships can suffer when attempts to regulate the diet of one individual have an adverse impact on mealtime that affects other family members. This can result in mealtime-associated stress if optimal family dynamics are not present. Patient Education is a cornerstone of treatment and has a tremendous impact on outcomes for those with impaired glucose regulation.

CLINICAL EXEMPLARS

Although much of the attention in this concept presentation has focused on diabetes, glucose regulation represents a number of other clinical exemplars that are categorized by hyperglycemic and hypoglycemic states and are presented in Box 15-2. Several of these exemplars

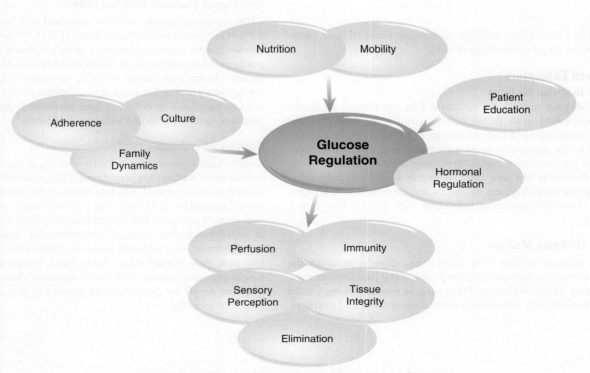

FIGURE 15-3 Glucose Regulation and Interrelated Concepts

BOX 15-2   EXEMPLARS OF IMPAIRED GLUCOSE REGULATION

Hyperglycemia

- Conditions of excess counterregulatory hormones: Cushing's syndrome
- Cystic fibrosis
- Diabetic Ketoacidosis
- Hyperosmolar Hyperglycemic Nonketotic Syndrome
- Type 1 diabetes
- Type 2 diabetes
- Overcorrection of hypoglycemia
- Rebound hyperglycemia ("Somogyi effect")
- Corticosteroid therapy
- Gestational diabetes
- Insulin resistance
- Polycystic ovary syndrome
- Hemochromatosis
- Pheochromocytoma
- Pancreatitis
- Stress response

Hypoglycemia

- Addison's disease
- Insulin treatment
- Gastroparesis
- Glycogen storage diseases
- Prematurity
- Starvation
- Large for gestational age infant
- Liver failure
- Nesidioblastoma
- Insulinoma

are briefly featured here. Detailed information about all these exemplars can be found in nursing textbooks.

Featured Exemplars

Type 2 Diabetes Mellitus

Type 2 diabetes mellitus is characterized by the features of insulin resistance paired with β cell failure resulting in hyperglycemia. Chronic hyperglycemia leads to damage of blood vessels and nerves, leading to the complications of retinopathy, nephropathy, neuropathy, and cardiovascular disease. Previously common in adults only, type 2 diabetes is now seen more commonly in children and adolescents due to increasing rates of obesity and overweight in this population. Ninety-five percent of individuals with diabetes have type 2 diabetes.

Type 1 Diabetes Mellitus

Type 1 diabetes mellitus is an autoimmune disorder in which the body's immune system destroys the β cells in the pancreas, resulting in absolute insulin deficiency. These patients require lifelong insulin replacement therapy to maintain normal metabolism and nutrition.

Most individuals with type 1 diabetes are thin or normal weight, and although it is more common in children and adolescents, approximately 13% of all newly diagnosed type 1 diabetes occurs in people ages 30–50 years.

Polycystic Ovary Syndrome (PCOS)

PCOS is the most common endocrine disorder in women of reproductive age. It is characterized by infrequent menses (longer than 35 days apart) and signs of higher than normal androgen levels (hirsutism, acne, and male pattern hair loss). Infertility is common due to lack of regular menses caused by anovulation. Women with PCOS are very insulin resistant, and approximately 40% of women with PCOS who are obese or overweight will have diabetes or prediabetes before the age of 40 years; therefore, diabetes prevention efforts in these women are crucial.[47]

Diabetic Ketoacidosis (DKA)

DKA is an acute event that results from insulin deficiency and is sometimes the presenting symptom of type 1 diabetes. The combination of hyperglycemia, ketosis, and acidosis leads to dehydration, and fluid resuscitation and insulin therapy are needed to correct this state. Other symptoms include abdominal pain, vomiting, poor skin turgor, tachycardia, and hypotension. Stress is a frequent trigger for DKA.

Hyperosmolar Hyperglycemic Nonketotic Syndrome (HHNS)

HHNS is a state characterized by hyperglycemia, hyperosmolarity, and dehydration without acidosis. HHNS is more common in elderly patients and can present with glucose levels greater than 600 mg/dL. This condition accounts for less than 1% of hospital admissions, and treatment is centered around correction of dehydration and lowering of blood glucose with insulin. HHNS typically has a trigger of stress or illness, and treatment of the underlying cause is a priority of care.

Gestational Diabetes Mellitus (GDM)

GDM is a hyperglycemic condition associated with pregnancy seen in 9.2% of pregnancies in the United States in 2014.[48] Placental hormones increase insulin resistance, especially as the pregnancy progresses, and postprandial hyperglycemia is the common presentation. Risk factors include obesity, past history of GDM, age older than 25 years, and family history of type 2 diabetes. Approximately 5–10% of women who develop gestational diabetes will have persistent hyperglycemia after pregnancy and be diagnosed with type 2 diabetes.[10]

Cushing's Syndrome

Cushing's syndrome is a rare disorder resulting in excessive corticosteroid secretion leading to hyperglycemia. This condition can be primary (caused by corticosteroid-secreting tumor of the adrenal cortex), secondary (caused by ACTH-secreting pituitary tumor or ectopic ACTH secretion), or iatrogenic (when symptoms are related to administration of supraphysiological doses of corticosteroids). Symptoms include hyperglycemia, elevated blood pressure, hypokalemia, central fat distribution, dark purple striae, ruddy facial complexion, hirsutism, weight gain, easy bruising, and muscle weakness. Only 10–15 of every 1 million people are diagnosed with primary or secondary Cushing's syndrome annually.

CASE STUDY

Source: diego cervo/iStock/Thinkstock

Case Presentation

Raymond Ramirez is a 66-year-old Latino male who presents to his health care provider in follow-up for diabetes management. He has a 10-year history of type 2 diabetes, hypertension, and hyperlipidemia. He retired 1 year ago after working as a lab technician for a local hospital for more than 30 years. He lost his wife 2 months ago from cancer and was her primary caregiver for the last 8 months of her life. He lives alone but has two adult children who live a few miles away from him. He has missed some of his checkups with his primary care provider in the past year due to his wife's illness. His HgbA1$_c$ 1 year ago was 8.1%. His current medications include metformin ER 2000 mg daily, exenatide 10 μg twice daily, ramipril 10 mg daily, atorvastatin 20 mg daily, and aspirin 81 mg daily. He has no allergies. He has not been checking his glucose levels at home very often, and he reports eating regular meals although he does not like to cook. He has not exercised for months, but he had been walking 3 miles a day prior to his wife's illness. Vital signs are as follows: weight, 88 kg; height,

70 in.; body mass index, 28.7; temperature, 98.4°F; pulse, 84 beats/minute; respiratory rate, 20 breaths/minute; and blood pressure, 140/82 mm Hg. Lab results are as follows: HgbA1C, 10.1%; glucose, 234 mg/dL; sodium, 135; blood urea nitrogen, 22; creatinine, 1.1; total cholesterol, 186 mg/dL; triglycerides, 325 mg/dL; HDL, 53; and LDL, 69.

Case Analysis

The laboratory tests and history confirm that Mr. Ramirez currently has poorly controlled diabetes. The challenges in his personal life are contributing factors to his lack of exercise and diet. Despite taking maximum doses of metformin and exenatide, he still has high glucose levels. He is probably going through a normal grieving process, and it may not be easy for him to work on health goals right now without assistance. The stress he has been experiencing during the past months may also be contributing to high glucose levels due to release of counterregulatory hormones.

He will need insulin to normalize his glucose levels because he has been experiencing "glucose toxicity," in which glucose levels are consistently high and thus insulin secretion from the pancreas is minimal. He will need education regarding insulin injections and how to recognize hypoglycemia as well as clear instructions on who to call should hypoglycemia occur. He will need frequent SMBG to assess his reaction to insulin therapy and need for dose adjustment. Mr. Ramirez should also be encouraged to resume his walking routine due to the effect of exercise on improving insulin resistance. He also may benefit from some nutritional advice because his eating and cooking habits may have drastically changed in the past several months. His triglyceride levels are elevated as a reflection of poor glucose control, and normalization of his glucose levels may result in improved triglyceride levels. Mr. Ramirez has several risk factors for depression, including recent loss of a spouse, living alone, and the diagnosis of diabetes, and he should be assessed for symptoms of depression. By helping him improve his glycemic control, he can reduce his risk for complications from diabetes and enjoy a higher quality of life during his retirement years.

ACCESS EXEMPLAR LINKS IN YOUR GIDDENS EBOOK

REFERENCES

1. DeFronzo R: Pathogenesis of type 2 diabetes mellitus. *Med Clin North Am* 88:787–825, 2004.
2. Kruger DF, Martin CL, Sadler C: New insights into glucose regulation. *Diabetes Educ* 32:221–228, 2006.
3. Bornfeldt K, Tarbas I: Insulin resistance, hyperglycemia and atherosclerosis. *Cell Metab* 14(5):575–585, 2011.
4. Noto H, Goto A, Tsujimoto T, et al: Cancer risk in diabetic patients treated with metformin: A systemic review and meta-analysis. *PLoS ONE* 7(3):e003341, 2012.
5. Scherrer U, Randin D, Vollenweider P, et al: Nitric oxide release accounts for insulin's vascular effects in humans. *J Clin Invest* 94:2511–2515, 1994.
6. Chaudhary K, Buddineni JP, Nistala R, et al: Resistant hypertension in the high-risk metabolic patient. *Curr Diab Rep* 11(1):41–46, 2010.
7. Appel LJ, Sacks FM, Carey VJ, et al, OmniHeart Collaborative Research Group: Effects of protein, monounsaturated fat, and carbohydrate intake on blood pressure and serum lipids: Results of the OmniHeart randomized trial. *JAMA* 294(19):2455–2464, 2005.

8. Shah M, Adams-Huet B, Garg A: Effect of high-carbohydrate or high-monounsaturated fat diets on blood pressure: A meta-analysis of intervention trials. *Am J Clin Nutr* 85(5):1251–1256, 2007.
9. Lam DC, Lam KS, May SM: Obstructive sleep apnea, insulin resistance and adipocytokines. *Clin Endocrinol* 82(2):165–177, 2015.
10. Centers for Disease Control and Prevention: National diabetes statistics report. Retrieved from <http://www.cdc.gov/diabetes/pubs/statsreport14/national-diabetes-report-web.pdf>, 2014.
11. Singleton JR, Smith AG, Bromberg MB: Increased prevalence of impaired glucose tolerance in patients with painful sensory neuropathy. *Diabetes Care* 24:1448–1453, 2001.
12. Pasquel FL, Umpierrez GE: Hyperosmolar non-ketotic state: A historical review of clinical presentation, diagnosis and treatment. *Diabetes Care* 37:3124–3134, 2014.
13. Venkatraman R, Singhi SC: Hyperglycemic hyperosmolar non-ketotic state. *Ind J Pediatrics* 73(1):55–60, 2006.
14. Beaser RS: *Joslin's diabetes deskbook: A guide for primary care providers*, ed 3, Boston, 2013, Joslin Diabetes Center.
15. McCoy RG, Van Houten HK, Ziegenfuss JY, et al: Increased mortality of patients with diabetes reporting severe hypoglycemia. *Diabetes Care* 35(9):1897–1901, 2012.
16. Feinkohl I, Phyu PA, Keller M, et al: Severe hypoglycemia and cognitive decline in older people with type 2 diabetes: The Edinburgh Type 2 Diabetes Study. *Diabetes Care* 37(2):507–515, 2014.
17. Vinik AI, Maser RE, Mitchell BD, et al: Diabetes autonomic neuropathy. *Diabetes Care* 26(5):1553–1579, 2006.

18. Seaquist ER, Anderson J, Childs B, et al: Hypoglycemia and diabetes: A report of a workgroup of the American Diabetes Association and the Endocrine Society. *Diabetes Care* 36(5):1384–1395, 2013.

19. American Diabetes Association: Standards of medical care in diabetes, 2014. *Diabetes Care* 37(Suppl 1):s14–s80, 2014.

20. Maayan-Metzger A, Lubin D, Kuint J: Hypoglycemia rates in the first days of life among term infants born to diabetic mothers. *Neonatology* 96(2):80–85, 2009.

21. Gong Z, Muzumdar RH: Pancreatic function, type 2 diabetes and metabolism in aging. *Int J Endocrinol* 2012:320482, 2012.

22. Ning F, Pang ZC, Dong YH, et al: Risk factors associated with the dramatic increase in the prevalence of diabetes in the adult Chinese population in Qingdao, China. *Diabet Med* 26(9):855–863, 2009.

23. Patterson CC, Dahlquist GG, Gyürüs E, et al: Incidence trends for childhood type 1 diabetes in Europe during 1989–2003 and predicted new cases 2005–20. *Lancet* 373(9680):2027–2033, 2009.

24. Shaikh SB, Haji IM, Doddamani P, et al: Study of autoimmune polyglandular syndrome (APS) in patients with type1 diabetes mellitus (T1DM) followed up at a tertiary care hospital. *J Clin Diagn Res* 8(2):70–72, 2014.

25. McCarthy MI: Dorothy Hodgkin lecture 2010: From hype to hope? A journey through the genetics of type 2 diabetes. *Diabet Med* 28(2):132–140, 2011.

26. DeFronzo R: Pathogenesis of type 2 diabetes mellitus. *Med Clin North Am* 88:787–825, 2004.

27. Gambineri A, Patton L, Paola A, et al: Polycystic ovary syndrome is a risk factor for type 2 diabetes: Results from a long-term prospective study. *Diabetes* 61(9):2369–2374, 2012.

28. Zhu Y, Hu Y, Zhang Y, et al: High uric acid directly inhibits insulin signaling and induces insulin resistance. *Biochem Biophys Res Commun* 447(4):707–714, 2014.

29. Kayaniyl S, Vieth R, Retnakaran R, et al: Association of vitamin D with insulin resistance and β-cell dysfunction in subjects at risk for type 2 diabetes. *Diabetes Care* 33(6):1379–1381, 2010.

30. Courbebaisse M, Souberbielle JC, Prié D, et al: Nonphosphocalcic actions of vitamin D. *Med Sci (Paris)* 26(4):417–421, 2010.

31. Aronsohn RS, Whitmore H, Van Cauter E, et al: Impact of untreated obstructive sleep apnea on glucose control in type 2 diabetes. *Am J Respir Crit Care Med* 181(5):507–513, 2010.

32. Nouwen A, Winkley K, Twisk J, et al: Type 2 diabetes as a risk factor for the onset of depression: A meta-analysis. *Diabetologia* 53:2480–2486, 2010.

33. Bonora E, Tuomilehto J: Pros and cons of diagnosing diabetes with A1C. *Diabetes Care* 34(Suppl 1):s184–s190, 2011.

34. Herman WH, Ma Y, Uwaifo G, Haffner S, et al: Differences in A1c by race and ethnicity among patients with impaired glucose tolerance in the Diabetes Prevention Program. *Diabetes Care* 30:2453–2457, 2007.

35. Diabetes Prevention Program Research Group: Reduction in incidence of type 2 diabetes with lifestyle intervention or metformin. *N Engl J Med* 346(6):393–403, 2002.

36. Ogden CL, Carroll MD, Kit BK, et al: Prevalence of childhood and adult obesity in the United States, 2011–2012. *J Am Med Assoc* 311(8):806–814, 2014.

37. Richter EA, Hargreaves M: Exercise, GLUT4 and skeletal muscle glucose uptake. *Physiol Rev* 93(3):99301017, 2013.

38. Colberg SR, Sigal RJ, Fernhall B: Exercise and type 2 diabetes: The American College of Sports Medicine and American Diabetes Association: A joint position statement. *Diabetes Care* 33(12):e147–e167, 2010.

39. U.S. Department of Health and Human Services: *Healthy People 2020*, Washington, DC, 2014, U.S. Department of Health and Human Services.

40. Diabetes Control and Complications Trial/Epidemiology of Diabetes Interventions and Complications (DCCT/EDIC) Research Group: Modern-day clinical course of type 1 diabetes mellitus after 30 years' duration: The Diabetes Control and Complications Trial/Epidemiology of Diabetes Interventions and Complications and Pittsburgh Epidemiology of Diabetes Complications Experience (1983–2005). *Arch Intern Med* 169(14):1307–1316, 2009.

41. American Diabetes Association: Implications of the United Kingdom Prospective Diabetes Study. *Diabetes Care* 25(Suppl 1):s28–s32, 2007.

42. Inzucchi SE, Bergenstal RM, Buse JB: Management of hyperglycemia in type 2 diabetes: A patient-centered approach. *Diabetes Care* 35(6):1364–1379, 2012.

43. Stone N, Robinson J, Lichtensten AH, et al: 2013 ACC/AHA guideline on the treatment of blood cholesterol to reduce atherosclerotic cardiovascular risk in adults: A report of the American College of Cardiology/American Heart Association Task Force on Practice Guidelines, Circulation published online November 2013: doi: 10.1161/01.cir.0000437738.63853.7a.

44. Bu D, Griffin G, Lichtman AH: Mechanism for anti-inflammatory effects of statins. *Curr Opin Lipidol* 22(3):165–170, 2011.

45. Godar DA, Kumar DR, Schelzer KM, et al: The impact of serum glucose on clinical outcomes in patients hospitalized with community-acquired pneumonia. *Wisconsin Med J* 30(9):244–250, 2013.

46. Van den Berghe G, Wouters P, Weekers F, et al: Intensive insulin therapy in critically ill patients. *N Engl J Med* 345(19):1359–1367, 2001.

47. Moran LJ, Misso ML, Wild RA, et al: Impaired glucose tolerance, type 2 diabetes and metabolic syndrome in polycystic ovary syndrome: A systematic review and meta-analysis. *Hum Reprod Update* 16(4):347–363, 2010.

48. DeSisto CL, Kim SY, Sharma AJ: Prevalence estimates of gestational diabetes mellitus in the United States, Pregnancy Risk Assessment Monitoring System (PRAMS), 2007–2010. *Prev Chronic Dis* 11:130415, 2014.

Nutrition

Sylvia Escott-Stump

Nutrition encompasses the process by which food and nutrients affect growth and development, cellular function and repair, health promotion, and disease prevention. As a science, nutrition delineates the requirements as well as the functions of macro- and micronutrients for optimal physiological functioning. Most nutrients are needed on a daily basis to achieve short-term and long-term health goals. Nutritional status impacts a variety of health conditions and disorders. In turn, many diseases adversely affect nutritional status by altering the ability to ingest, digest, absorb, and metabolize nutrients in their intact form or at the cellular level. Because nutrition and health are directly linked, this represents a fundamental concept for nursing practice.

DEFINITION

The concept of nutrition is complex, involving a number of physiological processes. For the purpose of this concept presentation, nutrition is defined as *the science of optimal cellular metabolism and its impact on health and disease.* Several other terms are essential to an understanding of this concept that merit definition. *Macronutrients* are the *kilocalorie (kcal)* energy-containing sources of carbohydrates, proteins, and fats. Alcohol also provides kilocalories, but it is not considered a macronutrient because it cannot support or maintain bodily functions. Vitamins and minerals are *micronutrients* because they are required in minute amounts. Some minerals are needed in such small amounts that they are called "ultra" trace mineral requirements. Water is the final product considered to be an essential nutrient. *Phytochemicals* is a term that refers to plant compounds that have antimicrobial, antioxidant, anti-inflammatory, and immune-boosting properties. Examples of phytochemicals include lutein (associated with the green color of vegetables) and lycopene (found in high amounts in tomato products).

SCOPE

Nutritional status can be viewed as either *optimal* or *suboptimal.* An optimal nutritional status is one in which all nutrients are available in balanced amounts for cellular metabolism and physiological function for the individual. A suboptimal state (or malnourished state) reflects either insufficient or excessive quantity or quality of macronutrients or micronutrients. The scope of this concept is represented as a continuum with malnutrition on both ends (insufficient nutrition and excess nutrition) and optimal nutrition in the middle (Figure 16-1).

The continuum representation is important because nutritional status has the potential to change in either direction due to a number of factors and can be corrected with successful measures. Nutritional health status is also an issue of balance or imbalance. Poor nutritional status negatively impacts health, and poor health can negatively impact nutritional status (Figure 16-2).

NORMAL PHYSIOLOGICAL PROCESS

Oral Intake

Normal intake requires appropriate ingestion of necessary foods to meet macronutrient, micronutrient, and fluid needs. Required macronutrients and micronutrients are presented in Table 16-1. The amount of nutrient intake needed for optimal function changes across the lifespan. National guidelines for recommended intake, referred to as Dietary Reference Intakes (DRIs), are available on the U.S. Department of Agriculture website (http://fnic.nal.usda.gov).

Adequate oral intake of nutrients (and water) involves access to food sources, informed food choices, and efficient chewing (mastication) and swallowing abilities. In general, the philosophy is "if the gut works, use it." Evidence shows that much immunity begins in the intestine, so it is important to provide nutrients through the gastrointestinal (GI) tract whenever possible.

Digestion

Digestion is the process of mechanical and chemical breakdown of food matter and complex forms of macronutrients. Mechanical breakdown includes chewing in the mouth, as well as the mixing motions and muscular (peristaltic) action of propelling food through the stomach and intestines. Digestive enzymes are responsible for the chemical breakdown of food matter; this process is most efficient when consumed food is thoroughly chewed, thus increasing the surface of food particles for enzyme action.

Chemical breakdown begins in the oral cavity. Saliva is a mucous-like fluid that contains the digestive enzyme amylase, which assists with the process of food breakdown and aids in the chewing and swallowing process. In the stomach, gastric enzymes begin to digest proteins into amino acids and carbohydrates into simple sugars. Pancreatic enzymes finalize digestion in the small bowel, with fats being converted into fatty acids. Bile, produced in the liver and stored in the gallbladder, is involved in fat digestion by modifying dietary fats into emulsions for better absorption.

FIGURE 16-1 Scope of Nutrition Concept

FIGURE 16-2 Interrelationship between Nutritional Status and Health Status

TABLE 16-1	Required Nutrients		
Macronutrients and Primary Role	**Fat-Soluble Vitamins**	**Water-Soluble Vitamins**	**Major Minerals**
Carbohydrates	Vitamin A	Vitamin C	Calcium
Primary source of	Vitamin D	B Vitamins	Phosphorus
fuel and energy	Vitamin E	Thiamin	Magnesium
Protein	Vitamin K	Riboflavin	Sodium
Facilitates growth		Niacin	Potassium
and repair of		Pyridoxine	Chloride
tissues; energy		Pantothenic	
source		Biotin	
Fat		Folate	
Source of fatty		Cobalamin	
acid, necessary			
for growth and			
development;			
energy			

Absorption

Once food matter has been digested, the microscopic hairlike projections (villi) that line the intestinal tract absorb nutrients into capillaries which are then transported by the vascular system. The upper portion of the small intestinal tract (duodenum) is the primary site for absorbing trace minerals. The middle section (jejunum) is the primary site for absorbing water-soluble vitamins and proteins. The lower section (ileum) is the site of fat and fat-soluble vitamin absorption. Water is primarily absorbed in the colon.

Elimination

Large food particles and undigested fibers are not absorbed—they are eliminated through the colon. A healthy GI tract with efficient peristaltic action is required for optimal elimination. Bulky stools, from adequate fiber intake, stimulate peristalsis. Elimination is enhanced with adequate fluid, fiber intake, and physical activity.

Cellular Metabolism

Cellular metabolism includes the hormonal and enzymatic processes that occur within cell structures that allow proteins, carbohydrates, or fats to be used for energy or made into new products or tissues. Adequate intake of both macro- and micronutrients is required for optimal

cellular metabolism. Proteins (in the form of essential amino acids) must be consumed for cells to manufacture other proteins, such as carrier proteins, and to enable tissue growth and repair. Adequate carbohydrate intake provides the energy for protein to do its many jobs. Carbohydrates are also required to provide glucose for the unique fuel needs of the brain, the neurologic system, and the red blood cells. Essential fatty acids maintain the integrity of the phospholipid-based cell membranes, found around every cell. Many metabolic enzymes assist in cellular metabolism. Zinc and magnesium are each part of more than 200 different metabolic enzymes. Both zinc and folic acid are critical in the production of proteins and cellular structures; without these micronutrients, growth and tissue repair are severely impaired.

Age-Related Differences

Although the general physiological process of nutrition is consistent throughout life, there are specific age-related considerations worth noting.

Infants and Children

Significant changes in growth and development occur in the first year of life. Birth weight triples, and length increases by an average of 50%. Infants have very different nutrient needs (compared to adults) to support this rapid growth. Due to the lack of teeth, chewing capability, and immature GI tract, the nutritional intake of infants should be limited to breast milk (or formula) and water for the first 6 months of life. Newborn infants depend on a strong suck–swallow reflex for adequate nutritional intake. As the child's GI tract develops, solid foods that do not require chewing can be gradually introduced (ideally starting at 6 months of age). As teeth emerge, the older infant and young child can be offered foods with various textures. The small orophyarx places young children at risk of choking; thus, the need to provide foods in small bites is particularly important. Specific nutrient requirements for infants and children can be found by referring to DRIs.

Pregnancy and Lactation

Significant changes in nutrition needs occur during pregnancy and lactation to account for the body composition changes during pregnancy (hormonal, metabolic, and anatomic), growing fetus (before birth), and the production of breast milk after delivery. Increases in carbohydrates, proteins, fats, and most micronutrients are recommended. Expected weight gain during pregnancy ranges from 15 to 40 pounds, depending on prepregnancy weight and stature. Specific nutrient requirements for pregnant women and during lactation can be found by referring to DRIs.

Older Adults

Physiologically, the effects of aging can be associated with a reduced ability to ingest, absorb, and metabolize nutrients. In the mouth, reduced chewing ability, reduced saliva production, and reduced sense of taste are common. The esophagus may be elongated (due to kyphosis), and atrophic changes occur, particularly in the lower esophagus. Atrophic changes and intestinal microflora occur in aging, resulting in reduced efficiency in absorption. In the absence of disease, the liver, gallbladder, and pancreas continue to function, although there is a decrease in metabolic efficiency.

VARIATIONS AND CONTEXT

Malnutrition is a comprehensive term that refers to two major categories of nutritional conditions: insufficient nutrition and excess nutrition. Within each of these two categories, nutritional problems are represented by the specific nutrient or nutrients involved. The causes of problems vary widely and include problems with access, intake, absorption, and metabolism.

Insufficient Nutrition

Insufficient nutrition occurs when there is inadequate intake, impaired nutrient absorption, or ineffective nutrient utilization occur, leading to a state of malnutrition. The malnutrition can be associated with insufficient calorie intake leading to unintended weight loss and/or insufficient intake of one or more nutrients leading to a number of nutritional deficiencies. The state of being underweight is described as a body mass index (BMI) less than 18.5. *Starvation-related malnutrition* describes conditions such as anorexia nervosa, whereas *acute disease-related malnutrition* occurs after burn injury or trauma. The third type of adult malnutrition (*chronic disease-related malnutrition*) is exemplified by sarcopenic obesity or pancreatic cancer.

Excess Nutrition

At the opposite end of the spectrum is the situation in which excessive nutritional intake progresses to weight gain or nutritional toxicities. The most common form of excess nutrition is associated with excessive calorie intake leading to weight gain. Standardized categories, based on BMI, are used to describe overweight and obesity. For adults, overweight is described as a BMI between 25.0 and 29.9. Three classes of obesity are class I (BMI of 30–34.9), class II (BMI of 35–39.9), and class III (BMI >40). Child obesity is described in terms of BMI compared to percentiles on standardized growth charts. A child who's BMI is between the 85th and 95th percentile for children of the same age and sex is classified as overweight; obesity is defined as a BMI greater than the 95th percentile.

Excess micronutrient intake most often occurs with high-dose fat-soluble vitamin and mineral supplements or when consuming foods that have 100% of the DRI levels of a nutrient, plus an oral supplement, and a liquid enhanced beverage all in the same day. The outcomes of excessive food or supplement intake on physiological processes can be detrimental, especially if prolonged over time.

CONSEQUENCES

A number of physiological consequences occur associated with a poor nutritional state on both ends of the spectrum: nutritional deficiencies and nutritional excess. These are best understood by considering the specific nutrients involved. Malnutrition is highly devastating for infants and children because it limits their growth, brain development, ability to learn, and, later, their ability to participate effectively in society.

Nutritional Deficiencies
Macronutrient Deficiencies

Protein is a component of every cell of the body. Thus, protein deficiency has diverse consequences, and the effects can be subtle or dramatic, depending on the severity, amount of inflammation, and length of time. In children, an inadequate intake of protein and kilocalories (*marasmus*) impairs growth and development, stunting height and brain development most evidently. The condition in which the insufficiency is protein alone, with adequate energy (*kwashiorkor*), is seen in developing countries after an infant is weaned to a diet that contains mostly grains. At any age, inadequate protein intake will adversely impact the body's ability to repair or replace body tissues or produce other constituents such as immune factors. In older adults, the loss of muscle mass (in sarcopenia) is difficult to replace. A spiraling decline in health may occur if not corrected through rapid and effective interventions. Insufficient circulating protein in the blood (hypoalbuminemia) can also lead to anasarca (severe generalized edema).

Inadequate carbohydrate intake can alter cellular metabolism and results in the use of dietary protein as a fuel substrate, diminishing cell growth and repair. Ultimately, if inadequate carbohydrate intake continues, there is a shift to use body fat catabolism and protein for energy resulting in weight loss and accumulation of ketones, especially if insulin is also limited.

Essential fatty acid deficiency affects all cellular membranes and is particularly a problem with premature infants. Docosahexaenoic acid (DHA) and eicosapentaenoic acid (EPA) are long-chain omega-3 fatty acids that support retinal development, neurotransmitter production, and brain function.

Vitamin and Mineral Deficiencies

Deficiency of vitamin C was one of the first recognized nutrient deficiency diseases, with the severe form (scurvy) being a cause of death among early sea voyagers. British sailors were called "limeys" because their intake of limes while onboard sea vessels prevented this condition. In the early twentieth century, processed grains were becoming popular. Soon, a mysterious syndrome appeared as the "4 D's": dermatitis on sun-exposed areas, diarrhea, dementia, and death. This condition (pellagra) was determined to be from a B vitamin deficiency. The government mandated that processed white flour products had to be enriched with the nutrients that were removed during processing—vitamins B_1, B_2, and B_3 (thiamine, riboflavin, and niacin, respectively).

The role of folate in the development of the central nervous system had been known for decades, but not until the 1990s did it become clear that most neural tube defects (NTDs) could be prevented by fortifying grains. Folic acid is now added to flour processed in the United States and in many countries; an important reduction in NTDs has been shown in these countries.

Lutein and zeaxanthin are carotenoids found in yellow and orange foods (cantaloupe, corn, carrots, salmon, and egg yolks) that help to prevent macular degeneration. The intact form of vitamin A is also essential for vision; deficiency begins with loss of night vision and progresses to total blindness.

Vitamin D insufficiency is known to lead to osteoporosis, hip fracture, and hyperparathyroidism. Studies also suggest links with cardiovascular disease, cancer, multiple sclerosis, tuberculosis, and muscular and immune system disorders. Table 16-2 summarizes key nutrient deficiency and toxicity concerns.

TABLE 16-2   Common Vitamin and Mineral Deficiencies and Toxicities

Nutrient	Consequences of Deficiencies	Consequences of Toxicities
Vitamin A	Night blindness	Loss of appetite, bone pain, hypercalcemia
Vitamin B$_1$ (thiamine)	Wernicke's encephalopathy with neurodegeneration	Toxicity rare
Vitamin B$_3$	Pellagra with 4 D's: dermatitis, diarrhea, dementia, death	Abnormal glucose metabolism, flushing, nausea and vomiting
Vitamin B$_{12}$	Pernicious anemia, psychiatric disorders	Toxicity unknown
Biotin	Hair loss	Toxicity unknown
Vitamin C	Bleeding tendency, scurvy	Inhibits zinc absorption, urinary stones
Vitamin D	Rickets, bone disease, muscle pain, falls	Hypercalcemia, renal stones, calcification of soft tissues
Copper	Anemia, skin lesions, neurologic disease, bone fragility	Found in Wilson's disease; neuron and liver cell damage
Iron	Anemia, fatigue, poor growth	Hemochromatosis (genetic) with liver, pancreatic, and cardiac damage
Magnesium	Hypertension, dysrhythmia, preeclampsia	Increased calcium excretion
Zinc	Dermatitis, impaired taste, impaired growth, low level of alkaline phosphatase enzyme	Copper deficiency, renal damage, nausea and vomiting, diarrhea

Nutritional Excess

Malnutrition also occurs from excess macronutrient (energy) intake that leads to weight gain. Often, obese individuals may have micronutrient insufficiency but macronutrient excesses.

The consequences of excessive weight have been well documented and can include type 2 diabetes, coronary heart disease, hypertension, stroke, fatty liver disease, gallbladder disorders, sleep apnea, asthma and other respiratory problems, musculoskeletal disorders, as well as some cancers. With more children and teens becoming obese, many of these medical conditions are seen at young ages, with similar challenges and high risks for early mortality.

RISK FACTORS

All individuals have a potential risk for malnutrition. Some risk factors are common in population groups or during certain life stages, but individual choices and circumstances also have influence.

Populations at Risk
Age or Life Stage

At the beginning of life and again at the later stages, nutritional deficits are a significant concern. Pregnancy is a very important stage because of the long-term effects on health of the infant and the mother. The very young are at risk because of immature organ development and total dependence on others for feeding. Particularly at risk are premature infants because of impaired oral intake. With parenteral or tube feeding, the use of breast milk may be impossible, eliminating the benefits of cost savings, immunological protection, ideal nutrient content, and microbial support.[1,2]

Senior citizens are also at high risk for nutritional inadequacies. Factors such as reduced organ function, limited income, interactions between nutrients and medications, isolation, decreased interest in meal preparation, changes in appetite, fatigue, and altered taste sensations are common. Those elderly who are institutionalized are at even greater risk. Severe dietary restrictions, rigid mealtimes, generally poor health status, and feeding dependency can lead to inadequate oral intake. Physiological risk factors include frailty, low BMI (BMI <21 is associated with a high risk of mortality despite nutritional intervention), and neurologic deficits from a stroke or Alzheimer's disease.[3–5]

Ethnicity/Race

Nutritional deficits and genetic predispositions have triggered many chronic diseases of the modern world.[6] Vitamin D deficiency is more frequently found among Hispanics and Americans of African heritage than those of European heritage.[7,8] Diseases more common in European heritage include type 1 diabetes, celiac disease, and neurodegenerative disorders such as Huntington's disease and multiple sclerosis.[9]

The Poor and Underserved

As a population group, those of low socioeconomic status are at risk for malnutrition because of food insecurity and food availability. Lack of access to healthy foods because of insufficient funds, distance to supermarkets, limited options for food preparation, high prices of quality foods, cheap prices of fast food, and limited transportation are some of the reasons why individuals with low incomes may eat poorly and become obese.[10] Where access to healthy, affordable food is limited, the community is designated as a "food desert." Creative approaches are often needed to help families learn to budget their food dollars wisely and nutritiously. The homeless who experience food insecurity on a daily basis and over a prolonged period of time are particularly at risk.

Individual Risk Factors
Genetics

Many conditions that impact nutrition are linked to genetics. Inherited metabolic defects include phenylketonuria (PKU), a deficiency in the enzyme responsible for the metabolism of the amino acid phenylalanine. PKU allows phenylalanine to accumulate in the brain, blood, and tissues leading to cognitive dysfunction unless the affected individual follows a low-phenylalanine diet for life. Other rare inherited metabolic defects include galactosemia and maple syrup urine disease. In cystic fibrosis (CF), thick secretions block pancreatic ducts, eventually leading to impaired digestion and absorption of fats and fat-soluble vitamins.

Lifestyle and Patterns of Eating

How one chooses foods, shops, plans, and prepares meals ultimately affects his or her nutritional status. Factors that influence these decisions include interpersonal relationships, learned stress-coping mechanisms, and alterations in mood. Weight gain can occur when food habits change to match those of the partner, such as during dating and marriage.

Family food offerings can positively or negatively influence nutritional intake. Mothers who avoid high-fat, high-sugar foods but emphasize a variety of vegetables, fruits, whole grains, lean meats, and low-fat milk can send the right message to their family. Family influences that may negatively impact nutritional status include lack of home-prepared meals, eating meals on the go, restricting multiple food groups because of allergies or dislikes, or limited choices because of financial challenges.

The influence of peers is common among adolescents. Skipping meals, following fad diets, choosing salty and sugary snacks over healthy foods, eating super-sized portions, and drinking alcohol are examples. Here, mood swings dominate. Coping mechanisms often include eating large amounts of sweets or comfort foods or reducing intake altogether during periods of depression. Peer influences are especially strong among young people with lower self-esteem.[11]

Personal Food Choices

Personal choice is the major internal influence over food intake. Women tend to experience cravings around their menstrual periods and during pregnancy.[12] If they give in to these cravings regularly, obesity may result. Occasionally, individuals may experience nutritional disorders because of erroneous understandings or perceptions about foods.

If a vegan diet is undertaken without adequate knowledge, the intake may be insufficient for essential amino acids, calcium, zinc, and vitamins D and B_{12}. Inadequate vitamin B_{12} has been associated with anemia and with neurologic damage, especially dangerous in children.[13] Calcium and vitamin D levels tend to be low unless fortified foods or supplements are used. Without adequate planning of foods containing the various amino acids, protein deficiency can occur. Fortunately, a carefully planned vegan diet offers protection against obesity, hypertension, type 2 diabetes, and cardiovascular disease, especially in men.[14]

Underlying Medical Conditions

A wide range of medical conditions place individuals at risk for various nutritional problems. Some of these are shown in Table 16-3.

Impaired oral intake. Adequacy of oral intake is associated with the ability to chew and swallow. Thus, the inability to chew or swallow properly can easily lead to malnutrition. Pain from dental caries, poorly fitting dentures, and loss of teeth can impair the ability to chew and limit diet quality. Cleft palate impacts an infant's sucking ability, thereby limiting successful breast-feeding. Difficulty swallowing (dysphagia) is common in neurologic conditions, especially after a stroke. Not all patients require altered food consistency, but patients should be seated as upright as possible to prevent aspiration. In conditions such as Parkinson's or Alzheimer's disease, the sense of smell diminishes, also leading to decreased food intake. Unbalanced food intake also occurs in mental health conditions such as anorexia nervosa, mood disorders, anxiety, and depression.

Impaired digestion and absorption. Many conditions interfere with digestion or absorption and place the affected individual at risk for malnutrition. Examples of such conditions include lactose intolerance, gastroparesis, gastric surgery, intestinal resection, and inadequate gastric acidity. Some genetic conditions lead to defects in metabolism of nutrients, such as PKU (mentioned previously). Impaired digestion and absorption can also occur as an adverse effect from some medications.

Increased metabolic demand. A variety of conditions increase metabolic rate and energy needs, thus increasing the risk for protein–calorie malnutrition. Examples include cancer, chronic obstructive pulmonary disease, Parkinson's disease, trauma (including burns), stroke, and HIV/AIDS. Depending on the severity of the disease state, it may be difficult to meet the increased nutrient needs without enteral or parenteral nutrition support.

Altered organ function. The failure of organs involved in digestion and metabolism are associated with nutritional deficiencies. Hepatic disease adversely impacts the ability to reassemble amino acids into the various proteins needed for physiological function. A damaged liver will also be unable to metabolize and excrete drugs properly, thus altering nutrient absorption and utilization even further. In chronic kidney disease (CKD), nutritional status is adversely impacted through a variety of mechanisms. Protein is lost through the urine and can lead to impaired skin integrity, slow wound healing, suppressed immunity, sarcopenia, and altered osmotic pressure. As CKD progresses, phosphorous levels can increase and lead to hypocalcemia. Renal disease further reduces nutrient levels, especially vitamin D because the kidney metabolizes vitamin D_2 into the bioactive D_3 form. With lowered vitamin D status, bone health is impacted because vitamin D is required to absorb calcium.

The kidneys are involved in producing red blood cells; therefore, in patients with CKD, anemia can develop that is unresponsive to iron intake due to an insufficient level of erythropoietin, a protein-based hormone. Even nutrition therapy can have adverse nutritional consequences; limited fluid or food intake and phosphorus/protein/potassium restrictions can be challenging. This is especially true when CKD is compounded by an acute illness. Thus, organ damage and illnesses can seriously impact nutritional status, as shown in Table 16-3.

ASSESSMENT

All nurses should know how to perform a basic assessment of nutritional status. Maintaining an awareness of the risk factors helps to focus the interview and examination.

History

In the interview of the patient or family members, it should be remembered that food has a strong emotional component. Actual food or eating practices may not be revealed unless there is trust and rapport. This is especially true when interviewing parents of a child whose growth and development are not within expected ranges. Generally, adults respond more openly to health providers if they are aware of the rationale for the questions. Mentioning some potential nutritional complications of a condition, or asking about the individual's personal health concerns, allows for focused interviewing.

The basic elements of a history include nutritional intake, diet restrictions, changes in appetite and intake, changes in weight, medical history, current medical conditions, current medications and treatments, allergies, family history, and social history. In addition, it is important to consider the chief complaint/presenting symptoms because they might relate to nutrition and may warrant a symptom analysis. The most important screening problems or presenting symptoms include the following: unplanned changes in weight, changes in appetite or intake, nausea and/or vomiting, difficulty chewing or swallowing, abdominal pain or discomfort, changes in bowel habits, and recent history of constipation or diarrhea.

Examination Findings

Several techniques are used to assess nutritional status, including general observation, anthropometric measurements, and other various clinical findings from systems' assessment. Measuring height and weight, and determining body mass index (BMI) are the initial steps

TABLE 16-3   Impact of Medical Conditions on Risk for Malnutrition

Medical Conditions or States	Impact on Nutritional Status
Oral/GI problems with limited protein–calorie intake (e.g., sensory issues, allergies, dental problems, dysphagia) Impaired intestinal absorption of proteins (diarrhea/malabsorption: e.g., celiac disease, Crohn's disease, short-bowel syndrome, bariatric surgery) Hepatic disease with impaired protein synthesis Chronic kidney disease with proteinuria Nephrotic syndrome Cancer with increased metabolic needs Burns with loss of protein in body fluids	Hypoalbuminemia/impaired protein nutrition
Hypoalbuminemia (lack of carrier proteins) Hyperphosphatemia (in chronic kidney disease, end stage) Malabsorption/diarrhea Hypoparathyroidism Hypomagnesemia Vitamin D deficiency	Hypocalcemia
Hyperparathyroidism Hyperthyroidism Adrenal insufficiency Cancer Hypervitaminosis A and D	Hypercalcemia
Wound healing protocol with excess supplementation of zinc	Copper deficiency anemia
GI bleed	Iron deficiency anemia/microcytic anemia
Hemochromatosis Hepatic disease	Iron overload
Gastrectomy Pernicious anemia/lack of intrinsic factor Primary hypothyroidism Achlorhydria	Vitamin B_{12} deficiency
Epilepsy with use of antiseizure medications Chronic kidney disease (end stage) and dialysis treatments Edema/hypertension with K^+-depleting diuretics Malabsorption/diarrhea Hepatic disease Pancreatitis	Folic acid deficiency/megaloblastic anemia Hypomagnesemia
Chronic kidney disease with limited ability to convert to active form Malabsorption	Vitamin D deficiency
Hypoalbuminemia Chronic kidney disease (end stage) and dialysis treatments Alcoholic cirrhosis/hepatic disease Inflammatory bowel disease Sickle cell anemia	Zinc deficiency

in assessing nutritional status. General goals and interpretation guidelines for BMI are presented in Table 16-4. If BMI is within normal limits and weight has been stable, it is still important to have at least a brief assessment of oral intake to verify that macronutrients and micronutrients are being consumed in appropriate amounts. If there is any suspicion of poor nutritional status, lab work should be ordered by the attending provider to help assess status more completely.

General physical appearance, level of orientation, and demeanor will give insight into health and nutritional status. Assess skin integrity and turgor. The skin should be smooth and elastic without cracks or bruising. The hair should be shiny and not brittle. Nail beds should be smooth, pink, and firm. The teeth should be free of cavities, and the oral tissues should be moist, pink, and firm. Mucous membranes around the eyes should be pink, moist and free of lesions; the sclera should be white. The cornea should be clear and shiny.

Diagnostic Tests

Nurses need to understand common nutrition-related tests, and they need to know when to alert the physician or dietitian if malnutrition is suspected.

Laboratory Tests

Serum albumin and pre-albumin. Serum albumin measures circulating protein in the blood. Low albumin can reflect protein-calorie malnutrition. However, other conditions (such as inflammation, blood loss, fluid status) can also cause low serum albumin levels. Low albumin levels predict severity of illness and are also predictors of mortality in adults older than age 60 years.[15] Pre-albumin reflects recent dietary protein intake. Thus, low pre-albumin is generally associated with nutritional intake as opposed to other conditions.

TABLE 16-4 Interpreting BMI in Children and Adults

Age Group and Approach	BMI	Interpretation
Children (percentile) BMI percentile for children: Apply calculated BMI (weight in pounds/ height in inches/height in inches × 703) to percentile growth chart (see http://www.cdc.gov/growthcharts)	<5th	Underweight; may be acceptable if bone growth is adequate and child "follows the curve"; promote increased kilocalorie intake as needed if weight curve is declining.
	5th to 85th	Optimal weight; still important to "follow the curve" and meet goals for bone growth.
	85th to 95th	Overweight; goal to prevent obesity without causing risk to bone growth or emotional development.
	≥95th	Childhood obesity; goal for young children is not to exceed percentile growth curve; promote physical activity and healthy eating to help "grow into weight."
Adults (calculated BMI) BMI calculated by weight in pounds/ height in inches/height in inches × 703	<19	Underweight; severe level <15 indicative of anorexia.
	19–24.9	Optimal body weight composition; elderly persons should strive for BMI >21.
	25–29.9	Overweight; may be appropriate given health status.
	30–34.9	Class I obesity; slow weight loss advised to promote permanent weight loss; not appropriate for elder population to lose weight.[19-21]
	35–39.9	Class II obesity; slow weight loss advised; may be a candidate for bariatric surgery if comorbidities present and not able to achieve long-term weight loss through diet and exercise.
	≥40	Class III or "extreme" obesity (formerly known as morbid obesity); may be a candidate for bariatric surgery based on health status, age, and level of obesity and history of not being able to achieve long-term weight loss through diet and exercise.

Blood glucose and hemoglobin A1c. Blood glucose reflects metabolism of carbohydrates, and this test is generally used to screen or monitor impaired glucose metabolism. Hypoglycemia may suggest inadequate caloric intake and hyperglycemia may be an indication of diabetes mellitus. Hemoglobin A_{1c} is a test that shows average blood glucose levels over time and is used in the management of diabetic patients. indicates how well glucose levels are controlled. Note that for anemia or renal disease, false readings of the A_{1c} level may occur; for this reason finger-stick glucose tests may be preferable in these situations.

Lipid profile. A lipid profile includes several tests that assess lipid metabolism and serve as important indicators of risk for cardiovascular disease. Tests included are low-density lipoprotein (LDL), high-density lipoprotein (HDL), cholesterol, and triglycerides. Triglyceride levels generally reflect hyperinsulinemia although an individual with newly diagnosed type 1 diabetes may have temporary elevations of triglycerides.

Electrolytes. Electrolytes provide information about general health status including specific information about micronutrients including sodium, potassium, calcium, magnesium, and phosphorus. These are usually ordered as part of a chemistry profile blood test. Electrolytes can become imbalanced with inadequate dietary intake or many other conditions such as renal disease, liver disease, and diabetes. See the Fluid and Electrolytes concept for further information.

Hemoglobin and hematocrit. Hemoglobin (Hgb) and hematocrit (Hct) is a blood test that examines red blood cells (including the number, size, shape, and color) to diagnose anemia caused by dietary deficiency such as iron, folate, and vitamin B12. Hgb and Hct also provide information about the hydration status of the patient.

CLINICAL MANAGEMENT

Primary Prevention

Primary prevention measures are aimed at preventing the onset of disease through risk reduction and behavior modification. The foundation of primary prevention efforts, as it relates to this concept, includes healthy eating and physical activity.

Healthy Eating

A person who follows the current *Dietary Guidelines for Americans* and MyPlate (see ChooseMyPlate.gov) can achieve a healthy diet. The inclusion of the minimum number of servings in MyPlate will meet the DRI micronutrient and macronutrient needs for general health needs. The *Dietary Guidelines* are aimed more at preventing chronic health diseases associated with excess intake of macronutrients, especially solid fats (saturated/trans fats), sugar, and salt. Food labels with DRI values reinforce the *Dietary Guidelines*. Food labels also state four marker nutrients: calcium, iron, vitamin A, and vitamin C. Generally, if these micronutrients are included in adequate amounts from foods naturally high in them, the other needed micronutrients will also be obtained.

Breast-feeding is recommended for optimal nutrition of infants for the 4–6 months of life. Breast milk contains all the essential nutrients and has immunologic benefits that protect the infant from acute and chronic disease.

Physical Activity

Physical activity helps to prevent obesity. The general goals include 30 minutes of physical activity on most days of the week or 150 or more minutes weekly. Weight loss may require at least twice this amount of exercise. However, guidelines for exercise need to be individualized. A sedentary person or one who has sarcopenia or cardiovascular disease needs limited time intervals of exercise more frequently.

Secondary Prevention (Screening)

Secondary prevention involves screening tests to detect disease. Screening for nutritional status in the general population is limited primarily to lipid screening, blood glucose screening, and BMI. Blood glucose screening is advised for persons with evidence of insulin resistance, such as central obesity found with metabolic syndrome. Lipid screening is also recommended, particularly for those with specific risk factors. Although not an essential nutrient, it often becomes necessary to supplement coenzyme Q10 with long-term statin use.

For infants, routine screening that occurs at birth includes the following: glucose levels; at least 40 different genetically linked metabolic disorders, including phenylketonuria and maple syrup urine disease, that are related to an inability to metabolize certain amino acids or to errors in fatty acid metabolism; carbohydrate disorders, including galactosemia; other congenital disorders that can affect nutritional status, including cystic fibrosis; and HIV. The number of screenings will vary from state to state.

Collaborative Interventions

There are several interventions for nurses to manage individuals who have nutritional-related health conditions. Interventions are classified into the following major groups: dietary interventions, pharmacologic agents, and surgical interventions. Coordination of care often involves working with the registered dietitian nutritionist, with home care services, or with a community agency (e.g., referral to Meals-On-Wheels for home-delivered meal services). Discharge planning is an essential team effort on behalf of the patient.

CLINICAL NURSING SKILLS RELATED TO NUTRITION

Assessment
- Physical signs of malnutrition
- Weight and height records—accuracy, frequency; scale calibrations

Education: Basic nutrition and modified diet guidance

Feeding-dependent patient assistance
- Dysphagia management
- Hydration, intake–output records
- Nursing assistant training

Nutrition support
- Enteral nutrition: Tube feedings
  - Nasogastric tube
  - Gastrostomy tube
  - Jejunostomy tube
- Parenteral nutrition

Nourishment administration
- Documentation

Red flags: Referral to the registered dietitian–nutritionist
- Pressure ulcers, weight loss
- Inadequate oral intake or changes in appetite
- NPO, nausea or vomiting >3 days

Dietary Interventions

As part of the health care team, nurses often work with other health professionals for optimal nutritional outcomes. *Registered dietitian nutritionists* (RDNs) are health professionals who have a background in biochemistry and metabolism, with knowledge about the macronutrient and micronutrient contents of foods and how the body uses them. Another health professional, the *dietetic technician*, assists the RDN with menu planning, nutrition education, and management of food services. Nutrition therapy is a term used to describe the typical services of the RDN or registered dietetic technician, whereas medical nutrition therapy is a legal term for reimbursable services provided by the RDN. The nutrition care process includes standardized language and codes within the profession of dietetics. Complex assessments, nutrition diagnosing, and diet therapy interventions are the role of the RDN. A qualified RDN may have diet order-writing privileges as determined by competency assessment, licensure laws, and facility protocols. Thus, the RDN can adjust a patient's meal plan so that it is appropriate for health goals, realistic, economical, and feasible for the family. Nurses should understand basic modified diets to reinforce messages provided by the RDN and encourage referrals as needed.

The concept of *personalized nutrition* is replacing the old paradigm that "one diet fits all" through the science of nutrigenomics—in other words how genetics influence nutritional intervention. Individuals differ in how nutrients are assimilated, metabolized, stored, and excreted; these differences are often significant. Further, individualized dietary plans are needed to address unique dietary needs of patients based on their age, calorie needs, and underlying health condition. For example, not all hypertensive individuals respond to sodium (salt) restriction, not all individuals with high serum cholesterol levels respond to a low saturated fat diet, and sugar alone is not the culprit in diabetes management.

Another aspect of dietary interventions is ensuring that the food provided matches the patient's ability to eat. A patient who has his or her original teeth (none missing) and good oral hygiene, or well-fitting dentures and adequate saliva, represents the best scenario for chewing all kinds of foods. Unfortunately, many hospitalized or aging patients require assistance because they have missing teeth or dentures or because their dentures no longer fit. Nurses can make note of these concerns early in treatment so that altered diets may be ordered or oral health services can be provided.

Enteral Nutrition

Nurses administer nutrition support via tube feedings. Tube feedings are indicated for an individual who is unable to eat or swallow but has an intact/functional GI tract. Feeding tubes are inserted directly into the stomach or small intestine for the delivery of enteral feedings. A specific formula is selected by the physician and RDN based on patient needs. In some hospitals, the RDN may be qualified to write the diet orders or even to insert the tube. The tube feeding is administered either by gravity or through a feeding pump. A common form of tube feeding is percutaneous endoscopic gastrostomy (PEG) feeding. A PEG tube requires a small incision into the stomach. Fortunately, the procedure is relatively safe, simple, and reversible. Although unused formula must be discarded after 24 hours, the tubes can be maintained longer with strict infection control procedures according to facility protocols.

Parenteral Nutrition

Parenteral nutrition is used to provide either total or supplemental nutrition intravenously. These intravenous feedings are generally used for patients who have intestinal failure and cannot be fed orally or by enteral feeding. Here, nutrition consists of a glucose-based intravenous solution (various dextrose concentrations) with electrolytes, minerals, and amino acids. Fat emulsions (lipids) may also be included or administered as a separate solution.

Because parenteral nutrition is indicated for individuals who are unable to process nutrients via the GI tract for more than 4 or 5 days, therapy can be short term or long term. For short term, it may be administered peripherally, whereas for long term, it can be administered centrally. Sepsis and electrolyte and metabolic imbalances can occur; thus, meticulous nursing care of the vascular access is required. Excessive infusion of enteral or parenteral nutrition solutions can be dangerous. The critically ill patient is vulnerable because metabolic shifts occur throughout each day from sepsis and various procedures. Ideally, indirect calorimetry is used to determine energy needs so overfeeding can be avoided. Extra caution should be used in pediatric and neonatal units.

Surgical Interventions

The most common surgical intervention affecting nutrition is bariatric surgery. It is increasingly being used to control obesity and diabetes. Generally, bariatric surgery has demonstrated good success for weight loss, improved glucose level, and normalized blood pressure. However, complications include macro- and micronutrient deficiencies that are not easily managed, either because of lack of adherence to dietary and supplement guidelines or because of limited knowledge of actual

FIGURE 16-3 Nutrition and Interrelated Concepts

needs.[16] In addition, weight gain can still occur if the patient is noncompliant with calorie control. The most malabsorptive bariatric surgical procedure is the Roux-en-Y gastric bypass. In this procedure, most of the stomach and the proximal small intestine are bypassed, with food entering a Y-shaped reconnection between the upper stomach and the distal portion of the duodenum or jejunum. Lap-band procedures are much less invasive, although nutritional deficits are still possible.

Pharmacologic Agents

A number of supplements are used to enhance the nutritional status of individuals, and most are available over the counter. Supplement examples include vitamin supplements (e.g., multivitamins, niacin, B vitamins, and Vitamin C), mineral supplements (e.g., iron and calcium folic acid), and protein and nutrient supplements (Ensure, nutrition bars, etc.).

In regard to pharmacologic agents for obesity management, research continues. There have been complications with previous forms of weight loss medications, and currently all of these medications have limitations on duration of use. Statins (e.g., atorvastatin, fluvastatin, lovastatin, pravastatin, and rosuvastatin) are the drugs of choice for treatment of lipid and cholesterol reduction because of their ability to inhibit the synthesis of cholesterol, leading to reductions in LDL and HDL. There are a variety of pharmacologic agents that address other nutrient-based problems, including dietary supplements, statins to control lipid levels, and agents to control glucose levels (see Concept 15 Glucose Regulation).

INTERRELATED CONCEPTS

Nutrition is interrelated with nearly all of the health and illness concepts as a preventive or disease management intervention. In addition, nutrition has an interrelated role with many body functions, as presented in Figure 16-3. **Glucose Regulation** (closely linked to **Hormonal Regulation**) is dependent on caloric intake and is critical to adequate metabolism of nutrients; glucose regulation is much like a subconcept of nutrition. Nutrition influences other metabolic processes, such as **Immunity**, **Clotting**, **Tissue Integrity**, and **Thermoregulation**; these all depend on adequate nutrients for optimal functioning. **Development**, **Culture**, and **Spirituality** are also

---

BOX 16-1 EXEMPLARS OF IMPAIRED NUTRITION

Conditions Associated with Insufficient Nutrition
- Anorexia nervosa
- Bulimia
- Fat malabsorption syndrome
- Iron deficiency anemia
- Protein–calorie malnutrition
- Vitamin deficiencies (A, B-complex, C, D, K)
- Zinc deficiency

Conditions Associated with Excessive Nutrition
- Obesity
- Hyperlipidemia
- Obesity-related conditions
  - Metabolic syndrome
  - Type 2 diabetes mellitus
  - Heart diseases
  - Stroke
  - Hypertension
  - Colon and hormonal cancers (prostate, breast)

Conditions Associated with Altered Digestion/Metabolism
- Lactose intolerance
- Celiac disease
- Gastroesophageal reflux
- Phenylketonuria

---

interrelated based on the influence of these concepts on dietary patterns and preferences.

CLINICAL EXEMPLARS

Clinical exemplars of nutrition represent conditions associated with insufficient nutrition and excessive nutrition. Although it is beyond the scope of this concept to list all possible conditions that have a link to nutrition, Box 16-1 presents common exemplars seen in clinical practice. A brief discussion of a few common clinical exemplars follows.

For detailed explanations and the nursing care for exemplars, see nutrition, medical–surgical, pediatric, and gerontology textbooks.

Featured Exemplars
Protein–Calorie Malnutrition

Protein–calorie malnutrition (PCM) refers to an extended state of insufficient protein and calorie intake. PCM is one of the most common nutritional deficiency conditions associated with insufficient intake, wasting disease, or a combination of both, and it has multisystem effects. This can affect individuals of all ages, but it especially affects patients with extended hospitalization with acute illness or injury or the institutionalized elderly. Among children, protein–calorie deficiencies are serious concerns because of the potential for delays in cognitive and physical development. PCM is characterized by muscle wasting, loss of subcutaneous fat, and protein deficiency.

Anorexia Nervosa

Anorexia nervosa is one of a group of psychiatric conditions associated with a fear of weight gain and distortion of body image. It is characterized by an avoidance of food consumption often combined with excessive exercise with the intent to lose weight. Untreated, patients with anorexia nervosa experience extreme weight loss and muscle wasting, representing a condition of insufficient nutrition. This condition is most common among adolescent females, but it is seen in both genders and can occur in childhood and adulthood.

Celiac Disease

Celiac disease is thought to be an autoimmune disorder whereby an inflammatory reaction occurs in the intestine when the mucosa is exposed to gluten, a protein found in wheat. Among the most commonly reported symptoms are abdominal discomfort, bloating, diarrhea, and nausea. The long-term consequence involves dietary deficiencies due to malabsorption of nutrients (as a result of the intestinal inflammation).[17] It is diagnosed based on the presence of flattened villi as well as specific antibodies in the blood. Less severe forms of gluten sensitivity have fewer symptoms, but there is still an autoimmune response to the proteins found in wheat, rye, and barley that requires lifelong use of a strict gluten-free diet.

Obesity

The most common form of excessive nutrition, obesity occurs when there is a greater intake of calories than energy expenditure. Obesity is caused by a number of factors and can include overeating, inactivity, and genetics. Obesity is thought to be associated with systemic, chronic low-grade inflammation and conditions related to the metabolic syndrome.[18] Consequences such as type 2 diabetes, heart disease, and stroke affect individuals of all ages and can lead to medical complications or a shortened lifespan. It is estimated that more than 66% of the U.S. population (including adults and children) is classified as overweight or obese. Overweight is defined as having a BMI greater than 25; obesity is associated with a BMI greater than 30, or being more than 20% over ideal body weight.

Hyperlipidemia

Another example of excess nutrition is hyperlipidemia, characterized by an elevation of serum lipids (cholesterol, triglycerides, and/or phospholipids). Individuals are thought to have a genetic predisposition to hyperlipidemia, but a dietary intake high in dietary fat is another contributing factor. Hyperlipidemia primarily affects adults (an estimated 100 million in the United States) but can occur associated with childhood obesity. Hyperlipidemia places an individual at significant risk for cardiovascular disease, including acute myocardial infarction and stroke.

CASE STUDY

Source: berna namoglu/iStock/Thinkstock

Case Presentation

Mary Williams is a 62-year-old female who has stage 4 CKD, poorly controlled type 2 diabetes, and class II obesity. She was "chunky" as a child and adolescent, with a lifetime habit of having consumed a relatively high-fat, high-calorie diet. As she recalls, her entire family was overweight, and she believed she had little control over the obesity.

After marriage, she gained excess weight with each of her three pregnancies and was never able to lose all the weight. Throughout her career, she worked as a legal assistant. She spent most of her free time watching her children do various activities or watching television, and she freely admits she has not really exercised since high school. Following the recent death of her husband, Mary lives in a one-bedroom apartment within a long-term senior health care center.

Soon after moving to her new residence, she experienced acute heart failure, which was subsequently resolved. She was also told her kidneys were "on the verge of failing." The episode of acute heart failure and the realization that she could have renal failure frightened Mary, so she has become very engaged in her care, making an effort to follow medical recommendations. Since that time, she has been advised to follow a controlled carbohydrate diet with a protein limit of 1 g of protein/kg and moderate intake of sodium, potassium, and phosphorus. She was also switched to a basal/bolus insulin regimen. She takes insulin at mealtimes based on the percentage of meal intake corresponding to the insulin-to-carbohydrate ratio. For 3 months, she has successfully adhered to the treatment strategies, maintaining optimal blood glucose levels, meeting dietary goals, and maintaining a stable weight.

Case Analysis

Mary has come to realize the adverse effects of chronic obesity and uncontrolled diabetes as reflected in heart failure and CKD. Her recent interest in following treatment recommendations is associated with the hope of avoiding further complications. Continuing to follow the treatment plan improves her overall health outlook. This case illustrates the complexity of this concept from the standpoint of the long-standing effects of overweight and obesity starting in childhood. Her family history, sedentary lifestyle, lifelong eating habits, and the subsequent complications are very typical for an individual with long-standing obesity.

ACCESS EXEMPLAR LINKS IN YOUR GIDDENS EBOOK

REFERENCES

1. Herrman K, Carroll K: An exclusively human milk diet reduces necrotizing enterocolitis. *Breastfeed Med* 9(4):184–190, 2014.
2. Su BH: Optimizing nutrition in preterm infants. *Pediatr Neonatol* 55(1):5–13, 2014.
3. Martone AM, Onder G, Vetrano GL, et al: Anorexia of aging: A modifiable risk factor for frailty. *Nutrients* 5(10):4126–4133, 2013.
4. Cereda E, Pedrolli C, Zagami A, et al: Body mass index and mortality in institutionalized elderly. *J Am Med Dir Assoc* 12(3):174–178, 2011.
5. Wirth R, Smoliner C, Jager M: Guideline clinical nutrition in patients with stroke. *Exp Transl Stroke Med* 5(1):14, 2013.
6. Collins J, Bertrand B, Hayes V, et al: The application of genetics and nutritional genomics in practice: An international survey of knowledge, involvement and confidence among dietitians in the US, Australia, and the UK. *Genes Nutr* 8(6):523–533, 2013.
7. Batai K, Murphy AB, Shah E, et al: Common vitamin D pathway gene variants reveal contrasting effects on serum vitamin D levels in African Americans and European Americans. *Hum Genet* 133(11):1395–1405, 2014.
8. Taksler GB, Cutler DM, Giovanucci EL, et al: Vitamin D deficiency in minority populations. *Public Health Nutr* 15:1–13, 2014.
9. Hollingworth S, Walker K, Page A, et al: Pharmacoepidemiology and the Australian regional prevalence of multiple sclerosis. *Mult Scler* 19:1712–1716, 2013.
10. Ghosh-Dastidar B, Cohen D, Hunter G, et al: Distance to store, food prices, and obesity in urban food deserts. *Am J Prev Med* 47(5):587–595, 2014.
11. Bevelander KE, Anshutz DJ, Creemers DH, et al: The role of explicit and implicit self-esteem in peer modeling of palatable food intake: A study on social media interaction among youngsters. *PLoS ONE* 8(8):72481, 2013.
12. Orloff NC, Hormes JM: Pickles and ice cream! Food cravings in pregnancy: Hypotheses, preliminary evidence, and directions for future research. *Front Psychol* 23(5):1076, 2014.
13. Demir N, Koc A, Ustoyl L, et al: Clinical and neurological findings of severe vitamin B_{12} deficiency in infancy and importance of early diagnosis and treatment. *J Paediatr Child Health* 49(10):820–824, 2013.
14. Le LT, Sabate J: Beyond meatless, the health effects of vegan diets: Findings from the Adventist cohorts. *Nutrients* 6(6):2131–2147, 2014.
15. Hannan JL, Radwany SM, Albanese T: In-hospital mortality in patients older than 60 years with very low albumin levels. *J Pain Symptom Manage* 43(3):631–637, 2012.
16. Freeland-Graves JH, Lee JJ, Mousa TY, et al: Patients at risk for trace element deficiencies: Bariatric surgery. *J Trace Elem Med Biol* 28(4):495–503, 2014.
17. Volta U, Villanacci V: Celiac disease: Diagnostic criteria in progress. *Cell Mol Immunol* 8(2):96–102, 2011.
18. Everard A, Cani PD: Diabetes, obesity and gut microbiota. *Best Pract Res Clin Gastroenterol* 27(1):73–83, 2013.
19. Rejeski WJ, Marsh AP, Chmelo E, et al: Obesity, intentional weight loss and physical disability in older adults. *Obes Rev* 11(9):671–685, 2010.
20. Zanni GR, Wick JY: Treating obesity in older adults: Different risks, different goals, different strategies. *Consult Pharm* 26(3):142–148, 153–154, 2011.
21. Chapman IM: Weight loss in older persons. *Med Clin North Am* 95(3):579–593, 2011.

Elimination

Carolyn McKenzie

limination is a concept that has various applications across multiple disciplines, including mathematics, economics, chemistry, and biology. From a biological perspective, elimination is a concept applicable to all living organisms—from the smallest of microbes to plants, animals, and humans. This concept presentation focuses on elimination as a physiological concept as it applies to humans and includes normal or expected elimination patterns and problems associated with elimination.

DEFINITION

Broadly speaking, the term *elimination* refers to the removal, clearance, or separation of matter. From a human physiological perspective, the term elimination is defined as *the excretion of waste products.*[1] The human body eliminates various forms of waste through the skin, kidneys, lungs, and intestines. This concept presentation focuses on elimination of waste from the urinary system and the gastrointestinal system. Specific definitions for each follow. Bowel elimination is defined as *the passage of stool through the intestinal tract and dispelling the stool by means of intestinal smooth muscle contraction.*[1] Urinary elimination is defined as *the passage of urine through the urinary tract by means of the urinary sphincter and urethra.*[2,3] Other terms related to elimination include *defecation* (bowel) and *micturition* or *urination* (urine). The term *continence* refers to the purposeful control of urinary or fecal elimination. Bowel movements may be referred to as *stool* or *feces*. Other terms related to urination include *anuria* (absence of urine), *dysuria* (painful urination), *polyuria* (multiple episodes of urination, as with diabetes), urinary *frequency* (multiple episodes of urination with little urine produced in a short period of time), and urinary *hesitancy* (the urge to urinate exists, but the person has difficulty starting the urine stream).

SCOPE

The scope of this concept includes the normal or expected physiological process of waste formation and excretion by the gastrointestinal and renal systems as well as problems associated with this process (Figure 17-1). The process of waste formation in the renal and gastrointestinal systems is very different. The kidneys are responsible for the removal of metabolic waste and other elements from the blood in the form of urine, and the gastrointestinal tract is responsible for the removal of digestive waste in the form of stool. The excretion of urine

and stool normally occurs under voluntary control. The scope of this concept also includes an impairment of elimination. A wide range of problems and conditions contribute to impaired elimination. These are explored in greater detail in the sections that follow.

NORMAL PHYSIOLOGICAL PROCESS

An overview of the normal physiological process of elimination is presented, followed by the problems and consequences of abnormal elimination patterns. Critical attributes and antecedents to bowel and bladder elimination are presented in Table 17-1.

Normal Urinary Elimination

Urinary elimination involves the process of waste formation (production of urine) and the excretion of urine involving several specific structures. The kidneys, ureters, bladder, and urethra must all function adequately for normal urination to occur.

Formation of Urine

The formation of urine is complex and involves three main processes: glomerular filtration, tubular reabsorption, and tubular secretion. The main functional unit of the kidneys is the nephron; each kidney has more than 1 million nephrons. Each nephron is composed of two parts—blood vessels and renal tubules (Figure 17-2). Optimal physiological effect of the kidneys depends on continuous perfusion of a large volume of blood (an average of 1 L per minute) to the kidneys and functioning nephrons.

Blood enters the kidney through the renal artery. Upon entering the kidney, the renal artery branches into progressively smaller arteries, arterioles, and finally to a cluster of capillaries known as the glomerulus. The glomerulus is a semipermeable membrane that serves to filter blood into a C-shaped structure of the renal tubule known as the Bowman's capsule. This process (*glomerular filtration*) represents the beginning of urine formation.

The filtrate contains water, electrolytes, and waste that have been removed from the blood. As the filtrate passes through a sequence of renal tubules (from the Bowman's capsule to the proximal convoluted tubule, the Loop of Henle, and the distal convoluted tubule), a network of capillaries surrounding the renal tubules reabsorb most of the water, electrolytes, and other necessary elements back into the blood. This process is referred to as *tubular reabsorption*. The third process, *tubular secretion*, involves a secondary process for small amounts of select

Waste Formation

Waste Excretion

FIGURE 17-1 Scope of Elimination

TABLE 17-1   Critical Attributes and Antecedents Associated with Concept of Elimination

Category	Critical Attributes	Antecedents
Bowel elimination (normal)	Presence of stool/feces Passage of stool Form of stool Color of stool Frequency of stool passage Retention of stool	Urge to defecate Possible intestinal cramping or feeling of fullness in rectum
Bladder elimination (normal)	Presence of urine Passage of urine Retention of urine Color of urine Frequency of urination Amount of urine	Urge to urinate Feeling of fullness or possible contraction of bladder

substances (e.g., potassium, hydrogen, ammonia, and drugs) to be moved from the blood in the capillaries surrounding the tubules into the tubules. The amount of water and electrolytes reabsorbed into the blood or excreted in the renal tubules is controlled by several hormones, particularly aldosterone, antidiuretic hormone, parathyroid hormone, renin, and atrial natriuretic factor.

Excretion of Urine

Urine formed in the renal tubules moves into the collecting duct and then into the renal pelvis, the ureter, and the bladder, where it is stored until urination occurs. The bladder holds approximately 300–500 mL before the pressure increases enough for stretch receptors in the bladder to signal the need for urination. An internal sphincter, composed of smooth muscle, contracts involuntarily to prevent urine from leaking out of the bladder. The external sphincter, located just below the internal sphincter and surrounding the upper part of the urethra, is composed of skeletal muscle and is voluntarily controlled. Thus, the process of urination involves a series of nerve signals between the bladder and spinal cord to trigger the micturition reflex; this causes the internal sphincter muscles to relax and bladder wall contraction. With the voluntary relaxation of the external urinary sphincter, urine passes out of the body through the urethra. The external urinary sphincter must be under the individual's control in order for urinary control (continence) to be successful.

Normal Bowel Elimination
Digestion and the Formation of Stool
The gastrointestinal system has two overarching functions: the breakdown and absorption of nutrients from foods ingested and the elimination of waste from this process. The gastrointestinal system extends

from the esophagus to the anus. The first part of the gastrointestinal tract (esophagus, stomach, and small intestines) is involved in the digestion and absorption of nutrients, a process that also involves other digestive organs, including the liver, gallbladder, and pancreas. The digestive process is described further in Concept 16 Nutrition.

The process of waste formation occurs in the colon. Smooth muscles within the intestinal tract stimulate peristalsis, which helps to move the waste product known as stool or fecal matter. The large intestine, which is 5 or 6 feet long and approximately 2 inches in diameter, has four parts: the cecum (and appendix), the colon, the rectum, and the anus. The function of the large intestine is to absorb water and electrolytes as fecal matter moves through its walls. Mucus in the intestine helps lubricate the walls and aids in the expulsion of the stool. If there is excessive peristalsis and the stool moves through the large intestine quickly, less water is absorbed, resulting in a loose stool. If the peristalsis is reduced, feces pass through the large intestine slowly, resulting in greater absorption of water and a harder stool.[3]

Elimination of Stool
When the stool reaches the rectum, pressure stimulates the urge to defecate through stimulation of the intestinal smooth muscle and its stretch response. The urge to defecate can be suppressed until an appropriate environment is obtained.

Age-Related Differences
Infants, Toddlers, and Children
Patterns of elimination change in the first few years of life. Infants and toddlers initially lack control over the sphincters and muscles that control urination and bowel elimination, but control is attained during early childhood as a normal developmental milestone. Children are typically 18–24 months of age before they are able to identify the urge to urinate and defecate.[4] Toilet training by the parent or caregiver helps the child obtain conscious control of his or her bowel and bladder functions.

Pregnant Women
Pregnancy can affect elimination patterns because the presence of the fetus in the abdominal cavity affects both bowel and bladder function. As the fetus grows, increased pressure is placed on the bladder, and frequent urination is required. The woman will have larger volumes of urine because she has a larger blood volume during the gestation. The growing fetus can also interfere with intestinal peristalsis and can cause constipation. The use of prenatal vitamins with iron can also contribute to constipation in the pregnant female.[5]

Older Adults
A number of physiological changes associated with aging affect elimination. By age 80 years, renal blood flow reduces to an estimated 600 mL/minute, and the kidneys lose up to 50% of functioning nephrons for a variety of reasons, including changes in size of the kidney and sclerosis. In the absence of disease, this does not change the older adult's ability to produce urine sufficiently to maintain normal

Renal corpuscle ⎱ Bowman's capsule
⎰ Glomerulus

Efferent arteriole

Juxtaglomerular (JG) apparatus

Afferent arteriole

Distal convoluted tubule (DCT)

Artery and vein

Peritubular capillaries

Ascending limb of loop of Henle

Descending limb of loop of Henle

Proximal convoluted tubule (PCT)

Peritubular capillaries

Collecting duct (CD)

FIGURE 17-2 The Nephron Modified from Patton KT, Thibodeau GA: The human body in health and disease, ed 6, St Louis, 2014, Mosby.

composition of body fluids, although it represents reduced renal reserve, making the older adult more susceptible to fluid and electrolyte imbalances and kidney damage due to medications. Although the bladder retains tone with age, the volume of urine that can be held reduces, leading to urinary frequency. In many older adults, muscles around the urethra become weak, thus increasing the risk of incontinence.

Age-related changes affecting bowel elimination include atrophy of smooth muscle layers in the colon and reduced mucous secretions. Reduced tone of the internal and external sphincter as well as reduced neural impulses (reducing the sensation of bowel evacuation) can make the older adult more susceptible to constipation or incontinence.

VARIATIONS AND CONTEXT

Alterations in elimination can occur with urinary or gastrointestinal function and represent a wide spectrum of problems. Most problems and conditions can be grouped by common themes and include incontinence, retention, discomfort, infections and inflammation, neoplasms, and organ failure. The interrelationships of some of these categories are shown in Figure 17-3.

Incontinence

Incontinence refers to the loss of control of either urine or bowel elimination. With "control issues," both urinary and bowel incontinence may be exhibited by involuntary loss of stool or urine through normal routes. Control issues arise as a result of undeveloped elimination mechanisms, malfunctions in the mechanism of elimination, or alterations in cognition. Almost 25% of Americans may experience either fecal or urinary incontinence during their lifetime.[2] Individuals who are incontinent are at risk for skin breakdown (particularly if bedridden) and can potentially experience changes in daily activities, functional activities, and social relationships.

Urinary Incontinence

Urinary incontinence is a disruption in the storage or emptying of the bladder with involuntary release of urine usually associated with

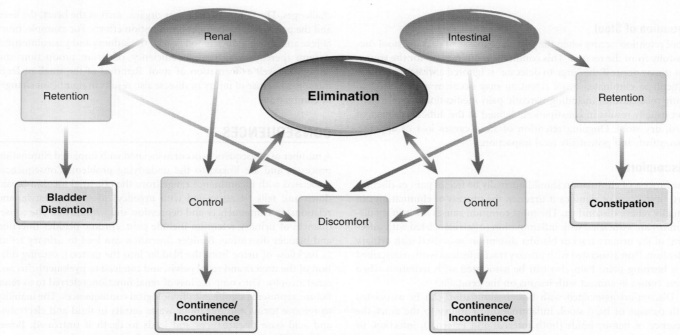

FIGURE 17-3 Problems Associated with Elimination: Control, Retention, and Discomfort

dysfunction of the external and/or internal urinary sphincters. It can range from light urine leakage when coughing or laughing (stress incontinence) to full loss of continence. Factors affecting urinary incontinence may be psychological or physical, such as depression, anxiety, cognitive impairments, or acute injury or surgical procedures. Types of urinary incontinence are listed in Table 17-2.

Bowel Incontinence

Bowel incontinence is the involuntary passage of stool and ranges from an occasional leakage of stool while passing gas (flatus) to a complete loss of bowel control. Bowel incontinence can occur with diarrhea, particularly when it is associated with forceful intestinal peristalsis (cramping). Complete incontinence usually occurs from a loss of sphincter control—usually as a result of traumatic injury, pathologic changes to the rectum, or from neurologic injury. Changes and/or loss of cognition can also result in bowel incontinence.

Retention

Retention refers to the unintentional retention of urine or stool and can occur at any age. The primary mechanisms causing retention are usually associated with obstructions, inflammation, or ineffective neuromuscular activation within the bladder or the gastrointestinal tract.

Urinary Retention

Urinary retention occurs as either incomplete emptying of the bladder after urination or a complete inability to urinate and is caused by a number of factors. Incomplete emptying can occur due to malfunction in nervous system innervation to the bladder or mechanical change in the shape of the bladder that causes retention.[6] For example, women may experience urinary retention if there is hard stool that presses against the bladder or rectoceles or cystoceles that cause prolapse of the bladder and trapping of urine. Retention can also occur when an obstruction blocks the passage of urine (e.g., an enlarged prostate) or when the external sphincter of the bladder does

TABLE 17-2	Types of Urinary Incontinence
Type of Incontinence	**Description**
Stress	Leakage of small amounts of urine during physical movement (coughing, sneezing, exercising)
Urge	Leakage of large amounts of urine at unexpected times, including during sleep
Overactive bladder	Urinary frequency and urgency, with or without urge incontinence
Functional	Untimely urination because of physical disability, external obstacles, or cognitive problems that prevent person from reaching toilet
Overflow	Unexpected leakage of small amounts of urine because of full bladder
Mixed	Usually occurrence of stress and urge incontinence together
Transient	Leakage that occurs temporarily because of a situation that will pass (infection, taking a new medication, colds with coughing)

not relax, allowing the urine to be expelled from the bladder. Medications that may cause urinary retention include antidepressants, anticholinergics, and antihistamines.[6] Postoperative patients may have problems with urinary elimination as a result of the effects of anesthetics or the use of catheters during the surgical procedure. Psychosocial factors (e.g., fear or anxiety) may also affect the ability to successfully void.

Retention of Stool

Stool retention occurs when the person is unable to pass the stool successfully from the rectum. This condition is not normal for the young, but it may occur if the "urge to defecate" is ignored and stool becomes difficult to eliminate.[7] Stool retention may occur as a side effect to many medications, including narcotic pain medications. Stool retention usually results in constipation, defined as the difficult passage of hard, dry stool. Ongoing retention of stool causes loss of appetite, discomfort, and potentially fecal impaction.[7]

Discomfort

The process of elimination should normally be free of pain or discomfort; in the case of significant urgency, the process of elimination can actually relieve discomfort. The most common causes for urinary discomfort are associated with inflammation (often associated with infection) of the urinary tract or bladder distention associated with urinary retention. Pain associated with urinary tract infection is often described as a burning pain. Pain also can be associated with irritation when urine comes in contact with lesions on the genitalia.

Discomfort associated with bowel elimination can be associated with passage of hard stool, inflammation or injury to the anus, the presence of hemorrhoids (both internal and external), infection, or irritation of the intestinal lining attributable to frequent passage of stool. In children, there can be telescoping of the bowel back into itself (intussusception) that can result in abdominal pain from obstruction and retention of stool.[4] Chronic conditions such as colitis or irritable bowel syndrome and excessive flatus can also be painful. Bowel irritability that is characterized especially by constipation or diarrhea, cramping abdominal pain, and the passage of mucus in the stool can cause discomfort. Pain also can be associated with lesions such as an anal fissure or hemorrhoids.

Infections and Inflammation

Elimination problems also can be caused by inflammatory or infectious conditions. Infection in the urinary system is often referred to as urinary tract infection, but specific structures in the urinary system can become inflamed or infected, including the kidney (nephritis), the renal pelvis (pyelonephritis), and the bladder (cystitis). Acute intestinal inflammation and infection are most commonly associated with viral infections or food poisoning. Chronic inflammatory conditions of the intestinal tract include colitis and diverticulitis, and these are associated with severe abdominal pain, discomfort, and nutritional deficits.

Neoplasms

Neoplasms are tumors and can have an effect on urinary and bowel elimination. Benign and malignant neoplasms of the prostate often lead to blockage of urinary flow in men. Tumors can also occur in the kidney or bladder, but these are less common. Neoplasms in the intestinal tract are also common and include benign growths (e.g., polyps) and cancerous lesions in the intestine, colon, or rectum.[8]

Organ Failure

One additional category of problems related to elimination is organ failure. The most obvious organ that comes to mind is the kidney. Renal failure can occur suddenly, usually associated with an injury to the kidney (referred to as acute kidney injury), or it can occur as a slow, chronic process (referred to as chronic kidney disease) whereby the kidneys lose functional capacity over months to years. The inability to remove metabolic waste and fluid creates significant physiological

challenges. The failure of other key organs, such as the heart, the liver, and the pancreas, also hampers elimination efforts. For example, heart failure and shock reduce blood flow to the kidneys and gastrointestinal system, thereby reducing the efficiency of urine production and removal as well as formation of stool. Removal of the small or large intestines because of injury or disease also results in significant changes in elimination.

CONSEQUENCES

A number of consequences occur associated with impaired elimination processes and are linked to the underlying problem. Consequences associated with incontinence range from the potential for skin breakdown and falls (if associated with urgency) to social, lifestyle, and relationship consequences and depression and withdrawal. The consequences of urinary retention include pain, chronic bladder infection and bladder distention. Bladder distention can lead to urinary reflux (a backflow of urine from the bladder into the ureters), causing dilation of the ureters and renal pelvis, and can lead to pyelonephritis and renal atrophy. The complete loss of renal function, referred to as renal failure, represents significant physiological consequences. The inability to remove toxins and metabolic waste results in fluid and electrolyte and acid–base disturbances and leads to death if untreated. Bowel retention leads to constipation, pain, loss of appetite, nausea, and vomiting. An ileus refers to a loss of peristaltic activity in the gastrointestinal tract. This can occur subsequent to abdominal trauma or surgery and is associated with nausea, vomiting, and distention. Although rare, rupture of the colon can occur, representing a life-threatening situation.

RISK FACTORS

Because elimination represents normal physiological function, this concept applies to all individuals and problems with the elimination of urine and stool and can affect any person regardless of age, gender, or race.

Risk Factors for Altered Urinary Elimination

Populations at risk for urinary incontinence include children younger than age 3 years , the elderly, pregnant women, and women who are menopausal.[9] The prevalence of urinary incontinence ranges from 19% in women age 45 years or younger to 49% in women age 80 years or older.[2] Men are more likely to experience urination difficulties as they age because of changes (hyperplasia) in the prostate gland that may cause either urinary retention or increased urinary frequency due to incomplete emptying of the bladder. There are many reasons why incontinence increases with age in both genders, including pelvic floor muscle weakness in women and neurologic problems in men. Medications such as diuretics can also contribute to the involuntary loss of urine in both men and women.

Individual risk factors include conditions that result in neurologic impairment, altered mobility, cognitive impairment, and immunologic impairment or infection. Persons with trauma to the brain or spinal cord may experience bladder and bowel impairment attributable to interruption of bowel and bladder innervation by the spinal cord. If messages cannot be sent along the nervous system pathways, the anus and bladder are unable to function normally.

Several medical conditions can place an individual at risk for alterations in urinary elimination, including cerebrovascular accidents (CVAs), spinal cord injury, diabetic neuropathy, dementia (including Alzheimer's disease), and AIDS or other autoimmune diseases.

Conditions that are specific to the urinary system are urinary calculi, enlarged prostate (benign prostatic hypertrophy), acute infection,[3] and chronic infections; some congenital defects can impair urinary elimination function, such as defects of the spinal cord or brain and bladder defects.

Risk Factors for Altered Bowel Elimination

Bowel or fecal incontinence occurs in approximately 8% or 18 million Americans.[2] Bowel problems occur in men and women from both acute neurologic injury and progressive neurologic changes with advanced age. Excessive use of medications such as laxatives can contribute to incontinence issues in both genders. Persons at highest risk for incontinence are those with cognitive impairment; those who are exposed to radiation for treatment purposes; and those who take multiple medications, consume excessive amounts of caffeine, or have limited access to toilet facilities because of immobility or environmental or sociocultural factors.[10,11] Risk factors that place individuals at risk for stool retention include lack of adequate fluids, fiber, or exercise, as well as use of medications that dry the system, such as diuretics, narcotics, antidepressants, or anxiolytics. Pregnancy increases risk for stool retention because of the pressure of the fetus on the bowel.

Many medical conditions can place an individual at risk for alterations in bowel elimination, including CVAs, spinal cord injury, diabetic neuropathy, dementia (including Alzheimer's disease),[12] and AIDS or other autoimmune diseases. Some conditions specific to the gastrointestinal system associated with risk include irritable bowel syndrome, Crohn's disease, and food allergies or intolerance, such as celiac disease.[13] Several congenital defects impair bowel elimination function, such as defects of the spinal cord or brain, colon, and rectal defects.

ASSESSMENT

Assessment of elimination includes taking a history, conducting a physical examination, and performing diagnostic testing when problems are identified.

History

Conducting a history is the first step to understanding problems associated with elimination. Ask about patterns of urinary and bowel elimination, including frequency, appearance of stool and urine, and associated symptoms. Common symptoms directly related to elimination include alterations in elimination patterns; changes in the appearance, frequency, or quality of stool or urine; or discomfort and difficulty associated with elimination. A symptom analysis approach is helpful to fully understand the symptom. Determine if there have been changes in diet, recent changes in health status (e.g., cognition, mobility, functional ability, or other medical conditions), and if there are new medications or changes in medications. Voluntary or involuntary (incontinence) emptying of the bowel or bladder also must be assessed to determine the impact of the condition on the individual.[14] Adults of all ages should be asked about urinary continence because it is an underreported phenomenon.[11]

Examination Findings

Physical assessment incorporates four examination techniques: inspection, auscultation, palpation, and percussion.

Inspection

The abdomen is inspected for contour; abdominal or bladder distention is an abnormal finding. The genitalia are also inspected to examine the urinary meatus for evidence of redness, lesions, or discharge.

Discharge from the urinary meatus is an abnormal finding and may suggest infection, especially if the patient reports pain with voiding. Observe the perianal area. The area should be free from redness or lesions; the presence of hemorrhoids or an anal fistula may be observed if the patient complains of pain with defecation.

Inspection also includes looking at a stool or urine sample if available. Urine should be clear and yellow with mild odor. Very dark urine may be indicative of dehydration, may be a side effect of medication, or may indicate the presence of blood. Stool should be brown and formed. Stools that are black and tarry in appearance often signal gastrointestinal bleeding. Loose stools or diarrhea may be associated with diet, inflammation, or infection.

Auscultation

Auscultation is limited to the abdomen to listen to bowel sounds. Bowel sounds should be heard in all four quadrants. An absence of bowel sounds may be associated with paralytic ileus; hyperactive bowel sounds may be noted with gastrointestinal inflammation or with an intestinal obstruction.[15] Auscultation is not indicated in urinary assessment.

Palpation

Abdominal palpation is a physical examination technique for both urinary and bowel elimination. The abdomen should be soft and nontender with palpation over the entire abdomen and over the urinary bladder. Abdominal or urinary distention is considered an abnormal finding and may be associated with reduced peristalsis or retention of stool or urine.

Rectal palpation is done to assess the rectal sphincter and to examine for the presence of masses, lesions, or impacted stool. Digital palpation is also part of the prostate examination.[15] Although this is not directly an examination associated with elimination, prostate enlargement can result from a tumor (benign or malignant) or inflammation; both can contribute to urinary retention.

Percussion

Abdominal percussion may be performed to help identify masses or excessive intestinal gas. Direct fist percussion over the costovertebral angle (over the kidney) should be painless; if sharp pain is produced, it could signal the presence of a kidney infection.[15]

Diagnostic Tests

There are a number of diagnostic tests associated with elimination. In general, the diagnostic tests are classified into one of three categories: laboratory, radiographic, and direct observation.

Laboratory Tests

Urinalysis. A urinalysis is one of the most common of all laboratory tests. It is useful for screening a number of conditions not associated with a problem in elimination and is obtained with either a sterile urine specimen or a clean-catch specimen. Bacteria indicate infection, whereas blood may indicate damage from infection or trauma to the urinary system. Urinary analysis that indicates the presence of bacteria or blood components in the urine may require further assessment of the urinary tract by a physician specialist in the field of urology.

Renal function tests. Laboratory tests assessing renal function include blood urea nitrogen, blood creatinine, and creatinine clearance tests. Creatinine and blood urea nitrogen are excreted entirely by the kidneys and therefore provide a measure of renal function.

Culture. Urine and stool cultures are relatively common laboratory tests. When a urinary tract infection is suspected, a urine culture determines the presence and type of organism causing the urinary infection. Stool cultures are indicated when a parasitic infection is suspected.

Occult blood. When blood is suspected in stool, an occult blood test is indicated. It also represents a basic screening that should be performed as part of a rectal examination. The presence of blood in the stool could be related to a gastrointestinal bleed (inflammation and infection), hemorrhoids, or tumors.

Pathology

A biopsy is a sample of tissue or cells that undergoes pathologic evaluation. A biopsy can be taken from the rectum, colon, bladder, or kidney. Biopsies provide information associated with tumors or with general organ function.

Radiographic Tests and Scans

Numerous radiographic tests are used to assess elimination. Common radiographic tests include x-rays, computerized tomography, magnetic resonance imaging, and ultrasound. These are used to detect a variety of problems, including the presence of an intestinal tumor, a congenital renal abnormality, or kidney stones. Angiography is used to assess renal blood flow and can detect renal artery stenosis.

Direct Observation Tests

The ability to directly observe internal organs can be accomplished with scopes. With regard to the concept of elimination, scopes can be used to visualize the colon (*colonoscopy*), the sigmoid colon (*sigmoidoscopy*), the bladder (*cystoscopy*), or the urethra or ureters (*uroscopy*).

Direct visualization of the colon is done for screening or diagnostic purposes for polyps, cancer, and inflammatory conditions such as Crohn's disease. Direct visualization of the bladder or ureters is done with a special scope as part of diagnostic or surgical procedures.

Other Diagnostic Tests

Several special tests are available to evaluate urinary elimination, including bladder stress testing, uroflowmetry and other urine flow studies, and postvoid residual measurement through use of bladder scans or postvoid catheterization.

CLINICAL MANAGEMENT

Primary Prevention

The prevention of problems with elimination occurs with individual application of prevention measures based on the person's normal bowel and bladder habits. By maintaining healthy bowel and bladder function with the intake of a healthy diet and adequate fluids, each person can promote the elimination of stool and produce the quality and quantity of urine that supports a healthy urinary system. Primary prevention through public education should occur regarding activities to promote bladder health, such as the following: encouraging adequate hydration, emptying the bladder with the first urge, maintaining normal body mass index, refraining from smoking, limiting intake of caffeinated beverages, and adhering to regular elimination habits and a consistent exercise program.

Environmental Factors

Avoidance of contaminated water and foods can assist in maintaining consistent bowel habits. Bacteria in water or food can cause diarrhea and colitis. Parasites can be present in water or food that is not properly prepared. Parasites not only can cause elimination problems but also can affect overall health. Laboratory testing can determine if parasites

are present in the gastrointestinal system that may be causing problems with bowel elimination.

Maintaining Hydration

Water is a key element for prevention of bowel and urinary elimination problems. Water is absorbed by the stool to soften it and promote intestinal motility, which assists in the elimination of stool. Water serves the urinary system in that it increases volume, reduces bladder irritation, and helps eliminate toxins from the body. Fluids that may create difficulty in both bowel and bladder elimination include those with caffeine, which may cause an increase in frequency of elimination. Any substances that irritate the bowel or bladder will cause alterations in normal elimination patterns.

Dietary Fiber

Fiber intake has been shown to assist in the prevention of stool retention, especially when implemented with adequate water intake and exercise.[16] Fiber creates enough friction along the bowel surface that it can assist in the production of a bowel movement. Adequate fluid intake with the fiber is imperative. Fiber should be slowly added to the diet to prevent abdominal discomfort and excessive gas formation in the intestine. The American Dietetic Association[16] recommends 14 g of fiber per 1000 kcal intake.

Maintenance of Regular Toileting Practices

Maintaining a consistent time of defecation is important in the regulation of bowel movements.[3] The use of familiar toileting facilities may also encourage defecation. Avoidance of foods that cause discomfort during digestion and absorption or are known to cause constipation can also help maintain regular patterns of bowel elimination. To prevent urinary incontinence or retention, there should be timely and complete emptying of the bladder. Holding urine should be discouraged because this encourages bacterial growth in the bladder and consequent urinary tract infection.

Secondary Prevention (Screening)

Two common screening tests associated with elimination are screening for occult blood and colonoscopy—both are considered effective for the detection of colon cancer. The U.S. Preventive Services Task Force (USPSTF) recommends occult blood testing, sigmoidoscopy, or colonoscopy for adults beginning at age 50 years until 75 years of age.[17] These tests allow visualization of the colon and removal of precancerous lesions, averting the development of colon cancer. Screening for occult blood is performed annually or as a component of all digital rectal examinations. Screening associated with urinary elimination includes prostate cancer screening. The USPSTF does not recommend routine screening for bladder cancer.[18]

Collaborative Interventions

Problems with elimination represent a wide range of conditions involving two major body systems—the gastrointestinal system and the urinary system. For the purposes of this concept, common interventions are only briefly described; detailed information is available in various nursing textbooks.

Pharmacologic Agents

Antibiotics. Infections of the kidney and urinary tract are treated with antibiotics. Antibiotics are usually selected based on the provider's best judgment and based on the results of culture and sensitivity testing. Although a variety of agents are used, trimethoprim, trimethoprim with sulfamethoxazole, or nitrofurantoin are commonly prescribed for urinary tract infections; parenteral antibiotics are indicated

CLINICAL NURSING SKILLS FOR ELIMINATION

- Assessment
- Urinary catheterization
- Suprapubic catheter care
- Catheter irrigation
- Enema
- Nasogastric tube for gastric decompression
- Ostomy care
- Medication administration

for more severe infections such as pyelonephritis. Antibiotics may also be used prophylactically with urinary retention or recurrent urinary tract infection.

Diuretics. Diuretics increase the volume of urine produced along with excreting sodium and potassium from the body by affecting the water resorption in the renal tubules. Loop diuretics prevent reabsorption of sodium in the Loop of Henle. Thiazide diuretics prevent sodium from being reabsorbed at the beginning of the distal convoluted tubules. Potassium-sparing diuretics stop the extensive loss of potassium at the distal convoluted tubules. Excessive use to treat certain conditions requires careful monitoring and frequent lab testing of the electrolytes.

Antispasmodics. Anticholinergics are often used to relieve smooth muscle spasms in the bowel or bladder. Bladder spasms can occur as a consequence of neurologic injury. Anticholinergics can reduce bladder spasms and can provide relief from urinary incontinence. Bowel spasms commonly occur with irritable bowel syndrome. Some antispasmodic medications, such as Imodium (loperamide), are effective for the treatment of diarrhea because they cause a reduction in peristalsis and slow the passage of stool.

Agents to manage constipation. Pharmacologic management to treat stool retention includes both prescribed and over-the-counter versions of laxatives, bulk-forming agents, bowel stimulants, lubricants, stool softeners, saline laxatives, and enemas. The drawback in using these medications is that the bowel can become dependent on laxatives and stimulants for the impulse to defecate. Medications for stool retention should be a last resort and discontinued as soon as the bowel elimination is achieved.

Analgesics. Analgesics are indicated for relief of mild discomfort to severe pain for select urinary or bowel elimination conditions. Examples of conditions causing pain with elimination include kidney stones, cystitis, urinary tract infections, bladder spams, hemorrhoids, and rectal fissures.

Incontinence Management

Multidisciplinary management of the person with alterations in elimination must occur in order to successfully control the condition. The need for retraining the bowel and bladder is of paramount importance. Providing a regular toileting schedule, managing fluid intake, modifying the environment, avoiding indwelling catheters, providing high-quality skin care and assessment, and avoiding medications that contribute to incontinence are nursing actions that will promote urinary continence. Personal absorbent pads or bed-protecting pads may be used to catch episodes of incontinence in both mobile and immobile individuals. Biofeedback may be used to assist the person in gaining improved control over the muscles of elimination. Biofeedback involves placement of sensors onto the affected area of bowel so that the person can receive feedback regarding which muscles are being used to control bowel function.[19] Among those with dementia, toilet assistance (including timed voiding and prompted voiding) along with protective pads and skin care are standard interventions.[12]

Invasive Procedures and Surgical Interventions Involving Urinary Elimination

A variety of procedures are performed as treatment for urinary elimination problems. The benefits must outweigh the risks for utilization of these interventions because they can be invasive and sometimes lifestyle-altering procedures.

Dialysis. Dialysis is indicated for acute or chronic renal failure. It involves filtration of the blood to remove toxins through an external process. Two types of dialysis are hemodialysis and peritoneal dialysis. A dialysis machine is used in hemodialysis to filter a patient's blood to remove excess toxins and water. The blood is circulated from the patient to the dialysis machine and then back to the patient over several hours. In peritoneal dialysis, a dialysate solution is introduced into the peritoneal cavity that absorbs the toxins over several hours; the solution and waste are then removed.

Procedures relieving urinary retention. The most common procedure to relieve urinary retention is urinary catheterization.[20] This can be intermittently performed with a straight catheter, or an indwelling catheter can be inserted. Measures must be taken to prevent complications (e.g., infection) when urinary drainage systems are used for long periods of time.[21]

Surgical intervention may be needed to treat other forms of obstructions, including surgery on the bladder, prostate, or ureters. Many procedures are conducted through a cystoscope. Stents, which are rigid tubes that provide an opening that is not normally present, may be used internally in the urethra and externally as part of anastomosis procedures performed for bladder cancer. Stents maintain the patency of pathways for urinary elimination.

Renal calculi. Renal calculi (also known as kidney stones) often require surgical intervention if the stones are unable to pass through the urinary tract. A variety of surgical procedures are available to treat renal calculi, including *lithotripsy* (fragmentation of the stones through sound wave technology); *endourologic procedures* (insertion of a ureteroscope and crushing the stones with a surgical instrument called a lithotrite); or open procedures (*nephrolithotomy, pyelolithotomy, ureterolithotomy*, or *cystotomy*), in which an incision is made and the stone is surgically removed.

Nephrectomy. Occasionally, surgical removal of the kidney is required, as with renal cancer. Other conditions, such as polycystic kidney disease, may also require surgical intervention.

Prostate surgery. An enlarged prostate can cause significant urinary obstruction. A transurethral resection of the prostate is a surgical procedure done for benign prostate hypertrophy when other noninvasive treatment measures have failed. Prostatectomy refers to the removal of the prostate and is usually performed among younger men diagnosed with prostate cancer, particularly if diagnosed in early disease stage.

Bladder surgeries. Surgical interventions of the bladder include a wide variety of procedures to treat many types of conditions, such as prolapsed bladder or bladder cancer. Surgical treatment options include laser surgery, transurethral resection, and partial or total cystectomy. If the bladder is removed, urinary diversion is required.

Urinary diversion. Urinary diversion procedures involve diverting the ureters to a urinary stoma on the skin (usually on the abdomen). There are multiple types of diversion procedures that are described in greater detail in many nursing textbooks. Urinary diversion is required with a cystectomy and is also used in the treatment of other conditions, such as bladder cancer, neurogenic bladder, or trauma to the bladder. Maintenance of skin integrity at the stoma site is of great importance.

FIGURE 17-4 Elimination and Interrelated Concepts

External urinary pouches are used in many cases to collect urine in these types of situations.

Invasive Procedures and Surgical Interventions Involving Bowel Elimination

Surgical procedures for bowel elimination problems are primarily associated with the colon, rectum, and anus, and they treat pathologic conditions or traumatic injury.

Colectomy. A colectomy (also referred to as a colon resection) involves removing a portion of the bowel. This may be done because of disease to a portion of the bowel (e.g., a cancerous tumor) or as treatment for traumatic injury. The two ends of the colon are reattached (anastomosed).

Colostomy/ileostomy. Diversion of the intestines (colon or small intestine) through a stoma on the skin is occasionally needed temporarily or permanently as a result of injured or diseased intestine, colon, or rectum. The use of external devices (e.g., a colostomy pouch) is required for the collection of stool. Maintenance of skin integrity around the stoma is of utmost importance.[14]

Rectal prolapse repair. Rectal prolapse is a condition that occurs when the rectum falls down into or through the anal opening. This is most common among young children and the elderly. Prolapse can occur from weak pelvic floor muscles or from excessive straining during bowel movements, as with chronic constipation. Surgical repair is indicated if prolapse occurs regularly or is associated with significant discomfort.

Hemorrhoidectomy. This procedure involves the excision of internal or external hemorrhoids. Hemorrhoids may require surgical intervention if topical treatments and changes in diet do not eliminate their associated discomfort. Thus, this procedure is usually only performed for patients with severe pain and multiple thrombosed hemorrhoids or when there is significant prolapse.

Fecal collection systems. A fecal collection system uses a flexible tube inserted into the rectum that is used to collect liquid stool in patients with incontinence who are not candidates for bowel retraining or have clostidium deficile and its resulting diarrhea. These are fecal management systems for liquid stool only and help prevent skin breakdown in cases of severe diarrhea.

INTERRELATED CONCEPTS

A number of concepts presented in this text are all interrelated and work together to ensure normal elimination. When any of these

factors are depleted or impaired, problems with elimination may occur (Figure 17-4).

As mentioned previously, Nutrition has a close interrelationship with bowel and urinary elimination. The types of foods and fluids ingested impact stool formation and urinary elimination. The kidneys play a vital role in maintaining homeostasis of Fluid and Electrolytes and Acid–Base Balance. Under the direction of hormones, the kidneys retain or eliminate water and electrolytes, which are critical for these balances to be maintained. Also, changes in electrolyte balance can interfere with smooth muscles, thus reducing or increasing intestinal peristalsis.

A lack of Mobility can result in both urinary and bowel elimination problems. Mobility helps with stimulation of peristalsis. Immobility, particularly when an individual is in a supine position, can lead to ineffective bladder emptying. Finally, changes in Cognition increase the potential for complications in both elimination mechanisms and can result from the inability to obtain and maintain adequate food and fluid intake. They can also lead to an inability to recognize cues for elimination—thus leading to incontinence.

CLINICAL EXEMPLARS

Exemplars of alterations in urinary elimination include conditions across the lifespan—ranging from bed-wetting, which may occur as a child is learning to control urinary elimination, to incontinence, which may occur as a person ages and the muscles supporting the bladder become less efficient.

Bowel function also spans the life cycle; a variety of issues may affect function as an infant, such as structural problems in the bowel (e.g., strictures and fissures), whereas functional issues such as constipation may occur as a person advances in age. Box 17-1 presents common exemplars of conditions associated with the concept of elimination.

Featured Exemplars
Urolithiasis

Urolithiasis refers to the presence of stones called calculi within the urinary tract. Although it is not entirely clear how stones are formed, most contain calcium. Stones can form in the kidney (nephrolithiasis) or within the ureters (ureterolithiasis). The stones are associated with severe pain when they move down the ureter, into the bladder, and through the urethra (referred to as passing the stone).[3] Hematuria

■■ ■ BOX 17-1   EXEMPLARS OF IMPAIRED ELIMINATION

Incontinence
- Bed-wetting
- Stress incontinence
- Urge incontinence
- Fecal incontinence

Retention
- Benign prostatic hyperplasia
- Bladder cancer
- Bowel obstruction
- Colorectal cancer
- Constipation
- Fecal impaction
- Prostatitis
- Prostate cancer
- Spinal cord injury
- Urethral stricture

Discomfort
- Anal fissure
- Anorectal abscess
- Hemorrhoids
- Interstitial cystitis

- Pilonidal cyst
- Urolithiasis

Infections and Inflammation
- Crohn's disease
- Diarrhea
- Gastritis
- Gastroenteritis
- Glomerulonephritis
- Pyelonephritis
- Ulcerative colitis
- Urinary tract infection

Renal Failure
- Acute kidney injury
- Chronic kidney disease

Neoplasms
- Benign prostate hyperplasia
- Bladder cancer
- Colorectal cancer
- Prostate cancer
- Renal cancer

---

is a common finding. If the stone becomes lodged in the ureter, a blockage can occur, leading to hydronephrosis and impaired kidney function.

Benign Prostatic Hyperplasia

Benign prostatic hyperplasia is an enlargement of the prostate gland commonly seen among older men. It is estimated that 30% of men age 60 years have moderate symptoms and 50% of men age 80 years or older have symptoms.[22] If untreated, the enlarging prostate, which surrounds the urethra at the base of the bladder, can obstruct urine flow, creating urinary retention. Common symptoms include frequency of urination, increased frequency of urinating at night, difficulty starting urinary flow, and a weak urinary stream. Chronic retention of urine can lead to urinary tract infection.

Urinary Tract Infection

Urinary tract infection (UTI) is caused by an infection in the urinary tract, representing the second most common bacterial infection in individuals. The symptoms associated with UTI include nausea and vomiting, chills, suprapubic or low back pain, bladder spasms, dysuria, burning with urination, frequency, urgency, hesitancy, or nocturia. UTIs are seen more frequently in pregnant women, females, and older men and women. These infections may cause sepsis and can result in death if not treated, especially in the elderly.[3]

Renal Failure

Renal failure occurs when there is a partially or complete cessation of kidney function. Renal failure can be acute or chronic. Acute kidney injury (AKI) is associated with a loss of renal function over a few days and can typically be reversed. Chronic kidney disease (CKD) involves a process of renal failure that occurs over a long period of time. It is

characterized by a gradual decrease in renal functioning and a gradual increase in metabolic waste. Regardless of the cause, untreated renal failure results in fluid overload, electrolyte imbalances, and metabolic acidosis and ultimately leads to death.

Constipation

Constipation refers to difficulty passing stool and is usually associated with the passage of hard, dry stool. Constipation may be painful due to the bloating and flatus that may occur and also with trying to pass the stool itself. Chronic constipation may be caused by a lack of dietary fiber, certain medications (narcotic pain medications), chronic decreased intestinal peristalsis, or decreased fluid intake.[3]

Diarrhea

Diarrhea is the frequent passing of watery, liquid, or loose stools. It can be acute or chronic. Acute diarrhea is usually associated with inflammation within the gastrointestinal tract due to a virus or bacteria and usually resolves in a few days. Chronic diarrhea persists for a longer period of time, such as several weeks. Because diarrhea is associated with the loss of water and electrolytes, dehydration and electrolyte imbalance may occur quickly, particularly among infants, children, and older adults.[3]

Colorectal Cancer

Colorectal cancer is the third leading cause of cancer in men and women in the United States, estimated to cause 49,700 deaths in 2015.[23] Colorectal incidence and mortality rates are highest among African American men and women. Colorectal screening can prevent the development of cancer by removing precancerous colon polyps and has been credited with reducing the incidence and mortality during the past decade.

CASE STUDY

Case Presentation

Source: Hemera Technologies/
AbleStock.com/Thinkstock

Ms. Amanda Doyle is a 61-year-old white female with a history of type 1 diabetes and has been bothered by osteoarthritis for the past several years. Her diabetes is well controlled with diet and insulin. Recently, she began taking over-the-counter ibuprofen 400 mg twice a day to manage the arthritis.

For the past 6 weeks, Ms. Doyle has experienced abdominal pain and increased frequency of bowel movements. Her stools are loose and not formed; quite frequently, they are a liquid consistency. Her life has been altered by the frequency of having to access a toilet because of the diarrhea. She has rectal bleeding and irritation from the frequent bowel movements, and she is suffered from abdominal pain at night as well as during the day. She reported these symptoms to her primary care provider, who referred her to a gastroenterologist for evaluation.

An occult blood test showed blood in her stool. A stool culture was done to rule out parasitic infections; this was negative. Because it had been 9 years since her last colonoscopy, a colonoscopy was ordered to rule out pathology within the colon such as ulcerations or tumors. This screening test was also negative. The nurse practitioner suggested that Ms. Doyle change her arthritis medication from ibuprofen to celecoxib. Within 2 weeks, Ms. Doyle has normally formed bowel movements and no abdominal pain.

Case Analysis

The symptoms described by Ms. Doyle are consistent with abnormal patterns of elimination. The diagnostic tests performed are routine given the symptoms and the time frame since the last screening tests. Nonsteroidal anti-inflammatory drugs (NSAIDs) cause gastrointestinal distress, bleeding, and diarrhea, particularly in high doses and when not administered with food or milk. Celecoxib is a COX-2 inhibitor and is indicated for osteoarthritis, particularly when gastrointestinal inflammation is experienced with other NSAIDs.

ACCESS EXEMPLAR LINKS IN YOUR GIDDENS EBOOK

REFERENCES

1. Venes D, editor: *Taber's cyclopedic medical dictionary*, ed 21, Philadelphia, 2013, Davis.
2. National Institute of Diabetes and Digestive and Kidney Diseases: Fecal incontinence, 2013. Retrieved from <http://www.niddk.nih.gov/health-information/health-topics/digestive-diseases/fecal-incontinence/Pages/facts.aspx>.
3. Lewis S, Dirksen S, Heitkemper M, et al: *Medical–surgical nursing*, ed 9, St Louis, 2013, Mosby.
4. Hockenberry MJ, Wilson D: *Wong's pediatric nursing*, ed 9, St Louis, 2012, Mosby.
5. National Center for Biotechnology Information: Treating constipation during pregnancy, 2012. Retrieved from <http://www.ncbi.nlm.nih.gov/pmc/articles/PMC3418980>.
6. National Kidney and Urologic Diseases Information Clearinghouse: Urinary retention, 2014. Retrieved from <http://kidney.niddk.nih.gov/kudiseases/pubs/UrinaryRetention>.
7. National Digestive Disease Information Clearinghouse NDDIC: Colonoscopy, n.d. Retrieved from <http://www.niddk.nih.gov/health-information/health-topics/diagnostic-tests/colonoscopy/Pages/diagnostic-test.aspx>.
8. Centers for Disease Control and Prevention: Colorectal (colon) cancer, 2015. Retrieved from <http://www.cdc.gov/cancer/colorectal/index.htm>.
9. National Kidney and Urologic Diseases Information Clearinghouse: Urinary incontinence in women, 2012. Retrieved from <http://kidney.niddk.nih.gov/kudiseases/pubs/uiwomen/index.aspx>.
10. Wang K, Palmer MH: Women's toileting behavior related to urinary elimination: Concept analysis. *J Adv Nurs* 66(8): 1874–1884, 2010.
11. Palmer MH: Urinary incontinence. In Carreri-Kohlman V, Lindsey AM, West CM, editors: *Pathophysiological phenomena in nursing: Human responses to illness*, ed 3, Philadelphia, 2003, Saunders.
12. Hägglund D: A systematic literature review of incontinence care for persons with dementia: The research evidence. *J Clin Nurs* 19(3–4):303–312, 2010.
13. National Digestive Diseases Clearinghouse: Celiac disease, 2012. Retrieved from <http://www.niddk.nih.gov/health-information/health-topics/digestive-diseases/celiac-disease/Pages/facts.aspx>.
14. Johns Hopkins Medicine: Bladder and bowel dysfunction, n.d. Retrieved from <http://www.hopkinsmedicine.org/healthlibrary/conditions/kidney_and_urinary_system_disorders/bladder_and_bowel_dysfunction_134,113>.
15. Wilson S, Giddens J: *Health assessment for nursing practice*, ed 5, St Louis, 2012, Elsevier.
16. Academy of Nutrition and Dietetics: Fiber, 2014. Retrieved from <http://www.eatright.org/resource/food/vitamins-and-supplements/nutrient-rich-foods/fiber>.
17. U.S. Preventive Services Task Force: Routine colorectal cancer: Screening, 2008. Retrived from <http://www.uspreventiveservicestaskforce.org/Page/Topic/recommendation-summary/colorectal-cancer-screening?ds=1&s=colorectal%20cancer%20screening>.
18. U.S. Preventive Services Task Force: Bladder cancer in adults: Screening, 2011. Retrieved from <http://www.uspreventiveservicestaskforce.org/Page/Topic/recommendation-summary/bladder-cancer-in-adults-screening?ds=1&s=bladder%20cancer%20screening>.
19. University of California, San Francisco: Biofeedback for incontinence, n.d. Retrieved from <http://www.ucsfhealth.org/education/biofeedback_for_incontinence/index.html>.
20. National Kidney and Urologic Disease Clearinghouse: Urinary retention, 2014. Retrieved from <http://kidney.niddk.nih.gov/kudiseases/pubs/urinaryretention/index.aspx>.
21. Newman DK: The indwelling catheter: Principles for best practice. *J Wound Ostomy Continence Nurs* 34(6):655–663, 2007.
22. Mayo Clinic: Benign prostatic hyperplasia (BPH), n.d. Retrieved from <http://www.mayoclinic.org/diseases-conditions/benign-prostatic-hyperplasia/basics/definition/CON-20030812>.
23. National Cancer Institute: Colorectal cancer, n.d. Retrieved from <http://www.cancer.gov/cancertopics/types/colorectal>.

Perfusion

Susan Wilson

All cells need a consistent blood supply to obtain oxygen and nutrients and to discard wastes. When the blood supply or perfusion is impaired, ischemia develops and can progress to necrosis, if prolonged. For this reason, perfusion is a critical concept for nurses to incorporate into practice. The purpose of this concept presentation is to help the nurse acquire an understanding about perfusion across the lifespan. In practice, nurses should be able to promote an individual's healthy behaviors that optimize perfusion, identify individuals at risk of impaired perfusion, recognize when individuals are experiencing an impairment of perfusion, and respond with appropriate interventions.

DEFINITION

For the purpose of this concept presentation, perfusion refers to *the flow of blood through arteries and capillaries delivering nutrients and oxygen to cells.* Perfusion is a normal physiological process that requires the heart to generate sufficient cardiac output to transport blood through patent blood vessels for distribution in the tissues throughout the body. Thus, maintaining cardiovascular health is essential to optimal perfusion. The extent of tissue damage from impaired perfusion depends on the size and location of the blood vessel and whether the blood supply is reduced or completely interrupted. When blood supply is available but decreased, the term *ischemia* is used. For example, when blood supply from coronary arteries to the myocardium is decreased but not absent, the term myocardial ischemia is used. Chest pain produced from this ischemia is called angina pectoris, and the function of myocardial cells is reduced, but cells do not die. However, prolonged ischemia of tissue leads to necrosis and eventually infarction if blood supply is not restored. Myocardial *infarction* indicates death of myocardial tissue with an inability to regenerate.

SCOPE

The concept of perfusion and problems associated with impaired perfusion represents a wide range of physiological processes and conditions. The scope of perfusion ranges from optimal perfusion to no perfusion (Figure 18-1). Various degrees of reduced perfusion lie between the two ends of the spectrum. Variations in perfusion are seen among individuals across the lifespan with multiple causative factors and a wide range of impact and duration from any cause. Changes in perfusion can be temporary, long term, or permanent. Disorders that lead to changes in perfusion include acute illnesses such as myocardial infarction or shock and chronic disorders such as hypertension, heart failure, and stroke. Conditions that specifically involve perfusion include neurologic (interfering with blood flow within the brain), pulmonary (impairing pulmonary blood flow), and cardiovascular (interfering with blood flow in heart, arteries, and veins). Conditions in these body systems can be caused by congenital defects, genetic conditions, injury, inflammation, and infections.

NORMAL PHYSIOLOGICAL PROCESS

From a conceptual lens, the process of perfusion can be thought of in two general categories: central perfusion and tissue perfusion. The normal physiological process of perfusion is presented from this perspective.

Central Perfusion

Central perfusion is generated by cardiac output—the amount of blood pumped by the heart each minute. Cardiac output is an outcome of coordinated effects of electrical and mechanical factors that move blood through the heart into the peripheral vascular vessels. This central perfusion propels blood to all organs and their tissues from patent arteries through capillaries and returns the blood to the heart through patent veins.

Central perfusion of blood begins when the heart is stimulated by an electrical impulse that originates in the sinoatrial (SA) node and travels to the atrioventricular (AV) node. From the AV node, the impulse moves through a series of branches (bundle of His) and Purkinje fibers in the myocardium, which causes the ventricles to contract. The phase of the cardiac cycle during which the ventricles contract is called systole. As the ventricles contract, they create pressure that closes the mitral and tricuspid valves, preventing the backflow of blood into the atria. This ventricular pressure forces the aortic and pulmonic valves to open, resulting in ejection of blood into the aorta (from the left ventricle) and the pulmonary arteries (from the right ventricle). As blood is ejected, the ventricular pressure decreases, causing the aortic and pulmonic valves to close. The ventricles relax to fill with blood. The movement of blood from the atria to the ventricles is accomplished when the pressure of the blood in the atria becomes higher than the pressure in the ventricles. The higher atrial pressures passively open the mitral and tricuspid valves, allowing blood to fill the ventricles. The phase of the cardiac cycle when ventricles fill with blood is called diastole.

FIGURE 18-1 The Scope of Perfusion Ranges from Optimal to Impaired and a Total Lack of Perfusion

Normal cardiac output ranges from 4 to 6 L/minute in the adult. The two variables that contribute to cardiac output are stroke volume (the amount of blood ejected with each contraction) and heart rate. Preload refers to the end diastolic volume in the heart (the amount of blood in the ventricles at the end of diastole) and is influenced by the stretch capacity of myocardial fibers and the amount of blood returned to the heart from the systemic circulation. Another factor that affects cardiac output is systemic vascular resistance (SVR) or the amount of resistance within the vasculature the heart pumps against (also referred to as afterload). SVR is moderated by the diameter of the blood vessels and blood volume. Figure 18-2 shows the flow of blood through the right and left sides of the heart.

Tissue Perfusion

Tissue perfusion refers to the volume of blood that flows through target tissues. This perfusion is supplied by blood flowing from arteries to capillaries. The force of ventricular contractions creates a pressure, called capillary hydrostatic pressure, that pushes blood through capillaries into the interstitial spaces allowing delivery of oxygen, fluid, and nutrients to cells.

Pressure generated from the myocardial contraction supplies blood to the peripheral vascular system. Arteries, capillaries, and veins provide blood flow to and from tissues. The tough and tensile arteries and their smaller branches, the arterioles, are subjected to remarkable pressure from the cardiac output. They maintain blood pressure by constricting or dilating in response to stimuli. The more passive veins and their smaller branches, the venules, are less sturdy but more expansible, enabling them to act as a reservoir for extra blood, if needed, to decrease the workload on the heart. Pressure within the veins is low

compared to that of arterial circulation. The valves in each vein keep blood flowing in a forward direction toward the heart.

Age-Related Differences
Infants
In infancy, the size of the heart in relation to the total body size is larger, and the heart occupies a larger space within the mediastinum. The systolic blood pressure after birth is low due to the weaker left ventricle of the neonate. The left side of the heart develops strength and the systolic pressure rises rather sharply during the first 6 weeks. Soon after puberty, the systolic pressure rises to adult levels. An increase in heart size occurs during the adolescent growth spurt with increase in blood pressure and decrease in heart rate. Arteries and veins lengthen to keep pace with growth.[1]

Older Adults
A number of cardiovascular changes occur with aging. Arterial stiffening contributes to an increase in blood pressure, which increases the workload of the myocardium. The cardiac output is decreased by 30–40%. A decrease in blood pressure upon standing (orthostatic hypotension) may contribute to falls.[2]

VARIATIONS AND CONTEXT

The two broad categories used to describe the normal physiological process of perfusion are also used to describe problems associated with perfusion: impaired central perfusion (mechanisms for blood delivery) and impaired tissue perfusion (actual amount of blood available to target tissues). Both of these categories are described further in the following sections.

Impaired Central Perfusion

Many conditions associated with impaired perfusion result in decreased cardiac output. As previously described, cardiac output refers to the volume of blood pumped by the heart each minute and is responsible for propelling blood to all organs and their tissues through the vascular system.

Various factors can reduce cardiac output. Inefficient mechanisms within the heart can occur from changes in myocardial conduction, problems with the heart values, disease to the heart muscle tissue, and congenital defects. Central perfusion problems can also result from increased SVR, attributed to vasoconstriction of the arteries or increased viscosity of the blood. An increased SVR requires the heart to increase contractile force and/or increase heart rate to maintain adequate cardiac output. The heart has limits to this compensatory effect; a sustained increase in SVR eventually leads to insufficient central perfusion. Likewise, cardiac output is affected by a reduction in SVR, attributed to vasodilation of the arteries or blood loss.

Regardless of the underlying cause, when central perfusion is impaired, clinical manifestations are systemic; in other words, the entire body is affected. Significant reduction of central perfusion results in shock, which occurs when blood supply to tissues is impaired because of inadequate cardiac output, significant blood loss, or vasodilation throughout the body. Specific examples of conditions that lead to impaired central perfusion are presented later.

Impaired Local/Tissue Perfusion

A number of conditions impair the volume of blood that flows through target tissues in the arteries to capillaries. Interference with tissue perfusion reduces blood flow through capillaries into the interstitial spaces allowing delivery of oxygen, fluid, and nutrients to cells.

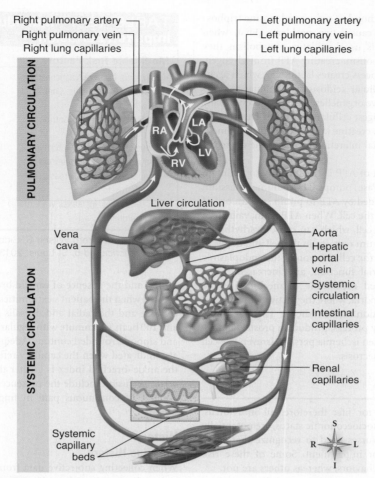

PULMONARY CIRCULATION

Right pulmonary artery
Right pulmonary vein
Right lung capillaries

Left pulmonary artery
Left pulmonary vein
Left lung capillaries

RA LA
LV
RV

SYSTEMIC CIRCULATION

Liver circulation

Vena cava

Aorta
Hepatic portal vein

Systemic circulation

Intestinal capillaries

Renal capillaries

Systemic capillary beds

FIGURE 18-2 Circulatory Routes. The pulmonary circulation routes blood flow to and from the gas exchange tissues of the lungs. The systemic circulation, on the other hand, routes blood flow to and from the oxygen-consuming tissues of the body. (Source: From Patton KT, Thibodeau GA: *Anatomy & physiology*, ed 9, St Louis, 2016, Mosby.)

Different organs and tissues require different volumes of blood to maintain adequate function. Some organs, such as the brain and intestines, require much larger volumes of perfused blood compared to skeletal tissue, for example. Inadequate tissue perfusion can result from poor central perfusion or from a mechanism within the organ itself, such as a blocked blood vessel leading to or from the tissue or from excessive edema within the tissue interfering with the cellular oxygen exchange or increased pressure and associated constriction or collapse of arterioles. Specific examples of conditions that lead to impaired central perfusion are presented later.

CONSEQUENCES

Consequences of Impaired Central Perfusion

Impairment of central perfusion occurs in conditions that decrease cardiac output or cause shock. Cardiac output is decreased when there is inadequate perfusion to the myocardium, inadequate impulse conduction through the heart, or malfunction of a heart valve. Any occlusion or constriction of coronary arteries that reduces blood flow to the myocardium can result in a myocardial infarction that decreases cardiac output. This impairment prevents the myocardium from performing the mechanical function of pumping blood to the body. Also, altered impulse conduction through the heart (from the SA node

through the AV node to the right and left bundle branches and Purkinje fibers) interrupts the electrical function necessary for the myocardium to contract and results in disorganized contraction. Finally, malfunction of heart valves, either stenosis or insufficiency, impairs flow of blood through the heart. Shock, the inability of central perfusion to supply blood to peripheral tissues, occurs when the heart is unable to act as a pump (cardiogenic shock), fluid is lost (hemorrhagic shock), or systemic vasodilation occurs (anaphylactic, neurogenic, or septic shock).

Consequences of Impaired Tissue Perfusion

Impairment of tissue perfusion is associated with occlusion, constriction, or dilation of arteries or veins. Atherosclerosis or thrombi can occlude arteries, and thrombi can occlude veins. Vasoconstriction can occur from frostbite. Examples of dilation are aneurysms in arteries and varicose veins. Impaired tissue perfusion interferes with blood flow, resulting in ischemia to localized tissue and, if uncorrected, cellular death.

Ischemia is *reversible* cellular injury that occurs when the demand for oxygen exceeds the supply because of a reduction or cessation of blood flow. This is an example of the interrelationship between the cardiovascular and respiratory systems because cells are deprived of oxygen from the lack of blood flow, from the lack of oxygen, or both.

Decreased oxygen to the mitochondria reduces adenosine triphosphate (ATP) production, which causes two problems. First, when oxygen is not available for the cells' usual oxidative metabolism, they are forced to use anaerobic metabolism, creating ATP from glycogen, to maintain cell function. This process creates lactic acid, which accumulates in the cell and causes cellular acidosis. The cellular acidosis causes lysosomes, the cell's digestive organelles, to swell and eventually release acidic enzymes that autodigest cellular structures. Destruction of tissues releases enzymes such as creatine kinase (CK); measurement of these enzymes after a myocardial infarction indicates the degree of damage to the heart muscle.[3]

The second problem with lack of ATP is the inability to maintain the adenosine triphosphatase (ATPase) pumps. The sodium–potassium pump normally uses energy provided by ATP to pump sodium out of the cell and allow potassium into the cell. When ATP is unavailable, a potassium deficit develops in the cell, which can cause dysrhythmias in myocardial tissue. Also, the sodium remains in the cell and draws in water, resulting in swelling within the cell, dilation of the endoplasmic reticulum, decreased mitochondrial function, and increased membrane permeability. The increased membrane permeability allows calcium ions to enter the mitochondria, where they activate lipases and proteases and increase the production of free radicals.[3] The membrane damage initiates the inflammatory process, producing prostaglandins, thromboxanes, and cytokines. When ischemia persists, irreversible cell injury or cell death occurs from necrosis.

RISK FACTORS

Adequate perfusion is required for life; therefore, all individuals, regardless of age, gender, race, or socioeconomic status, are potentially at risk for impaired perfusion. Nurses need to recognize that some individuals are at greater risk for impairment. Some of these risk factors are controllable lifestyle behaviors, whereas others are not.

Populations at Risk

Populations at greatest risk of impaired perfusion are middle-age and older adults, especially among males and African Americans. Also at risk are infants with congenital heart defects. Children and young adults commonly experience impaired perfusion as a result of trauma; this leads to central perfusion failure attributable to blood loss.

Individual Risk Factors

Adults in middle and old age are commonly affected by atherosclerosis involving the heart and peripheral vessels, myocardial disease, and other chronic conditions that negatively impact the cardiovascular system. Atherosclerosis is characterized by plaques of cholesterol and other lipids lining the inner layers of arteries, which obstruct blood flow. Older adults are at risk for impaired perfusion because of anatomic changes expected with advanced age, such as fibrosis and sclerosis of the sinoatrial node and mitral and aortic valves.

A number of modifiable and nonmodifiable risk factors linked to impaired perfusion are presented in Table 18-1.

ASSESSMENT

Sources of data come from the patient as well as from physical assessment and laboratory findings. Assessment of perfusion involves recognizing indications of adequate and inadequate perfusion. The presence of central perfusion is noted by heart rate and blood pressure measurements within normal limits. Cerebral tissue perfusion is indicated by the patient's orientation to time, place, person, and situation; expected bilateral movement and sensation; clear speech; the presence of carotid

TABLE 18-1 Individual Risk Factors for Impaired Perfusion

Modifiable Risk Factors	Unmodifiable Risk Factors
• Smoking: Nicotine vasoconstricts	• Age: Increases with age
• Elevated serum lipids: Contribute to atherosclerosis	• Gender: Men > women
• Sedentary lifestyle: Contributes to obesity	• Genetics: Family history
• Obesity: Increases risk for type 2 diabetes and atherosclerosis	
• Diabetes mellitus: Increases risk of atherosclerosis	
• Hypertension: Increases work of myocardium	

Source: Adapted from Wilson S, Giddens J: *Health assessment for nursing practice*, ed 5, St Louis, 2013, Elsevier.

pulses; and the absence of carotid bruit. Peripheral tissue perfusion is present when the patient's extremities are warm with color appropriate for race and the radial and dorsalis pedis pulse rates are between 60 and 100 beats per minute with regular rhythm, easily palpable upstroke, and smooth, rounded contour. Adequate peripheral tissue perfusion is also indicated when the capillary refill time is less than 2 seconds and the ankle–brachial index is greater than 0.9. Patients' reports of adequate perfusion include the presence of warm hands and feet and the absence of continuous pain in fingers and toes or leg pain when walking.[2]

History
Baseline History

When collecting subjective data from patients, nurses ask about lifestyle behaviors including diet, exercise, smoking, and alcohol consumption. A diet high in fat and carbohydrates together with minimal or infrequent exercise contributes to atherosclerosis and obesity. The nicotine present in cigarettes constricts blood vessels, contributing to hypertension and increasing the workload of the heart. Excessive alcohol intake is associated with dysrhythmias. Also, patients are asked about any chronic diseases, such as diabetes mellitus, renal failure, and hypertension. Nurses ask patients for a list of medications they take, both prescription and over-the-counter, including the reason for each medication and its effectiveness. Patients are also asked about use of recreational or street drugs such as cocaine, because it is associated with myocardial infarction and stroke.[2]

Problem-Based History

When providing their history, patients may describe pain, shortness of breath (dyspnea), edema (swelling), and fainting (dizziness). When these symptoms are reported, the nurse follows up with a symptom analysis to obtain additional data, including the onset of the symptom; the location, duration, and severity of the symptom; a description of the symptom; factors that alleviate or aggravate the symptom; other associated symptoms; and actions taken by the patient to relieve the symptom.[2]

Pain. A common symptom reported by patients with impaired tissue perfusion is pain. When there is inadequate perfusion to carry needed oxygen to meet tissue needs, patients experience ischemic pain. This type of pain occurs by the same process whether it is occurring in the coronary arteries or the femoral arteries.

Chest pain may be due to impaired blood flow to the myocardium or pulmonary emboli. Patients experience myocardial ischemia, also called stable angina, when there is an increased demand for oxygen on the heart. They often report a precipitating event, such as physical exertion, exposure to cold temperatures, or emotional stress. Patients with angina pectoris describe their chest pain as a constricting or squeezing sensation that is relieved with rest and/or by taking one or more nitroglycerin tablets. By contrast, patients with acute coronary syndrome (unstable angina advancing to myocardial infarction) report severe chest pain that is not relieved by rest or nitroglycerin; shortness of breath; radiating pain to the jaw or arms; and nausea, vomiting, and diaphoresis. Although men and women may experience the same symptoms, some women report atypical chest pain, shortness of breath, and fatigue as their only indications of myocardial infarction. Patients experiencing pulmonary emboli report varied and nonspecific symptoms. Classic symptoms of chest pain and shortness of breath are reported only by approximately 20% of patients. The pain onset varies from gradual to sudden. Pleuritic chest pain also is reported at the onset of a pulmonary embolus.[4,5]

Pain in the legs attributable to impaired perfusion may be caused by peripheral arterial disease (PAD) or a deep vein thrombus. Patients with PAD may report pain when walking that is relieved with rest, called intermittent claudication. This pain indicates an inadequate supply of blood to transport needed oxygen to meet the demands of the leg muscles. Thus, the pain stops when the increased demand of oxygen from walking stops. As the arterial occlusion increases, patients may report "rest pain," which is leg pain while walking that is not relieved with rest.

Dyspnea. Inadequate circulation of blood interferes with oxygen transport to tissues, making patients dyspneic or short of breath during activity. This symptom may be reported by patients with primary perfusion problems, such as heart failure, or by those with primary gas exchange problems, such as chronic obstructive pulmonary disease. Patients may report having to sleep sitting up or using several pillows to prop up during the night. Lightheadedness may be reported attributable to inadequate oxygen transport to the brain. Nurses inquire about the duration of patients' shortness of breath as well as if the dyspnea occurs on inhalation or exhalation or both. They ask what makes the dyspnea better and what makes it worse. Nurses ask if patients have any other symptoms occurring at the same time, such as chest pain or swelling of the feet and ankles.[2] When an infant is being evaluated for heart disease, the mother or caretaker may report the infant needing to stop sucking "to catch his or her breath" or the infant exhibited a bluish color around the lips when sucking.[6]

Edema (swelling). Patients may report their socks leaving an indentation around their legs or edema in their feet that is worse at the end of the day. This edema reflects excessive fluid in the interstitial spaces, which indicates a fluid overload or an accumulation of fluids. The excessive fluid may occur from renal disease when blood cannot be filtered by the kidneys. Right-sided heart failure is another cause of peripheral edema that develops if the right ventricle is unable to eject its usual volume of blood. Reflux of blood occurs from the right ventricle into the right atrium and then into the inferior and superior venae cavae. Because of the buildup of blood, the veins are unable to transport blood back to the heart, resulting in an accumulation of blood in the venous system that pushes fluid into the interstitial spaces, causing edema.

Dizziness or fainting. Patients may report feeling dizzy. Using a symptom analysis, nurses collect data to learn when this lightheadedness occurs as well as aggravating and relieving factors. If the dizziness occurs when the patient sits up suddenly, it is called orthostatic hypotension, which is defined as a 20- to 30-mm Hg drop in systolic blood pressure when a patient moves from a lying to a sitting or standing position. Nurses inquire about the duration of the dizziness. For many patients, the dizziness subsides if they sit for a few seconds before standing. In contrast, dizziness unrelated to position changes may be caused by inadequate blood flow to the brain. The carotid arteries may be obstructed from atherosclerosis, preventing adequate blood flow to the brain.

Examination Findings
Central Perfusion
When assessing patients experiencing inadequate *central perfusion*, nurses may notice changes in vital signs such as hypotension or tachycardia. When assessing for orthostatic hypotension, blood pressure is measured with the patient in three positions: lying, sitting, and standing. Nurses compare these three blood pressure readings to confirm position changes as a contributing factor to the dizziness or fainting. Auscultation of the patient's heart may reveal S_1 and S_2 heart sounds as expected as well as S_3 or S_4 abnormal heart sounds. Murmurs heard indicate turbulent blood flow through the heart. There may be a change in mentation reflecting impaired blood flow to the brain. Shortness of breath can result from insufficient oxygenation of the blood. Additional findings may include changes in heart rhythm indicating altered cardiac electrical function; peripheral edema can develop from fluid retention or inadequate cardiac output. Patients may have a sympathetic nervous system response causing diaphoresis or anxiety.

Infants may have low weight and failure to thrive attributable to a weak suck and dyspnea while feeding. Children may not be as active and may squat on the playground to compensate for impaired perfusion. Characteristic heart murmurs are heard in infants with congenital heart disorders such as atrial septal defect, ventricular septal defect, and patent ductus arteriosus. Infants with coarctation of the aorta have high blood pressure and bounding pulses in the arms but lower blood pressure, weak to absent pulses, and cool lower extremities.[1]

Tissue Perfusion
Manifestations of poor *tissue perfusion* are dependent on the tissues involved. When assessing patients with impaired blood flow to the lower extremities, the nurse may notice less hair on the legs and pale skin on inspection. Palpation reveals cool skin, diminished to absent dorsalis pedal or posterior tibial pulses, and slowed capillary refill time. An ankle–brachial index measurement of less than 0.9 indicates that the brachial blood pressure is stronger than the ankle blood pressure, confirming reduced perfusion to the lower extremities.

When ischemia involves the kidneys, such as in response to hemorrhagic shock, kidneys produce less urine because of lack of blood flow. The lack of perfusion stimulates the renin–angiotensin–aldosterone system, resulting in a relative increase in blood pressure because of the effects both of angiotensin II (vasoconstricts blood vessels) and of increases in aldosterone secretion (retains sodium and then water, causing peripheral edema).

When ischemia involves the brain, the manifestations produced depend on the extent of ischemia and the areas of the brain affected. For example, when mild atherosclerosis occludes the right carotid artery, patients experience a transient ischemic attack that may involve left-sided weakness and difficulty speaking—conditions that usually resolve within 24 hours. By contrast, if blood supply to the right anterior cerebral artery is reduced or absent, patients will have a reduce level of consciousness and paralysis of the left leg.

Diagnostic Tests
Blood Tests
Enzymes and markers. Enzymes released from damaged cells and circulating in the blood can be measured to confirm impaired perfusion:

- Creatine kinase (CK) is an enzyme present in myocardium (CK-MB), in muscle (CK-MM), and in brain (CK-BB) tissues. When enzymes are isolated, the level of CK-MB is elevated after a myocardial infarction.
- Lactate dehydrogenase (LDH) is an enzyme found in large amounts in the heart, liver, muscles, and erythrocytes. When enzymes are isolated, the level of LDH_1 isoenzyme is elevated after damage to the myocardium and erythrocytes.[7]
- Natriuretic peptides include two hormones. Atrial natriuretic peptide is a hormone secreted from right atrial cells when right atrial pressure increases; it is used to detect heart failure. Brain-type natriuretic peptide is a hormone secreted from cardiac cells in increased amounts when pressures are high; it is used to detect heart failure.[7]
- Troponin is a myocardial muscle protein released after myocardial injury. Increased blood levels of this protein are found in patients who have had a myocardial infarction. Troponin also can be used to predict the likelihood of future cardiac events.[7]
- Homocysteine (Hcy) is an amino acid produced during protein metabolism. Elevated levels of Hcy can be hereditary or acquired from dietary deficiencies such as vitamin B_6, vitamin B_{12}, or folate. The link to perfusion is that elevated levels of Hcy have been identified as a predictor of coronary artery disease (CAD), cerebrovascular accident, peripheral arterial disease, and venous thrombosis.[8] Hcy promotes atherosclerosis by causing endothelial damage, promoting deposits of low-density lipoproteins, and promoting vascular smooth muscle growth.[7] Testing for Hcy has been recommended in those patients with a familial predisposition for early cardiovascular disease or history of cardiovascular disease in the absence of other common risk factors.[8]
- C-reactive protein (CRP) is produced by the liver during acute inflammation and is emerging as an independent risk factor for CAD. Measurement of CRP using a high-sensitivity test (hsCRP) has been shown to predict the risk of future cardiac events in patients with unstable angina and myocardial infarction.[8]

Serum lipids. Serum lipids are measured to detect hyperlipidemia and include cholesterol lipoproteins (low-density lipoproteins, high-density lipoproteins, very low-density lipoproteins, and triglycerides). These provide information about risk factors and the possible presence of vessel disease.

Electrocardiogram

An electrocardiogram (ECG) is performed by placing 12 leads on the patient's chest and extremities to record the electrical impulses through the heart. The waveforms generated detect cardiac dysrhythmias by documenting on a screen or paper the electrical impulses generated by the heart during contraction and relaxation of atria and ventricles.[7] A 12-lead ECG is obtained to detect myocardial ischemia or infarction when patients complain of chest pain. An ECG also is used to continuously monitor the heart rhythm using one or more leads.[9]

Cardiac Stress Tests

Exercise cardiac stress test. The exercise cardiac stress test is one of the most common cardiac stress tests because it is relatively simple and noninvasive. The patient exercises on a treadmill with a progressive increase in speed and elevation. During the test, an ECG is recorded along with regular monitoring of heart rate and rhythm, blood pressure, and respiratory rate. If coronary artery disease is present, changes in electrical conduction or other symptoms such as chest pain may occur.

Pharmacologic stress test. Another common cardiac stress test involves the administration of certain pharmacologic agents that

stimulate the physiological effects of exercise. This is often done when patients are unable to perform the exercise stress test due to underlying conditions. Agents often administered include dobutamine and adenosine. ECG monitoring (or radionuclide imaging) is performed while the pharmacologic agents are given to detect problems with conduction, heart rate, or strength of contractions.[7]

Radiographic Studies

Chest x-ray. Chest x-rays provide visualization of the lungs, ribs, clavicles, vertebrae, heart, and major thoracic vessels. For patients with impaired perfusion, x-rays are taken to visualize the size of the heart and lung fields.[8]

Ultrasound. Doppler ultrasound uses a probe that directs high-frequency sound waves to indicate blood flow in the artery. Duplex imaging uses a color Doppler system to map the blood flow throughout the entire region of tan artery.[10]

Arteriogram. An arteriogram allows visualization of arteries by injecting radiopaque contrast into them so that the location and extent of occlusion can be identified. A cardiac catheterization is one type of arteriogram that allows visualization of coronary arteries and heart chambers. A catheter is passed into the heart through a peripheral vein or artery, depending on whether catheterization of the left or right side of the heart is being performed. Pressures are recorded through the catheter, and radiographic contrast is injected to visualize the patency of coronary arteries.[7]

CLINICAL MANAGEMENT

Clinical management associated with the perfusion concept involves the prevention of illness, early detection, and appropriate collaborative management of cardiovascular problems.

Primary Prevention

Primary prevention includes measures to promote health and prevent development of disease. There are several measures that prevent or diminish conditions that impair perfusion. Prevention measures are based on a heart-healthy lifestyle, which includes eating a healthy diet, exercising most days of the week, and not smoking. Recommendations by the American Heart Association[11] are presented in Box 18-1.

Secondary Prevention (Screening)

Secondary prevention includes screening and early diagnosis and prompt treatment of existing health problems. Its purpose is to shorten the duration and severity of consequences. Routine screening involves monitoring blood pressure and serum lipids.

Blood Pressure Screening

Blood pressure screening is a simple and cost-effective screening recommended across the lifespan. Beginning in infancy, blood pressure screening is recommended at every well-child visit and at least annually. Among adults, the U.S. Preventive Services Task Force (USPSTF)[12] recommends screening for high blood pressure in adults ages 18 years or older. For patients who have hypertension, the Joint National Committee on Prevention, Detection, Evaluation, and Treatment of High Blood Pressure[12] recommends screening every 2 years when blood pressures are less than 120/80 mm Hg. This same committee recommends screening every year when systolic blood pressures are 120–139 mm Hg or diastolic pressures are 80–90 mm Hg.

Lipid Screening

Recommendations for screening of lipids vary between men and women. The USPSTF strongly recommends screening men ages 35

BOX 18-1 American Heart Association Health Promotion Recommendations

1. Eat a variety of fruits, vegetables, grains, legumes, fat-free or low-fat dairy products, fish, poultry, and lean meats:
   - Reduce sodium (salt) intake to less than 1500 a day.
   - Reduce saturated and trans fats to less than 10% of calories.
2. Participate in physical activity:
   - Adults older than 20 years of age: At least 150 minutes/week of moderate-intensity activity
   - Children 12–19 years of age: At least 60 minutes of moderate intensity activity every day
3. Refrain from smoking and have no exposure to environmental tobacco smoke.
4. Maintain blood pressure:
   - Adults older than 20 years of age: <120/80 mm Hg
   - Children 8–19 years of age: <90th percentile
5. Maintain total cholesterol
   - Adults older than 20 years of age: <200 mg/dL
   - Children 6–19 years of age: <70 mg/dL
6. Maintain fasting blood glucose
   - Adults older than 20 years of age: <100 mg/dL
   - Children 12–19 years of age: <200 mg/dL
7. Achieve and maintain desirable weight
   - Adults older than 20 years of age: 25 kg/m^2
   - Children 12–19 years of age: <85th percentile

Source: Data from Lloyd-Jones DM, et al.: Defining and setting national goals for cardiovascular health promotion and disease reduction: The American Heart Association's strategy impact goal through 2020 and beyond, *Circulation* 121:586–613, 2010.

years or older for lipid disorders and screening men ages 20–35 years if they are at increased risk for coronary artery disease. For women, the USPSTF strongly recommends screening those ages 45 years or older for lipid disorders if they are at increased risk for coronary heart disease. Among younger women, ages 20–45 years, the USPSTF recommends lipid screening if they are at increased risk for coronary heart disease.[12]

Collaborative Interventions

The management of individuals with impaired perfusion is highly dependent on the specific condition. The following sections describe common interventions implemented in the treatment of conditions resulting in impaired perfusion.

Nutrition Therapy

Nutrition therapy should meet the recommendations described under Primary Prevention, but the goal of the heart-healthy diet is tertiary prevention—to lower serum lipid levels, lose weight, and maintain an optimal weight. For this reason, nutrition therapy is considered an intervention in both primary prevention and disease management.

Activity, Exercise, and Positioning

Activity and exercise are a regular part of any treatment regimen. Specifically, they are included in the following applications:
- For the purpose of weight loss and weight maintenance
- Cardiac rehabilitation after acute coronary syndrome[4]
- Progressive activity for patients with peripheral arterial disease

Smoking Cessation

Smoking cessation is also considered both primary prevention and collaborative intervention for disease management. For interventions directed at smoking cessation, refer to Concept 19 Gas Exchange.

Pharmacotherapy

Pharmacotherapy represents one of the most common collaborative interventions for individuals with conditions associated with cardiovascular disease. The following are the general classifications of drugs; there are many types of drugs within each of these categories:
- *Vasodilators* increase the diameter of blood vessels in a variety of ways that block normal mechanisms. For example, vasodilators can block the following: α-adrenergic receptors; calcium influx into vascular smooth muscle; formation of angiotensin II, which normally increases aldosterone concentration to retain sodium as well as vasoconstriction; and receptors that receive angiotensin II. Myocardial contractility is reduced for the purpose of lowering cardiac output by blocking calcium influx into the myocardium and blocking the β-adrenergic receptors in the heart.[13] Vasodilators are used to treat hypertension as well as angina. Common types of vasodilator agents include angiotensin-converting enzyme inhibitors (captopril, lisinopril, and losartan), nitrates (amyl nitrite, nitroglycerine, and nitroprusside), potassium channel activators (diazoxide and minoxidil), and smooth muscle relaxants (hydralazine).
- *Vasopressors* decrease the diameter of blood vessels by stimulating the α-adrenergic or dopamine receptors to effect the normal mechanism of vasoconstriction.[4] Examples include epinephrine, norepinephrine, and dobutamine.
- *Diuretics* reduce blood volume by preventing the reabsorption of sodium in the kidneys, which increases urine output. Common examples include furosemide, hydrochlorathiazide, triamterene, and spironolactone.
- *Antidysrhythmics* correct erratic electrical impulses to create regular cardiac rhythms. These agents act by blocking electrolytes that affect electrical conduction in the heart, such as sodium, potassium, and calcium (nifedipine, verapamil, and diltiazem), or by blocking β-adrenergic receptors (Lopressor, metoprolol, and Toprol).[4]
- *Cardioglycosides* have a positive inotropic effect with a lowering of heart rate to increase cardiac output and are used for the treatment of heart failure. The classic example is digoxin.[1]
- *Anticoagulants* prevent blood clotting at several locations in the clotting cascade to suppress the production of fibrin. They are most effective in preventing venous thrombosis. Common examples include heparin, exoprin, warfarin sodium, and ardeparin.
- *Antiplatelet* agents prevent platelets from aggregating to form clots. They are most effective in preventing arterial thrombosis. Two classes of antiplatelet agents are glycoprotein platelet inhibitors (tirofiban, eptifibatide, and abciximab) and platelet aggregation inhibitors (aspirin and ticagrelor).
- *Thrombolytics* disrupt blood clots that are impairing perfusion by lysing fibrin. Common examples include tissue plasminogen activator, alteplase, urokinase, and streptokinase.
- *Lipid-lowering agents* decrease the levels of lipids that contribute to atherosclerosis and result in blood vessel occlusion by reducing the synthesis of cholesterol. The primary group of drugs used are the statins (e.g., atorvastatin, fluvastatin, lovastatin, and pravastatin).

Procedures and Surgical Interventions

There are many procedures and surgical interventions that improve electrical conduction in the heart as well as perfusion.

Pacemaker insertion. A pacemaker is an electronic device used to increase the heart rate in severe bradycardia by electronically stimulating the myocardium. The basic pacing circuit consists of a battery-operated pulse generator and one or more conducting leads that pace the atrium and one or both ventricles. Pacemakers can be external (temporary) or surgically implanted (permanent).[9]

Electrical cardioversion. The use of electric energy is an intervention to treat select abnormal cardiac rhythms. Cardiac defibrillation is used for emergency treatment during cardiac arrest when ventricular fibrillation or ventricular tachycardia is present. Synchronized cardioversion is a therapeutic procedure used to convert an abnormal rhythm, such as ventricular tachycardia with a pulse or atrial fibrillation, to a normal sinus rhythm. The procedure for cardioversion is the same as that for defibrillation with a few exceptions. If synchronized cardioversion is performed on a nonemergent basis, the patient is sedated before the procedure. The initial energy needed for synchronized cardioversion is less than the energy needed for defibrillation. Synchronized cardioversion starts at levels of 50–100 J and is increased as needed.[9]

Intra-aortic balloon pump. An intra-aortic balloon pump (IABP) provides temporary circulatory assistance to the patient in the critical care unit who has a compromised heart. This pump reduces afterload to decrease the workload of the ventricles and augments the aortic diastolic pressure, resulting in improved coronary blood flow. Afterload is the force that the ventricles must exert to open the pulmonic and aortic valves. The IABP consists of a sausage-shaped balloon that is inserted percutaneously or surgically into the femoral artery. The balloon is advanced toward the heart and positioned in the descending thoracic aorta just below to the left subclavian artery and above to the renal arteries. A pneumatic device fills the balloon with helium at the start of diastole and deflates it just before the next systole. The ECG is the primary trigger used to initiate deflation on the upstroke of the R wave (of the QRS complex) and inflation on the T wave. IABP therapy is referred to as *counterpulsation* because the timing of the balloon is opposite that of ventricular contraction.[9]

Heart valve surgery. Heart valve surgery is a procedure to replace or repair one or more heart valves with a prosthetic valve. This surgery is indicated for patients with valves that have stenosis (do not open completely) or insufficiency (do not close completely). Valves may be mechanical or biological. Mechanical valves are constructed of metal alloys, pyrolytic carbon, and Dacron, whereas biological valves are constructed from bovine, porcine, or human (cadaver) cardiac tissue and usually contain some man-made materials.[14]

Cardiac transplant. A cardiac transplant is the transfer of a heart from one person after death to another person to treat a variety of terminal or end-stage heart conditions.[15]

Coronary artery bypass graft. Coronary revascularization is accomplished with a coronary artery bypass graft (CABG). This procedure surgically implants patent blood vessels to transport blood between the aorta and the myocardium distal to the obstructed coronary artery or arteries. The internal mammary artery, radial artery, and saphenous vein from the patient are used frequently as bypass grafts. CABG requires a sternotomy to gain access to the heart and cardiopulmonary bypass (CPB) to divert the patient's blood from the heart to the CPB machine. The CPB machine oxygenates the patient's blood and returns it to the patient, allowing the surgeon to operate on a nonbeating, bloodless heart while perfusion to organs is maintained.[16]

Peripheral artery revascularization. This procedure is accomplished using an autogenous vein or synthetic graft to bypass the lesion in the artery that is impairing perfusion. Femoropopliteal bypass is an example of this procedure in which a graft is attached to the femoral artery to divert blood around the occlusion and attached to the popliteal artery.[15] The femoral artery is clamped proximal to the insertion of the graft, allowing the surgeon to attach the graft to a bloodless artery.

Stent placement and angioplasty. A stent is an expandable mesh-like structure designed to expand in the artery to maintain patency.[16] Cardiac catheterization and coronary angiography provide images of coronary circulation to identify lesions blocking coronary arteries. If appropriate, revascularization can be performed using balloon angioplasty. During this procedure, a catheter equipped with an inflatable balloon tip is inserted into the affected coronary artery. When the blockage is located, the catheter is passed through it, the balloon is inflated, and the blockage (atherosclerotic plaque) is compressed, which dilates the artery. Intracoronary stents are often inserted into the artery during an angioplasty to hold the artery open.

Endarterectomy. Endarterectomy is a surgical procedure in which the artery is opened to remove obstructing plaque that is impairing perfusion.[10] The carotid artery is a common site for this procedure, resulting in improved perfusion to the brain and thereby preventing an ischemic stroke.

CLINICAL NURSING SKILLS FOR PERFUSION

- Assessment
- Cardiac monitoring
- Hemodynamic monitoring
  - Continuous arterial blood pressure monitoring
  - Pulmonary artery pressure monitoring
- Circulatory assist devices
  - Intra-aortic balloon pump
  - Ventricular assist device
- Medication administration
- Patient teaching

INTERRELATED CONCEPTS

Because all cells in the body depend on perfusion to carry oxygen and nutrients to cells, this concept is interrelated to nearly all of the health and illness concepts within this textbook. Concepts that most closely interrelate with perfusion are shown in Figure 18-3 and explained below.

Patients complain of **Pain** when perfusion is impaired by **Clotting**, whether it be in the coronary arteries, causing chest pain, or in the iliac or femoral arteries, causing leg pain when walking. Impaired tissue perfusion leading to ischemia creates lactic acid that contributes to pain. Because impaired tissue perfusion to the legs causes pain during walking, peripheral arterial disease reduces the **Mobility** of patients due to the pain they experience. Walking is beneficial to exercise the heart and improve central perfusion, an important health promotion behavior. **Nutrition** also is an important health promotion consideration for heart and vessel health—and adequate perfusion in the gastrointestinal system is necessary for the digestion and metabolism of nutrients. **Inflammation** occurs when there is tissue damage, which is linked to ischemia. Also, it is the inflammation that develops after damage to the endothelium of arteries that initiates atherosclerosis. Impaired perfusion results in impaired **Gas Exchange** because the blood carries oxygen from alveoli to cells and carbon dioxide away from cells to alveoli for exhalation. **Elimination** from the kidneys is an indirect indicator of cardiac output because blood flows from the heart through the aorta to the renal arteries and through nephrons that

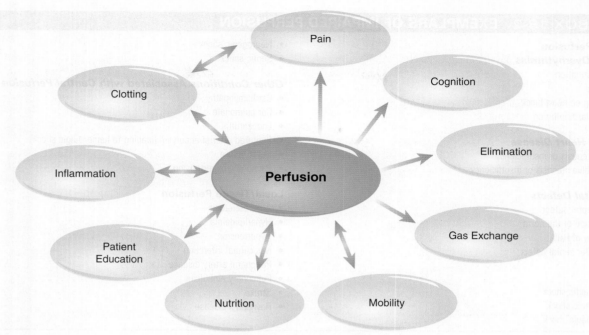

FIGURE 18-3 Perfusion and Interrelated Concepts

produce urine. **Cognition** is altered when perfusion to the brain is impaired. The neurons require a consistent supply of oxygen and glucose to maintain function. **Patient Education** is central to the prevention of cardiovascular disease as well as management of cardiovascular disease.

CLINICAL EXEMPLARS

Multiple conditions contribute to impaired perfusion—far more than are described in this text. Box 18-2 lists common conditions associated with impaired perfusion across the lifespan; further details about these conditions can be found in pathophysiology, medical–surgical, and pediatric nursing textbooks.

Featured Exemplars
Atrial Fibrillation
Atrial fibrillation is a disorganization of atrial electrical activity due to impulses triggering atrial contraction that are not initiated from the SA node. The result is ineffective atrial contraction, with atrial rates as high as 350–600 beats per minute. Because the ventricles do not have time to fill, cardiac output is reduced. The pulse rhythm is irregularly irregular. It occurs in approximately 3% of people older than age 65 years, and its prevalence increases with age. Clots form in the atria due to blood stasis, which can become emboli that flow to the brain causing strokes. Atrial fibrillation accounts for as many as 20% of all strokes.[9]

Heart Failure
Heart failure is associated with long-standing hypertension, coronary artery disease, and myocardial infarction and affects 1 out of every 100 older adults. These cardiac disorders impair the pumping and/or filling of the heart. In left-sided failure, the most common type, the impairment causes blood to back up into the left atrium and pulmonary veins. In right-sided failure, the blood backs up into the right atrium and venous circulation. Approximately 5 million people in the United States have heart failure, which represents the most common reason for hospital admission in adults older than age 65 years.[16]

Hyperlipidemia
Elevated blood levels of cholesterol and triglycerides indicate hyperlipidemia. Diets high in cholesterol and genetic inheritance are common causes of hypercholesterolemia. Triglycerides are a simple fat compound obtained from animal and vegetable fats. Both cholesterol and triglycerides circulate within lipoproteins and may increase the risk of thickening arterial walls in coronary or cerebral vessels, leading to myocardial infarction or stroke. An estimated 71 million American adults (33.5%) have high cholesterol, but in one-third of them, the condition is under control with medication, exercise, and diet.[17]

Hypertension
A persistent systolic blood pressure of 140 mm Hg or greater, a persistent diastolic blood pressure of 90 mm Hg or greater, or current use of antihypertensive medication is classified as hypertension.[18] Adequate blood pressure is needed to maintain tissue perfusion in rest and activity. Elevated blood pressure increases with workload of the heart and damages endothelium contributing to atherosclerosis. Because hypertension has no symptoms, people should routinely have their blood pressures measured. One in three adults in the United States has high blood pressure. The overall risk for hypertension increases with age.[19]

Myocardial Infarction
When perfusion from the coronary arteries is impaired, sustained ischemia causes irreversible myocardial cell death (necrosis) resulting in a myocardial infarction (MI). The MI is one part of acute coronary syndrome, which includes unstable angina caused by temporary ischemia to the myocardium as well as specific types of MI.[4] Most MIs are caused by a thrombus. Risk factors include high blood pressure, high cholesterol, and smoking. Chest pain, shortness of breath, and lightheadedness are common symptoms. The goal of care is to treat the MI as soon as possible to preserve cardiac muscle.[4] Coronary artery disease is the most common type of heart disease, with 720,000 Americans diagnosed with an MI and 380,000 dying annually.[20]

■■■ BOX 18-2   EXEMPLARS OF IMPAIRED PERFUSION

Central Perfusion

Cardiac Dysrhythmias
- Atrial fibrillation
- Asystole
- Third-degree heart block
- Ventricular fibrillation

Valvular Heart Disease
- Aortic stenosis or insufficiency
- Mitral valve stenosis or insufficiency

Congenital Defects
- Atrial septal defect
- Coarctation of the aorta
- Tetralogy of Fallot
- Ventricular septal defect

Shock
- Anaphylactic shock
- Cardiogenic shock
- Hemorrhagic shock

- Neurogenic shock
- Septic shock

Other Conditions Associated with Central Perfusion
- Cardiomyopathy
- Cor pulmonale
- Endocarditis
- Ruptured arterial aneurysm (leading to hemorrhagic shock)
- Heart failure
- Pulmonary hypertension

Local/Tissue Perfusion
- Atherosclerosis
- Hyperlipidemia
- Hypertension
- Myocardial infarction
- Peripheral artery disease
- Pulmonary embolism
- Stroke
- Raynaud's disease

Peripheral Artery Disease

Peripheral artery disease (PAD) involves the gradual thickening of artery walls, resulting in progressive narrowing in upper and lower extremities that reduces perfusion. The risk for PAD increases with age, and it typically appears in the sixth to eighth decades. Risk factors include tobacco use, hyperlipidemia, uncontrolled hypertension, and diabetes mellitus. Manifestations include decreased to absent peripheral pulses; cool skin temperature; loss of hair and thin, taut, shiny skin on affected extremities; and ischemic pain during exercise (intermittent claudication).[10]

Ventricular Septal Defect

This birth defect develops when the muscular wall (septum) separating the right and left ventricles does not fully form, creating a hole between the ventricles. This hole allows oxygenated blood to leak from the left ventricle to the right ventricle instead of flowing into the aorta and into the body.[21] Ventricular septal defect is the most common congenital heart defect, estimated to occur in 42 of every 10,000 infants.[22] It can lead to heart failure, pulmonary hypertension, endocarditis, dysrhythmias, and delayed growth. Small holes may heal on their own, whereas large holes may require surgical repair.[21]

CASE STUDY

Source: joyfnp/iStock/Thinkstock

Case Presentation

George Jones is a 59-year-old male who has arrived at the emergency department with chest pain. He had experienced this chest pain for 30 minutes, and it was not relieved after taking four nitroglycerin tablets 5 minutes apart. He reports the pain feels "like an elephant is sitting on my chest." He is diaphoretic and appears anxious. His vital signs are as follows: temperature, 99°F; blood pressure, 100/68 mm Hg; heart rate, 110 beats/minute; and respiratory rate, 24 breaths/minute. Mr. Jones is overweight and has type 2 diabetes mellitus, hyperlipidemia, and hypertension. He quit smoking last year after a 40-year history of smoking one pack of cigarettes a day. His troponin level is elevated, and the ECG shows ST segment elevation. The nurse administers oxygen and draws blood for arterial blood gas analysis. Mr. Jones is told he will have a cardiac catheterization to locate the blockage, determine its severity, and evaluate left ventricular function.

The cardiac catheterization revealed a 90% blockage in one coronary artery. The cardiologist performed a balloon angioplasty and placed a stent in Mr. Jones' blocked coronary artery to re-establish perfusion. Mr. Jones was admitted to the cardiovascular surgery unit and was ambulating within 24 hours after stent placement. The nurse's goals for Mr. Jones' plan of care are to maintain effective cardiac output, control pain, relieve anxiety, and balance physical activity with energy-conserving activities. The nurse also played a significant role in Mr. Jones' therapy by teaching him and his family about lifestyle changes, including diet and exercise, and the purpose of his prescribed medications, including adverse effects and the importance of following the medication regimen. Mr. Jones is referred for cardiac rehabilitation after discharge.

Case Analysis

This case exemplifies an impairment of local perfusion of the heart that could have developed into central impairment if Mr. Jones had not been treated. He had several risk factors, including obesity, which contributed to type 2 diabetes mellitus. The hyperlipidemia and diabetes mellitus contributed to the blockage of his coronary artery and his hypertension, which increased the workload of his heart. Mr. Jones' manifestations were consistent with impaired tissue perfusion to the myocardium. The stent re-established perfusion to the myocardium. Mr. Jones' recovery and prevention of further cardiovascular disease will be improved by his lifestyle changes.

ACCESS EXEMPLAR LINKS IN YOUR GIDDENS EBOOK

REFERENCES

1. Schroeder M, Delaney A, Baker A: The child with cardiovascular dysfunction. In Hockenberry M, Wilson D, editors: *Wong's nursing care of infants and children*, ed 10, St Louis, 2015, Elsevier, pp 1251–1321.

2. Wilson S, Giddens J: *Health assessment for nursing practice*, ed 5, St Louis, 2013, Mosby.

3. McCance K, Grey T: Altered cellular and tissue biology. In Huether S, McCance K, editors: *Understanding pathophysiology*, ed 5, St Louis, 2012, Elsevier, pp 59–97.

4. Bucher L, Castellucci D: Nursing management: Coronary artery disease and acute coronary syndrome. In Lewis S, editor: *Medical–surgical nursing: Assessment and management of clinical problems*, ed 8, St Louis, 2011, Mosby, pp 760–796.

5. Malone M: Nursing management: Lower respiratory problems. In Lewis S, editor: *Medical–surgical nursing: Assessment and management of clinical problems*, ed 8, St Louis, 2011, Mosby, pp 545–586.

6. Conlon P, Wilson D: The child with respiratory dysfunction. In Hockenberry M, Wilson D, editors: *Wong's nursing care of infants and children*, ed 10, St Louis, 2015, Elsevier, pp 1164–1250.

7. Pagana K, Pagana T: *Mosby's diagnostic and laboratory test reference*, ed 10, St Louis, 2011, Mosby.

8. DiSabatino A, Bucher L, et al: Nursing assessment: Cardiovascular system. In Lewis S, editor: *Medical–surgical nursing: Assessment and management of clinical problems*, ed 8, St Louis, 2011, Mosby, pp 715–737.

9. Bucher L: Nursing management: Dysrhythmias. In Lewis S, editor: *Medical–surgical nursing: Assessment and management of clinical problems*, ed 8, St Louis, 2011, Mosby, pp 818–840.

10. Wipke-Tevis D, Rich K, et al: Nursing management: Vascular disorders. In Lewis S, editor: *Medical–surgical nursing: Assessment and management of clinical problems*, ed 8, St Louis, 2011, Mosby, pp 866–896.

11. American Heart Association: Getting healthy, (n.d.). Retrieved from: <http://www.heart.org/HEARTORG/GettingHealthy/GettingHealthy_UCM_001078_SubHomePage.jsp>.

12. U.S. Preventive Services Task Force: Home, 2015. Retrieved from: <http://www.uspreventiveservicestaskforce.org>.

13. Lehne R: *Pharmacology for nursing care*, ed 7, Philadelphia, 2010, Saunders.

14. Bucher L, Seckel M, et al: Nursing management: Critical care. In Lewis S, editor: *Medical–surgical nursing: Assessment and management of clinical problems*, ed 8, St Louis, 2011, Mosby, pp 1681–1716.

15. Kupper N, Mitchell D, et al: Nursing management: Inflammatory and structural heart disorders. In Lewis S, editor: *Medical–surgical nursing: Assessment and management of clinical problems*, ed 8, St Louis, 2011, Mosby, pp 841–865.

16. Bouffard L, et al: Nursing management: Heart failure. In Lewis S, editor: *Medical-surgical nursing: assessment and management of clinical problems*, ed 8, St Louis, 2011, Mosby/Elsevier, pp 797–817.

17. Centers for Disease Control and Prevention: High cholesterol facts, 2015. Retrieved from: <http://www.cdc.gov/cholesterol/facts.htm>.

18. The seventh report of the Joint National Committee on Prevention, Detection, Evaluation, and Treatment of High Blood Pressure (JNC-7). *JAMA* 289:2560, 2003. Retrieved from: <http://www.nhlbi.nih.gov/guidelines/hypertension/index.htm>.

19. Bradley E: Nursing management: Hypertension. In Lewis S, editor: *Medical–surgical nursing: Assessment and management of clinical problems*, ed 8, St Louis, 2011, Mosby, pp 738–759.

20. Centers for Disease Control and Prevention: Heart disease facts, 2014. Retrieved from: <http://www.cdc.gov/heartdisease/facts.htm>.

21. Mayo Clinic: Congenital heart disease in adults, 2014. Retrieved from: <http://www.mayoclinic.org/diseases-conditions/congenital-heart-disease/basics/definition/con-20034800>.

22. Centers for Disease Control and Prevention: Facts about ventricular septal defect, 2014. Retrieved from: <http://www.cdc.gov/ncbddd/heartdefects/VentricularSeptalDefect.html>.

Gas Exchange

Susan Wilson

All cells depend on a consistent supply of oxygen and removal of waste. For this reason, gas exchange is a critical concept for nurses to understand and incorporate into practice. The purpose of this concept presentation is to help nurses acquire an understanding about gas exchange across the lifespan. In practice, nurses promote individuals' healthy behaviors that optimize gas exchange, identify individuals at risk of impaired gas exchange, recognize when individuals are experiencing impairment in gas exchange, and respond with appropriate interventions.

DEFINITION

Gas exchange is defined as *the process by which oxygen is transported to cells and carbon dioxide is transported from cells*. This normal physiological process requires interaction among the neurologic, respiratory, and cardiovascular systems. The lungs deliver oxygen to the pulmonary capillaries, where it is carried by hemoglobin to cells. After cellular metabolism, carbon dioxide is carried in hemoglobin to the lungs, where it is exhaled. Thus, adequate functioning of these systems is essential for optimal gas exchange. Several other terms are important as they relate to this concept. *Ischemia* is insufficient flow of oxygenated blood to tissues that may result in hypoxemia and subsequent cell injury or death. *Hypoxia* is insufficient oxygen reaching cells, whereas *anoxia* is the total lack of oxygen in body tissues. *Hypoxemia* is reduced oxygenation of arterial blood.[1,2]

SCOPE

The concept of gas exchange and problems associated with impaired gas exchange represent a variety of physiological processes. Variations in gas exchange are seen among individuals across the lifespan, with multiple causative factors and a wide range of impact and duration from any cause. From the broadest perspective, the scope of gas exchange represents a spectrum of optimal gas exchange and impaired gas exchange (Figure 19-1). The further gas exchange is impaired, the more compromised the body becomes due to insufficient oxygen (hypoxia). Cessation of gas exchange leads to anoxia.

NORMAL PHYSIOLOGICAL PROCESS

The process of gas exchange is presented in Figure 19-2. Breathing is involuntary because changes in ventilation rate and volume are stimulated and regulated automatically by the nervous system to maintain arterial blood gases within normal ranges. Chemoreceptors in the medulla sense carbon dioxide levels, and when carbon dioxide concentration is elevated, these receptors transmit impulses to the diaphragm and intercostal muscles to contract. As the diaphragm contracts, negative pressure pulls in 21% oxygen from the atmosphere. The nose warms and humidifies the air, which flows to alveoli through patent airways (trachea and bronchi). Alveolar walls are lined with a single layer of epithelial cells, called type I alveolar cells, that provide structure. In between these type I cells are thicker type II alveolar cells that produce surfactant—a lipoprotein that coats the inner surface of alveoli to keep them open. The high pressure of oxygen in alveoli causes it to diffuse into pulmonary capillaries, where it dissolves into the plasma and attaches to hemoglobin in erythrocytes to be transported (perfused) to cells. Oxygen dissolved in plasma is measured clinically by the partial pressure of oxygen in the artery or PaO_2. Oxygen attached to hemoglobin is measured clinically by the saturation of arterial hemoglobin or SaO_2. At the cellular level, oxygen is released from hemoglobin, which is called hemoglobin desaturation. Oxygen dissolves in plasma and diffuses into the interstitial space and then diffuses into cells to be used in metabolic processes.[1]

Carbon dioxide, a by-product of cellular metabolism, is transported to the atmosphere in the reverse order of oxygen and lowers the arterial carbon dioxide level. The high pressure of the carbon dioxide in cells causes it to diffuse into plasma, which is measured clinically by the partial pressure of carbon dioxide in the artery or $PaCO_2$. When the amount of $PaCO_2$ decreases, it turns off signals to the medulla to initiate inhalation until the carbon dioxide level rises again to repeat the gas exchange process.

The term gas exchange can be misinterpreted because the word "exchange" can mean "swap, substitute, or trade." However, as described by Dalton's law of partial pressures, the pressure exerted by each gas is independent of the pressure exerted by other gases. Oxygen diffuses from the alveoli to the pulmonary capillaries because the pressure of oxygen in the alveoli is higher than the pressure of oxygen in the capillaries. Gases diffuse from areas of high concentration to areas of low concentration.[1,2] The belief that oxygen diffuses based on the diffusion of carbon dioxide is incorrect. These two gases are independent; they do not exchange with each other.

Age-Related Differences

Babies born after 30 weeks of gestation have a sufficient surfactant to prevent alveoli from collapsing after every exhalation. Infants are obligate nose breathers until approximately 3 months. Should their nasal

FIGURE 19-1 Scope of Concept: Gas Exchange

passages become occluded, they may have difficulty breathing. Sneezing occurs commonly as a way to clear the nose. Respiratory patterns for newborns may be irregular, with brief pauses between breaths of no more than 10–15 seconds.[3]

For older adults, diminished strength of respiratory muscles reduces the maximal inspiratory and expiratory force. This may result in a weaker cough. The alveoli become less elastic and more fibrous, causing dyspnea more frequently. Older adults experience a reduction in erythrocytes, which increases their risk of anemia.[3]

VARIATIONS AND CONTEXT

Variations in gas exchange may occur in individuals across the lifespan with a wide range of impact. Problems with gas exchange may occur from babies born before 30 weeks of gestation when surfactant is not yet present to adults 100 years or older who experience expected changes due to cigarette smoke, air pollution, and aging. Changes in gas exchange can be temporary, long term, or permanent. Disorders that lead to changes in gas exchange include acute illnesses such as asthma or pneumonia and chronic disorders such as chronic obstructive pulmonary disease (COPD), which includes emphysema and

chronic bronchitis. Conditions that specifically involve gas exchange include neurologic (including those affecting the brain or spinal cord), cardiovascular (including blood flow in heart, arteries, and veins), and hematologic (including anemia). Conditions in these body systems can be caused from congenital defects, genetic conditions, injury, inflammation, infections, and malignant neoplasms. The three broad categories that represent problems associated with this concept are ventilation, transport, and perfusion.

Ventilation

Ventilation is the process of inhaling oxygen into the lungs and exhaling carbon dioxide from the lungs. Ventilation may be impaired by the unavailability of oxygen, such as at high altitudes, as well as by any disorder affecting the nasopharynx and lungs. Impaired ventilation may occur in the following situations:

- Inadequate bone, muscle, or nerve function to move air into the lungs, such as rib fracture that reduces inhalation due to pain, muscle weakness that prevents full thoracic expansion, or cervical spinal cord injury that limits movement of the diaphragm
- Narrowed airways from bronchoconstriction (e.g., in asthma) or from obstruction (e.g., in chronic bronchitis or cystic fibrosis)

FIGURE 19-2 Process of Gas Exchange

- Poor gas diffusion in the alveoli, such as in pulmonary edema, acute respiratory distress syndrome, or pneumonia

Clinical manifestations depend on the area affected, but individuals must work harder to breathe or must change the route by which air enters the lungs. When individuals have edema of the sinuses, they are unable to breathe through the nose; instead, they breathe through the mouth until the edema subsides.

Transport

Transport refers to the availability of hemoglobin and its ability to carry oxygen from alveoli to cells for metabolism and to carry carbon dioxide produced by cellular metabolism from cells to alveoli to be eliminated. *Altered transport of oxygen* occurs when an insufficient number or quality of erythrocytes is available to carry oxygen or when the amount of hemoglobin in the blood is low. This occurs when patients have anemia for any reason. Blood loss from acute or chronic causes reduces the number of erythrocytes, thus making hemoglobin unavailable to carry oxygen. Finally, destruction of erythrocytes occurs in hemolytic anemias when the spleen destroys these cells prematurely, such as in sickle cell crisis.

Perfusion

Perfusion refers to the ability of blood to transport oxygen-containing hemoglobin to cells and return carbon dioxide-containing hemoglobin to the alveoli. Inadequate or impaired perfusion can be caused by decreased cardiac output as well as by thrombi, emboli, vessel narrowing, vasoconstriction, or blood loss. (See Concept 18 Perfusion.)

CONSEQUENCES

When gas exchange is compromised for any reason, a reduction or cessation of oxygen occurs that affects the cells, triggering a number of physiological problems depending on the extent of impairment.

With mild impairment, an individual often experiences fatigue. This symptom actually helps the body compensate through rest—thus reducing oxygen demand. Heart rate and respiratory rate also may increase in an attempt to increase oxygen delivery to cells. When impaired gas exchange becomes more pronounced, a reduction of oxygen at the cellular level leads to reduced mitochondrial respiration and oxidative metabolism. Carbon dioxide transport from the cells to the alveoli leads to a buildup of acid. Thus, when the underlying problem is associated with ventilation, respiratory acidosis may result. Metabolic acidosis can occur if the underlying problem is associated with transport or perfusion. If the impairment is prolonged or severe, cellular ischemia and necrosis can occur. A complete cessation of gas exchange occurs when breathing or perfusion stops and quickly results in death.

RISK FACTORS

Because adequate gas exchange is required for life, all individuals—regardless of age, gender, race, or socioeconomic status—potentially are at risk for gas exchange impairment. Nurses need to recognize, however, that some individuals are at greater risk for impairment. Some of these risk factors are controllable due to lifestyle behaviors, whereas others are not.

Populations at Risk

Populations at greatest risk are infants, young children, and older adults. Infants are at risk because they have fetal hemoglobin. Fetal hemoglobin is present for the first 5 months of life and results in shortened survival of erythrocytes, causing physiological anemia by

age 2 or 3 months. Contributing to anemia at approximately 6 months of age is the lower level of hemoglobin caused by gradually diminishing maternal iron stores.[4] Infants and young children are at risk for impaired gas exchange because they have less alveolar surface area for gas exchange as well as narrow branching of peripheral airways that are easily obstructed by mucus, edema, or foreign objects.[5]

Older adults are at risk for impaired gas exchange because of anatomic and physiological changes that are expected with advanced age. The chest wall becomes stiffer with loss of elastic recoil. Respiratory muscles become weaker, reducing the effectiveness of coughing—normally a protective mechanism to prevent aspiration. Additional expected changes are dilation of alveoli, decreased surface area for gas diffusion, and decreased pulmonary capillary network. Finally, the ability to initiate an immune response to infection is decreased in older adults.[1]

Individual Risk Factors

A number of personal risk factors are linked to impairment in gas exchange. Nonmodifiable risk factors include age (as described under Populations at Risk), air pollution, and allergies. *Tobacco use* is the single most preventable cause of death and disease in the United States and is the most significant risk factor for impaired gas exchange. Boxes 19-1 and 19-2 present data about those who use tobacco. The percentages in each of the five categories in Box 19-2 have decreased over the last few years, indicating fewer people smoking. Risk for aspiration is increased during an altered state of consciousness such as from a chemical alteration (e.g., alcoholism, drug overdose, and anesthesia) or from a neurologic disorder (e.g., head injury, seizure, and stroke). Patients requiring tracheal intubation are at risk because of the bypassing of protective mechanisms for the alveoli. Bed rest and prolonged immobility reduce thoracic expansion, which can increase the risk for atelectasis and pneumonia. Chronic diseases, such as cystic fibrosis, COPD, or heart failure, increase risk because of mucus and fluid accumulation in the airways and alveoli. Immunosuppression alters the body's natural ability to fight infection, whether it is from a systemic disorder (e.g., aplastic anemia), a cancer (e.g., leukemia), or a treatment regimen (e.g., cancer chemotherapy).

ASSESSMENT

Nurses gather data from the patient's history, physical examination, and the patient's diagnostic test results. Assessment of gas exchange involves recognizing indications of adequate and inadequate ventilation, transport, and perfusion. Adequate ventilation is apparent when the following occur:

- Breathing is quiet and effortless at a rate appropriate for age.
- Oxygen saturation (SaO_2) is between 95 and 100%.
- Skin, nail beds, and lips are appropriate colors for the patient's race.
- Thorax is symmetric with equal thoracic expansion bilaterally.
- Spinous processes are in alignment; scapulae are bilaterally symmetric.
- Anteroposterior (AP) diameter of the chest is approximately a 1:2 ratio of AP to lateral diameter.
- Trachea is midline.
- Breath sounds are clear bilaterally.[3]

History
Baseline History

When collecting subjective data from patients, nurses ask about lifestyle behaviors, including diet, exercise, and smoking habits. Nurses ask about patients' work and home environments to identify potential respiratory irritants. Also, patients are asked about any chronic diseases

BOX 19-1   Use of Tobacco Products by Adults, Adolescents, and Children

Adults

- 20.6% of adults ages 18 years or older were current cigarette smokers in 2008 (age adjusted to the year 2000 standard population).
- 2.3% of adults ages 18 years or older were current users of snuff or chewing tobacco products in 2005 (age adjusted to the year 2000 standard population).
- 2.2% of adults ages 18 years or older were current cigar smokers in 2005 (age adjusted to the year 2000 standard population).

Adolescents

- 26.0% of adolescents in grades 9–12 used cigarettes, chewing tobacco, snuff, or cigars in the past 30 days in 2009.
- 19.5% of adolescents in grades 9–12 smoked cigarettes in the past 30 days in 2009.
- 8.9% of adolescents in grades 9–12 used smokeless (chewing tobacco or snuff) tobacco products in the past 30 days in 2009.
- 14.0% of adolescents in grades 9–12 smoked cigars in the past 30 days in 2009.

Children and Adolescents

- 7.8% of children and adolescents ages 12–17 years who had not previously used tobacco products in their lifetime first used tobacco products in the past 12 months in 2008.

Source: From *Healthy People 2020:* 2020 Topics and objectives. Retrieved from http://www.healthypeople.gov/2020/topics-objectives/topic/tobacco-use/objectives.

BOX 19-2   Characteristics of Smokers

By Gender

- 20.5% men
- 15.8% women

By Age

- 17.3% ages 18–24 years
- 21.6% ages 25–44 years
- 19.5% ages 45–64 years
- 8.9% ages 65 years or older

By Race/Ethnicity

- 21.8% of American Indians/Alaska natives
- 10.7% Asians
- 18.1% of blacks (non-Hispanic)
- 12.5% of Hispanics
- 19.7% of whites (non-Hispanic)
- 26.1% multiple-race individuals

By Education

- 24.7% adults with 12 or less years of education (no diploma)
- 41.9% adults with a General Educational Development (GED) diploma
- 23.1% of adults with a high school diploma
- 9.1% of adults with an undergraduate college degree
- 5.9% of adults with a postgraduate college degree

By Poverty Status

- 27.0% of adults who live below the poverty level
- 17.0% of adults who live at or above the poverty level

Source: From Centers for Disease Control and Prevention: Current cigarette smoking among adults in the United States, 2015. Retrieved from http://www.cdc.gov/tobacco/data_statistics/fact_sheets/adult_data/cig_smoking/index.htm.

as well as allergies that may affect the respiratory system. Nurses ask patients about medications they take, both prescription and over-the-counter, and the reason each medication is taken as well as its efficacy.[3]

Problem-Based History

The following symptoms are often reported by individuals experiencing gas exchange impairment: cough, shortness of breath, and chest pain. When a symptom is reported, a symptom analysis is conducted.

Cough. When a cough is reported or observed, the patient should be asked if the cough causes fatigue or interferes with sleep. The patient should also be asked if the cough is productive or nonproductive. Inquire about the color and consistency of productive coughs. Question the patient about factors that aggravate and alleviate the cough as well as any self-treatment measures taken to relieve the cough. Also, the patient should be asked about other symptoms that accompany the cough, such as fever or shortness of breath.[3]

Shortness of breath. Patients may report they have had to stop climbing stairs to "catch their breath." Others may report having to sleep sitting up or using several pillows to prop themselves up during the night. Lightheadedness may be reported as a result of inadequate oxygen transport to the brain. Inquire about what precipitated the shortness of breath and if it occurs during inhalation or exhalation or both. The patient should be asked what factors aggravate and alleviate the dyspnea and also if there are other symptoms, such as cough, chest pain, or swelling of the feet and ankles.[3]

Chest pain with breathing. The patient should be asked what activity is associated with the chest pain when it occurs and how long the pain lasts. Inquire if the onset of chest pain was gradual or sudden,

and ask for a description of the pain, such as sharp or dull, pain radiation, and severity.[3]

Examination Findings

Vital Signs

Inadequate gas exchange is noticed by changes in vital signs such as an increase in respiratory rate, decrease in SaO_2, increase in heart rate, and increase in temperature. An increased respiratory rate may be due to increased work of breathing. The SaO_2 value may drop below 95% when oxygen is not being transported by hemoglobin to cells. Tachycardia may occur either from anxiety caused by not being able to breathe well or from anemia. Temperature may be elevated because of an infection, such as pneumonia or respiratory syncytial virus.

Inspection

If a patient is having difficulty breathing, the nurse may notice the patient assuming a position to ease the work of breathing (e.g., sitting leaning forward). Patients with impaired gas exchange often appear anxious because of the sensation of not getting enough air or a feeling of suffocation. Low oxygen saturation may impair mentation as a result of lack of adequate oxygen supply to the brain. Patients may use accessory muscles on inspiration to help get air into the lungs. They may use pursed-lip breathing on exhalation to keep airways open longer. The skin and lips may appear pale because of anemia or hypoxemia. A late sign of hypoxemia is cyanosis. Clubbing of nails develops in patients with chronic hypoxic disorders such as cystic fibrosis or

COPD. When patients develop a barrel chest from air trapped in alveoli from emphysema, their anteroposterior to lateral diameter ratio changes from a normal of 1:2 to 1:1. The thorax may be asymmetric with unequal thoracic expansion unilaterally attributable to pneumothorax. Scoliosis is a curvature of vertebrae that creates asymmetric expansion of the thorax as well as malalignment of spinous processes and scapulae. The trachea shifts from midline away from the lung that is experiencing a tension pneumothorax.[3]

Additional assessment findings commonly noted in infants and young children with inadequate gas exchange are flaring of the nares, chest wall retractions on inspiration, grunting on inspiration, cyanosis around the lips when sucking, and the need to stop during feeding to breathe.[5]

Auscultation

During auscultation, narrowed bronchi may produce expiratory and/or inspiratory wheezing or stridor. Mucus or secretions in the bronchi may create rhonchi, and fluid in alveoli may generate crackles.[3]

Diagnostic Tests

There are a number of diagnostic tests associated with gas exchange that are used to assess for impairment.

Laboratory Tests

Arterial blood gases. Arterial blood gases reveal measurements of pH, oxygen, carbon dioxide, and bicarbonate concentrations in arterial blood. They are used to detect respiratory acidosis and alkalosis. Respiratory acidosis develops during hypoventilation when carbon dioxide is retained, such as in patients with COPD. Respiratory alkalosis develops during hyperventilation when excessive carbon dioxide is exhaled, such as during anxiety or hysteria. Arterial blood gases include the following measures:

- pH is inversely proportional to the actual hydrogen ion concentration. Normal values are between 7.35 and 7.45. pH values less than 7.35 indicate acidosis, and those greater than 7.45 indicate alkalosis.[6]
- SaO_2 is an abbreviation for "saturation of arterial oxygen" and represents the percentage of arterial hemoglobin that is saturated with oxygen. This value accounts for approximately 97% of arterial oxygen. The normal value for adults is 95–100% and for newborns 40–90%.[6]
- PaO_2 is an abbreviation for the "partial pressure of arterial oxygen" and represents the pressure of oxygen dissolved in arterial blood. This value accounts for approximately 3% of oxygen. The normal value for adults is 80–100 mm Hg and for newborns 60–70 mm Hg.[6]
- $PaCO_2$ is an abbreviation for the "partial pressure of arterial carbon dioxide" and represents the pressure of carbon dioxide dissolved in arterial blood. The $PaCO_2$ is a measurement of ventilation capability. The normal value for adults is 35–45 mm Hg and for children younger than age 2 years 26–41 mm Hg.[6]
- HCO_3 is an abbreviation for bicarbonate and represents most of the carbon dioxide in the blood. Normal values are 22–26 mEq/L. There is a direct proportional relationship between HCO_3 concentration and pH; thus, when HCO_3 concentration is above normal, the pH increases, indicating alkalosis. When the HCO_3 concentration is below normal, the pH decreases, indicating acidosis. The kidneys compensate for primary respiratory acid–base alterations. For example, in respiratory acidosis, the kidneys compensate by retaining HCO_3 in an attempt to regain acid–base balance. However, in respiratory alkalosis, the kidneys compensate by excreting HCO_3 in an attempt to regain acid–base balance.[6]

Complete blood count. The complete blood count is obtained from venous blood and includes measurements of red blood cell count (RBC) count, hemoglobin (Hb), hematocrit (Hct), and white blood cell (WBC) count:

- RBC count determines the oxygen-carrying capacity of the blood. Each RBC carries hemoglobin that transports oxygen to tissues and carbon dioxide from tissues. Patients who have anemia have decreased numbers of RBCs, which reduces the patient's oxygen-carrying ability.
- Hb level reflects the number of RBCs in the venous blood and determines the oxygen and carbon dioxide transport capability.
- Hct measures the percentage of venous blood volume that is composed of RBCs. The Hct closely reflects the Hb and RBC values.
- WBC count measures the number of leukocytes in venous blood. The WBC differential measures the percentage of each leukocyte (e.g., neutrophils, eosinophils, basophils, or monocytes) contained within the total number of WBCs. Elevations in total WBC count occur when there is inflammation, and often the inflammation is due to infection. Decreases in WBC count occur with certain cancers and as an adverse effect of chemical or radiation therapy to treat cancer. Patients with low WBC counts are at risk for newly acquired infection because the immune system is unable to respond optimally.[6] The WBC differential is helpful in suggesting a generalized cause of the abnormal value. For example, elevated neutrophils indicate an acute inflammation, whereas increased monocytes indicate a chronic infection. Eosinophils are elevated during allergies.

Sputum examination. Studying sputum specimens can help in the diagnosis of respiratory disorders. Culture and sensitivity are performed on a single specimen to detect bacteria and determine which antibiotic is most effective. Gram stain of sputum distinguishes gram-positive from gram-negative bacteria. Testing a series of three early morning sputum samples for acid-fast bacillus is diagnostic for tuberculosis. A single sputum specimen for cytologic examination is performed to detect a pulmonary malignancy.[7]

Skin tests. Mantoux screens for tuberculosis. A positive reaction to the skin test indicates that patients have developed antibodies to *Mycobacterium tuberculosis*. Allergies detected by skin tests may indicate causes of bronchoconstriction. The sweat chloride test screens for cystic fibrosis, which produces high levels of chloride in the sweat.

Pathologic analysis. Tissue from the lungs or bronchus may be taken for pathologic analysis, particularly if a malignant tumor is suspected.

Radiologic Studies

Chest x-ray. Chest x-ray films are very useful in detecting impaired ventilation because they provide visualization of the lungs, ribs, clavicles, vertebrae, heart, and major thoracic vessels. They are useful in identifying foreign bodies, infiltrations in pneumonia, tubercles in tuberculosis, tumors in cancer, or edema. In patients with COPD, chest x-rays show the flat diaphragm and barrel chest configuration of ribs and vertebrae. Also, chest x-rays can identify pleural effusion, pneumothorax, hemothorax, or empyema.[7]

Computed tomography. Computed tomography scans of the chest produce three-dimensional images of the lungs and are useful for detecting pulmonary densities, space-occupying tumors, and pulmonary emboli.[7]

Ventilation–perfusion scans. Ventilation–perfusion (V/Q) scans use radioactive particles to diagnose disorders involving both perfusion and ventilation. Radioactive particles are injected into peripheral veins to detect impaired perfusion to the lungs. Also, inhaled radioactive particles are used to detect impaired lung function. This scan is used to diagnose pulmonary emboli.[7]

Positron emission tomography. Positron emission tomography scans use intravenous injection of radioactive chemical compounds to distinguish benign from malignant pulmonary nodules.[7]

Pulmonary Function Studies

Pulmonary function tests assess the presence and severity of diseases in large and small airways. A spirometer measures the volume of air moving in and out of the lungs and then calculates the lung capacities.[7] One example of its use is for patients with asthma. Because their bronchoconstriction worsens, they exhale less air. This finding is reported as decreased forced expiratory volume.

Pulmonary function tests are also used to distinguish between obstructive and restrictive pulmonary diseases. Because air trapping increases for patients with obstructive lung disease such as cystic fibrosis or COPD, more air remains in their lungs, which is reflected as an increase in reserve volume. Obstructive lung diseases impair patients' ability to get air out of the lungs. By contrast, patients may develop restrictive lung diseases from intrapulmonary or extrapulmonary causes. Intrapulmonary causes include pulmonary fibrosis or empyema. Extrapulmonary causes include chest wall trauma or cervical spinal cord injury. Restrictive lung diseases impair the patient's ability to get air into the lungs, as reflected in a decreased tidal volume.

Endoscopy Examination

Bronchoscopy is an endoscopic examination in which a flexible fiber-optic bronchoscope is extended through the bronchi for the purpose of diagnosis, specimen collection, or tissue biopsy.[7]

CLINICAL MANAGEMENT

Clinical management related to gas exchange includes health promotion and the management of emerging or present conditions that compromise gas exchange. The ultimate goal is to optimize gas exchange.

Primary Prevention

Primary prevention includes measures to promote health and prevent development of disease. Several measures prevent conditions known to impair gas exchange.

Infection Control

One of the simplest primary prevention measures is infection control. Proper hand hygiene helps to prevent respiratory tract infections. All individuals should be taught the importance of hand hygiene and proper hand washing technique; in addition, individuals should be instructed to clean surfaces that are frequently touched, such as doorknobs and countertops. Coughing or sneezing into a tissue or into the elbow or sleeve reduces the particles delivered into the air. Avoiding large groups of people reduces the airborne transmission of microorganisms.

Smoking Cessation

Smoking cessation is important for both primary prevention, discussed here, and an intervention to treat disease. *Healthy People 2020* goals related to tobacco use include reducing tobacco use and initiation by adolescents and adults; adopting policies and strategies to increase access, affordability, and use of smoking cessation services and treatments; and establish policies to reduce exposure to secondhand smoke, increase cost of tobacco, restrict tobacco advertising, and reduce illegal sales to minors.[8]

Nicotine in tobacco products is the psychoactive drug that produces dependence, the most common form of chemical dependence in the United States. The American Lung Association and American Cancer Society have resources to help patients stop smoking.[9,10] Quitting smoking is difficult and may require multiple attempts. Smokers often report lack of success in smoking cessation because of stress, weight gain, and withdrawal symptoms, which include irritability, anxiety, difficulty concentrating, and increased appetite.

People who are successful at smoking cessation greatly reduce their risk for disease and premature death. In addition to nicotine, cigarette smoke contains at least 250 chemicals known to be toxic or carcinogenic.[11] Health benefits of smoking cessation include reducing the risk for lung and other cancers and reducing the risk for coronary heart disease, stroke, peripheral vascular disease, and COPD. When women in their reproductive years quit smoking, they reduce the risk for infertility. Smoking cessation in women who are pregnant reduces the risk of delivering a low-birth-weight infant.[11]

Immunizations

Immunizations prevent infection by bacteria or viruses, such as diphtheria, *Haemophilus influenzae* type b (Hib), H1N1 flu, influenza, measles, pneumococcal pneumonia, pertussis, and rubella. Schedules for these immunizations from infancy to adulthood are found on the Centers for Disease Control and Prevention website.[12]

Preventing Postoperative Pulmonary Complications

After a surgical procedure, patients are encouraged to deep breathe and cough at least every 2 hours and/or use an incentive spirometer to prevent pneumonia and atelectasis. This device encourages deep breathing for patients and measures the air inhaled as an outcome indicator that is useful for nursing assessment.

Preventing deep vein thrombosis is essential for all patients who are less active than usual so that pulmonary emboli are prevented. This includes patients after a surgical procedure or those whose disease process prevents them from ambulating as much as usual. One intervention is to subcutaneously administer an anticoagulant to reduce clotting of platelets. Another intervention is to apply elastic stockings to the legs or use intermittent compression devices to the lower legs to prevent venous stasis. A third intervention is to encourage ambulation as soon as possible.

Secondary Prevention (Screening)

Secondary prevention includes screening and early diagnosis and prompt treatment of existing health problems. Its purpose is to shorten the duration and severity of consequences. There are few routine screenings for problems associated with gas exchange. A Mantoux skin test may be administered to individuals who have exposure risks to tuberculosis.

Collaborative Interventions
Smoking Cessation

Although smoking cessation is typically considered primary prevention (to prevent respiratory illness), it is also considered an important intervention strategy among individuals who have a disease process because smoking exacerbates respiratory and cardiovascular disease.

Pharmacotherapy

Pharmacotherapy plays a very important role in managing individuals with impaired gas exchange. Agents can be used to open upper and lower airways to improve gas exchange by dilating airways, reducing edema, increasing a cough's effectiveness, and killing or limiting the growth of microorganisms. Depending on the pharmacologic agent, these drugs are administered through a number of routes, including oral, intravenous, and inhalation through inhalers or nebulizer (aerosol). Descriptions of general classifications of agents are presented next; consult a pharmacology textbook for further information about specific agents.

Drugs that affect upper airways. Antihistamines relieve symptoms of sneezing, rhinorrhea, and nasal itching experienced in allergic rhinitis. They are more effective when taken prophylactically. Antihistamines block the histamine$_1$ receptors to cause vasoconstriction and decreased capillary permeability of small arterioles and venules.[13]

Decongestants relieve congestion in passageways and sinuses. Intranasal glucocorticoids exert an anti-inflammatory effect to prevent or suppress major symptoms of allergic rhinitis such as congestion, rhinorrhea, sneezing, nasal itching, and erythema. Sympathomimetics act as decongestants by activating the α_1-adrenergic receptors on nasal blood vessels to cause vasoconstriction that shrinks edematous membranes, thereby reducing nasal drainage.[13]

Lower airway bronchodilators. Glucocorticoids reduce bronchial hyperreactivity that occurs in asthma by suppressing inflammation. Specifically, they decrease synthesis and release of inflammatory mediators such as leukotrienes, histamine, and prostaglandins; decrease infiltration of inflammatory cells such as eosinophils and leukocytes; and decrease edema of airway mucosa. They may be given by inhalation, orally, or intravenously.

Sympathomimetic agents are β_2 agonists that act on these receptors to relax the bronchial smooth muscle of the lung to relieve bronchospasm. These agents stimulate the normal sympathetic nervous system to open airways.[13]

Anticholinergics improve lung function by blocking muscarinic receptors in the bronchi, causing bronchodilation. These agents block the normal parasympathetic nervous system so it cannot stimulate constriction of airways.[13]

Agents to help cough up mucus. Mucolytics react directly with the mucus to make it more liquid. Expectorants cause the cough to be more productive by stimulating the flow of respiratory tract secretions.

Agents to suppress cough. Coughing is a protective mechanism and is useful to expectorate sputum. However, when coughing is chronic and nonproductive, it may prevent sleep or tire the patient, making cough suppression therapeutic. Most antitussives act within the central nervous system.

Antimicrobials. Respiratory tract infections are treated with antimicrobials to kill or limit growth of microorganisms.

Agents to aid smoking cessation. Many products available as first-line treatment for smoking cessation are used as nicotine replacement therapy (NRT). They are available in gum, lozenge, patch, inhaler, or nasal spray form. NRT allows smokers to substitute a drug source of nicotine for the nicotine in cigarettes and gradually withdraw the replacement nicotine to wean off nicotine completely.[13]

Oxygen Therapy

Delivery of humidified oxygen is a cornerstone of gas exchange intervention. Nurses collaborate with respiratory therapists to supply patients with oxygen and teach them how to use oxygen at home when applicable. Oxygen therapy is provided through a variety of delivery mechanisms when patients require more than 21% oxygen. A nasal cannula is used to deliver 24% oxygen (at flow rates of 1 L/min) to 44% oxygen (at flow rates of 4 L/min) through plastic nasal prongs. This is a safe and simple method that is used for long-term therapy. The cannula allows patients to eat, talk, and cough while wearing this device. Patients whose pulmonary disease causes retention of carbon dioxide, such as those with COPD, should not use oxygen levels greater than 3 L/min.[14] Their bodies have adjusted to chronically high levels of carbon dioxide (hypercapnea) so that carbon dioxide no longer acts

as the stimulant to breathe. For these patients, low blood oxygen levels become the stimulant to initiate breathing. Thus, giving these patients oxygen at more than 3 L/min can eliminate their stimulus to breathe, causing hypoventilation and, if prolonged, death.

Another oxygen delivery device is a simple face mask that covers the patient's nose and mouth. This mask delivers between 35 and 50% humidified oxygen at flow rates of 6–12 L/min and is used for short-term therapy because of its uncomfortable fit.[14]

Partial or non-rebreathing masks are used for short-term therapy when patients need higher levels of humidified oxygen between 60 and 90% at flow rates of 10–15 L/min. Oxygen flows into a reservoir bag and mask during inhalation. To attain these high levels of oxygen, the mask must fit snugly over the nose and mouth and may be uncomfortable.[14]

Venturi masks can deliver precise, high flow rates of humidified oxygen. These lightweight, cone-shaped devices are fitted to the face and are able to deliver 24, 28, 31, 35, 40, and 50% oxygen. These masks are used to deliver low-flow, constant oxygen concentrations to patients with COPD.[14]

Oxygen delivery devices such as a tracheostomy collar are available to provide humidified oxygen to patients with tracheostomy tubes.

Airway Management and Breathing Support

Patients with an acute disorder causing impaired gas exchange may need airway support. Before arrival of the emergency team, the nurse may insert an oropharyngeal airway to maintain the patient's breathing. Patients may require intubation using an endotracheal tube or tracheostomy tube. Humidified oxygen is delivered to the trachea and bronchi. When breathing support is needed, the patient's respiratory rate and volume are controlled by a ventilator.

Chest Physiotherapy and Postural Drainage

Chest physiotherapy and postural drainage are performed for the purpose of loosening and moving secretions into large airways where they can be expectorated. Chest physiotherapy includes percussion (cupping and clapping) and vibration to loosen secretions. Postural drainage involves positioning the patient in specific positions (e.g., head down, on left and right sides, and supine and prone) to use the benefit of gravity to remove secretions after they are loosened from specific segments of the lungs. Patients with cystic fibrosis use this procedure frequently to help remove the thick secretions formed by their disorder.

Invasive Procedures

There are a number of invasive therapeutic interventions. The nurse generalist does not perform these interventions but does provide care for patients during and after the procedures.

Chest tubes. Chest tubes are placed in the pleura to remove air (pneumothorax) and/or blood (hemothorax) so that the lungs can be re-expanded after thoracic surgery or trauma. Nurses monitor the amount and appearance of drainage from chest tubes and change the dressing around these tubes as ordered.

Thoracentesis. Thoracentesis is a procedure to relieve a pleural effusion by inserting a needle into the pleural space to remove fluid. Nurses assist physicians with this procedure and monitor the patient's vital signs, lung sounds, and pain level afterward.

Bronchoscopy. Bronchoscopy is a procedure that can be diagnostic or therapeutic. The procedure involves insertion of a bronchoscope through the trachea into bronchi. The diagnostic effect is directly visualizing the airway or taking tissue samples for biopsy. The therapeutic effects can include removing foreign objects and suctioning mucous plugs from airways or lavaging airways. Airway patency can also be accomplished using laser therapy, electrocautery, cryotherapy, and stents placed through a bronchoscope.[7]

Nutrition Therapy

Nutrition therapy is needed to provide energy for the increased work of breathing and to support the immune system. High-protein, high-calorie, nutritious foods and drinks meet the needs of these patients. Small meals are advised for patients who become dyspneic while eating. For patients with a productive cough, oral care should be offered before meals to reduce any lingering taste of sputum.[14]

Positioning

Two positions are important interventions for patients with impaired gas exchange. The first position is *sitting up*. Patients with acute or chronic impaired gas exchange breath more easily in high Fowler's position, Fowler's position, or semi-Fowler's position. These positions use gravity to move the diaphragm away from the lungs to reduce the work of breathing. Orthopnea refers to an abnormal condition in which a person must sit or stand to breathe comfortably. Patients with chronic pulmonary disease may use a tripod position or prefer sleeping while leaning forward over a table.

The second position is *lying horizontally*, which helps patients who are hypoxemic and have acute lung disease. The distribution of pulmonary capillary blood flow is affected by gravity in different body positions. The greatest volume of pulmonary blood flow occurs in the gravity-dependent areas of the lung. Thus, the areas of the lung that are most dependent become the best ventilated and perfused.[1] Although thoracic expansion of the dependent lung is reduced somewhat by the mattress, the gravity-dependent lung still has better ventilation and perfusion than the other lung.[15]

Other Interventions

Alternate activity with rest periods; for example, if the patient becomes dyspneic after a bath or shower, allow a rest period before a meal or exercise. Many patients with COPD perceive they can breathe easier when there is an increase in air circulation, which they accomplish by using an electric fan.

Patients' coping may be improved by encouraging them to express their feelings about their impaired gas exchange and how it has changed their lives. Nurses may be able to help patients locate needed resources.

CLINICAL NURSING SKILLS FOR GAS EXCHANGE

- Assessment
- Oxygen administration
- Positioning
- Peak expiratory flow rate
- Nebulizers
- Chest physiotherapy
- Airway suctioning
- Endotracheal tube and tracheostomy care
- Chest tube
- Mechanical ventilation
- Medication administration

INTERRELATED CONCEPTS

Gas exchange is interrelated with nearly all of the health and illness concepts within this textbook because all cells in the body depend on

gas exchange and removal of gases. Concepts that most closely interrelate with gas exchange are illustrated in Figure 19-3 and described below.

Acid–Base Balance is affected by gas exchange in several ways. Diseases that retain carbon dioxide, such as COPD, create increased levels of carbonic acid, which causes respiratory acidosis. Conversely, when excessive carbon dioxide is exhaled such as during an anxiety attack, less carbonic acid is formed, causing a respiratory alkalosis. Hypoxia attributable to inadequate **Perfusion**, such as from a myocardial infarction, causes lactic acid formation that causes metabolic acidosis. When patients experience breathlessness, such as during an asthma attack, they may experience anxiety due to the lack of oxygen. **Anxiety** also links to gas exchange because individuals who are unable to get sufficient oxygen become very anxious.

Mobility may be reduced when patients with impaired gas exchange become dyspneic when walking or climbing stairs. **Fatigue** is related to gas exchange in two different ways. When anemia is a cause of impaired gas exchange, fatigue may be a manifestation of the anemia. However, patients who must use accessory muscles and work hard to breathe, such as those with emphysema, exert significant energy to breath, which contributes to fatigue.

Nutrition is a concern for patients who expend more than usual energy to breathe, such as those with emphysema and cystic fibrosis. They require high-calorie, high-protein, and nutritious foods in small servings so they do not tire while eating. When dyspneic, patients focus on getting air in and are thus unable to eat. Patients with anemia need food high in iron to maintain or increase their hemoglobin levels.

CLINICAL EXEMPLARS

There are multiple conditions that contribute to impaired gas exchange—more than are described in this text. Box 19-3 lists common conditions associated with impaired gas exchange across the lifespan; further details about these conditions can be found in medical–surgical and pediatric nursing textbooks.

Featured Exemplars

Asthma

Asthma is a chronic disorder characterized by periods of reversible airflow obstruction. These *asthma attacks* are caused by hyperreactive airways leading to contraction of the muscles surrounding the airways and inflamed airways. Patients experience wheezing, coughing, dyspnea, and chest tightness. Factors involved in the development of asthma include genetics, inhalation of airborne allergens or pollutants, airway infections, exercise, or emotional stress. Asthma can be controlled with medications and avoidance of triggers for asthma attacks. Prevalence for adults is higher among females, people 18–24 years old, and multirace and black persons. Among children, prevalence is higher among males, children 5–9 years old, and multirace and black persons.[16]

Chronic Obstructive Pulmonary Disease

Chronic obstructive pulmonary disease (COPD) is characterized by chronic airflow limitation that is not fully reversible. COPD includes two obstructive airway diseases: chronic bronchitis and emphysema. *Chronic bronchitis* develops when hypersecretion of mucus obstructs the trachea and bronchi, caused by irritants such as cigarette smoke, air pollution, or respiratory infection. Symptoms are productive cough and dyspnea on exertion.[3] *Emphysema* develops when the alveolar walls are destroyed leading to permanent abnormal enlargement. The most common cause is cigarette smoking. Emphysemic patients are often underweight with a barrel chest and become short of breath with

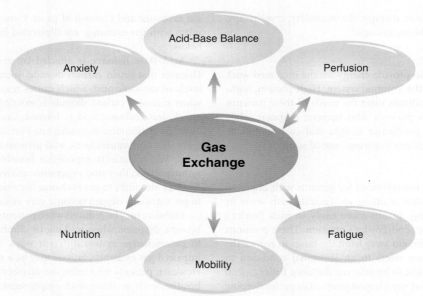

FIGURE 19-3 Gas Exchange and Interrelated Concepts

Impairment of Ventilation
- Acute respiratory failure
- Adult respiratory distress syndrome
- Asthma
- Atelectasis
- Chronic bronchitis
- Cystic fibrosis
- Emphysema
- Infant respiratory distress syndrome
- Lung cancer
- Pleural effusion
- Pneumonia
- Pneumothorax
- Respiratory syncytial virus
- Trauma and flail chest
- Tuberculosis

Impairment in Perfusion
- Aneurysm
- Heart failure
- Peripheral artery disease
- Pulmonary emboli
- Shock

Impairment in Transportation
- Aplastic anemia
- Folic acid deficiency anemia
- Hemolytic anemia
- Iron deficiency anemia
- Pernicious anemia
- Sickle cell anemia
- Thalassemia

minimal exertion.[14] COPD is typically diagnosed in adults approximately 50 years of age after a long history of smoking. It is the third leading cause of death in the United States.[17]

Lung Cancer

An uncontrolled growth of anaplastic cells in the lung describes lung cancer. Causes include cigarette smoke, asbestosis, ionizing radiation, or other inhaled toxins. The most common initial symptom is persistent cough. Lung cancer is the leading cause of cancer-related deaths in the United States, accounting for 28% of all cancer deaths. Incidence and mortality rates for men have declined in the past decade, but this trend has not occurred in women. Lung cancer has surpassed breast cancer as the leading cause of death in women.[18]

Pneumonia

An inflammation of terminal bronchioles and alveoli results in pneumonia. Microorganisms are the most frequent causes. Viral pneumonia tends to produce a nonproductive cough or clear sputum, whereas bacterial pneumonia causes a productive cough of white, yellow, or green sputum. Other manifestations include fever, chills, dyspnea on exertion, and sharp, stabbing chest pain in inspiration.[19] Rhonchi or crackles may be heard on auscultation. Children may experience retractions and nasal flaring. Viral pneumonias occur more frequently than bacterial pneumonia in children of all ages.[5] Older adults with pneumonia may experience confusion.[19]

Anemia

Oxygen moves from the alveoli to the cells attached to erythrocytes. When erythrocytes are in short supply, as occurs in anemia, oxygenation is less than optimal. Anemia is caused by disorders that interfere with the formation of erythrocytes (aplastic, folic acid, iron deficiency, pernicious anemia, and thalassemia), premature destruction of erythrocytes (sickle cell anemia), and loss of erythrocytes (hemolytic anemia). Despite the cause, common manifestations that occur in all anemias include weakness, fatigue, pallor, exertional dyspnea, dizziness, and lethargy.[20] Vitamin B_{12} deficiency may occur in 12% of older people due to inadequate dietary intake or malabsorption due to low stomach acid.[21]

Pulmonary Emboli

A blockage of pulmonary arteries by a thrombus, fat or air embolism, or tumor tissue creates a pulmonary embolism (PE). The embolus travels with blood flow through smaller blood vessels until it obstructs perfusion of alveoli. Most emboli arise from deep vein thrombosis (DVT) in the legs. Venous thromboembolism is the preferred terminology to describe the spectrum of pathology from DVT to PE. Manifestations are nonspecific, making diagnosis difficult. The classic triad of dyspnea, chest pain, and hemoptysis occurs in approximately 20% of patients. Hypoxemia with low arterial carbon dioxide is a common finding. The highest rate of DVT is seen in patients with spinal cord injury.[18]

CASE STUDY

Source: Stockbyte/Thinkstock

Case Presentation

Martha Moore is an 87-year-old woman with a history of osteoporosis and hypertension. She had an exploratory laparotomy for a small bowel obstruction 2 days ago. Before assessing this patient, the nurse noticed Mrs. Moore's hemoglobin level was 9 g and her SaO_2 was 90%. During this morning's assessment, Martha reports her cough kept her awake last night. Vital signs are as follows: temperature, 101°F; blood pressure, 150/78 mm Hg; heart rate, 100 beats/min; and respiratory rate, 24 breaths/min. On auscultation, the nurse hears crackles in both lungs. The patient reports a sharp pain in her chest when she took the deep breath. After the deep breath for auscultation, the patient has a productive cough, and the nurse notices the sputum is green with rust-colored tinting. Martha reports she tries not to cough because it causes abdominal pain at her incision site.

The nurse recognizes that Mrs. Moore has symptoms suggesting pneumonia as a postoperative complication. The nurse knows Mrs. Moore needs to deep breathe, increase activity as tolerated, and increase fluid intake. The nurse works with Mrs. Moore to implement the plan of care. The nurse asks Mrs. Moore to use the incentive spirometer and notices she is moving only 800 mL of air. The nurse emphasizes the importance of using the incentive spirometer approximately 10 times every hour while awake to help get air into Mrs. Moore's lungs. Together, they agree on a goal of moving 1500 mL using the spirometer. The nurse also talks with Mrs. Moore about giving her pain medication to relieve the abdominal pain. To further reduce pain when coughing, the nurse recommends that Mrs. Moore hold a pillow over her incision when she coughs to splint the incision site. After receipt of pain medication, Mrs. Moore is assisted to sit on the side of the bed and walk to a chair to eat the clear liquid breakfast. The nurse encourages Mrs. Moore to drink all of the liquids to help liquefy her secretions. When the surgeon makes rounds, the nurse reports the findings from Mrs. Moore's assessment and the plan of care initiated. The surgeon orders a chest x-ray, aspirin as needed for fever, an antibiotic, and iron tablets. After a bath, a nap, pain medication, and use of incentive spirometry with coughing, Mrs. Moore is assisted to walk in the hall. Before discharge, Mrs. Moore is taught about ways to treat her anemia with foods rich in iron and with the daily iron tablet. The outcome of this plan of care is that by discharge, Mrs. Moore will be able to move at least 1500 mL on the spirometer, have clear breath sounds bilaterally, have an SaO_2 greater than 95%, be afebrile, and be able to state the plan to treat her anemia.

Case Analysis

This case clearly exemplifies impairment in gas exchange in a number of ways. Mrs. Moore has several classic risk factors, including her age, a recent surgical procedure, and hesitancy to cough for fear of abdominal pain. The clinical presentation of Mrs. Moore's signs and symptoms is consistent with two types of gas exchange impairments: bacterial pneumonia, a very common exemplar of impaired gas exchange representing impairment of ventilation, and anemia, which impairs the oxygen-carrying capacity of the blood.

ACCESS EXEMPLAR LINKS IN YOUR GIDDENS EBOOK

REFERENCES

1. Brashers V: Structure and function of the pulmonary system. In Huether S, McCance K, editors: *Understanding pathophysiology*, ed 5, St Louis, 2012, Elsevier, pp 659–677.
2. Brashers V: Alterations of pulmonary function. In Huether S, McCance K, editors: *Understanding pathophysiology*, ed 5, St Louis, 2012, Elsevier, pp 678–706.
3. Wilson S, Giddens J: *Health assessment for nursing practice*, ed 5, St Louis, 2013, Elsevier.
4. Wilson D: Health promotion of the infant and family. In Hockenberry M, Wilson D, editors: *Wong's nursing care of infants and children*, ed 10, St Louis, 2015, Elsevier, pp 413–451.
5. Conlon P, Wilson D: The child with respiratory dysfunction. In Hockenberry M, Wilson D, editors: *Wong's nursing care of infants and children*, ed 10, St Louis, 2015, Elsevier, pp 1164–1250.
6. Pagana K, Pagana T: *Mosby's diagnostic and laboratory test reference*, ed 11, St Louis, 2012, Mosby.
7. Norris C: Nursing assessment respiratory system. In Lewis S, editor: *Medical–surgical nursing: Assessment and management of clinical problems*, ed 8, St Louis, 2011, Mosby, pp 497–518.
8. Healthy People 2020: Tobacco use. Retrieved from <http://www.healthypeople.gov/2020/topics-objectives/topic/tobacco-use>, 2015.
9. American Lung Association: Stop smoking. Retrieved from <http://www.lungusa.org/stop-smoking>.
10. American Cancer Society: Stay healthy, Guide to quitting smoking. Retrieved from <http://www.cancer.org/Healthy/StayAwayfromTobacco/GuidetoQuittingSmoking>, n.d..
11. Centers for Disease Control and Prevention: Quitting smoking. Retrieved from <http://www.cdc.gov/tobacco/data_statistics/fact_sheets/cessation/quitting>, 2015.
12. Centers for Disease Control and Prevention: Immunization schedules. Retrieved from <http://www.cdc.gov/vaccines/schedules/index.html>, 2015.
13. Lehne R: *Pharmacology for nursing care*, ed 8, Philadelphia, 2012, Elsevier.
14. Kaufman J: Nursing management: Obstructive pulmonary disease. In Lewis S, editor: *Medical–surgical nursing: Assessment and management of clinical problems*, ed 8, St Louis, 2011, Mosby, pp 587–640.
15. Yeaw E: How position affects oxygenation: Good lung down? *Am J Nurs* 92(4):27–29, 1992.

16. Centers for Disease Control and Prevention: Asthma facts: CDC's National Asthma Control Program Grantees. Retrieved from <http://www.cdc.gov/asthma/pdfs/asthma_facts_program_grantees.pdf>, 2013.

17. American Lung Association: Chronic obstructive pulmonary disease (COPD) fact sheet. Retrieved from <http://www.lung.org/lung-disease/copd/resources/facts-figures/COPD-Fact-Sheet.html>, 2014.

18. Malone MJ: Nursing management: Lower respiratory problems. In Lewis S, editor: *Medical–surgical nursing: Assessment and management of clinical problems*, ed 8, St Louis, 2011, Mosby, pp 545–586.

19. American Lung Association: Pneumonia, symptoms, diagnosis and treatment. Retrieved from <http://www.lung.org/lung-disease/pneumonia/symptoms-diagnosis-and.html>, n.d..

20. Schwartz A, Rote N, McCance K: Alterations of hematologic function. In Huether S, McCance K, editors: *Understanding pathophysiology*, ed 5, St Louis, 2012, Elsevier, pp 500–534.

21. Rome SI: Nursing management: Hematologic problems. In Lewis S, editor: *Medical–surgical nursing: Assessment and management of clinical problems*, ed 8, St Louis, 2011, Mosby, pp 661–713.

Clotting

Susan Wilson

All cells depend on a consistent supply of blood. When injury occurs to veins and arteries, the clotting process is initiated to stop the blood loss. This represents an important physiological protective mechanism allowing the body to maintain homeostasis when injury occurs. However, excessive clotting can impair perfusion, whereas inadequate clotting increases blood loss. For this reason, clotting is a critical concept for nurses to understand and incorporate into practice. Nurses should identify individuals at risk of impaired clotting, recognize when individuals are experiencing impaired clotting, and respond with appropriate interventions.

DEFINITION

For the purposes of this concept presentation, clotting is defined as *a physiological process in which blood is converted from a liquid to a semi-solid gel.* This is a normal and expected physiological event that usually starts when veins or arteries are injured.[1] Multiple coagulation factors interact in a sequence with fibrin and platelets to form a blood clot. The result of the clotting process is *hemostasis*, a term that refers to the stoppage of blood flow or bleeding.

The clotting process can become impaired in two ways. First, when clotting factors are not available, patients experience excessive bleeding. Alternatively, if blood clots form when they are not physiologically indicated, then a *thrombus* (blood clot) may obstruct blood vessels and interfere with blood flow. Effects of impaired clotting vary depending on the extent of impairment and the anatomic location.

SCOPE

The concept of clotting and problems associated with impaired clotting represent a variety of physiological processes. The scope of the concept represents a continuum ranging from excessive clotting beyond physiological need at one end of the spectrum to impaired clotting resulting in bleeding at the other end. Expected physiological clotting processes fall in the middle of this continuum. Both excessive clotting and ineffective clotting may occur locally or systemically. Figure 20-1 depicts the continuum of clotting as a concept.

NORMAL PHYSIOLOGICAL PROCESS

The homeostatic process is a protective mechanism to prevent excessive bleeding when vascular injury occurs and is achieved through a complex coagulation process. In a normal clotting process, the damaged vessels, platelets, and clotting factors work together to stop bleeding.

The first response is vasoconstriction, which reduces blood flow, allowing the clotting process to start. Bleeding is slowed further when accumulating blood surrounding the blood vessel creates pressure against the walls of the affected vessel.

The second response, triggered by the damaged blood vessel, is formation of a platelet plug. Platelets are activated and stick to the injured blood vessel because of a protein (called von Willebrand's factor) produced by the cells of the vessel wall. The platelet plug develops in 3–7 minutes.

Next, clotting factors are activated either from the intrinsic or from the extrinsic pathway and proceed in a coagulation cascade to the common final pathway. The difference between intrinsic and extrinsic pathways has to do with the initiation of the clotting factors. The intrinsic pathway is activated by collagen exposure when there is damage to the surface of the blood vessel (within the vessel). The extrinsic pathway is initiated when damaged tissues release tissue factor or tissue thromboplastic (external to the blood vessel).

Both intrinsic and extrinsic pathways converge to follow a common final pathway whereby thrombin stimulates fibrinogen to form insoluble fibrin that stabilizes the clot.[2] Figure 20-2 illustrates the coagulation cascade.

VARIATIONS AND CONTEXT

Variations in clotting may occur in individuals across the lifespan with a wide range of impact, and they represent conditions associated with excessive clotting or conditions associated with excessive bleeding. Variations in the normal clotting process occur in relation to the presence of clotting factors, the size of the vessel affected, the type of vessel (artery or vein), and the location of the bleeding. When there is an excess of clotting factors, thrombi may form; a deficit of clotting factors may produce bleeding. A significant difference results depending on whether the blood vessel is small or large. The pressure of blood is greater in arteries compared with veins. A simple paper cut of a finger can cause immediate bleeding from a vein in a small area of the body, whereas severing a major artery can result in severe blood loss and perhaps death. The location of the bleeding is another variable. For example, bleeding from a weakened artery within the brain can cause immediate neurologic deficits and perhaps death, whereas bleeding from veins injured by a skinned knee impairs the skin

FIGURE 20-1 Scope and Categories of Clotting Concept

integrity, causes some discomfort, and can be healed perhaps without a scar.

CONSEQUENCES

Pathophysiological Consequences of Excessive Clotting/Thrombi

Normal homeostatic processes can become impaired when excessive clotting factors lead to thrombus formation. A thrombus can form in arteries or veins. The impact of one or multiple thrombi can vary from partial obstruction to complete occlusion of the affected vessel(s).

Arterial Thrombosis

Arterial thrombi are associated with conditions that increase platelets or erythrocyte production or create turbulent blood flow with platelet adhesion. Another source of thrombi is atherosclerosis, which begins with injury to the endothelium. Causes of endothelial injury include hypertension from the increased pressure of blood in the arteries creating a shearing force. Other causes of endothelial injury include exogenous chemical agents such as toxins from cigarette smoke and endogenous agents such as cholesterol.

FIGURE 20-2 Coagulation Cascade Coagulation cascade showing steps in the intrinsic and extrinsic pathways. (Source: From Lewis S, et al, editors: *Medical–surgical nursing: Assessment and management of clinical problems*, ed 9, St Louis, 2014, Mosby.)

When a thrombus blocks an artery, it interrupts the flow of oxygenated blood to the tissue, leading to ischemia. If left untreated, this results in cell death; however, if adequate collateral circulation exists, it can compensate for the reduced blood flow and avert cell death. The pathologic consequence of such an event is determined by the artery location (e.g., coronary artery, cerebral artery, and femoral artery) and the size of the thrombus in relation to the size of the affected artery. A large thrombus in a small artery may stop the flow of blood, whereas a small thrombus in a large artery may create turbulent and slow blood flow. A thrombus that detaches from an artery becomes an embolus and can lodge in another artery. For example, a small arterial emboli flowing through a cerebral artery can cause transient ischemia, or a large arterial emboli can lodge in a cerebral artery creating a cerebrovascular accident (stroke).

Venous Thrombosis

Venous thrombosis is the formation of a blood clot in a vein—usually in association with inflammation within the vein. Superficial and deep veins may be affected. Three factors associated with the formation of venous thrombosis are hypercoagulability of the blood, injury to the vessel wall endothelium, and stasis of blood flow.[2] These three factors are commonly known as Virchow's triad (Figure 20-3). Endothelial damage of the vein initiates the release of clotting factors or activates platelets. Stasis of venous blood occurs when there is dysfunction of venous valves, inactivity of extremity muscles, or change in unidirectional venous blood flow.[3]

A thrombus that detaches from a vein becomes an embolus and can lodge in another vein. For example, a thrombus from a deep vein thrombus in the leg can lodge in pulmonary vessels, creating a pulmonary embolus.

Pathophysiological Consequences of Inadequate Clotting/Bleeding

Bleeding occurs after injury to arteries and veins, but it also can occur spontaneously when the factors needed for clotting are reduced. These clotting factors include platelets and clotting factors II (prothrombin), VII, VIII, IX, and X. The extent of bleeding can be as minor as bruising or as significant as hemorrhage. Thrombocytopenia is defined as a platelet count less than 150,000/mm^3, although the decrease is not considered significant unless the platelet count declines below 100,000/mm^3. When the platelet count declines below 50,000/mm^3, the risk for hemorrhage after minor trauma increases and petechiae, purpura, or ecchymosis may form. Spontaneous bleeding without trauma, such as a spontaneous nosebleed, occurs when the platelet count ranges from 10,000 to 15,000/mm^3. Liver disease, such as cirrhosis, impairs the liver's synthesis of clotting factors, including factors II, VII, IX, and X. Reduction in the amounts of these clotting factors prevents formation of clots after trauma or hemorrhage.

The impact of hemorrhage on an individual varies with the percentage of blood volume lost. After loss of 20% of blood volume, the person has tachycardia on exertion and sight postural hypotension. With the loss of 30%, the person has tachycardia at rest, postural hypotension, and flat neck veins in a supine position. With the loss of 40%, the manifestations are hypotension; tachypnea; and cold, clammy skin. With the loss of 50% of blood volume, there is hemorrhage shock and death.[3]

Hemolytic anemia can be a consequence of blood loss that affects several body systems. The effects on the respiratory system include increased respiratory rate and dyspnea on exertion. The cardiovascular system responds by increasing the heart rate and peripheral vasoconstriction. The effect on the nervous system is the

PATHOPHYSIOLOGY MAP

Virchow's triad

Venous stasis
- Dysfunctional vein valves
- Inactive extremity muscles
- Change in unidirectional blood flow

Endothelial damage
- Release of clotting factors
- Activation of platelets

Blood hypercoagulability
- Imbalance in clotting mechanism → coagulation
- Increase in fibrin production

- Platelets aggregate (especially at vein valve cusps)
- Clotting factors stimulated to produce fibrin
- Fibrin entraps RBCs, WBCs, and platelets and begins to adhere to vein wall

Thrombus formation

Clinical manifestations
- Unilateral leg edema, pain, and erythema
- Chronic venous insufficiency
- Embolism of thrombotic fragments

FIGURE 20-3 Virchow's Triad Virchow's triad showing the pathophysiology of venous thromboembolism. (Source: From Lewis S, et al, editors: *Medical–surgical nursing: Assessment and management of clinical problems*, ed 9, St Louis, 2014, Mosby.)

emergence of confusion, anxiety, dizziness, and fainting.[3] The skin and mucous membranes become pale. The person reports weakness and fatigue.

RISK FACTORS

Populations at Risk

Older adults have increased risk for clotting because of expected physiological changes that occur with advanced age such as increased platelet adhesiveness,[2] which promotes blood stasis.

Individuals of black race may have a genetic disorder called sickle cell anemia. When affected persons experience hypoxia, dehydration, low temperature, or metabolic acidosis, their red blood cells change to a shape of a sickle, which results in abnormal clotting in peripheral arteries, causing ischemia and pain.[4]

Individual Risk Factors

Impaired clotting affects all individuals regardless of age, gender, race, or socioeconomic status. Common risk factors are described in the following sections.

Genetics

Several genetic disorders are associated with hematologic conditions. The classic example is hemophilia, a recessive genetic disorder caused by the inability to produce adequate clotting factors needed for blood coagulation. Hemophilia A and hemophilia B are similar in that they are both recessive sex-linked genetic disorders in males whose affected clotting factor is defective or deficient. The difference between these types of hemophilia is the affected clotting factor. In hemophilia A, factor VIII is deficient, whereas in hemophilia B, factor IX is deficient. By contrast, von Willebrand's disease is a bleeding disorder that is an autosomal dominant genetic disorder affecting both genders; affected individuals have a deficiency in von Willebrand factor coagulation protein and factor VIII as well as a platelet dysfunction. Deficiencies of these clotting factors result in spontaneous bleeding, including nosebleeds and hematuria (blood in urine).[4]

Immobility

Immobility contributes to blood clot formation by slowing the return of venous blood to the heart. Slow blood flow results in stasis, a risk factor for thrombi formation. Immobility may occur as a result of paralysis or an unconscious or impaired cognitive state or from bed rest needed to recover from an illness, injury, or surgery. Individuals who are confined to a sitting position for long periods (e.g., on long airplane flights) are also susceptible to the formation of venous clots.

Smoking

Smoking is a known risk factor that contributes to hypercoagulability of the blood—a contributing factor to clot formation.

ASSESSMENT

Nurses gather data from the patient's history, physical assessment, and diagnostic test results. Adequate clotting is apparent when the patient forms a blood clot after endothelial damage. Peripheral pulses are present, capillaries refill within less than 2 seconds, and the skin is warm and dry without discolorations, such as bruises or the presence of edema. Also, blood pressure and heart rate are at expected rates for the patient's age.

History

The history includes current and past medical conditions. Nurses inquire about patients' chronic diseases. Many medical conditions are associated with bleeding or clotting disorders. Common conditions associated with clotting disorders are presented later (see Box 20-2).

Also included in the history are medications the patient is currently taking because many medications affect clotting.[5] Aspirin is taken daily by many people to reduce the potential for clot formation because of its antiplatelet effects. Warfarin (Coumadin) is a prescription drug taken to prevent blood clotting by interfering with the four vitamin K-dependent clotting factors (II, VII, IX, and X). Nurses also ask patients about over-the-counter medications or herbal and dietary supplements they take that may affect clotting. These supplements include bilberry, black cohosh, chamomile, chondroitin sulfate, feverfew, garlic, ginger, ginkgo biloba, ginseng, goldenseal, omega-3 fatty acids, melatonin, niacin, soy, and turmeric.[6]

Lifestyle behaviors are important to assess as part of the history. Questions include exercise habits, including the kind of exercise and how often it is performed and for what length of time, because exercise increases blood flow. Nurses ask patients about smoking habits because nicotine causes vasoconstriction and is a toxin that damages the endothelium, contributing to atherosclerosis.

Bleeding

The nurse should ask about abnormal bleeding from gums when brushing teeth, from the rectum after defecation, or after a minor trauma. Patients may describe bleeding that takes longer than usual to stop. Patients with bleeding problems may report bleeding in many forms and from various areas of the body, including nosebleeds; new bruises; black, tarry stools; blood from rectum (hematochezia); blood in the urine (hematuria); blood in emesis (hematemesis); coughing up blood (hemoptysis); or bleeding from the mouth. Indications of intracranial bleeding may include a headache, changes in vision, sudden difficulty talking, or weakness of one arm or leg. Patients may report fatigue or dyspnea from anemia caused by blood loss. When applicable, women are asked about the amount of blood lost during menses and whether the length of menses has increased.

Parents of children with hemophilia may report that the children bleed after minor trauma such as from a circumcision, during loss of deciduous teeth, or after a slight fall. Bleeding into a joint (hemarthrosis) may produce complaints of stiffness, tingling, or ache of knees, elbows, and ankles. Hematuria may be reported.[4]

Clotting

The nurse asks patients about recent prolonged sitting, such as on an airplane or in a car, or prolonged bed rest because these are risk factors for venous thrombosis. Nurses should inquire about swelling, redness, and pain in an extremity. They should also ask about a history of atrial fibrillation, which increases risk of atrial emboli into the cerebral circulation. A report of leg pain when walking may indicate arterial insufficiency of the lower extremities.

Examination Findings
Bleeding

When assessing patients with *prolonged bleeding*, nurses may notice petechiae, ecchymosis, and purpura during inspection of the skin that indicate localized bleeding in the subcutaneous tissue. For patients with hemophilia, subcutaneous and intramuscular hemorrhages are common. Hemarthrosis results in warmth, redness, edema, and severe pain of affected joints followed by decreased joint range of motion.[4] Bleeding into the brain produces varying manifestations of stroke depending on the amount of blood released and the area of the brain affected. When bleeding is excessive, changes to vital signs—specifically increased heart rate and decreased blood pressure—may be noted.

Clotting

When assessing patients with a thrombosis, nurses find different manifestations depending on the location and whether arteries or veins are affected. Clots within veins frequently develop in lower extremities, where they impair perfusion and cause pain, redness, and edema with an increased circumference of the affected extremity. The patient may have a palpable firm vein that is tender to touch. When venous thrombi become emboli, the emboli flow superiorly in the inferior vena cava and lodge in pulmonary capillaries. Manifestations produced from pulmonary emboli vary by location affected and size of the emboli; however, the classic triad includes dyspnea, chest pain, and hemoptysis.[7]

As mentioned previously, an arterial thrombus in the lower extremities impairs perfusion. Accompanying the common reported symptoms of *pain* and *paresthesia* may be other manifestations, such as *pulselessness, pallor*, and *poikilothermia* (cool skin temperature over the affected area). These are often referred to as "the five P's." Blood clots that travel as emboli through the carotid circulation can impair perfusion to the brain, producing manifestations of a brain attack that vary by location affected and size of the emboli.

Diagnostic Tests
Laboratory Tests

Prothrombin time. Prothrombin time (PT) measures the adequacy of the extrinsic system and common pathways in the clotting mechanism, which include clotting factors I (fibrinogen), II (prothrombin), V, VII, and X. When these clotting factors are found in decreased amounts, the PT is prolonged, meaning more time is needed for blood to clot. PT results are reported in seconds along with a control value. The patient's value should be approximately equal to the control. A normal finding is 11.0–12.5 seconds. The PT is used to monitor the therapeutic ranges of anticoagulants such as warfarin (Coumadin), and these therapeutic values are 1.5–2.5 times normal.[8]

International normalized ratio. The international normalized ratio (INR) was established by the World Health Organization to standardize the INR results regardless of the reagents or methods used to analyze the blood. The INR is used to monitor the effectiveness of anticoagulant therapy such as warfarin (Coumadin) that is given to inhibit the formation of blood clots. Normal values vary depending on the patient's disorder; for example, 1.5–2.0 is preferred for prophylaxis for deep vein thrombosis, 2.0–3.0 when treating deep vein thrombosis, and 3.0–4.0 when treating atrial fibrillation.[8]

Partial thromboplastin time. Partial thromboplastin time (PTT) measures the intrinsic system and common pathway of clot formation, which includes factors I (fibrinogen), II (prothrombin), V, VIII, IX, X, XI, and XII. Factors II, VII, IX, and X are vitamin K–dependent factors. When there are reduced amounts of these clotting factors, the PTT is prolonged, meaning more time is needed for blood to clot. Like the PT values, the PTT results are reported in seconds along with a control value. The patient's normal value should be approximately equal to the control. A normal finding is 60–70 seconds. Activators were added to PTT reagents to shorten normal clotting time and provide a narrow normal range. This shortened time is called activated PTT or APTT, with a normal value of 30–40 seconds. The PTT is used to monitor the therapeutic ranges of patients taking anticoagulants such as heparin, and these therapeutic values are 1.5–2.5 times normal.[8]

Fibrinogen. Fibrinogen (or clotting factor I) is part of the common pathway in the coagulation system. It is converted to fibrin by the action of thrombin during the coagulation process. Reduced fibrinogen level occurs in patients with liver disease, malnutrition states, and consumptive coagulopathies such as disseminated intravascular coagulation (DIC). Normal values for adults range from 200 to 400 mg/dL, and those for newborns range from 125 to 300 mg/dL.[8]

Platelet count. Platelet count is the number of platelets (thrombocytes) per cubic millimeter of blood. This test is performed on patients with suspected bleeding disorders or clotting disorders. Normal values are as follows: adults and children, 150,000–400,000 per mm^3; premature infants, 100,000–300,000 per mm^3; newborns, 150,000–300,000 per mm^3; and infants, 200,000–475,000 per mm^3.[8]

D-dimer. The D-dimer test assesses the activity of both thrombin, used to form blood clots, and plasmin, used to break down blood clots. While plasmin breaks down fibrin clots, fibrin degradation products and D-dimer are produced. The D-dimer assay provides a highly specific measurement of the amount of fibrin degradation that occurs as the clot is dissolved. Plasma normally does not have detectable amounts of fragment D-dimer. This test is used to confirm a diagnosis of DIC.[8]

Erythrocyte count, hemoglobin, and hematocrit. These measures are used to diagnose the presence of polycythemia and anemia. Patients with polycythemia have elevated levels of erythrocytes or red blood cells (RBCs), which increase risk of clotting. Patients may develop anemia due to blood loss, which is indicated by RBC, hemoglobin, and hematocrit values below normal.

Bone marrow examination. An examination of the bone marrow may be done to assess for evidence of hyper- or hypoproduction of platelets and RBCs. This test may be indicated for polycythemia or thrombocytopenia.

Radiologic Tests

Three common radiographic tests to evaluate vessels are useful in the diagnosis of individuals with clotting or bleeding tendencies. In all cases, the test produces an image of the vessel.

Noninvasive venous studies. Ultrasound is used as a noninvasive approach for evaluation for venous thrombosis.

Arteriograms. Arteriograms allow visualization of arteries by injecting radiopaque contrast into them so that the location and extent of occlusion or dilation can be identified.[8]

Venograms. Venograms of the lower extremities allow visualization of veins by injecting radiopaque contrast into them so that the location and extent of thrombi can be identified.[8]

CLINICAL MANAGEMENT

Clinical management related to clotting includes health promotion and the management of emerging or present conditions that compromise clotting. The ultimate goal is to optimize the clotting process. The *Healthy People 2020* objectives for bleeding and clotting are summarized in Box 20-1.[9]

Primary Prevention

Primary prevention includes measures to promote health and prevent disease. For problems associated with excessive bleeding, the only true primary prevention measure is genetic counseling. Genetic counseling is advised for couples who have a family history of bleeding disorders and want to start a family. Genetic counseling will assist couples to comprehend the medical facts, understand risks and options, and make an informed decision. Measures to prevent bleeding as a complication of a disease process or medical treatments for other conditions are discussed in the collaborative care section.

For this concept, most primary prevention measures relate to prevention of blood clots. Strategies for prevention include minimizing the risks for blood stasis, increased blood viscosity, and vessel injury. Patients at risk for venous stasis or those with clotting disorders are encouraged to enhance blood flow by performing leg exercises, engaging in regular walking, or wearing compression stockings. High-risk patients (e.g., those following knee or hip replacement surgery) are administered anticoagulant therapy as a prophylactic measure. These agents are further discussed later. Women with an increased risk for clots may be advised to avoid taking birth control pills because of their adverse effect on clotting. Teaching patients about the importance of smoking cessation is a priority because nicotine both causes vasoconstriction, which contributes to stasis of blood flow, and damages the endothelium, contributing to atherosclerosis. Maintaining adequate hydration reduces the potential for increased blood viscosity.

Secondary Prevention (Screening)

Secondary prevention includes screening, early diagnosis, and prompt treatment of existing health problems. There are no routine screening tests indicated for the general public related to this concept.

Collaborative Interventions for Bleeding Disorders
Prevention and Control of Bleeding

Prevention and control of bleeding are the cornerstones for management of individuals with bleeding disorders. Patients must learn to recognize signs and symptoms of bleeding and to notify the health care provider when indications of bleeding occur. They also must be taught strategies to minimize risk for trauma. Patients with bleeding disorders or individuals who are taking anticoagulants are taught to avoid taking drugs that contribute to bleeding, such as any drugs containing aspirin. They are encouraged to avoid situations that could cause injury resulting in bleeding, such as participation in contact sports. Nurses may teach strategies designed to avoid bleeding. For example, patients learn to use a soft bristle toothbrush to avoid bleeding from gums while brushing teeth. They use an electric razor rather than a blade razor to avoid nicks to the skin. Patients are encouraged to avoid blowing their nose forcefully to reduce the likelihood of nosebleeds. They should avoid getting tattoos and body piercings. Women who are menstruating should count the number of pads or tampons they use daily and notify the health care provider if that

number increases. Patients should understand the importance of notifying health care personnel before seemingly benign invasive procedures such as teeth cleaning, manicure, or pedicure.[10]

Medications given by injection should be avoided if possible to prevent the needle stick that causes bleeding. When an injection is unavoidable, nurses use the smallest size needle possible.[10] In addition, nurses monitor laboratory tests such as INR to assess risk and to provide direction in medication management.

Management of Bleeding Episodes

During episodes of active bleeding, the obvious goal is to control hemorrhage. Direct pressure over bleeding sites is indicated. The use of topical agents (e.g., Gelfoam or fibrin foam) might also help to slow the bleeding. Ice applications are also indicated for topical bleeding or bleeding within a joint space. Pharmacologic agents (discussed next) and the provision of supportive care, such as volume replacement and oxygen support, may be needed to prevent the progression of bleeding to the point of hemodynamic instability.

Pharmacotherapy

Clotting factor replacement or stimulating agents. Several agents are used to replace factor VIII and factor IX—the deficient clotting factors associated with hemophilia. Desmopressin acetate is a synthetic vasopressin agent that stimulates release of factor VIII and von Willebrand factor. This agent is useful for milder forms of hemophilia.[10]

Platelet replacement agents. Several pharmacologic agents are used to increase the number of platelets. Platelet growth factor agents (e.g., oprelvekin, romiplostim, and eltrombopag) stimulate bone marrow production of platelets. A transfusion of platelets is also a way to increase a patient's platelet volume, but this is generally performed to treat life-threatening hemorrhage.

Collaborative Interventions for Clotting Disorders

Because there are several conditions that can lead to clotting, collaborative interventions are dependent on the underlying cause.

Pharmacotherapy

Several groups of drugs are used to treat individuals with clotting disorders and to prevent the formation of clots among high-risk individuals. Refer to Figure 20-2 for assistance with understanding drug actions.

Anticoagulants. Two common anticoagulant agents used to prevent the formation of blood clots are warfarin and heparin. Warfarin (Coumadin) acts by decreasing the production of four vitamin K-dependent clotting factors: II (prothrombin), VII, IX, and X. Coumadin is the only oral anticoagulant currently available.[11] People taking warfarin need periodic INR blood tests to determine the adequacy of the anticoagulant therapy and are taught to avoid foods high in vitamin K such as spinach that interfere with the action of the drug. Heparin acts by inactivating clotting factors, primarily thrombin and factor Xa. Low-molecular-weight heparin drugs, such as enoxaparin (Lovenox) and dalteparin (Fragmin), are the most commonly used agents in this category.

Two oral anticoagulants are available that do not require blood tests or restrict diet. One is dabigagran (Pradaxa), which acts by inhibiting thrombin and preventing platelet aggregation and thrombus formation by preventing the conversion of fibrinogen to fibrin. Another anticoagulant is rivaroxaban (Xarelto), which acts by inhibiting coagulation factor Xa.[12]

Antiplatelets. Agents such as aspirin or clopidogrel (Plavix) act as antiplatelets by preventing platelet aggregation.

Direct thrombin inhibitors. These synthetic agents act as anticoagulants by directly inhibiting thrombin. An example of a drug in this category is bivalirudin (Angiomax).[12]

Thrombolytic agents. Thrombolytic agents such as streptokinase (Streptase), alteplase (a tissue plasminogen activator), and tenecteplase (TNKase) are used to dissolve blood clots. These agents act by digesting fibrin in clots and breaking down plasmin and other clotting factors. All of these agents have risks of serious bleeding.[11]

Invasive Procedures

Phlebotomy. Phlebotomy, or the removal of blood, is a common treatment to prevent clots for individuals with polycythemia. The goal of this treatment is to reduce blood volume, blood viscosity, and bone marrow activity. Phlebotomy may be needed as often as every 2 or 3 months.

Thrombectomy. A thrombectomy is the removal of a thrombus from a vessel. This can be accomplished through a catheter placed percutaneously or as an open surgical procedure (e.g., direct arteriotomy or venous thrombectomy) in which the vessel is opened to remove the thrombus.

Filters. Filter devices are used to prevent pulmonary embolism for individuals with clotting disorders who are unable to take anticoagulant agents or have a history of pulmonary emboli. Filters (also known as vena cava interruption devices) are inserted percutaneously through the right femoral vein or right internal veins and floated into the vena cava, where they block blood clots from reaching the pulmonary capillaries.

Nutrition Therapy

Warfarin (Coumadin) is an anticoagulant that acts by interfering with vitamin K-dependent clotting factors (VII, IX, X, and II (prothrombin)). The dosage of this drug is adjusted regularly to maintain the INR between 2 and 3. Patients taking warfarin should keep their vitamin K intake consistent to maintain the therapeutic effects of the drug. If the dietary intake of vitamin K increases, then the dose of warfarin must be increased as well and vice versa. Sources of vitamin K include green, leafy vegetables such as spinach or kale, mayonnaise, canola oil, and soybean oil.[11]

Positioning

Positioning affects blood flow and comfort. Patients with a deep venous thrombosis (DVT) (also known as venous thromboembolism) in a lower extremity are taught to elevate the affected leg when lying or sitting to facilitate venous return to the heart. By contrast, patients with an arterial thrombus of a lower extremity are taught to position the affected leg in a dependent position to use gravity to improve perfusion to the feet. During the acute phase after a brain attack, patients are positioned with the head of the bed elevated at least 30 degrees to facilitate venous blood flow from the brain to help prevent cerebral edema. Positioning for all patients prescribed bed rest includes preventing pressure ulcers by repositioning patients as needed to maintain perfusion in dependent areas. Bed rest patients wear sequential compression devices to stimulate venous return to the heart.

INTERRELATED CONCEPTS

Concepts that are closely interrelated with clotting are illustrated in Figure 20-4 and described further below.

Perhaps the closest interrelated concept is Perfusion. Perfusion of blood through blood vessels is impaired when blood clots slow or stop blood flow. In addition, uncontrolled bleeding and hemorrhage can lead to excessive blood loss. Excessive blood loss threatens adequate volume of blood needed to perfuse oxygenated blood to all body tissues.

Clotting is interrelated with Gas Exchange because inadequate perfusion (noted previously) is linked to inadequate gas exchange in the peripheral tissues. Also, gas exchange is impaired when pulmonary emboli reduce pulmonary capillary blood available to carry oxygen from alveoli to cells.

Because the brain is highly dependent on the steady perfusion of oxygenated blood, Intracranial Regulation is also interrelated with clotting. Interruption of cerebral blood flow either due to cerebral blood clots or due to cerebral hemorrhage can lead to brain tissue injury or death. Examples of such problems include stroke, aneurysm, traumatic brain injury, and communicating hydrocephalus.

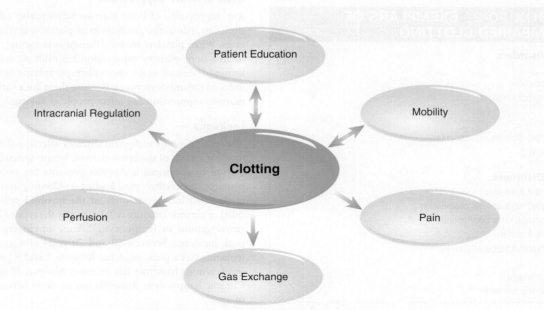

FIGURE 20-4 Clotting and Interrelated Concepts

Individuals with clotting disorders can experience impaired **Mobility** due to illness or recovery from surgery. This immobility increases the risk for DVT. Treatment for DVT is bed rest, which further impairs mobility.

Pain is a common symptom experienced by patients from an arterial thrombus or constriction impairing perfusion to a lower extremity as well as by hemorrhage in a joint space. Individuals with venous clots also experience pain.

Another closely interrelated concept is **Patient Education**. This concept links to clotting as a way to enhance primary prevention strategies as well as to help patients manage their bleeding or clotting disorders. Individuals with clotting disorders require extensive patient education; likewise, inadequate education can lead to complications.

CLINICAL EXEMPLARS

Multiple conditions contribute to impaired clotting—more than are described in this text. Box 20-2 lists common conditions associated with impaired clotting across the lifespan. Some of these disorders are acute, whereas others are chronic; some are preventable, others are not. Further details about these conditions can be found in medical–surgical and pediatric textbooks.

Featured Exemplars
Venous Thromboembolism

This is a condition associated with the formation of a blood clot or thrombus in a vein. Two primary conditions are associated with venous thromboembolism: DVT and pulmonary embolism (PE). DVT occurs when a blood clot forms within a large deep vein (most commonly in the lower leg, thigh, or pelvis). A PE occurs if the clot or a piece of the clot breaks free, travels through the circulatory system, and lodges in the pulmonary vasculature. An estimated 300,000–600,000 individuals each year have DVT, with it most commonly affecting older adults.

■■■ BOX 20-2 EXEMPLARS OF IMPAIRED CLOTTING

Clotting Disorders
Local
- Arterial embolism
- Venous thromboembolism

Systemic
- Disseminated intravascular coagulation
- Polycythemia

Bleeding Disorders
- Bone marrow depression
- Disseminated intravascular coagulation
- Heparin-induced thrombocytopenia
- Hemophilia A and B
- Immune thrombocytopenia purpura
- Leukemia
- Thrombocytopenia
- von Willebrand's disease

Sudden death occurs in an estimated 25% of individuals who experience a PE.[13]

Arterial Embolism

An arterial embolism results when a clot forms in an artery, causing a complete or partial blockage of blood flow. Obstruction of blood flow in an artery is an emergency because of a reduction or loss of oxygenated blood reaching tissues; the outcome is dependent on the degree, length of time, and location of the obstruction. An arterial thrombosis can occur in any artery, but the three most common sites are the vessels of the heart (leading to cardiac ischemia or infarction), the brain (leading to ischemic stroke), and the vessels in the legs.

Disseminated Intravascular Coagulation

DIC is a condition that represents both excessive clotting and bleeding. The primary disorder initiates generalized clotting forming numerous thrombi resulting in multiple organ failure. The abnormal number of thrombi consume and deplete platelets and coagulation factors, leading to hemorrhaging. Thrombotic manifestations are a result of fibrin or platelet deposits in microvasculature and include cyanosis, paralytic ileus, and kidney damage. Bleeding manifestations include oozing blood, upper gastrointestinal bleed, and hematuria. The causes are numerous, including septicemia, severe trauma, and neoplasms, and DIC may affect people at any age. Diagnosis is based on the presence of degradation products as detected by the D-dimer test.[10]

Hemophilia

Hemophilia represents a group of inherited bleeding disorders caused by a gene mutation leading to the absence of or ineffective production of clotting protein factors. The severity of the condition is determined by the level of clotting factor. The two most common types of hemophilia are factor VIII deficiency (hemophilia A) and factor IX deficiency (hemophilia B). This genetic recessive disorder of the X chromosome affect only males, although females can be carriers of the hemophilia gene. It is estimated that approximately 20,000 males in the United States have hemophilia, accounting for approximately 1 in every 5000 male births.[14]

Bone Marrow Suppression

Any suppression of bone marrow activity, also called myelosuppression, can reduce the production of platelets, erythrocytes, and leukocytes. When platelets are low (thrombocytopenia), abnormal bleeding occurs. Bone marrow suppression has multiple causes, including leukemia (discussed next), chemotherapy, aplastic anemia, and heparin-induced thrombocytopenia. Because there are a variety of causes, bone marrow suppression can affect people at any age.

Leukemia

This is a group of malignant diseases affecting the blood and blood-forming tissues of the bone marrow, lymph system, and spleen. Proliferation of abnormal leukocytes prevents the normal production of platelets and erythrocytes, leading to bleeding and anemia. Leukemia is classified by the maturity of the involved cell—acute (immature cells) or chronic (mature cells)—and by the type of leukocytes involved (myelogenous or lymphocytic). Acute myelogenous leukemia has a peak incidence between 60 and 70 years of age. Acute lymphocytic leukemia has a peak incidence between 2 and 9 years of age. Chronic myelogenous leukemia has an onset between 25 and 60 years of age. Chronic lymphocytic leukemia has an onset between 50 and 70 years of age.[10]

CASE STUDY

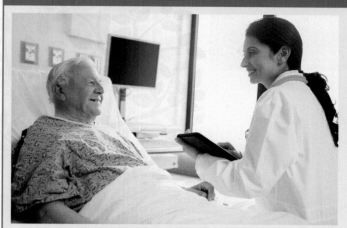

Source: monkeybusinessimages/iStock/Thinkstock

Case Presentation

Arthur Rosen is a 78-year-old widower who lives alone. He has a history of atrial fibrillation and has a prescription for warfarin 5 mg once a day. Arthur finished his Coumadin prescription 3 weeks ago and did not have an opportunity to obtain the refill. He was admitted to the hospital for treatment of an ischemic stroke attributable to cerebral emboli. His manifestations were paralysis and anesthesia of the left leg. During the morning assessment, the nurse notices Arthur's left thigh is red and edematous. Arthur tells the nurse his left upper leg feels achy. The circumference of the right leg is 51 cm, whereas the circumference of the left leg is 53 cm. Arthur has no feeling in his left leg. His vital signs are as follows: temperature, 98°F; blood pressure, 140/72 mm Hg; heart rate, 86 beats/min and irregularly irregular; and respiratory rate, 18 breaths/min. Based on these recent changes, the nurse suspects a DVT and notifies the physician of these changes. An ultrasound of the extremity is performed and confirms a DVT. Arthur is prescribed immediate full bed rest, and a new order for intravenous heparin is started until his INR is 2.0 or greater for 24 hours. Also, the nurse notifies the physical therapist of the suspected DVT so that therapy can be rescheduled. The nurse elevates Arthur's left leg on two pillows and does not perform the passive range-of-motion exercises of the lower extremities she had earlier planned.

Case Analysis

This case exemplifies impairment of clotting in several ways. Arthur had a history of atrial fibrillation. This disorder causes stasis of blood in the left atrium, which can cause clot development. These clots can dislodge, allowing emboli to travel to the cerebral circulation. The emboli lodged in the right anterior cerebral artery, impairing blood flow to the right frontal and parietal lobes. This lack of perfusion caused the paralysis and anesthesia of the left leg. Arthur's therapy is bed rest with limited mobility until he becomes stronger. Immobility is a risk factor for the development of thrombi, particularly in the lower extremity.

ACCESS EXEMPLAR LINKS IN YOUR GIDDENS EBOOK

REFERENCES

1. Porth C: *Essentials of pathophysiology*, ed 3, Philadelphia, 2011, Lippincott Williams & Wilkins.
2. Rote N, McCance K: Structure and function of the hematologic system. In Huether S, McCance K, editors: *Understanding pathophysiology*, ed 2, St Louis, 2012, Elsevier, pp 477–499.
3. Schwartz A, Rote N, McCance K: Alterations of hematologic function. In Huether S, McCance K, editors: *Understanding pathophysiology*, ed 5, St Louis, 2012, Elsevier, pp 500–534.
4. Kline N: Alterations of hematologic function in children. In Huether S, McCance K, editors: *Understanding pathophysiology*, ed 5, St Louis, 2012, Elsevier, pp 535–555.
5. Wilson S, Giddens J: *Health assessment for nursing practice*, ed 5, St Louis, 2013, Elsevier.
6. Wipke-Tevis D, Rich K: Nursing assessment: Vascular disorders. In Lewis S, Dirksen SR, Heitkemper MM, et al, editors: *Medical–surgical nursing: Assessment and management of clinical problems*, ed 8, St Louis, 2011, Elsevier, pp 866–896.
7. Malone M: Nursing management: Lower respiratory problems. In Lewis S, Dirksen SR, Heitkemper MM, et al, editors: *Medical–surgical nursing: Assessment and management of clinical problems*, ed 8, St Louis, 2011, Elsevier, pp 545–586.
8. Pagana K, Pagana T: *Mosby's diagnostic and laboratory test reference*, ed 10, St Louis, 2011, Elsevier.
9. *Healthy People 2020*: Goals for bleeding and clotting. Retrieved from <http://www.healthypeople.gov/2020/default.aspx>.
10. Rome SI: Nursing assessment: Hematologic problems. In Lewis S, Dirksen SR, Heitkemper MM, Bucher L, editors: *Medical–surgical nursing: Assessment and management of clinical problems*, ed 8, St Louis, 2011, Elsevier, pp 661–713.
11. Lehne R: *Pharmacology for nursing care*, ed 8, Philadelphia, 2012, Saunders.
12. Skidmore-Roth L: *Mosby's 2014 nursing drug reference*, ed 27, St Louis, 2014, Elsevier.
13. Centers for Disease Control and Prevention: Deep vein thrombosis/pulmonary embolism, Retrieved from <http://www.cdc.gov/ncbddd/dvt/data.html>, 2014.
14. Centers for Disease Control and Prevention: Hemophilia, Retrieved from <http://www.cdc.gov/ncbddd/hemophilia/facts.html>, 2014.

CONCEPT
21

Reproduction

Kathleen Bell and Nancy Jallo

The creation of all life occurs as a result of reproduction. As a foundational concept in the biological sciences, reproduction has been studied extensively. Two main types of reproduction described are sexual and asexual reproduction. With asexual reproduction, an organism can create genetic copies of itself. Viruses, bacteria, fungi, and some plants reproduce through such a process. Sexual reproduction is a biological process in which a combination of genetic material from two sources is needed. Mammals, fish, reptiles, and most plants reproduce through this process. The purpose of this concept analysis is to present the concept of reproduction as it applies to humans and in the context of nursing from the formation of reproductive cells and the creation of a pregnancy through birth.

DEFINITION

There are multiple definitions of human reproduction in the literature. However, the foundational principle of human reproduction is that it is the process by which human beings produce a new individual. Sexual intercourse between a man and a woman may result in the conception of a child. The sex glands or gonads (ovaries in the female and testes in the male) produce the germ cells (oocytes and spermatozoa) that unite and grow into a new individual.

During sexual intercourse, the interaction between the male and female reproductive systems may result in fertilization of the woman's ovum by the man's sperm. Fertilization of the ovum may also be achieved outside the uterus without sexual intercourse using a process known as assisted reproductive technology (ART). This includes procedures such as *in vitro* fertilization and intrauterine insemination. Childbirth follows a typical gestation period of 40 weeks. For the purpose of this concept presentation, reproduction is defined as *the total process by which organisms produce offspring*. In humans, the concept is referred to as human reproduction.[1]

SCOPE

In the broadest sense, the scope of reproduction for a woman or a couple falls into one of two states—the non-pregnant state and the pregnant state (Figure 21-1). However, significant complexity underlies this simplistic dichotomous perspective.

Non-Pregnant State

The majority of the life of a female is spent in a non-pregnant state. All individuals in a non-pregnant state represent one of two variables: (1) not pregnant by choice or (2) not pregnant, not by choice. *Not pregnant by choice* is a relatively simple variable, represented by a man, a woman, and/or a sexually engaged couple who are capable of creating a pregnancy and take specific measures to avoid a pregnancy. Pregnancy avoidance behavior is achieved through contraceptive measures or sexual abstinence. By contrast, *not pregnant, not by choice* represents individuals or couples who are unable to create a pregnancy—regardless if pregnancy is desired or not. Three categories representing this variable are (1) individuals who have not yet reached sexual maturity, (2) individuals who have reached sexual maturity and are infertile (including women who have reached menopause), and (3) those who have reached sexual maturity but are fertile and partnerless (or lack resources to create a pregnancy by other means).

Pregnant State

The other state is pregnancy and represents individuals or couples who intentionally create a pregnancy and those experiencing an unplanned pregnancy. The pregnant state begins at conception and is sustained until birth or ends with a premature cessation of the pregnant state. Not surprisingly, the range of emotion and acceptance of a pregnancy ranges from significant joy and celebration to worry and stress (particularly if the pregnancy was unplanned or if complications arise).

NORMAL PHYSIOLOGICAL PROCESS

In order for normal human reproduction to occur, the following complex developmental and physiological events must occur sequentially: the formation of reproductive cells, the menstrual cycle, conception, and pregnancy. Although the majority of this discussion focuses on the female, the male role in reproduction is not to be minimized.

Formation of Reproductive Cells

A physiological discussion of reproduction starts with the formation of reproductive cells known as germ cells. These cells carry the genetic materials needed for conception and the diverse genetic material needed to perpetuate the species.[2] Gametogenesis is a term that refers to the formation and development of germ cells, oocytes, and spermatocytes.[1] A specialized form of cell division called meiosis produces cells with a haploid number of 23 chromosomes. Two sequential meiotic cell divisions occur during gametogenesis. Homologous chromosomes pair during prophase and separate during anaphase. The first

Not Pregnant		Pregnant	
By Choice	Not by Choice	Unplanned	Planned
• Contraceptive measures • Abstinence	• Sexual maturity not reached • Infertility • Partnerless	Conception to birth or pregnancy termination.	

FIGURE 21-1 Scope of Reproduction

meiotic division is a reduction division in which each new cell forms a secondary oocyte or spermatocyte retaining the haploid number of chromosomes. In the second meiotic division, each chromosome divides to form two chromatids that are drawn to a different pole of the cell. The daughter cells that are produced contain a haploid number of chromosomes representative of each pair.[2] The primary spermatocyte contains one X and one Y chromosome; thus, during the first reduction division, two secondary spermatocytes are produced—one X and one Y. Therefore, spermatocytes have either X or Y chromosomes. Because the primary oocyte contains two X chromosomes, all oocytes have X chromosomes.

Oogenesis

In females, the process of egg formation (ovum) begins during fetal life and is known as oogenesis. The ovaries at birth contain all the cells that may undergo meiosis during a woman's reproductive stage of life. Only 400–500 ova out of 2 million oocytes will mature during a woman's reproductive years. Primary oocytes begin their first meiotic division before birth but remain suspended in prophase until puberty. At puberty, at the onset of menarche, monthly cycles begin, and usually one oocyte matures and completes the first meiotic division. The second meiotic division begins at ovulation but progresses only to metaphase when division is arrested. If the zona pellucida (inner layer) is penetrated by a sperm, the second meiotic division is completed.[3]

Spermatogenesis

In males, the formation of a germ cell to a sperm cell is known as spermatogenesis. This process begins at puberty under the influence of testosterone and continues throughout adult life. Spermatogenesis takes place in the seminiferous tubules within the testes. As sperm cells are produced, they travel through efferent tubules to the epididymis, where they mature. Once mature, sperm cells move to the ejaculatory duct through the vas deferens, where they wait until ejaculation.

Menstrual Cycle and Ovulation

The female menstrual cycle represents a physiological preparation for conception. It is regulated by hormonal levels controlled by the hypothalamus, anterior pituitary, and ovaries and occurs in four stages that repeat every 28 days. Stage I (menstrual phase) occurs with the shedding of the endometrium (caused by decreases in estrogen and progesterone), triggering menstrual bleeding. Stage II (follicular phase) is the preovulation phase, whereby the ovary and follicle prepare for the release of an ovum through the influence of follicle-stimulating hormone and estrogen. In stage III (ovulation phase), ovulation occurs, which is the process in which the ovum is expelled from the follicle (triggered by a sharp rise in estrogen and luteinizing hormone) and is drawn into the fallopian tube. During

stage IV (luteal phase), cilia in the fallopian tubes are stimulated by high estrogen levels, which propel the ovum toward the uterus. The follicle transforms into the corpus luteum during this phase and releases progesterone, which causes the uterine wall to thicken in anticipation of supporting a fertilized egg. If an ovum is not fertilized within 24 hours of ovulation by a sperm, it is usually reabsorbed by the woman's body.[3] The corpus luteum degenerates and estrogen and progesterone decrease, thus triggering the shedding of the uterine wall and starting the next cycle.

Pregnancy

Pregnancy is considered a normal physiological process that occurs without incident in the large majority of cases. Regardless of whether the pregnancy is planned or unplanned, it is an expected outcome among women of childbearing years who have sexual intercourse in the absence of contraceptive measures or when contraceptive measures fail. Each year in the United States, almost 625,000 women ages 15–19 years become pregnant.[4] Pregnancy begins with conception and, in the absence of complications, involves a 40-week gestation period (measured from the first day of the last menstrual period) and results in a live birth.

Fertilization

During sexual intercourse, sperm is ejaculated through the penis and into the vagina. Because of their mobility, sperm travel through the cervix into the uterus and into the fallopian tubes in search of an ovum. Fertilization of an ovum by sperm usually occurs in the lower third of the fallopian tube (Figure 21-2) when a sperm penetrates the ovum membrane. The sperm and ovum are enclosed in a process called the cortical reaction; this prevents other sperm from entering the ovum. The ovum nucleus becomes the female pronucleus, and the second meiotic division is completed. The head of the sperm enlarges to form the male pronucleus and the tail degenerates.

Fertilization results in a new cell called the zygote, which has two sets of chromosomes; half of the zygote genetic material is obtained from the ovum and half is obtained from the sperm.[2] A female develops through the fertilization of the ovum by an X-bearing sperm, producing an XX zygote; a male is produced through the fertilization of a Y-bearing sperm, producing an XY zygote. Therefore, at fertilization, chromosomal sex is established.[1]

Within the fallopian tube, a membrane-like sac, known as the zona pellucida, forms around the zygote. Approximately 30 hours after fertilization, division of the zygote (a process known as cleavage) begins. The zygote divides and two blastomeres are produced; soon thereafter, these divide again to form four blastomeres. Rapid cellular division occurs while the blastomeres travel down the reproductive tract. Although there is an increase in the number of cells, there is no increase in mass. Approximately 3 days after fertilization, a cell mass of 12–16 blastomeres known as the morula enters the woman's uterus.[3]

FIGURE 21-2 Fertilization and Implantation (Source: From National Institutes of Health: Blastocyst implantation picture, 2010. Retrieved from http://stemcells.nih.gov/info/scireport/pages/appendixA.aspx.)

Implantation

A cavity is formed within the morula 4 days after fertilization. It becomes a blastocyst and floats freely within the uterus for 2 days. Spaces form between the central cells of the morula and fluid passes through the zona, collecting in these spaces. The cells then separate into an outer layer know as a trophoblast and an inner layer known as an embryoblast. The blastocyst receives nourishment from the endometrial glands in the uterus, including carbohydrates, pyrimidines, purines, and amino acids, by active and passive transport. While the blastocyst implants into the endometrium at 6 days following fertilization, the zona pellucida lyses and degenerates (see Figure 21-2). By 9.5 days following ovulation, the blastocyst is completely imbedded into the endometrium, where it is provided nourishment for growth. The idea that the human implantation window is narrow has been challenged. Evidence obtained from *in vitro* fertilization programs suggests that the window for implantation may be 2 or even 3 days later than expected, but the issue is still being studied.[3]

Embryonic Period

The embryonic period is the stage between weeks 3 and 8 after conception. During this time, differentiation of body systems and organs occurs. Teratogenicity is a major concern during this period because all external and internal structures are developing (Figure 21-3). A pregnant woman should avoid exposure to all potential toxins during pregnancy, especially alcohol, tobacco, radiation, and other sources of infection during embryonic development. At the end of this period, the embryo has human features and is referred to as a fetus.[3]

Fetal Period

The fetal period represents the final stage of development beginning on the ninth week after fertilization until birth. This is a period of significant fetal growth; in fact, the normal human fetus grows approximately 1.5% per day. Because differentiation of major organs occurs during the embryonic period, the fetus is less susceptible to congenital malformations. The process of human development presented by stages is shown in Figure 21-3.

VARIATIONS AND CONTEXT

A number of problems are associated with the concept of reproduction and essentially can be categorized in two major areas: infertility and problems sustaining a pregnancy to term gestation. In addition, for some individuals and couples who were not seeking a pregnant state, unplanned pregnancy could be considered a problem.

Infertility

Infertility is defined as not being able to get pregnant despite having unprotected sex for at least 1 year. Although difficult to calculate for a number of reasons, it is estimated that infertility affects approximately 15% of reproductive-age couples in the United States and worldwide.[5,6] In addition, human reproduction may be inefficient with as many as 30% of pregnancies, resulting in spontaneous losses or "miscarriage."[6]

A number of conditions and factors cause infertility. Contributing factors can originate in both males and females, such as genetic problems (e.g., Turner's syndrome or Klinefelter's syndrome). Ovarian

FIGURE 21-3 Critical Periods in Human Development (Source: From Moore K, Persaud T: *Before we are born: Essentials of embryology and birth defects*, ed 7, Philadelphia, 2008, Saunders.)

factors affecting female fertility include developmental anomalies, primary or secondary anovulation, pituitary or hypothalamic hormone disorder, adrenal gland disorder, congenital adrenal hyperplasia, disruption of hypothalamic–pituitary–ovarian axis, amenorrhea after discontinuing oral contraceptive pills, premature ovarian failure, and increased prolactin levels. Uterine, tubal, and peritoneal factors affecting female fertility include developmental anomalies, reduced tubal motility, tubal inflammation, tubal adhesions, endometrial and myometrial tumors, uterine adhesions, endometriosis, chronic cervicitis, pelvic inflammatory disease, and inadequate cervical mucus. Other factors affecting female fertility include nutritional deficiencies such as anemia, obesity, thyroid dysfunction, and idiopathic conditions.[6]

Hormonal disorders affecting male fertility include low testosterone levels, hypopituitarism, and endocrine disorders. Structural and anatomical complications affecting male fertility include testicular damage caused by mumps, undescended testes, hypospadias, varicocele, obstructive lesions of the vas deferens or epididymis, or retrograde ejaculation. Other factors affecting male fertility include sexually transmitted infections; exposure to environmental hazards such as radiation or toxic substances; exposure of the scrotum to high temperatures; nutritional deficiencies; obesity; the presence of anti-sperm antibodies; substance abuse; changes in sperm motility; decrease in libido; and impotence caused by alcohol, antihypertensive medications, and idiopathic conditions.[6] With age, male testes become smaller and softer. Sperm shape, quality, quantity, and motility decline. There is also an increased risk of genetic defects in the sperm.[1] Patients with infertility are usually referred to a reproductive endocrinologist or obstetrician who specializes in infertility.

Maintaining a Pregnancy and Optimizing Fetal Growth and Development

There are a multitude of reproduction problems characterized by failure to maintain a pregnancy. These problems are related to maternal/fetal complications and are categorized by trimester. First-trimester complications may include maternal/fetal infections such as rubella or toxoplasmosis, ectopic pregnancy, trauma, or spontaneous abortion (miscarriage). Spontaneous abortion in the first trimester usually results from chromosomal abnormalities.

Complications of pregnancy that become evident during the second and third trimesters include fetal congenital and chromosomal anomalies, maternal systemic conditions (e.g., gestational diabetes, gestational hypertension, and preeclampsia), and infections. Many other complications can occur later in pregnancy, such as preterm labor, premature rupture of the membranes, placenta previa, abruptio placentae, trauma, fetal distress, and intrauterine fetal death.[7]

Unplanned Pregnancy

Pregnancy is considered an expected event among persons who engage in intercourse without contraceptive measures. Unplanned pregnancy occurs when contraceptive efforts fail, when consensual or nonconsensual sexual intercourse occurs without contraceptive measures, or when people lack education regarding conception and pregnancy.

CONSEQUENCES

The consequences of reproductive problems are highly variable and can affect the woman, her partner, and the fetus. Consequences of infertility are generally associated with stress, anxiety, and grief, particularly if the treatment options are not successful. Such consequences can be debilitating to individuals and couples.

Complications of pregnancy can lead to several consequences as well, depending on the type of problem and the stage of pregnancy or labor at which the complications occur. Fetal consequences can range from fetal stress to long-term health problems for the infant (e.g., genetic and congenital defects) and fetal demise. Fetal distress may be caused by any number of physiological or mechanical insults; for example, a pregnant woman involved in a motor vehicle collision may sustain abdominal trauma that could then cause fetal distress. Premature infants often have long-term physiological consequences, including developmental and intellectual disabilities or delays, cerebral palsy, or problems with sensory integration. In cases of severe prematurity or fetal distress, fetal death may occur in the intrapartum setting.

Physiological consequences to a mother can range from lacerations sustained to the perineum during childbirth to postpartum hemorrhage and death. For example, if postpartum bleeding or hemorrhage is severe enough, the mother may require surgical intervention to stop the bleeding, such as a hysterectomy.

RISK FACTORS

Despite the complexity of human reproduction, this process occurs without incident in the majority of individuals. However, as discussed previously, problems do occur, and reproduction does not always progress as expected. This section identifies common risk factors for problems associated with reproduction. Risk factors affecting successful human reproduction and fertility transcend all races and nations, with Third World developing countries largely affected because of poverty.

Populations at Risk

The adolescent population worldwide is a reproductive high-risk group. Adolescent pregnancy concerns and complications include impaired nutrition, anemia, infections, depression, social isolation, preeclampsia, protracted labor, cephalopelvic disproportion, premature birth, and cesarean section. The impact on the woman is lifelong and includes the risks of higher dropout rates, completing school later or not at all, lower income and dependence on government assistance, and living in poverty. In 2010 the U.S. teen pregnancy rate was 57.4 pregnancies per 1000 women ages 15–19 years.[4] By comparison, western Europe and other countries have considerably lower teen pregnancy rates (United Kingdom, 25.8:1000; Canada, 14.5:1000; Ireland, 8.2:1000; Sweden, 6.5:1000; The Netherlands, 6.2:1000; France, 5.7:1000; and Japan, 5.4:1000). There are also differences between ethnicities, with the 2010 birth rates for U.S. blacks at 99.5:1000, Hispanics at 83.5:1000, and whites at 37.8:1000. Although teen pregnancy rates among black women have decreased, they still remain higher than those of other ethnicities and are more than twice the teenage pregnancy rate of white, non-Hispanic teenagers.[8] The disparity has existed for decades and may be due to differences in approaches to contraceptive education and availability.[9]

Individual Risk Factors

There are numerous risk factors for women and men affecting reproductive health and pregnancy outcomes. These can be categorized into biophysical, psychosocial, sociodemographic, and environmental factors. Some of the risk factors for human reproduction fit into multiple categories.

Biophysical Factors

Genetic concerns encompass altered or mutated genes, inherited disorders, chromosomal anomalies, multiple gestation, large fetal size, and ABO incompatibilities. Nutritional concerns include malnutrition, diets, young age, pre-pregnancy obesity, inadequate or excessive weight gain, and anemia. Medical and obstetric disorders encompass complications of past or current pregnancies, obstetric illnesses, and previous pregnancy losses.[1,10] Although changes in fertility and sexual functioning occur in males as they grow older, there is no maximum age at which a man can father a child.

Psychosocial Factors

Psychosocial factors include smoking, excessive caffeine intake, alcohol consumption, drug abuse, spousal abuse, and addictive lifestyles. In addition, maternal emotional well-being has been found to influence reproductive health.[1,10] For example, negative affective states such as stress, anxiety, and depression during pregnancy are risk factors for shortened gestation and preterm birth.[11] Conversely, positive affect during pregnancy may be beneficial for outcomes related to the length of gestation.[12]

Sociodemographic Factors

Sociodemographic factors include low income, inadequate prenatal care, age at both ends of the reproductive years (younger than age 15 years and older than age 35 years), parity, marital status, geographic location (urban vs. rural), and race/ethnicity.[3,10] It is beyond the scope of this concept presentation to discuss every ethnic group worldwide. However, a disproportionate number of nonwhite women die of pregnancy-related causes annually compared to white women (a 3:1 ratio). African-American newborns have the highest rate of prematurity, low birth weight, and infant mortality.[1]

Environmental Factors

Environmental factors affecting reproductive health and pregnancy outcomes include industrial pollution, radiation, chemical exposure, bacterial and viral infections, drugs (over-the-counter, therapeutic, and illicit), and stress.[1,10]

ASSESSMENT

The assessment of human reproduction involves history, examination, and diagnostic testing. Nurses should have a basic understanding of the elements of an assessment; they should also be able to recognize abnormal findings and understand common diagnostic tests related to normal reproduction.

History

Elements of a reproductive and sexual health history include inquiring about sexual history (including number and sex of partners), contraceptive history (including methods previously used and reasons for discontinuation), relevant surgical history (i.e., removal of polyps, fibroids, or neoplasms of the genitourinary system), alterations in pelvic support (including uterine displacement, uterine prolapse, cystocele, or rectocele), Papanicolaou history (including normal and abnormal results), and menstrual history. Additional pertinent history includes immunization status (including, but not limited to, hepatitis B, rubella, and tetanus), mental health history, dietary history (including any history of deficiency or disordered eating), alcohol and caffeine intake, drug use (both prescribed and nonprescribed), and known genetic familial disorders. Positive findings that are not expected would alert the nurse that additional testing, screening, or monitoring may be needed.[10,13]

Subjective assessment of the pregnant woman data may reveal fatigue, nausea, and vomiting for 4–12 weeks of gestation due to increasing levels of human chorionic gonadotropin.[7] Increased levels of estrogen and progesterone can cause breast enlargement, fullness, tenderness, and heightened sensitivity, as well as increased urinary frequency. As the pregnancy progresses, the pregnant woman may feel Braxton Hicks contractions starting at 16 weeks and palpable, "obvious" fetal movements at approximately 20 weeks.[1,13]

Examination Findings

When conducting a physical examination on a pregnant woman, normal vital signs are expected, including normotension, afebrile state, and normal respiration and pulse. In addition, although many pregnant women experience some degree of varying discomfort during their pregnancy due to musculoskeletal changes, significant pain or discomfort is not expected. Weight gain is expected to be within normal limits depending on the patient's pre-pregnancy body mass index, pre-pregnancy nutritional status, and current pregnancy. For example, a woman who is underweight or overweight before pregnancy will have specific dietary requirements and should also be under the care of a dietician or nutritionist during the pregnancy. A woman pregnant with twins has a significantly higher daily caloric requirement than a woman carrying a single fetus. Benign physical findings are expected as each body system is examined, including the cardiovascular, respiratory, gastrointestinal, and lymph systems. These findings may be altered based on the woman's past medical history and current state of health. Expected physical changes of the breasts and genitourinary systems are outlined next.[13]

Typical objective data gathered during an examination of the genitourinary system reflect the following expected and normal changes: softening and compression of the lower uterine segment (Hegar's sign), softening of the cervical tip (Goodell's sign), and a violet blue vaginal mucosa and cervix at 6 weeks (Chadwick's sign).[10] The breasts will also enlarge to prepare for lactogenesis, or the production of breast milk for infant nutrition, and the areola and nipples may darken. The pregnant woman should be reassured that these findings are normal and her body's way of preparing for birth and subsequent breast-feeding.

Objective assessment data also include visualization of the fetus by real-time ultrasound at 5 weeks, fetal heart activity observed at 6 weeks via transvaginal ultrasound, fetal heart tones auscultated at approximately 8 weeks by external Doppler, and palpable fetal movement by approximately 19 weeks. It is important to reassure women that these times are merely averages. A woman's previous pregnancy history, gestational age, and state of health may alter each of these values.[3,13]

Diagnostic Tests

Several diagnostic tests are performed during pregnancy and for reproductive health. Table 21-1 shows commonly ordered laboratory tests, screening tests, and other diagnostic studies throughout the pregnancy. Not all women need every test listed, and some may choose to defer various tests or screening procedures based on personal belief or need. For example, some women may choose not to have any diagnostic screening that would alert them to the risk of a child with Down's syndrome or other trisomy. The type and frequency of testing and screening should be determined with the woman, keeping in mind her values and priorities for her health and pregnancy. Also, based on various risk factors, some women may have additional screening tests done throughout the pregnancy. For example, a woman who is

TABLE 21-1 Routine, Screening, and Diagnostic Tests Performed in Pregnancy

First Trimester	Second Trimester	Third Trimester
• Urine or serum pregnancy test	• Repeat CBC at approximately 24–26 weeks gestation	• Group B strep testing at approximately 36+ weeks of gestation
• CBC with differential	• 1–Hour glucose tolerance test	• Screening and diagnostic ultrasound
• Blood type and Rh factor	• MSAFP screen	• Emotional well-being
• Rubella titer	• Amniocentesis as needed	
• Hepatitis B titer	• Emotional well-being	
• Syphilis test (RPR or VDRL)		
• HIV test		
• Urinalysis and culture		
• Pap test		
• Gonorrhea and chlamydia cultures[a]		
• Nuchal translucency screening at 10–12 weeks		
• Amniocentesis as needed		
• Emotional well-being		

[a]Gonorrhea and chlamydia cultures may be repeated at any time exposure is suspected, as well as HIV testing.
CBC, complete blood count; RPR, rapid plasma reagin; VDRL, Venereal Disease Research Laboratory. MSAFP, maternal serum α-fetoprotein.

morbidly obese or who has a history of diabetes will require earlier glucose screening.[10]

Various screening tests assess fetal health and development *in utero*. The maternal serum α-fetoprotein (MSAFP) test analyzes a sample of maternal blood and searches for abnormally high or low hormonal levels that may be indicative of trisomy 21, trisomy 18, or neural tube defects. These values are determined based on the mother's age, ethnicity, and gestational age. Because this test may be done only between 16 and 18 weeks of gestation, it is imperative to have an accurate gestational age when conducting this screening. Amniocentesis is another form of genetic analysis available to pregnant women. A sample of amniotic fluid is collected and the fetal karyotype is analyzed, providing definitive diagnosis. It is often used as a follow up to an abnormal screening test, such as the nuchal translucency or MSAFP.[2] If any testing reveals abnormal findings, treatment and further monitoring may be necessary to ensure the health of the woman and her fetus.

Pregnancy Monitoring

During the first and second trimesters, the woman is usually seen once a month. The third trimester (starting at 28 weeks) begins with visits every 2 weeks. At 36 weeks, the visits are weekly until birth. The individual needs of the child-bearing family are considered, and the pregnant woman may need fewer or more frequent visits depending on her health status.[3,13] Prenatal visits are not only important for the health and well-being of the developing child but also important to ensure the mother's health and adjustment to the pregnancy and impending birth, as well as the health and well-being of her partner.

CLINICAL MANAGEMENT

The health management related to reproduction includes using interventions to prevent problems and optimize health, screening for problems, and providing collaborative interventions if problems arise. The levels of care related to the concept of human reproductive health are discussed next; for the pregnant female, prenatal care is the cornerstone to nursing care.

Primary Prevention

Primary prevention refers to health-promotion activities that further health and well-being. An example of primary prevention is teaching a group of high school students about reproductive health. Topics to discuss may include abstinence; the importance of safe sex; contraceptive options; tobacco, alcohol, and drug cessation; avoidance of environmental toxins; folic acid supplementation; and the need for preconception counseling and prenatal care throughout pregnancy.[14]

Nurses should be instrumental in providing anticipatory guidance to women and childbearing families by providing instruction in human sexuality and maternal and newborn care; offering parenting classes; and promoting healthy lifestyles through education about proper nutrition, exercise, and stress management. Education provided during teachable moments—at the right place and time—can change the course of a woman's life and positively affect her reproductive health.

The use of contraceptive agents is also primary prevention, and it is the intentional prevention of pregnancy during sexual intercourse.[3] The effectiveness of contraception varies and depends on both the method and user characteristics. For example, oral contraceptive pills (OCPs) are 99% effective in preventing pregnancy if taken as directed. To achieve this level of effectiveness, however, the user must remember to take the OCPs each day at the same time. Other methods of contraception include abstinence, natural family planning, coitus interruptus, spermicides, male and female condoms, diaphragms, cervical caps, vaginal sponges, vaginal contraceptive rings, transdermal patches, injectable and implantable progestins, intrauterine devices, and surgical sterilization of either the male or the female.

Secondary Prevention (Screening)

Secondary prevention refers to early detection of disease and disease sequelae. An example of secondary prevention relating to reproductive health is continuing prenatal care in the second trimester of pregnancy. The purpose of prenatal care is to determine the gestational age of the fetus, identify risk for and minimize reproductive complications, define the health status of the fetus and the mother, provide education and counseling, and perform the normal screening done at prenatal clinic visits.[3,13] Screening includes complete blood count; blood type and Rh; rubella titer; TB skin test; urinalysis; urine culture; Pap smear; glucose tolerance test; and tests for gonorrhea, chlamydia, syphilis, human papilloma virus, and HIV. In addition, each visit provides a valuable opportunity to screen for the mother's emotional health and well-being (early warning signs of depression), as well as the emotional health of her partner or support people. In addition, each visit should include screening for domestic violence and abuse.

Collaborative Interventions

Collaborative interventions in this specific population include routine pregnancy care. Table 21-2 presents common pharmacologic agents

TABLE 21-2   Pharmacologic Agents Commonly Used in Pregnancy and the Peripartum

Pharmacologic Agents	Indications for Usage
Analgesics (e.g., acetaminophen)	Pain
Antibiotics (e.g., ampicillin, clindamycin, cefazolin, metronidazole, gentamicin, penicillin, erythromycin)	Infections
Antidepressants (e.g., sertraline, escitalopram)	Mood disorders
Antiemetics (e.g., promethazine, ondansetron)	Nausea/vomiting of pregnancy
Folic acid	Prevention of neural tube defects
Ferrous sulfate (iron)	Important for transfer of iron to fetus and to expand maternal red blood cell mass; used to treat iron deficiency
Flu vaccine	Prevention of influenza
Laxative/stool softeners (e.g., docusate)	Constipation
Magnesium sulfate	Prevention of seizures in preeclamptic patients and fetal neurologic protection in women experiencing preterm labor
Prenatal vitamins	Support maternal nutrition and optimal fetal growth
Progesterone	Support early intrauterine pregnancy; promote uterine relaxation in those at risk for preterm labor
$Rh_o(D)$ immune globulin (e.g., Rhogram)	Used to prevent hemolytic disease of newborn
Tocolytics (e.g., nifedipine)	Suppress uterine contractions in those with preterm labor

used during pregnancy. Collaborative interventions also include the management and treatment of pregnancy-related conditions or complications. This may include prescribing antibiotics for a sexually transmitted infection or following up with serial ultrasounds to measure fetal growth in an infant diagnosed with a congenital condition or referral for mental health services for issues related to maternal distress. More common examples are treatment for gestational diabetes, preeclampsia, and premature cervical dilation. Other collaborative interventions include assistive reproductive technology and abortion.

CLINICAL NURSING SKILLS FOR REPRODUCTION

- Assessment
- Education, support, and anticipatory guidance
- Fetal monitoring
- Breast-feeding education and support
- Contraception education
- Medication administration

Management of High-Risk Pregnancy

Women experiencing a high-risk pregnancy are often managed by an obstetrician/gynecologist or a perinatologist. Factors related to high-risk childbearing are categorized as biophysical, psychosocial, sociodemographic, and environmental. *Biophysical factors* include genetics, nutritional status, and obstetric-related illnesses including gestational diabetes and preeclampsia. *Psychosocial factors* include effects of nicotine, caffeine, alcohol, and drugs on the developing fetus and maternal psychological status. *Sociodemographic factors* include low income, lack of prenatal care, pregnant adolescents or older mothers, parity, marital status, residence, and race/ethnicity. *Environmental factors* related to high-risk pregnancy may include infections, radiation exposure, chemical exposures such as to lead or mercury, therapeutic and/or illicit drugs, cigarette smoke, industrial pollutants, poor diet, and stress.[3,13,15]

Collaborative interventions for the management of high-risk pregnancy include ongoing assessment of maternal and fetal well-being, which includes maternal weight, blood pressure, and the presence of protein in the urine. Ongoing fetal assessment may include ultrasound to assess fetal growth and fetal monitoring for heart rate.

Assisted Reproductive Technologies

The inability to conceive a child is a reproductive dilemma that affects more than 15% of all couples worldwide. Couples who are unable to conceive naturally may consult specialists and seek ART procedures such as *in vitro* fertilization–embryo transfer, gamete intrafallopian transfer, zygote intrafallopian transfer, therapeutic donor insemination, or intracytoplasmic sperm injection.[1] See other resources for discussion of these procedures.

Abortion

Abortion is the elective termination of pregnancy. Indications may include (1) a woman's request, (2) genetic disorders of a fetus, (3) incest or rape, and (4) preserving the health of a woman. The most common planned clinic abortion procedure is vacuum aspiration. It is used up to 16 weeks after a woman's last menstrual period. Other types of abortion procedures include dilation and curettage, in which the cervix is dilated and the products of conception are removed from the uterus, and dilation and extraction, which is typically used in later-aged gestations. This is usually performed later than 16 weeks after a woman's last menstrual period.[16] The women's health nurse needs to be familiar with state-specific laws regarding abortion for the state(s) in which he or she practices.

INTERRELATED CONCEPTS

Figure 21-4 shows the interrelationships of major concepts that influence or are influenced by the process of human reproduction. Sexuality and Hormonal Regulation are obviously closely related to reproduction. The entire reproductive cycle is influenced by hormones, as noted previously. Hormonal balance is often an underlying factor in reproductive problems. The discussion of the effects of proper Nutrition on human reproduction and pregnancy outcomes is prevalent in the literature. In the 1950s, researchers concluded that prenatal folic acid supplementation prevented pregnancy-induced megaloblastic anemia. In the 1990s, further research studies confirmed that periconceptual folic acid supplementation (400 μm per day) and folic acid food fortification decreased the incidence of neural tube defects.[17]

Adequate Perfusion of maternal blood to the growing fetus is absolutely essential, as is adequate Gas Exchange. A female who smokes tobacco may reduce oxygenation to her developing fetus, which can lead to a number of complications. Smoking cessation has been recognized as the most important preventable risk factor for improving reproductive and pregnancy outcomes worldwide.[18]

Understanding the interrelationships of these major concepts helps nurses recognize risk factors and their potential effect on the human reproductive process and pregnancy outcomes. These are important steps in providing anticipatory guidance, clinical judgment, and screening when planning for reproductive health needs of adolescents and childbearing families.

CLINICAL EXEMPLARS

The concept of reproduction represents many clinical situations, from pregnancy prevention to conception and pregnancy. A comprehensive

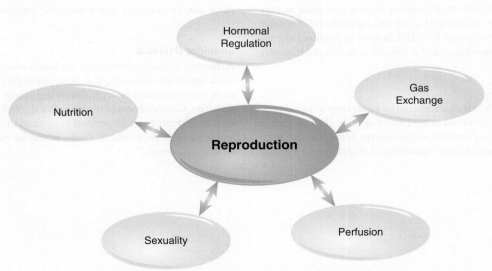

FIGURE 21-4 Reproduction and Interrelated Concepts

BOX 21-1 EXEMPLARS OF REPRODUCTION

Normal Reproductive Health

Contraception
- Hormonal contraception
- Natural family planning
- Intrauterine device
- Cervical cap
- Contraceptive sponge
- Condoms and spermicides

Pregnancy
- Planned, uncomplicated pregnancies
- Unplanned, uncomplicated pregnancies

Problems Associated with Reproduction

Conception
- Infertility

Gestational Conditions
- Gestational diabetes
- Gestational hypertension
- Iron deficiency anemia
- Preeclampsia

- Eclampsia
- HELLP syndrome
- Hyperemesis gravidarum
- Spontaneous abortion or "miscarriage"
- Premature dilation of the cervix
- Ectopic pregnancy
- Abruptio placentae
- DIC
- Sexually transmitted infections
- Preterm labor
- Dystocia
- Prolapsed umbilical cord
- Uterine rupture
- Postpartum hemorrhage

Fetal Complications/Genetic Congenital Defects
- Neural tube defects (spina bifida)
- Other genetic anomalies
- Intrauterine growth restriction
- Impaired fetal brain development/anencephaly
- Fetal alcohol syndrome
- Premature delivery

DIC, disseminated intravascular coagulation; HELLP syndrome, syndrome of hemolysis, elevated liver enzymes, and low platelet count.

discussion related to all these factors is beyond the scope of this concept, and it is best left to other textbooks devoted to sexual and reproductive health. Box 21-1 presents common exemplars related to reproductive conditions seen in clinical practice.

Featured Exemplars
Gestational Diabetes Mellitus

Gestational diabetes mellitus (GDM) is defined as carbohydrate intolerance of variable severity with onset or first recognition during pregnancy that is often a consequence of the altered maternal metabolism due to changing maternal hormonal levels.[13] Because GDM complicates approximately 3–10% of all pregnancies, every pregnant woman should be assessed for risk of GDM at the first prenatal visit.[13] Women at high risk should be screened for GDM as soon as possible, whereas those of average risk are often tested at the end of the second trimester, typically 24–28 weeks.[13]

Preeclampsia

Preeclampsia is a syndrome characterized by an increase in blood pressure after 20 weeks of gestation accompanied by renal changes such as proteinuria in a previously normotensive woman possibly due to alternations in vascular remodeling, endothelial dysfunction, an immune response to paternal antigens, and/or an exaggerated systemic inflammatory response.[13] In the United States, preeclampsia complicates approximately 3–8% of all pregnancies and can lead to numerous maternal and fetal morbidities as well as death.

Postpartum Hemorrhage

A postpartum hemorrhage occurs when a mother loses a significant amount of blood after the delivery of the fetus. Although definitions vary between textbooks or among health care providers, the typically accepted definitions are a blood loss of 500 mL or more after a vaginal birth and 1000 mL or more after a cesarean section delivery. Hemorrhage may be managed with a variety of uterotonic drugs.

Shoulder Dystocia

A shoulder dystocia occurs when the fetus's anterior shoulder becomes stuck under the maternal pubic bone preventing vaginal birth. This is most commonly seen in larger infants (e.g., those born to mothers with diabetes). Consequences of prolonged or unresolved shoulder dystocia include increased risk of perineal trauma to the mother and hypoxia and acidosis in the newborn. Dystocia may be managed with a variety of fetal maneuvers.[19]

CASE STUDY

Source: Antonio_Diaz/iStock/Thinkstock

Case Presentation

Katherine Cordova, a 25-year-old female, gravida 4, para 2, with a history of one spontaneous abortion at 8 weeks, presents with her male partner to the community women's clinic for her first prenatal appointment. Last week, she took a urine pregnancy test at home, and it was positive. The nurse at the clinic estimates her current gestational age based on Katherine's last menstrual period at approximately 10 weeks and 2 days.

The couple has been together for 4 years; her partner is the father of her other children. Both Katherine and her partner are social drinkers, but they do not smoke cigarettes. They are weight appropriate for height, although Katherine does not engage in regular cardiovascular exercise. She estimates that she exercises perhaps twice a week for approximately 20 minutes each time. Both she and her partner work outside the home full-time; she is a teacher's aide in a second-grade elementary school class, and her partner works as a police officer. They both have health insurance, and Katherine denies financial concerns at this time. In addition, Katherine denies domestic violence, and she states that they have support of their extended family and friends. This is a planned pregnancy about which she and her partner are excited.

At this time, she reports slight nausea and vomiting in the mornings, but otherwise she is having no other symptoms of pregnancy. Her medical history is grossly noncontributory, although she has a history of genital herpes simplex virus (HSV), diagnosed at the age of 20 years. She denies recent or current outbreaks, and she is not experiencing prodromal symptoms.

Katherine is prescribed prenatal vitamins that include folic acid 400 μg daily. She is also educated on proper diet for pregnancy, which includes a diet high in grains and fiber, as well as fruits and vegetables and lean proteins. Katherine is given anticipatory guidance by the nurse practitioner in the clinic that at 36 weeks of gestation, she will need to begin suppressive therapy to help prevent HSV outbreaks during the last 4 or 5 weeks of pregnancy.

Case Analysis

This case study illustrates an example of a first prenatal care appointment for a newly diagnosed pregnancy. By beginning her prenatal care early, Katherine is helping to ensure optimal pregnancy outcomes for herself, her baby, and her family. In addition, by getting appropriate anticipatory guidance throughout the pregnancy, Katherine is able to anticipate and plan for expected changes and therapies that will be prescribed to her.

ACCESS EXEMPLAR LINKS IN YOUR GIDDENS EBOOK

REFERENCES

1. Perry SE: Conception and fetal development. In Lowdermilk DL, Perry SE, Cashion K, et al, editors: *Maternity & women's health care*, ed 10, St Louis, 2012, Mosby, pp 270–288.
2. Lewis R: *Human genetics: Concepts and applications*, Boston, 2008, McGraw-Hill.
3. Beckmann C, Ling FW, Herbert W, et al: *Obstetrics and gynecology*, ed 7, Philadelphia, 2014, Lippincott Williams & Wilkins.
4. United Nations Statistics Division: Adolescent fertility rate (births per 1,000 women ages 15–19), 2014. Retrieved from: <http://data.un.org/Data.aspx?q=birth+rate&d=WDI&f=Indicator_Code%3aSP.ADO.TFRT>.
5. World Health Organization: Global prevalence of infertility, infecundity and childlessness, 2013. Retrieved from: <http://www.who.int/reproductivehealth/topics/infertility/burden/en>.
6. Gingrich PM: Infertility. In Lowdermilk DL, Perry SE, Cashion K, et al, editors: *Maternity & women's health care*, ed 10, St Louis, 2012, Mosby, pp 194–210.
7. Moore MC: Maternal and fetal nutrition. In Lowdermilk DL, Perry SE, Cashion K, et al, editors: *Maternity & women's health care*, ed 10, St Louis, 2012, Mosby, pp 307–328.
8. Kost K, Henshaw S: U.S. teenage pregnancies, births and abortions, 2010: National and state trends by age, race and ethnicity. Retrieved from: <http://www.guttmacher.org/pubs/USTPtrends10.pdf>.
9. American Society for Reproductive Medicine: Age and fertility: a guide for patients, 2012. Retrieved from: <http://www.reproductivefacts.org/uploadedFiles/ASRM_Content/Resources/Patient_Resources/Fact_Sheets_and_Info_Booklets/agefertility.pdf>.
10. Zdanuk JL: Assessment and health promotion. In Lowdermilk DL, Perry SE, Cashion K, et al, editors: *Maternity & women's health care*, ed 10, St Louis, 2012, Mosby, pp 307–328.
11. Dunkel Schetter C, Tanner L: Anxiety, depression and stress in pregnancy: Implications for mothers, children, research, and practice. *Curr Opin Psychiatry* 25(2):141–148, 2012.
12. Voellmin A, Entringer S, Moog M, et al: Maternal positive affect over the course of pregnancy is associated with the length of gestation and reduced risk of preterm delivery. *J Psychosom Res* 75:336–340, 2013.
13. Davidson MR, London ML, Ladewig PA: *Maternal–newborn nursing & women's health across the lifespan*, ed 9, Boston, 2012, Pearson.
14. Johnson K, Posner SF, Viermann J, et al: CDC/ATSDR Preconception Care Work Group, Select Panel on Preconception Care: Recommendations to improve preconception health and health care—United States: A report of the CDC/ATSDR Preconception Care Work Group and the Select Panel on Preconception Care. *Morbid Mortal Weekly Rep* 55(RR-6):1–23, 2006.
15. Reece EA, Hobbins JC: *Handbook of clinical obstetrics: The fetus and mother*, Malden, MA, 2007, Blackwell.
16. Planned Parenthood: In-clinic abortion procedures, 2011. Retrieved from: <www.plannedparenthood.org/health-topics/abortion/in-clinic-abortion-procedures-4359.asp>.
17. Tsunenobu T, Picciano MF: Folate and human reproduction. *Am J Clin Nutr* 83(5):993–1016, 2006.
18. Cnattingius S: The epidemiology of smoking during pregnancy: Smoking prevalence, maternal characteristics, and pregnancy outcomes. *Nicotine Tobacco Res* 6(Suppl 2):S125–S140, 2010.
19. Piotrowski KA: Labor and birth complications. In Lowdermilk DL, Perry SE, Cashion K, et al, editors: *Maternity & women's health care*, St Louis, 2012, Elsevier, pp 779–823.

Sexuality

Sue Goebel

I n general, human sexuality is how people experience and express themselves as sexual beings. It includes our body parts and sex. It is that sense of being "girl" and feminine and "male" or masculine, regardless of the "parts." It includes how we express that sense of gender, whom we are attracted to, and who is attracted to us. It is the nature of relationships with ourselves and others. Sexuality is unique to the individual, is core to who we are, and is dynamic throughout a lifetime. Learning about human sexuality and the sexual well-being of patients is an important part of providing holistic patient-centered nursing care.

DEFINITION

For the purpose of this concept presentation, the World Health Organization provides a working definition of sexuality as follows:

> *A central aspect of being human throughout life encompasses sex, gender identities and roles, sexual orientation, eroticism, pleasure, intimacy and reproduction. Sexuality is experienced and expressed in thoughts, fantasies, desires, beliefs, attitudes, values, behaviors, practices, roles and relationships. While sexuality can include all of these dimensions, not all of them are always experienced or expressed. Sexuality is influenced by the interaction of biological, psychological, social, economic, political, cultural, legal, historical, religious and spiritual factors.[1]*

The word "sexuality" has its roots in the word "sex." The word sexuality, meaning the action or fact of being sexual, is documented as early as 1789. In 1879, sexuality was further defined to include being capable of sexual feelings, and by 1980 the definition included the idea of sexual identity and sexual orientation.[2] In 2001, the Surgeon General of the United States issued a "Call to Action" to promote sexual health and responsible sexual behavior;[3] sexual health is a function of sexuality and, thus, needs to be defined. The Centers for Disease Control and Prevention (CDC) offers the following encompassing definition of sexual health:

> *A state of well-being in relation to sexuality across the lifespan that involves physical, emotional, mental, social and spiritual*

> *dimensions. Sexual health is an intrinsic element of human health and is based on a positive, equitable, and respectful approach to sexuality, relationships and reproduction, that is free of coercion, fear, discrimination, stigma, shame, and violence.[4]*

Other related terms are defined in Box 22-1.

SCOPE

The scope of sexuality as a concept ranges from sexual well-being to sexual ill-being; these can be a measure of sexual function and dysfunction (Figure 22-1). Well-being is defined as the state of being happy, healthy, or successful (function), and ill-being is defined as a condition of being deficient in health, happiness, or prosperity (dysfunction).[5] Although it is a simplistic definition, sexual well-being can be evidenced by the presence of positive attitudes, the absence of negative emotions, and an "overall satisfaction with life, fulfillment, and positive functioning."[6]

NORMAL PHYSIOLOGICAL PROCESS

Sexuality is more complex than one might initially imagine. To fully understand the physiological process of sexuality, three perspectives are presented: sexual response, age-related considerations, and sexual attitudes and behaviors.

Sexual Response

The human sexual response cycle, first described by Masters and Johnson in 1966, was based on physiological measures of heart rate, blood pressure, changes in genital size, and genital lubrication during stimulation and orgasm.[7] Four consecutive phases were identified to describe human sexual response: excitement, plateau, orgasmic, and resolution phases. Since then, other human sexual response models have been formulated to consider psychological and sociological factors as well, most notably the notions of sexual motivation and desire. The original works of Masters and Johnson continue to inform present-day models of sexual response. Although aspects of each model may vary slightly, the general phases are the same and include motivation, arousal, genital congestion, orgasm, and resolution.[7–10]

FIGURE 22-1 Scope of Sexuality

BOX 22-1 Definitions Related to the Concept of Sexuality

- *Sex:* One of four primary drives that also include thirst, hunger, and avoidance of pain.
- *Sexual acts:* Occur when behaviors include genitalia and erogenous zones.
- *Sexuality:* Is the result of biological, psychological, social, and experiential factors that mold an individual's sexual development, self-concept, body image, and behavior. Sexuality depends on four interrelated psychosexual factors:
  1. *Sexual identity:* Whether one is male or female based on biological sexual characteristics
  2. *Gender identity:* How one views one's gender as masculine or feminine, socially derived from experiences with the family, friends, and society
  3. *Sexual orientation:* How one views one's self in terms of being emotionally, romantically, sexually, or affectionally attracted to an individual of a particular gender
  4. *Sexual behavior:* How one responds to sexual impulses and desires

Source: From Shives L: *Basic concepts of psychiatric mental health nursing,* Philadelphia, 2008, Wolters Kluwer.

Motivation

The desire to engage in sexual activity is also known as libido or sex drive. Libido is biological, psychological, sociological, and spiritual in nature. It can be impacted by medical conditions, medications, personality, temperament, personality, lifestyle, relationships, and environmental stressors.

Arousal

Sexual arousal is the physiological response to the release of neurotransmitters that stimulate specific areas of the brain involved in cognition, emotion, motivation, and organization of genital congestion. An awareness of being sexually aroused is described as sexual excitement. Human sexuality is a sensual matter; consider the notion that someone can be "turned on" or "turned off" sexually by varying stimuli of sight, smell, sound, taste, and touch. The stimulus–response can be excitatory or inhibitory in action; dopamine, norepinephrine, and melanocortins are excitatory neurotransmitters, whereas serotonin, prolactin, and GABA are inhibitory neurotransmitters.[7–10]

Genital Congestion

Genital congestion is a reflexive autonomic response facilitated by the parasympathetic and inhibited by the sympathetic nervous system responses. This vasocongestion can occur within seconds of a sexual stimulus and results in increased blood flow to the genital area. In a female, clitoral swelling and vulvar engorgement will occur, along with an increase in vaginal lubrication. In a male, this neurovascular response will result in an erection of the penis. Concurrently, flushing of skin throughout the body may occur and can be seen as pinking of the skin in areas of the face, torso, genitals, and even hands and feet.[7–10]

Orgasm

Generally a pleasurable sensation, orgasm produces rapid contractions of the muscles in the genital and anal area and, for some humans, throughout the body; it is the mechanism by which pelvic congestion is relieved slowly. The physical process of orgasm is similar for both sexes. In females, contractions occur in the lower part of the vagina, in the uterus, anus, and pelvic floor. Approximately 10% of women also ejaculate a clear fluid from the urethra at orgasm; the fluid originates from the Skene's glands in the wall of the urethra and is much like the prostate fluid found in male ejaculate. In males, the pelvic floor muscle contractions result in a pulsatile ejaculation of seminal fluid. Ejaculation with orgasm is much more common in men than in women. Most of the time, a man will have an orgasm at the same time he ejaculates, but occasionally men have an orgasm without ejaculating or ejaculate without having an orgasm.[7–10]

Resolution

Resolution is described as a sense of well-being, muscular relaxation throughout the body, or fatigue that generally follows orgasm; sexual arousal need not result in orgasm for resolution to occur. Resolution is believed to be directly related to the neurotransmitters prolactin, ADH, and oxytocin that are released during orgasm. In a female, relief of pelvic congestion will occur slowly, and the sense of pelvic and genital fullness will abate. In a male, the penis will decrease in size and return to its flaccid state as pelvic congestion is relieved.[7–10]

Age-Related Differences

Human sexuality can be described as a developmental process, beginning at conception and ending at death. Our early awareness of sexual self as an aspect of self-identity begins in infancy and is influenced by the dynamic combination of *biological, societal, cultural,* and *familial* factors (Figure 22-2). The development of human sexuality can be observed through the socially defined stages of childhood, preadolescence, adolescence, and adulthood. Three common attributes of sexual development—gender identity, sexual response, and the capacity for meaningful, intimate relationships—are essential as we move from infancy through adulthood.[11]

FIGURE 22-2 Factors Influencing the Development of Sexuality (Source: From Brown RT, Brown JD: Adolescent sexuality, *Prim Care Clin Office Pract* 33:373–390, 2006.)

Childhood (Birth to 7 Years)

The physiological capacity for sexual response is first observed in infancy: Baby boys get erections and baby girls exhibit increased vaginal lubrication, a result of genital congestion. Infants of both sexes have been observed fondling their own genitals, a natural form of sexual expression and arousal. Attitudes and behaviors conveyed by a child's family during childhood are key in shaping sexuality as each child begins to form a gender identity—the sense of maleness and femaleness. Sexual interest and activity are observed as young children begin to model adult behaviors while they "play house" or "play doctor" as part of their natural curiosity. Facilitated by positive physical contact, the quality of relationships during early childhood is instrumental in shaping sexual and emotional relationships later in life.[11]

Preadolescence (8–12 Years)

During this stage, there is often a general social division of boys and girls into separate groups and, thus, sexual curiosity and learning occurs between children of the same sex. Research indicates that many children engage in masturbation during this stage, with as many as 40% of females and 38% of males in a sample of college students reporting this activity prior to starting puberty.[12]

Adolescence (13–19 Years)

During adolescence, the physical changes associated with puberty become evident. Although these physical changes associated with sexual maturation signal the possibility of adult-like sexual activity, psychosocial factors can facilitate or inhibit such sexual expression. During adolescence, two developmental tasks present: learning to manage physical and emotional aspects of sexuality in order to form intimate relations and resolving the conflict between identity and role confusion.[13] Further development of gender identity, just as sexual identity, emerges as well. Sexual identity, a sense of being attractive and being attracted to others, is described in terms of being heterosexual, homosexual (lesbian and gay), bisexual, and transgendered.[11]

Adulthood (20 Years and Older)

The process of sexual maturation continues throughout a lifetime. Two major developmental tasks for adults are learning to effectively communicate in intimate relationships and making informed decisions about sexual health, such as issues of family planning and prevention of sexually transmitted infections. Attitudes and behaviors related to sexuality are further defined as adults experience varying lifestyles and social influences. Sexual lifestyle options include celibacy, long-term monogamy, serial monogamy, and polyamory. Although many factors contribute to changes in sexual function, sexual interest and desire may continue well into late adulthood.[11]

Positive Sexual Attitudes and Behaviors

Practitioners often equate positive sexual functioning with Masters and Johnson's sexual response cycle rather than considering the psychological and emotional components of what truly makes an optimal sexual encounter.[14] Recent research has identified six components of optimal sexuality.

The most predominant component is that of *being present*—in the moment and fully attentive,[14] described as "utter immersion and intensely focused attention" in which they are fully embodied in the experience and able to allow thinking to stop and arousal to take over.[14] Being present is inextricably linked with a second component of *authenticity*, described as "feeling free to be themselves with their partner."[14] A third theme is *intense emotional connection*, described as heightened intimacy during the sexual encounter. Many couples felt that intimacy needed to be present both inside and outside of the bedroom, whereas others noted that "great sex" also occurred in new relationships, with friends or "play partners." Another component of optimal sexuality is *sexual and erotic intimacy*, described as a deep sense of caring for one another regardless of the length of the relationship. Excellent *communication* is also crucial to the success of any sexual encounter, which includes not only verbal communication but also empathy and making one's needs known through touch.[14] The sixth component is *transcendence*, a combination of heightened mental, emotional, physical, relational, and spiritual states of mind.[14] This picture of "great sex" that is painted by these six attributes is certainly different from that touted by mass media. These findings illustrate that optimal sexuality is not necessarily about technique or skill but, rather, about attitude, positive behaviors, and healthy relationships.

VARIATIONS AND CONTEXT

Many individuals experience sexual problems, but it is also important to acknowledge the wide variation, based on individual perceptions and expectations. For example, one individual's desire to have sex daily and another's to have sex every few months does not delineate function versus dysfunction; the difference is not a dysfunction unless it results in a self-identified source of personal or relational distress. As noted by Herdman et al., "The perception of the patient is a critical factor in determining whether the diagnosis is within the domain of nursing and amenable to nursing intervention in the form of teaching and counseling."[15] Recall that the word "normal" in scientific context generally means "average," and there is limited ability to define average when it comes to human sexuality.

Etiology of Sexual Disorders

A number of underlying situations can lead to sexual disorders or sexual dysfunction (SD), including physiological, psychological, maturational, and environmental factors, or some combination thereof. Specifically, categories include sexually transmitted infections, SD, and intimate partner violence. Alterations in sexuality and sexual function can be further categorized as lifelong versus acquired, situational versus generalized, and organic versus psychogenic. These are not necessarily discrete categories; instead, SD is often multifactorial with an overlap between categories.[9,10,16]

Physiological Factors

An alteration in physiological function of a body system(s) (i.e., cardiovascular, respiratory, musculoskeletal, neurological, and endocrine) can result in SD. An acute illness, infection, surgery, trauma, medications, loss of mobility, decreased activity tolerance, hormonal changes, and alcohol or substance abuse are physiological conditions that can contribute to alterations in sexual function.[8] Pregnancy and the process of aging, although not pathological conditions, can also result in SD.

Psychological Factors

Any stressor that impacts the human psyche has the potential to result in SD. Psychological and emotional factors such as fear, anxiety, fatigue, reproductive health concerns, and adverse childhood events can result in SD. Alterations in body image and self-image, role confusion, and personal conflicts (religion, culture, and values) can also contribute to SD. Furthermore, mental health conditions such as psychosis or alterations in cognition related to dementia will impact sexuality.[9,10,16]

Maturational

For some, SD can be a result of a knowledge deficit with regard to sexuality, birth control, safer sex practices, and changes associated with aging. Lack of general social skills can interfere with establishing intimate and social relationships necessary in the growth and development of one's own sexuality.[9,10]

Environmental

There is increasing evidence that environmental pollutants and chemicals can depress sexual function. Situational factors that influence the patient's environment include social isolation and the absence or lack of a partner, disallowing persons to experience the wholeness of their sexuality. Lack of privacy or an appropriate environment in which to be sexual can contribute to SD.[9,10]

Sexually Transmitted Infections

Among the most common sexuality problems are sexually transmitted infections (STIs). These are infections transmitted through sexual contact and can include protozoa, parasites, and viral and bacterial infections. Some STIs are associated with symptoms that cause an individual to seek medical attention, and other STIs can be asymptomatic but lead to longer term problems, such as complications with pregnancies and increased cancer risk. Some STIs (e.g., chlamydia) are curable with treatment, and others (e.g., genital herpes) are chronic.

Female Sexual Disorders

According to the National Institute of Health, as many as 40% of women in America suffer from sexual dysfunction, and it can affect a woman at any age.[17] Although SD may involve many physiological factors (diabetes, neuropathy, paralysis, and hormones), the majority of research and clinical trials on SD in women have focused on psychological causes (stress, anxiety, depression, and anger). In keeping with the stages of the human sexual response cycle of motivation, arousal, genital congestion, orgasm, and resolution, various sexual dysfunctions have been described. The condition of SD includes the medical diagnoses of hyposexual activity disorder, sexual aversion disorder, sexual arousal disorder, orgasmic disorder, sexual pain disorder, and persistent genital arousal disorder; the general nature of the SD can be presumed simply by its name.[9,10,16]

Male Sexual Disorders

Although men can experience sexual dysfunction related to sexual desire (libido), arousal, and pain, the two widely recognized conditions specific to men are erectile dysfunction and ejaculatory disorders. Erectile dysfunction is an inability to develop or maintain an erection of the penis during sexual activity. Ejaculatory dysfunction is characterized by reduced or absent semen volume, which may be the result of a psychological condition, a medical condition, a medication, or a surgery. Stress, diabetes, antidepressants, antihypertensive medications, and prostate surgery can affect ejaculatory function. Four categories of ejaculatory disorders are premature ejaculation, delayed ejaculation, retrograde ejaculation, and anejaculation/anorgasmia (no ejaculation/no orgasm).[10]

CONSEQUENCES

A number of consequences can occur as a result of sexual disorders and are based on physiological and psychological concerns. Physiological consequences can include, but are not limited to, unfulfilled sexual desire, unsatisfactory sexual responses, pain, STI infection as a result

of a sexual encounter, inability to create a pregnancy, and complications with pregnancies. Psychosocial consequences include problems with relationships (particularly if sexual responses between a couple have changed), low self-esteem, anxiety, and depression. The significance of the consequences is also dependent on the patient's age, interest in sex, and whether the underlying sexual disorder is a temporary or chronic condition.

RISK FACTORS

It is important for nurses to be aware that some groups of patients will be more vulnerable to and at increased risk for alterations in sexual well-being.

Populations at Risk
Adolescents

Addressing adolescent sexuality includes considering critical factors that may influence their behavior: socioeconomic status, family structure, future perspectives for education, and lived experiences. Life certainty, defined as living beyond age 21 years and surviving to at least age 35 years,[18] is correlated with a reduction in sexual risk-taking behaviors and highest levels of sexual knowledge. Many adolescents are at risk for HIV, STIs, unintended pregnancy, and sexual violence. According to the 2013 U.S. Youth Risk Behavior Surveillance System, 7.3% of students reported having been physically forced to have sexual intercourse when they did not want to, and the prevalence of physical dating violence was reported as 9.4%. Although unintended pregnancy remains a risk factor, the pregnancy rate is at its lowest point in 30 years at 67.8 per 1000, and the birth rate at its lowest point in 70 years at 39.1 births per 1000 adolescent females.[18]

Disabilities: Cognitive, Developmental, and Physical

Sexuality and its expression has long been overlooked as an essential aspect and an inherent right of people with disabilities; there exists an underlying assumption that these individuals are asexual and have no need of sexual fulfillment. All people, including those with disabilities, are entitled to move toward both sexual and social maturity in the same manner.[19] For some with disabilities, ignorance will place them at further risk because sexual behavior is a result of poor decision making, loneliness, manipulation, or even force instead of being a healthy expression of their sexuality.

Newly Unpartnered

A unique population at increased risk for negative sequelae are those adults who have recently separated—unpartnered—from their long-term partners because of death or divorce and are now exposed to an entirely new sexual paradigm. These adults may begin dating and suddenly have several new and unknown sexual partners.[20] Depending on their age, HIV, AIDS, and other STIs may not have been of concern when these adults were initially partnered. Although HIV/AIDS infections in the United States are now considered to be chronic conditions, all parties who have intercourse must be cognizant of their risk for exposure to these and other diseases and receive appropriate health education.[20]

Sexual Orientation: Lesbian, Gay, Bisexual, Transgender

In comparison to their heterosexual counterparts, gay, lesbian, and bisexual youths have been found to engage in more high-risk sexual practices.[21] Young women who primarily have sex with women also report that they are likely to engage in sexual activity with men who are homosexual, bisexual, or injection drug users.[21] Adolescent boys who participate in sexual activity with bisexual men are at significantly

---

BOX 22-2 Common Medications That Reduce Sexual Desire or Response

- Antihypertensives (ACE inhibitors, β blockers, β agonists, diuretics)
- Antiulcer medications (cimetidine, omeprazole)
- Antidepressants
- Antipsychotics
- Anticonvulsants
- Diuretics
- Narcotics

---

increased risk for possible transmission of HIV and AIDS.[21] New cases of HIV diagnosis are increasing among men who have sex with men (particularly those of racial minorities) perhaps because of the "glamorization" of anal intercourse, misperceptions that partners are at low risk, and the belief that medical advances in the treatment of AIDS have eliminated the need for appropriate protection during sexual activity.[21–23]

Individual Risk Factors
High-Risk Behaviors
Although sexual activity is considered a normative process, some individuals inadvertently place themselves at increased risk for sexual health problems—primarily those who engage in sexual activity with multiple and casual partners and/or refrain from "safe sex" practices.[20] According to the most recent surveys, these individuals are composed of young people (particularly lesbian, gay, bisexual, and transgender youth) and men who have sex with men regardless of race.[21,23,24]

Of secondary importance is the influence of nonsexual high-risk behavior, such as the use of alcohol, marijuana, or other illicit substances. Prior research has shown that when these substances are ingested close to the time of sexual activity, the rate of sexual risk-taking increases.[22,25] The abuse of alcohol or drugs most often results in impaired judgment and consequently less thoughtfulness related to the sexual act.[20]

Underlying Medical Conditions and Medications
A number of underlying medical conditions, particularly chronic health conditions, and/or medications used to treat underlying conditions can place an individual at risk for sexual disorders. Some of the most common conditions that increase risk include acute or chronic pain, chronic fatigue, anxiety, depression, cardiovascular disease, diabetes, and chronic respiratory conditions. Likewise, many medications can affect sexual health. Common medications that can affect sexual function are presented in Box 22-2.

ASSESSMENT

A majority of nurses believe that sexual assessment is part of their professional responsibility in providing nursing care. In practice, however, most nurses rarely or never address sexuality as a health issue, even though patients have identified it as an expected and appropriate behavior in the nurse–patient relationship.[26–30] Application of the nursing process in identifying and addressing problems related to sexuality is essential to promoting sexual well-being of individuals, couples, families, and communities.[15,31]

History
A sexual history is elicited as an essential part of a routine health history during an initial visit and annual visits thereafter. Despite the

importance of sexual health and patients' expressed desire to be queried about sexual issues, questions related to sexual health are infrequently raised during routine examinations.[32] Barriers identified by nurses include personal discomfort, lack of training, and lack of time; those identified by patients include personal discomfort and beliefs that their concerns would be dismissed and that it is the provider's responsibility to initiate the dialogue.[29,30,32]

The CDC drafted guidelines for sexual history taking and incorporates five areas that should be broached with patients; these are known as the "the five P's."[33] These stand for partners, practices, protection from infection, past history of infection, and prevention of pregnancy. Partners includes the number and gender of the patient's sexual partners. Practices refers to safe sex practices. If the patient reports more than one partner in the past 12 months or if the patient has had sex with a partner who has other sex partners, the nurse should inquire about condom use. Protection refers to questions assessing measures that the patient takes to protect himself or herself from STIs. This may include exploring about abstinence, monogamy, and the patient's perception of his or her own risk or his or her partner's risk. These questions are helpful in assessing patient risk for STIs.

Typical health history questions for females include those about menarche, menstruation, pregnancy, contraception, and menopause; for males, questions include those about contraception, penile discharge or lesions, scrotal pain or swelling, and alterations in urine elimination and andropause. Questions about practices for both sexes include those regarding safer sex knowledge and practice, frequency of intercourse, number of partners/lifetime partners, sexual behaviors, preferences, sexual response, and personal safety.

Examination Findings
The physical examination is guided by the sexual history and the patient's age, gender, and pertinent needs. A physical examination may or may not be a necessary component of nursing care as it relates to sexuality. For example, the report of genital pain will rely on the assessment techniques of history, inspection, and palpation, whereas a report of an alteration in sexual motivation or desire may not warrant physical examination.

Knowledge of the physical changes associated with normal growth and development is essential, and those associated with milestones such as puberty, pregnancy, menopause, and andropause are of particular interest as they relate to sexuality. Described as a sequence of physical changes, sexual maturation can be estimated based on the observed changes of primary and secondary sex characteristics: in females, breast development and pubic hair, and in males, genital development, along with pubic hair. Relying on a scale first suggested in the 1960s as an aide to quantify these physical changes is commonly referred to as "Tanner staging," named after the physician who first proposed it.[34]

Female Physical Examination
The first genital exam should occur at birth with the infant girl in a supine position; it is a relatively easy and noninvasive assessment. A general assessment of the vulva will include inspection of the labia majora, labia minora, clitoris, urethral opening, introitus, hymen, perineum, and anus. The initial assessment should confirm the sex of the infant and the patency of the urethra and anus; this is baseline data. Nurses observe for the passage of urine and meconium to confirm patency of the urethra and anus. Throughout childhood, the sexual history will guide the appropriate physical examination.

The gynecologic examination, generally associated with puberty and beyond, includes inspection and palpation of the external genitalia, internal inspection of the vagina per speculum, collection of specimens as indicated (swabs for cervical smears and STI screening), and bimanual palpation (pelvic exam) if indicated; a rectal exam may be performed if indicated. Physical findings might include the following: healed scars from childbirth or trauma, hymenal tags, bulges (cystoceles or rectoceles), thinning of the vaginal wall, fistulas, masses, lesions, and inflammation. An annual gynecological exam typically includes a clinical breast exam as well.

Male Physical Examination

The first genital exam should occur at birth with the infant male in a supine position. A general assessment will include inspection of the penis, testes, scrotum, perineum, and anus. The initial assessment will confirm the sex of the infant, patency of the anus, and the location of the urinary meatus with any deviation (epispadias and hypospadias) documented; this is baseline data. Throughout childhood, the sexual history will guide the appropriate physical examination.

A general assessment of the male examination includes inspection and palpation of the penis, scrotum, testicles, perineum, and perianal area; a digital rectal examination (DRE) for assessment of the prostate may be indicated. The nurse should begin by examining the penis, scrotum, and testicles. The penis is inspected for discharge and lesions; the scrotum is inspected for lesions and contour. The testicles within the scrotal sac are palpated for size, texture, and tenderness, which may reveal such findings as hydrocele, masses, nodules, tenderness, or inflammation.[35]

Diagnostic Tests

Based on the patient's history and needs, a number of laboratory tests and diagnostic procedures may be indicated. Specimen collection from a variety of sources includes serum, urine, genital discharge/secretions, lesions, and semen. Diagnostic procedures include tissue biopsy, aspiration, ultrasound, x-ray, laparoscopy, colposcopy, and colonoscopy. Diagnostic testing may be performed for screening of genetic issues (ambiguous genitalia noted at birth), cancers (cervical, ovarian, prostate, and anus), infections (chlamydia, gonorrhea, syphilis, HPV, and HIV), hormonal states (hypogonadism and pregnancy); the type of testing is best determined individually for each patient.

CLINICAL MANAGEMENT

Primary Prevention

Patient education, counseling, and referral are essential components of health promotion and disease prevention for optimal sexual well-being. Focused areas of discussion include abstinence, contraception, safer sex practices, STIs, healthy relationships, and community resources. Although a great diversity of opinion exists regarding how to address sexuality issues in the United States, two common themes have been identified that support a communication framework for sexual health. The first theme is about protecting health through making good choices with regard to sexual behavior.[36] The second theme supports broadening sexual health programs to go beyond disease control prevention to include wellness-related approaches to promote sexual health.[36]

Human papilloma virus (HPV) can be prevented by HPV vaccination. There are currently three U.S. Food and Drug Administration-approved HPV vaccines available; each is a three-dose series. Vaccination is routinely given at 11 or 12 years of age to both girls and boys. HPV vaccination is considered to be safe and effective, and it offers protection from genital warts and cancers caused by HPV, including that of the female cervix.[37]

Secondary Prevention (Screening)

In contrast to primary prevention strategies, secondary prevention attempts to diagnose an existing disease in its earliest stages. This is referred to as screening with a goal of reducing morbidity and mortality and preserving quality of life.

Screening for Sexually Transmitted Infection

There is limited consistency in the literature regarding screening recommendations. The U.S. Preventive Services Task Force (USPSTF) recommends screening based on level of risk.[38] Level of risk is based on sexual behavior and includes unprotected intercourse, having sex with multiple partners, adolescent-onset intercourse, sharing of intravenous needles, and history of STIs. Individuals in a mutually monogamous relationship are considered low risk. For individuals who are at increased risk, periodic screening for chlamydia, gonorrhea, syphilis, and HIV is recommended; specific screening intervals vary, but it is common for screenings to occur as part of an annual pelvic examination.

Screening for Intimate Partner Violence

The USPSTF recommends that all women of childbearing age (14–46 years) be screened for intimate partner violence (IPV), whereas others advocate for universal screening of patients across the lifespan.[39] Available screening instruments, including the Hurt, Insult, Threaten, Scream (HITS) screening tool, have been determined to be valid and reliable in the detection of current, past, and risk for abuse in clinical settings. Adequate evidence supports that effective interventions can reduce violence, abuse, and physical or mental harms for women of reproductive age.

Collaborative Interventions

A number of interventions are indicated for individuals experiencing a wide range of sexual problems and disorders.

Pharmacotherapy

Antibiotics. Infections of the reproductive tract are usually caused by STIs. A wide range of antibacterial, antiviral, and antiprotozoal agents are used in the treatment of STIs depending on the microorganism involved.

Hormone Replacement Therapy. Hormone replacement therapy (HRT) is often used to treat the symptoms of menopause, most notably hot flashes and vaginal dryness. HRT may be given as low-dose estrogen (for women who have had a hysterectomy) or combination therapy (estrogen and progesterone) for women who still have their uterus.

Phosphodiesterase-5 Inhibitors. Two phosphodiesterase-5 (PDE-5) drugs (sildenafil and vardenafil) represent the first-line treatment for erectile dysfunction (ED). These drugs act by relaxing smooth muscles in the corpora cavernosa of the penis to increase blood flow and compressing the veins in the corpora to reduce outward blood flow. These combined actions result in penile erection with sexual stimulation.

Surgical Procedures

There are indications for surgical procedures for men and women who are experiencing certain sexual problems.

Hysterectomy. A hysterectomy is the surgical removal of the uterus and may be indicated for a variety of uterine conditions, including menorrhagia, pelvic pain from endometriosis, prolapse of the female reproductive organs (uterus, cystocele, and rectocele), uterine fibroids, myomas, and cancer.

Penile Implant Surgery. Penile implant surgery is the insertion of an inflatable device in the penis with a reservoir placed in the scrotum. The device is inflated by squeezing the reservoir. This procedure has become much less common since the introduction of pharmacotherapy for ED.

Minor Procedures. Other surgical procedures include removal of genital lesions (e.g., warts or polyps) or incision and drainage for cysts or abscess.

Cognitive–Behavioral Therapy

For some individuals, cognitive–behavioral therapy (CBT) and sexual counseling have proven effective in the treatment of sexual problems with psychological origins, including some cases of ED. Many psychological and emotional factors, such as fear, anxiety, fatigue, and reproductive health concerns, can impair sexual performance. Individuals with sex addictions may also benefit from CBT.

Other Interventions

An alternative to PDE-5 in the treatment of ED is the vacuum construction device. This is an external cylinder-like device that fits over the penis and uses a vacuum effect to draw blood into the penis to gain an erection. A tension band is placed at the base of the penis to maintain the erection once the cylinder is removed, allowing the individual to have sex. The ring is removed within 1 hour.

INTERRELATED CONCEPTS

The concept of sexual health represents the "integration of somatic, emotional, intellectual and social aspects of sexual being in ways that are enriching and enhance personality, communication and love."[1] Sexuality and interrelated concepts are presented in Figure 22-3. This model illustrates some concepts that may be impacted by normative sexual functioning and/or have an impact on sexuality.

Reproduction (and reproductive health) are highly interrelated to sexuality. By definition, they include topics of puberty, contraception, STIs, safer sex practices, fertility, infertility, and sexuality. Additional considerations for females are breast and cervical cancer screening, menstruation, preconceptual counsel and screening, pregnancy, and menopause.

One barrier to healthy sexual expression and function is Pain. Regardless of the source or type of pain the patient experiences, it can contribute to sexual dysfunction; pain can be chronic or acute, physical, psychological, or spiritual. For those in pain, sometimes the pain itself makes having sex not possible. It is noteworthy that both positive touch and sexual intimacy are known to stimulate the release of endorphins, the body's natural painkillers.

Medical conditions that lead to alterations in Gas Exchange (e.g., chronic obstructive pulmonary disease, cystic fibrosis, interstitial lung disease, and asthma) can lead to shortness of breath, fatigue, depression, and feelings of anxiousness and thus can inhibit the human sexual response and can result in sexual dysfunction.[40] Individuals who rely on supplemental oxygen may experience impaired body image.

"Being present" is identified as a positive attribute of sexuality; Anxiety can preoccupy the mind, body, and spirit. Patients with anxiety often present with concerns related to sexual dysfunction; those who seek care for SD often report feelings of anxiety. Anxiety is often linked to stress. If a patient is undergoing extreme Stress from other life issues, this may have a negative impact on sexual function. Anxiety stimulates the sympathetic nervous system—the stress response is that of fight–flight–freeze—and negatively impacts the sexual response cycle.[41]

CLINICAL EXEMPLARS

Any number of exemplars could be chosen to effectively illustrate the concept of human sexuality. Those presented in Box 22-3 address a continuum of concerns that have a significant impact on a person's sexual health and well-being across the lifespan.

Featured Exemplars
Erectile Dysfunction

ED is estimated to affect 18–30 million men in the United States; it is believed to be an underreported disease process as a result of embarrassment, shame, and lack of understanding of the condition. ED affects men of all ages and can be chronic or transient in nature. ED is positively correlated with age, cardiovascular conditions, risk factors, physical inactivity, alcohol use, smoking, and obesity; these conditions impact vascular perfusion, which is necessary for penile erection. For some men, there is an associated alteration in body image, self-concept,

FIGURE 22-3 Sexuality and Interrelated Concepts

BOX 22-3 EXEMPLARS OF IMPAIRED SEXUALITY

Disorders Affecting Sexual Response
- Anorgasmia
- Coital incontinence
- Dysfunctional uterine bleeding
- Ejaculatory disorders
- Endometriosis
- Erectile dysfunction
- Hyposexual activity disorder
- Menopause
- Orgasmic disorder
- Pelvic organ prolapse
- Persistent genital arousal disorder
- Sexual arousal disorder
- Sexual aversion disorder
- Sexual pain disorder
- Vaginismus
- Vulvovaginitis

Sexually Transmitted Infections
Protozoa
- Trichomoniasis

Viruses
- Cytomegalovirus
- Hepatitis A and hepatitis B
- Herpes simplex virus 1 and 2 (HSV)
- HIV
- Human papillomavirus (HPV)

Bacteria
- Chancroid
- *Chlamydia*
- Genital mycoplasmas
- Gonorrhea
- Group B *Streptococcus*
- Syphilis

Other Exemplars
- Intimate partner violence
- Sexual violence
- Intersex

and self- esteem, all of which can be negatively impacted by a perceived loss of manhood.[42]

Menopause

Menopause is associated with the cessation of ovulation. The age of onset is variable, with the average age at 51 years. Common symptoms include hot flashes, night sweats, impaired sleep, headaches, changes in memory, loss of sexual desire, urinary concerns, mood alterations, and dryness of skin and vaginal tissues.[43] In addition to managing symptoms, issues to be addressed include nutrition, bone health, heart disease prevention, weight management, hormonal balance, and cancer screening, along with psychosocial concerns of relationships, retirement, and available community support systems. Nurses have the ability to provide accurate information to patients regarding the physiology of menopause and its effect on sexuality.[36]

Pelvic Organ Prolapse

Symptoms of sexual dysfunction and altered body image often coexist with prolapse of the female reproductive organs (uterus, cystocele, and rectocele). Approximately 50% of women experience some degree of prolapse by the time they reach the age of 40 years.[44] Intercourse may be painful or embarrassing and associated with fecal or urinary incontinence. Conservative management includes lifestyle changes—such as losing weight, avoiding constipation, and reducing high-impact exercise (e.g., running)—and pelvic muscle floor training (Kegel exercises),[44] although surgical intervention may be necessary for advanced cases.

Intimate Partner Violence

IPV is a serious, preventable public health issue that affects millions of Americans. The CDC defines IPV as

actual or threatened physical, sexual, psychological, emotional, or stalking abuse by an intimate partner. An intimate partner can be a current or former spouse or nonmarital partner, such as a boyfriend, girlfriend, or dating partner. Intimate partners can be of the same or opposite sex.[45]

It is clearly documented that IPV during adolescence is associated with negative biopsychosocial health effects, poor school performance, and a predisposition for sexual ill-being and problems in future relationships throughout life.[45]

Sexual Violence

Sexual violence is a public health issue throughout the world and is detrimental to the sexual well-being of an individual, a family, and a community. The CDC defines sexual violence as

nonconsensual completed or attempted penetration of the vagina or anus, nonconsensual completed or attempted oral sex, nonconsensual intentional touching of a sexual nature, or nonconsensual non-contact acts of a sexual nature such as voyeurism and verbal or behavioral sexual harassment.[18]

Sexual violence includes child sexual abuse, intimate partner violence, incest, drug-facilitated sexual assault, sexual harassment, sexual exploitation, stalking, voyeurism, exhibitionism, frottage, and unwanted exposure to pornography.

Intersex

Intersex represents a group of conditions in which an infant's external genitals do not appear distinctly male or female or the external genitalia may not match the internal sex organs or genetic sex of the infant. This condition is confusing and distressing for families, as well as challenging for the health care team, which may have limited experience with and understanding of the condition. Medical care includes chromosomal analysis, endocrine studies, and radiologic studies to assist in guiding gender assignment. Physiological complications of the condition of intersex include infertility and an increased risk of certain types of cancer.[46,47]

CASE STUDY

Source: bbevren/iStock/
Thinkstock

Case Presentation

Anna Garner is a 44-year-old married white female who has an appointment to see her nurse practitioner (NP) for her annual examination. As part of her annual physical, Anna will be having a pelvic examination including a Papanicolau test in order to screen for cervical cancer. Anna has three teenage daughters, all born by spontaneous vaginal delivery. Several years ago, Anna returned to work full-time at a rather sedentary job. Anna has found her weight to be increasing during these past few years and is now carrying 160 pounds at 5 feet, 4 inches tall. Throughout the years, Anna and her NP have developed a trusting and therapeutic relationship. As part of the history-taking process, the NP asks Anna if there have been any changes in the past year related to the sexual relationship that she has with her partner. Anna appears somewhat embarrassed; however, with some encouragement, she goes on to explain that in the past she and her husband have always enjoyed intercourse two or three times a week and that this is a very important part of their marriage. Anna states that for the past 9 or 10 months, she has begun to "lose urine" during intercourse. Sometimes this occurs during foreplay, and on other occasions it will happen during orgasm. Anna reports that she often interrupts their sexual activity to go to the bathroom.

Recently, she has been finding excuses to avoid sex altogether and is concerned that she is driving her husband away. The NP explains to Anna that this condition is referred to as "stress or coital incontinence" and may be the result of childbearing, aging, and her recent weight gain. Education is provided regarding the necessity for urodynamic evaluation and the possible treatment modalities available. Anna is instructed on how to perform Kegel exercises. The NP reassures Anna that although this condition is neither uncommon nor life-threatening, if left untreated it may result in other unanticipated symptomatology, including depression, loss of self-esteem, altered body image, worsening of incontinence, reduced social interaction, and decreased sexual interest and activity. Anna is very reassured by this education and agrees to the treatment plan.

Case Analysis

This case study illustrates a patient-centered relationship founded on established trust and rapport. Relying on her assessment skills of the patient's appearance and behavior in response to the interview questions, the NP pursues the history as it relates to the patient's sexual relationship with her husband. The NP discovers the patient's reticent demeanor is related to her stress incontinence and the subsequent feelings of embarrassment, shame, and a lack of understanding regarding the condition. This is interfering with the patient's sexual well-being and her intimate relationship with her husband that the patient values. The NP takes the opportunity to provide appropriate patient education with regard to stress incontinence, and while not minimizing the concern, she instead normalizes the condition for the patient. The NP has provided a tangible intervention that the patient can do with ease by instructing about Kegel exercises. In addition, the NP has reinforced for Anna that she is safe to discuss her sexuality with her health care provider and that it is an important part of her health care.

ACCESS EXEMPLAR LINKS IN YOUR GIDDENS EBOOK

REFERENCES

1. World Health Organization: *Defining sexual health: Report of a technical consultation on sexual health, Jan 28–31, 2001, Geneva*, Geneva, 2006, World Health Organization.
2. Online Etymology Dictionary: Sex, 2013. Retrieved from: <http://www.etymonline.com/index.php?allowed_in_frame=0&search=sex&searchmode=none>.
3. Office of the Surgeon General: *The Surgeon General's call to action to promote sexual health*, Rockville, MD, 2001, Office of the Surgeon General; and Centers for Disease Control and Prevention. Sexual health. Retrieved from: <http://www.cdc.gov/sexualhealth/Default.html>.
4. Centers for Disease Control and Prevention: Intimate partner violence, 2015. Retrieved from: <www.cdc.gov/ViolencePrevention/intimatepartnerviolence>.
5. Merriam–Webster: Well-being, n.d. <Retrieved from: <http://www.merriam-webster.com/dictionary/well-being>.
6. Merriam–Webster: Ill-being, n.d. <Retrieved from: <http://www.merriam-webster.com/dictionary/ill-being>.
7. Masters WH, Johnson VE: *Human sexual response*, Boston, 1966, Little, Brown.
8. Bancroft J: Biological factors in human sexuality. *J Sex Res* 30(1):15–21, 2002.
9. Basson R, Leiblum S, Brotto L, et al: Definitions of women's sexual dysfunction reconsidered: Advocating expansion and revision. *J Psychosom Obstet Gynecol* 24:221–229, 2003.
10. Merck: Merck manuals: Sexual dysfunction: Overview of male sexual function, 2010. Retrieved from: <http://www.merckmanuals.com/professional/genitourinary-disorders/male-sexual-dysfunction/overview-of-male-sexual-function>.
11. DeLamateur J, Friedrich WN: Human sexual development. *J Sex Res* 39(1):10–14, 2002.
12. Bancroft J, editor: *Sexual development in childhood*, Bloomington, IN, 2003, Indiana University Press.
13. Kneisl CR, Trigoboff E: *Contemporary Psychiatric–Mental Health Nursing*, ed 3, New York, 2013, Pearson.
14. Kleinplatz PJ, Menard AD: Building blocks toward optimal sexuality: Constructing a conceptual model. *Family J* 15:72–78, 2007.
15. Herdman TH, North American Nursing Diagnosis Association: *NANDA-I nursing diagnoses: Definitions & classification, 2009–2011*, Oxford, 2008, Wiley–Blackwell.
16. Berman JR: Physiology of female sexual function and dysfunction. *Int J Impotence Res* 17:S44–S51, 2005.
17. Sobczak JA: Female sexual dysfunction: Knowledge development and practice implications. *Perspect Psychiatr Care* 45(3):161–172, 2009.
18. Conklin K: Adolescent sexual behavior, 2012. Retrieved from: <http://advocatesforyouth.org>.
19. Ailey SH, Marks BA, Crisp C, et al: Promoting sexuality across the lifespan for individuals with intellectual and developmental disabilities. *Nurs Clin North Am* 38:229–252, 2003.
20. Lowdermilk DL, Perry SE, Cashion K, et al, editors: *Maternity & women's health care*, ed 10, St Louis, 2012, Mosby.
21. Brown RT, Brown JD: Adolescent sexuality. *Prim Care Clin Office Pract* 33:373–390, 2006.
22. Dowshein N, Garofalo R: Optimizing primary care for LGBTQ youth. *Contemp Pediatr* 26(10):2009.
23. Sanders SA, Reece M, Herbenick D, et al: Condom use during most recent vaginal intercourse event among a probability sample of adults in the United States. *J Sex Med* 7(Suppl 5):362–373, 2010.
24. Fenton KA: Time for change: Rethinking and reframing sexual health in the United States. *J Sex Med* 7(Suppl 5):250–252, 2010.

25. Herbenick D, Reece M, Schick V, et al: An event-level analysis of the sexual characteristics and composition among adults ages 18 to 59: Results from a national probability sample in the United States. *J Sex Med* 7(Suppl 5):346–361, 2010.

26. Gott M, Galena E, Hinchliff S, et al: "Opening a can of worms": GP and practice nurse barriers to talking about sexual health in primary care. *Fam Pract* 21:528–536, 2004.

27. Hoekstra T, Lesman-Leegte I, Couperus MF, et al: What keeps nurses from the sexual counseling of patients with heart failure? *Heart Lung* 41(5):492–499, 2012.

28. Palmer H: Exploring sexuality and sexual health in nursing. *Professional Nurse* 14(1):15–17, 1998.

29. Reynolds KE, Magnan MA: Nursing attitudes and beliefs toward human sexuality. *Clin Nurse Specialist* 19(5):255–259, 2005.

30. Zillotto GC, Marcolan JF: Perception of nursing professionals on sexuality in people with mental disorders. *Acta Paul Enferm* 26(1):86–92, 2013.

31. Ayaz S: Sexuality and nursing process: A literature review. *Sexuality Disability* 31:3–12, 2013.

32. Shifren JL, Johannes CB, Monz BU, et al: Help-seeking behavior of women with self-reported distressing sexual problems. *J Women's Health* 18(4):461–468, 2008.

33. Centers for Disease Control and Prevention: A guide to taking a sexual history, 2014. Retrieved from: <http://www.cdc.gov/std/treatment/sexualhistory.pdf>.

34. Quigley BH, Palm ML, Bickley L: *Bates' nursing guide to physical examination and history taking*, Philadelphia, 2012, Wolters Kluwer.

35. Ignatavicius DD, Workman ML: *Medical–surgical nursing*, ed 7, St Louis, 2013, Elsevier.

36. Robinson SJ, Stellatu A, Stephens J, et al: On the road to well-being: The development of a communication framework for sexual health. *Public Health Rep* 128:43–52, 2013.

37. Centers for Disease Control and Prevention: 2015 STD treatment guidelines. Retrieved from: <http://www.cdc.gov/std/tg2015/default.htm>.

38. U.S. Preventive Services Task Force: USPSTF recommendations for STI screening, 2014. Retrieved from: <http://www.uspreventiveservicestaskforce.org/Page/Name/uspstf-recommendations-for-sti-screening>.

39. U.S. Preventive Services Task Force: Intimate partner violence and abuse of elderly and vulnerable adults: Screening, 2013. Retrieved from: <http://www.uspreventiveservicestaskforce.org/Page/Topic/recommendation-summary/intimate-partner-violence-and-abuse-of-elderly-and-vulnerable-adults-screening>.

40. McCoy K, Jones N: Is COPD ruining your sex life? 2012. Retrieved from: <http://www.everydayhealth.com/copd/copd-and-your-sex-life.aspx>.

41. Corretti G, Baldi I: The relationship between anxiety disorders and sexual dysfunction. *Psychiatric Times* 2007.

42. Selvin E, Burnett A, Platz E: Prevalence and risk factors for erectile dysfunction in the U.S. *Am J Med* 120(2):151–157, 2007.

43. Northrup C: *The wisdom of menopause: Creating physical and emotional health and healing during the change*, rev ed, New York, 2012, Random House.

44. Richardson K, Hagen S, Glazener C, et al: The role of nurses in the management of women with pelvic organ prolapse. *Br J Nurs* 18(5):294–296, 298–300, 2009.

45. Centers for Disease Control and Prevention: Intimate partner violence, 2015. Retrieved from: <http://www.cdc.gov/ViolencePrevention/intimatepartnerviolence>.

46. Sanders C, Carter B, Goodacre L: Parents need to protect: Influences, risks, and tensions for parents of pre-pubertal children born with ambiguous genitalia. *J Clin Nurs* 21:3315–3323, 2012.

47. Parker L: Ambiguous genitalia: Etiology, treatment and nursing implications. *J Obstet Gynecol Neonatal Nurs* 27:15–22, 1998.

Immunity

Carolyn Sabo

The ability of the human body to sustain health within the environment requires multiple protective mechanisms. One of the most complex protective mechanisms is the immune response. When immune processes are functioning optimally, the body has the ability to mount an efficient defense in response to the invasion of foreign substances. Such a response is critical to maintaining health. It is reasonable, then, to conclude that multiple health problems occur in the absence of a normal immune response. Although this concept presentation describes the concept of immunity from the perspective of both normal and abnormal functioning, the primary focus is on that of abnormal function because of the multitude of health-related problems that result.

DEFINITION

Immunity is commonly defined as a physiological process that provides an individual with protection or defense from disease. It is a characteristic that allows one to be resistant to a particular disease or condition; the term is derived from the Latin word *immunis*, meaning exempt.[1,2] Immunity is accomplished through the actions of the immune system, which is a body-wide, complex, interrelated group of cells, tissues, and organs that work within a dynamic communication network to protect the body from attacks by foreign antigens, typically proteins. These foreign antigens may include microorganisms (bacteria, viruses, parasites, or fungi), but they may also be proteins found in pollens; foods; bee, snake, or spider venom; vaccines; transfusions; and transplanted tissues.[3] As noted previously, this concept includes abnormal function leading to health problems. For the purpose of this concept presentation, a broader definition of immunity is used: *the normal physiological response to microorganisms and proteins as well as conditions associated with an inadequate or excessive immune response.*

Additional terms are used to differentiate the type of immunity protection. *Innate immunity* (also referred to as natural or native) is the immunity present at birth; it provides nonspecific response not considered antigen specific. *Acquired immunity* refers to immunity protection that is gained after birth either actively or passively. *Active acquired immunity* develops after the introduction of a foreign antigen resulting in the formation of antibodies or sensitized T lymphocytes. For example, active immunity may be obtained artificially through the immune response to an immunization, or it may be obtained naturally through the immune response to exposure to infectious pathogens

such as varicella–zoster virus. *Passive acquired immunity* occurs by the introduction of preformed antibodies—either from an artificial route, such as a transfusion of immunoglobulin (Ig), or from a natural route, such as from a mother to her fetus through placental blood transference or through colostrum transfer during breast-feeding.[1,4–6]

SCOPE

The complexity of immunity often makes it a difficult topic to fully understand from a traditional presentation. From a conceptual perspective, it is useful to think about what this concept represents from a very broad view and consider the context of patient-related issues. The scope of immunity and related immunity problems are described as optimal and abnormal responses (Figure 23-1). An optimal response represents an immune system that protects the body from the invasion of microorganisms, removes dead and damaged tissue and cells, and recognizes and removes cell mutations. Abnormal function includes a suppressed immune response and exaggerated immune response.[7–9]

To the far left of the immune response spectrum (see Figure 23-1) is a hypo- or suppressed immune response. Individuals who have suppressed immune responses are referred to as immunocompromised or are considered to be in a state of immunodeficiency. Individuals with suppressed immune responses are at significant risk for infection, or if immunosuppression occurs over time, they are at risk for cancer because of the loss or removal of mutating cells.[8–11]

To the far right of the immune response spectrum (see Figure 23-1) is a hyperimmune or exaggerated immune response. Hyperimmune responses range among allergic reactions, cytotoxic reactions, and autoimmune reactions. A critical component of the immune system is its ability to differentiate between "self" and "non-self." When this recognition fails, the immune system may begin attacking host cells in an exaggerated immune response. This process leads to the development of autoimmune diseases and disorders.[8–11]

NORMAL PHYSIOLOGICAL PROCESS

The immune response involves the following three primary protective functions:
1. Protects the body from invasion of microorganisms and other antigens
2. Removes dead or damaged tissue and cells

FIGURE 23-1 Scope of Immunity Concept

3. Recognizes and removes cell mutations that have demonstrated abnormal cell growth and development

To accomplish these functions, the immune system reacts with three lines of defense. The first line of defense is the skin boundary surfaces, including mucous membranes, enzymes, natural microbial flora, and complement proteins. The second line of defense is accomplished by the activities of phagocytes, natural killer T lymphocytes, granulocytes, and macrophages providing innate, nonspecific immunity. Finally, the third line of defense comes from antibodies derived from B lymphocytes and the T lymphocytes resulting from learned or acquired specific immunity.[8–11]

Recognition of the "self" and recognition of foreign proteins are the hallmarks of a properly functioning immune system. The individual must be able to differentiate between host and foreign proteins in order to respond appropriately. With the invasion of foreign proteins, a protective response is needed; failure to respond appropriately (immunosuppression or immunodeficiency) results in infection or disease. Likewise, the body must maintain the ability to recognize host proteins and not initiate an immune response. When this recognition fails, the immune system launches an attack on host cells (autoimmune response) or initiates a hyperactive immune response such as occurs in asthma (hyperimmune response).

Major Histocompatibility Complex Proteins

Surface proteins called major histocompatibility complex (MHC) proteins are divided into two classes, with class I being found on all cells and class II on specialized cells. MHC proteins function, in part, to differentiate cells of the self/host from foreign proteins. Substances that are "non-self" are capable of initiating an immune response. A foreign antigen may be a whole cell, a virus, a bacterium, an MHC marker protein, or a small portion of a larger foreign protein. Epitopes are the markers on foreign antigens that cause the immune response in individuals.[3] The MHC provides what has been termed a "scaffold" that presents the foreign antigen to the immune cells. The empty MHC scaffold, also termed a self-marker scaffold, of a foreign cell from a donor organ may be introduced into the host during a transplant. These MHC self-marker scaffolds are the individual's tissue type or human leukocyte antigen.[3,12]

Organs Comprising the Immune System

Organs of the immune system are spread throughout the body. They are termed lymphoid organs and include the bone marrow, thymus gland, spleen, tonsils, adenoids, and appendix. From these organs, the lymphocytes are formed, grow, mature, and are released into the body. The body's lymphatic system provides the network by which organs of the immune system are connected. The blood also provides a connection among the organs and provides the route for lymphocyte movement throughout the body.

Origin of Cells in an Immune Response

A variety of components work together to provide an immune response. All cells in the immune system are derived from stem cells in the bone marrow and begin as either myeloid progenitor or lymphoid progenitor cells. Myeloid progenitors include neutrophils, monocytes (which become macrophages in body tissues), eosinophils, basophils, and mast cells. Lymphoid progenitor cells include B lymphocytes (which become plasma or memory B cells), mature T lymphocytes, and natural killer cells.[13,14]

B and T Lymphocytes

During fetal development, B and T lymphocytes are produced in large numbers. All immune cells begin as immature stem cells in the bone marrow and grow into specific immune cell types such as B or T lymphocytes and phagocytes. Preprocessing and maturation of the B lymphocytes occur in the liver during mid-fetal life and in the bone marrow during late fetal life and after birth. Maturation of T lymphocytes occurs in the thymus gland. This process is called generation of clonal diversity. As a person is challenged by the presence of foreign antigens during life, *specificity* of lymphocytes to a specific antigen emerges—a process termed clonal selection.[8,9] On re-exposure to the same antigen, the person will have a more rapid and efficient immune response, indicating a *memory* capacity for the immune system.

Antibody Production

Antibodies are secreted by B lymphocytes. Antibodies or immunoglobulins are formed after a B lymphocyte encounters and engulfs an antigen and then interacts with helper T lymphocytes; the B lymphocyte then begins producing identical copies of a specific antibody. Researchers have identified nine classes of antibodies or immunoglobulins (four forms of IgG, two forms of IgA, and one form each of IgE, IgM, and IgD). Immunoglobulins are found in various concentrations at different sites throughout the body:[8,9,15]

- IgG: Primary immunoglobulin in the blood (80–85% of circulating immunoglobulins); may enter tissue spaces; selectively crosses the placenta; coats antigen for more effective and efficient presentation for an immune response; binds to macrophages and neutrophils for increased phagocytosis
- IgD: Found within the cell membrane of B lymphocytes
- IgE: Responsible for allergy symptoms and increases in the presence of parasitic worms; normally found in trace amounts
- IgA: Protects entrances to the body; found in high concentrations in body fluids (tears, saliva, and secretions of the respiratory and gastrointestinal tracts)
- IgM: Remains in the blood and efficiently kills bacteria; largest of the immunoglobulins; first antibody produced with an initial (primary) immune response

Phagocytes

Phagocytes are found throughout the body and are usually responsible for recognizing and ingesting foreign antigens as they enter the body. Macrophages and neutrophils are the primary phagocytic cells responsible for this first line of defense during an immune response. Macrophages are the primary defensive cells against antigen entry to the body, when awaiting the need for phagocytic activity, large numbers of macrophages are stored in connective tissue, the spleen and liver, and the lining of the gastrointestinal and respiratory tracts. Neutrophils remain circulating in the blood.[3,8,9]

Phagocytosis is the process of ingesting cellular material and involves the ability of phagocytes to be selective in recognizing cells that must be ingested and discarded. Healthy cells of the self tend to be smooth and covered with a smooth protein coat that normally functioning phagocytes tend to ignore. Antibody–antigen complexes have rougher surfaces and are particularly susceptible to phagocytic functioning. Although both neutrophils and macrophages are phagocytes, in an immune response the macrophages are more effective than neutrophils.[8]

Complement System

The complement system works to enhance the immune response and to help rid the body of antibody–antigen complexes. The complement system is composed of 25 major proteins that circulate in an inactive form in the blood and are engaged in a cascade of interactions when the first protein molecule (C1) encounters an antigen–antibody complex. The complement cascade is also responsible for the dilation and ultimate leaking of fluid from the vascular system, leading to the redness and swelling during the inflammatory process that are associated with an immune response.[3,8,9]

Lymphocyte Function in an Immune Response

A general overview of immune system development and maturation leading to an immune response to a foreign antigen is presented in Figure 23-2.

B Lymphocyte Response

McCance and colleagues[9] differentiate immunoglobulins as all molecules that have specificity to an antigen and an antibody as one particular set of immunoglobulins with specificity against a known antigen. Immunoglobulin, or antibody, is a glycoprotein produced by B lymphocyte plasma cells in response to the presentation of an antigen. Plasma cells are B lymphocytes that have differentiated into plasma cells and memory cells from exposure to an antigen. The major classes of immunoglobulins and areas of focus in an immune response have been previously identified. Immunoglobulins are primarily responsible for the body's response to invading bacteria and viruses and provide the humoral immunity component of an immune response.[13,14]

T Lymphocyte Response

T lymphocytes undergo differentiation on exposure to a foreign antigen, developing into subtypes of cells that may directly attack the antigen or stimulate the activation of other leukocytes. Cytotoxic T lymphocytes attack and kill antigens directly, with preference for viruses or mutated cells that have become cancerous. This type of innate immunity is termed cellular or cell-mediated immunity.[3,8,9,14,15]

Several types of T lymphocytes (or T cells) may be classified into three primary groups: helper T cells, cytotoxic T cells, and suppressor T cells. Helper T cells (CD4 cells) comprise approximately 75% of all T lymphocytes. They help in the functions of the immune system by regulating most of the system's functions via the protein mediators, lymphokines. They help direct and encourage other T cells and also help to activate B lymphocytes. Cytotoxic T cells, also termed killer cells, directly kill foreign antigens and may kill cells of the self. Suppressor T cells suppress the function of both helper and cytotoxic T cells in order to prevent hyperimmune responses.[9,16]

Complement System Response

The 25 primary proteins of the complement system contribute to an immune response by amplifying and increasing the efficiency and efficacy of the other components of the immune system. The complement system also contributes to the inflammatory response. The primary activities resulting from activation of the complement cascade include increasing bacterial susceptibility to phagocytosis, lysing some types

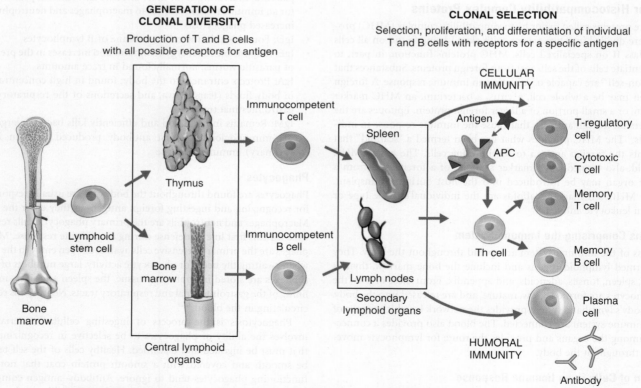

GENERATION OF CLONAL DIVERSITY

Production of T and B cells with all possible receptors for antigen

CLONAL SELECTION

Selection, proliferation, and differentiation of individual T and B cells with receptors for a specific antigen

Bone marrow

Lymphoid stem cell

Thymus

Bone marrow

Central lymphoid organs

Immunocompetent T cell

Immunocompetent B cell

Spleen

Lymph nodes

Secondary lymphoid organs

CELLULAR IMMUNITY

Antigen

APC

Th cell

T-regulatory cell

Cytotoxic T cell

Memory T cell

Memory B cell

Plasma cell

HUMORAL IMMUNITY

Antibody

FIGURE 23-2 Overview of Immune Response (Source: From McCance KL, Huether SE, Brashers VL, et al.: *Pathophysiology: The biologic basis for disease in adults and children*, ed 7, St Louis, 2014, Mosby.)

of bacteria and foreign antigens, producing chemotactic substances, increasing vascular permeability, and increasing smooth muscle contraction.

Dendritic Cell Function in an Immune Response

Dendritic cells are potent cells in asserting control from initiation to termination of the immune response. Dendritic cells have a "sentinel" function throughout the body as they look for foreign antigens and alert lymphocytes to the presence of injury or infection. They are also considered *antigen-presenting cells*; they bind to antigens and then process and present them to both B and T lymphocytes in an immune response. They have been found to directly activate helper and killer T cells and present cancer cells to cytotoxic T cells, which respond by killing mutant cells.[15,17–21]

VARIATIONS AND CONTEXT

Problems associated with immunity may occur in individuals across the lifespan with a range of impact from minor symptoms such as a runny nose to life-threatening consequences. Variations may occur as a result of diminished or exaggerated immune functioning or responses to autoimmune situations in which the immune system is attacking the "self."

Suppressed Immune Response

An inadequately functioning immune system leaves the individual immunocompromised. Immunodeficiency is either classified as primary or secondary.

Primary immunodeficiency (PI) is a situation in which the entire immune defense system is inadequate and the individual is missing some, if not all, of the components necessary for a complete immune response. The National Institutes of Health (NIH) has identified more than 70 different types of immunodeficiencies.[22,23] Ten warning signs of primary immunodeficiency were also identified by the NIH, with PI suspected if 2 or more of the signs are evident.[24] The 10 warning signs include the following: four or more new ear infections within 1 year; two or more serious sinus infections within 1 year; 2 or more months of taking antibiotics with little effect; two or more pneumonias within 1 year; failure of an infant to gain weight or grow normally; recurrent, deep skin or organ abscesses; persistent thrush in mouth or fungal infection on skin; need for intravenous antibiotics to clear infections; two or more deep-seated infections including septicemia; and a family history of primary immunodeficiency. Common variable

immunodeficiency is one of the most prevalent PI diseases and is manifest with a defect in antibody formation following a defect in B lymphocytes that interferes with the ability of the cells to differentiate into plasma (antibody-producing) cells.[25]

Secondary immunodeficiency is a loss of immune functioning (in a person with previously normal immune function) as a result of an illness or treatment. A depressed immune system may be created with medication in order to avoid rejection of transplanted tissue, or it may be induced as a result of treatment for various types of cancer. In the treatment of some types of leukemia, destruction of the bone marrow is necessary before healthy stem cells may be reintroduced and a healthy immune system regrows. Throughout the treatment process, the immune system is partially destroyed, leaving the individual immunocompromised. Conversely, some cancers, such as multiple myeloma, Hodgkin's disease, and non-Hodgkin's lymphoma, may directly lead to immune system dysfunction and immunocompromise.

Exaggerated Immune Response

An exaggerated immune response will generally be classified as one of four classes of hypersensitivity disorders: type I, IgE-mediated or atopic ("allergic"); type II, tissue-specific or cytotoxic; type III, immune complex-mediated; and type IV, cell-mediated or delayed hypersensitivity. Hypersensitivity may be defined as "an abnormal condition characterized by an exaggerated response of the immune system to an antigen … hypersensitivity reaction is inappropriate and excessive."[1] The pathology associated with hypersensitivity reactions is summarized in Table 23-1.

Exaggerated immune responses may be localized or they may affect all body systems. A bee sting may cause a localized type I allergic reaction or it may cause a systemic anaphylactic reaction. Systemic anaphylactic reactions caused by a number of foreign antigens are also considered type I hypersensitivity reactions. Type II tissue-specific reactions may lead to myasthenia gravis, hyperacute graft rejection with transplanted tissues, or autoimmune-based hemolytic anemia. Type III immune complex-mediated responses are the basis for rheumatoid arthritis or systemic lupus erythematosus (SLE). Type IV cell-mediated responses are seen with transplant rejection or poison ivy allergic responses.[9,10,26,27]

In cases of exaggerated immune response, the individual may be damaged or otherwise harmed by a response that is supposed to be protective or curative as is seen in the presence of anaphylaxis. Autoimmune responses may result in the development of type 1 diabetes mellitus, SLE, or rheumatoid arthritis.

TABLE 23-1 Immunologic Mechanisms of Tissue Destruction

Type	Name	Rate of Development	Class of Antibody Involved	Principal Effector Cells Involved	Complement Participation	Examples of Disorders
I	IgE-mediated reaction	Immediate	IgE	Mast cells	No	Seasonal allergic rhinitis
II	Tissue-specific reaction	Immediate	IgG IgM	Macrophages in tissues	Frequently	Autoimmune thrombocytopenic purpura, Graves' disease, autoimmune hemolytic anemia
III	Immune complex-mediated reaction	Immediate	IgG IgM	Neutrophils	Yes	Systemic lupus erythematosus
IV	Cell-mediated reaction	Delayed	None	Lymphocytes, macrophages	No	Contact sensitivity to poison ivy and metals (jewelry)

Ig, immunoglobulin.

Source: From McCance KL, Huether SE, Brashers VL, et al.: *Pathophysiology: The biologic basis for disease in adults and children*, ed 7, St Louis, 2014, Mosby.

CONSEQUENCES

Consequences of Immunosuppression

A number of serious health problems develop for the immunocompromised individual. Some problems include an increase in the incidence of infection by bacteria and viruses, the development of superinfections such as methicillin-resistant *Staphylococcus aureus* (MRSA) or *Clostridium difficile* (*C. difficile* or *C. diff.*), or the development of treatment-resistant fungal infections secondary to antibiotic treatment for primary bacterial infections.[28–31] In situations in which a suppressed immune response is evident, the individual may not be able to mount a sufficient response to avoid or repair a diseased body organ or system. For example, cancer, particularly in the elderly, has been associated with an immunocompromised state and a diminished ability to recognize and destroy mutant cells.

Consequences of an Exaggerated Immune Response

Multisystem or single system disease may result from an initiating hypersensitivity response. Cardiovascular diseases may emerge as a consequence of autoimmune disorders such as Graves' disease or SLE. Renal failure may result from chronic glomerulonephritis or polycystic kidney disease. HIV disease weakens the immune system, and a variety of opportunistic diseases and infections will ultimately result.[32]

Autoimmune disorders occur when the immune system attacks and destroys healthy cells following a breakdown of what has been termed "self-tolerance." With more than 80 autoimmune disorders already identified, an individual may have more than one autoimmune disorder simultaneously.[33] This type of immune disorder is associated with three potential outcomes: destruction of one or more types of body tissues, abnormal organ growth, or changes in organ function. The degree of destruction and functional loss varies dramatically and depends on the type of immune disorder, age, overall physical and nutritional health, and treatment. Some of the more commonly occurring autoimmune diseases include rheumatoid arthritis, SLE, muscular sclerosis, Graves' disease, and diabetes mellitus. Genetic predisposition is an important factor in the development of autoimmune diseases, with manifestation of the disease often associated with some type of environmental trigger, such as bacterial or viral infections, or physiological or environmental stressors.[8,9,34–37]

RISK FACTORS

People from all age, socioeconomic, and racial/ethnic groups can potentially have impaired immune systems. However, some population groups and individuals are at greater risk than others. Risk factors for suppressed and exaggerated immune function are presented separately in the following sections.

Suppressed Immune Response

Age

In the very young, the immune system is immature with inadequate lymphocyte function, particularly T lymphocyte deficiency. Newborns rely on immune protection from the mother through placental blood transfer and from the high levels of immunoglobulin found in colostrum during breast-feeding. During the next few months, maternal antibodies are slowly destroyed, with the rate of catabolism exceeding the rate of newborn immunoglobulin production.[38] This mild hypogammaglobulinemia contributes to the increased risk of infection in the newborn.

In the elderly, loss of immune effectiveness occurs in part because of the physiological aging and shrinking of the thymus gland, leaving it at approximately 15% of its maximum size by middle age and

decreasing the ability of T lymphocytes to mature in the gland over time.[38] Research has also demonstrated that elderly people have fewer T lymphocytes, produce fewer immunoglobulins, experience a delayed and diminished hypersensitivity response, and demonstrate an increase in autoantibodies.[8,9,38] B lymphocyte function is diminished secondary to a decrease in circulating memory cells that evolve after approximately 60 years of age.

Nonimmunized State

Individuals who are not immunized are susceptible to a number of infections, including rubella, measles, mumps, tetanus, diphtheria, and hepatitis. Many of these diseases can be fatal to the very young, the elderly, or those who are immunocompromised as a result of disease processes or their treatment and other environmental factors.

Environmental Factors

Environmental factors such as poor nutrition, exposure to pollutants (including tobacco smoke) or heavy metals, and other stressors may depress immune functioning.[23,39–41] Unsafe sanitary conditions, food and water contamination, and poor hand hygiene also contribute to disease transmission and are particularly dangerous to the very young or elderly and those with other chronic illnesses. Some of these situations are easily remedied by the individual, whereas others require more of a community-focused attention to solving the problem.

Chronic Illnesses

Depressed immune function can develop as a result of chronic illness or treatments for medical conditions. In addition to primary immunodeficiency conditions that directly impair the immune system (e.g., HIV), many chronic conditions (e.g., diabetes mellitus, chronic obstructive pulmonary disease, malnutrition, and cancer) also lead to reductions in immune function as a secondary consequence to the disease or its treatment.

Medical Treatments

Medical treatments may be implemented specifically to inhibit a normal immune response or an autoimmune response, or they may lead to immunosuppression as a consequence of the treatment. For instance, in the case of tissue graft or tissue/organ transplantation, medication is administered to induce a state of immunosuppression so that the body does not mount a normal immune response and cause rejection of the graft tissue. Conversely, pharmacologic treatments for autoimmune hypersensitivity reactions, such as SLE or multiple sclerosis, include treatment regimens that inhibit the immune response. Immunosuppression is a common side effect of cancer treatment. The stress associated with many medical treatments, both psychological and physical, places an added burden on the immune system and may leave the individual vulnerable to illness.

Genetics

An individual's genetic base, overall health, and history of exposure to potential antigens influence immune functioning.[42] A number of genetic diseases may lead to depressed or absent functioning of parts or all of the immune system. As a group, complement deficiencies are comparatively rare, and their prevalence varies depending on the specific deficiency and the age of a person. Another immune deficiency, common variable immunodeficiency, is one of the most prevalent primary immunodeficiency diseases, with an estimated 1 case per 30,000 population.[40] Allergies to food or environmental stimuli and type 1 diabetes mellitus are also considered a type of immune dysfunction. The incidence of those diseases is widespread in both children and adults of all ethnic origins, with variations depending on geography and ethnicity.

High-Risk Behaviors and Substance Abuse

A number of high-risk behaviors have been associated with the development of a dysfunctional immune system. Transmission of HIV and hepatitis virus may be directly related to high-risk sexual behaviors and sharing needles among intravenous drug abusers. According to Waldschmidt and colleagues,[43] excessive alcohol consumption leads to compromised immunity (innate and acquired), dysfunction of components of the immune system, and increased risk of infection.

Pregnancy

Immunity is influenced by pregnancy, creating a situation in which the mother is immunocompromised. The developing fetus exists in what has been termed a "privileged" immunity environment in which fetal antigens from the father do not stimulate an immune response and rejection of the graft created by the fetus–placenta connection and the mother. The placental barrier between mother and fetus is open to communication between mother and fetal cells. It has been found that fetal cells may remain in the mother's tissues for long periods of time, creating a situation termed *microchimerism* or a mixing of cells of different origins. A microchimerism may also be created in the fetus, and research is investigating the role that this may play in the development of autoimmune diseases.[9]

Exaggerated Immune Response
Gender, Race, and Ethnicity

Some hypersensitivity disorders have higher incidence and prevalence by virtue of gender, race, or ethnicity. For example, SLE occurs more often in women than in men by a 10:1 ratio, and African-Americans are eight times more likely than white non-Hispanics to contract the disease.[9]

Genetics

Genetics is often responsible for the formation of an exaggerated immune response. An exaggerated reaction may be minor and serve more as an annoyance, such as seen with some environmental or food allergies, or may lead to destruction of normal tissue, loss of organ function, or death. In some cases, the genetic basis for the development of hyperimmune disorders requires that the gene or chromosome be carried by both parents (or sometimes only one parent), and some disorders require an environmental or physiological trigger (e.g., hormonal changes seen in puberty) in addition to the predisposition to a hyperimmune disorder created by genetics.

Environmental or Medication Exposure

Environmental or medication exposure to a foreign antigen may elicit an exaggerated immune response. Foods, drugs, pollens, dust, molds, bee venom, vaccines, or serum may all evoke hypersensitivity reactions (types I, II, or III), and some may evoke more than one type of hypersensitivity.[5,8,9] Generally, these hypersensitivity reactions do not occur on first exposure to the foreign antigen but, rather, on reexposure. However, genetic predisposition, exposure by the mother during fetal development, or other contributing factors may cause an exaggerated response on first presentation of the pathogen. In many cases, individuals who manifest an allergic type of exaggerated response to one type of pathogen (e.g., pollen) will demonstrate a similar reaction to other antigens in the same or similar class.

Medication exposure may act similarly to environmental exposure in inducing an exaggerated response. Some individuals report an allergic type of exaggerated reaction on first exposure to some medications (e.g., penicillin). In some individuals, a previously expressed exaggerated immune response may be amplified further in the presence of specific medications. For example, cancer treatment that includes the use of monoclonal antibodies has triggered exaggerated hypersensitivity reactions in some patients even though a more mild reaction to the same pathogen was experienced in the past.

ASSESSMENT

Assessment of immune response and dysfunction begins with a thorough health history and physical examination. Basic laboratory and diagnostic testing procedures are followed with more specific tests depending on the individual's history and current presenting symptoms. Genetic testing may also be important to confirm a diagnosis, to determine appropriate counseling concerning the person's prognosis, or to make reproduction recommendations.[44]

History

The health history is useful to determine a patient's risk for an altered immune response and to determine if symptoms are described that link to problems with the immune system. The history should include current and past medical problems including treatments, especially the presence of conditions associated with immune problems (see Box 23-1 later in the chapter). The patient should be asked about allergies to substances, including the response that occurs with exposure. Also included are current medications taken by the patient and the vaccination history. Ask questions related to general health status including energy levels, nutritional status including normal dietary intake, and recent changes in weight and wound healing. Associated health topics of concern include health problems during pregnancy, conditions causing significant or consistent psychological stress, exposure to environmental agents or stressors, physical trauma, and a history of exposure to microorganisms that may cause immunosuppression (Epstein–Barr virus, HIV, cytomegalovirus, herpes simplex virus type 6, hepatitis B virus, etc.).

Examination Findings

Examination findings indicative of immune status are presented from the perspective of normal (optimal) immune functioning, suppressed immune functioning, and exaggerated immune functioning.

Clinical Findings Indicative of Optimal Immune Functioning

Clinical indicators of optimal immune functioning reveal an individual who generally appears well and is well nourished. Vital signs are within normal parameters for age; lymph nodes should be soft, movable, and nontender (although lymph nodes are often not palpable among older adults). Wounds that may be present are healing within a time frame normal for the type of wound.

Clinical Findings: Suppressed Immune Function

Clinical indicators of suppressed immune functioning may be mild or widespread, and they may be indicative of impending immune system failure. Vital signs may or may not be within normal parameters for age depending on the amount of suppression and the degree to which the host is immunocompromised. The individual may not appear to be well nourished, may present with weight loss or wasting syndrome, and may complain of generalized fatigue or malaise. Impaired wound healing is present, and with sufficient immune system suppression, opportunistic infections and diseases may also be present. As a result of inflammation and infection within the central nervous system, psychological evaluation should be included because it may disclose a change in cognitive functioning or depression. The presence of seizure activity or changes in motor behavior should also be determined. Should the individual present with clinical manifestations indicating significant immunocompromise, a more thorough evaluation related to specific opportunistic infections and diseases would be appropriate.

Clinical Findings: Exaggerated Immune Function

Clinical findings associated with an allergic response may vary from typical mild symptoms (sneezing, watery eyes, and nasal congestion) to severe responses (rashes, swelling, and shock syndrome). They may produce a minor decrease in quality of life or be life-threatening.

Clinical manifestations of autoimmune disorders are often vague and less obvious while often affecting multiple organ systems. Symptoms may become more apparent when system function is impaired. For example, cardiovascular symptoms may include pericarditis, congestive heart failure, pulmonary or peripheral edema, and anemia. Renal symptoms will range from no symptoms to glomerulonephritis and from acute to chronic renal failure and end-stage renal disease. Musculoskeletal manifestations can include joint pain or the inability to control movements, including walking, as seen with multiple sclerosis. Some autoimmune disorders have classic findings. For example, a subtle butterfly rash across the nose and cheeks is a common finding associated with SLE.

Diagnostic Tests
Primary Testing

Laboratory and diagnostic testing begins with basic blood tests to determine red blood cell and white blood cell counts with differential evaluation. A fluorescent antinuclear antibody test is standard in the evaluation of potential autoimmune diseases. Screening tests—C-reactive protein (CRP) and erythrocyte sedimentation rate (ESR)—may also be completed. CRP is used to determine inflammation in the body and not to diagnose a specific immune dysfunction. It may also be used to follow the progress of and response to treatment for diseases such as rheumatoid arthritis, SLE, and other autoimmune disorders. An ESR is useful in monitoring inflammatory or cancerous diseases, rheumatoid arthritis and other autoimmune diseases, and tuberculosis.[45–47]

Allergy Testing

Allergy testing is often important in diagnosis, and it may necessitate a skin test, an allergen-specific immunoglobulin (IgE) blood test, or both. Skin testing helps determine allergens to which the individual is sensitive, and the IgE blood test measures the amount of IgE in the blood—higher levels are associated with a more severe allergic response. Circulating blood levels of IgM and IgA may also be measured.

Advanced or Disease-Specific Testing

More specific blood testing includes cytogenic analysis to detect chromosomal instability, indicative of chromosomal disorders; DNA analysis to detect genetic mutations; and enzyme-linked immunosorbent assay (ELISA) to determine blood levels of IgG subclasses and diagnose IgG deficiency. T lymphocyte levels and proliferative response to antigen introduction testing aids in determining T cell capacity in an immune response and provides another avenue for information. Rheumatoid factor is a blood test to determine the presence of antibodies against immunoglobulins and is evaluated in combination with other blood tests on the immune system.[2,48] The ELISA and confirmatory Western blot tests are done to confirm the presence of antibodies to HIV infection. The TORCH antibody panel searches for the presence of antibodies to cytomegalovirus, herpes simplex, rubella, and toxoplasmosis.[48] Complement system testing is done to determine the

presence of deficiencies or abnormalities in complement proteins, addressing both quality and activity of the proteins. Deficiencies contribute to increased incidence and severity of infections and autoimmune dysfunction.

Tests of Organ Function

Tests are often performed to aid in assessing specific organ function or to monitor the effectiveness of treatment regimens. These tests include hemoglobin A_{1c} levels in diabetes mellitus management, hepatic function tests, and thyroid screening panels. In most cases, serial laboratory testing is recommended to assess both progression of disease and effectiveness of treatment strategies.

CLINICAL MANAGEMENT

The clinical management of individuals with immunosuppression or hyperimmune conditions varies widely depending on the type of condition, severity, and attribute variables such as age, health status, and underlying medical conditions. Such variables must be considered when making clinical management decisions.

Primary Prevention

The cornerstone of primary prevention for immune system disorders is based on recommended vaccinations across the lifespan. The CDC's Advisory Committee on Immunization Practices has established recommended vaccination schedules for children, adolescents, and adults, in addition to a "catch-up" schedule.[49,50] Schedules and updates are easily found on the CDC website. Primary prevention also includes reduction of modifiable risk factors noted previously. This includes avoiding high-risk behaviors, minimizing exposure to environmental triggers, eating a proper diet, and engaging in regular exercise. Research has demonstrated that achieving the daily recommended doses of vitamins and minerals contributes to a properly functioning immune system. New research is addressing the role of vitamins A and D in protecting and supporting the immune response and may serve a valuable contribution to many medical treatment regimens in addition to their usefulness in one's daily diet for health maintenance.[8,9]

Secondary Prevention (Screening)

Secondary prevention focuses on screenings for the presence or emergence of immune system disorders. There are few screenings specifically directed at immune system dysfunction for the general public. However, some screenings (e.g., HIV screening) are recommended for high-risk groups. Advances in genomic testing may prove useful in developing screening tests for more diseases affecting the immune system in the future.

Collaborative Interventions

Collaborative treatment strategies vary depending on whether the immune dysfunction is one of deficiency or an exaggerated response. Thus, interventions may range from supporting an inadequate immune response to diminishing the consequences of an exaggerated response. An overview of selected clinical management strategies for the treatment of immune system diseases or dysfunction is provided in Table 23-2.

INTERRELATED CONCEPTS

The concept of immunity is closely related to the concepts of Inflammation and Infection. There exists overlap among the concepts in the areas of pathology, laboratory and diagnostic tests, clinical manifestations, nursing interventions, and clinical outcomes. A

TABLE 23-2 Interventions in the Clinical Management of Immune Dysfunction

Management of Clinical Manifestations	Clinical Outcomes
Suppressed Immune Response	
Infection	Normal gastrointestinal transit time
Clinical management of infection and opportunistic diseases is typically an	Resolution of infection
important part of clinical care; interventions and clinical outcomes are discussed	Adequate hydration
in Concept 25 Infection	Adequate nutrition
Gastrointestinal dysfunction	Resolution of skin rash
Pharmacologic treatment of diarrhea, candidiasis, and fluid and electrolyte loss	Restoration of adequate nutrition, body weight, and BMI
Skin disorders	
Pharmacologic treatment of skin rash	
Nutrition	
Multiple vitamin and mineral supplements	
Dietary supplements such as Ensure or equivalent	
Evaluation of weight and BMI	
Exaggerated Immune Response	
Anaphylaxis	Adequate ventilation
Support of airway, breathing, and circulation: Subcutaneous epinephrine if type 1	Restoration of blood pressure and pulse to pre-reaction normal levels
reaction; other bronchodilators; intubation and ventilator support, circulatory	Adequate urine output indicating adequate circulatory volume
volume expanders, and vasopressors to maintain blood pressure and circulating	Modulation of hypersensitivity responses
volume	Management of pain experience
Pharmacotherapy: Epinephrine and bronchodilators as described previously	Maintenance of joint and muscle mobility; self-care for ADLs where
Education: Avoiding contact with pathogen initiating anaphylactic response; proper	possible; restoration or maintenance of adequate levels of physical
use of an EpiPen for self-administration of epinephrine	activity
Immunosuppression	
Pharmacotherapy: Corticosteroids, chemotherapeutic agents, NSAIDs,	
immunomodulators	
Pain management	
Pharmacotherapy: NSAIDs, corticosteroids	
Hypothermia or hyperthermia treatments as appropriate	
Maintenance of mobility and physical activity	

ADLs, activities of daily living; BMI, body mass index; NSAIDs, nonsteroidal anti-inflammatory drugs.

discussion of the concepts inflammation and infection is found in Concept 24 Inflammation and Concept 25 Infection, respectively. Tissue Integrity is also closely aligned to immunity because a defect in tissue integrity will cause the body to invoke an immune response and may lead to both inflammation and infection. Stress has been discussed as a pathologic influence that both may initiate an immune response and may lead to immune dysfunction. Stress may also lead to an alteration in Glucose Regulation. Resultant elevated blood glucose levels can exaggerate both inflammation and infection situations. Both inadequate Nutrition and extreme or prolonged Fatigue are stressors to the body, either of which may cause the individual to become immunocompromised or cause the individual to have an exaggerated preexisting immune response. These concepts were previously discussed as methods by which an individual may become immunocompromised. Interrelationships are demonstrated in Figure 23-3.

CLINICAL EXEMPLARS

Examples of diseases that may develop with immune system diseases represent cases of B or T lymphocyte dysfunction, hypersensitivity reactions, complement dysfunction, or dysfunction of more than one component. Many examples have been introduced throughout this concept presentation. Box 23-1 provides a brief

overview of some of the more common diseases that may lead to immunocompromise.

When considering an immune response, it is most important to remember that the response is a complex interaction between a foreign antigen and a wide variety of differing cells and is also dependent on genetic, environmental, and overall health parameters that are unique to each individual. The presence and progress of immune responses and the development of immunocompromise are unique to each individual and require a thorough review of health history, presenting symptoms, and laboratory and diagnostic data when determining nursing care strategies.

Featured Exemplars
Hodgkin's and Non-Hodgkin's Lymphoma

Hodgkin's and non-Hodgkin's lymphoma are types of cancer that originate in the lymphatic system and represent a suppressed immune state. Non-Hodgkin's lymphoma is more common than Hodgkin's lymphoma, and it may arise from either the B cells or the T cells. Symptoms for both types of lymphoma include swollen lymph nodes in the neck, axilla, or groin; abdominal pain; persistent fatigue; fever and chills; night sweats; and weight loss. Most people diagnosed with non-Hodgkin's lymphoma have no obvious risk factors. Some factors that may increase the risk include medications that suppress the immune system, infection with selected bacteria or viruses, pesticides, or older age (>60 years).[51,52]

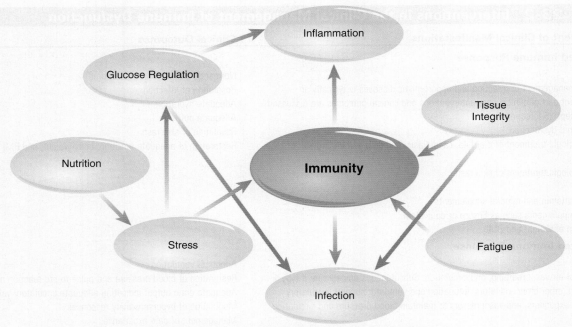

FIGURE 23-3 Immunity and Interrelated Concepts

■■■ BOX 23-1 EXEMPLARS OF INEFFECTIVE IMMUNITY

Suppressed Immune Response
- Classic complement pathway deficiency
- Deficiencies of immunoglobulin A, G, D, or M
- DiGeorge syndrome
- HIV
- Hodgkin's and non-Hodgkin's lymphoma
- Plasma cell disorders
- Primary immunodeficiency
- Severe combined immunodeficiency

Exaggerated Immune Response
Allergic Responses
- Allergic reaction
- Allergic rhinitis
- Anaphylaxis
- Asthma

Autoimmune Responses
- Autoimmune thrombocytopenic purpura
- Crohn's disease
- Diabetes mellitus (type 1, insulin-dependent)
- Glomerulonephritis
- Graves' disease
- Multiple sclerosis
- Myasthenia gravis
- Rheumatoid arthritis
- Systemic lupus erythematosus
- Ulcerative colitis

HIV Disease

Infection with the retrovirus, HIV, leads primarily to destruction of CD4+ T cells, leaving the person with an immune deficiency and a diminishing ability to fight other opportunistic diseases and infections. CH4+ or "helper" T cells are critical in the overall functioning of the immune response by signaling other cells in the immune system to perform their designated function. HIV-mediated destruction of lymph nodes and lymph organs also contributes to immune system dysfunction. Ultimately, CD4+ destruction results in the development of AIDS, the third and final stage of HIV disease.[53–55]

Anaphylaxis

Anaphylaxis is an extreme, exaggerated allergic response to foods, medication, stinging insects, and exercise. Anaphylaxis may involve a few or multiple body organs or systems, with symptoms ranging from non-life-threatening (sneezing, hives, itching, and diarrhea) to life-threatening with restriction of breathing and circulation. Symptoms can occur from minutes to hours after exposure to the allergen, with the reaction being one of three types: single reaction occurring immediately after exposure; double reaction with the first reaction minutes to hours after exposure and a second reaction 8–72 hours after the first reaction; and a single long-lasting reaction that may last hours to days.[56]

Allergic Rhinitis

Allergic rhinitis, commonly referred to as "hay fever" or "pollen allergy," may also be associated with food allergies, atopic dermatitis (eczema), or asthma. Allergic rhinitis is common in all age groups and in approximately 10% of children younger than age 18 years. The condition is often seasonal, and symptoms typically include inflammation of the nasal passages resulting in a runny nose, sneezing, congestion of the nose, and itchy, red, watery eyes. Hyposensitization by injection of a diluted form of the antigen may be a necessary part of the treatment regimen.[1,57]

Systemic Lupus Erythematosus

SLE is a chronic, inflammatory autoimmune disease that affects multiple body organs and systems, including joints, skin, kidneys, blood cells, brain, heart, and lungs. The most obvious sign of SLE is a butterfly-shaped facial rash that spreads across the cheeks and bridge of the nose. This rash is present in most, but not all, cases of SLE. As an autoimmune disease with an exaggerated response, cells of the immune system begin to attack cells of the "self," damaging or destroying multiple organs with periods of flare and remission. There is no cure for SLE; treatment is directed at managing symptoms.[58]

Type 1 Diabetes Mellitus

Type 1 diabetes mellitus, another autoimmune disease, typically manifests in young people, although it can occur in adults, presenting with hyperglycemia as a result of the β cells in the pancreas either not producing or not producing enough insulin because the immune system has attacked and destroyed the insulin-producing cells. Heredity plays a major role in determining susceptibility to β

cell destruction. The most common presenting symptoms include hyperglycemia, polydipsia, polyuria, and metabolic acidosis. If uncontrolled, chronic high glucose levels lead to damage to the vascular and microvascular system, peripheral neuropathy, kidney damage, and hypertension.[59]

Multiple Sclerosis

Multiple sclerosis is a neurologic disease that ranges from being relatively benign to overwhelmingly disabling as the immune system attacks the nerve-insulating myelin sheaths and disrupts communication between nerves and muscles. The first symptoms generally occur between the ages of 20 and 40 years and include a combination of blurred vision, blindness in one eye, muscle weakness, balance or coordination impairment, paresthesias, numbness or tingling, speech impediments, dizziness, or hearing loss. Over time, many people experience cognitive impairment, difficulty with concentration or memory, poor judgment, and depression. Although there is no cure, some medications are demonstrating promise in reducing the number of exacerbations and slowing the progression of physical disability.[60]

CASE STUDY

Source: Fuse/Thinkstock

Case Presentation

Jonathan Eckert is a 22-year-old white male who has been involved in a number of high-risk sexual behaviors. Three months ago, he developed a 4-day course of fever and chills, malaise, lethargy, night sweats, diarrhea, and anorexia. He believed he had acquired the flu (influenza) and self-medicated with acetaminophen, vitamin C, and increased fluid intake. He became increasingly concerned about his health because he had friends who were infected with HIV, so he contacted his primary care provider to obtain a blood screening test for HIV and hepatitis B and C.

Jonathan's screening test for hepatitis B and C was negative, and the HIV screening tests—ELISA and confirmatory Western blot—both returned positive for HIV infection. Additional laboratory testing was done to assess his red blood cell count, white blood cell count with differential, and CD4 and CD8 lymphocyte counts (lymphocyte immunophenotyping). All of his blood tests were within the normal range. Serologic testing for hepatitis B and C was negative, skin testing for tuberculosis returned negative, and a chest x-ray was unremarkable.

Jonathan was given information on, and demonstrated understanding of, the need to maintain a healthy lifestyle with appropriate nutrition, physical activity, stress management, avoidance of cigarettes and other forms of tobacco, maintenance of appropriate vaccinations including an annual influenza vaccination, and adherence to safer sexual practices to avoid reinfection with a potentially more virulent strain of the virus and transmission of the virus to others. He was given information on community support groups and a referral to a care provider specializing in HIV/AIDS care. New research on the advantages of beginning treatment for HIV within the first year of exposure to the virus and seroconversion were discussed with him, and Jonathan and his provider are considering this option.

Case Analysis

Jonathan has developed an infection with HIV and is currently asymptomatic. His immune system has responded to the pathogen invasion by producing antibodies to the virus, and cytotoxic T lymphocytes are also responding to the viral infection. At this time, he would not typically be a candidate for highly active antiretroviral therapy (HAART); however, he must continue to monitor his immune functioning.

ACCESS EXEMPLAR LINKS IN YOUR GIDDENS EBOOK

REFERENCES

1. Mosby: *Mosby's dictionary of medicine, nursing, and health professions,* ed 9, St Louis, 2013, Mosby.
2. Venes D, editor: *Taber's cyclopedic medical dictionary,* ed 22, Philadelphia, 2013, Davis.
3. National Institutes of Health: Immune system, 2014. Retrieved from: <http://www.niaid.nih.gov/topics/immuneSystem/pages/overview.aspx>.
4. Centers for Disease Control and Prevention: Immunity types, 2009. Retrieved from: <http://www.cdc.gov/vaccines/vac-gen/immunity-types.htm>.
5. National Institutes of Health, U.S. National Library of Medicine: Immune response, 2014. Retrieved from: <http://www.nlm.nih.gov/medlineplus/ency/article/000821.htm>,

6. National Institutes of Health, National Institute of Allergy and Infectious Diseases: Immune system: Immune cells, 2014. Retrieved from: <http://www.niaid.nih.gov/topics/immunesystem/Pages/immuneCells.aspx>.

7. University of Hartford: Immune system, 2001. Retrieved from: <http://uhaweb.hartford.edu/BUGL/immune.htm>.

8. Hall JE: *Textbook of medical physiology*, ed 12, Philadelphia, 2011, Saunders.

9. McCance KL, Huether SE, Brashers VL, et al, editors: *Pathophysiology: The biologic basis for disease in adults and children*, ed 6, St Louis, 2010, Mosby.

10. National Institutes of Health, National Institute of Allergy and Infectious Diseases: Immune system: Disorders of the immune system, 2014. Retrieved from: <http://www.niaid.nih.gov/topics/immuneSystem/Pages/immuneDisorders.aspx>.

11. National Institutes of Health, U.S. National Library of Medicine: Immune response. Retrieved from: <http://www.nlm.nih.gov/medlineplus/ency/article/000821.htm>.

12. Kimball J: Histocompatibility molecules, 2011. Retrieved from: <http://users.rcn.com/jkimball.ma.ultranet/BiologyPages/H/HLA.html>.

13. Kimball J: B cells and T cells, 2013. Retrieved from: <http://users.rcn.com/jkimball.ma.ultranet/BiologyPages/B/B_and_Tcells.html>.

14. Kimball J: Helper T cells, 2014. Retrieved from: <http://users.rcn.com/jkimball.ma.ultranet/BiologyPages/T/Th1_Th2.html>.

15. National Institutes of Health, National Institute of Allergy and Infectious Diseases: Immune system: B cells. Retrieved from: <www.niaid.nih.gov/topics/immuneSystem/immuneCells/Pages/bcells.aspx>.

16. Tang W, Wang H, Claudio E, et al: The oncoprotein and transcriptional regulator Bcl-3 governs plasticity and pathogenicity of autoimmune T cells. *Immunity* 41:555–566, 2014.

17. Steinman R: Introduction to dendritic cells, 2015. Retrieved from: <http://lab.rockefeller.edu/steinman/>.

18. Steinman R: Dendritic cells initiate the immune response, 2015. Retrieved from: <http://lab.rockefeller.edu/steinman/dendritic_intro/immuneResponse>,

19. Steinman R: Dendritic cells and immune tolerance, 2015. Retrieved from: <http://lab.rockefeller.edu/steinman/dendritic_intro/immuneTolerance>.

20. Leon B, Ardavin C: Monocyte-derived dendritic cells in innate and adaptive immunity. *Immunol Cell Biol* 86:320–324, 2008.

21. Maason F, Mount AM, Wilson NS, et al: Dendritic cells: Driving the differentiation programme of T cells in viral infections. *Immunol Cell Biol* 86:333–342, 2008.

22. National Institutes of Health, U.S. National Library of Medicine: Immune system and disorders, 2010. Retrieved from: <http://www.nlm.nih.gov/medlineplus/immunesystemanddisorders.html>.

23. National Institutes of Health, National Library of Medicine: Immunodeficiency disorders. Retrieved from: <http://www.nlm.nih.gov/medlineplus/ency/article/000818.htm>.

24. National Primary Immunodeficiency Resource Center: 10 Warning signs of primary immunodeficiency, 2009. Retrieved from: <http://info4pi.org/aboutPI/index.cfm?section=aboutPI&content=warningsigns>.

25. Park CL: Common variable immunodeficiency, 2010. Retrieved from: <http://emedicine.medscape.com/article/885935>.

26. Winfield JB: Fibromyalgia, 2010. Retrieved from: <http://emedicine.medscape.com/article/329838-overview>.

27. Heib V, Becker M, Taube C, et al: Advances in the understanding of mast cell function. *Br J Haematol* 142:683–694, 2008.

28. Mayo Clinic: MRSA infection, 2010. Retrieved from: <http://www.mayoclinic.com/health/mrsa/DS00735>.

29. Davis C: MRSA infection, 2008. Retrieved from: <http://www.emedicinehealth.com/script/main/art.asp?articlekey=86302&>.

30. Mayo Clinic: C. difficile *infection*, 2010. Retrieved from: <http://www.mayoclinic.com/health/c-difficile/DS00736>.

31. Centers for Disease Control and Prevention: *Clostridium difficile* infection, 2010. Retrieved from: <http://www.cdc.gov/HAi/organisms/cdiff/Cdiff_infect.html>.

32. Iwami S, Miura T, Nakaoka S, et al: Immune impairment in HIV infection: Existence of risky and immunodeficiency thresholds. *J Theor Biol* 260:490–501, 2009.

33. National Institutes of Health, U.S. National Library of Medicine: Autoimmune disorders, 2009. Retrieved from: <http://www.nlm.nih.gov/medlineplus/ency/article/000816.htm>.

34. Copstead LC, Banasik JL: *Pathophysiology*, ed 4, St Louis, 2010, Saunders.

35. Milner JD, Vogel TP, Forbes L, et al: Early-onset lymphoproliferation and autoimmunity caused by germline STAT3 gain-of-function mutations. *Blood* 125:591–599, 2015.

36. Arizona Center for Advanced Medicine: Autoimmune diseases—Overview, 2013. Retrieved from: <http://arizonaadvancedmedicine.com/autoimmune-diseases>.

37. National Institutes of Health, National Institute of Allergy and infectious Diseases: Immune system: Immune tolerance, 2014. Retrieved from: <http://www.niaid.nih.gov/topics/immunesystem/Pages/immuneTolerance.aspx>.

38. National Institutes of Health, U.S. National Library of Medicine: Aging changes in immunity, 2012. Retrieved from: <http://www.nlm.nih.gov/medlineplus/ency/article/004008.htm>.

39. Burns CE, Dunn AM, Brady MA, et al: *Pediatric primary care*, ed 4, St Louis, 2009, Saunders.

40. Arizona Center for Advanced Medicine: Immune system dysfunction, 2013. Retrieved from: <http://arizonaadvancedmedicine.com/articles/immune_system_dysfunction.html>.

41. Chaganti RK, Schwartz RA: Complement deficiencies, 2009. Retrieved from: <http://emedicine.medscape.com/article/135478>.

42. Nolan D, Gaudieri S, Mallal S: Host genetics and viral infections: Immunology taught by viruses, virology taught by the immune system. *Curr Opin Immunol* 18:413–421, 2006.

43. Waldschmidt TJ, Cook RT, Kovacs EJ: Alcohol and inflammation and immune responses: Summary of the 2006 Alcohol and Immunology Research Interest Group (AIRIG) meeting. *Alcohol* 42:137–142, 2007.

44. National Institutes of Health: Clinical exome sequencing detects disease-causing glitches, 2014. Retrieved from: <http://www.nih.gov/researchmatters/november2014/11032014exome.htm>.

45. Shiel WC: Antinuclear antibody test (ANA), 2015. Retrieved from: <http://www.medicinenet.com/antinuclear_antibody/article.htm>.

46. National Institutes of Health, U.S. National Library of Medicine: ESR, 2009. Retrieved from: <http://www.nlm.nih.gov/medlineplus/ency/article/003638.htm>.

47. National Institutes of Health, U.S. National Library of Medicine: C-reactive protein, 2009. Retrieved from: <http://www.nlm.nih.gov/medlineplus/ency/article/003356.htm>.

48. Pagana KD, Pagana TJ, Pagana J: *Mosby's diagnostic and laboratory test reference*, ed 12, St Louis, 2014, Mosby.

49. Centers for Disease Control and Prevention: Immunization schedules: Birth–18 years & "catch-up" immunization schedules, 2014. Retrieved from: <http://www.cdc.gov/vaccines/schedules/hcp/child-adolescent.html>.

50. Centers for Disease Control and Prevention: Immunization Schedules: Adult immunization schedules, 2014. Retrieved from: <http://www.cdc.gov/vaccines/schedules/hcp/adult.html>.

51. Mayo Clinic: Non-Hodgkin's lymphoma, 2013. Retrieved from: <http://www.mayoclinic.org/diseases-conditions/non-hodgkins-lymphoma/basics/definition/con-20027792>.

52. Mayo Clinic: Hodgkin's lymphoma, 2014. Retrieved from: <http://www.mayoclinic.org/diseases-conditions/hodgkins-lymphoma/basics/definition/CON-20030667>.

53. National Institutes of Health, National Institute of Allergy and Infectious Diseases: How HIV Causes AIDS, 2012. Retrieved from: <http://www.niaid.nih.gov/topics/HIVAIDS/Understanding/howHIVCausesaids/Pages/cause.aspx>.

54. National Institutes of Health: AIDS Information: HIV overview, 2014. Retrieved from: <http://aidsinfo.nih.gov/education-materials/fact-sheets/19/46/the-stages-of-hiv-infection>.

55. National Institutes of Health: AIDS information: The HIV lifecycle, 2014. Retrieved from: <http://aidsinfo.nih.gov/education-materials/fact-sheets/19/73/the-hiv-life-cycle/>.

56. National Institutes of Health, National Institute of Allergy and Infectious Diseases: Anaphylaxis, 2014. Retrieved from: <http://www.niaid.nih.gov/topics/anaphylaxis/Pages/default.aspx>.

57. National Institutes of Health, National Institute of Allergy and Infectious Diseases: Allergic diseases, 2014. Retrieved from: <http://www.niaid.nih.gov/topics/allergicdiseases/Pages/default.aspx>.

58. Mayo Clinic: Lupus, 2014. Retrieved from: <http://www.mayoclinic.org/diseases-conditions/lupus/basics/definition/con-20019676?reDate=17072015>.

59. National Institutes of Health, National Diabetes Information Clearinghouse: Your guide to diabetes: Type 1 and type 2, 2014. Retrieved from: <http://www.diabetes.niddk.nih.gov/dm/pubs/type1andtype2/index.aspx>.

60. National Institutes of Health, National Institute of Neurological Disorders and Stroke: NINDS multiple sclerosis information page, 2014. Retrieved from: <http://www.ninds.nih.gov/disorders/multiple_sclerosis/multiple_sclerosis.htm>.

Inflammation

Carolyn Sabo

Inflammation is a normal and expected physiological response to cellular injury. The response is protective in that it provides an opportunity for the body to heal and repair the injury. This biophysical concept is foundational to patient care across the lifespan.

DEFINITION

The term *inflammation* is derived from the Latin *inflammare*—to set on fire. As a concept, *inflammation* is defined as *an immunologic defense against tissue injury, infection, or allergy.* The Centers for Disease Control and Prevention (CDC) has defined inflammation as "the body's reaction to injury, irritation, or infection characterized by redness, swelling, warmth, and/or pain; caused by accumulation of immune cells and substances around the injury or infection."[1] Inflammation is a protective process initiated to minimize or remove the pathologic agent or stimulus triggering the inflammation and to promote healing. Although inflammation is always present with infection, inflammation may also occur in the absence of infection. Inflammation is the body's physiological response to injury—not the agent causing the injury as is seen with infection. The inflammatory process is very similar regardless of the cause of cellular injury; however, there is variability in the degree of response depending on the severity and scope of injury and the physiological capacity of the affected individual.[2–5]

SCOPE

The scope of inflammation ranges from no inflammation to active inflammation. Active inflammation is classified as acute, chronic, or repair/restorative (Figure 24-1). The scope also reflects an inflammation as localized or systemic.

An initial injury leading to an inflammatory response may be from various sources, including mechanical trauma (e.g., laceration, splinter, and crushing); thermal, electrical, or chemical injury; radiation damage; or biological assault (viral, bacterial, or fungal infections). Acute inflammation is the immediate response to tissue injury and is short in duration (minutes to days). The role of an acute inflammatory response is to eradicate the harmful stimuli from the body and initiate repair. Inflammation that continues for weeks to years after initial injury is termed chronic; tissue is repeatedly being destroyed and repaired, thus impairing healing. Localized

chronic inflammation results in the formation of a granuloma—an accumulation of macrophages, fibroblasts, and collagen—as seen with untreated *Mycobacterium tuberculosis.* Systemic chronic inflammation may result from many diseases or may be the consequence of disease processes, including autoimmune diseases such as the inflammatory bowel diseases ulcerative colitis (UC) and Crohn's disease.[5] Chronic inflammation may be a complication of the inflammatory process, or it may be a consequence of disease, as seen in rheumatoid arthritis.[1–9]

NORMAL PHYSIOLOGICAL PROCESS

The functioning of the immune system and the primary activities of an immune response, both acute and chronic, were presented in Concept 23 Immunity. An inflammatory response is often directly linked to the activities of the immune system, demonstrating an overlap and interplay of physiological processes between the two systems (immune and inflammatory) providing protection to the host. It has also been noted that an inflammatory process has two primary functions directed at a positive outcome for the individual: (1) restitution of normal functioning cells following injury or (2) fibrous repair when functional cells cannot be restored.

Inflammation is a process involving white blood cells (WBCs) and a number of different chemicals that serve to protect the body against invading pathogens or cellular/tissue trauma. WBCs are attracted to an area of inflammation by chemotaxis. Chemotaxis is a complex process involving more than a dozen different chemicals whose release is initiated by stimuli that may generally be classified into four categories: (1) bacterial or viral exotoxins, (2) degenerative by-products of inflammation, (3) products of complement system activation, and (4) reactive products of plasma clotting in the inflamed area.

Proinflammatory hormones are mediating factors in the inflammatory response and are critical to the effective implementation of the response. There are three major hormone groups: prostaglandins, cytokines, and histamines. In general, the proinflammatory hormones increase blood flow to the injured area, increase vascular membrane permeability, activate various components of an immune response including the complement system of proteins, attract leukocytes to the area of injury, promote angiogenesis, stimulate growth of connective tissue, and cause fever.[1,2] Specific actions of selected proinflammatory, mediating hormones are listed in Table 24-1.

FIGURE 24-1 Scope of Inflammation

TABLE 24-1 Effects of Proinflammatory Mediators

Proinflammatory Factor	Source	Effect on Inflammatory Response
Prostaglandins Leukotrienes	Phospholipids from mast cell and other cell membranes; derived from arachidonic acid in cell membrane	Mediate late stages of acute inflammatory response Increase vasodilation Increase vascular permeability Active in anaphylactic hypersensitivity reactions
Bradykinins	Plasma protein Kinins	Increase vascular permeability Increase vasodilation Responsible for pain production
Complement proteins	Macrophages Liver endothelium	Primarily from proteins C3a, C4a, and C5a: initiate chemotaxis of neutrophils and macrophages Activate mast cells and basophils to release histamine, heparin, and other chemicals Result in increased blood flow, increased vascular permeability, and leaking of plasma proteins to extracellular fluid
Histamine Serotonin	Mast cells Basophils	Mediates early acute inflammatory response Increases vasodilation Increases vascular permeability
IL-1	Macrophages Neutrophils B lymphocytes Dendritic cells Other antigen-presenting cells	Promotes T lymphocyte proliferation and differentiation Promotes release of acute-phase inflammatory proteins Promotes neutrophil adhesion to endothelial cell walls Promotes development of fever
IL-8	T lymphocytes Monocytes (blood) Macrophages (tissue)	Chemotaxic factor for neutrophils Chemotaxic factor for T lymphocytes
IL-17	Helper T lymphocytes (Th17 cells)	Increases chemotaxis of neutrophils Increases chemotaxis of macrophages Increases epithelial cell chemokine production
Platelet-activating factor	Platelets	Promotes secretion of chemical mediators Promotes vasodilation and increased permeability Activates neutrophils
Transforming growth factor-β	T lymphocytes Activated macrophages Fibroblasts	Inhibits T and B lymphocyte activity Chemotaxic factor for macrophages Increases macrophage IL-1 production Inhibits macrophages
TNF-α	Activated macrocytes Selected lymphocytes	Promotes cellular proliferation Increases phagocytosis Increases leukocytosis Induces fever Promotes neutrophil adhesion to endothelial cell walls Toxic to some tumor cells

Source: Adapted from Venes D: *Taber's cyclopedic medical dictionary*, ed 21, Philadelphia, 2009, Davis; Hall JE: *Textbook of medical physiology*, ed 12, Philadelphia, 2011, Saunders; McCance KL, Huether SE, Brashers VL, Rote NS, editors: *Pathophysiology: The biologic basis for disease in adults and children*, ed 6, St Louis, 2010, Mosby; and Copstead LC, Banasik JL: *Pathophysiology*, ed 4, St Louis, 2010, Saunders.

Acute Inflammation

The pathologic processes associated with acute inflammation are complex but sequential, as shown in Figure 24-2. They involve a constant interaction with various components of the immune system and are regulated by feedback systems. The primary steps in an acute inflammatory response have the following sequence:

1. Injury to or death of tissue and release of chemical mediators
2. Vasodilation and increased blood flow to the small vessels surrounding the area of injury
3. Swelling and partial retraction or separation of activated endothelial cells
4. Increased vascular permeability and leakage of water, salts, fibrinogen (later becoming fibrin), and other small plasma proteins into the surrounding tissue
5. "Walling off" of the area from surrounding tissues to delay the spread of the pathogen and toxic products from the pathogen
6. Margination and migration of polymorphonucleocytes, monocytes, lymphocytes, and macrophages (later) to the endothelial cell walls and out of the vascular system to the area of injury; margination of endothelial cell walls by neutrophils is possible because of the increased level of cellular adhesiveness created by activation of the endothelial cell.
7. Exudates exiting the vascular system fill spaces left by damaged, necrotic tissue
8. Movement of glucose and oxygen to the area in support of removal of necrotic tissue and cellular repair

9. Release of nitric oxide and prostacyclin, endothelin, thromboxane A_2, angiotensin II, growth factor, and chemokines from activated endothelial cells

Neutrophils are of significant importance in an acute inflammatory response. Movement of neutrophils is mediated by several chemotaxic factors that arise from the area of tissue damage. The chemotaxic factors bind to the surface of the neutrophils and cause them to release additional factors, resulting in pathogen breakdown from lysosomal cytoplasmic enzymes. The neutrophils are also directly involved in phagocytosis after they bind to antibodies already connected to the antigen. In preparation for the neutrophil, opsonization has occurred with either the antibody or the complement proteins; then neutrophil lysosomal granules can be released to begin phagocytosis. Note that during the process of phagocytosis, reactive oxygen species (ROS) are created by the neutrophils and macrophages. ROS bind with the lysosomes to help kill the invading pathogen.[10,11]

Neutrophil blood counts increase fourfold to fivefold within a few hours after the onset of acute severe inflammation, making more neutrophils available to continue the inflammatory response. Neutrophils comprise the primary WBC component of exudate created during an acute inflammatory response to bacterial invasion. Band cells, or immature neutrophils, may also be present in the blood to achieve the increased numbers of neutrophils required of the severe response. The bone marrow will also significantly increase production of both granulocytes and monocytes; however, it takes 3 or 4 days before these cells are mature and ready to leave the bone marrow.[3]

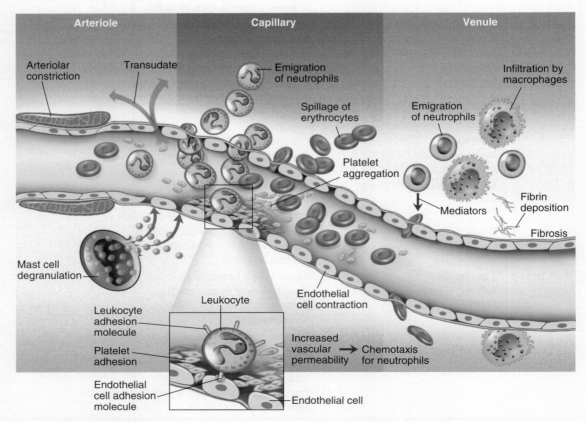

FIGURE 24-2 Acute Inflammation Response (Source: From McCance KL, Huether SE, Brashers VL, Rote NS, editors: *Pathophysiology: The biologic basis for disease in adults and children*, ed 7, St Louis, 2014, Mosby.)

Lymphocytes are most prominent in inflammatory responses to viral antigens. They are also important in combination with monocytes and macrophages in situations of chronic inflammation. Eosinophils are most evident in inflammatory responses to parasitic infections and in association with allergic hypersensitivity immune reactions. Mast cells and basophils release histamine, which contributes to the increased vascular permeability seen in an inflammatory response.[2,12]

An acute inflammatory response may last minutes to days, with the majority of activity taking place in the first 12–24 hours after tissue injury. The response may be localized or systemic. Localized inflammatory responses begin when damaged tissue or invading organisms activate the immune system. Complement system proteins and cytokines begin a cascading sequence of events that lead to the classic signs and symptoms associated with the immune response. Autoimmune reactions may cause systemic activation of the inflammatory response with the body being attacked by its own cells. In most people, the inflammatory response may last up to 5 days while invading pathogens are destroyed, phagocytosis of antigens and necrotic tissue occurs, and fibroblasts begin the process of tissue healing.

Chronic Inflammation

Macrophages are critical in a chronic inflammatory response. They release tissue thromboplastin to facilitate hemostasis and to promote fibroblast activity. They are instrumental in removing necrotic tissue and foreign pathogen material from the area of injury (debridement), allowing for repair and healing. Macrophages and lymphocytes will comprise the majority of the WBCs found in the exudate during a chronic inflammatory response. Unfortunately, when inflammation is chronic, healing processes may be interrupted by reinjury or renewed inflammation and immune system activity with the inflammatory cycle being reactivated.

Chronic inflammation may also be subclinical, manifesting with elevated levels of nonspecific blood markers such as C-reactive protein (CRP) or an increased erythrocyte sedimentation rate (ESR) with no obvious overt symptoms. A WBC scan, or inflammatory scan, may be required to identify areas of inflammation. Low-grade chronic inflammation has been associated with systemic manifestations including body aches and pains, frequent infections, diarrhea, dry eyes, and shortness of breath.[13–17]

Regardless of whether the inflammation is acute or chronic, a number of systemic manifestations result. Localized symptoms depend on the degree of injury and the resistance of the host to injury. Systemic responses include neutrophilia, fever, malaise, loss of appetite, and muscle catabolism. The liver will respond by releasing a number of proteins, called acute phase proteins, that include complement system proteins, clotting factors, and protease inhibitors. The acute phase proteins also stimulate an increase in the level of fibrinogen, promoting hemostasis. CRP and serum amyloid are also released by the liver. CRP assists in opsonization of the foreign pathogen to facilitate phagocytosis.[3–5,11,18]

VARIATIONS AND CONTEXT

Variations in inflammation may occur in individuals across the lifespan, with a range of impact from minor symptoms such as mild redness of the skin to life-threatening consequences. Variations may occur as a result of an acute or a chronic inflammatory response or an autoimmune response as is seen in rheumatoid arthritis. An acute inflammatory response following tissue insult or injury may evolve into a chronic condition, as demonstrated by the development of

chronic sinusitis or cirrhosis following an acute inflammatory response to an antigen with continued tissue damage. An acute response may lead to additional tissue injury beyond the initial insult. For example, if inadequately treated, a mildly sprained ankle with tendon or ligament damage may lead to additional tissue injury and cellular death if post-injury swelling is not controlled. Chronic cirrhosis may also be the result of an acute infection with hepatitis C virus. Autoimmune diseases may also manifest with chronic inflammation, as is seen with rheumatoid arthritis.

CONSEQUENCES

Although inflammation has significant physiological benefit, negative consequences are also possible and may include an overly severe immune response to stimuli resulting in additional tissue damage or an inadequate response leading to infection or chronic inflammation and illness.[2] Spinal cord injuries are an example of one type of trauma in which the inflammatory response may cause significant additional tissue damage if swelling to the damaged region is not controlled. The physiological response to injury that an inflammatory response provides, in this case with increased blood flow, increased vascular permeability, and the movement of exudate to the damaged tissue may cause additional compression-based trauma to an already damaged spinal cord.

Excessive stimulation of the inflammatory response and the development of chronic inflammation may also be a consequence of hypersensitivity reactions by the immune system, including allergies and autoimmune diseases such as asthma, rheumatoid arthritis, multiple sclerosis, and systemic lupus erythematosus. In these diseases, an initial immune response and resultant inflammatory response trigger a sequence of cyclic physiological responses that result in a pathologic disease process.

Systemic pathology may also result from an inflammatory response. Wisse[19] studied the metabolic effects of obesity and identified the potential role of inflammation within fat cells as a basis in generating metabolic syndrome. The role of cytokines secreted by adipose tissue in modulating an immune response and promoting a chronic inflammatory condition was discussed. Research on the role of reducing inflammation by altering selected dietary fatty acid intake and thus reducing the amount of arachidonic acid levels in cell membranes is ongoing. Because arachidonic acids play a role in the production of proinflammatory molecules, altering the level of this acid may influence the severity of an inflammatory response.[20]

Multisystem organ failure associated with sepsis or septic shock invokes both a strong immune response and a strong inflammatory response. One of the negative consequences of inflammatory activity in the presence of shock is that inflammatory mediators instigate activation of coagulation inhibitors of fibrinolysis and may cause diffuse endovascular injury, organ dysfunction, or death. Widespread inflammation may also lead to hypovolemia, pleural effusion, respiratory distress, renal failure, and death.[21–23]

Chronic inflammation has been linked to a number of systemic diseases or diseases with systemic consequences if the affected individual is compromised. For example, recent studies have examined the role of inflammation in coronary artery calcification, a critical component in the development of coronary atherosclerosis.[24–27] Silverstein discussed the relationship between chronic renal disease, the proinflammatory state that exists in individuals with this disease, and the need to mediate the inflammatory process to prevent consequential tissue damage.[28–30] Batool and colleagues' research indicated that inflammation and susceptibility to infection and parasitic diseases may be directly linked to the nutritional status of the host.[31] Research is ongoing on the relationship between inflammation and blood–brain barrier dysfunction, with suggestions that inflammatory challenges that occur during brain development may have consequences later in life for a variety of neurologic disorders. Similarly, interrelationships among autoimmune diseases such as asthma and diabetes mellitus, cancer, and inflammation are no longer considered theoretical.[3–5,32–38]

RISK FACTORS

Populations at Risk

Individuals of all ages, genders, ethnic and socioeconomic groups, geographic locations, and prior health histories are susceptible to an acute or chronic inflammatory process. Age plays a role in the development of more severe inflammatory responses. For the very young, an immature immune system may lead to a more severe inflammatory response because the immune system is unable to control a minor pathogen and infection may be severe. For the elderly, the immune system becomes less able to respond to foreign pathogens, resulting in a stronger inflammatory response than might have been encountered earlier in life. Those who are uninsured or underinsured are at increased risk because they may not have access to sufficient or early health care intervention and a comparatively simple inflammatory response to injury may escalate to one with more severe injury or to a chronic inflammatory state.[39–44]

Individual Risk Factors

Individual risk factors for an inflammatory response include the presence of autoimmune diseases and allergies, exposure to pathogens with or without resultant infection, and being very young or elderly with a compromised immune system. Genetics plays a role in the emergence of chronic inflammatory processes because many autoimmune diseases have a genetic basis for predisposition and involve an inflammatory response. Certain chronic disease processes such as atherosclerosis, rheumatoid arthritis, diabetes mellitus, and cancer may lead to or be the result of chronic inflammation. Research is also underway evaluating the role of obesity and vitamin D and magnesium deficiency in the development of chronic inflammation.[3–5,14,15,45–48]

Any process that weakens the immune system increases the potential for what might have been a mild inflammatory response to develop into an acute severe inflammation or chronic inflammatory process.[49,50] The absence of effective hand hygiene procedures, the sharing of personal hygiene or grooming material and equipment, poor sanitation, poor nutrition, and living or congregating in tight spaces with large numbers of people increase the risk for infection and accompanying inflammation. Within the health care system, inadequate use of standard precautions increases the individual's risk for infection, with a resulting inflammatory response. Environmental factors, such as pollution and smoking or exposure to repeated trauma, also increase the risk of stimulating an inflammatory response.

ASSESSMENT

As with any other pathologic process, the basis and extent of disease must be assessed in order to guide appropriate treatment interventions to either eradicate or manage inflammation, whether acute or chronic. Assessment of an individual for the presence of inflammation includes asking appropriate questions to elicit a history and conducting a physical examination. In addition, laboratory and diagnostic testing aids in the diagnosis. Common clinical findings associated with inflammation are featured in Table 24-2.

TABLE 24-2   Clinical Manifestations of Inflammation

Local Manifestations	Systemic Manifestations
Swelling	Fever
Pain	Leukocytosis
Heat	Increase in plasma proteins
Redness	Malaise
Exudate	Fatigue
Serous exudate	
Fibrinous exudate	
Purulent exudate	
Hemorrhagic exudate	

History

The history should be focused on determining the nature of the inflammatory trigger (e.g., recent injury and exposure to allergens and infectious agents) and the patient's physiological ability to respond or, specifically, the risk for an ineffective inflammatory response. The nurse should also inquire about the presence of symptoms commonly associated with inflammation, including swelling, pain, and fatigue. It is also important to determine the duration of the inflammatory process and the treatment measures, if any, that have already been initiated.

Examination Findings

Several classic findings are associated with inflammation. Obvious trauma or minor wounds will likely appear red, be warm to the touch, and be associated with some degree of pain. Swelling may be present with or without an open wound, such as would be seen with a strained or sprained joint. Drainage or pus may be evident from a laceration or other injury in which the skin or mucosal surface has been broken. Any time an infection is evident, some degree of inflammation will also be present. Inflammation associated with an immune response, but without external trauma, will present with some combination of swelling, pain, fever, and decreased or absent functioning of the tissue or organ. Severe inflammation may be associated with shock syndrome or multiorgan failure, significant hyperthermia, seizure, coma, or death.

Diagnostic Tests

Laboratory testing and diagnostic data collection will be determined by the clinical presentation of the individual, evidence of obvious trauma, likelihood of exposure to infection-causing pathogens, and health history particularly as related to immune dysfunction or deficiency or a history of any chronic illnesses.

Blood Tests

Blood testing for WBC counts with differential is helpful in determining if neutrophil, lymphocyte, or macrophage cell counts are elevated, indicating bacterial or viral infection and acute or chronic inflammation. CRP and ESR blood testing are nonspecific tests that will confirm the presence of inflammation but not the location or cause. Various serologic tests for viruses or antibodies against pathogens, such as hepatitis, HIV, Epstein–Barr, severe acute respiratory syndrome, herpes simplex, syphilis, methicillin-resistant *Staphylococcus aureus*, *Clostridium difficile*, and *Helicobacter pylori*, will be helpful in determining the cause of inflammation and guide treatment regimens to eradicate or control infection and minimize damage from inflammation.[17]

Radiographic and Other Testing

Computer-assisted tomography, magnetic resonance imaging, proton emission tomography scans, or colonoscopy are useful in determining the location and extent of inflammation within the body.

CLINICAL MANAGEMENT

Primary Prevention

Preventing inflammation is directed at reducing risk for injury and infection. Although many injuries occur as a result of accidents with an associated inflammatory response being unavoidable, some precautions can be taken. Following appropriate hand hygiene precautions can significantly decrease the risk of pathogen transmission between people, thus reducing the potential for an inflammatory response. Similarly, keeping wounds clean and covered will help accelerate the healing process, potentially decreasing the total or duration of an inflammatory response. Using designated safety equipment when involved in sports or other physical activity can also minimize the incidence of injury. In addition, being aware of food and water safety standards and any issues that may arise from contamination can prevent the transmission of pathogens and avoid potential inflammation associated with an immune response.

Secondary Prevention (Screening)

There are no routine screening procedures for inflammation, making primary prevention strategies critical in reducing the incidence and severity of inflammatory responses.

Collaborative Interventions

The clinical management of inflammation is directed at mediating the inflammatory process to promote repair and healing and avoid an excessive inflammatory response that may lead to further tissue injury. Some general guidelines to treatment can be made depending on the cause of the inflammation. If inflammation is due to infection, the underlying cause of the infection must be eradicated. If inflammation is due to a hypersensitivity-type immune response, such as allergies, asthma, or autoimmune diseases, management of inflammation must be combined with management of the immune response and the pathologic consequence of immune dysfunction (e.g., diabetes mellitus, inflammatory bowel syndrome, rheumatoid arthritis, or muscular sclerosis). If inflammation is due to an uncomplicated strain or sprain, the standard treatment regimen of *rest*, *ice*, *compression*, and *elevation* (RICE) combined with nonsteroidal anti-inflammatory drugs (NSAIDs) will help with both management of pain and moderation of the inflammatory response.

Chronic inflammatory responses to disease require careful monitoring to prevent or slow the process of tissue damage that may result in organ failure. Treatment of the underlying cause of the disease, support for ongoing tissue function, and prevention of organ or limb dysfunction or deformity are all important areas of clinical management. Sometimes treatment is aimed at finding alternative routes to achieve physiological outcomes, such as providing insulin to the individual with type 1 diabetes mellitus, replacing endogenous insulin that is no longer being manufactured in the pancreas.

Rest, Ice, Compression, and Elevation

RICE represents a set of activities directed at minimizing the swelling associated with a sprain or strain. As described previously, swelling of the tissues immediately surrounding an area of injury is a part of the normal inflammatory response. By minimizing swelling, the injured tissue and surrounding tissue will be protected from additional damage

resulting from the swelling itself. The first 24–48 hours after the injury is the critical period when RICE measures will be most beneficial. Typically, icing of the sprain or strain for 20 minutes at a time every 2 or 3 hours is indicated, and leaving the ice in place for a longer period of time may cause additional tissue damage. Compression of the damaged area also helps to minimize swelling; the compression wrap must be snug but not so tight as to impede circulation (be alert to fingers or toes becoming cool, tingling, or turning blue in color). Whenever possible, elevation of the injured area above the level of the heart is useful in helping to minimize swelling.[51]

Immobilization Devices

Immobilization devices such as splints or slings contribute to the ability to rest the injured area. Wheelchairs, walkers, or crutches may also be useful in minimizing weight bearing to an injured extremity. If bed rest is indicated, leg exercises or pneumatic compression devices should be considered to protect against thrombus formation in the legs.

Pharmacologic Agents

Pharmacologic intervention options are diverse and depend on the cause of inflammation. Three major goals of treatment include reducing inflammation, managing fever, and providing pain relief. For this reason, many pharmacologic agents prescribed for the treatment of inflammation have one or more of these properties.

Steroidal agents. Glucocorticoids (e.g., prednisone) are steroids used to suppress the immune system and thus suppress an inflammatory response. They are particularly effective in reducing the swelling and pain that accompany inflammation. Steroids such as prednisone are used in a wide range of inflammatory conditions—from swelling secondary to trauma to inflammation found in allergies and autoimmune diseases such as rheumatoid arthritis or systemic lupus erythematosus.[52]

Nonsteroidal anti-inflammatory drugs (NSAID). NSAIDs, such as ibuprofen or naproxen, are important in the management of pain, fever, and inflammation. These medications may be found as over-the-counter products, or they may be combined with narcotics (e.g., hydrocodone or oxycodone) and require a prescription. Significant inflammation may require the use of cyclooxygenase (COX) inhibitors. COX-1 is produced by all tissues and promotes a number of protective functions. COX-2 is produced primarily at sites of tissue injury and acts to mediate inflammation and to sensitize receptors to painful stimuli. It is also found in the brain, where it helps to mediate fever and assist the brain in pain perception. Inhibition of COX-2 is important in treating an inflammatory response because the medication triggers processes that lead to suppression of inflammation, control of pain, and reduction of fever. First-generation NSAIDs inhibited both COX-1 and COX-2, and newer-generation NSAIDs (e.g., celecoxib) are able to inhibit COX-2 only.[52]

Recombinant DNA and monoclonal antibodies. Recombinant DNA and monoclonal antibody development has produced an entirely new line of pharmacologic treatment for inflammation. Interleukin-1 (IL-1) antagonists inactivate IL-1 receptors, whereas tumor necrosis factor-α (TNF-α) inhibitors prevent IL-1 from producing its inflammatory actions but leave the individual more susceptible to infection. Recombinant protein C helps the body dissolve microvascular clots formed during inflammation, and although infliximab (Remicade) is a TNF inhibitor, it has been key to more recent treatments of lymphoma, rheumatoid arthritis, and inflammatory bowel diseases.[52]

Antipyretics. Fever is a common physiological response to an inflammation. For this reason, antipyretics are often administered for fever management. Antipyretic agents, such as acetaminophen, aspirin,

Causes

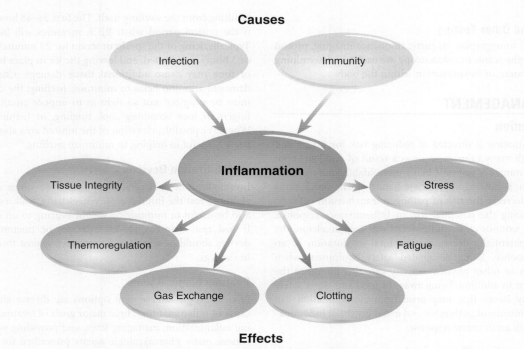

FIGURE 24-3 Inflammation and Interrelated Concepts

and NSAIDs (described previously), reduce fever by inhibiting cyclo-oxygenase. These are often administered in combination with opioid analgesic agents.

Analgesics. Nonopioid analgesic agents, such as acetaminophen or aspirin, are the most common type of analgesic used for pain relief caused by inflammation. NSAIDs are also considered analgesics because a reduction in inflammation tends to also relieve associated pain. Opioid analgesic agents are used when inflammatory pain is severe.

Antimicrobials. Antibiotics, antivirals, and other antimicrobials are important in treating the underlying cause of infection leading to inflammation. Antimicrobials encompass a wide variety of medications that are required to treat diseases associated with immune and inflammatory responses. These are discussed further in Concept 25 Infection.

INTERRELATED CONCEPTS

Several concepts featured in this textbook are interrelated to inflammation (Figure 24-3).

Immunity and Infection are probably the most closely related concepts. Many of the pathophysiological processes associated with inflammation are also found in both immunity and infection, with pathology from one process overlapping those of the other two processes or with one process triggering another. This can be seen with hypersensitivity reactions of the immune system triggering an inflammatory response or infection stimulating an inflammatory response.

Tissue Integrity is at risk in an inflammatory response, as is impaired mobility and pain associated with an initial injury and with the consequences (swelling) of an inflammatory response. Thermoregulation may be influenced by inflammation depending on the severity of the response to tissue injury. Gas Exchange may be insufficient in the presence of inflammation-induced pleural effusion.

Hemostasis alterations in the form of microvascular Clotting may also be a consequence of inflammation, particularly if it is chronic.

Both Fatigue and Stress are often associated with injury and recovery from an acute inflammatory response or may be prolonged during the chronic inflammation from an autoimmune hypersensitivity reaction.

CLINICAL EXEMPLARS

Exemplars for the concept of inflammation are presented in Box 24-1. These examples are divided into conditions that represent acute inflammation, chronic inflammation, or inflammation based on the presence of an autoimmune hypersensitivity response. Note that overlap often occurs between acute and chronic inflammation, with chronic inflammatory conditions having acute exacerbations and acute inflammatory responses developing into chronic conditions. Thus, some artificial division among the three types of inflammation is unavoidable. It is beyond the scope of this concept to provide details for each of these exemplars, but some of the most common are briefly described here. Additional information about these exemplars can be easily found in a variety of nursing textbooks.

Featured Exemplars
Bronchitis

Bronchitis is inflammation of the bronchial tubes and may begin as an acute irritation and progress to chronic infection. Bronchitis is commonly seen after introduction of a cold virus or other respiratory infection. Acute bronchitis typically presents with symptoms such as cough, increased production of thick mucus that may be clear or discolored, shortness of breath, fever and chills, and chest tightness on inspiration. The cough associated with acute bronchitis may persist for days or weeks after resolution of the initial infection. Should chronic bronchitis develop over time, it would be considered a COPD.[11,53]

BOX 24-1 EXEMPLARS OF INFLAMMATION

Acute Inflammation
- Acute infection (bacterial, viral, fungal, parasitic)
- Bronchitis
- Burn
- Bursitis
- Foreign body injury
- Insect bite or sting
- Joint sprain or strain
- Nephritis
- Rheumatic fever
- Tendonitis
- Traumatic injury

Chronic Inflammation
- Atherosclerosis
- Chronic infection
- Chronic obstructive pulmonary disease
- Cirrhosis
- Diverticulitis
- Fibromyalgia
- Gingivitis
- Inflammatory bowel disease
- Myocarditis
- Osteoarthritis
- Psoriasis
- Vasculitis

Autoimmune-Based Inflammation
- Asthma
- Crohn's disease
- Goodpasture's syndrome
- Grave's disease
- Multiple sclerosis
- Myasthenia gravis
- Rheumatoid arthritis
- Systemic lupus erythematosus

Gastroenteritis

Gastroenteritis is inflammation of the stomach and intestines. It may be caused by a variety of viruses, contaminated water or food, as a side effect of medications, and in infants it may present with the introduction of allergens within new foods. Symptoms generally last for a few days and include nausea or vomiting, abdominal cramps and diarrhea, or a low-grade fever. The course of the inflammation is usually self-limiting, but it may require more aggressive treatment if symptoms persist for more than 2 days. Dehydration is a common manifestation and can be life-threatening if undetected and untreated.[11,54,55]

Atherosclerosis

Atherosclerosis is a disease characterized by the buildup of plaque on the intimal layer of arteries and represents a chronic inflammatory process. Plaque is made up of fat, cholesterol, calcium, and other substances that harden and narrow the lumen of arteries over time. Artherosclerosis can affect every artery in the body, including those in the heart, peripheral arteries, brain, and kidneys. Atherosclerosis of the coronary arteries leads to coronary artery disease and myocardial infarction, whereas atherosclerosis of the carotid arteries may lead to stroke. Chronic kidney disease and end-stage renal disease or kidney failure are consequences of atherosclerosis of the renal arteries.[11,18,56-60]

Cirrhosis

Cirrhosis is a disease state that results from the destruction of healthy liver tissue and replacement with scar tissue. Chronic cirrhosis may evolve from an acute injury or be the result of chronic liver tissue insult. The scar tissue may block blood flow through the liver or cause the transformation of sufficient healthy functioning cells to scarred cells and nonfunctional tissue, which the liver is not able to sufficiently provide the metabolic support to maintain homeostasis. Cirrhosis results in disturbance of many systems because of the diminished ability of the liver to produce clotting factors, immune factors, and bile and to remove the waste products of metabolism and medications.[11,61]

Asthma

Asthma represents an autoimmune-based inflammation. The National Asthma Education and Prevention Program Expert Panel defined asthma as "a common chronic disorder of the airways that is complex and characterized by variable and recurring symptoms, airflow obstruction, bronchial hyperresponsiveness, and an underlying inflammation. The interaction of these features determines the clinical manifestations and severity of asthma."[62] Airway inflammation leads to airway obstruction and the development of bronchoconstriction, airway hyperresponsiveness to stimuli, and airway edema with hypersecretion of mucus. Asthma may be caused by innate immunity, genetics, or environmental factors (e.g., airborne antigens or viral infections). The relationship between exposure to tobacco smoke (*in utero* or after birth) is also being investigated.[62,63]

Rheumatoid Arthritis

Rheumatoid arthritis (RA) is an autoimmune disease causing inflammation to the joints and is characterized by periods of "flares" and "remission." Although the exact cause of RA is unclear, research has demonstrated links among genetics, the environment, and some hormones. There is no cure for RA, but it has been documented to flare and then go into complete remission with no long-term sequelae. Treatment involves pain management, control of joint swelling, and retention of joint function. Recent research is directed at immunotherapies to restore immune tolerance of the "self" and the critical immunopathogenic pathways seen in RA.[11,64,65]

CASE STUDY

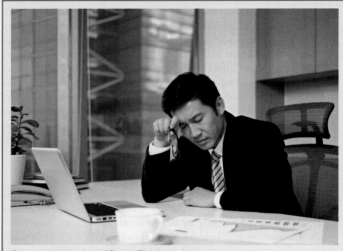

Source: imtmphoto/iStock/Thinkstock

Case Presentation

Chris Shomni is a 40-year-old male in a stressful, professional position. He was recently diagnosed with ulcerative colitis (UC) after developing abdominal pain and cramping and bloody diarrhea intermittently (although more frequently recently) during the past several weeks. He has lost 10 pounds in the past 4 weeks and has complained of nausea and fatigue. A colonoscopy demonstrated the presence of significant inflammation and ulcers in the colon and rectum. No strictures, perforations, or areas of paralysis of the colon were noted. Biopsy and further evaluation of the colonoscopy confirmed the presence of UC and ruled out Crohn's disease. He has no family history of inflammatory bowel disease. Assessment of the skin revealed the presence of erythema nodosum lesions, which are characteristic of UC. Laboratory testing further identified the presence of lowered red blood cell (RBC) and hemoglobin levels, elevated platelet count, and normal white blood cell count. Serum total protein and albumin levels were low.

Diagnosis of UC was made, with complications of anemia and hypoalbuminemia. Mr. Shomni was also demonstrating impaired nutrition as a result of impaired nutrient absorption and diarrhea and anemia secondary to inflammation of the bowel and loss of fluid, protein, and RBCs. Pain from inflammation and abdominal cramping was present but not significant, and he was at risk for fluid volume deficiency. It was determined that the bowel needed to be rested, that bowel resection surgery was not indicated at this time, and that inflammation must be reduced. Mr. Shomni was admitted to the hospital to begin treatment for inflammation, rest the bowel, reduce his diarrhea, and balance his fluid and electrolyte levels.

Overall goals of treatment for Mr. Shomni include controlling colon inflammation, ensuring adequate nutrition and hydration, and relieving pain and diarrhea. With control of inflammation and diarrhea, it is expected that the anemia and hypoalbuminemia will resolve. Pharmacologic intervention included aminosalicylates containing 5-aminosalicylic acid (5-ASA) to control inflammation. Corticosteroids to reduce inflammation will only be used if Mr. Shomni has an exacerbation of his UC and his disease becomes severe and nonresponsive to 5-ASA. If Mr. Shomni does not respond sufficiently to the 5-ASA or corticosteroids, immunomodulators such as 6-mercaptopurine or monoclonal antibodies such as infliximab (Remicade) may have to be introduced in the future. With chronic inflammatory bowel disease, at some point in his life, Mr. Shomni may need to have surgery for a colostomy or ileostomy because tissue damage to the intestinal tract may be so severe that it no longer functions.

Mr. Shomni was discharged after 3 days with new medications and instructions to avoid enteric and time-released medications, an understanding of dietary changes to include specifically prescribed bacterial probiotic cultures, strategies for stress reduction, and actions to be taken should signs and symptoms of an inflamed or infected bowel be evident.

Case Analysis

Inflammatory bowel disease encompasses two primary inflammatory processes: ulcerative colitis and Crohn's disease. UC is a chronic inflammatory disease with symptoms that may range from mild to severe. Chris Shomni's case provides a classic example of chronic inflammation with symptoms including abdominal pain and cramping, bloody diarrhea, weight loss, nausea, and fatigue. Clinical symptoms included significant inflammation and ulcers in the colon and rectum evident during his colonoscopy and erythema nodosum lesions on his skin. Primary treatment regimens were directed at reducing and controlling Mr. Shomni's colon inflammation, relieving pain and diarrhea, and enhancing his nutrition and hydration status.

ACCESS EXEMPLAR LINKS IN YOUR GIDDENS EBOOK

REFERENCES

1. Centers for Disease Control and Prevention: Inflammation, 2014. Retrieved from: <http://www2a.cdc.gov/nip/isd/ycts/mod1/scripts/glossary.asp?item=inflammation>.
2. Venes D, editor: *Taber's cyclopedic medical dictionary*, ed 22, Philadelphia, 2013, Davis.
3. Hall JE: *Textbook of medical physiology*, ed 12, Philadelphia, 2011, Saunders.
4. McCance KL, Huether SE, Brashers VL, et al, editors: *Pathophysiology: The biologic basis for disease in adults and children*, ed 6, St Louis, 2010, Mosby.
5. Copstead LC, Banasik JL: *Pathophysiology*, ed 4, St Louis, 2010, Saunders.
6. Kimball J: Inflammation, 2010. Retrieved from: <http://users.rcn.com/jkimball.ma.ultranet/BiologyPages/I/Inflammation.html>.
7. Mosby: *Mosby's dictionary of medicine, nursing, and health professions*, ed 9, St Louis, 2013, Mosby.
8. Kahn MA, Solomon LW: Acute inflammation, wound healing & repair I, 2007. Retrieved from: <http://.ocw.tufts.edu/data/51/551512.pdf>.
9. National Institutes of Health, National Library of Medicine: Inflammation, 2010. Retrieved: <http://ghr.nlm.nih.gov/glossary=inflammation>.
10. Kimball J: Reactive oxygen species (ROS), 2010. Retrieved from: <http://users.rcn.com/jkimball.ma.ultranet/BiologyPages/R/ROS.html>.
11. Kumar V, Abbas AK, Aster JC: *Robbins and Cotran pathologic basis of disease*, ed 9, Philadelphia, 2014, Saunders.
12. Humpath.com: Acute inflammation, (n.d.). Retrieved from: <http://www.humpath.com/spip.php?article3575>.
13. McAuley JL, Tate MD, MacKenzie-Kludas CJ, et al: Activation of the BLRP3 inflammasome by IAV virulence protein PB1-F2 contributes to severe pathophysiology and disease. *PLoS Pathog* 9(5):e1003392, 2013.
14. Pick M: What is chronic inflammation? 2010. Retrieved from: <https://www.womentowomen.com/inflammation/whatischronicinflammation.aspx>.
15. Pick M: C-reactive protein (CPR and hs-CRP)—are you on fire? 2010. Retrieved from: <https://www.womentowomen.com/understandyourbody/tests/crp.aspx>.
16. Aronson D, Avizohar O, Levy Y, et al: Factor analysis of risk variables associated with low-grade inflammation. *Atherosclerosis* 200(1):206–212, 2008.

17. Pagana KD, Pagana TJ, Pagana J: *Mosby's diagnostic and laboratory test reference*, ed 12, St Louis, 2014, Mosby.

18. Golias C, Batistatou A, Bablekos G, et al: Physiology and pathophysiology of selectins, integrins, and IgSF cell adhesion molecules focusing on inflammation: A paradigm model on infectious endocarditis. *Cell Commun Adhes* 18:19–32, 2011.

19. Wisse BE: The inflammatory syndrome: The role of adipose tissue cytokines in metabolic disorders linked to obesity. *J Am Soc Nephrol* 15:2792–27800, 2004.

20. Clifton P: Dietary fatty acids and inflammation. *Nutr Dietet* 66:7–11, 2009.

21. Al-Khafaji AH, Sharma S, Eschun G: Multisystem organ failure of sepsis, 2010. Retrieved from: <http://emedicine.medscape.com/article/169640-print>.

22. Dellinger RP, Cinel I, Sharma S, et al: Septic shock, 2010. Retrieved from: <http://emedicine.medscape.com/article/168402-print>.

23. Rubins J: Pleural effusion, 2010. Retrieved from: <http://emedicine.medscape.com/article/299959-print>.

24. Knorr M, Munzel T, Wenzel P: Interplay of NK cells and monocytes in vascular inflammation and myocardial infarction. *Front Physiol* 5:295, 2014.

25. Chistiakov DA, Orekhov AN, Sobenin IA, et al: Plamacytoid dendritic cells: Development, functions, and role in atherosclerotic inflammation. *Front Physiol* 4:279, 2014.

26. Muller II, Muller KAL, Schonleber H, et al: Macrophage migration inhibitor factor is enhanced in acute coronary syndromes and is associated with the inflammatory response. *PLoS ONE* 7(6):e38376, 2012.

27. Blann AD, Kuzniatsova N, Lip GYH: Inflammation does not influence arterial stiffness and pulse-wave velocity in patients with coronary artery disease. *J Hum Hypertens* 27:629–634, 2013.

28. Pearson TA, Mensah GA, Hong Y, et al: AHA conference proceedings—CDC/AHA workshop on markers of inflammation and cardiovascular disease: Application to clinical and public health practice: Overview. *Circulation* 110:e543–e544, 2004.

29. Li JJ, Zhu CG, Yu B, et al: The role of inflammation in coronary artery calcification. *Ageing Res Rev* 6:263–270, 2007.

30. Silverstein DM: Inflammation in chronic kidney disease: Role of the progression of renal and cardiovascular disease. *Pediatr Nephrol* 24:1445–1452, 2009.

31. Batool R, Butt MS, Sultan MT, et al: Protein–energy malnutrition: A risk factor for various ailments. *Crit Rev Food Sci Nutr* 55(2):242–253, 2015.

32. Stolp HB, Dziegielewska KM: Review: Role of developmental inflammation and blood–brain barrier dysfunction in neurodevelopmental and neurodegenerative diseases. *Neuropathol Appl Neurobiol* 35:132–146, 2009.

33. Ferguson LR: Chronic inflammation and mutagenesis. *Mutat Res* 690:3–11, 2010.

34. Buck I, Morceau F, Grigorakaki C, et al: Linking anemia to inflammation and cancer: The crucial role of TNF. *Biochem Pharmacol* 77:1572–1579, 2009.

35. Murdoch JR, Lloyd CM: Chronic inflammation and asthma. *Mutat Res* 690:24–39, 2010.

36. Garcia C, Feve B, Ferre P, et al: Diabetes and inflammation: Fundamental aspects and clinical implications. *Diabetes Metab* 36(5):327–338, 2010.

37. Jacobs M, van Greevenbroek MMJ, van der Kallen CJH, et al: Low-grade inflammation can partly explain the association between the metabolic syndrome and either coronary artery disease or severity of peripheral arterial disease: The CODAM study. *Eur J Clin Invest* 39:437–444, 2009.

38. Medenwald D, Girndt M, Loppnow H, et al: Inflammation and renal function after a four-year follow-up in subjects with unimpaired glomerular filtration rate: Results from the observational population-based CARLA cohort. *PLoS ONE* 9(9):e108427, 2014.

39. Wadley AJ, Veldhuijzen van Zanten JJCS, Aldred S: The interactions of oxidative stress and inflammation with vascular dysfunction in ageing: The vascular health triad. *Age (Omaha)* 35:705–718, 2013.

40. Nowakowski A: Chronic inflammation and quality of life in older adults: A cross-sectional study using biomarkers to predict emotional and relational outcomes. *Health Qual Life Outcomes* 12:141, 2014.

41. Trollor JN, Smith E, Agars E, et al: The association between systemic inflammation and cognitive performance in the elderly: The Sydney Memory and Ageing Study. *Age (Omaha)* 34:1295–1308, 2012.

42. Lee AR, Pechenino AS, Dong H, et al: Aging, estrogen loss and epoxyeicosatrienoic acids (EETs). *PLoS ONE* 8(8):e70719, 2012.

43. Macaulay R, Akbar AN, Henson SM: The role of the T cell in age-related inflammation. *Age (Omaha)* 35:563–572, 2013.

44. Arranz E, Pena AS, Bernardo D: Mediators of inflammation and immune responses in the human gastrointestinal tract. *Mediators Inflamm* 2013:865638, 2013. Retrieved from: <http://dx.doi.org/10.1155/2013/865638>.

45. Pick M: Inflammation—The key to chronic disease? 2010. Retrieved from: <https://www.womentowomen.com/inflammation/default.aspx>.

46. Challem J: The dangers of inflammation, 2005. Retrieved from: <http://www.seabuckthorn.com/The%20dangers%20of%20inflammation.pdf>.

47. Nielsen FH: Magnesium, inflammation, and obesity in chronic disease. *Nutr Rev* 68:333–340, 2010.

48. Ferrante AW: Obesity-induced inflammation: A metabolic dialogue in the language of inflammation. *J Intern Med* 262:408–414, 2007.

49. Lopes-Virella MF, Carter RE, Gilbert GE, et al: Risk factors related to inflammation and endothelial dysfunction in the DDCT/EDIC cohort and their relationship with nephropathy and macrovascular complications. *Diabetes Care* 31:2006–2012, 2008.

50. Chung HY, Cesari M, Anton S, et al: Molecular inflammation: Underpinnings of aging and age-related diseases. *Ageing Res Rev* 8:18–30, 2009.

51. Quinn E: RICE—Rest, ice, compression and elevation soft tissue injury first aid, 2010. Retrieved from: <http://sportsmedicine.about.com/cs/rehab/a/rice.htm>.

52. Adams M, Holland N, Urban C: *Pharmacology for nurses: A pathophysiologic approach*, ed 4, Boston, 2014, Pearson.

53. Mayo Clinic: Bronchitis, 2014. Retrieved from: <http://www.mayoclinic.org/diseases-conditions/bronchitis/basics/definition/con-20014956>.

54. Mayo Clinic: Gastroenteritis: First aid, 2012. Retrieved from: <http://www.mayoclinic.org/first-aid-gastroenteritis/basics/art-20056595>.

55. Mayo Clinic: Viral gastroenteritis (stomach flu), 2014. Retrieved from: <http://www.mayoclinic.org/diseases-conditions/viral-gastroenteritis/basics/definition/con-20019350>.

56. National Institutes of Health, National Heart, Lung, and Blood Institute: What is atherosclerosis? 2014. Retrieved from: <http://www.nhlbi.nih.gov/health/health-topics/topics/atherosclerosis>.

57. National Institutes of Health, National Heart, Lung, and Blood Institutes: What causes atherosclerosis? 2014. Retrieved from: <http://www.nhlbi.nih.gov/health/health-topics/topics/atherosclerosis>.

58. National Institutes of Health, National Heart, Lung, and Blood Institutes: At a glance: Atherosclerosis, 2009. Retrieved from: <http://www.nhlbi.nih.gov/files/docs/public/heart/atherosclerosis_atglance.pdf>.

59. Evani SJ, Murthy AK, Mareedu N, et al: Hydrodynamic regulation of monocyte inflammatory response to an intracellular pathogen. *PLoS ONE* 6(1):e14492, 2011.

60. Churton S, Brown L, Shin TM, et al: Does treatment of psoriasis reduce the risk of cardiovascular disease? *Drugs* 74:169–182, 2014.

61. National Institutes of Health, National Institute of Diabetes and Digestive and Kidney Diseases: Cirrhosis, 2014. Retrieved from: <http://www.niddk.nih.gov/health-information/health-topics/liver-disease/cirrhosis/Pages/facts.aspx>.

62. National Institutes of Health, National Heart, Lung, and Blood Institutes: Guidelines for the diagnosis and management of asthma: Expert panel report 3, 2007. Retrieved from: <https://www.nhlbi.nih.gov/files/docs/guidelines/asthgdln.pdf>.

63. Centers for Disease Control and Prevention: Asthma's impact on the nation: Data from the CDC national asthma control program, (n.d.). Retrieved from: <http://www.cdc.gov/asthma/impacts_nation/asthmafactsheet.pdf>.

64. Law SC, Benham H, Reid HH, et al: Identification of self-antigen-specific T cells reflecting loss of tolerance in autoimmune disease underpins preventative immunotherapeutic strategies in rheumatoid arthritis. *Rheum Dis Clin North Am* 40:735–752, 2014.

65. National Institutes of Health, National Institute of Arthritis and Musculoskeletal and Skin Diseases: What is rheumatoid arthritis? 2014. Retrieved from: <http://www.niams.nih.gov/Health_Info/Rheumatic_Disease/rheumatoid_arthritis_ff.asp>.

Infection

Carolyn Sabo

Microorganisms are found throughout the environment. As a consequence, humans are constantly exposed to a multitude of microorganisms at any moment. Although many microorganisms do not pose a health threat to humans, some microorganisms cause human disease and are known as pathogens. Our bodies are constantly confronted with pathogens in the forms of bacteria, viruses, parasites, or fungi. These pathogens are routinely found on the skin; the mucous membranes; the linings of the respiratory, gastrointestinal, and urinary tracts; and the mouth and eyes.[1] Typically, an individual's immune system is able to rid the body of pathogens without developing an infection. An infection occurs when a susceptible host is invaded by a pathogen that multiplies and causes disease. This concept presentation provides an overview of the infection concept, including identifying individuals most at risk, recognizing signs and symptoms of infection, and understanding ways to treat or manage an infection.

DEFINITION

For the purposes of this concept presentation, infection is defined as *the invasion and multiplication of microorganisms in body tissues, which may be clinically unapparent or result in local cellular injury due to competitive metabolism, toxins, intracellular replication, or antigen–antibody response.* Several additional terms are important to understand. When an infection occurs, it may be *acute* (resolving in a few days or weeks) or *chronic* (an infection that typically lasts longer than 12 weeks and in some cases is noncurable). Terms are also used to describe the extent of spread in the body. A *localized infection* is limited to a specific body area. *Disseminated* is a term used to describe a spread of infection from an initial site to other areas of the body. The term *systemic* is used to describe an infection that affects the body as a whole or has spread throughout the body. *Sepsis*, a common type of systemic infection, is the presence of pathogens in the blood or other tissues throughout the body.

Two additional terms that are significant to the concept of infection are epidemic and pandemic. The term *epidemic* is used to describe a situation in which there are more cases of an infectious disease than is normal for the population or geographic area. A *pandemic* is a worldwide epidemic of a disease.[2] The global nature of our modern world presents challenges because people with asymptomatic infections can travel from home to virtually anyplace in the world in less than 24 hours. Professional conferences, worldwide sporting events, and gatherings for various types of entertainment can bring people together from all over the world. They are often transported to and from the events in confined airplanes and participate in events in close proximity of others. Exposure to infection leads to the spread of disease before returning to their homes.

SCOPE

Infections may be categorized in several ways, including on the basis of the multiple variables involved such as mode of transmission, trajectory of illness, and body systems affected. The most common way to categorize and discuss infections is based on the classification of the causative microorganism (Figure 25-1).

The most common microorganisms initiating an infection are bacteria, viruses, fungi, and parasites or protozoa. Table 25-1 identifies common pathogens for each of these microorganism categories. The type of invading organism influences the immune response. B lymphocytes and T lymphocytes take "leadership" roles depending on whether it is a bacterial or viral invasion, the complement system is always present to enhance the immune response, and dendritic cells will help to modulate the immune response.[3–8]

Bacterial Infections

Bacteria are one-celled organisms without a true nucleus or cellular organelles. They synthesize deoxyribonucleic acid (DNA), ribonucleic acid (RNA), and proteins and can reproduce independently, but they require a host for a suitable environment for multiplication. Bacteria cause cellular injury by releasing toxins that are either exotoxins (enzymes released by gram-positive bacteria into the host) or endotoxins (part of the bacterial cell wall of gram-negative bacteria that can cause damage to the host even if the bacteria are dead). Diseases caused by bacterial invasion depend on the type of bacterial pathogen and the area of the body that is primarily invaded.[9]

Viral Infections

A virus is a pathogen with a nucleic acid within a protein shell and requires invasion of a host for replication. An invading virus may immediately cause disease or may remain relatively dormant for years. The virus causes cellular injury by blocking its genetically prescribed protein synthesis processes and using the cell's metabolic processes for the reproduction of the virus. Diseases develop as a result

TABLE 25-1   Common Pathogens

Bacteria	Virus	Fungus	Parasite or Protozoa
Methicillin-resistant *Staphylococcus aureus*	HIV	Tinea pedis	Giardiasis
Clostridium difficile	Hepatitis A, B, C, or E virus	Candidiasis	Trichinosis
Vancomycin-resistant *Enterococci*	Human papillomavirus	Histoplasmosis	Toxoplasmosis
Streptococcus pyogenes (group A)	Ebola virus	Lobomycosis	Malaria
Corynebacterium diphtheria	Hantavirus	Cryptococcosis	Ascariasis
Escherichia coli	SARS-associated coronavirus	Aspergillosis	Pediculosis
Mycobacterium tuberculosis	Respiratory syncytial virus	Coccidioidomycosis	Cryptosporidiosis
Pseudomonas aeruginosa			*Pneumocystis jirovecii* pneumonia
Neisseria gonorrhoeae			
Clostridium tetani			

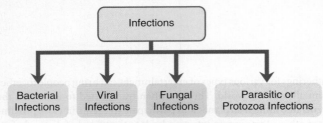

FIGURE 25-1 Scope of Infection

of interference of normal cellular functioning of the host, with destruction of the virus by the immune system also requiring death of the host cell.[9]

Fungal Infections

A fungus is a microorganism belonging to the kingdom Fungi, which includes yeasts, molds, and mushrooms. They may grow as single cells (yeasts) or as multicellular filamentous colonies (molds or mushrooms). In an otherwise healthy individual, fungi do not cause disease and are contained by the body's natural flora. Fungi causing disease are termed fungi imperfecti, and in the immunocompromised individual they can result in infections that lead to death.[9] Other fungal infections, such as tinea pedis (athlete's foot) or ringworm, may also develop in the individual with a competent immune system.

Protozoa/Parasitic Infections

Protozoa include a subcategory termed parasitic protozoa and, with few exceptions, generally infect individuals with compromised immune responses. They are typically found in dead material in water and soil and are spread by the fecal–oral route by ingesting food or water that is contaminated with the parasitic spores or cysts. Disease may develop in an otherwise healthy individual when the spores invade organs and stimulate an immune response, interfering with normal functioning of the organ system.[9]

Other Types of Infections

Sometimes an infection will develop that begins as one type and after an additional pathogen is introduced, a secondary infection occurs. Fungal infections may develop when treatment for a bacterial infection decimates the body's natural flora, or bacterial infections may arise while a debilitated body is treated for a viral infection. When considering bacterial infections, some bacteria are always pathogenic, are never part of the normal flora, but may cause subclinical infection (*Mycobacterium tuberculosis*); some bacteria are part of the normal flora but can become pathogenic (*Escherichia coli*); some are part of the normal

flora but can cause infection if they reach deep tissues, perhaps by surgery (*Staphylococcus epidermidis*); and some bacteria are part of the normal flora and become pathogenic when the individual is immunocompromised (*Acinetobacter*).[9]

An increase in morbidity and mortality secondary to infections has been seen from the emergence of previously unknown infections and the reemergence of infections that were considered controlled in various areas of the world.[10] As these infections manifest, globalization of travel and increased ease of introducing new infections into a geographic area have contributed to changes in morbidity and mortality.

Health care-acquired and community-acquired infections have emerged as a significant public health concern. Although methicillin-resistant *Staphylococcus aureus* (MRSA), *Clostridium difficile* (C. diff.), and vancomycin-resistant *Enterococci* (VRE) are debilitating health care-acquired diseases, community-acquired MRSA is even more prevalent in some areas.[11] Hospitals and other health care centers have been proactive in providing alcohol-based solutions for hand hygiene in both patient care rooms and public areas, but this same attention to infection prevention has not translated nearly as extensively to sporting arenas, areas where children gather for sporting and other group events, restaurants, food stores and other shopping facilities, movie theaters, and other group activity locales.[12–14]

NORMAL PHYSIOLOGICAL PROCESS

Pathogens may be highly virulent and able to cause disease when small numbers invade the body. Other pathogens are weakly virulent and able to cause disease only when an excess number invade the body or the host body is already weakened by disease, malnutrition, excessive fatigue, or other stresses. Opportunistic infections cause disease when the host immune system is severely compromised, such as seen in HIV infection leading to AIDS.

Some diseases are communicable before symptoms are evident in the carrier (herpes simplex virus, varicella–zoster virus, human papillomavirus, influenza, or poliomyelitis), whereas others remain communicable after initial symptoms have subsided (HIV and Epstein–Barr virus). Some infections remain dormant within the host and may resurface as the same or as a different disease; an example is the varicella–zoster virus (VZV), which first presents as chickenpox and later may manifest as shingles.[15–17] The "iceberg" concept of infectious disease has also emerged. This concept postulates that there are three levels of infection: The vast majority of a population may, at any given time, carry an infection wherein they are asymptomatic or undiagnosed. This group is thought to be the largest section

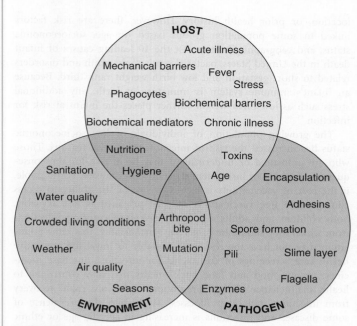

FIGURE 25-2 Process of Infection: Interactions of Host, Pathogens, and the Environment (Source: Modified from Copstead LC, Banasik JL: *Pathophysiology*, ed 5, St Louis, 2013, Saunders.)

of individuals, the part of the iceberg that is underwater. A smaller population group presents with an infection that manifests as less severe, symptomatic disease; the smallest group presents with classical, clinical symptoms of disease, and is at the very tip of the iceberg. Epidemiology is important in the study of infection because it is concerned with the manner in which a disease spreads through groups or a population and the application of this information to the control of health problems.[9]

Infection Process

An infection involves an interface with a person, the environment, and a pathogen (Figure 25-2). The process of infection requires the following six elements, all of which must be present for the infection to develop: pathogen, susceptible host, reservoir, portal of exit (from the reservoir), mode of transmission, and portal of entry (to the susceptible host). The reservoir is anywhere the pathogen may live and multiply, either in the body or on objects contaminated with the organism (e.g., door handles, stagnant water, and health care equipment). Portals of exit for a pathogen include urine or feces, saliva, blood, skin, or the gastrointestinal tract. Portals of entry include broken skin, intimate sexual contact, mouth, respiratory tract, gastrointestinal tract, and contaminated food or water. The spread of infection is dependent on a reliable mode of transmission.

Pathogen Invasion

When a pathogen invades the body, a number of immune system responses are initiated to minimize tissue and organ damage. B lymphocytes are activated to differentiate into plasma cells for the production of antibodies and memory cells in preparation for a future re-exposure. T lymphocytes directly kill the invading organism, secreting lymphokines that attract and stimulate the activity of macrophages. Macrophages and monocytes initiate phagocytosis. The complement system is activated to enhance the entire immune response. Some tissue damage will occur as a result of endotoxins

released by the pathogen that kill host cells, neurotoxins that affect nerve impulse transmission, or enterotoxins that damage cells of the gastrointestinal tract. The physiological effect of endotoxins may be mild (fever, chills, weakness, and malaise) or severe (shock syndrome or disseminated intravascular coagulation). Some injuries leading to infection will also manifest with swelling and tenderness at the site, drainage from a wound, or red streaks on the skin leading away from the injury. These manifestations are associated with an inflammatory response.[1]

Infections remain a significant cause of morbidity and mortality as a result of the emergence of antibiotic-resistant bacteria, the development of infections that have become resistant to multiple antibiotics, and the occurrence of both infections that had previously been controlled and newly discovered infections. Some bacteria are able to adapt, with the ability to produce toxins and extracellular enzymes that destroy phagocytic cells, coat part of an antibody to prevent its activation of the complement system, or degrade and suppress an immune response.[10] Exotoxins released by bacteria may act locally at the site of infection or enter the blood and produce symptoms throughout the body. Symptoms associated with release of exotoxins from various pathogens include profuse diarrhea (cholera), spastic paralysis (tetanus), phagocyte death (gangrene), and prevention of nerve impulse transmission (botulism). Severe exotoxin release may cause septic shock syndrome, which if not controlled rapidly can lead to death.

VARIATIONS AND CONTEXT

Infections vary by severity, location, host response to treatment, and potential for debilitating consequences or sequela. Variations such as these can affect individuals of any age, gender, ethnicity, socioeconomic status, geographic location, or prior health history. Infections may occur singularly or in combination, such as bacterial infections superimposed on an existing viral infection (e.g., *Streptococcus pneumoniae* following infection with a cold virus), a new viral infection occurring secondary to an existing viral infection (e.g., cytomegalovirus and HIV), or a fungal infection developed during treatment for a bacterial infection (e.g., development of *Candida albicans* following antibiotic administration). Infections may also be mild and self-limiting, as is often observed when an infection develops in a simple cut or abrasion requiring first-aid treatment, or the infection may be life-threatening, as is the case with systemic septicemia requiring hospitalization.

CONSEQUENCES

Infections that are severe, poorly responsive to therapy, or initially untreated may challenge the body's restorative and compensatory responses, leading to the development of septic shock syndrome and multisystem organ failure or multiorgan dysfunction syndrome. Symptoms of failure may include hypotension, tachycardia, tachypnea, oliguria or anuria, hypoxia, hypercapnia, seizures, or coma. The pathologic processes leading from uncontrolled infection or septicemia to multisystem failure and the symptoms just identified involve a complex interaction among a number of body systems. A bacterial infection is described as the foundation for this potential progression.

Unresponsive or Untreated Infection

When a bacterial pathogen invades the body and initiates an immune response, lymphocytes (to produce antibodies), the complement system, and phagocytes will respond aggressively. Following invasion, bacteria will cause cellular injury by the release of exotoxins or endotoxins or both into the host and initiate an inflammatory response. Exotoxins released during bacterial growth damage host cells, as do endotoxins released after bacterial cell death. In some cases, a combination of the relative virulence of the bacteria and the immunocompromised status of the host may allow for the bacterial infection to overwhelm the immune system and cause significant host damage before the mounting of an effective defense against the bacteria. When this happens, the host will initiate compensatory actions to support vital functions, but these actions will eventually fail without supportive treatments, leading to death of the host.

Vascular, Renal, and Nervous System Compensation

An inflammatory response to the invading bacteria will initiate the host defense mechanisms. This response will trigger a complement system response and all of the activities inherent in that type of response. Vascular permeability will increase and allow for the shift of fluid from the intravascular compartment to the extravascular/extracellular spaces in the tissues, leading to hypovolemia and hypotension. The nervous system will attempt to compensate for the hypotension with peripheral vascular constriction and shunting of blood from nonessential to essential organs such as the brain, heart, and lungs. Acute systemic hypoperfusion may ensue and result in increased heart rate and cardiac contractility in an effort to maintain the cardiac output. In this early period, inadequate tissue perfusion may have caused organ damage despite a hyperdynamic cardiovascular state.

The renal system will initially attempt to compensate by creating a vasodilatory response of the glomeruli in an attempt to maintain an internal degree of pressure to continue filtration. Continued hypoperfusion of the kidneys leads to decreased urine output to retain cardiovascular volume, resulting in oliguria or anuria. Peripheral vasoconstriction may lead to increased cardiac ventricular preload. Should the myocardium become compromised, an increase in ventricular afterload may challenge the pulmonary vascular system with excess fluid that the ventricles cannot eject.

Respiratory Compensation

The respiratory system will attempt to compensate for inadequate tissue perfusion (oxygenation) or hypoxemia by increasing the rate of respiration. This process may well be hampered by cardiovascular decompensation, leading to decreased cardiac output and resultant fluid accumulation and pulmonary edema. Inadequate tissue perfusion (hypoxia) and hypercapnia will result, leading to central nervous system decompensation as evidenced by an early change in mental status progressing to seizures, stupor, and coma.

Multisystem Failure

Without effective treatment, the bacterial invasion leads to the development of septic shock syndrome with multiorgan failure. Eventually, the consequences of inadequate tissue perfusion, overextended compensatory mechanisms, and host cell damage will result in irreversible organ failure and death of the host.[10,18] Figure 25-3 provides an overview of the primary pathologic processes and consequences of a bacterial infection leading to septic shock syndrome.

RISK FACTORS

Populations at Risk

Infectious diseases may cause health concerns for all individuals regardless of age, ethnicity, gender, socioeconomic status, geographic location, or prior health history. However, there are risk factors linked to some population groups based on age, socioeconomic status, and geographic location. Of the 10 leading causes of infant death in the United States, bacterial sepsis ranks ninth and disorders related to short gestation and low birth weight rank third. Because an infant's immune system is immature at birth, any additional stress such as low birth weight further places the infant at risk for infection.[19–21]

The growing population of individuals of low socioeconomic status has increased the risk of infection for several reasons. Those who are uninsured or underinsured may be at risk for the consequences of absent or insufficient preventive health care. For example, if the cost of vaccinations is too expensive or the ability to access clinics where free vaccinations may be provided is not available, both children and adults can be at risk for acquiring infections from which they should be protected. Furthermore, this same population may not have the resources available to travel for preventive health care screenings or treatments for infection; purchase medicines; or buy food and food supplements that may contribute to health maintenance, disease prevention, and more rapid recovery from infections and other illnesses. Meanwhile, the prevalence of some diseases and infections is increasing in specific age or ethnic groups (HIV) or in geographic locations worldwide (cholera and malaria), all of which influence the prevalence of infection in the United States.

Individual Risk Factors

Individual risk factors for infection are influenced by a number of variables. The immune status of the host is a very important risk factor, as is the type and dose of exposure to microorganisms.

Compromised Host Because of Immunodeficiency

Individual risk factors for infection include being very young or elderly because these individuals have immune systems that are immature or become less responsive and efficient with age. Those who are immunocompromised are also at increased risk for infection. An immunocompromised state may develop as a result of genetic factors (primary immunodeficiency), malnutrition, preexisting infection with other pathogens (e.g., HIV or Epstein–Barr virus), acute or chronic psychological or environmental stress, use of medications that induce immunosuppression, and the presence of or treatment for cancer. These processes associated with immunodeficiency were discussed in Concept 23 Immunity.

Compromised Host Because of Chronic Disease

Chronic illness and associated treatments increase the risk for infection. In the United States, infections accounted for 4 of the top 10 leading causes of adult deaths in 2010, including chronic lower respiratory tract diseases, influenza and pneumonia, and nephritis.[21,22] Diseases such as diabetes mellitus, inflammatory disorders, cancers, and hepatic or respiratory disorders challenge the immune system and increase individual vulnerability to infection. Pathologic changes within these body systems may alter the structural integrity of the system and create an environment conducive to infection while treatment regimens are imposed that may also increase the risk of infection. Treatment strategies requiring the introduction of invasive lines (parenteral or other catheters), immunosuppressive medications (corticosteroids), antibiotics or antivirals, surgery, or intubation and mechanical ventilation all expose the body to avenues of entry for pathogenic organisms. In association with chronic illness-derived immunosuppression, required treatment regimens may only serve to enhance the risk of individual infection.

FIGURE 25-3 Pathophysiological Process of Septic Shock (Source: From Copstead LC, Banasik JL: *Pathophysiology*, ed 5, St Louis, 2013, Saunders.)

Environmental Conditions

Exposure to unsafe sanitary conditions may also make an individual vulnerable to a multitude of pathogens. These pathogens may directly cause infection or challenge the immune system and increase the potential for infection upon future introduction of other microorganisms. Crowded living conditions increase the likelihood of the spread of disease and may also contribute to less than optimal sanitation, both of which increase the potential for infection. Other environmental factors influence the individual's susceptibility to infection and include the presence or absence of clean food and water, conditions involving food preparation, and sufficiency of air ventilation.

ASSESSMENT

History

A health history includes questions to assess an individual's risk for infection, recognize symptoms associated with infection, and appreciate factors associated with a presenting infection. Questions include the incidence of injury, known exposure to pathogens, and a history of prior infections. Current or immediate past treatment for cancer, recent surgical procedures, the presence of autoimmune or immunodeficiency disease, and use of immunosuppressant medication regimens must also be assessed. Travel should also be evaluated, particularly outside of the United States or to underdeveloped areas of the world that may expose the individual to pathogens in air, food, and water or to pathogens that are generally not found in the United States, such as smallpox. Other avenues of inquiry may include assessing incidences of interaction with larger groups of people, such as attending entertainment or sporting events where the close proximity of others may facilitate the transmission of infectious pathogens.

Symptoms of infection are those verbalized by the patient and are often caused by the inflammatory response to infection, such as pain, swelling, or redness (see Concept 24 Inflammation); other clinical manifestations may be those associated with the effect of the infectious process on the body system. Specific symptoms are often influenced by the affected organ, such as a cough with an infection of the respiratory system. Some symptoms are a result of generalized stress to the host, such as fatigue or malaise.

Examination Findings

Physical examination findings of particular importance in assessing for the presence of infection include fever, swelling, chills, malaise, redness or drainage in or around a wound, pain, and respiratory congestion.[10,18,23–25] In general, clinical manifestations associated with infection parallel those of inflammation. Should infection with *Clostridium difficile* (*C. diff.*) or parasites be suspected, the presence of watery diarrhea, loss of appetite, nausea, and abdominal pain or tenderness should also be evaluated because these symptoms may be indicative of infection with these pathogens.[22]

Diagnostic Tests

Laboratory and diagnostic studies are foundational to the diagnostic process for infections. Laboratory studies may be done on any type of body fluid or tissue and can prove the presence of infection. Radiographic diagnostic tests provide additional information to understand the location and extent of infections.

Laboratory Tests

Complete blood count. The complete blood count with a white blood cell (WBC) differential count is one of the most critical laboratory tests to evaluate the presence of infection. Elevated levels of B and T lymphocytes, neutrophils, and monocytes are indicative of infection, particularly a bacterial or viral infection. Neutrophil counts are significantly elevated with bacterial infections and may lead to an increase in the number of band cells (immature neutrophils) when an infection is acute. Parasitic infections may result in an increase in the number of basophils and eosinophils; however, these two WBCs are not elevated in the presence of bacterial or viral infections.

Culture and sensitivity. A culture and sensitivity (C&S) test is done to identify the invading pathogen and to determine the antimicrobial most likely to be effective in treatment. This test can be done on any body fluid, tissue, or exudates and is critical in the management of infections. Some of the most common specimens for C&S are obtained from the genitourinary tract (urine culture), respiratory tract (sputum culture), oropharynx (throat culture), blood, wounds, and spinal fluid. Specimens may also be obtained from within the body during invasive procedures or surgeries or from invasive equipment such as intravenous lines, feeding tubes, endotracheal tubes, and indwelling urinary catheters. Nurses are often responsible for the collection of specimens for C&S, and it is critical that correct collection procedures are followed to avoid sample contamination leading to incorrect pathogen identification. Details of collection procedures are typically outlined in textbooks about laboratory and diagnostic procedures.

Other laboratory tests. Several other blood and body fluid screening tests are used to determine the presence of or evaluate an infection. These include C-reactive protein, erythrocyte sedimentation rate (ESR), and various serologic tests for the detection of a virus or antibodies against pathogens such as hepatitis, HIV, Epstein–Barr virus, severe acute respiratory syndrome (SARS), herpes simplex virus, syphilis, MRSA, *C. diff*, and *Helicobacter pylori*.[26]

Radiographic Tests

Radiographic tests typically do not lead to an affirmative diagnosis of infection by themselves because this requires confirmation through clinical pathology analysis (gained through laboratory testing). Radiographic tests are useful in visualizing certain body tissues to gain insight to the possibility of an infection (if not yet diagnosed) and/or the extent and scope of some confirmed infections. Chest x-rays, computer-assisted tomography scans, magnetic resonance imaging scans, positron emission tomography scans, and indium (indium-111) scans are examples of radiographic testing procedures that are useful in identifying areas of infection and inflammation within the body.[27]

CLINICAL MANAGEMENT

Success in the prevention and treatment of infections has progressed dramatically during the past century with the introduction of antibiotics, the modernization of sanitation practices, the development of public health initiatives, and the spread of immunization programs. Morbidity and mortality rates for many infections have decreased substantially, with some infections being nearly eradicated worldwide. In the United States, smallpox vaccinations are no longer recommended and poliomyelitis is nearly eradicated with widespread vaccination protocols. Progress is being made in the development of vaccines for other diseases such as HIV, and a combined vaccination for smallpox and anthrax is being investigated.[2,10,28–35]

Success gained in the prevention and treatment of infections must also be tempered by the following facts: (1) Some community- or hospital-acquired bacterial infections are now difficult to treat because of emerging antibiotic resistance (e.g., MRSA and VRE), (2) the prevalence of hospital-acquired infections is increasing in the form of both MRSA and *C. diff.*, (3) tuberculosis remains one of the world's leading causes of death, and (4) foodborne and waterborne bacteria (*Salmonella* and *Campylobacter*) continue to cause debilitating diarrheal disease throughout the world. Following Alexander Fleming's discovery of penicillin in 1928, 85 years of using increasingly more potent antimicrobials has resulted in bacteria and viruses that are resistant to even the most potent weapons in our arsenal. The National Institute of Allergy and Infectious Diseases (NIAID) issued a statement of concern about the increasingly difficult process of disease management given the microbial resistance that has emerged against some of the most powerful antimicrobials. NIAID particularly expressed concern related to treating staphylococcal infection, tuberculosis, influenza, gonorrhea, *Candida* infection, and malaria.[10,22,36–38] Continued research to find more powerful antimicrobials, while teaching the population about the consequences of overuse or inappropriate use of antimicrobials, will challenge health care providers and researchers for years to come.

Primary Prevention

Primary prevention involves a wide variety of infection control measures. Infection control has been defined by the World Health Organization as measures aimed at the protection of those who might be vulnerable to acquiring an infection, including both individuals residing in the community and persons receiving care for health care problems within a wide variety of settings. The basic tenant of infection control is identified as *hygiene* and encompasses such topics as patient safety, infection control and prevention in health care, injection safety, and food safety.[39]

Hand Hygiene and Standard Precautions

Following basic hand hygiene principles and adhering to Standard Precautions are the most effective methods of blocking transmission of infection in community and health care settings. The Centers for Disease Control and Prevention (CDC) has published guidelines for infection control and hand hygiene within health care settings, as well as guidelines related to health care-associated infections.[40–50] The guidelines are updated periodically and serve as excellent resources for ensuring adherence to infection control principles.[51,52]

The following are some recommendations for infection control proposed by the CDC[53]: Keep hands clean by washing thoroughly with soap and water (for at least 20 seconds) or using an alcohol-based hand rub (for at least 15 seconds; not as effective if hands are visibly dirty or greasy), keep cuts and scrapes clean and covered with a bandage until healed, avoid contact with other people's wounds and bandages, and refrain from sharing personal items such as towels or razors. In athletic settings, participants should shower immediately after participation and before using whirlpools. Uniforms should be washed and dried after each use. In health care settings, prevention of infection requires following accepted principles of hand hygiene, Standard Precautions, and contact precautions. Visitors should follow hand hygiene principles and avoid touching wound dressings, catheters, or wound sites of an infected person.[54–57]

Immunizations

Another significant primary prevention measure is the administration of vaccinations. Worldwide, health care organizations have demonstrated various levels of success in providing vaccinations in an effort to eradicate some of the more devastating infectious diseases, such as polio and smallpox.[28–31] Standard vaccinations in the U.S. arsenal to control the spread of disease through prevention of initial infection include those for human papillomavirus (HPV); hepatitis A and hepatitis B; varicella; measles, mumps, and rubella (MMR); influenza (annual); pneumococcus; tetanus, diphtheria, pertussis (Td/Tdap); and polio. Research continues worldwide to discover an effective vaccine for HIV.[32–34] Vaccinations are recommended for individuals across the lifespan; specific vaccination schedules are readily available from the CDC website (http://www.cdc.gov/vaccines/schedules/).

Secondary Prevention (Screening)

Secondary prevention through disease screening is less effective in controlling infection, but represents an opportunity to identify an infection with the intent for earlier treatment and reducing transmission.

The areas of screening most strongly supported are those for the identification of sexually transmitted diseases such as bacterial infections (*Chlamydia trachomatis*, *Neisseria gonorrhoeae*, or group B *Streptococci*), viral pathogens (HIV, herpes simplex virus, hepatitis virus, or HPV), fungal pathogens (*Candida albicans*), or protozoa (*Giardia lamblia*). Pap smears for sexually active women can be used as screening tools not only for cancer cells but also for the presence of HPV.

Collaborative Interventions

Management of infections requires both treatment of the infectious process itself and support for the affected body systems. The goal of treatment is to eradicate the infection, prevent secondary infections, and limit damage to the body. Many interventions are related to supporting affected body systems. The following infection control measures are critical for a rapid recovery and are universal in that they apply to infection treatment regardless of the system involved: Know and follow the principles of effective hand hygiene, clean and disinfect environmental surfaces, and avoid close contact with infected individuals or crowded conditions in which bacterial or viral infections may be easily disseminated.[40–42]

Antimicrobials

Interventions in the treatment of various infections begin with the use of antibiotics, antivirals, and other antimicrobials. The laboratory and

---

CLINICAL NURSING SKILLS FOR INFECTION

- Hand hygiene
- Personal protective equipment
  - Gloves
  - Mask
  - Protective eyewear
  - Gown
  - Cap
- Isolation precautions
- Sterility
- Collecting specimens for culture
- Medication administration

---

diagnostic testing identified previously helps to direct the health care provider to the appropriate antimicrobial. Instructing the infected individual to complete the full course of antimicrobial therapy helps to avoid a secondary infection or re-emergence of infection because of inadequate initial treatment.

Antibiotic agents. There are several classifications of antibiotics based on bacterial spectrum and activity (bactericidal or bacteriostatic). Spectrum refers to the number of organisms affected by the antibiotic (i.e., broad-spectrum or narrow-spectrum antibiotic). Activity refers to the way in which the antibiotic kills bacteria. Bactericidal agents attack and kill the bacteria directly, whereas bacteriostatic agents interfere with replication of the pathogen. The common classifications of antibiotics are presented in Table 25-2. Antibiotics within a structural class generally have similar patterns of effectiveness, toxicity, and allergic potential.

Antiviral agents. Like antibiotics, antiviral agents either kill viruses or suppress their replication, preventing their ability to multiply and reproduce. These agents are primarily used to minimize the severity of illness by limiting the viral spread. Common classifications of antiviral agents are presented in Table 25-2.

Antifungal agents. Antifungal agents kill fungal organisms. Because there are various types of fungi that cause infection, multiple classifications of antifungal agents are available and include polyenes, imidazoles, triazoles, thiazoles, allylamines, and echinocandins.

Nutrition and Fluids

Replacement of fluids and electrolytes (oral or parenteral) is critical in the presence of fever, vomiting, or diarrhea. Adequate rest and nutrition provide the body with energy needed for optimal functioning of the immune system and resolution of infection. Allowing time for rest

---

TABLE 25-2 Classification of Antibiotic and Antiviral Agents

Antibiotics	Antiviral Agents
Penicillin	Adamantane
Cephalosporins	Antiviral chemokine receptor agonist
First generation	Antiviral interferon
Second generation	Neuraminidase inhibitors
Third generation	Non-nucleoside reverse-transcriptase inhibitors
Fourth generation	Nucleoside reverse-transcriptase inhibitors
Fluoroquinolones	Protease inhibitors
Tetracyclines	Purine nucleosides
Macrolides	
Aminoglycosides	

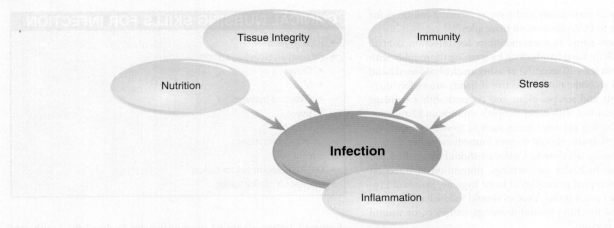

FIGURE 25-4 Infection and Interrelated Concepts

and ensuring adequate fluids and nutritional intake are equally important.

INTERRELATED CONCEPTS

The concept of infection is closely aligned with several concepts featured in this textbook. These interrelated concepts are presented in Figure 25-4.

Immunity is critical in providing a level of surveillance for early identification of pathogen entry into the body. The immune system is the first line of defense against infection and the body's primary method of response to an invading organism. Inflammation is part of the body's response to a foreign antigen, with many of the symptoms of infection being those of the body's inflammatory response (redness, swelling, and pain). Tissue Integrity is critical to avoiding infection, with the skin being the largest component of the immune system. Intact tissues are less vulnerable to pathogen entry and form natural barriers to infection. As noted previously, Stress—whether physical, emotional, or environmental—challenges the immune system and makes it more vulnerable to damage, less able to respond effectively and efficiently to pathogen invasion, and more difficult for the body to respond to treatment for an infection. Finally, maintaining adequate Nutrition and rest is also necessary for the body to respond to active infection treatment regimens and support the work of an immune response.

CLINICAL EXEMPLARS

Table 25-1 identifies examples of common pathogens that cause infection. A variety of infections have been presented as recurring, emerging, resistant, and global infections. Box 25-1 presents some of the more commonly occurring infections by body systems. Some of the most common or important exemplars briefly described in the section that follows.

Featured Exemplars

Pneumonia

Pneumonia is an infection in the lungs that may range from mild to severe and occurs in people of any age, gender, or ethnicity. Worldwide, it is the leading cause of death in children younger than age 5 years.[59] One's potential for developing pneumonia is diminished with proper hand hygiene and by disinfecting regularly touched surfaces, being a nonsmoker, not having underlying diseases such as diabetes mellitus or heart disease, and being vaccinated with the pneumonia vaccine.

Pneumonia symptoms include chest tightness, shortness of breath, difficulty breathing, cough, and fever, and the disease is treated with antibiotics and antiviral drugs.[59,60]

Conjunctivitis

Commonly called "pink eye," conjunctivitis is characterized by redness and swelling of the conjunctiva, thick discharge from the eye with crusting on the eyelids or lashes, and itchy, inflamed eyes. Pain is not typically associated with the infection. Conjunctivitis is common in children and adults, easily spread from one person to another, and when one child in a family is diagnosed with conjunctivitis, all children are commonly treated as a prophylactic measure. In the newborn, conjunctivitis occurring within the first 3 weeks of life is often caused by gonococcal or chlamydial infections of the mother and, if left untreated, may lead to blindness.[61-63]

Otitis Media

Otitis media may be classified into one of three types: acute otitis media (AOM), otitis media with effusion (OME), and otitis externa (Swimmer's ear). Guidelines require differentiation of OME and AOM, and the patient's age, to determine appropriate antibiotic use. AOM is usually painful and often requires treatment with antibiotics. Other symptoms include redness of the tympanic membrane, pus, and fever. OME is a buildup of fluid in the middle ear without symptoms of infection and is often caused by viral upper respiratory infections and allergies, generally resolving on its own. Swimmer's ear is an infection of the ear and outer ear canal. Treatment with antibiotics is usually required.[64,65]

Hepatitis

Hepatitis is inflammation of the liver and generally refers to one of three viral causative agents: hepatitis A, hepatitis B, and hepatitis C. It is the leading cause of liver cancer and the most common cause of liver transplantation. The CDC estimates that 4.4 million Americans are living with chronic hepatitis and do not know they are infected.[66] Since 1990, effective vaccination strategies have led to a decrease in the incidence of acute hepatitis B virus (HBV); however, the incidence of acute hepatitis C virus (HCV) has been on the rise since 2006. Furthermore, significant underreporting of HBV and HCV is acknowledged due to asymptomatic infections. Acute onset of symptoms is discrete and includes nausea and vomiting, fever, malaise, dark urine, and jaundice. Ascites develops later in disease progression.[67]

Human Papillomavirus

HPV is the most common sexually transmitted infection, with more than 40 types, and is typically passed through genital contact during vaginal, anal, or oral sex. Symptoms may develop years after exposure and may lead to genital warts and cancer. HPV tests can be used to screen for cervical cancer. A vaccination is available to men and women against the types of HPV that most often lead to cancer and is given at the age of 11 or 12 years. HPV is so common that the CDC estimates that most sexually active men and women will get at least one type of HPV sometime in their life.[68,69]

■■■ BOX 25-1 EXEMPLARS OF INFECTION

Neurologic
- Encephalitis
- Meningitis

Respiratory
- Pneumonia
- Respiratory syncytial virus

Cardiovascular
- Endocarditis
- Myocarditis

Eyes
- Conjunctivitis

Ears
- Otitis media

Skin
- Cellulitis
- Methicillin-resistant *Staphylococcus aureus*
- Pressure ulcers
- Surgical wounds

Gastrointestinal
- *Clostridium difficile*
- Gastroenteritis
- Hepatitis
- Tapeworm

Genitourinary
- Cystitis
- Pyelonephritis
- Urinary tract infection

Reproductive
- *Candida albicans*
- *Chlamydia trachomatis*
- Group B *Streptococci*
- Herpes simplex virus
- Human papillomavirus
- *Neisseria gonorrhoeae*

Systemic
- HIV
- Measles
- Mumps
- Sepsis

CASE STUDY

Source: Medioimages/Photodisc/ Thinkstock

Case Presentation

Mrs. Bovier is a 72-year-old woman who recently spent 5 days in the hospital for pneumonia, where she received intravenous antibiotics and respiratory therapy. She was discharged 1 week ago and has been at home with her elderly husband, who assists in her care. She has arthritis and typically is not very physically active.

Mrs. Bovier returned to her primary care provider for a checkup and complained of increasing difficulty breathing, headache, and coughing up yellowish-colored sputum. On examination, she was found to have a low-grade fever, chest auscultation revealed areas of atelectasis, oxygen saturation (PaO_2) was 91%, and she was diaphoretic. A sputum specimen was obtained for culture and sensitivity that later revealed the presence of MRSA. Chest x-ray confirmed pulmonary congestion and atelectasis. Laboratory analysis showed an elevated WBC count, the presence of band cells (immature neutrophils), and an elevated ESR.

Mrs. Bovier was again hospitalized because of the severity of her respiratory distress, the need for intravenous antibiotics to manage the MRSA pulmonary infection and pulmonary therapy to assist in resolving her pulmonary congestion, and the need for contact isolation because of her recurrent pneumonia and MRSA infection. Mrs. Bovier's age and lack of physical activity are complications that may influence MRSA treatment, requiring a more watchful course of initial therapy.

Hospital care for Mrs. Bovier included instruction in methods to improve the productivity of her cough, humidified oxygen to assist with loosening secretions while improving ventilation, and respiratory therapy to help with expectoration and to facilitate lung expansion and air exchange. She received intravenous vancomycin, mucolytic agents, a bronchodilator, and expectorants to treat her pulmonary disease and assist in breathing.

On discharge, Mrs. Bovier received instructions in the proper technique for effective hand hygiene; the importance of avoiding large crowds of people as well as areas where people are smoking, to diminish her exposure to irritating respiratory stimuli; and the need to increase her physical activity, including frequent ambulation in her home, to help stimulate deep breathing and avoid peripheral vascular clot formation. She demonstrated understanding of her medication regimen and the need to maintain adequate food and fluid intake to support her immune system and provide energy while healing. The need for rest to promote healing was also emphasized. Finally, Mrs. Bovier was instructed on warning signs of recurring pulmonary disease or dysfunction.

Case Analysis

Health care-acquired MRSA is the most severe form of MRSA, with life-threatening infections such as bacteremia, surgical site infections, pneumonia, septic arthritis, toxic shock syndrome, and endocarditis as consequences. People at risk for acquiring MRSA infections include patients and visitors of patients in health care settings.

Mrs. Bovier met a number of the criteria that put her at risk for the development of MRSA. She was elderly, had been hospitalized with pneumonia (foreign pathogen), and had received intravenous antibiotics (invasive port of entry for MRSA). When she sought follow-up care to her hospitalization for pneumonia, she was found to have pulmonary congestion, hypoxemia, and fever. Diagnostic data revealed atelectasis on chest x-ray, an elevated white blood cell count, and immature neutrophils indicating the presence of a bacterial infection. These are classic clinical findings associated with infection. Diagnosis and treatment measures were consistent with the standards of care.

ACCESS EXEMPLAR LINKS IN YOUR GIDDENS EBOOK

REFERENCES

1. Hall JC: *Textbook of medical physiology*, Philadelphia, 2011, Elsevier.
2. Ross AL, Brave A, Scarlatti G, et al: Progress towards development of an HIV vaccine: Report of the AIDS Vaccine 2009 Conference. *Lancet Infect Dis* 10(5):305–316, 2010.
3. National Institutes of Health: Immune system. Retrieved from: <http://www.niaid.nih.gov/topics/immunesystem/Pages/default.aspx>, 2008.
4. Steinman R: Introduction to dendritic cells, 2015. Retrieved from: <http://lab.rockefeller.edu/steinman/>.
5. Steinman R: Dendritic cells initiate the immune response, 2015. Retrieved from: <http://lab.rockefeller.edu/steinman/dendritic_intro/immuneResponse>.
6. Steinman R: Dendritic cells and immune tolerance, 2015. Retrieved from: <http://lab.rockefeller.edu/steinman/dendritic_intro/immuneTolerance>.
7. Leon B, Ardavin C: Monocyte-derived dendritic cells in innate and adaptive immunity. *Immunol Cell Biol* 86:320–324, 2008.
8. Maason F, Mount AM, Wilson NS, et al: Dendritic cells: Driving the differentiation programme of T cells in viral infections. *Immunol Cell Biol* 86:333–342, 2008.
9. Venes D, editor: *Taber's cyclopedic medical dictionary*, ed 22, Philadelphia, 2013, Davis.
10. McCance KL, Huether SE, Brashers VL, et al: *Pathophysiology: The biologic basis for disease in adults and children*, St Louis, 2010, Mosby.
11. Centers for Disease Control and Prevention: Frequently asked questions about *Clostridium difficile* for healthcare providers, 2012. Retrieved from: <http://www.cdc.gov/HAI/organisms/cdiff/Cdiff_faqs_HCP.html>.
12. Cohen SH, Gerding DN, Johnson S, et al: Clinical practice guidelines for *Clostridium difficile* infection in adults: 2010 update by the Society for Healthcare Epidemiology of America (SHEA) and the Infectious Diseases Society of America (IDSA). *Infect Control Epidemiol* 31(5):431–455, 2010.
13. Centers for Disease Control and Prevention: *Clostridium difficile* infection, 2013. Retrieved from: <http://www.cdc.gov/HAI/organisms/cdiff/Cdiff_infect.html>.
14. Centers for Disease Control and Prevention: Vancomycin-resistant Enterococci (VRE) in healthcare settings, 2010. Retrieved from: <http://www.cdc.gov/HAI/organisms/vre/vre.html>.
15. Centers for Disease Control and Prevention: Chickenpox (varicella): Clinical overview, 2013. Retrieved from: <http://www.cdc.gov/chickenpox/hcp/clinical-overview.html>.
16. Centers for Disease Control and Prevention: Conducting varicella surveillance, 2012. Retrieved from: <http://www.cdc.gov/chickenpox/hcp/conducting-surveillance.html>.
17. Centers for Disease Control and Prevention: People at high risk for complications, 2014. Retrieved from: <http://www.cdc.gov/chickenpox/hcp/high-risk.html>.
18. Copstead LC, Banasik JL: *Pathophysiology*, ed 4, St Louis, 2010, Saunders.
19. Xu J, Kochanek KD, Murphy SL, et al: Deaths: Final data for 2007. *CDC Natl Vital Stat Rep* 58(19):1, 2010.
20. National Institutes of Health, National Library of Medicine, Aging changes in immunity, 2008. Retrieved from: <http://www.nlm.nih.gov/medlineplus/ency/article/004008.htm>.
21. Heron M: Deaths, leading causes for 2010. *Natl Vital Stat Rep* 62(6):1, 2013.
22. Centers for Disease Control and Prevention: Information for healthcare providers, 2005. Retrieved from: <http://www.cdc.gov/ncidod/dhqp/id_CdiffFAQ_HCP.html>.
23. Centers for Disease Control and Prevention: About MRSA. 2008. Retrieved from: <http://www.cdc.gov/mrsa/mrsa_initiative/skin_infection/index.html>.
24. Jernigan J, Kallen A: Methicillin-resistant Staphylococcus aureus (MRSA) infections, presentation at the Nevada State Health Division Conference on "MRSA, Healthcare-Associated Infections," Las Vegas, NV, November 16, 2010.
25. National Institutes of Health News: Stop the spread of superbugs: Help fight drug-resistant bacteria, 2014. Retrieved from: <http://newsinhealth.nih.gov/issue/Feb2014?Feature1>.
26. Pagana KD, Pagana TJ, Pagana J: *Mosby's diagnostic and laboratory rest reference*, ed 12, St Louis, 2014, Elsevier.
27. National Institutes of Health, National Library of Medicine: WBC scan, 2012. Retrieved from: <http://www.nlm.nih.gov/medlineplus/ency/article/003834.htm>.
28. Merkel TJ, Perera PY, Kelly VK, et al: Development of a highly efficacious vaccinia-based dual vaccine against smallpox and anthrax, two important bioterror entities. *Proc Natl Acad Sci USA* 107(42):18091–18096, 2010.
29. Centers for Disease Control and Prevention: Course: "Smallpox: Disease, prevention, and intervention," 2014. Retrieved from: <http://emergency.cdc.gov/agent/smallpox/training/overview>.
30. Centers for Disease Control and Prevention: What is polio? 2014. Retrieved from: <http://www.cdc.gov/polio/about/index.htm>.
31. Centers for Disease Control and Prevention: Who we are: CDC and the global polio eradication initiative, 2013. Retrieved from: <http://www.cdc.gov/polio/who/index.htm>.
32. National Institutes of Health, National Institute of Allergy and Infectious Diseases: HIV/AIDS: HIV vaccine design and strategies, 2012. Retrieved from: <http://www.niaid.nih.gov/topics/hivaids/research/vaccines/Pages/strategies.aspx>.
33. National Institutes of Health, National Institute of Allergy and Infectious Diseases: NIH grantees sharpen understanding of antibodies that may cut risk of HIV infection, 2014. Retrieved from: <http://www.niaid.nih.gov/news/newsreleases/2014/Pages/RV144Correlate.aspx>.
34. National Institutes of Health, National Institute of Allergy and Infectious Diseases: Study of antibody evolution charts course toward HIV vaccine, 2014. Retrieved from: <http://www.niaid.nih.gov/news/newsreleases/2014/Pages/V1V2HIVantibodyevolution.aspx>,
35. Centers for Disease Control and Prevention: HIV in the United States: At a glance, 2014. Retrieved from: <http://www.cdc.gov/hiv/statistics/basics/ataglance.html>.
36. National Institutes of Health, National Institute of Allergy and Infectious Diseases: Bacterial infections, 2010. Retrieved from: <http://www.niaid.nih.gov/topics/bacterialinfections/pages/default.aspx>.
37. Centers for Disease Control and Prevention: Methicillin-resistant *Staphylococcus aureus* (MRSA) infections, 2014. Retrieved from: <http://www.cdc.gov/mrsa>.
38. National Institutes of Health, National Institute of Allergy and Infectious Diseases: Antimicrobial (drug) resistance, 2009. Retrieved from: <http://www.niaid.nih.gov/topics/antimicrobialresistance/understanding/pages/default.aspx>.
39. World Health Organization: WHO guidelines on hand hygiene in health care, 2009. Retrieved from: <http://www.who.int/gpsc/information_centre/hand-hygiene-2009/en>.
40. Rutala WA, Weber DJ: HICPAC: Guideline for disinfection and sterilization in healthcare facilities, 2008. Retrieved from: <http://www.cdc.gov/hicpac/pdf/guidelines/Disinfection_Nov_2008.pdf>.
41. Centers for Disease Control and Prevention: Guideline for hand hygiene in health-care settings. *Morbid Mortal Wkly Rep* 51:1–45, 2002. Retrieved from: <http://www.cdc.gov/mmwr/PDF/rr/rr5116.pdf>.
42. Centers for Disease Control and Prevention: Guideline for isolation precautions: Preventing transmission of infectious agents in healthcare settings, 2007. Retrieved from: <http://www.cdc.gov//ncidod/dhqp/pdf/isolation2007.pdf>.
43. Centers for Disease Control and Prevention: Type of healthcare-associated infections, 2010. Retrieved from: <http://cdc.gov/HAI/infectionTypes.html>.
44. Centers for Disease Control and Prevention: Preventing healthcare-associated infections, 2010. Retrieved from: <http://www.cdc.gov/HAI/prevent/prevention.html>.
45. Centers for Disease Control and Prevention: Monitoring healthcare-associated infections, 2010. Retrieved from: <http://www.cdc.gov/HAI/surveillance/monitorHAI.html>.
46. Centers for Disease Control and Prevention: First state-specific healthcare-associated infections summary data report: CDC's national healthcare safety network (NHSN), January–June, 2009 Q and A, 2010. Retrieved from: <http://www.cdc.gov/HAI/surveillance/QA_stateSummary.html>.

47. Centers for Disease Control and Prevention: Guidelines: Hand hygiene in healthcare settings, 2011. Retrieved from: <http://www.cdc.gov/handhygiene/Guidelines.html>.

48. Centers for Disease Control and Prevention: Hand hygiene basics, 2014. Retrieved from: <http://www.cdc.gov/handhygiene/Basics.html>.

49. Centers for Disease Control and Prevention: Top CDC recommendations to prevent healthcare-associated infections, 2012. Retrieved from: <http://www.cdc.gov/HAI/pdfs/hai/top-cdc-recs-factsheet.pdf>.

50. Centers for Disease Control and Prevention: Healthcare associated infections (HAIs): Research, 2013. Retrieved from: <http://www.cdc.gov/HAi/research/research.html>.

51. Centers for Disease Control and Prevention: Healthcare associated infections (HAIs): Types of healthcare-associated infections, 2014. Retrieved from: <http://www.cdc.gov/HAi/infectionTypes.html>.

52. Centers for Disease Control and Prevention: Healthcare associated infections (HAIs): Data and statistics, 2014. Retrieved from: <http://www.cdc.gov/HAi/surveillance/index.html>.

53. Centers for Disease Control and Prevention: Handwashing—Clean hands save lives: When and how to wash your hands, 2013. Retrieved from: <http://www.cdc.gov/handwashing/when-how-handwashing.html>.

54. Centers for Disease Control and Prevention: General information about MRSA in healthcare settings, 2013. Retrieved from: <http://www.cdc.gov/mrsa/healthcare>.

55. Centers for Disease Control and Prevention: MRSA information for coaches, athletic directors, and team healthcare providers, 2013. Retrieved from: <http://www.cdc.gov/mrsa/community/team-hc-providers/index.html>.

56. Centers for Disease Control and Prevention: General information about MRSA in the community, 2013. Retrieved from: <http://www.cdc.gov/mrsa/community/index.html>.

57. Centers for Disease Control and Prevention: MRSA tracking, 2013. Retrieved from: <http://www.cdc.gov/mrsa/tracking/index.html>.

58. National Institutes of Health, National Institute of Allergy and Infectious Diseases: Basic vaccine discovery, 2012. Retrieved from: <http://www.niaid.nih.gov/topics/hivaids/research/vaccines/Pages/default.aspx>.

59. Centers for Disease Control and Prevention: Pneumonia, 2014. Retrieved from: <http://www.cdc.gov/pneumonia>.

60. Goulding J, Godlee A, Vekaria S, et al: Lowering the threshold of lung innate immune cell activation alters susceptibility to secondary bacterial superinfection. *J Infect Dis* 1(October):1086–1094, 2011.

61. *Mosby's dictionary of medicine, nursing, and health professions*, ed 9, St Louis, 2013, Mosby.

62. Centers for Disease Control and Prevention: Conjunctivitis (pink eye), 2014. Retrieved from: <http://www.cdc.gov/conjunctivitis/index.html>.

63. Centers for Disease Control and Prevention: Conjunctivitis (pink eye): Causes, 2014. Retrieved from: <http://www.cdc.gov/conjunctivitis/about/causes.html>.

64. Centers for Disease Control and Prevention: Otitis media; Physician information sheet (Pediatrics), 2013. Retrieved from: <http://www.cdc.gov/getsmart/campaign-materials/info-sheets/child-otitismedia.html>.

65. Centers for Disease Control and Prevention: Ear infections, 2013. Retrieved from: <http://www.cdc.gov/getsmart/antibiotic-use/URI/ear-infection.html>.

66. Centers for Disease Control and Prevention: Viral hepatitis, 2014. Retrieved from: <http://www.cdc.gov/hepatitis/index.htm>.

67. Centers for Disease Control and Prevention: Surveillance for viral hepatitis—United States, 2012. 2014. Retrieved from: <http://www.cdc.gov/hepatitis/Statistics/2012Surveillance/Commentary.htm>,

68. Centers for Disease Control and Prevention: What is HPV? 2013. Retrieved from at: <http://www.cdc.gov/hpv/whatishpv.html>.

69. Centers for Disease Control and Prevention: Genital HPV infection—Fact sheet, 2014. Retrieved from: <http://www.cdc.gov/std/HPV/HPV-factsheet-March-2014.pdf>.

Mobility

Jean Giddens

The 10-month-old child taking his first steps, the 6-year-old girl riding a bicycle, the high school athlete "dunking" the basketball, the newly married couple dancing at their wedding, the 40-year-old neighbor walking his dog, and the 76-year-old grandmother knitting a scarf are all examples of mobility accomplished through functions of the musculoskeletal and nervous systems. As a basic physiological process, mobility is required for optimal health. Changes in mobility can significantly affect biophysical health, psychosocial health, and functional status. Nurses should be familiar with interventions to promote optimal mobility, prevent situations leading to immobility, and minimize complications when immobility occurs.

DEFINITION

Mobility refers to purposeful physical movement, including gross simple movements, fine complex movements, and coordination. Mobility is dependent on the synchronized efforts of the musculoskeletal and nervous systems as well as adequate oxygenation, perfusion, and cognition. Specifically, mobility requires adequate energy, adequate muscle strength, underlying skeletal stability, joint function, and neuromuscular coordination to carry out the desired movement. For the purposes of this concept analysis, mobility is defined as a *"state or quality of being mobile or movable."*[1,p1479] There are many variations on the term mobility seen throughout the literature worth mentioning. The term *immobility* refers to an inability to move. *Impaired physical mobility* describes a state in which a person has a limitation in physical movement but is not immobile.[2] Although immobility is typically considered a negative state, there are times when immobility or immobilization is therapeutic. For example, the immobilization of a shoulder if it has been dislocated provides desired rest, recovery, and comfort.

The term *deconditioned* is used to describe a loss of physical fitness. This applies not only to an athlete who fails to maintain an optimal level of training but also to an individual who does not maintain optimal physical activity. In the context of health care, this term applies to patients who experience extended immobility (e.g., following prolonged bed rest), resulting in an overall deconditioned state of the musculoskeletal and cardiopulmonary systems. This is particularly a problem among older adults. Another similar term, *the disuse syndrome*, first proposed more than 30 years ago by Bortz, describes the predictable adverse effect on body tissues and functions associated with sedentary lifestyle and inactivity.[3] Identifying characteristics of the disuse syndrome, as defined by Bortz, included cardiovascular vulnerability, obesity, musculoskeletal fragility, depression, and premature aging.

SCOPE

The scope of mobility as a concept ranges on a continuum from full mobility to partial mobility (also referred to as impaired mobility) and complete immobility (Figure 26-1). Mobility can be considered on a micro or macro perspective. Mobility and immobility may refer to a particular part of the body (e.g., an arm or a leg), or they can refer to the entire body. Thus, mobility and immobility are not mutually exclusive; for example, a patient with an immobilized extremity can be mobile. Also, because mobility is on a continuum, a change in mobility may be temporary.

NORMAL PHYSIOLOGICAL PROCESS

Optimal mobility relies on bones, joints, articular cartilage, tendons and ligaments, skeletal muscle, and the mechanics of muscle contraction. Underlying these functions is an intact neurologic system whereby signals for all movement are communicated to and from the brain through nerve impulses.

Neurologic System

All movement is coordinated by the brain through a complex process of sensing internal and external data signals, integrating these data signals, and responding by triggering motor activity. The motor cortex in the frontal lobe of the brain is responsible for voluntary motor activity through a series of nerve impulses sent from the brain, through the spinal cord and peripheral nerves, to the target muscle. The cerebellum, located at the base of the brain, coordinates movement, equilibrium, muscle tone, and proprioception.

Musculoskeletal System
Bones

The skeleton has three overarching roles as related to mobility: It acts as the structural foundation for the body and as leverage to move body parts, supports and protects tissues and internal organs, and provides attachment sites for muscles and ligaments. Bones also serve as a

| Complete Immobility | Partial Mobility | Complete/Full Mobility |

FIGURE 26-1 Scope of Mobility as a Concept

storage center for calcium and as a production center for red blood cells within the bone marrow.[4] The human body has 206 bones classified into two groups: the axial skeleton (bones that comprise the skull, thorax, and spinal column) and the appendicular skeleton (bones that comprise the upper and lower extremities).

All structures designed for use over time require ongoing maintenance and intermittent repair. The same is true for the skeletal system. Remodeling is a term that describes an ongoing maintenance of bone tissue through a process in which new bone tissue replaces existing bone tissue in bone-remodeling units.[5] The remodeling process also provides the mechanism to repair injured bones (e.g., a fracture). Remodeling requires adequate nutrition, hormonal regulation, and blood supply. The severity of the bone injury and the availability of remodeling elements influence the rate or speed at which injured bone heals.

Joints

Bones come together at joints. Joints provide stability to bones and allow skeletal movement. Mobility is impacted by the degree of joint freedom; joints allow for skeletal positioning to carry out the desired action. The various types of movement provided by joints include flexion, extension, rotation, adduction, abduction, supination, and pronation. Some of the most common problems associated with mobility arise as a result of joint pain and/or changes in joint function.

Three classifications of joints (based on stability and movement) include synarthrosis joints (nonmovable), amphiarthrosis joints (slightly movable), and diarthrosis joints (freely movable).[5] Joints are also classified by structure. Fibrous joints serve to hold bones together in place with connective tissue. For example, the tibia and fibula are held together by a fibrous ligament. Cartilaginous joints feature cartilage material that holds the joint together and provides some movement. For example, ribs are attached and held to the sternum by cartilaginous material, allowing movement for the process of breathing but providing chest stability required for the breathing process. Joints that allow the most movement are also the most complex. Synovial joints have multiple elements, including a joint capsule, synovial membrane, joint cavity, synovial fluid, and articular cartilage. Articular cartilage acts as a cushion by distributing joint loads over a wide area, thereby reducing prolonged compression of articulating bones within the joint. Without cartilage, significant friction and pain result from joint movement.

Muscles

Skeletal muscle differs from other types of muscle in the body in many ways, but one of the most important differences is that it is under voluntary control.[4] Optimal skeletal muscle function depends on the following five factors: nerve impulses reaching the muscle, muscle fibers' response to nerve stimulus, proprioception, mechanical load, and joint mobility. Impairment of any one of these factors negatively impacts purposeful movement.

Nerve impulses reach skeletal muscle from the spinal cord and peripheral nerves via motor neurons. The motor neurons innervate a group of muscle fibers known as the motor or muscle unit. There are many different types of muscle fibers within a muscle unit depending on the function and type of responsiveness required. Muscles that maintain body posture do not have the same need for quick responsiveness as do the ocular muscles, for example, but are less sensitive to fatigue.

Muscle movement occurs in response to nerve stimulation of the muscle fibers triggering muscle contraction. On a cellular level, the functional units of muscle contraction are myofibrils. Movement occurs in a reciprocal manner among muscle groups. If one group contracts, another group must relax. For example, flexion of the elbow to move the forearm up requires contraction of the biceps muscles and relaxation of the triceps muscles; likewise, extension of the elbow joint requires contraction of the triceps muscles and relaxation of the biceps muscles. If both are contracted at the same time, no movement occurs.

Proprioception is the mechanism that provides a sense of position and movement; this process allows for accuracy in the degree of movement with muscle contraction. Mechanical load of movement is associated with having adequate strength within the muscle group to carry out the desired task. For example, most humans would struggle to pick up a 250-pound object and walk 50 feet with it. However, such a feat is entirely possible for individuals who are well conditioned for this.

Age-Related Differences

Significant changes to the musculoskeletal system occur throughout infancy and childhood as a function of growth and development. The appendicular skeleton (extremities) grows faster than the axial skeleton (head, thorax, and spine)—partly because the appendicular skeleton is disproportionately shorter than the axial skeleton. Throughout infancy, childhood, and adolescence, bones change in composition, grow in length and diameter, and undergo changes in rotation and alignment. Similarly, the size and composition of muscles undergo changes as a result of physical growth and development throughout childhood, and they are a major factor in weight gain during adolescence.[5,6]

A number of musculoskeletal changes occur with aging. In the spinal column, a thinning of vertebral disks, shortening of the spinal column, and onset of kyphosis with spinal column compression occur. Bone density decreases and becomes brittle (particularly in females), leaving older adults more susceptible to fracture. Cartilage becomes rigid and fragile, and there is a loss of resilience and elasticity of ligaments. Muscle mass and tone reduce significantly in late adult years. Cumulatively, these changes result in mobility impairment attributable to reduced range of motion and pain in joints, reduced muscle strength, and increased risk for bone fracture.[4]

VARIATIONS AND CONTEXT

Variations in mobility are seen among individuals across the lifespan with multiple causative factors and a wide range of degree of impact and duration. Changes in mobility can be temporary, long term, or permanent and are influenced by general health status, with specific conditions associated with the neurologic or musculoskeletal system (Figure 26-2). Restrictions in mobility may also be indicated following a medical procedure or diagnostic test.

An individual's general health status has significant influence on mobility. Many conditions lead to changes in mobility, including acute illness or injury (e.g., influenza), debilitating chronic conditions

FIGURE 26-2 Categories Leading to a Change in Mobility

TABLE 26-1	Consequences of Immobility
System Affected	**Physiological Effect and Potential Complications**
Cardiovascular system	Reduced cardiac capacity Decreased cardiac output Orthostatic hypotension Venous stasis Deep vein thrombosis
Respiratory system	Recued lung expansion Atelectasis Pooling of respiratory secretions
Musculoskeletal system	Reduction in muscle mass and atrophy Contracture of joints Bone demineralization
Integumentary system	Skin breakdown
Gastrointestinal system	Reduced peristaltic motility Constipation
Urinary system	Renal calculi Urinary stasis Infection

(particularly cardiovascular and pulmonary conditions leading to fatigue), and conditions involving end-of-life care (e.g., cancer or dementia). Conditions that specifically lead to mobility impairment include neurologic (including the brain, the spinal cord, and the peripheral nerves), musculoskeletal (bones, joints, and muscles), or a combination of both (neuromuscular conditions). Conditions in these three categories can be caused by congenital defects, genetic conditions, injury, inflammation, infection, autoimmune disorders, and neoplasms. Medical procedures (e.g., surgery) and diagnostic tests may require temporary restrictions on mobility to reduce complications.

CONSEQUENCES

Attaining and/or maintaining mobility is paramount to health. The human body was designed to move; thus, when movement is limited, consequences occur. The degree of consequence is largely dependent on the degree of mobility impairment and length of time the impairment exists. As a general rule , the greater the extent and length of time, the greater the physiological consequences. A state of complete immobility has a significant impact on the entire body; literally all body systems are affected (Table 26-1).

Cardiovascular Complications

Cardiovascular complications occur both with central and with peripheral perfusion. A lack of physical activity results in reduced cardiac capacity. According to one study, a 15% reduction in muscle mass will occur after 12 weeks of complete immobility.[7] This translates to reduced force of cardiac contraction and a reduction in cardiac output. The loss of endurance and the deconditioned state present challenges when the resumption of physical activity is desired.

Problems also occur within the vascular system. Decreased efficiency of orthostatic neurovascular reflexes and diminished vasopressor mechanism cause orthostatic hypotension intolerance when an individual attempts to attain an upright position because of blood pooling in the extremities.[5] Adequate perfusion and venous return depend on skeletal muscle contraction and frequent changes in body position. Because muscular contraction (particularly in the legs) facilitates venous return, venous stasis occurs during periods of inactivity. Slowed blood flow provides an opportunity for the formation of blood clots. Deep vein thrombosis is a relatively common complication associated with immobility.

Respiratory Complications

Physical activity is associated with full lung expansion, particularly among those engaging in exercise. Immobility contributes to reduced lung expansion and eventually leads to atelectasis (an airless state of the alveoli) and reduced capacity for gas exchange. Pooling of respiratory secretions, coupled with a reduced cough effort, places the immobilized patient at risk for stasis pneumonia.

Musculoskeletal Complications

Muscle tone, joint movement, and maintenance of bone density require active skeletal contraction and weight bearing. Skeletal muscle adapts to nonuse by reducing mass. Thus, prolonged immobility leads to significant reductions in muscle mass and atrophy; in fact, an average loss of 25% muscle mass occurs with permanent immobility.[7] The lack of activity leads to contracture in the joint, primarily as a result of muscle shortening. Muscle atrophy and joint contraction are particularly concerning because together these negatively affect functional ability.[8]

The lack of weight bearing leads to bone demineralization and calcium loss from the skeletal system. The degree of bone demineralization and calcium depletion is related to the severity and duration of immobility as well as the degree of weight-bearing ability. Over time, osteoporosis can develop in response to immobility.

Integument System

Sustained pressure on the skin reduces perfusion to the tissues. A reduced flow of oxygenated blood causes hypoxia of the tissues and increases the risk for skin breakdown. Individuals who lack the ability to move in bed have increased risk not only because of pressure but also because of shearing forces that often accompany certain positions or occur during transfers. These problems are further exacerbated if the patient has a poor nutritional status and is incontinent. Development of pressure ulcers commonly results.

Gastrointestinal Complications

Constipation is a frequently reported complication of immobility for several reasons. First, not being able to assume an optimal upright position makes having a bowel movement more challenging; for many people, relying on the assistance of others to have a bowel movement is embarrassing and may lead to reluctance in acting on the urge. From a physiological standpoint, the gastrointestinal tract slows during states of immobility, resulting in reduced peristaltic motility. Constipation, reduced appetite, and anorexia negatively impact nutritional status.

Urinary Complications

Immobility leads to three common problems that occur within the urinary system: renal calculi, urinary stasis, and infection. Renal calculi result from stasis of urine in the renal pelvis and because of increased circulating serum calcium levels (as a result of bone reabsorption mentioned previously). The bladder loses tone, making it difficult to completely empty the bladder, particularly in a lying position for voiding. This often results in urinary tract infection because the presence of urinary stasis provides an optimal environment for the growth of bacteria.

Psychological Effects

Acute and chronic psychological conditions that result from immobility include boredom, depression, feelings of helplessness/hopelessness, grieving, anxiety, anger, disturbed body image, and decreased verbal and nonverbal communication. Individuals who are unable to work or are even unable to meet basic activities of daily living often experience a loss of self-worth or value associated with the role change. Social isolation and mood disturbances are common.

Psychological effects of immobility are especially concerning among children. For children, physical activity is integral to daily activity. Not only is it essential for physical growth and development but also it is central to expression, communication, and making sense of the world around them. Immobilization can interfere with intellectual and psychomotor function. Emotional responses range from anger and aggressive behavior to passive quiet demeanor and withdrawal. Developmental regression is common. Children often become less communicative and may experience depression; in some cases, hallucinations occur.[6]

RISK FACTORS

Populations at Risk

All individuals are potentially at risk for altered mobility regardless of age, ethnicity, race, or socioeconomic status. Because of the effects of aging, the population group at greatest risk for impaired mobility is older adults. These changes predispose older individuals to a greater incidence of falls and greater challenges regaining full mobility following a period of impaired mobility. An estimated 90% of hip fractures are a result of falling; 76% of hip fractures occur among elderly women.[9]

Individual Risk Factors

Individual risk factors for changes in mobility are often attributed to acute and chronic conditions, chronic pain, and injury/trauma. Specifically, individuals with orthopedic injury, congenital deformities, neurologic disorders, strokes, head injury, spinal injury or deformities, nutritional deficiencies, cardiopulmonary conditions, and end-stage cancer are particularly susceptible. Side effects and adverse effects of many medications (e.g., corticosteroids and chemotherapy) and medical treatments can also affect mobility.

ASSESSMENT

History

The history, as it relates to the concept of mobility, includes general health information (past health history, medications, and surgery/treatments) and social history (lifestyle, employment, family assessment, and activities of daily living) as a starting point.[10] In addition, the history includes an investigation of specific symptoms experienced by the patient. Areas of questions specific for mobility include the following:

- Presence of pain with movement
- Recent changes in mobility or problems with balance
- Presence of fatigue
- Recent falls
- Recent changes in ability to complete activity of daily living

Examination Findings

Objective data regarding the assessment of the musculoskeletal system include an assessment of gait and body posture; joints; size, symmetry, and strength of muscles; and range of motion of joints.[10] Pediatric assessment also involves observation of motor activities as related to developmental milestones.[6]

Expected findings include erect posture and symmetry of extremities. Gait should be smooth, coordinated, and balanced. The spine should be straight with expected curvatures. Muscles and joints should be assessed for size, symmetry, strength, range of motion, and stability. Comparisons are made between right and left sides.[10] Assessment of muscle strength is done utilizing a muscle strength scale (0 = no detection of muscular contraction; 5 = full muscle strength). Findings considered abnormal include observed deformity of bone or joint, edema, ecchymosis, localized warmth and redness, a loss of function, numbness, guarding (due to pain), and limitations in movement or mobility. Further information related to conducting an assessment of the musculoskeletal system can be found in physical assessment textbooks.

Diagnostic Tests

Many diagnostic tests are used to evaluate musculoskeletal disorders. These are briefly described next.

Radiographic Diagnostics

- The x-ray evaluates the integrity of bones and joints and is the most common radiographic test used to diagnose fractures.
- Computed tomography scan identifies soft tissue and bony abnormalities and evaluates musculoskeletal trauma.
- Magnetic resonance imaging uses radio waves and magnetic fields to provide an image of soft tissue. This is used most efficiently to evaluate soft tissues, such as a vertebral disk, tumor, ligaments, and cartilage.[11]
- Myelogram is a radiographic study of the spinal cord and nerve root using a contrast dye. This is particularly useful in the evaluation of individuals with back pain.
- Arthrography (arthrogram) is a visualization of a joint by injection of a radiopaque substance into the joint cavity, allowing for the evaluation of bones, cartilage, and ligaments. This is most commonly performed on the knee and shoulder joints, but it also can be done on hips, ankles, and wrists.[11]
- Bone mineral density is a diagnostic test used to determine the core mineral content and the density of bone. This test is used for the diagnosis of osteoporosis and osteopenia.
- Bone scan evaluates the bone uptake of a radionuclide material; the uptake is related to the metabolism of the bone. The primary indication of this test is to detect metastatic cancer in the bone,[11] but it is also used to evaluate avascular necrosis or unexplained bone pain.

Other Diagnostic Tests

- Arthroscopy is a procedure that allows direct visualization of the interior of a joint through an endoscope. This procedure is most commonly performed on the knee, but it can be done on other joints as well.

- Electromyography is an evaluation of electrical activity generated within the muscle. This is used to determine the quality of neuromuscular innervation.

- Laboratory tests can be used to provide various types of information about the functional state of muscles, bones, or joints. Types of tests include blood tests (e.g., alkaline phosphatase, calcium, phosphorus, uric acid, creatine kinase, blood urea nitrogen, creatinine, and myoglobinuria), analysis of joint fluids, and pathologic analysis of biopsied tissue (e.g., a muscle biopsy or bone biopsy).

CLINICAL MANAGEMENT

Primary Prevention

Regular physical activity is associated with multiple health benefits and is foundational to primary prevention measures.[12,13] Prevention of problems associated with mobility is relatively simple—that is, maintaining the highest level of regular physical activity possible along with optimal nutrition, keeping an ideal body weight, and getting adequate rest. Taking measures to prevent injury and trauma are also considered primary prevention strategies.

Nutrition, as a primary prevention strategy, links to musculoskeletal development. During infancy, childhood, and adolescence, adequate protein and calcium in the diet are critical for the musculoskeletal development described previously. Adequate calcium intake is also necessary to prevent osteoporosis among older individuals. Maintaining a healthy body weight prevents excessive joint strain and is associated with fewer problems with back pain. Falls represent one of the most common mobility problems among older adults; thus, fall prevention is an important aspect of primary prevention. Strategies include participating in regular physical activity (to maintain muscle strength and balance), making the environment safer (e.g., avoiding hazards, using hand rails, wearing sturdy shoes with nonslip soles, and having adequate lighting), and optimizing vision.[9]

Secondary Prevention (Screening)

The primary areas to highlight related to mobility and screening are osteoporosis, mobility screening, and fall risk assessment. For osteoporosis screening, the U.S. Preventive Services Task Force (USPSTF) recommends screening of women age 65 years or older as well as younger women who have increased fracture risk; dual-energy x-ray absorptiometry of the hip and spine is the recommended method to measure bone density. There is no recommendation for the screening interval.[14] Furthermore, USPSTF concludes that evidence is insufficient to recommend screening for men.[14]

A large number of mobility and fall risk assessment screening tools are available. Scott and colleagues reviewed 38 different fall and mobility assessment tests for use among older adults and concluded that most are reliable. However, they were unable to conclude whether one screening test was better than another because of the wide range of settings for use.[15] One of the most common screening tests is the Timed Get Up and Go test, which measures mobility in people who are able to walk on their own (assistive devices allowed).[16] Another common screening is the Performance-Oriented Mobility Assessment test,[17] which aids in the identification of gait and balance impairments. Mobility scales, such as the Greenville Early Mobility Scale, are used in inpatient settings to track the status and progress of a patient's mobility, thus enhancing the effectiveness of mobility interventions among interdisciplinary teams.[18]

CLINICAL NURSING SKILLS FOR MOBILITY

- Assessment
  - General assessment
  - Mobility assessment
- Patient handling/transfers
- Positioning
- Range-of-motion exercises
- Continuous passive motion
- Sequential compression device and elastic stockings
- Ambulation
- Assistive devices
  - Cane
  - Crutches
  - Walker
  - Wheelchair
- Patient handling technology
  - Mats
  - Slings
  - Lifts
- Traction
- Heat and cold therapy
- Immobilization devices
- Medication administration

Collaborative Interventions

Numerous interventions for the care of individuals with limitations in mobility exist and are usually presented based on the underlying medical condition or diagnosis. Interventions specific for a health condition associated with changes or loss in mobility often overlap. From a conceptual perspective, a general discussion of interventions delivered by various members of the health care team that address mobility impairments includes several categories, such as care of the immobilized patient, exercise therapy, pharmacologic agents, surgical interventions, immobilization, and assistive devices.

Patients with impaired mobility are at risk for injury when interventions are not carried out properly. Likewise, health care workers caring for patients with mobility impairment are at risk for occupational injury—often caused by manually moving a patient. National standards for safe patient handling and mobility, released by the American Nurses Association in 2013, are designed to improve the safety of patients and health care workers. The standards were developed by an interprofessional working group and are intended to provide a blueprint to adopt a safe patient handling and mobility program that can be adapted to any health care setting and with any patient population. Included in the standards are establishing a culture of safety, education and training, application of ergonomic principles in the care environment, patient-centered assessment, and integration of safe patient handling technology in the care environment.[19]

Care of Immobilized Patient

An important overarching principle to emphasize is the need for early mobility. Early mobility requires a cultural mindset among interdisciplinary teams to overcome challenges and barriers associated with patient mobility. Barriers to early mobility include patient factors (excessive sedation or delirium, morbid obesity, and multiple invasive devices) and care delivery factors (fragmented care, availability of adequate equipment, time constraints, adequate number of providers, and concerns for patient safety).[20]

Many nursing interventions are incorporated into care for the immobilized patient, regardless of the underlying condition. Progressive mobility refers to the application of a mobility plan involving a series of gradual progressive interventions and activities that include positioning, turning, continuous lateral rotation therapy (CLRT), range-of-motion exercise, head elevation, tilt table, chair position, dangling, and ambulation. First, the patient should be positioned with appropriate *body alignment*. This is important to prevent injury to extremities and joints and is critical to prevent pulmonary complications. For example, pillows are commonly used to support the body alignment of a patient placed in a Sims position. The patient should be *repositioned* at least once every 2 hours. Principles of safe patient handling should be applied when patients are moved for repositioning. The patient dependent on caregivers for positioning is at significant risk for skin breakdown because of prolonged pressure over bony prominences. Thus, *skin care* is a priority for immobilized patients; the skin should be kept clean, dry, and protected to prevent skin breakdown. The skin is regularly monitored and examined for evidence of adequate circulation.

Because immobilized patients are at risk for stasis pneumonia, coughing and deep breathing are part of the standard treatment plan. Patients with adequate cognition are encouraged to use an incentive spirometer every hour to maintain ventilator capacity. Rotational bed therapy and CLRT have been shown to reduce the incidence of pneumonia among patients receiving mechanical ventilation in intensive care settings.[21,22]

Bed exercises should be encouraged to the extent possible to minimize atrophy and maintain joint movement. Many types of exercise can be done, including flexion and extension of the foot to promote venous blood return and prevent venous stasis.[23] If a patient has a trapeze bar over the bed, pull-up exercise should be encouraged if he or she is able. Range-of-motion (ROM) exercise is critical to promote circulation and to minimize complications to the joints.[23] Active ROM is performed by the patient; assisted ROM involves a patient doing most of the exercise but under the guidance/assistance of a health professional. Passive ROM involves the nurse taking each affected joint through the full range of motion. It is important not to force the joints past the point of resistance. If tolerated, patients should be encouraged to stand at the side of the bed to promote weight bearing. Doing this a few times a day for a few minutes helps to reduce bone demineralization.

Exercise Therapy

Exercise therapy is a cornerstone intervention in the management of individuals with impairments in mobility. Several forms of exercise therapy exist, including the following: Exercise Therapy: Ambulation, Exercise Therapy: Joint Mobility, Exercise Therapy: Stretching, and Exercise Therapy: Balance. Exercise therapy is performed by nurses or physical therapists in acute care, community-based, and home care settings. The goal of exercise therapy is rehabilitative or preventive, and it is often done in multiple combinations. There are many examples of exercise therapy, such as ROM exercises mentioned previously, water exercise, and gait training. Specific exercise therapy interventions are created based on patient needs in collaboration with physicians, nurses, physical therapists, and occupational therapists.

Pharmacologic Agents

Many of the drugs used to treat mobility problems are for the relief of pain or inflammation or to treat underlying conditions. It is beyond the scope of this concept presentation to describe each drug separately, but general categories are briefly presented.

Anti-inflammatory agents. Inflammation is a common primary or secondary finding among conditions leading to changes in mobility, from an underlying autoimmune condition to a traumatic injury. Anti-inflammatory agents, such as corticosteroids and nonsteroidal anti-inflammatory drugs (NSAIDs), are by far the most commonly used. Another group of agents used to reduce inflammation are the immunomodulators. These function to weaken or modulate the activity of the immune system, thereby decreasing the inflammatory response.

Analgesics and muscle relaxants. Although a reduction in inflammation provides some relief of discomfort associated with inflammation, analgesic agents are an important component of drug therapy. Agents that are specific for analgesia include opioids (e.g., morphine), NSAIDs, and aspirin. Although not considered analgesics, muscle relaxants provide relief from discomfort by eliminating muscle spasms.

Supplements. In addition to adequate dietary intake, nutritional supplementation with vitamin D and calcium is a useful prevention and treatment measure for osteoporosis, particularly for postmenopausal women. Bisphosphonates are antiresorptive agents that slow or stop the reabsorption of calcium from the bone, resulting in maintained or increased bone density and strength. These agents are used to treat osteoporosis.

Surgical Interventions

Many conditions that affect mobility are treated with surgical intervention. Surgical intervention can be either curative or palliative, depending on the underlying cause.[23] Examples of surgical interventions related to mobility/immobility include arthroscopic procedures, open and/or closed reduction of a fracture with or without external and/or internal fixation, amputation, synovectomy, osteotomy, debridement, arthroplasty, arthrodesis, diskectomy, and spinal fusion. Specific details about these procedures can be found in medical–surgical textbooks.

Immobilization

Following an injury or surgery, immobilization of a joint or bone is often necessary to provide stability and hold the appendage in place so that healing can occur. Following a fracture, for example, bone remodeling takes several weeks before the fracture is stable. Immobilization is necessary to enhance the healing process, protect the bone from further injury, and provide comfort to the patient. Common examples of immobile devices include casts, splints, abductor pillows, shoulder restraints, braces, and traction. Assessment to verify adequate perfusion (the presence of pulse and/or rapid capillary refill in nail beds), movement, and sensation is critical. Another indication for immobilization is to prevent injury. For example, for all patients with suspected spinal injury, spinal immobilization is routinely applied in the prehospital setting by strapping the patient on a backboard and using a cervical collar to prevent head rotation.[24]

Assistive Devices and Patient Handling Technology

Assistive devices are objects to provide assistance with a task. Many types of assistive devices are commonly used in patient care, including assistive devices for ambulation and assistive devices for activities of daily living. Common ambulation assistive devices include canes, crutches, walkers, wheelchairs, and prostheses.[25] Patients must be taught to use these devices correctly to avoid injury.

Patient handling technology refers to a variety of equipment in the care environment designed to assist with the handling and movement of patients. Examples include transfer mats, slings, and lifts. Education and training on indications and use of these devises, including assessment and decision algorithms for equipment selection, are essential to ensure the safety of the patient and the health care providers.

Causes

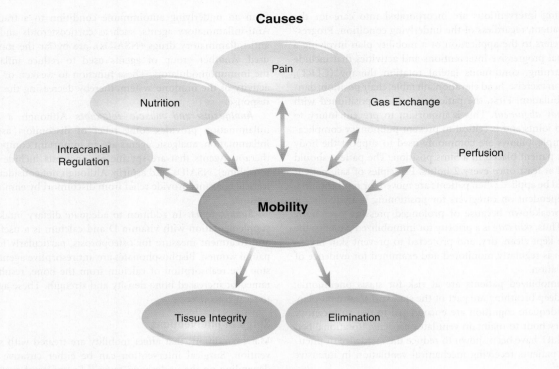

FIGURE 26-3 Cause-and-Effect Model: Mobility and Interrelated Concepts

INTERRELATED CONCEPTS

Mobility links to numerous concepts. Those considered most important are shown in Figure 26-3 and discussed further.

Individuals who have inadequate **Gas Exchange** may experience reduced mobility because of excessive fatigue. Immobile patients are at risk of developing complications associated with gas exchange, such as stasis pneumonia due to reduced lung expansion. The brain controls movement, coordination, and balance. Thus, optimal mobility is dependent on an intact neurologic system. Individuals who have problems associated with **Intracranial Regulation** may become immobile as a result of unsteadiness, imbalance, or the inability to initiate or execute purposeful movement to the arms, legs, or trunk. Individuals who are immobile may be unable to purchase, prepare, and/or consume adequate **Nutrition**; likewise, individuals with inadequate nutrition may have decreased mobility because of excessive fatigue. Malnutrition can lead to muscle wasting and bone loss. In addition, individuals experiencing extended immobility often experience reduced appetite. **Pain** (acute or chronic) may interfere with mobility. For example, an individual with chronic pain associated with cancer or back pain may experience changes in mobility as a pain management strategy. Likewise, some conditions that are directly associated with immobility (e.g., a fracture) are very painful. Individuals who have impaired **Perfusion** are less able to be mobile because of reduced oxygenated blood reaching peripheral tissues. Among individuals who are immobile, perfusion is less effective because of reduced venous return (which increases the risk for venous clots) and because of extended pressure on tissue. Immobility is a significant risk factor for impaired **Tissue Integrity**. Extended pressure on bony prominences reduces the perfusion of oxygenated blood (especially on the sacrum, hips, elbows, and heel), and skin sheering from movement and transfers may occur, particularly with

extended immobility. Individuals who are immobile may have changes to their pattern of **Elimination** or be at risk of experiencing problems such as constipation or urinary retention. This often leads to discomfort and reduced appetite that could negatively affect nutritional intake.

CLINICAL EXEMPLARS

Many clinical exemplars related to mobility and impaired mobility exist and are seen in all population groups. The following featured exemplars provide a brief explanation of classic conditions causing immobility. Detailed explanations and the nursing care for these conditions are presented in medical–surgical, pediatric, and gerontology resources. Box 26-1 presents additional common exemplars across the lifespan.

Featured Exemplars

Osteoarthritis

Osteoarthritis (OA) is caused by gradual degenerative changes of the joint (cartilage, joint lining, ligaments, and bone), usually affecting weight-bearing joints (hips, knees, and vertebra) and hands. These changes lead to pain, swelling, and reduced mobility of the joint. It most commonly affects middle-aged and older adults and typically begins after age 40 years; OA is estimated to affect 33% of adults older than age 65 years.[26]

Rheumatoid Arthritis

Rheumatoid arthritis (RA) is a systemic autoimmune condition with genetic predisposition that creates an inflammatory process in the synovial membrane of the joints and other body tissues. Over time, the joint inflammation leads to erosion of the membrane and cartilage, causing pain, swelling, and joint deformity; significant

BOX 26-1 EXEMPLARS OF IMPAIRED MOBILITY

Congenital Defects
- Club foot
- Developmental dysplasia of the hip
- Metatarsus adductus
- Spina bifida
- Syndactyly

Skeletal Conditions
- Amputation
- Fracture
- Fibrosarcoma
- Osteosarcoma
- Osteomyelitis
- Osteoporosis
- Osteogenesis imperfecta
- Rickets

Muscle Conditions
- Disuse atrophy
- Fibromyalgia
- Myotonia

- Myositis
- Rhabdomyoma
- Rhabomyosarcoma

Back and Spine Conditions
- Spinal cord injury
- Herniated disk
- Low back pain (acute/chronic)
- Scoliosis
- Spinal stenosis

Neuromuscular Dysfunction
- Amyotrophic lateral sclerosis
- Cerebral palsy
- Guillain–Barré syndrome
- Huntington's disease
- Multiple sclerosis
- Muscular dystrophy
- Myasthenia gravis
- Parkinson's disease

Joint and Connective Tissue Conditions
- Sprains
- Tendonitis
- Joint dislocation
- Osteoarthritis
- Rheumatoid arthritis
- Juvenile idiopathic arthritis
- Gout

---

impairment in mobility can result. Affecting less than 1% of the general population, RA is most common among women and individuals older than age 60 years.[26]

Juvenile Idiopathic Arthritis

Juvenile idiopathic arthritis (JIA) represents a group of diseases characterized by chronic inflammation of joints from autoimmune conditions. Depending on severity and duration, JIA can cause significant disability, with joint deformity, mobility impairments, and physical disability. It affects children younger than age 16 years, with a peak onset between ages 1 and 2 and girls affected at a rate twice that of boys. Although JIA eventually becomes inactive in the majority of cases, nearly 30% of children affected will have progressive arthritis into adulthood.[26]

Bone Fracture

Bone fracture refers to a partial or complete disruption in the bone structure. Interruption of bone structure leads to a reduction or loss in movement and pain. Although fractures are usually the result of traumatic injury, spontaneous fractures can occur in the presence of bone disease (e.g., osteoporosis or a neoplasm). Fractures occur at any age, but they are unusual during infancy. Most fractures occur in children and adolescents and adults older than age 65 years (wrist and hip fractures as a result of falls).

Parkinson's Disease

Parkinson's disease (PD) is a neurologic disorder associated with a loss of dopamine production in the brain. This disorder leads to changes in mobility resulting from muscular tremor, rigidity of the extremities and trunk, slowness of movement, and impaired coordination and balance. Mobility impairment increases with disease progression. Typically, PD affects adults older than age 50 years, with a higher incidence among men than women.

Spinal Cord Injury

Spinal cord injury (SCI) is an injury to the spinal cord that runs through the spinal column. Depending on the degree of injury, SCI may result in temporary or permanent neurologic impairment and mobility. The primary cause of SCI is traumatic injury from motor vehicle accidents, falls, sports injury, or personal violence. SCI can occur at any age, but males between ages 15 and 30 years account for the highest percentage of those affected.[27]

Low Back Pain

Low back pain is one of the most common conditions affecting mobility; nearly all individuals experience low back pain at some point during their life. Back pain generally is caused by muscle, bone, or nerve irritation from a variety of conditions, including muscle strain or spasm, degenerative conditions (e.g., arthritis, stenosis, or intervertebral disc disease), and trauma; it is also a common symptom in late-term pregnancy. Severe back pain can be debilitating and can significantly impair mobility. Back pain can occur in all age groups, but it is most common between ages 30 and 50 years.

CASE STUDY

Case Presentation

Source: Stockbyte/Digital Vision/ Thinkstock

Mrs. Lydia Martin, an 88-year-old widow, lives alone independently in her single-story home. During the middle of the night, Mrs. Martin fell in her home while walking to the bathroom. Unable to get up, she crawled to reach her phone and dialed 911. She was transported to the emergency department and underwent diagnostic tests including hip and femur x-ray and computerized tomography, which confirmed a left femoral neck fracture. Her past medical history includes anxiety, osteoporosis, arthritis, and cataracts.

Mrs. Martin underwent an open reduction internal fixation procedure. Following surgery, she had a compression dressing with ice to the left hip, a Foley catheter, anti-embolism stockings, a sequential compression device, and an order to use the incentive spirometer every hour while awake. Her medications included hydrocodone bitartrate 7.5 mg/acetaminophen 750 mg (Vicodin ES) two tabs by mouth every 4 hours as needed for pain and enoxaparin (Lovenox) 40 mg daily subcutaneously.

The day after surgery, the physical therapist began to work with Mrs. Martin; the goal of the session was to get her out of bed to a chair. During the attempted transfer, Mrs. Martin's surgical site was painful, and her Foley catheter was pulled, causing pelvic pain. She screamed in pain and refused to continue the process. Mrs. Martin was anxious and fearful of pain and also became worried that she would never walk again and would end up in a nursing home. She was unwilling to move and declined physical therapy the next 3 days. Mrs. Martin became constipated and lost her appetite. She also developed a stage 2 pressure ulcer over her sacrum. Eventually, on post-op day 4, Mrs. Martin agreed to work with the physical therapist. By this time, she experienced significant weakness and fatigue and was unable to move independently. Mrs. Martin was later transferred to a rehabilitation center to continue regaining her mobility.

Case Analysis

This case exemplifies the concept of mobility in many ways. Mrs. Martin's age and injury were significant risk factors for a fall and hip fracture. Following surgery, she was immobile for several days because of pain and experienced several consequences of immobility, including constipation, loss of appetite, poor nutrition, and impaired skin integrity.

ACCESS EXEMPLAR LINKS IN YOUR GIDDENS EBOOK

REFERENCES

1. Venes D, editor: *Taber's cyclopedic medical dictionary*, ed 22, Philadelphia, 2013, Davis.
2. Ackley BJ, Ladwig GB: *Nursing diagnosis handbook*, ed 9, St Louis, 2010, Mosby.
3. Bortz WM: The disuse syndrome. *Western J Med* 141:691–694, 1984.
4. Copstead LC: *Pathophysiology*, ed 5, St Louis, 2013, Saunders.
5. McCance KL, Huether SE: *Pathophysiology: The biologic basis for disease in adults and children*, ed 7, St Louis, 2014, Elsevier.
6. Hockenberry MJ, Wilson D: *Wong's essentials of pediatric nursing*, ed 9, St Louis, 2013, Mosby.
7. Hill J: Cardiac plasticity: Mechanisms of disease. *N Engl J Med* 358:1370–1380, 2008.
8. Kasper CE: Skeletal muscle atrophy. In Carrieri-Kohlman V, Lindsey AM, West CM, editors: *Pathophysiological phenomena in nursing*, St Louis, 2003, Saunders.
9. Centers for Disease Control and Prevention: Hip fractures among older adults, 2014. Available at <http://www.cdc.gov/homeandrecreationalsafety/falls/adulthipfx.html>.
10. Wilson S, Giddens J: *Health assessment for nursing practice*, ed 5, St Louis, 2013, Elsevier.
11. Pagana KD, Pagana TJ: *Mosby's manual of diagnostic and laboratory tests*, ed 5, St Louis, 2014, Elsevier.
12. U.S. Department of Health and Human Services: Healthy People 2020, 2010: Available at <http://www.healthypeople.gov>.
13. Pender N, Murdaugh C, Parsons MA: *Health promotion in nursing practice*, ed 7, Upper Saddle River, NJ, 2015, Pearson.
14. U.S. Preventive Services Task Force: The guide to clinical preventative services, 2014. Accessed at <http://www.uspreventiveservicestaskforce.org>.
15. Scott V, Votova K, Scanlan A, et al: Multifactorial and functional mobility assessment tools for fall risk among older adults in community,

home-support, long-term and acute care settings. *Age Aging* 36(2): 130–139, 2007.
16. Wall JC, Bell BS, Campbell S, et al: The timed get-up-and-go test revisited: Measurement of component tasks. *J Rehabil Res Dev* 37(1): 109–111, 2000.
17. Tinetti ME: Performance-oriented assessment of mobility problems in elderly patients. *J Am Geriatr Soc* 34:119–126, 1986.
18. Czaplijski T, Marshburnm D, Hobs T, et al: Creating a culture of mobility: An interdisciplinary approach for hospitalized patients. *Hosp Top* 92(3):74–79, 2014.
19. American Nurses Association: *Safe patient handling and mobility: Interprofessional national standards across the care continuum*, Washington, DC, 2013, Author.
20. Morris PE: Moving our critically ill patients: Mobility barriers and benefits. *Crit Care Clin* 23(1):1–20, 2007.
21. Goldhill DR, Imhoff M, McLean B, et al: Rotational bed therapy to prevent and treat respiratory complications: A review and meta-analysis. *Am J Crit Care* 16(1):50–61, 2007.
22. Wanless S, Matthew A: Continuous lateral rotation therapy—A review. *Nurs Crit Care* 12(1):28–35, 2011.
23. Lewis SL, Bucher L, Heitkemper M: *Medical–surgical nursing: Assessment and management of clinical problems*, ed 9, St Louis, 2014, Elsevier.
24. Peery CA, Brice J, White WD: Prehospital spinal immobilization and the backboard quality assessment study. *Prehosp Emerg Care* 11(3):293–297, 2007.
25. Kedlaya D: Assistive devices to improve independence, 2008: Retrieved from Medscape Reference, <http://emedicine.medscape.com/article/325247-overview>.
26. Centers for Disease Control and Prevention: Arthritis, 2014. Retrieved from <http://www.cdc.gov/arthritis>.
27. Centers for Disease Control and Prevention: Spinal cord injury fact sheet, 2014. Retrieved from <http://www.cdc.gov/TraumaticBrainInjury/scifacts.html>.

Tissue Integrity

Debra Hagler

The skin, the largest organ of the body, supports critical life functions, including management of temperature, conservation of fluid, and protection from infection.[1] Maintenance of skin and tissue integrity is a fundamental component of nursing care. Not only do nurses play a pivotal role in maintaining skin and tissue integrity but they also contribute independently and collaboratively to the care management when that integrity is disrupted.

DEFINITION

Tissues are organized groups of cells with common functions. Of the four types of tissues—muscle, neural, connective, and epithelial—the concept of tissue integrity is most closely aligned with epithelial tissue. The term *impaired skin integrity* is specifically focused on damage to the epidermal and dermal layers of epithelial tissue, but deep damage to skin integrity is associated with disruption of underlying tissues. For the purposes of this concept, tissue integrity is defined as *the state of structurally intact and physiologically functioning epithelial tissues such as the integument (including the skin and subcutaneous tissue) and mucous membranes.* The term *impaired tissue integrity* reflects varying levels of damage to one or more of those groups of cells.[2,3]

SCOPE

The concept of tissue integrity ranges from an intact state serving as the body's protective barrier to some level of disrupted or impaired surface. Disrupted tissue integrity ranges from superficial or partial-thickness injury of the epidermis to deep or full-thickness injury of the dermis and deeper tissues (Figure 27-1). Individuals at all points across the lifespan experience disruptions to tissue integrity.

NORMAL PHYSIOLOGICAL PROCESS

Epithelial cells join to cover nearly every internal and external surface of the body, providing protection from the external environment, absorption of needed substances, secretion into body cavities, and excretion of wastes from the body. The skin, as an external surface, protects other body tissues and organs from mechanical trauma, fluid loss, chemical disruption, and infectious organisms. The nerves in the skin layer provide a safety mechanism as sensations of pain, temperature, and touch inform a person about the environment and reveal the need to take actions that prevent or limit damage to the body. The integument is made up of the two layers commonly known as skin—the epidermis and the dermis—and the underlying subcutaneous or fat tissue (Figure 27-2). Sweat glands and the small muscles in the dermal layer that control piloerection (goosebumps) help to maintain body temperature in a fairly narrow range despite air temperature changes. Subcutaneous tissue, under the dermal layer, contains fat cells and additional sweat glands that assist in temperature regulation.

Mucous membranes are epithelial tissues continuous with the skin that line the eyelids, nose and mouth, ears, genital area, urethra, and anus. Some, but not all, mucous membranes secrete thick, slippery mucus that helps protect the body from infection.[4]

Age-Related Differences
Infants, Children, and Adolescents

Skin texture and function change over the course of the lifespan. Infants have thinner, more permeable skin with less subcutaneous fat than older children and adults, which leads to a greater potential for fluid loss and less effective temperature regulation. The skin texture of infants and young children is smooth and dry. Apocrine glands are nonfunctional until puberty. Adolescents experience increased apocrine sweat glands and sebaceous gland activity, resulting in more oily skin and acne.[5]

Older Adults

Several changes to the skin occur as a result of the aging process. The skin becomes thin with a decrease in strength, moisture, and elasticity. A decrease in underlying supportive structures such as lean muscle mass and subcutaneous fat often results in skin hanging loosely over other tissues. A diminished perception of pain may prevent early recognition of injury, and reduced arterial and venous blood flow to the tissues not only make skin more prone to injury but also may result in slow wound healing when a disruption of skin occurs. In addition, hair and nail growth slow with aging, and a decrease in sebaceous gland activity can result in rough, dry, and itchy skin.[4] The aging process of skin is partly due to genetics and race, but it is also largely

FIGURE 27-1 Scope of Concept Tissue integrity ranges from intact skin to partial-thickness injury and full-thickness injury.

associated with environmental exposure—particularly sun and wind exposure.

VARIATIONS AND CONTEXT

Six major categories of impaired tissue integrity are trauma/injury, loss of perfusion, immunologic reaction, infections and infestations, thermal or radiation injury, and lesions. Within each of these categories, partial- or full-thickness injury can occur.

Trauma/Injury

Tissue trauma or injury includes intentional and unintentional damage that can range from a superficial abrasion or scrape to a deep wound penetrating the skin and subcutaneous layers, with possible extension to muscle, internal organs, and bone. In areas where there is little or no subcutaneous tissue (e.g., the back of the hand, top of the foot, or the skull), a relatively minor blunt or penetrating injury may extend directly through the skin layers to the muscle or bone. A surgical incision is an example of an intentional injury to the skin, inflicted to reach deeper structures for a therapeutic purpose.

Loss of Perfusion

All tissue requires a continuous supply of oxygenated blood. The skin is relatively tolerant of poor circulation compared to other organs, and in times of shock it even survives a temporary shunting of oxygenated blood away from the skin to protect the perfusion of other organs such as the heart and brain. However, prolonged poor perfusion or a short period of no perfusion can lead to tissue necrosis. Examples of impaired tissue integrity resulting from a chronic state of poor perfusion include ulcerations, necrosis, and loss of digits. Examples of short-term or temporary disruption of perfusion to tissue caused by unrelieved pressure are dermal or pressure ulcers. Dermal ulcers are also described as bedsores, pressure sores, and pressure ulcers. Dermal ulcer is a more general term than pressure ulcer; dermal tissue damage may be caused by a number of factors, including excessive pressure on tissue, but a dermal ulcer is not necessarily caused by pressure.[2]

Immunologic Reaction

The skin is a visible indicator of an allergic response to a foreign substance, and the presence of redness, rash, or hives is a common way that allergies are first noted. Common substances that lead to skin irritation and/or local allergic response are soaps, detergents, cleaning products, fragrances, and metals such as nickel, silver, and copper.[4] In addition, many common skin disruptions, such as psoriasis, are thought to be chronic immune responses to unknown antigens. In rare cases, a hypersensitivity response to a medication can cause extensive tissue sloughing. Severe hypersensitivity disorders such as Stevens–Johnson syndrome or toxic epidermal necrolysis involve large areas of epidermal tissue sloughing with a high risk for life-threatening fluid loss, hypothermia, and infection.[1]

Infections and Infestations

Skin and mucous membrane infections can be the result of bacteria, fungi, or viruses. Live arthropods can cause tissue disruption by burrowing under the skin or attaching to skin structures such as hair shafts.

Bacterial Infection

Bacteria normally present on the skin generally cause no harm, but pathogenic bacteria can cause superficial or deep infection. A small abrasion or lesion can provide a portal for opportunistic or pathogenic infectious organisms to infect deeper tissues. Superficial skin infections involve only the dermis, but deeper bacterial infection causes cellulitis, an inflammation of the subcutaneous and potentially muscle tissues. Impetigo, caused by staphylococci or β-hemolytic streptococci, is the most common superficial bacterial infection, and it spreads easily among small children on contact. A common bacterial infection of the skin seen in adolescents is acne vulgaris.

Fungal Infections

The fungi that cause superficial fungal infections live on the dead skin cells of the epidermis. *Candida albicans* and other *Candida* species thrive in warm, moist areas of the skin and mucous membranes, particularly the mouth, the vagina, and the skin folds. In the absence of normal flora's bacterial protection on the skin or mucous membranes, *Candida* grow more readily. It is common for a person to experience a fungal infection with *Candida* after a course of antibiotics for a bacterial infection has decreased the normal protective flora and allowed the *Candida* to flourish. Tinea refers to a group of diseases caused by a fungus that vary in skin sites and the types of fungal species, such as tinea capitis on the head and tinea pedis (athlete's foot) on the feet.[4]

Viral Infections

Several viruses are known to cause a disruption in skin integrity. A common form of skin virus is the verruca, or wart. Although warts most commonly occur on the skin of the hands and feet, they also can be found on the genitalia. Herpes simplex virus (HSV) can infect the skin and mucous membranes; HSV type 1 (HSV-1) is more common on the face and mouth, whereas HSV-2 is more common on genital mucosa.[4]

Infestations

The skin can be infested with live arthropods such as mites and lice. The scabies mite burrows into the epidermis and lays eggs. Mites are transmitted person-to-person or through infested sheets or clothing, where they can live for up to 2 days. Lice most commonly infect the body, head, or pubic hair. Lice lay eggs along the hair shafts and are transmitted by personal contact, clothing and bedding, and shared hair care items or hats.

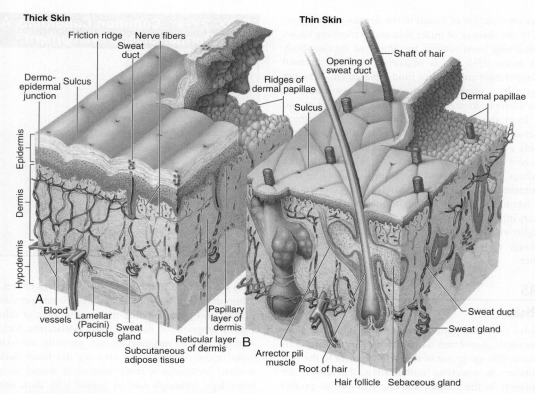

Thick Skin

Friction ridge — Nerve fibers
Sweat duct
Dermo-epidermal junction — Sulcus
Epidermis
Dermis
Hypodermis
A
Blood vessels — Lamellar (Pacini) corpuscle — Sweat gland
Subcutaneous adipose tissue — Reticular layer of dermis

Thin Skin

Opening of sweat duct — Shaft of hair
Ridges of dermal papillae
Sulcus — Dermal papillae
Papillary layer of dermis
B — Arrector pili muscle
Root of hair
Hair follicle — Sebaceous gland
Sweat duct
Sweat gland

FIGURE 27-2 Diagram of Skin Structure A, Thick skin, found on surfaces of the palms and soles of the feet. B, Thin skin, found on most surface areas of the body. In each diagram, the epidermis is raised at one corner to reveal the papillae of the dermis. (Source: From Patton KT, Thibodeau GA: *Anatomy and physiology*, ed 9, St Louis, 2016, Mosby.)

Thermal or Radiation Injury

Thermal and radiation injuries to the skin range from the common sunburn to extensive scald burns and radiation burns. Sunburn appears after the epidermis is exposed to excessive ultraviolet (UV) radiation. It appears as redness and inflammation, and it may extend to blistering with chills, fever, and pain, followed by peeling skin. Burns resulting from a scald with hot liquids or contact with flame/heated items cause a series of chemical and mechanical events at the tissue level. Radiation therapy, used to treat some forms of cancer, requires careful monitoring and skin care to prevent burns. The initial tissue response to burns is inflammation and vasoconstriction; edema at the site of a burn can last for several days. Later, fibroblasts produce the proteins collagen and elastin, which restore some structure and elasticity to the wound. Macrophages remove bacteria and foreign substances to clean the wound. New vascular networks form and new epithelial cells grow and cover the open area from the wound edges to the center as the wound begins to contract.[4]

Lesions

Lesions can range from benign skin growths and vascular lesions to invasive malignant tumors. The most common types of skin cancers are melanoma, basal cell, and squamous.[6] Benign skin growths may cause concern if they cause pressure on or displacement of other structures or change the person's appearance in a distressing way.

Expected Physiological Process for Wound Healing

Tissue injuries and wounds heal by processes of primary, secondary, or tertiary intention. Primary intention healing occurs when wound margins are well approximated, as in a sutured surgical incision or a simple laceration, and takes place more rapidly than the other types of healing. Secondary intention healing processes occur when wounds such as ulcerations have distant edges and granulation tissue gradually fills the gap to close the wound. Tertiary intention healing processes occur when a wound is sutured closed much later, resulting in more scarring than that which occurs for wounds closed with primary intention. Tertiary closure is used when a wound must stay open until infection or wound contamination is resolved; later, the clean wound is sutured to facilitate continued healing.

There are three phases of wound healing: inflammatory, granulation, and maturation. The inflammatory phase lasts 3–5 days while blood clots form at the site of injury and platelets release growth factors to begin the healing process. A matrix of cells and debris forms at the site and is later removed by macrophages. During the granulation phase, new vessels and collagen structures are formed, resulting in a very vascular pink wound. White blood cells continue to remove debris while epithelium begins to grow from the edges toward the center of the wound. The maturation phase of collagen fiber remodeling and scar contraction may continue for months or years.[7,8]

CONSEQUENCES

When tissue integrity is impaired, a number of body functions are affected, including thermoregulation, elimination, fluid and electrolyte balance, protection from infection, safety, comfort/pain, and body image. The skin normally regulates body temperature within a narrow range through the constriction or relaxation of piloerector muscles, vasodilation or vasoconstriction of vessels in the dermis, and the production of sweat. In the absence of intact skin and underlying tissue, such as an overwhelming burn surface, the ability to regulate body heat and prevent excess fluid loss is impaired, requiring external maintenance of temperature and massive fluid replacement. Whether the skin is disrupted by a small abrasion or a massive wound, that loss of the skin as a barrier means that underlying structures are no longer protected from the environment's infectious and chemical dangers. Even a small open wound provides a portal that could lead to an overwhelming infection if the person is immunocompromised or the infectious agent is particularly virulent. Loss of deep structures such as nerve endings prevents normal sensation that provides cues about the environment and helps promote safety during movement. Because the skin has many sensory nerve endings, particularly over the hands and face, injuries and lesions can be painful. Skin conditions are often highly visible to the individual and others, potentially affecting body image and provoking psychological distress about physical appearance.[2]

RISK FACTORS

Age-Related Risks

Some risk factors for skin disruptions are related to age or developmental level. For example, diaper rash is a common rash among infants and toddlers; likewise, this age group is at risk for injuries to the skin and mucosa secondary to uncertain mobilization, the affinity for placing various objects in the mouth, and the inability to protect themselves from environmental dangers. Communicable skin infections such as impetigo are more commonly transmitted where there is frequent skin-to-skin contact, such as in childcare centers or on playgrounds. School-age children may experience frequent minor tissue injuries such as abrasions, bruises, and small lacerations that occur during active play.

The changes to skin associated with aging are actually a result of sun and environmental damage over a long period of time, leading to a wrinkled and leathery appearance. Exposure of the skin to sun over an extended period of years increases the risk of skin cancers.[6] Older adults are also more prone to skin tears that can occur with minimal contact or pressure as a result of the thin, fragile texture.[7]

Individual Risk Factors

Many individual risk factors for tissue disruption are associated with underlying health conditions. Health conditions associated with poor peripheral perfusion, malnutrition, obesity, fluid deficit or excess, impaired physical mobility, and immunosuppression increase the risk of tissue disruption. In addition, exposure to chemical irritants, radiation, excessively hot or cold temperatures, and mechanical damage may cause a loss of tissue integrity. Individuals who have undergone medical treatments, surgical procedures, or invasive procedures have disruptions to skin and tissue integrity as a result of those procedures.

Genetics

A number of skin disorders are inherited and are often associated with an underlying metabolic condition or a chronic condition that affects many body systems. Examples of inheritable skin conditions include ichthyosis vulgaris, xeroderma pigmentosa, albinism, epidermolysis, ectodermal dysplasia, and incontinentia pigmenti.

Skin Cancer Risk

Basal cell skin cancer usually occurs in areas that have been exposed to the sun, such as the face, and is the most common skin cancer in light-skinned persons. Squamous cell skin cancer is usually found in

> **BOX 27-1   Common Conditions Associated with Dermal Ulcer Development**
>
> Spinal cord injury
> Stroke
> Traumatic brain injury
> Trauma
> Skeletal fractures
> Neuromuscular disorders
> Rheumatoid arthritis
> Parkinson's disease
> Multiple sclerosis
> Alzheimer's disease
> Heart failure
> Peripheral arterial disease
> Chronic obstructive pulmonary disease
> Diabetes (type 1 and type 2)

areas less exposed to the sun, such as the legs or feet, and is the most common type of skin cancer in dark-skinned persons. Melanoma is a virulent and potentially life-threatening form of skin cancer that has a good prognosis if detected early. Melanoma, which begins in the pigment cells or melanocytes, can grow on any skin surface and is found most commonly in men on the head, neck, and torso. In women, melanoma is more commonly found on the torso or the lower legs. Although rare in people with dark skin, when it does develop, melanoma is found under the nails and on the palms and soles. Fair-skinned men and women older than 65 years, persons with atypical moles, and those with more than 50 moles are at substantially increased risk for melanoma. Other risk factors for skin cancer include family history and a considerable history of sun exposure and sunburns.[9]

Dermal Ulcer Risk

In 2007, approximately 1 of every 100 residents of nursing homes was reported to have one or more pressure ulcers.[10] Risk factors for dermal ulcers include those with impaired cognition or sensory perception, immobility, friction and shearing, poor nutrition, impaired perfusion or oxygenation, impaired sensation, and incontinence/moisture. Certain medical conditions (many of which are associated with these risk factors) also are associated with increased risk (Box 27-1).

ASSESSMENT

The assessment of skin involves taking a history, conducting a skin examination, and performing diagnostic testing.

History

The health history begins with questions related to past and current conditions, medications, known allergies, and family history. Medications may cause rashes through an allergic reaction, a side effect, or by inducing hypersensitivity to sunlight. Box 27-2 lists specific information about tissue integrity to discuss during the health history.

Examination Findings
Inspection

Examination of the skin starts with inspection, which includes color and the presence of lesions. Normal adult skin is a consistent color, ranging for individuals from light pink to olive tones and deep brown, with relatively darker shades in areas of sun exposure. Oral and eye mucosa may appear pale pink to darker pink, red, or brown. Skin findings may vary by natural skin color; for example, cyanosis may appear

BOX 27-2 Health History Related to Tissue Integrity

- Previous history of skin disease
- Change in pigmentation
- Change in mole
- Change in nails
- Hair loss
- Excessive dryness or moisture
- Pruritus
- Excessive bruising
- Rash or lesion
- Self-care behaviors
- Medications
- Environmental or occupational hazards

Source: From Jarvis CL: *Physical examination and health assessment,* ed 7, Philadelphia, 2016, Saunders.

as a blue-gray color in light-skinned persons, whereas it appears as an ashen gray color in dark-skinned persons and is particularly visible in the nail beds and mucosa. The more visible areas for identifying generalized changes in skin color for a dark-skinned person are those with the least pigmentation, particularly the subglossal mucosa, the buccal mucosa, the palpebral conjunctiva, and the sclera.[5]

There is a wide range of types of skin lesions, including both normal variations and lesions that indicate possible disease. A bright light, a ruler, and a magnifying glass are helpful tools for skin inspection. Describe the lesions' location, size, shape, color, elevation, consistency, and pattern. Describe the grouping of multiple lesions in rings, lines, or diffusely scattered arrangements and the color, odor, and consistency of any exudates.[5]

Palpation

The skin should be smooth and intact with an even surface and minimal perspiration or oiliness except after exercise or heat exposure. There should not be dryness, peeling, or cracking, although there may be calluses over the hands, feet, elbows, and knees. Skin folds should not be excessively moist or macerated. Skin mobility and turgor are assessed by picking up and slightly pinching the skin on the forearm or under the clavicle. The skin should move easily when lifted and should return to place immediately when released. Checking for skin turgor using the older adult's hand may give a false impression of dehydration, so turgor should be checked in the forearm or under the clavicle instead. The loss of subcutaneous tissue in the hands causes an appearance of skin tenting even when hydration is normal.

Wound Assessment

Wounds may be caused by direct or indirect tissue injury. Assess the wound location, size, shape, and color as well as the color, odor, and consistency of any drainage or exudate.[7,8] Redness of the surrounding tissue, foul odor, or purulent drainage may indicate wound infection.

A surgical wound may be left open to the air or covered with a dressing to protect the wound site and absorb drainage. Covered wounds should be carefully assessed when the wound is exposed during dressing changes. If there is a wound drainage tube or system present, the amount and character of drainage can be described.[11]

Assessment of dermal ulcers. Dermal ulcers, a specific type of wound, are assessed for size and depth, as well as for level of tissue injury. Pressure ulcers are classified by four stages, presented in Box 27-3. If the dermal ulcer is covered with eschar, a dry scab covering, it is not possible to determine the stage of the wound. The eschar

BOX 27-3 NPUAP Pressure Ulcer Stages/Categories

Category/Stage I: Non-blanchable erythema
Intact skin with non-blanchable redness of a localized area usually over a bony prominence. Darkly pigmented skin may not have visible blanching; its color may differ from the surrounding area.
Category/Stage II: Partial thickness
Partial thickness loss of dermis presenting as a shallow open ulcer with a red pink wound bed, without slough. May also present as an intact or open/ruptured serum-filled or sero-sanguinous filled blister.
Category/Stage III: Full thickness skin loss
Full thickness tissue loss. Subcutaneous fat may be visible but bone, tendon or muscle are not exposed. Slough may be present but does not obscure the depth of tissue loss. May include undermining and tunneling.
Category/Stage IV: Full thickness tissue loss
Full thickness tissue loss with exposed bone, tendon or muscle. Slough or eschar may be present. Often includes undermining and tunneling.
Unstageable/Unclassified: Full thickness skin or tissue loss—depth unknown
Full thickness tissue loss in which actual depth of the ulcer is completely obscured by slough (yellow, tan, gray, green or brown) and/or eschar (tan, brown or black) in the wound bed.
Suspected Deep Tissue Injury—depth unknown
Purple or maroon localized area of discolored intact skin or blood-filled blister due to damage of underlying soft tissue from pressure and/or shear. The area may be preceded by tissue that is painful, firm, mushy, boggy, warmer or cooler as compared to adjacent tissue.

Source: From National Pressure Ulcer Advisory Panel: Pressure ulcer stages/categories revised by NPUAP, 2007. Used with permission of the National Pressure Ulcer Advisory Panel August 2015. Retrieved from http://www.npuap.org/resources/educational-and-clinical-resources/npuap-pressure-ulcer-stagescategories/

may have to be removed through pharmacologic, mechanical, or surgical debridement to allow for accurate assessment and to promote healing.

Diagnostic Tests

Only a few common diagnostic tests are linked to the concept of tissue integrity:

- *Patch testing:* This is a test used to identify specific allergens causing dermatitis. One or many potential allergens can be tested simultaneously by applying a small amount of the substance to a marked area of the skin, usually on the back.
- *Wound cultures:* Cultures identify the organisms causing infection. Because some bacteria are present on healthy skin, normal skin flora may be identified in wound cultures along with any pathogenic bacteria.
- *Tissue biopsy:* Various types of biopsies—such as punch, incision, excision, and shave—are conducted for pathologic evaluation of tissue when skin lesions are suspected to be malignant. The type and depth of biopsy are based on the lesion and the location.
- *Woods lamp:* Use of a Woods lamp (black light) or immunofluorescence enhances inspection with magnification and special lighting. It is used to identify the presence of infectious organisms and proteins.[7]

CLINICAL MANAGEMENT

Primary Prevention

Primary prevention measures guard against development of disease. Primary measures to prevent disrupted tissue integrity include hygiene, nutrition, and protection from excessive sun exposure or other environmental hazards.

General Skin Hygiene

Basic skin hygiene prevents many common skin irritations and infections. Infants and toddlers need frequent cleansing of hands and face to remove food residue and frequent perineal care to prevent irritation from urine and stool. During adolescence, sebaceous and sweat glands become more active; therefore, more frequent bathing becomes necessary to reduce body odors and oils. In older adults, sebaceous and sweat glands become less active again and skin loses some of its moisture and elasticity. Older adults may find that a complete daily bath with soap can cause excessively dry skin, and they may prefer to bathe less frequently and use a gentle moisturizing cleanser.

Hygiene practices are often linked to cultural norms and rituals. Although in North America it is common to bathe or shower daily and to use deodorant, people of a variety of cultures may prefer to bathe less frequently or not bathe when they are ill or after childbirth.[11]

Nutrition

Adequate protein, calories, minerals, vitamins, and hydration are needed for maintenance of healthy skin. In the chronic absence of adequate nutrition, skin becomes dry and flaky, hair appears dull, and subcutaneous fat disappears. Even a short period of poor nutrition, such as being unable to eat before and after surgery, can damage tissue integrity and delay wound healing.[8]

Sun Exposure

Box 27-4 lists National Cancer Institute[6] recommendations for skin cancer prevention through protection from sun exposure. Population-based interventions designed to increase sun-protective behaviors in recreational settings include offering culturally relevant educational materials and reminders at the entrances to the setting; providing sun-safety training for, and role modeling by, lifeguards, aquatic instructors, recreation staff, parents, and children; increasing the availability of shaded areas; and having sunscreen readily available.[12]

Burn Prevention

Smoke alarms should be installed and maintained to help prevent burns in the home setting. Hot-water temperature should be set at a maximum of 120°F to avoid scald burns. Infants and toddlers are at particular risk for burns. Parents should be advised not to carry an infant and hot liquids or foods at the same time. Milk and formula should not be heated in the microwave because the uneven temperatures can scald the infant's mouth. Young children should be kept away from hot oven doors, irons, wall heaters and grills, electrical cords, and cups or dishes of hot food. Older children should be taught stovetop and microwave oven safety.[13] Adults with decreased temperature sensation, such as in peripheral neuropathy, should test bath water with a thermometer before stepping in.

Dermal Ulcer Prevention

Prevention of pressure ulcers requires initial assessment and daily re-evaluation and documentation for inpatients at risk of pressure ulcer development using a tool such as the Braden Scale for Predicting Pressure Sore Risk.[14] The Braden scale consists of six subscales based on common causes of dermal ulcers: sensory perception, moisture, activity, mobility, nutrition, and friction and shear. Adults scoring less than 18 of 23 possible points on the Braden scale are considered at risk for dermal ulcers. The scale is often completed as part of a health care facility admission assessment and periodic reassessment. Persons found to be at higher risk should have more intensive preventive measures instituted. Those at risk in home settings can be taught to assess their own skin with the assistance of family members or caregivers. Prevention interventions include minimizing or eliminating friction and shear (e.g., sliding on sheets), minimizing pressure through frequent repositioning and use of pressure-relieving devices, managing moisture on skin surfaces, and maintaining adequate nutrition and hydration.[15]

Secondary Prevention (Screening)

Malignant melanoma is a particularly virulent type of skin cancer, but early detection and treatment improves the outcome. Use the mnemonic ABCDEF to remember the early signs of melanoma during a skin assessment, and teach the mnemonic to patients to guide their own comprehensive monthly skin self-assessments:[6]

- *Asymmetry*: The shape of one half does not match that of the other half.
- *Border that is irregular*: The edges are often ragged, notched, or blurred in outline. The pigment may spread into the surrounding skin.
- *Color that is uneven*: Shades of black, brown, and tan may be present. Areas of white, gray, red, pink, or blue may also be seen.
- *Diameter*: There is a change in size, usually an increase. Melanomas can be tiny, but most are larger than the size of a pea (larger than 6 mm or approximately ¼ in.).
- *Evolving*: The mole has changed during the past few weeks or months.

Collaborative Interventions
Pharmacotherapy

Medications for skin disorders include topical and oral or parenteral antibiotics, steroids, topical moisturizers, and anticancer agents or immunosuppressive chemotherapy.

BOX 27-4 Recommendations for Protection from Sun Exposure

- Avoid outdoor activities during the middle of the day. The sun's rays are the strongest between 10 AM and 4 PM. When you must be outdoors, seek shade.
- Protect yourself from the sun's rays reflected by sand, water, snow, ice, and pavement. The sun's rays can go through light clothing, windshields, windows, and clouds.
- Wear long sleeves and long pants. Tightly woven fabrics are best.
- Wear a hat with a wide brim all around that shades your face, neck, and ears. Keep in mind that baseball caps and some sun visors protect only parts of your skin.
- Wear sunglasses that absorb UV radiation to protect the skin around your eyes.
- Use sunscreen lotions with a sun protection factor (SPF) of at least 15. (Some doctors suggest using a lotion with an SPF of at least 30.) Apply the product's recommended amount to uncovered skin 30 minutes before going outside, and apply again every 2 hours or after swimming or sweating.
- Sunscreen lotions may help prevent some skin cancers. It is important to use a broad-spectrum sunscreen lotion that filters both *UVB* and *UVA radiation*. However, you still need to avoid the sun during the middle of the day and wear clothing to protect your skin.

Source: From National Cancer Institute: *What you need to know about melanoma and other skin cancers*, NIH Publication No. 10-7625, Bethesda, MD, 2010, Author.

Antibiotics. When a specific organism is identified through culture, topical or parenteral antibiotics may be prescribed. Common fungal infections such as athlete's foot may be treated with over-the-counter antifungal creams or sprays. When arthropod infestations appear in the skin, an antibiotic is commonly administered in a shampoo or lotion form applied to the affected area.

Steroids. Topical steroids are often used to treat allergic dermatitis and the irritating symptom of pruritus (itching). Oral or parenteral steroids may be used when urticaria (hives) manifests on the skin, indicating a systemic allergic reaction.

Emollients. Lotions, creams, and ointments may be used to retain moisture in the skin or as a base for other medications. Gels and powders are used when there already is excessive moisture present.

Chemotherapy agents. When skin lesions are malignant, cancer chemotherapy and systemic adjunct therapy may be used.[7]

CLINICAL NURSING SKILLS FOR TISSUE INTEGRITY

- Assessment
- Skin hygiene
- Wound care
- Medication administration
- Patient teaching

Wound Care

Cleansing. The goal of wound cleansing is to promote wound healing by removing debris and excessive exudates. Shallow wounds that appear healthy are generally cleaned with mild soap and water, and deeper but healthy wounds are cleaned gently with normal saline. Harsh solutions such as diluted bleach, acetic acid, or hydrogen peroxide can break down the cell walls of the newly formed tissues, so those solutions are reserved for use in heavily contaminated wounds.

Dressings. Wounds may be mechanically protected to promote healing in a moist but not soggy environment using a simple adhesive bandage or more complex dressings. Dry dressings are used to absorb excessive exudates, whereas moist dressings are used to maintain a slightly damp environment to promote tissue repair. Nonadherent dressings are useful when the wound drainage is slight and may dry between dressing changes, causing the dressing to stick to the fragile wound surface and then disrupt the wound during dressing removal. Occlusive and semiocclusive dressings are used for clean wounds that have minimal drainage but need to be protected from environmental pathogens, such as a central intravenous catheter puncture site. Hydrocolloid, hydrogel, and alginate dressings are used to absorb exudates while maintaining a therapeutically moist wound surface to promote healing. Vacuum-assisted closure systems are special dressings for complex wounds attached to a device that maintains negative pressure at the wound surface, aiding in removal of large amounts of exudates.[8]

The Institute for Clinical Systems Improvement[16] suggests that, when treating a person with a pressure ulcer, multiple aspects of care be integrated with the wound management (Box 27-5).

Phototherapy

Some skin disorders, such as psoriasis and atopic dermatitis, respond to controlled phototherapy with UV light. Protection from excessive UV exposure is important to prevent tissue damage.

BOX 27-5 Integrating Care for a Person with a Pressure Ulcer

- Establishing the treatment goal
- Moist wound healing
- Cleansing the wound
- Choosing appropriate topical wound care products
- Wound debridement
- Consideration of adjunct therapy
- Pain management
- Management of nutrition
- Surgical consultation
- Patient and staff education
- Discharge plan or transfer of care
- Documentation of all items in patient's medical record

Source: From U.S. Department of Health & Human Services Agency for Healthcare Research and Quality. Pressure ulcer prevention and treatment protocol. Health care protocol. Retrieved from http://www.guideline.gov/content.aspx?id=36059.

Surgical Treatment

Excisions—scalpel or laser. Surgical removal is indicated for benign lesions such as deep plantar surface warts unresponsive to other therapy and malignant lesions such as squamous, basal cell, and melanoma skin cancers. Surgical excision of primary melanoma includes not only removal of the lesion but also removal of an additional margin around the lesion to ensure eradication of malignant cells. For example, a 4-mm lesion would be removed along with an additional 2-cm margin around the lesion, which means that the resulting wound would be 4.4 cm in diameter—much larger than the size of the original lesion.[17]

Debridement. Wounds covered with a dry, leathery eschar surface may not heal until the eschar is removed. Surgical debridement enables rapid removal of the eschar and debris, whereas debridement using topical collagenase or wet to dry dressings is done slowly over a longer period of time. Collagenase ointment breaks down the peptide bonds in necrotic ulcer or burn wound tissues without damaging the healthy tissue.[18]

Skin grafts. When there is extensive damage associated with large or deep burns, wound excision and skin grafting are required to cover and heal the wounds. Grafts may be taken from other areas of the person's skin, from living or nonliving donors, or as porcine grafts. In addition to grafts, skin substitutes and bioengineered skin coverings are available.[8]

Nutrition. Tissue maintenance and repair is dependent on adequate nutrition. Protein and vitamins A and C are particularly critical for collagen synthesis in wound healing. In the absence of adequate nutrition, wound healing is delayed and infection is more likely. Early enteral or parenteral nutrition is important to consider for patients at risk.[8]

INTERRELATED CONCEPTS

Multiple concepts have a close interrelationship with tissue integrity. Adequate Perfusion with oxygen- and nutrient-enriched blood (Gas Exchange) promotes tissue integrity; in the absence of oxygen or sufficient Nutrition, the tissues can be suffocated and/or starved, leading to atrophy or necrosis. Adequate Sensory Perception and Mobility provide the stimulus and action needed to prevent prolonged pressure from limiting the perfusion to a specific tissue area. The nerves of the skin provide feedback about temperature and

Causes

Effects

FIGURE 27-3 Tissue Integrity and Interrelated Concepts This is a cause-and-effect model showing the concepts that impact tissue integrity and those concepts that are negatively impacted when tissue integrity is disrupted.

pressure that serve as a safety mechanism for the person negotiating the environment. Unrelieved pressure on a body tissue eventually causes injury.

In the presence of tissue integrity, the skin functions to maintain balance of Fluid and Electrolytes and has a role in Thermoregulation. Production of sweat, which includes both water and electrolytes, serves to cool the excessive body temperatures that could lead to organ damage, and it also serves to remove wastes. Altered Elimination through urinary or bowel incontinence can also contribute to impairment of tissue integrity through skin contact with caustic excretions. A loss of tissue integrity often results in Pain because the skin is laden with sensory nerve endings reactive to the irritation of the local damage. The skin and mucous membranes provide a barrier to most organisms and many toxic substances in the environment. A break in the barrier provided by intact skin and mucous membranes provides a portal for Infection with environmental organisms. These interrelationships are depicted in Figure 27-3.

CLINICAL EXEMPLARS

There are a large number of clinical exemplars related to tissue integrity. Box 27-6 presents common clinical conditions associated with tissue integrity impairment by categories noted previously: trauma/injury, loss of perfusion, immunologic conditions, infections, thermal/radiation, and lesions. In this section, several exemplars are featured because of their importance or frequency seen in practice. Also, a case study is presented illustrating the concept in a specific clinical context.

Featured Exemplars

The following featured exemplars provide a brief explanation of common conditions causing impaired tissue integrity. For detailed explanations and suggested nursing care for these conditions, consult specific medical–surgical, pediatric, and gerontology resources.

Abrasion/Laceration

Abrasions and lacerations are superficial traumatic injuries to the epidermis, dermis, and subcutaneous layers or to mucous membranes. Superficial injuries to highly vascular areas such as the scalp and oral mucosa may bleed extensively. The major risk of epidermal and dermal injury is the loss of a protective barrier, increasing the possibility of infection by contact with pathogens.

Dermal Ulcer

Unrelieved pressure can disrupt perfusion and oxygenation to tissue cells, leading to dermal or pressure ulcers. Dermal ulcers represent tissue necrosis of varying depths, from superficial to bone deep. Individuals who have decreased sensation or mobility are at greater risk for dermal ulcers. Recognition of risk factors (see Box 27-1) and prevention are critical for meeting the *Healthy People 2020* goal of reducing pressure ulcer prevalence by 10% from the 2007 rate.[10]

Psoriasis

Psoriasis is a recurrent inflammatory skin disease that affects and estimated 7.5 million Americans (or 2.2% of the population in the United States).[19] Individuals most commonly develop psoriasis between ages 15 and 35 years. Although most cases involve mild silvery scales and redness over a small percentage of the body, individuals with severe psoriasis and extensive lesions may feel isolated and withdraw from social contact. Psoriatic arthritis, a painful joint inflammation, is present in 10–30% of those with psoriasis.[20]

Bacterial Infection: Cellulitis

Cellulitis is inflammation of the skin and subcutaneous tissues, often caused by *Staphylococcus aureus* or streptococcal infection following a break in skin integrity such as a minor laceration or surgical incision. A hot, tender, reddened area of local infection develops at the site of injury. The individual may experience generalized responses to infection such as fever and malaise.[7]

■■■ BOX 27-6 EXEMPLARS OF IMPAIRED TISSUE INTEGRITY

Trauma/Injury
- Abrasion
- Blister
- Chemical irritant
- Ecchymosis
- Hematoma
- Laceration
- Surgical incision

Loss of Perfusion
- Dermal ulcer
- Diabetic foot ulcer

Immunologic Disorders
- Atopic dermatitis
- Psoriasis
- Scleroderma

- Stevens–Johnson syndrome
- Systemic lupus erythematosus
- Toxic epidermal necrolysis

Infection
Bacterial
- Cellulitis
- Impetigo

Fungal
- Tinea pedis (athlete's foot)
- Vaginitis

Viral
- HSV-1 (usually oropharyngeal)
- HSV-2 (usually genital)
- Verruca (warts)

Infestations
- Lice
- Scabies

Thermal/Radiation
- Burns
- Frostbite
- Radiation burns
- Sunburn

Lesions
- Basal cell carcinoma
- Benign tumors
- Malignant melanoma

Fungal Infection: Tinea Pedis (Athlete's Foot)

Tinea pedis, a fungal infection of the foot, causes scaling and maceration between the toes and may cause red scales and blisters across the plantar surface. Tinea pedis is contagious and commonly acquired in shared facilities such as locker rooms or dormitory showers. Treatment includes application of an antifungal agent.[7]

Sunburn

Sunburn can range from a mild redness to blistering or deep tissue damage. The following increase the risk of sunburn: direct exposure of the skin to the sun; use of tanning booths or sunlamps; or being near snow, water, or at high altitude. Sunburn and recurrent thermal damage to the skin is a risk factor for skin cancers.[7]

Malignant Melanoma

Malignant melanoma, a tumor that develops from melanin-producing skin and mucosal cells, is the most common cause of skin cancer deaths, and rates continue to rise. The risk of death from melanoma is greatest for people who have light-colored hair, eyes, and skin. White individuals are 10 times more likely than African-Americans to die of melanoma.

Individuals should consult a health care provider immediately if moles or lesions show a sudden or progressive change in size, shape, or color. Melanoma cells can metastasize to other organs.[21]

CASE STUDY

Source: diego cervo/iStock/Thinkstock

Case Presentation

Mrs. Ramona Garcia, a 76-year-old female, is admitted to a medical respiratory unit with pneumonia after 4 days of increasing difficulty breathing, fever, and a productive cough with purulent sputum. She reports that she has been sleeping sitting upright in a chair because she could not breathe well lying down. When Mrs. Garcia's breathing becomes comfortable enough for her to be turned briefly for a full skin assessment, the nurse notes a 4-cm red area on the buttock over the left ischial tuberosity that does not blanch to pressure. Recognizing the reddened area as a stage I dermal ulcer likely related to the prolonged pressure from sitting, the nurse collaborates with the patient, family, and health team on a plan for prevention of further tissue breakdown including frequent movement and positioning, adequate nutrition, hygiene for prevention of moisture collection from sweat or urine that might lead to skin maceration, and use of pressure-relieving devices.

Case Analysis

Mrs. Garcia has a serious medical problem that has kept her in a sitting position struggling for airflow over several days. Continuously sitting up to improve her air exchange has prevented her from relieving the pressure on her ischium, which she would normally have done by changing her position when she noticed discomfort. Poor perfusion from the near constant pressure on her ischium and a low capillary oxygen level from her respiratory illness have begun to cause damage at the tissue level. Mrs. Garcia's nurse identifies a reddened area of skin that does not blanch to touch as a stage I dermal ulcer and realizes that any further injury to the area could result in deep tissue damage and an open wound. In order to promote tissue healing and prevent further injury, the nurse begins tissue integrity interventions promptly. The nurse recognizes that helping Mrs. Garcia maintain more comfortable air exchange is essential in encouraging her to position herself without pressure on the dermal ulcer.

ACCESS EXEMPLAR LINKS IN YOUR GIDDENS EBOOK

REFERENCES

1. McCance KL, Huether SE: *Pathophysiology: The biologic basis for disease in adults and children*, ed 7, St Louis, 2015, Elsevier.

2. Carpenito-Moyet LJ: *Nursing diagnosis: Application to clinical practice*, ed 14, Philadelphia, 2012, Wolters Kluwer.

3. Venes D, editor: *Taber's cyclopedic medical dictionary*, Philadelphia, 2013, Davis.

4. Grossman C, Porth CM: *Porth's Pathophysiology: Concepts of altered health states*, ed 9, Philadelphia, 2014, Wolters Kluwer.

5. Wilson S, Giddens J: *Health assessment for nursing practice*, St Louis, 2009, Mosby.

6. National Cancer Institute: *What you need to know about melanoma and other skin cancers*, NIH Publication No. 10–7625, Bethesda, MD, 2010, Author. Available at: <http://www.cancer.gov/publications/patient-education/wyntk-skin-cancer>.

7. Lewis SL, Dirksen S, Heitkemper M, et al, editors: *Medical–surgical nursing: Assessment and management of clinical problems*, ed 9, St Louis, 2014, Mosby.

8. Barbul A, Efron DT: Wound healing. In Brunicardi FC, editor: *Schwartz's principles of surgery*, New York, 2010, McGraw-Hill.

9. U.S. Preventive Services Task Force (USPSTS): Screening for skin cancer: USPSTS recommendation statement. *Ann Intern Med* 150:188, 2009.

10. U.S. Department of Health and Human Services: Healthy People 2020: The road ahead, 2010. Retrieved from: <http://healthypeople.gov>.

11. Potter PA, Perry AG, Stockert P, et al: *Basic nursing*, ed 7, St Louis, 2011, Mosby.

12. Guide to Community Preventive Services: Preventing skin cancer: Education and policy approaches in outdoor recreation settings, 2014. Retrieved from: <http://www.thecommunityguide.org/cancer/skin/education-policy/outdoorrecreation.html>.

13. American Academy of Pediatrics: Treating and preventing burns, 2015. Retrieved from: <http://www.healthychildren.org/English/health-issues/injuries-emergencies/Pages/Treating-and-Preventing-Burns.aspx>.

14. Bergstrom N, Braden BJ, Laguzza A, et al: The Braden scale for predicting pressure sore risk. *Nurs Res* 36(4):205–210, 1987.

15. Boltz M: *Evidence-based geriatric nursing protocols for best practice*, New York, 2012, Springer.

16. Institute for Clinical Systems Improvement (ICSI): *Pressure ulcer prevention and treatment protocol*, Bloomington, MN, 2014, Author.

17. American Society of Plastic Surgeons: *Evidence-based clinical practice guideline: Treatment of cutaneous melanoma*, Arlington Heights, IL, 2007, Author.

18. Ramundo J, Grey M: Collagenase for enzymatic debridement: A systematic review. *J Wound Ostomy Continence Nurs* 36(6):S4, 2009.

19. National Psoriasis Foundation: Psoriasis statistics prevalence, (n.d.). Retrieved from:: <https://www.psoriasis.org/research/science-of-psoriasis/statistics>.

20. National Psoriasis Foundation: About psoriasis, (n.d.). Retrieved from: <https://psoriasis.org/about-psoriasis>.

21. American Cancer Society: Melanoma skin cancer, 2014. Retrieved from: <http://www.cancer.org/cancer/skincancer-melanoma/index>.

Sensory Perception

Beth Hopkins and Jean Giddens

Sensory perception represents a complex physiological process that allows humans to interact efficiently within the environment. These senses provide the basis for social interactions, communication, and learning. Sensory perception also provides a level of protection through detection and reaction to dangers within the environment. Impairment in any of the five senses can lead to significant challenges that can negatively impact development, health, and well-being with consequences that are potentially significant. This concept presentation provides an overview of the concept, including recognizing who is most at risk for impairment in sensory perception and possible treatment when impairment occurs.

DEFINITION

To describe the concept of sensory perception, it is important first to define both sensation and perception. *Sensation* is the ability to perceive stimulation through one's sensory organs such as the nose, ears, and eyes. This stimulation can be internal, from within the body, or external, from outside the body, and includes feelings of pain, temperature, and light. External stimuli are commonly received and processed through the five senses: vision, hearing, taste, smell, and touch. *Perception* is defined as the process by which we receive, organize, and interpret sensation. Sensory perception can then be defined as *the ability to receive sensory input and, through various physiological processes in the body, translate the stimulus or data into meaningful information.*[1]

SCOPE

Both sensation and perception occur within various parts of body systems and through a complex interaction of both sensory receptors and the nervous system. For persons to interact fully with the environment in which they live, it is important that these systems are as functional as possible. This concept represents five senses:
- Vision
- Hearing
- Taste
- Smell
- Touch

With each of these senses, the level of function ranges from optimal functioning to impairment (Figure 28-1). For the purposes of this concept presentation, impairment of sensory perception includes altered function or perceptual ability but does not include psychiatric applications such as auditory, visual, or tactile hallucinations or psychosis.

NORMAL PHYSIOLOGICAL PROCESS

Vision

Vision requires functioning of the visual system, which includes the eyes; surrounding optic muscles; and cranial nerves II (optic), III (oculomotor), IV (trochlear), V (trigeminal), and VI (abducens). The eyelid, conjunctiva, lacrimal gland, and eye muscles all comprise the external eye, which helps to regulate and control the visual input as well as protect the eye, aid with tear production, and move the eye when desired. The internal eye consists of three separate layers: the outer sclera and cornea; the middle layer that houses the choroid, ciliary body, and iris; and the innermost layer, which is the retina.[2] The iris allows light to enter the eye and regulates the amount of light entering the eye at any given time. The lens bends entering light rays so that they can properly fall on the retina. The ciliary body, which consists of ciliary muscles, is fed by the choroid, a highly vascular structure (Figure 28-2). The innermost area of the eye is the retina, which transforms light impulses into electrical impulses that are transmitted to the optic nerve. The optic nerve, in turn, communicates with the brain to produce vision.[2] Cranial nerves II–VI all have important roles in eye function (Table 28-1).

Hearing

Hearing, which involves the body's auditory system, is composed of the peripheral and central auditory systems. The peripheral system involves the external, middle, and inner ear and is concerned with hearing and processing sound. The external ear includes the auricle and external auditory canal and functions primarily to collect and transmit sound to the tympanic membrane and to protect the inner ear (Figure 28-3).[3]

The middle ear is an air-filled space that is located in the temporal bone. It connects to the throat/nasopharynx by the Eustachian tube, whose primary function is to equalize air pressure on both sides of the eardrum. The Eustachian tube opens to allow airflow when chewing

FIGURE 28-1 Scope of Sensory Perception Scope of sensory perception ranges from optimal functioning to impairment for vision, hearing, taste, smell, and tactile perception.

and swallowing. Vibrations of the tympanic membrane (or eardrum), which separates the external ear from the middle ear, cause the auditory ossicles to further amplify the sound waves and transmit these airborne sound waves to the fluid-filled inner ear.

The inner ear consists of a bony labyrinth surrounding a membrane. Within this structure is the cochlea, closely connected to hearing ability, and the vestibular system, which helps control balance.[4] Sound waves stimulate this series of actions, and once these waves reach the inner ear, the hair cells or sensory receptor cells of the cochlea pick up the vibrations. These cochlear cells, by means of a complex series of mechanical wave activities, innervate impulses that are carried by nerve fibers to cranial nerve VIII (vestibulocochlear) to the brain, where the cerebellum receives the signals and helps to maintain a sense of balance, and further reaching the auditory area of the temporal lobe for hearing.[5]

Taste

A person's gustatory system, or sense of taste, involves various cranial nerves and is directly related to the ability of the mouth and tongue to detect chemicals in the foods, also referred to as tastants, that we eat. These taste signals are initiated by chemical stimulation of the taste buds primarily located on the surface of the tongue and in the pharynx. Sensory receptor stimulation, conducted via cranial nerves VII, IX, and X, is then transmitted to the nucleus of the solitary tract in the medulla of the brain and also sent to other areas within the brain. Messages about smell converge here along with visceral sensory fibers from the esophagus, stomach, intestines, and the liver, which allow taste and odor signals to initiate digestive activity.[6]

Smell

Sense of smell is controlled primarily by cranial nerve I (olfactory) and is critical in the desire to eat and maintain a healthy nutritional state.[6] Smell depends on sensory receptors located in the mucous membranes of the upper and posterior parts of the nasal cavity that respond to airborne chemicals. These airborne chemicals bond to the cilia receptors in the nose, which trigger a series of reactions that eventually lead to signals traveling along the olfactory nerve to the brain. The brain then processes this information and makes a determination as to the type of smell. In healthy young adults, it is estimated that approximately 10,000 different chemicals can be identified by smell.[6]

Touch

The perception of sensation originates in the sensory receptors throughout the body and by means of complex travel pathways ultimately converges in the somatosensory cortex. This somatic organization allows for the precise localization of signals related to fine and crude touch, vibration, pressure, temperature, itch, and pain.[7]

Age-Related Differences
Infants and Children

Significant changes occur during growth and development in early infancy that primarily affect visual acuity and hearing perception. Although the eyes are physically developed by the eighth month *in utero*, making the fetus capable of opening its eyes, the development of gross visual ability to recognize objects, perform purposeful eye movement, and color recognition primarily occurs during the first year of life. The 1-year-old typically has developed 20/50 vision or is able to see at 20 feet what an individual with normal vision can see at approximately 50 feet. Most research suggests that visual acuity progressively improves in early childhood, reaching 20/30 or better by age 5 years, as is generally required for passing mandatory state vision standards upon entry into primary school.[8,9] The ear structures and the ability to hear sounds are developed during the early part of embryonic life; thus, hearing is fully developed at birth. Infants have the ability to detect a few distinct odors, such as the mother's milk; however, refined taste discrimination is limited until infants reach approximately 3 months of age.[10] Infants also have a well-developed sense of touch and are able to show response to peripheral tactile stimulation at birth.[10] This ability to distinguish tactile stimulation rapidly develops from a tight hand grasp at 1 month of age to pincer grasp, holding a cup, and walking steadily by 1 year of age.

Older Adults

Research illustrates that a decline in sensory function occurs with aging. This is increasingly prevalent among the older population and is believed to be due in part to prescribed treatments for other age-related conditions (e.g., medications used for treatment of cardiovascular disease).[11] The National Social Life, Health, and Aging Project began a major research study in 2005 that is exploring the health and social factors of older Americans as they age. This is the first national study attempting to provide a comprehensive assessment of sensory function among older adults. The study has examined more than 3000 people ages 57–85 years, and the data show declines in all five senses within this population.[12]

Age-related changes in vision begin in middle age when reduced elasticity of the lens occurs, making it difficult to focus on near objects (presbyopia).[13] Age-related hearing loss (presbycusis) is caused by changes in the inner ear or in the nerve pathways from the inner ear to the brain. This results in a decreased ability to hear and process sound, although the degree of hearing loss is variable.[14] Another physiological change with aging is reduced olfactory epithelium along with a decreased number of nasal cilia receptors available to assist in sending olfactory signals to the brain. Not only is the ability to smell decreased with aging but also the ability to distinguish between various smells is greatly affected.[6] Reduced sense of smell typically begins at approximately age 60 years, with increasing loss into the seventies and eighties. A study of more than 90 people age 45–84 years showed olfactory impairment in approximately 25% of the subjects, and impairment increased with age in both genders.[15] It is unknown why one's sense of taste tends to decline with age. It is thought to be related to both the decrease in olfaction and the potential chewing problems and tooth loss.[16] Furthermore, decreased levels of certain hormones, such as

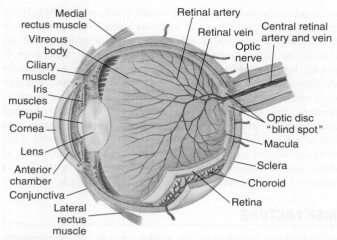

FIGURE 28-2 Structures of the Eye (Source: From Ball J, Dains J, Flynn J, et al: *Seidel's guide to physical examination*, ed 8, St Louis, 2015, Mosby.)

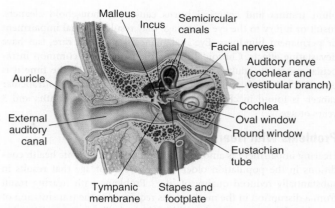

FIGURE 28-3 Structures of the Ear (Source: From Ball J, Dains J, Flynn J, et al: *Seidel's guide to physical examination*, ed 8, St Louis, 2015, Mosby.)

TABLE 28-1	Cranial Nerves and Function
Cranial Nerve	**Function**
I: Olfactory	Smell reception and interpretation
II: Optic	Visual acuity and visual fields
III: Oculomotor	Raising eyelids, extraocular movements, and papillary constriction
IV: Trochlear	Downward and inward eye movement
V: Trigeminal	Jaw opening and closing; sensation to eye, forehead, nose, mouth, teeth, ear, and face
VI: Abducens	Eye movement laterally
VII: Facial	Controls most facial expressions; taste with anterior two-thirds of tongue; excretion of tears and saliva
VIII: Acoustic	Hearing and equilibrium
IX: Glossopharyngeal	Swallowing and speaking; sensation of nasopharynx, gag reflex, and taste to posterior third of tongue; secretion of salivary glands and carotid reflex; certain speech sounds and swallowing
X: Vagus	Sensation behind ear and portion of external ear canal; secretion of digestive enzymes; peristalsis; carotid reflex; heart, lungs, and digestive processes
XI: Spinal accessory	Turn head and shrug shoulders
XII: Hypoglossal	Tongue movement, speech, and swallowing

Source: Modified from Ball J, Dains J, Flynn J, et al: *Seidel's guide to physical examination*, ed 8, St Louis, 2015, Mosby.

testosterone, in the older adult population can contribute to a decrease in cell growth, including taste cells located in taste buds. The decrease in the number of taste cells thus leads to a decrease in the sense of taste.[6] Evidence suggests that aging, dementia-related diseases such as Alzheimer's disease, and Parkinson's disease can lead to decline in olfactory detection and recognition abilities.[17]

Tactile thresholds (perceptibility to the sense of touch) tend to increase with aging. An example of this is a delay in the process of sensing a wrinkled sheet under the back or a slight prick from a small needle, thus resulting in potential injuries. In addition, certain tests that measure the ability to accurately assess tactile sensation tend to show a decline in function that corresponds with aging—a decline of 1% per year between the ages of 20 and 80 years.[18] Sensation at the fingertips and toes declines faster, especially with heat and cold, which can lead to problems with burns and potential frostbite in the older adult population.[6] A study comparing sensation thresholds of older (mean age, 93 years) and younger (mean age, 28 years) subjects found that older subjects required two to more than five times the tactile stimulation required by the younger group.[19]

VARIATIONS AND CONTEXT

A number of problems and conditions are represented by this concept and are grouped by problems with vision, hearing, smell, taste, and tactile perception. Common to all senses, conditions affecting sensory perception can be primary problems or secondary problems, representing both acute and chronic change, caused by congenital abnormality, primary and chronic conditions, treatment-related negative effects, and acute injury.

Problems with Vision

Problems with vision are seen across the lifespan. Although most individuals experience changes in vision associated with the normal aging process (previously discussed), there are many medical conditions that affect vision. Poor vision is defined as best-corrected visual acuity of less than 20/40 in the better seeing eye, and blindness is considered corrected visual acuity of 20/200 in the better seeing eye. Visual problems can occur as primary eye disorders (e.g., cataracts, glaucoma, retinal detachment, and macular degeneration), as secondary disorders caused by systemic chronic conditions such as diabetes or hypertension (diabetic retinopathy), or be congenital (e.g., a congenital cataract).[20] As of 2004, blindness or low vision affected more than 3 million Americans ages 40 years or older.[3] This number is predicted to double by 2030 because of the increasing epidemics of diabetes and other chronic diseases as well as the rapidly aging population.

Ocular infection in the first few weeks of life is increasingly more common among newborns and commonly caused by previously untreated maternal-induced infection by *Neisseria gonorrhoeae* and/or *Chlamydia*. Younger children are at risk for eye injury from accidental blunt trauma and chemical burns caused by household cleaners. Insult or injury to the eye at any age may result in visual impairment or permanent blindness. Eye malignancies, although rare, can have devastating effects. Choroidal melanoma is the most common intra-ocular cancer in adults and often has metastasized by the time it is detected.[21] Retinoblastoma, the second leading cause of intraocular cancer, is found in children between the ages of 14 months and 3 years of age.[21]

Problems with Hearing

Hearing impairment is among the most prevalent chronic health conditions in the population older than 65 years of age that results in substantially reduced quality of life.[22] Problems with hearing result from a disruption in the mechanisms required for the transmission of sound and/or nerve impulse within the ears. Sensorineural hearing loss, the most prevalent type of hearing loss, occurs when there is disruption in the afferent nerves necessary to transmit impulses. Conductive hearing loss results when there is disruption in the transmission of sound or vibration in the outer ear canal and middle ear structures. Some individuals may experience some degree of both types of hearing loss, described as a mixed hearing loss. Many subtypes of sensorineural hearing loss exist, including congenital hearing loss, genetic hearing loss, noise-induced hearing loss, presbycusis, sudden sensorineural hearing loss, and autoimmune hearing disorders.[22] Conductive hearing loss can be a result of cerumen impaction in the ear canal or the more serious consequences of an acute ear infection leading to a tympanic membrane perforation or rupture. Hearing loss at birth or congenital hearing loss occurs in 1–6 per 1000 newborns, of which 50% is suspected to be genetic related and 25% is nongenetic in origin.[23] Other genetic syndromes (such as Down and Alport syndromes) are often associated with hearing loss as one of their symptoms.[24]

Problems with Taste and Smell

Multiple factors influence the perception of smell and taste across the lifespan. These changes can be sudden and temporary when associated with an acute viral upper respiratory infection or long term when associated with the untoward effects of chemotherapeutic cancer-related treatment.[6,11] Some chronic conditions of adulthood, such as dementias, strongly correlate with loss of smell.[11] Among infants and children, problems with taste and smell are usually associated with direct injury or trauma to the olfactory ciliary receptor sensory and neural pathways, or they are associated with congenital abnormalities.

Problems with Tactile Sensation

Acute injury or trauma to the head, spinal cord, or peripheral appendages may result in disruption of sensory perception. Nontraumatic changes associated with the sense of touch are most common and are frequently caused by the progression of comorbid disease. Normal aging affects touch, as is experienced with the other senses as well. Studies indicate that it is likely that both central nervous processing of stimuli and a peripheral component contribute to diminishing touch sensation as people age.[24]

CONSEQUENCES

A number of consequences potentially occur with impaired sensory perception, and these depend on the type, extent, and number of impairments and also adjustments made to the impairment. Sensory-perceptual impairments share many of the same types of consequences including a reduced overall quality of life. There is significant risk for many types of injury as a result of impairments in sensory perception such as falls, burns, cold, or pressure, and the inability to smell or taste spoiled food or to smell toxic gases or smoke. Impaired vision and hearing can contribute to significant developmental delay and learning disabilities among infants and children and a loss of functional ability for adults. Psychosocial consequences can include difficulty establishing vocations, impaired interpersonal relationships, social isolation, depression, anxiety, and loss of self-worth. Another consequence less easily measured is the financial burden many of these impairments represent—both in direct cost of treatments and assistive devices and in the loss of income if the impairment represents an inability to work.

RISK FACTORS

All individuals, regardless of age, gender, ethnicity, or socioeconomic status, are at risk for disturbances in sensation and perception. However, there are certain populations and individual factors associated with increased risk.

Populations at Risk

The population at the highest risk is the elderly population as a result of changes in sensory perceptual functioning associated with the aging process (previously described). There are no significant population risk factors accountable to race/ethnicity, gender, or socioeconomic status associated with a decline in sensory perception in older adults.[25] Visual acuity begins to decline in the fourth decade of life, and by the sixth decade, most individuals will experience some degree of declining visual acuity.[21] Hearing loss related to aging affects an estimated 50% of individuals older than age 75 years.[25]

Individual Risk Factors

Significant individual risk factors include genetic predisposition, adverse effects of medications, chronic medical conditions, lifestyle choices, and occupation.

Congenital Conditions and Genetics

Congenital conditions that may result in detrimental long-term effects on the newborn infant's vision perception, if not detected early in life, include congenital glaucoma, congenital cataracts, and retinoblastoma (intraocular malignancy).[21] Congenital hearing loss is commonly the result of congenital malformations in the structure or functional components of the auditory system, although more than half of infants born with hearing loss have no significant risk factors.[26] Hearing loss at birth may be associated with maternal infection during pregnancy (e.g., measles) or family history of childhood hearing loss. Additional risk factors for congenital hearing loss include history of meningitis, low Apgar score, intensive care unit admission, and elevated bilirubin.[21]

Adverse Reactions and Side Effects of Medications

Changes in sensory perception function are a common side effect or adverse effect of many medications, particularly when taken for a long time, such as with chronic illness (Table 28-2). Visual disturbances are among the most common undesirable side effects associated with medication therapy. Examples include blurred vision, papillary constriction, retinal toxicity, halo effects, and dry eyes.[6] Ototoxicity, as an adverse medication effect, can result in permanent or temporary inner ear problems that can affect hearing, balance, and speech. This represents one of the main preventable causes of deafness.[27]

TABLE 28-2 Common Medications That Can Affect Sensation and Perception

Drug Classification	Possible Side Effects
Antihistamines (loratadine, diphenhydramine)	Blurred vision, dry mouth
Antihypertensives (β-blockers, calcium channel blockers, ACE inhibitors)	Blurred vision, alterations in taste and smell
Miotic eye drops (pilocarpine, carbachol)	Changes in vision, increase in near-sightedness, blurred vision
Antiseizure drugs (topiramate, acetazolamide)	Numbness in hands and feet, dry mouth, tinnitus (ringing in ears), blurred vision, eye pain, metallic taste
Diuretics (furosemide)	Hearing loss, tinnitus, alterations in taste and smell
Chemotherapeutic drugs	Alterations in taste and smell, paresthesia
Antibiotics	Alterations in taste and smell, ototoxicity

ACE, angiotensin-converting enzyme.

Many drugs also affect both taste and smell. In fact, medications (especially chemotherapy agents) are the most common cause of taste disturbances.[28] It is often reported that up to half of all cancer patients experience changes in their taste and/or smell perception.[29,30] Alterations in taste and smell that are considered severe are associated with poor nutrient intakes, food enjoyment, and quality of life.[31] Other drugs that cause taste disturbances include antimicrobial drugs, antivirals, antihypertensives, calcium channel blockers, and diuretics. If it is possible for the medication to be discontinued, the person's sense of smell and taste is often restored; however, some medications induce long-term changes in taste and smell, and occasionally produce permanent loss.[31]

Paresthesia, can also be caused by various medications, including select antineoplastic agents. Certain anticonvulsants can cause paresthesia in the hands, feet, face, and lips, which does not tend to improve until the medication is discontinued.

Acute Injury

Accidental and nonaccidental trauma to the eye in childhood is common. Ocular damage is dependent on the type of impact, with high-velocity impacts often causing extensive damage. Nonaccidental inflicted neurotrauma (formerly known as shaken baby syndrome) occurs in an estimated 1300 children annually, resulting in death within the first 3 days in approximately 20% of cases.[21] In the younger children who survive, many develop traumatic retinoschisis as a result of retinal damage.

Chronic Medical Conditions

A number of medical conditions place an individual at risk for sensory perception impairment as a matter of the disease sequela. Some of the most common medical conditions leading to sensory perception impairments are presented in Box 28-1.

Brain tumors, cancers, head injuries, infectious diseases, stroke, and some cardiovascular diseases, such as hypertension, are risk factors for

BOX 28-1 Medical Conditions or Treatments Leading to Sensory Perception Change

Vision
- Retinopathy of prematurity
- Diabetes and hypertension-induced retinopathy
- Eye infection
- Foreign body of eye
- Corneal abrasion
- Traumatic eye injury

Auditory
- Acute suppurative otitis media
- Otitis media with effusion
- Tympanic membrane perforation
- Traumatic ear injury
- Foreign body

Olfactory
- Sinus and other upper respiratory infections
- Brain injury or trauma
- Parkinson's disease
- Alzheimer's disease
- Medications and chemical exposure
- Head and neck radiation
- Growths or tumors of nasal cavity

Gustatory
- Head and neck surgery
- Radiation to head and neck
- Head injury
- Oral abscess and other dental problems
- Brain
- Exposure to chemicals and medication
- Burning mouth syndrome

Somatosensory
- Systemic sclerosis
- Raynaud's syndrome
- Cerebral vascular accident or stroke
- Third-degree burns
- Spinal cord injury
- Peripheral vascular disease

vision and auditory problems.[6] Sinus and upper respiratory tract infections, seasonal allergies, and also dental problems can alter both the sense of smell and the sense of taste. In addition, nasal polyps and exposure to certain environmental chemicals can cause disturbances in both smell and taste.

Cerebrovascular accident (CVA) or stroke can affect many aspects of sensation and perception in the body. Alterations in taste sensation, balance issues, and visual disturbances can result from a stroke, depending on the area of the brain affected. Children and adults with autism report sensory disturbances such as insensitivity to pain as well as unusual sensory responses to visual, auditory, tactile, and olfactory stimulation. Although many children with developmental delays have sensory perception impairments, these problems tend to be more prevalent in children with autism.[32]

Lifestyle Choices and Occupation

Certain lifestyle choices can increase the risk of sensory and perceptual alterations. Smoking creates an increased risk for alterations in both smell and taste primarily because it damages the taste receptors on the tongue and sensory receptors in the nose. However, when a smoker who experiences a decreased sense of smell and taste stops smoking, both senses typically return to their proper level of functioning.[33] Individuals exposed to loud noise at work or for recreation have risk for hearing deficit because such loud vibrations damage the small hairlike cells in the inner ear. This loss can be spontaneous or occur over time, typically when sound is at or exceeds 85 decibels; once damage has occurred, it is typically irreversible.[34] Individuals who work where flying debris is commonly present, such as miners and steelworkers, and those who work with certain chemicals are at high risk for eye injuries, especially when not wearing protective equipment.

ASSESSMENT

A comprehensive health assessment is essential to determining current health status, identifying present health risks, predicting future health risks, and identifying appropriate health-promoting activities. An assessment includes conducting a history and examination as well as diagnostic testing when sensory perceptual conditions are suspected.

History and Physical Examination

When performing any type of physical assessment, a thorough health history (including past medical, surgical, family, and social history) is taken. For infants, it is important to ask about prenatal and maternal history. Because of the potential for adverse effects with medications, a list of all medications (prescription and over-the-counter) used by the patient should be included. Health history questions should also specifically ask about sensory perceptual symptoms/problems for each of the categorical areas. A physical examination, particularly related to symptoms, is crucial. Common symptoms that suggest impairments are described for each category.

Vision

Ask the patient about changes in vision (blurred vision, difficulty seeing close up and/or far away), peripheral visual changes, and eye pain. For the infant and toddler, ask caregivers if tracking of the eyes has been observed when the child is watching movement and to ensure that the eyes have been observed moving in synchrony.

Examination of the eyes starts by inspecting external eye structures, including the eyebrows, eyelashes, and eyelids, paying attention to symmetry, size, and extension. In addition, the nurse should palpate both the eyelid and the eye and inspect the conjunctiva—the thin membrane that covers the inner eyelid and sclera—closely for redness and irritation. The sclera should be predominantly white, and the lens should be transparent.

Visual acuity (a measure of how well a person sees) is also included in the examination. Infants and young children are challenging to test for visual acuity; however, it is essential to do a thorough penlight examination of the cornea. At approximately 6 months of age, the cover test is helpful to screen for possible visual loss. Once a child reaches the age of 3 years, visual testing is achieved using the Snellen letter chart. Visual acuity is recorded as a fraction in which the numerator shows the distance that the patient was from the chart, typically 20 feet, and the denominator represents the distance that the average eye can read that same line of the chart.[2] For example,

20/60 means a patient can see clearly at 20 feet what the average eye sees at 60 feet.

Eye movement is typically controlled by cranial nerves III, IV, and VI and by six extraocular muscles and is tested by having the patient follow the examiner's finger, keeping the head stationary as the finger moves through the six cardinal fields of gaze.[2] A person's inability to follow through all the fields can indicate a host of visual disorders. Nystagmus—a rapid, involuntary movement of the eye—can often be detected during this part of the visual assessment.

The internal eye exam allows for visualization of the optic disc, arteries, veins, and retina. This is done using an ophthalmoscope, and often following dilation of the pupils, although this is not always necessary. Some unexpected findings include hemorrhages, optic disc swelling (referred to as papilledema), or cotton wool spots, which are poorly defined yellow areas on the retina and often are related to damage of the nerve fibers.[2] Checking pupils for response to light should be evaluated in both the adult and the pediatric population.

Hearing

Difficulty hearing, tinnitus, and ear pain are common complaints that prompt a patient to have the auditory system evaluated by a health care professional. For the pediatric population, frequent problems with otitis media are common and can include symptoms such as ear drainage, pain, and fever.

Inspection of the outer portion of the ear, or auricle/pinna, includes noting the symmetry, size, shape, and possible discharge. Inspecting the inner ear is performed using an otoscope. The nurse should look for cerumen (earwax), noting its color and any odor if present.[2] The tympanic membrane (see Figure 28-2) should be translucent with a pearly, gray color. Abnormal findings include a bulging or retracted tympanic membrane (or eardrum) and/or perforations of the tympanic membrane. Evaluating hearing is usually done by assessing the patient's ability to hear during general conversation. If hearing deficit is suspected, further diagnostic studies are indicated.

Taste

The most common complaint associated with the sense of taste is a lack of one. Most patients who think they have a taste disorder actually have a problem with smell.[35] Obtaining a complete list of current medications is especially important because many medications can cause alterations in taste.

Inspect the tongue and oral cavity, searching for any abnormalities such as an atrophied tongue or a tongue that does not appear red and moist.[2] Overgrowth of yeast or ulcerations or nodules should be noted. However, patients with taste disturbances often have normal-appearing, well-functioning tongues. Several validated taste tests[36] are available; however, they are costly to obtain and timely to perform. Thus, it is prudent to first ensure that a patient has a good sense of smell before doing further testing.

Smell

Assessing the sense of smell is first done by obtaining a detailed history, including medications the patient is taking, and assessing for recent upper respiratory tract complaints such as sinus infections, allergies, and nasal polyps. Examination includes inspection of the nose, searching for abnormalities such as nasal discharge or blockages, and evaluation of the color and size of the nasal passages. If discharge is observed, the nurse should note the color, consistency, odor, and amount. Nasal breathing is assessed by pinching one naris or one nostril and asking the patient to breathe in and out with his or her mouth closed, alternating nostrils. Breathing through each unobstructed side of the nasal passage should be quiet and effortless.[2]

Touch

Touch and balance are largely regulated by the body's neurologic system. Alterations in perception can often manifest as balance disturbances. Balance is routinely tested by the Romberg test, which involves asking patients to stand with their feet together and arms at their sides with their eyes first open and then to shut their eyes. Some slight swaying is normal, but the patient should be able to stand still for the most part. The nurse should also observe the patient's gait for abnormal findings, such as shuffling, staggering, and asymmetric stride.

Evaluating sensory function is accomplished by having the patient identify stimuli affecting the major peripheral nerves including the hands, arms, feet, legs, and abdomen. Cranial nerve VII, the trigeminal nerve, is most closely associated with sensory function. The patient should be able to correctly identify if a stimulus feels sharp or dull and the location of the sensation. In addition, the patient should be able to properly differentiate temperature (hot/cold), the location of the stimulus, and the correct side of the body that is being stimulated.[2] Monofilament testing is a common way to assess for peripheral neuropathies that cause decreased sensation to the extremities. Monofilaments are single-fiber nylon threads that are placed on the patient's skin, typically on the feet. An abnormal finding is that the patient will not be able to detect the presence of the filament.[37]

Diagnostic Tests

After a basic history and a physical assessment are completed, occasionally further diagnostic testing is warranted. This is described by sensory classification.

Vision

Some common visual diagnostic tests include evaluating peripheral vision by testing visual fields with automated perimetry. A patient looks straight ahead into a device with a concave dome while small flashes of light are shown sporadically in all visual fields. The patient then pushes a button every time he or she sees a light. Decreased visual field acuity could be indicative of glaucoma, optic nerve damage, and other visual problems. Another example is noncontact tonometry, or the puff-of-air test. This involves an eye's resistance to a puff of air from a small handheld jet, which calculates a range of intraocular pressure (IOP). Elevations in IOP can be indicative of glaucoma. Radiographic examinations of the brain may be indicated if a tumor is suspected of causing visual disturbances.

Hearing

If hearing loss is suspected, a referral to a licensed audiologist is often done for further testing. A pure-tone air conduction audiometric test, which determines the faintest tones a person can hear at selected frequencies ranging from low to high. Typically, earphones are worn so that information can be obtained for each ear separately.[38] Other common screening methods used often with infants are otoacoustic emissions (OAEs) and auditory brain stem response (ABR). OAEs are sounds from the inner ear after the cochlea has been stimulated by a sound, and these are measured by using a small probe in the ear canal. Those with hearing loss do not produce such sounds. The ABR test is performed by placing electrodes on the head to record brain wave activity in response to sounds.[38]

CLINICAL MANAGEMENT

Primary Prevention

Many measures exist to prevent injury and disease to the eyes, ears, mouth, and nose. Basic measures to protect the eyes and ears include the use of protective devices; patient education related to these practices is essential. Safety goggles are recommended for selected sporting activities and work activities in which small particles (e.g., sawdust, wood chips, metal pieces, and vegetation debris) are present in the air. More than 2000 workers in the United States receive medical treatment each year because of eye injuries that occur on the job.[39] The use of earplugs or other ear protection is also a requirement in many work settings involving loud machinery and is suggested for other activities such as attending loud concerts. Wearing helmets when riding a bicycle, skiing, or participating in contact sports can prevent brain injury—another cause of sensory disturbances.

Primary prevention extends beyond wearing protective devices. Newborns receive erythromycin eye ointment in their eyes at the time of their birth to help reduce the chance of the mother passing on certain sexually transmitted diseases. Reinforcing the importance of proper oral hygiene to prevent diseases to the mouth is essential to reducing the risk for changes in ability to discriminate taste or smell.

Secondary Prevention (Screening)

Screening tests are common for vision and hearing. There are no routine screenings to evaluate the sense of smell or taste. Screening for sensory function is often performed as part of the physical assessment.

Vision

Vision screens are recommended across the lifespan. Starting in the newborn period, a pediatric eye evaluation is recommended at each well-child visit. Eye evaluations for children up to age 3 years should occur at all well-child checkups and include history, assessment, external inspection of the eyes and lids, ocular motility assessment, pupil examination, and red reflex examination.[40] After age 3 years, the evaluation should also include age-appropriate visual acuity measurement and an attempt at ophthalmoscopy. Any abnormal findings would warrant a referral to a pediatric ophthalmologist.

Adults up to age 40 years should receive an eye exam at least every 2 years.[41] The same recommendation is applicable for middle-age adults, those up to age 60 years; however, special attention should be paid to individuals with chronic conditions such as diabetes, heart disease, and hypertension, who would then be considered to be high risk for the development of visual problems. In addition, this is the time frame in which presbyopia often begins to develop.

For adults older than age 60 years, yearly eye exams are recommended to screen for simple vision loss related to aging as well as age-related eye disorders such as glaucoma and macular degenerative disease.[41] Eye examination with dilation and careful inspection can often diagnose these problems, but tonometry is necessary when considering glaucoma, a disease in which fluid pressure in the eye is consistently elevated, causing damage to the optic nerve and leading to loss of vision. Tonometry involves the use of a covered probe to gently touch the corneal surface several times to record the average intraocular pressure. The cornea is anesthetized first with eye drops before the pressures are measured. Normal IOP is 10–22 mm Hg, and pressures greater than 22 mm Hg are considered abnormal. Those with ongoing pressures greater than 27 mm Hg are at a higher risk of glaucoma.[4]

Hearing

Screening for hearing is recommended for all neonates by 1 month of age and, if abnormal, to be repeated by 3 months of age.[26] Hearing tests are usually done within 48 hours of birth in the hospital setting. Infants who fail the hearing test are referred to their local Early Hearing Detection and Intervention program for follow-up. However, sometimes the failure is due to external ear canal vernix or middle ear fluid resulting in temporary hearing loss.[42] The two common screening methods used with infants are OAEs and ABR, which have already been discussed. Outer and inner ear inspection, with the use of an otoscope, is typically done with each well-child visit; however, for adults, otoscopic inspection is usually completed only when the patient reports a hearing problem.

Collaborative Interventions: Vision

For many visual problems, especially those associated with decreased visual acuity, corrective lenses (glasses and contact lenses) are a relatively easy and inexpensive treatment.

Surgery

There are a number of surgical procedures performed to treat conditions of the eye. Laser-assisted *in situ* keratomileusis (LASIK) is a surgical procedure that involves cutting a small flap in the cornea and then retracting the flap. Pulses from a computer-controlled laser then remove small parts of the cornea, permanently reshaping its surface. The reshaped cornea can better focus light onto the eye and onto the retina, allowing for improved vision.[35] The most common treatment for cataract is surgical removal, which may be an option for macular degenerative disease although not curative. In addition to surgery, those with macular degeneration also have the option of injectable drug treatments and photodynamic therapy.[31] Microsurgical procedures and laser procedures are also available to treat many other visual disorders and are being done more frequently.[43]

Pharmacotherapy

Certain visual disorders can be initially treated with β-adrenergic eye drops, which decrease production of aqueous humor. Other types of eye drops prescribed include prostaglandin analogs, adrenergic agonists, and carbonic anhydrase inhibitors. In addition, oral forms of carbonic anhydrase inhibitors can also be prescribed. In addition to surgery, those with macular degeneration also have the option of injectable drug treatments and photodynamic therapy.[44] Other common forms of ophthalmic pharmacotherapy include antibiotic, steroidal, and analgesic agents.

Collaborative Interventions: Hearing

Surgery

For recurrent otitis media in children, unresolved by antimicrobial use, surgical intervention may become necessary. A myringotomy involves a small incision made in the tympanic membrane, removal of fluid, and the insertion of a small tube. This surgery is typically done as an outpatient procedure with the patient being administered a general anesthetic.[45]

Cochlear implants are devices that are surgically implanted to provide direct electrical stimulation to the auditory nerve. Children as young as 2 years of age and adults with profound hearing loss may have success with these implants. Although a cochlear implant may not restore hearing, it may allow for the perception of sound.[7]

Adaptive Methods

Adaptive methods provide additional options for hearing and vision problems and include braille, guide dogs, sign language, closed caption television, assistive listening, and newer technologies. As previously mentioned, if a person is experiencing sensory loss from medication therapy, it is likely that discontinuing the therapy may result in the deficit being restored.

Collaborative Interventions: Smell and Taste

Individuals with disorders of the nose, sinuses, and mouth that affect taste and smell may require surgical intervention or use of medication therapy to improve or restore sensory perception.

Surgery

Surgical removal of nasal polyps, chronically inflamed sinus tissue, and retained secretions is performed to restore normal sense of smell. Oral and dental surgical procedures to remove diseased tissue or teeth aim to restore normal flora and function.

Pharmacotherapy

The use of an intranasal corticosteroid spray is recommended to reduce or eliminate inflammation in the nasal and sinus passages. Further use of medications such as antihistamines is effective for the treatment and control of allergic rhinitis, which often causes chronic sinus congestion and polyposis.

Adaptive Methods

Avoidance measures to reduce or eliminate environmental chemicals and toxins and allergens with the use of masks and filtration systems are advised, furthering the preservation of the sense of smell and taste.

Collaborative Interventions: Touch

Loss of the sense of touch is most often associated with comorbid disease; therefore, treatment with surgery and/or medications will be aimed at control or elimination of the primary cause.

Adaptive Methods

For individuals with impairment in their sense of touch, adaptive devices aimed at and ensuring safety in the home and injury prevention are imperative. This can be achieved in many ways, from setting the hot water heater to a lower temperature to prevent unintentional burns to the wearing of proper footwear to prevent trauma to the feet when walking and gain better balance control. Protecting the fingertips during cold temperatures is imperative for individuals with Raynaud syndrome and other peripheral vascular problems to prevent frostbite.

CLINICAL NURSING SKILLS FOR SENSORY PERCEPTION

- Assessment
  - General assessment
  - Assessment of senses
- Irrigation of eye and ear
- Medication administration
- Oral hygiene demonstration/teaching
- Prevention strategies for occupational and recreational exposure to hazards
  - Eye protection
  - Hearing protection
  - Other proper protective equipment
- Foreign body removal
- Age-appropriate teaching strategies for safety in the home (e.g., childproof cupboard locks and hot water heater setting)
- Assistive devices
  - Hearing aide
  - Eyewear
  - Cane/walker/wheelchair
  - Prosthetics (e.g., eye and lower limb)

INTERRELATED CONCEPTS

As previously mentioned, the concept of sensory perception is interrelated with several other health and illness concepts discussed in this textbook but especially Intracranial Regulation, Pain, Mobility, Nutrition, Development, and Functional Ability (Figure 28-4).

The brain is an amazing organ with more than 100 billion cells that regulate sensory input and output. For this reason, Intracranial Regulation is highly interrelated to this concept. This is most notable in the presence of brain disturbances, when presenting symptoms are seen with changes in sensory function. Pain is a sensation that most people do not want to experience; however, sometimes pain is necessary to provide the brain with the signals needed to cause action to remove the pain source. Certain disorders, especially neurologic disorders, have the potential to alter sensation and perception and affect Mobility. For example, when a person has suffered a neurologic impairment such as a CVA, often mobility is impaired due to paralysis and paresthesia of an arm or leg.

The inability to taste and smell reduces the desire to eat because these senses have a vital role in initiating the digestive process and can lead to Nutrition impairment. For example, patients undergoing chemotherapy often experience taste disturbances that decrease their desire for food, leading to nutritional deficiencies.

Development can be significantly affected among children with limitations in hearing and vision. Such problems can lead to delays in speech, language, and communication skills. Adaptation to special methods of communication must begin early in life to ensure progression throughout this critical developmental period to avoid isolation, reduced academic achievement, and poor self-concept.[46] Among adults, Functional Ability may be impeded when an individual experiences either diminished or complete loss of sensory perception, leading to changes in functional ability. Adequate sensory perception allows humans to interact efficiently within the environment and provides the basis for social interactions, communication, and learning. Impairment at any age or stage of life can have detrimental effects on the ability to enjoy this human interaction and impacts quality of life and well-being. As individuals age, age-related decline in hearing and vision occurs, often leading to depression, anxiety, and social isolation.[47]

CLINICAL EXEMPLARS

The concept of sensory perception represents the five senses; therefore, a multitude of exemplars exist. Box 28-2 details several exemplars that may occur across the lifespan. Note that an overlap of one or more acute and/or chronic conditions affecting sensory perception often occurs in one's lifetime. Detailed explanations and the nursing care for these conditions are presented in a variety of medical–surgical, pediatric, and gerontology resources. Brief explanations of several classic conditions are described next.

Featured Exemplars

Presbycusis

Age-related hearing loss, called presbycusis, is typically sensorineural (caused by pathologic changes in the inner ear or in the nerve pathways from the inner ear to the brain) and refers to a decrease in the ability to hear and process sound that is associated with aging and cannot be explained by the patient's genetic history, other diseases, or injury to the auditory system.[14] Presbycusis is present in approximately 35% of individuals 65–75 years of age, and it is present in 50% of individuals older than age 75 years.[25]

Otitis Media

Otitis media is the second most common illness diagnosed in children. Children younger than age 7 years are particularly vulnerable because of their immature immune system, and this illness is further complicated by poor functioning Eustachian tubes. Persistent or prolonged otitis media can lead to repeated use of antimicrobial therapy, conductive hearing loss and associated developmental delay in speech and language, disseminated infection, disruption of the tympanic membrane, and surgery.[48]

Nasal Polyps

Nasal polyps are known to be associated with several immunologic conditions, infection, and aspirin sensitivity. Although the etiology for the development of nasal polyposis is unclear, the condition appears to be directly related to chronic inflammation in the nose and nasal passages. Patients with nasal polyps frequently experience significant changes in their ability to smell, often leading to partial (hyposmia) or

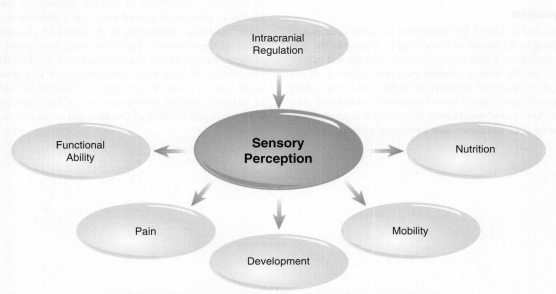

FIGURE 28-4 Sensory Perception and Interrelated Concepts

<table>
<tr><td colspan="3">■■ ■■ ■ BOX 28-2 EXEMPLARS OF IMPAIRED SENSORY PERCEPTION</td></tr>
</table>

Congenital Exemplars
- Deafness
- Cleft palate/lip
- Structural ear anomalies
- Congenital cataracts
- Retinopathy of prematurity

Visual Exemplars
- Amblyopia
- Blindness
- Presbyopia
- Cataract
- Retinal detachment
- Macular degenerative disease
- Glaucoma

Auditory Exemplars
- Sensorineural hearing loss
- Conductive hearing loss
- Mixed hearing loss
- Neoplasm and cholesteatoma
- Meniere's disease

Gustatory Exemplars
- Ageusia
- Hypogeusia
- Dysgeustia
- Burning mouth syndrome

Olfactory Exemplars
- Anosmia
- Hyposmia
- Parosmia
- Phatosmia
- Tobacco use disorder

Somatosensory Exemplars
- Peripheral neuropathy
- Peripheral artery disease
- Raynaud's syndrome
- Systemic sclerosis

---

complete loss of smell (anosmia). The presence of nasal polyps is also associated with exacerbation of or poorly controlled asthma. Treatment is generally with the use of oral or intranasal corticosteroids. Treatment of severe nasal polyposis is often surgical, although recurrence is common.[49]

Meniere's Disease

Meniere's disease is characterized by episodic unilateral temporary hearing loss often accompanied by ringing (tinnitus) and a sensation of ear fullness or congestion in the affected ear and severe dizziness (vertigo). Patients often experience these symptoms in clusters of varying severity and duration with interspersed complete remission. Meniere's disease is thought to be caused by a dysfunction of the endolympatic system in the inner ear resulting in interference with balance and hearing. Because there is no cure, treatment is focused on symptom control, with low-sodium diet, diuretic therapy, vestibular suppressant, cognitive therapy, pulse pressure treatment, and, in rare case, ear surgery.[17]

Raynaud's Syndrome

Raynaud's syndrome is caused by vasospasms of distal arteries and arterioles resulting in limitation of blood supply, leading to the skin turning white (pallor) and then blue (cyanosis). Patients will experience numbness, prickly feeling, stinging pain, and coldness of the hands and feet that is generally triggered by sudden cold temperature exposure. Raynaud's syndrome is more common in individuals who reside in colder climates and occurs more frequently in women. Treatment is primarily cold avoidance and protective clothing, tobacco avoidance, and, if needed, medications to dilate blood vessels and promote circulation.[21]

Chemotherapy-Induced Alteration in Taste

It is reported that nearly three-fourths of patients who receive chemotherapy experience alterations in taste.[29] These changes can range from a sweet, sour, or bitter taste in the mouth to complete loss of taste perception. Patients also often experience inflammation in the oral mucosa (stomatitis), oral thrush, dry mouth, and other changes associated with cancer treatment. Changes in taste perception occur in approximately 50% of patients receiving chemotherapy and may result in food aversion, subsequent weight loss, and malnutrition.[29] Diminished quality of life and social isolation may occur as a result, further challenging the resolve of the cancer patient.

Diabetic Retinopathy

Diabetic retinopathy is the leading cause of blindness among adults in America.[22] The effects of diabetic retinopathy are often already present in patients diagnosed with type 2 diabetes at age 30 years or older.[22] Diabetic retinopathy is the result of changes to the blood vessels of the retina that occur over time. Patients are often unaware of these changes during the early stages of development; however, as the damage becomes more extensive, vision loss ensues. Prevention is the primary focus of care with good control of blood sugar levels. In addition, surgical procedures such as laser treatment and vitrectomy to control bleeding of the damaged retina and restore sight may be used.

CASE STUDY

Source: Juanmonino/iStock/Thinkstock

Case Presentation

Mr. Robert Holton is a retired 74-year-old male who spent his entire working career as a self-employed carpenter. He has a 22-year history of type 2 diabetes; he also has hypertension and emphysema. He is an active smoker (52-pack year smoking history), although he has attempted to stop smoking on several occasions. He wears a hearing aid in each ear because of hearing loss as a result of working around machinery for several years.

Robert presents for a routine 3-month visit with the nurse practitioner accompanied by his wife. Mrs. Holton reports that Robert's feet smell very bad, but he does not seem to notice the odor. The nurse practitioner removes Robert's shoes and socks; a large infected foot ulcer is observed on the bottom of the foot. Robert is surprised that he was unaware of the wound. When asked about other changes, Robert does not respond. Mrs. Holton reports that he recently failed his visual acuity test for driver's license renewal and now must depend on her for transportation. She adds that he has become increasingly withdrawn during the past 6 months and does little to communicate with her or others and is not interested in leaving the house. She asks the nurse practitioner if he is depressed.

Case Analysis

This case illustrates many aspects of this concept. Mr. Holton is an older adult with diabetes, a chronic condition known to lead to changes in vision (attributable to diabetic retinopathy) and peripheral sensation (attributable to peripheral neuropathy). Along with the natural changes associated with aging, Mr. Holton's smoking history has contributed to his reduced sense of smell. The loss of tactile and olfactory sensation contributed to his lack of awareness of a diabetic foot ulcer that had developed. Mr. Holton's hearing loss can be attributed to his age and past work history with machinery. A common response to hearing and vision loss is social isolation—particularly when independence is lost—such as with the loss of his driver's license.

ACCESS EXEMPLAR LINKS IN YOUR GIDDENS EBOOK

REFERENCES

1. Day A: Sensation, perception, and cognition. In Daniels R, editor, *Nursing fundamentals: Caring and clinical decision making*, Florence, KY, 2008, Delmar Cengage Learning.
2. Seidel H, Dains J, Flynn J, et al: *Mosby's guide to physical examination*, St Louis, 2015, Elsevier.
3. Centers for Disease Control and Prevention: Vision health initiative, 2009. Retrieved from <http://www.cdc.gov/visionhealth>.
4. Smith S, Neely S: Visual and auditory systems. In Lewis S, Heitkemper M, Dirksen S, et al., editors, *Medical–surgical nursing: Assessment and management of clinical problems*, St Louis, 2007, Mosby.
5. Copstead LC, Banasik JL: *Pathophysiology*, ed 4, St. Louis, 2010, Saunders.
6. Schiffman SS: Critical illness and changes in sensory perception, *Proc Nutr Soc* 66:331–345, 2007.
7. American Speech Language Hearing Association: Cochlear implants, (n.d.). Retrieved from <http://www.asha.org/public/hearing/Cochlear-Implant>.
8. Burns CE, Dunn AM, Brady MA, Starr NB, Blosser CG: *Pediatric primary care*, ed 5, Philadelphia, 2013, Saunders.
9. The University of the State of New York, the State Education Department Student Support Service Team: School vision screening guidelines, April 2011. Available at <http://www.p12.nysed.gov/sss/schoolhealth/schoolhealthservices/VisionScreeningGuidelines2011.pdf>.
10. D'Amico D, Barbarito C: *Health & physical assessment in nursing*, ed 2, Upper Saddle River, NJ, 2012, Pearson.
11. Institute of Medicine (U.S.) Food Forum: *Providing healthy and safe foods as we age: Workshop summary*, Washington, DC, 2010, National Academies Press.
12. Schumm L, McClintock M, Williams S, et al: Assessment of sensory function in the national social life, health, and aging project. *J Gerontol B Psychol Sci Soc Sci* 64:i76, 2009.
13. Schiffman S: Sensory impairment: Taste and smell impairments with aging. In Wales C, Ritchie C, editors, *Handbook of clinical nutrition and aging*, ed 2, Totowa, NJ, 2009, Humana Press.
14. Bance M: Hearing and aging. *Can Med Assoc J* 176:925, 2007.
15. Murphy C, Schubert C, Cruickshanks K, et al: Prevalence of olfactory impairment in older adults. *JAMA* 288:2307, 2007.
16. Boyce J, Shone G: Effects of ageing on smell and taste. *Postgrad Med J* 82:239, 2006.
17. Lalwani AK: *Diagnosis & treatment in otorhinolaryngology—Head & neck surgery*, New York, 2004, McGraw-Hill.
18. Wickremaratchi M, Llewelyn J: Effects of ageing on touch. *Postgrad Med J* 82:301, 2005.
19. Craig J, Rhodes R, Busey T, et al: Aging and tactile temporal order. *Attention Percept Psychophys* 72:226, 2010.
20. Sharts-Hopko N: Lifestyle strategies for the prevention of vision loss. *Holist Nurs Pract* 24:284, 2010.
21. Rakel RE, Rakel DP: *Textbook of family medicine*, ed 8, Philadelphia, 2011, Saunders.
22. Harris LL, Huntoon MB: *Core curriculum for otorhinolaryngology and head–neck nursing*, ed 2, New Smyrna Beach, FL, 2008, Society of Otorhinolaryngology and Head–Neck Nurses.
23. American Speech Language Hearing Association: Hearing loss at birth (congenital hearing loss), 2015. Retrieved from <http://www.asha.org/public/hearing/Congenital-Hearing-Loss>.
24. Wickremaratchi MM, Llewelyn JG: Effects of ageing on touch. *Postgrad Med J* 82(967):301–304, 2006.
25. Freedman V, Martin L, Schoeni R: Recent trends in disability & functioning in older adults in the United States. *J Am Med Assoc* 228(24):3137–3146, 2002.
26. U.S. Preventive Services Task Force: Clinical summary: Hearing loss in newborns, 2008. Retrieved from <http://www.uspreventiveservicestaskforce.org/Page/Topic/recommendation-summary/hearing-loss-in-newborns-screening>.
27. Yorgason J, Fayad J, Kalinec F: Understanding drug ototoxicity: Molecular insights for prevention and clinical management. *Expert Opin Drug Saf* 5:383, 2006.
28. Madnani N, Khan K: Doc, I can't taste my food! *Indian J Dermatol Venerol Leprol* 76:296, 2010.
29. Wasserman A: Management of chemotherapy-induced dysgeusia, 2012. Retrieved from <http://www.oncolink.org/resources/article.cfm?id=1047>.
30. Hutton J, Baracos V, Wismer W: Chemosensory dysfunction is a primary factor in the evolution of declining nutritional status and quality of life in patients with advanced cancer. *J Pain Symptom Manag* 33:156, 2007.
31. Doty R, Bromley S: Effects of drugs on olfaction and taste. *Otolaryngol Clin North Am* 37:1229, 2004.
32. Leekam S, Nieto C, Libby S, et al: Describing the sensory abnormalities of children and adults with autism. *J Autism Dev Disord* 37:894, 2007.

33. Vennemann M, Hummel T, Berger K: The association between smoking and smell and taste impairment in the general population. *J Neurol* 255:1121, 2008.

34. National Institute on Deafness and Other Communication Disorders: Noise-induced hearing loss, 2014. Retrieved from <http://www.nidcd.nih.gov/health/hearing/pages/noise.aspx>.

35. U.S. Department of Health and Human Services: Lasik, 2014. Retrieved from <http://www.fda.gov/MedicalDevices/ProductsandMedicalProcedures/SurgeryandLifeSupport/LASIK/default.htm>.

36. National Institute on Deafness and Other Communication Disorders: Smell disorders, 2014. Retrieved from <http://www.nidcd.nih.gov/health/smelltaste/pages/smell.aspx>.

37. Dros J, Wewerinke A, Bindels P, et al: Accuracy of the monofilament testing to diagnose peripheral neuropathy: A systematic review. *Ann Fam Med* 7:556, 2009.

38. American Speech Language Hearing Association: Hearing screening and testing, (n.d.). Retrieved from <http://www.asha.org/public/hearing/Hearing-Testing>.

39. HealthyPeople.gov: Vision, 2015. Retrieved from <https://www.healthypeople.gov/2020/topics-objectives/topic/vision>.

40. American Academy of Pediatrics: Eye examination in infants, children, and young adults by pediatricians. *Pediatrics* 111:902, 2003.

41. American Optometric Association: Comprehensive eye and vision examination, 2015. Retrieved from <http://www.aoa.org/patients-and-public/caring-for-your-vision/comprehensive-eye-and-vision-examination?sso=y>.

42. Doyle KJ, Burggraaff B, Fujikawa S, et al: Neonatal hearing screening with otoscopy, auditory brain stem response, and otoacoustic emissions. *Otolaryngol Head Neck Surg* 116:597–603, 1997.

43. Dahl A: Glaucoma, 2015. Retrieved from <http://www.medicinenet.com/glaucoma/article.htm>.

44. Mayo Clinic Staff: Cataracts, 2015. Retrieved from <http://www.mayoclinic.org/diseases-conditions/cataracts/basics/definition/con-20015113>.

45. Cunha J: Ear tubes, 2015. Retrieved from <http://www.medicinenet.com/ear_tubes/article.htm>.

46. American Speech–Language–Hearing Association: Effects of hearing loss on development, 2015. Retrieved from <http://www.asha.org/public/hearing/Effects-of-Hearing-Loss-on-Development>.

47. Heine C, Browning CJ: Communication and psychosocial consequences of sensory loss in older adults: Overview and rehabilitation directions. *Disability & Rehabilitation* 24(15):763–773, 2002.

48. Rosenfeld RM, Schwartz SR, Pynnonen MA, et al: Clinical practice guideline: Tympanostomy tubes in children. *Otolaryngol Head Neck Surg* 149(Suppl 1):S1–S35, 2013.

49. Newton JR, Ah-See KW: A review of nasal polyposis. *Ther Clin Risk Manag* 4(2):507–512, 2008.

Pain

Angela Starkweather

Across the lifespan, pain is one of the most common reasons people seek health care, a frequent reason for taking medication, and a major cause of disability.[1] In the United States, common chronic pain conditions affect more than 100 million people and cost more than $560 billion annually in direct medical treatment and lost productivity.[2] Although the field of pain management has experienced rapid growth in technology and research during the past several years, pain continues to be undertreated across care settings. Aligned with ethical standards for health care professionals regarding the provision of measures to minimize pain and suffering, adequate assessment and management of pain is viewed as a human right.[3] As the only health care professionals who provide 24-hour presence 7 days a week, nurses play an important role in the management of pain and can be instrumental in ensuring their patients receive the best possible pain relief available.

DEFINITION

The International Association for the Study of Pain defines *pain* as *"an unpleasant sensory and emotional experience associated with actual or potential tissue damage, or described in terms of such damage."*[4,p209] This definition describes pain as a complex phenomenon with multiple components that impact a person's psychosocial and physical functioning. The accepted clinical definition of pain, which was proposed by Margo McCaffery in 1968, is accepted worldwide and reinforces that pain is a highly personal and subjective experience: *"Pain is whatever the experiencing person says it is, existing whenever he says it does."*[5,p8] This is why all accepted guidelines consider the patient's report to be the most reliable indicator of pain.[6]

SCOPE

Pain is a universal experience, although each person may experience pain in a different way. Conceptually, pain is a multidimensional symptom that can influence virtually every aspect of a person's life—the physical, psychological, emotional, social, and spiritual realms. The scope of pain as a concept may be viewed as a normal physiological response to tissue injury or as a pathological symptom associated with a disease process or alteration of the somatosensory system. Normally, pain serves as a protective mechanism that is meant to alert the brain to potential or actual bodily harm or tissue damage, such as pain that results from an ankle sprain or fractured limb. However, pain that

persists after the usual time for healing to take place serves no useful purpose and is viewed as pathologic. The concept of pain also ranges across several descriptive continuums, including location, intensity, frequency, and duration. In terms of location, pain may be well localized, such as in a joint, or widespread, occurring all over the body. The intensity continuum of pain ranges from none to minimal, moderate, and severe pain (Figure 29-1). The frequency of pain may be intermittent, occurring every few minutes, hourly, or daily with episodes of no pain, or it may be constant without any breaks at all. Pain may be acute, such as pain that occurs directly after an injury and that dissipates with time as the injury heals. However, pain can also be chronic when it is associated with a disease process or when it persists after injury and may last for months, years, or a lifetime.

NORMAL PHYSIOLOGICAL PROCESS

The sensations that we experience in our body are orchestrated by an eloquent network of cells, fibers, and organs, known as the somatosensory system, which receives, transmits, and interprets sensory information. Specialized sensory receptor cells carry specific types of sensory information (vision, hearing, touch, heat/cold, proprioception, and pain) along different anatomical pathways depending on the information carried.[7] The cells of free nerve endings in the skin and peripheral organs that are somatosensory receptors for the sensation of pain are known as nociceptors. Nociceptors are found in all tissues except the central nervous system (CNS). Tissue injury activates nociceptors to transmit pain information through the somatosensory system, a process known as nociception. When the brain receives and interprets the information as an unpleasant painful sensation, it is known as nociceptive pain, which is a protective mechanism to alert the brain to potential or actual tissue damage.[5] Although nociceptive pain requires the occurrence of nociception, nociception does not always result in nociceptive pain. The brain has a powerful influence on how we perceive sensory information and may filter or block pain information from awareness or change our perception of the sensory information.[8] First proposed in 1965 by Melzack and Wall, the gate control theory is considered to be one of the most influential theories of pain because of its focus on a neural basis of pain.[9] The gate control theory asserts that non-noxious input can close the "gate" to the CNS, thereby preventing painful input from reaching the brain. In this manner, non-painful stimulation is able to suppress pain. Since that time, it has become well recognized that pain is a complex condition involving

FIGURE 29-1 Scope of Pain

numerous areas of the brain and is influenced by emotional, cognitive, and environmental elements.

Neurological System

Pain is a conscious experience that requires an awareness of sensations via an intact CNS to receive sensory information and interpret the information as an unpleasant and painful sensation. The mechanisms that lead to the perception of nociceptive pain are described here and illustrated in Figure 29-2.

Transduction

Tissue damage results in the release of chemical mediators from damaged cells that activate nociceptors. These chemical mediators include prostaglandins, bradykinin, serotonin, substance P, and histamine.[10] When the chemical mediators attach to the membrane of the nociceptor, this can result in the opening of sodium channels that activate the nociceptor and cause the generation of an action potential.

Transmission

The action potential subsequently moves from the site of nociceptor activation along specialized afferent nerve fibers that carry pain impulses, known as Aδ and C fibers, to the spinal cord. Aδ fibers are thinly myelinated sensory fibers that send pain impulses faster than unmyelinated C fibers. Due to the myelin covering the Aδ fibers, they are capable of transmitting sharp, stabbing pain sensations, whereas C fibers transmit aching burning-type pain sensations. Substance P and other neurotransmitters allow the action potential to proceed across the cleft to the dorsal horn of the spinal cord, where it ascends the spinothalamic tract to the thalamus and midbrain.

Perception

Fibers from the thalamus send the nociceptive message to the somatosensory cortex, frontal and parietal lobe, as well as the limbic system, where pain is perceived and interpreted based on past experience, beliefs, attitudes, and meaning.

Modulation

Activation of the midbrain results in the release of substances such as endorphins, enkephalins, serotonin, and dynorphin from neurons that descend to the lower areas of the brain and spinal cord, stimulating the release of endogenous opioids that inhibit transmission of pain impulses at the dorsal horn.

Age-Related Differences

The mechanisms of nociceptive pain are normally present at birth and remain functional throughout the adult lifespan. The presence of acute pain remains approximately the same across the adult lifespan; however, there is an age-related increase in the prevalence of chronic pain, which affects more than 50% of older persons living in the community and greater than 80% of nursing home residents.[11] Although chronic pain

is prevalent among older adults, it is not a normal part of aging.[12] Clinical studies have shown that elderly individuals are more vulnerable to chronic pain and that the ability to tolerate severe pain decreases with age.[2]

VARIATIONS AND CONTEXT

Acute and Chronic Pain

Pain is usually described as being *acute* or *chronic* (*persistent*).[4] Acute pain is of sudden onset and is typically clearly linked to a specific event injury or illness. For example, tissue damage as a result of surgery, trauma, or burns produces acute pain, which is expected to be relatively short-lived and to diminish with normal healing. However, there may be variations in the intensity, frequency, and duration of pain between individuals after having the same surgical procedure or injury. This is why the subjective report of pain is so important; the experience of pain is highly individualized. However, when referring to acute pain, it is expected to dissipate with time along with the normal healing process.

In contrast, chronic pain is defined as pain lasting more than 3 months and may last for years.[4] Chronic pain may result from underlying medical conditions (pathology), such as cancer pain from tumor growth or osteoarthritis pain from joint degeneration. Chronic pain may also develop from an injury, medical treatment, inflammation, or unknown causes that alter the somatosensory system, in the periphery, spinal cord, or brain. As an advancement from the gate control theory, which describes the origins of pain, the neuromatrix theory posits that pain is the output of the neural network that is "genetically determined and modified by sensory experience" throughout life.[13] This theory has promoted new thinking about chronic pain conditions, such as fibromyalgia, that do not have an obvious cause but are associated with changes in the CNS. Chronic pain can persist throughout a person's lifespan and varies in intensity, frequency, and duration. In addition, patients may experience both acute and chronic pain, such as when a patient with chronic cancer pain experiences acute pain after undergoing a painful procedure related to cancer treatment.

Pain Classification

Pain is most often classified by its inferred mechanism as being either *nociceptive pain* or *neuropathic pain*.[4] Nociceptive pain refers to normal functioning of the somatosensory system in response to noxious stimuli (tissue injury) that is perceived as being painful. Simply stated, nociception means "normal" pain transmission. Normal transduction of pain sensation by nociceptors is also known as eudynic pain. Examples of nociceptive pain include pain from a sunburn, surgery, or trauma. Patients often describe this type of pain as "aching," "cramping," or "throbbing." Nociceptive pain may also be categorized as somatic or visceral. Somatic pain is characterized as sharp pain that is well localized to a specific area of injury. Visceral pain arises from within the body cavity, most commonly the thorax, abdomen, and pelvis. Pain receptors in the visceral cavities respond to stretching,

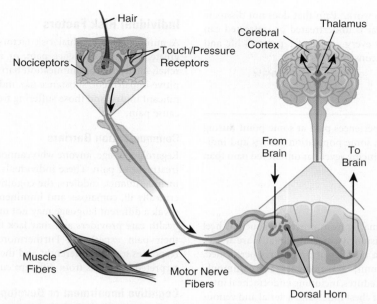

FIGURE 29-2 Pain Pathways from the Periphery to the Brain and Back

swelling, and oxygen deprivation, and the pain may radiate to other locations in the back or chest.

Although the normal mechanisms of nociceptive pain occur from stimulation of nociceptors, pain may also occur as neuropathic pain, which results from a pathology or disease of the somatosensory system.[4] Simply stated, neuropathic pain is pathologic. Examples of neuropathic pain include postherpetic neuralgia, diabetic neuropathy, phantom pain, complex regional pain syndrome, trigeminal neuralgia, and poststroke pain syndrome. Patients with neuropathic pain use very distinctive words to describe their pain, such as "burning," "sharp," and "shooting." Other forms of neuropathic pain are described by the mechanism involved. Sympathetically mediated pain is accompanied by evidence of edema, changes in skin blood flow, and abnormal sensations such as allodynia, hyperalgesia, and hyperpathia. Deafferentation pain is chronic and results from the loss of afferent input to the CNS. The pain may arise in the periphery from a peripheral nerve avulsion or in the CNS from spinal cord lesions or multiple sclerosis. Neuralgia pain is lancinating and associated with nerve damage or irritation along the distribution of a single nerve. Central pain arises from a lesion in the CNS, usually involving the spinothalamic cortical pathways, such as a thalamic infarct. The pain is usually constant with a burning, electrical quality. It is exacerbated by activity, and hyperesthesia and hyperpathia and/or allodynia are usually present.

Some patients have a combination of nociceptive and neuropathic pain. For example, a patient may have nociceptive pain as a result of a peripheral tumor that is growing and activates nociceptors around actual tissue damage; if the tumor is pressing against a nerve plexus, the patient may also report radiating sharp and shooting neuropathic pain. Some painful conditions and syndromes are not easily categorized and thought to be unique with multiple underlying and poorly understood mechanisms. These are referred to as *mixed pain syndromes* and include fibromyalgia and some low back and myofascial pain.

CONSEQUENCES

Pain triggers a number of physiological and psychosocial responses and can produce a cascade of harmful effects in all body systems.

Physiological Consequences

The stress response causes the endocrine system to release excessive amounts of hormones, such as cortisol, catecholamines, and glucagon. Insulin and testosterone levels decrease.[14] Increased endocrine activity in turn initiates a number of metabolic processes, particularly accelerated carbohydrate, protein, and fat destruction (catabolism), which can result in weight loss, tachycardia, increased respiratory rate, shock, and even death.[15] The immune system is also affected by pain, as demonstrated by research showing a link between unrelieved pain and a higher incidence of nosocomial infections[16] and increased tumor growth.[17,18]

Unrelieved pain impacts the respiratory system, causing small tidal volumes and decreases in functional lung capacity, which can lead to pneumonia, atelectasis, and an increased need for mechanical ventilation.[19,20] Effects on the cardiovascular system include increased postoperative blood loss[21] and hypercoagulation,[22] which can lead to myocardial infarction and stroke. Increased heart rate and blood pressure are autonomic responses to acute pain.

Pain can affect a patient's level of physical functioning. When pain is experienced with movement or mobility, the patient may associate the movement with pain. In this situation, it is very important for patients to understand that nonuse of the affected area and immobility can lead to muscle atrophy and joint contraction, which further promotes pain and impairs physical functioning. Sympathetic nervous system activation caused by acute pain decreases the release of digestive enzymes in the gastrointestinal tract and slows peristalsis. When mobility is not restored after surgery or trauma, this can further impair gastrointestinal function.[23] In turn, many opioid medications used to treat pain can cause constipation, making it necessary to have routine stool softeners along with the opioid medications.

Psychosocial Consequences

Along with the array of physical consequences that can develop due to pain, chronic pain in particular may be associated with significant psychological and social consequences, including fear, anger, depression, anxiety, and reduced ability to maintain relationships, engage in normal activities, and continue to work.[2] Pain that does not dissipate with normal healing and pain that is undertreated or untreated can have a negative impact on nearly every aspect of a person's life and result in psychological and social consequences.

RISK FACTORS

With rare exception, everyone experiences pain at some point during the course of a lifetime. However, some population groups and individuals are at higher risk of experiencing severe or unrelieved pain than others.

Populations at Risk
Infants and Children

Neonates are at risk for pain, primarily from procedures such as heel sticks, venipuncture, and circumcision.[2] Critically ill infants are at very high risk for pain due to the high number of procedures performed. In the neonatal intensive care unit, sick neonates are commonly exposed to numerous painful procedures, including endotracheal intubation and suctioning, insertion of chest tubes, and arterial and venous punctures.[2] Infants, toddlers, and developmentally preverbal children do not have the cognitive skills to report and describe pain; thus, other indicators besides self-report must be used to recognize and treat pain.

Older Adults

Although not all older adults experience pain, the incidence of pain increases with age, placing this population at higher risk for pain than younger individuals.[11] Pain has been shown to be very common in the older adult in the inpatient acute care setting and in the outpatient setting, such as nursing homes.[12] This is in large part because older adults suffer many of the conditions associated with pain, including musculoskeletal disorders such as degenerative spine conditions and arthritis. They are frequent recipients of surgical procedures and at increased risk of injury from falls and trauma, all of which can result in pain.[11] Some pain syndromes, such as postherpetic neuralgia, poststroke pain, and diabetic neuropathy, are more prevalent in the older population.[12] Cancer is more common in older adults than in younger adults, and as many as 80% of cancer patients experience pain as a consequence of the disease process as well as its treatment. The older adult is at high risk for undertreatment of pain as well. Many are reluctant or unable to report their pain because of illness or cognitive impairment.[8] Research shows that clinicians fail to provide adequate analgesia based on the misconception that analgesics are not needed or fears that analgesics may cause adverse effects, such as confusion and respiratory depression.[12]

Other Population Groups

Other risk factors for pain or undertreatment of pain include sex, race, and ethnicity.[24] Across settings, women report a higher prevalence of chronic pain than men, which may relate to the various chronic pain syndromes that occur exclusively or predominantly in women, such as endometriosis and fibromyalgia. In experimental studies, women report lower pain thresholds (the amount of stimulus at which pain begins to be felt) and less tolerance for pain (the maximum level of pain that a person can tolerate).[2] Such gender differences are linked in part to hormone levels. Social factors that have an influence on access to pain treatments include income and education and geographic location. Cultural and/or religious convictions may pose a barrier to reporting pain. In addition, as a population group, military veterans have increased vulnerability to pain due to the high risk of combat-related injury or trauma.[2]

Individual Risk Factors

A number of individual risk factors exist that place individuals at greater risk to experience pain, or risk for having insufficient pain relief, including communication barriers, genetic predisposition, cognitive impairment, substance use, individuals who have sustained significant injury, and those suffering from conditions that are known to cause pain.

Communication Barriers

Regardless of age, anyone who cannot report pain is at risk for undertreatment of pain. These individuals are referred to as *nonverbal* and include infants, toddlers, the cognitively impaired, and anesthetized, critically ill, comatose, and imminently dying patients. Patients who speak a different language may not understand the questions asked by health care providers and may lack the ability to adequately describe their pain experience. Furthermore, they may exhibit behavioral responses to pain differently, and these cues may be missed or misinterpreted by nurses from different cultural backgrounds.

Cognitive Impairment or Developmentally Disabled

The prevalence and burden of pain is higher in cognitively impaired or developmentally disabled children and adults compared to healthy individuals. Although a majority of individuals with cognitive impairment or developmental disability are verbal and can use a self-report pain assessment tool, behavioral pain tools should be used as well for initial and ongoing assessments.

Mental Health Conditions

Patients with a history or current use of illicit substances may be perceived as trying to obtain pain medication as part of their addiction. However, individuals with addictive disease also experience pain, and their report of pain should be addressed through multimodal therapies.[2] Mental illness is a common comorbidity with chronic pain.[2] A preexisting psychiatric illness may affect pain severity. In addition, patients with chronic pain may develop depression or anxiety disorders, particularly when they feel powerless or view their condition as hopeless. When patients present with mental illness and pain, both conditions should be addressed.

Injury or Conditions Associated with Pain

Some of the most obvious risk factors for pain are traumatic injury, critical illness, surgical procedures, or other conditions associated with pain. Acute and chronic medical conditions that are classically associated with severe pain include fractures, cluster headaches, passing kidney stones, trigeminal neuralgia, pancreatitis, shingles, herniated disc, and late stages of cancer. Critically ill patients of all ages experience a significant amount of pain from underlying painful pathologic conditions and the repetitive painful procedures to which they are exposed during the course of care.[15,19] Research has shown that the most painful procedure in the intensive care unit is turning,[20,21] which underscores the high prevalence of pain in the critical care setting.

ASSESSMENT

In a national agenda for improving pain assessment and management, the Joint Commission adopted the concept of "pain as the fifth vital sign," emphasizing the need for frequent assessment and re-assessment of pain.[2] Precise and systematic assessment is required to determine the areas affected by pain, likely contributing factors, and most effective treatment plan for patients who present with pain. In addition, the location and description of pain can serve as a diagnostic clue for underlying pathology. The past medical history should be obtained, including relevant health conditions that may affect pain, past surgeries and injuries, psychiatric illnesses and chemical dependence, and prior problems with pain and treatment outcomes. Current stressors that the patient is facing can also help to identify psychosocial issues affecting the pain. The health of family members and family history of pain or illness should be obtained.

Conducting a Pain Assessment

The gold standard of pain assessment is the patient's subjective report of the pain experience.[4–6] A thorough pain assessment is obtained by asking the patient a number of questions, and it serves as the foundation for effective pain management. It is used to establish the initial treatment plan and determine when changes are needed.[6] The components of a comprehensive pain assessment are presented here.

Location(s) of Pain

Ask the patient to point to the area(s) of pain on the body.

Intensity

Ask the patient to rate the intensity of pain using a reliable and valid pain assessment tool. A number of scales in several language translations have been evaluated and made available for use in clinical practice and for educational purposes.[6] The following scales are most commonly used:

- Numeric rating scale (NRS): The NRS is most often presented as a horizontal 0- to 10-point scale, with word anchors of "no pain" at one end of the scale, "moderate pain" in the middle of the scale, and "worst possible pain" at the end of the scale.
- Faces Pain Scale–Revised (FPS-R): The FPS-R has six faces to make it consistent with other scales using the 0–10 metric. The faces range from a neutral facial expression to one of intense pain and are numbered 0, 2, 4, 6, 8, and 10. Patients are asked to choose the face that best describes their pain. The FPS-R is valid and reliable for use in children and adults, including cognitively intact and impaired elders.[25] Although young children may be able to select a face on a faces scale, they are unable to optimally quantify pain (identify a number) until approximately 8 years of age.[26]
- Wong–Baker FACES Pain Rating Scale: The FACES scale consists of six cartoon faces with word descriptors, ranging from a smiling face on the left for "no pain (or hurt)" to a frowning, tearful face on the right for "worst pain (or hurt)." The faces are most commonly numbered using a 0, 2, 4, 6, 8, 10 metric; however 0–5 can also be used. Patients are asked to choose the face that best describes their pain. The FACES scale is used in adults and children as young as age 3 years.[27]
- Verbal descriptor scale (VDS): A VDS uses a series of different words or phrases to describe the intensity of pain, such as "no pain," "mild pain," "moderate pain," "severe pain," "very severe pain," and "worst possible pain." The patient is asked to select the phrase that best describes his or her pain intensity. The scale can be presented horizontally or vertically and can be helpful for patients with difficulty using a numeric scale.[28]

Quality

Ask the patient to describe how the pain feels. Descriptors such as "burning" or "shooting" may identify the presence of neuropathic pain.

Onset and Duration

Ask the patient when the pain started, what activities he or she was performing when it began, as well as whether it is constant or intermittent.

Alleviating and Relieving Factors

Ask the patient what makes the pain better and what makes it worse. The answers help to determine which pain medications and nonpharmacologic interventions are effective and which are not.

Effect of Pain on Function and Quality of Life

Ask the patient to describe medication side effects (e.g., constipation, nausea, and sedation) and difficulty sleeping or eating. Assess for comorbidities, such as anxiety and depression. It is particularly important to ask patients with chronic pain about how pain has affected their lives; what could they do before the pain began that they can no longer do, or what do they want to do but cannot do because of the pain.

Comfort–Function (Pain) Goal

Discuss the expectation of functional goal achievement. For example, tell surgical patients that they will need to deep breathe, cough, turn, and ambulate or participate in physical therapy after surgery. Patients with chronic pain can be asked to identify their unique functional or quality-of-life goals, such as being able to work, walk the dog, or garden. Ask the patient to identify (using a 0–10 scale) a level of pain that will allow accomplishment of the identified functional or quality-of-life goals with reasonable ease. A realistic goal for most patients is 2 or 3, and pain intensity ratings that are consistently above the goal warrant further evaluation and consideration of an intervention and possible adjustment of the treatment plan.[6]

Breakthrough Pain

An important part of the pain assessment is to determine whether the patient is experiencing *breakthrough pain* and if its treatment is effective. Breakthrough pain (also called *pain flare*) is a transitory exacerbation of pain in a patient who has relatively stable and adequately controlled baseline pain.[8] When breakthrough pain is brief and precipitated by a voluntary action, such as movement, it is referred to as *incident pain*. Another type of breakthrough pain called *idiopathic pain* is not associated with any known cause and often lasts longer than incident pain. Episodes of pain that occur before the next analgesic dose is due are called *end-of-dose failure pain*. A fast-onset, short-acting formulation of a first-line analgesic, such as morphine, oxycodone, hydromorphone, or fentanyl, is used to manage breakthrough pain. Analgesic doses or the frequency of their administration is adjusted as needed to minimize the occurrence of breakthrough pain.[8]

Reassessment

Following initiation of the pain management plan, pain is reassessed and documented on a regular basis as a way to evaluate the effectiveness of the treatments. At a minimum, pain should be reassessed with each new report of pain and before and after the administration of analgesics.[29] The frequency of reassessment depends on the stability of the patient's pain and is guided by institutional policy. For example, in the acute care hospital setting, reassessment may be necessary as often as every 10 minutes when pain is unstable during the titration phase (gradual increases in dose to establish analgesia) and every 8 hours in patients with stable pain. Findings that warrant further evaluation or notification of the prescriber include pain ratings that continue to be higher than the patient's comfort–function goal, a change in the location or quality of pain, and the development of medication-induced side effects that do not respond to treatment. Nurse monitoring of side effects is essential to ensure patient safety during analgesic administration. Life-threatening opioid-induced respiratory depression is the most serious of the opioid side effects; however, nurses can be key to preventing this complication by performing systematic assessments of their patients' sedation levels.[8] Less opioid is required to produce sedation than to produce respiratory depression, a characteristic that makes sedation a particularly sensitive indicator of impending respiratory depression. Gradual increases in sedation level warrant prompt reduction of opioid dose and increased frequency of nurse monitoring until the patient demonstrates an acceptable level of sedation.[30]

Challenges in Assessment

Many patients are unable to provide a report of their pain because they are cognitively impaired or too young (infants and small children) to use customary self-report pain assessment tools. Other patients who present challenges in pain assessment are the critically ill (intubated and unresponsive) and those who are receiving neuromuscular blocking agents or are sedated from anesthetics and other drugs given during surgery. All of these patients are collectively referred to as "nonverbal" patients.[31]

When patients are unable to report pain using traditional methods, an alternative approach based on the Hierarchy of Importance of Pain Measures is recommended.[6,31,32] The key components of the hierarchy are to (1) attempt to obtain self-report, (2) consider underlying pathology or conditions and procedures that might be painful (e.g., surgery), (3) observe behaviors, (4) evaluate physiological indicators, and (5) conduct an analgesic trial.

Diagnostic Tests

Diagnostic tests, such as x-rays, computed tomography, magnetic resonance imaging, or ultrasound, may be used to examine the areas of pain to identify a potential etiology. However, these should not delay appropriate treatment of pain.

CLINICAL MANAGEMENT

For most of the health and illness concepts presented in this text, clinical management includes all phases of health promotion, including primary and secondary prevention. However, for the concept of pain, the relevant focus of clinical management involves interventions to treat pain.

Collaborative Interventions
Pharmacologic Strategies

Because pain is a complex phenomenon involving multiple underlying mechanisms a multimodal regimen, which combines drugs with different underlying mechanisms, is often indicated. This allows lower doses of each of the drugs in the treatment plan, thereby reducing the potential for adverse effects[11,33] and can result in comparable or greater pain relief than can be achieved with any single analgesic.[11] Guidelines recommend the use of multimodal analgesia for all types of pain.[33-35]

Analgesics. There are three major analgesic groups:
- Nonopioid analgesics
- Opioid analgesics
- Adjuvant analgesics

Figure 29-3 shows the first-line analgesics in each group.

Nonopioid analgesics are appropriate alone for mild to some moderate nociceptive-type pain and are added to opioid analgesics as part of a multimodal analgesic regimen for more severe nociceptive pain.[10,36] For example, unless contraindicated, all surgical patients should routinely be given acetaminophen and a nonsteroidal anti-inflammatory drug (NSAID) in scheduled doses throughout the postoperative course. Opioid analgesics are added to the treatment plan to manage moderate to severe postoperative pain. A local anesthetic is sometimes administered epidurally or by continuous peripheral nerve block. An anticonvulsant may be added to the treatment plan as well to control severe pain or prevent a chronic postsurgical pain syndrome, such as post-thoracotomy or postmastectomy pain.[36]

Anticonvulsants and antidepressants are first-line analgesics for neuropathic pain.[37] These analgesics require a period of several days to weeks of dose titration to determine efficacy and safety and to achieve adequate pain control. Lidocaine patch 5% is used for well-localized peripheral neuropathic types of pain, such as postherpetic neuralgia (shingles-related pain). Long-term opioid therapy can be effective for some individuals with neuropathic pain as well.[11] It is not unusual to find a multimodal pain treatment regimen for a person with neuropathic pain that includes an antidepressant, anticonvulsant, local anesthetic, and an opioid.

Routes of administration. A variety of routes of administration is used to deliver analgesics. A principle of pain management is to use

FIGURE 29-3 Pharmacologic Management of Pain This figure shows the three analgesic groups and examples of first-line options within each group.

the oral route of administration whenever feasible.[11] All of the first-line analgesics used to manage pain are available in short-acting and long-acting formulations. For patients who have continuous pain, a long-acting analgesic, such as modified-release oral morphine, oxycodone, hydromorphone, or transdermal fentanyl, is used to treat the persistent baseline pain. A fast-onset, short-acting analgesic (usually the same drug as the long-acting) is used to treat breakthrough pain if it occurs.[11]

When the oral route is not possible, other routes of administration are used, including intravenous (IV), subcutaneous, transdermal, and rectal. Opioids are often given by IV patient-controlled analgesia (PCA). Patients who use PCA must be able to understand the relationships between pain, pushing the PCA button, and pain relief. They must also be able to cognitively and physically use the PCA equipment.[11] Other routes for pain administration include intraspinal analgesia and continuous peripheral nerve block infusions with or without PCA capability. Nurses play a key and extensive role in the successful management of these therapies, and the American Society for Pain Management Nursing (http://aspmn.org) provides guidelines for care.[34] As more information is gathered regarding how genetic factors influence the metabolism of medications used to treat pain and the side effects produced, a more patient-centered pain management approach may be used.[33]

Invasive or Surgical Strategies

Regional anesthetic strategies for pain management include epidural steroid injections to treat radicular pain, joint injections, nerve blocks, and implantation of intrathecal analgesic delivery systems. More invasive measures may include spinal cord stimulators, rhizotomy or neurectomy, nerve decompression, and joint replacement therapies. These invasive procedures are typically performed after other treatment modalities have failed to provide pain relief.

Nonpharmacologic Strategies

Nonpharmacologic strategies encompass a wide variety of nondrug treatments that may contribute to comfort and pain relief. These include the body-based (physical) modalities, such as massage, acupuncture, and application of heat and cold, and the mind–body methods, such as guided imagery, relaxation breathing, and meditation. In addition, psychological therapies such as cognitive–behavioral treatment, biofeedback, and hypnosis may be used along with other therapies to help manage pain. There are also biologically based therapies, which involve the use of herbs and vitamins, and energy therapies such as reiki and tai chi.[35]

Nonpharmacologic methods may be effective alone for mild to some moderate-intensity pain and are used to complement, but not replace, pharmacologic therapies for more severe pain.[38] The effectiveness of nonpharmacologic methods can be unpredictable, and although not all have been shown to relieve pain, they offer many benefits (such as facilitating relaxation and reducing stress) to patients with pain.[35–38] Many patients find that the use of nonpharmacologic methods helps them cope better with their pain and feel greater control over the pain experience.[39] The following list provides examples of nonpharmacologic measures that are noninvasive and relatively easy to incorporate into daily clinical practice. They can be used individually or in combination with other nondrug therapies:

- Proper body alignment achieved through proper *positioning* and regular repositioning can help prevent or relieve pain. Pillows can be used to maintain the position and support the patient's back and extremities.[40]
- Thermal measures such as the *application of localized, superficial heat and cooling* may relieve pain and provide comfort by

decreasing sensitivity to pain and muscle spasms and alleviating joint and muscle aches. The two measures are often used interchangeably.[39]

- *Mind–body therapies* are designed to enhance the mind's capacity to affect bodily function and symptoms[39] and include music therapy, distraction techniques, meditation, prayer, hypnosis, guided imagery, relaxation techniques, and pet therapy.[39,41]

CLINICAL NURSING SKILLS FOR PAIN

- Pain assessment
- Nonpharmacologic pain management
- Massage
- Splinting
- Relaxation and guided imagery
- Distraction
- Pharmacologic pain management
- Oral medications
- Intravenous medications
- Epidural analgesia
- Patient-controlled analgesia
- Local anesthesia

INTERRELATED CONCEPTS

Pain is connected to numerous concepts, with those considered more relevant listed here. These are presented in Figure 29-4.

The expression and interpretation of pain varies widely across cultural groups, thus **Culture** is an important interrelated concept. Having an awareness of such differences is critical for nurses so that an accurate pain assessment can be conducted and appropriate pain interventions can be implemented. The expression of pain may also be influenced by one's **Spirituality**. A person may be more accepting and tolerant of pain gained through spiritual strength. An individual's level of **Development** impacts how pain is interpreted by the individual and the ability of that individual to communicate his or her pain. Nociceptive pain is typically associated with altered **Tissue Integrity**. Acute pain associated with compromised tissue integrity is expected to dissipate with the normal healing process. **Mobility** is an important interrelated concept because severe pain can be immobilizing to individuals, and, in fact, some of the most disturbing effects of unrelieved pain are seen in the musculoskeletal system with impaired muscle, skeletal, or joint function. Inadequately managed pain can affect **Functional Ability**. This is often seen in the postoperative setting where the patient's ability to ambulate and participate in important physical therapy activities,[42] prolongs recovery,[43,44] and is associated with a higher incidence of complications including long-term disability.[45] In the outpatient setting, individuals with poorly managed chronic pain report inability to complete even the simplest of activities of daily living, which can result in loss of independence and greater reliance on family, friends, and the health care system.[46,47] Patients with poorly managed chronic pain frequently report **Sleep** disturbances,[48] and sleep disturbances can contribute to increased pain perception, as well as a reduced ability to cope with pain. Pain also leads to **Fatigue**, particularly when sleep is impaired. Increased levels of fatigue along with pain can further impair mobility and functional ability. Pain also affects **Mood and Affect**. Patients with severe pain are more likely to rate their general health as poor,[49] and describe having suicidal

FIGURE 29-4 Pain and Interrelated Concepts

■■■■ BOX 29-1 EXEMPLARS OF PAIN

Nociceptive Pain
Somatic Pain
- Ankylosing spondylitis
- Cancer pain (tumor growth) and pain associated with bony metastases
- Labor pain (cervical changes and uterine contractions)
- Osteoarthritis pain
- Osteoporosis pain
- Pain of Ehlers–Danlos syndrome
- Rheumatoid arthritis pain
- Surgical trauma/postoperative pain
- Pain from traumatic injuries
  - Wounds
  - Burns
  - Fractures
  - Deep tissue bruising

Visceral Pain
- Crohn's disease
- Irritable bowel syndrome
- Organ-involved cancer pain
- Pancreatitis
- Ulcerative colitis

Neuropathic Pain
Centrally Generated Pain
- Complex regional pain syndrome
- Pain following spinal cord injury
- Phantom pain as a result of peripheral nerve damage
- Poststroke pain

Peripherally Generated Pain
- Alcohol–nutritional neuropathy
- Diabetic neuropathy
- Nerve root compression, nerve entrapment
- Pain of Guillain–Barré syndrome
- Postherpetic neuralgia
- Some types of neck, shoulder, and back pain
- Trigeminal neuralgia

Mixed Pain
- Fibromyalgia
- Myofascial pain
- Pain associated with HIV
- Pain associated with Lyme disease
- Some headaches
- Some types of neck, shoulder, and back pain

thoughts. Research has even shown that severe chronic pain is associated with increased mortality, independent of sociodemographic factors such as income, age, and gender.[50]

CLINICAL EXEMPLARS

As mentioned previously, most individuals experience pain across the lifespan and in many different ways. Thus, the nurse will encounter multiple situations that will require pain assessment and interventions. A discussion of each situation is beyond the scope of this concept analysis; however, Box 29-1 presents the most common pain conditions in the context of the major categories of pain.

Featured Exemplars
Osteoarthritis Pain

Osteoarthritis is a condition that causes the cartilage in a joint to become stiff and lose elasticity. As this occurs, the cartilage can wear away, causing tendons and ligaments to stretch and bones to rub against one another, resulting in pain. Osteoarthritis commonly affects the hands as well as weight-bearing joints and is more frequent in women than in men. Osteoarthritis pain is an example of nociceptive, somatic pain.

Trigeminal Neuralgia

Also known as tic douloureux, trigeminal neuralgia is a form of neuropathic pain arising from the trigeminal (fifth) cranial nerve. It causes extreme, sporadic burning or shocklike facial pain that can last seconds to minutes per episode. The intensity of pain can be physically and mentally incapacitating.

Postherpetic Neuralgia

Another type of neuropathic pain is postherpetic neuralgia, which develops after a case of shingles caused by the herpes zoster virus. Typically, thin blisters associated with shingles disappear within a few weeks, but when the pain continues after the blisters have disappeared, the burning pain is known as postherpetic neuralgia. The incidence of postherpetic neuralgia increases with age.

Poststroke Pain

More than half of all stroke survivors report some form of poststroke pain. It can occur immediately following a stroke or weeks to months afterwards and may affect any area of the body. Patients typically describe burning pain or unpleasant and painful "pins-and-needles" sensation.

Complex Regional Pain Syndrome

Complex regional pain syndrome (CRPS) is a form of neuropathic pain that affects one of the limbs (arm, leg, hand, or foot) after an injury or trauma of the limb. CRPS is characterized by prolonged or excessive pain and mild to dramatic changes in skin color, temperature, and swelling of the affected area. It is more frequent in women.

Fibromyalgia

Fibromyalgia is a mixed pain disorder that is associated with widespread musculoskeletal pain, fatigue, sleep disturbances, and cognitive and mood disorders. Symptoms often begin after physical trauma, surgery, infection, or significant psychological stress and accumulate over time. Fibromyalgia is more common in women.

Phantom Pain

Phantom pain feels like it is coming from a body part that is no longer there.[2] Although phantom pain most often develops after removal of an arm or a leg, with up to 75% of patients developing pain within the first few days after limb amputation, it can also occur after removal of other body parts. Many factors are thought to influence the risk of phantom pain, particularly pre-amputation pain and genetic factors; however, phantom pain is thought to originate in the brain. Multimodal therapies are often required to reduce pain, although most patients experience a decrease in pain over time.

CASE STUDY

Source: Siri Stafford/Digital Vision/Thinkstock

Case Presentation

Jenny Alvers is a 38-year-old otherwise healthy female who has been admitted directly to the intensive care unit (ICU) after an automobile accident and emergency abdominal surgery. In addition to surgery, she has deep face, neck, and chest lacerations and contusions. Jenny is on a ventilator and somewhat disoriented and restless with elevated blood pressure and heart rate. She is unable to provide a report of pain, but based on her pathologic condition, the nurse assumes that Jenny has pain and consults with the surgeon about orders for a continuous IV opioid infusion. Knowing that Jenny will be subjected to painful procedures such as endotracheal suctioning and wound care during her stay in the ICU, the nurse also requests supplemental IV opioid doses to administer prophylactically. Jenny's sister reported that Jenny has no allergies but experienced severe nausea when she was given IV morphine following an appendectomy 3 years ago. The surgeon prescribes an IV infusion of hydromorphone at a dosage appropriate for an adult with moderate to severe pain and supplemental IV hydromorphone bolus doses every hour as needed. Scheduled doses of IV acetaminophen and IV ibuprofen are also ordered.

The nurse suspects that Jenny's restlessness could be related to unrelieved pain and therefore administers an IV hydromorphone loading dose before initiating the infusion. Infusions of IV ibuprofen followed by IV acetaminophen are also administered. An aqua pad circulating cool water is placed over Jenny's chest to provide additional analgesia. The nurse reduces the external stimuli in the room as much as possible and provides Jenny with calm reassurance and orientation while caring for her. Within 45 minutes of these interventions, Jenny is no longer restless, her vital signs are within normal limits and stable, and she appears to be resting comfortably.

Case Analysis

Pain assessment in Jenny is a challenge because she is unable to report pain using customary assessment tools. According to the Hierarchy of Pain Measures, when self-report of pain cannot be obtained, clinicians should assume pain is present based on the existence of painful pathology. Behaviors, if present, may also be observed as possible indicators of pain. The nurse correctly suspected that Jenny's restlessness might be due to unrelieved pain and administered analgesia promptly. It is important to note that elevated vital signs, which often accompany restlessness, are not reliable measures of pain, but they are sometimes used to further support the assumption that acute pain may be present. When Jenny recovers enough to provide a report of pain, self-report tools such as the NRS or FPS-R will be introduced and used to assess her pain.

The type of pain is used to determine the appropriate treatment approach. Jenny has experienced surgery as well as significant trauma-related tissue damage, both of which yield nociceptive pain. The first-line analgesics for moderate to severe nociceptive pain include opioids and nonopioids, such as acetaminophen and NSAIDs. Because Jenny is on a ventilator, the analgesics are administered by the IV route. Fortunately, several opioid and some nonopioid analgesics are available in IV formulation. Administration of a loading dose (IV bolus in this case) before initiation of the maintenance analgesic (IV infusion) is recommended to establish rapid analgesia. When Jenny is able to take oral fluids, analgesics will be given orally.

ACCESS EXEMPLAR LINKS IN YOUR GIDDENS EBOOK

REFERENCES

1. Nicholas MK: Expanding patients' access to help in managing their chronic pain. *IASP: Pain Clin Updates* 23:1–8, 2015.

2. Institute of Medicine: *Relieving pain in America: A blueprint for transforming prevention, care, education and research*, Washington, DC, 2011, National Academies Press.

3. International Association for the Study of Pain: *Desirable characteristics of national pain strategies*, Washington, DC, 2014, IASP Press.

4. International Association for the Study of Pain: Part III: Pain terms, a current list with definitions and notes on usage. In Mersky H, Bogduk N, editors: *Classification of chronic pain*, ed 2, Seattle, 1994, IASP Press, pp 209–214.

5. McCaffery M: *Nursing practice theories related to cognition, bodily pain, and man–environment interactions*, Los Angeles, 1968, University of California.

6. McCaffery M, Herr K, Pasero C: Assessment. In Pasero C, McCaffery M, editors: *Pain assessment and pharmacologic management*, St Louis, 2011, Mosby, pp 13–176.

7. Haines DE: *Fundamental neuroscience for basic and clinical applications*, ed 4, New York, 2012, Saunders.

8. Pasero C, Portenoy RK: Neurophysiology of pain and analgesia and the pathophysiology of neuropathic pain. In Pasero C, McCaffery M, editors: *Pain assessment and pharmacologic management*, St Louis, 2011, Mosby, pp 1–12.

9. Moayedi M, Davis KD: Theories of pain: From specificity to gate control. *J Neurophysiol* 109(1):5–12, 2013.

10. Starkweather AR, Pair VE: Decoding the role of epigenetics and genomics in pain management. *Pain Manag Nurs* 14:358–367, 2013.

11. American Geriatrics Society: Pharmacological management of persistent pain in older persons. *J Am Geriatr Soc* 57:1331–1346, 2009.

12. Herr K: Pain in older adult: An imperative across all health care settings. *Pain Manag Nurs* 11(2):S1–S10, 2010.

13. Melzack R: Evolution of the neuromatrix theory of pain. *Pain Pract* 5:85–94, 2005.

14. Grace PM, Hutchinson MR, Maier SF, et al: Pathological pain and the neuroimmune interface. *Nat Rev Immunol* 14:217–231, 2014.

15. Cata JP, Bauer M, Sokari T, et al: Effects of surgery, general anesthesia, and perioperative epidural analgesia on the immune function of patients with non-small cell lung cancer. *J Clin Anesth* 25(4):255–262, 2013.

16. Kaye AD, Patel N, Bueno FR, et al: Effect of opiates, anesthetic techniques and other perioperative factors on surgical cancer patients. *Ochsner J* 14(2):216–228, 2014.

17. Pei L, Tan G, Wang L, et al: Comparison of combined general–epidural anesthesia with general anesthesia effects on survival and cancer recurrence: A meta-analysis of retrospective and prospective studies. *PLoS ONE* 9(12):e114667, 2014.

18. Verma V, Sheikh Z, Ahmed AS: Nociception and role of immune system in pain. *Acta Neurol Belg* 12(1):120–128, 2014.

19. Erb J, Orr E, Mercer D, et al: Interactions between pulmonary performance and movement-evoked pain in the immediate postsurgical period: Implications for perioperative research and treatment. *Reg Anesth Pain Med* 33(4):312–319, 2008.

20. Panretou V, Toufektzian L, Siafaka I, et al: Postoperative pulmonary function after open abdominal aortic aneurysm repair in patient with chronic obstructive pulmonary disease: Epidural versus intravenous analgesia. *Ann Vasc Surg* 26(2):149–155, 2012.

21. Guay J: Postoperative pain significantly influences postoperative blood loss in patients undergoing total knee replacement. *Pain Med* 7(6):476–482, 2006.

22. Bigeleisen PE, Goehner N: Novel approaches in pain management in cardiac surgery. *Curr Opin Anaesthesiol* 28(1):89–94, 2015.

23. Vincent HK, Adams MC, Vincent KR, et al: Musculoskeletal pain, fear avoidance behaviors, and functional decline in obesity: Potential interventions to manage pain and maintain function. *Reg Anesth Pain Med* 38:481–491, 2013.

24. Barr DA: *Health disparities in the United States: Social class, race, ethnicity and health*, Baltimore, MD, 2008, Johns Hopkins University Press.

25. Ware L, Epps DE, Herr K, et al: Evaluation of the revised faces pain scale, verbal descriptor scale, numeric rating scale and Iowa pain thermometer in older minority adults. *Pain Manag Nurs* 71:117–125, 2006.

26. Spagrud LJ, Piira T, Von Baeyer CL: Children's self-report of pain intensity: The Faces Pain Scale–Revised. *Am J Nurs* 103(12):62–64, 2003.

27. Herr KA, Spratt KF, Mobily PR, et al: Pain intensity assessment in older adults: Use of experimental pain to compare psychometric properties and usability of selected pain scales with younger adults. *Clin J Pain* 20:207–219, 2004.

28. Miaskowski C, Cleary J, Burney R, et al: *Guideline for the management of cancer pain in adults and children*, Glenview, IL, 2005, American Pain Society.

29. Pasero C: Assessment of sedation during opioid administration for pain management. *J Perianesth Nurs* 24(3):186–190, 2009.

30. Nisbet AT, Mooney-Cotter F: Selected scales for reporting opioid-induced sedation. *Pain Manag Nurs* 10(3):154–164, 2009.

31. Herr K, Coyne PJ, McCaffery M, et al: Pain assessment in the patient unable to self-report: Position statement with clinical practice recommendations. *Pain Manag Nurs* 12(4):230–250, 2011.

32. Pasero C: Challenges in pain assessment. *J Perianesth Nurs* 24(1):50–54, 2009.

33. Pasero C, Quinn TE, Portenoy RK, et al: Opioid analgesics. In Pasero C, McCaffery M, editors: *Pain assessment and pharmacologic management*, St Louis, 2011, Mosby, pp 277–622.

34. Ashburn MA, Caplan RA, Carr DB, et al: Practice guidelines for acute pain management in the perioperative setting: An updated report by the American Society of Anesthesiologists task force on acute pain management. *Anesthesiology* 100(6):1573–1581, 2004.

35. Dworkin RH, O'Connor AB, Backonja M, et al: Pharmacologic management of neuropathic pain: Evidence-based recommendations. *Pain* 132(3):237–251, 2007.

36. National Heart, Lung and Blood Institute: Managing chronic complications of sickle cell disease. In *Evidence-based management of sickle cell disease*, Bethesda, MD, 2014, Author, pp 55–70.

37. Pasero C, Polomano RC, Portenoy RK: Adjuvant analgesics. In Pasero C, McCaffery M, editors: *Pain assessment and pharmacologic management*, St Louis, 2011, Mosby, pp 623–818.

38. Pasero C, Portenoy RK, McCaffery M: Nonopioid analgesics. In Pasero C, McCaffery M, editors: *Pain assessment and pharmacologic management*, St Louis, 2011, Mosby, pp 177–276.

39. Gatlin CG, Schulmeister L: When medication is not enough: Nonpharmacologic management of pain. *Clin J Oncol Nurs* 11:699, 2007.

40. Allred KD, Byers J, Sole ML: The effect of music on postoperative pain and anxiety. *Pain Manag Nurs* 11:15, 2010.

41. National Center for Complementary and Integrative Health: Complementary, Alternative, or Integrative Health: What's in a Name? 2015. Retrieved from: <https://nccih.nih.gov/health/integrative-health>.

42. Morrison RS, Magaziner J, McLaughlin MA, et al: The impact of post-operative pain on outcomes following hip fracture. *Pain* 103:303–311, 2003.

43. Kehlet H, Wilmore DW: Evidence-based surgical care and the evolution of fast-track surgery. *Ann Surg* 248(2):189–198, 2008.

44. Pavlin DJ, Chen C, Penaloza DA, et al: Pain as a factor complicating recovery and discharge after ambulatory surgery. *Anesth Analg* 95(3):627–634, 2002.

45. Pavlin DJ, Chen C, Penaloza DA, et al: A survey of pain and other symptoms that affect the recovery process after discharge from an ambulatory surgery unit. *J Clin Anesth* 16(3):200–206, 2004.

46. Rudy TE, Lieber SJ: Functional assessment of older adults with chronic pain. In Gibson SJ, Weiner DK, editors: *Pain in older persons*, Seattle, 2005, IASP Press, pp 153–173.

47. Simmonds MJ, Novey D, Sandoval R: The differential influence of pain and fatigue on physical performance and health status in ambulatory patients with human immunodeficiency virus. *Clin J Pain* 21(3):200–206, 2005.

48. Turk DC, Cohen MJM: Sleep as a marker in the effective management of chronic osteoarthritis pain with opioid analgesics. *Semin Arthritis Rheum* 39(6):477–490, 2010.

49. Mantyselka PT, Turunen JHO, Ahonen RS, et al: Chronic pain and poor self-rated health. *JAMA* 290(18):2435–2442, 2003.

50. Torrance N, Elliott AM, Lee AJ, et al: Severe chronic pain is associated with increased 10 year mortality: A cohort record linkage study. *Eur J Pain* 14:380–386, 2010.

Fatigue

Kathy Fletcher

Fatigue is a common symptom reported by people seeking health care. It is experienced by individuals across the lifespan and populations.[1] If fatigue is left unchecked, it can significantly impact a person's school or work performance and impact family and social relationships. Fatigue can become so pervasive in a person's life that it can impair their ability to physically and emotionally care for themself, resulting in a decreased quality of life. Despite its pervasive nature and prevalence, fatigue has traditionally failed to elicit the same level of attention from health care professionals as symptoms such as pain. As such, the scientific knowledge of fatigue, pathogenesis, techniques for assessment, and treatment are not as well developed.[2] Nurses can play a pivotal role in early recognition of this detrimental problem and initiation of care management strategies to mitigate its effects.

DEFINITION

Many authors have tried to define the true nature of fatigue, but there is no widely accepted definition. For the purposes of this concept presentation, fatigue is defined as a *"subjective lack of physical and/or mental energy that is perceived by the individual or caregiver to interfere with usual and desired activities."*[3,p2] This definition highlights the subjective nature of the concept that makes it so difficult to detect by others as well as the interference it can cause with normal life functioning. This definition also describes fatigue in a broader manner, indicating that it has both physical and psychological dimensions. Markowitz and Rabow[4] suggest that fatigue has three defining characteristics:

1. A perception of generalized weakness, resulting in inability to initiate certain activities
2. Easy fatigability and the reduced capacity to maintain performance
3. Mental fatigue resulting in impaired concentration and loss of memory and emotional stability

The definition and defining characteristics allow the nurse to recognize fatigue more easily in the assessment.

SCOPE

The scope of fatigue is presented on a continuum of having vitality and energy with no fatigue at one end to a feeling of exhaustion at the other end (Figure 30-1).[5] A continuum is a useful representation of this symptom because it is not fixed and is highly variable. The scope considers two factors—the severity and frequency of symptoms. The degree or severity of fatigue experience varies in all individuals, in part due to the underlying health status but also based on how the symptoms are interpreted and expressed. The frequency of fatigue is influenced by underlying health status and includes those who rarely experience fatigue and those who experience fatigue on a regular basis. The severity and frequency of fatigue influence the effect the symptom has on the individual's functional ability. Moderate fatigue to exhaustion makes completion of daily activities a significant challenge.

NORMAL PHYSIOLOGICAL PROCESS

Fatigue can be considered an expected symptom experienced by healthy individuals, but it is not considered a normal or expected finding when fatigue is persistent or severe. Individuals in a healthy state have the mental and physical strength to initiate and sustain actions in order to take care of life needs. This inner strength and the ability to maintain performance support a positive outlook that motivates the person to psychologically stay focused to achieve goals. Healthy individuals experience fatigue intermittently when they have overexerted themselves physically and/or mentally; in these situations, fatigue serves as a useful physiological signal as the need to rest. In healthy individuals, fatigue is relieved by physical and/or cognitive rest.

VARIATIONS AND CONTEXT

When fatigue is persistent and impairs normal life functioning, it is considered a health problem. For fatigue to be recognized as a significant health problem, it needs to be a prominent symptom for at least 2 consecutive weeks.

Classifications of Fatigue

Most sources describe three general classifications of fatigue that are delineated by cause: physiological, secondary, and unknown etiology (Figure 30-2). Within each of these general classifications, fatigue can be further categorized as temporary or chronic depending on its duration. Although there is not total agreement about the duration, many define chronic fatigue as persisting greater than 6 months.[6] Physiological fatigue occurs when there is an imbalance between exercise, other activity, sleep, and diet.[6] This type of fatigue is not caused by an underlying medical condition. Secondary fatigue is caused by an underlying medical condition or treatment and will usually be resolved or decreased if the underlying problem is addressed.[6] The last type of

No Fatigue
Full functional status

Mild Fatigue

Moderate Fatigue

Exhaustion
Impaired functional status

FIGURE 30-1 Scope of Fatigue as a Concept

fatigue includes those with an unknown etiology. Chronic fatigue syndrome (CFS) and idiopathic chronic fatigue are two examples of this type of fatigue. Diagnostic criteria for CFS are presented in Box 30-1.[7] Idiopathic chronic fatigue persists greater than 6 months, has no identifiable medical cause, and does not fit the criteria for CFS.

Causes of Fatigue

Although fatigue is associated with many conditions, the actual pathogenesis remains uncertain. There are many models or theories to explain what happens within the body to cause fatigue, but no single theory completely explains this multidimensional concept. Three leading theories are waste product accumulation, insufficient supply of substances, and an inflammatory process.

Waste Product Accumulation

Some forms of fatigue result from the accumulation of waste products within the body.[8] For example, patients with end-stage renal disease experience extreme fatigue and have difficulty concentrating on tasks of daily living. It is postulated that this fatigue is rooted in the accumulation of waste products from poor kidney function. As these toxic waste products build up, they cause chemical alterations that produce the symptoms of fatigue.

Insufficient Supply of Substances

Fatigue can also result from insufficient supply of necessary substances (e.g., carbohydrates, fat, protein, adenosine triphosphate, protein, and oxygen) for optimal metabolism and bodily function. For example, individuals who have anemia have decreased oxygen-carrying capacity, resulting in reduced oxygenation to tissues. The poor oxygenation supply triggers a number of physiological challenges and typically causes generalized fatigue.[9]

Inflammatory Process

Another general cause of fatigue is thought to be associated with an inflammatory process causing central nervous system (CNS)-mediated fatigue.[10,11] The hypothalamus and the basal ganglia of the brain are involved, and this process involves a complex interaction of neurotransmitters and immune factors. The inflammatory process provokes the CNS to cause fatigue as well as changes in sleep, appetite, and social behavior.

FIGURE 30-2 Classifications of Fatigue

CONSEQUENCES

Fatigue can cause significant changes in a person's life that result in the loss of a job, loss of relationships, and inability to care for oneself. Experiencing these losses can lead to significant psychological consequences, particularly depression. Although fatigue does not cause death or organ failure, mortality from suicide was higher in patients with chronic idiopathic fatigue than in the general population.[12] There is also a poorer prognosis associated with those with fatigue who are older, have a chronic illness, a comorbid psychiatric disorder, or believe that physical causes are responsible for the fatigue.[13] Chronic fatigue is resistant to treatment. Approximately 2% of patients with chronic fatigue report complete long-term resolution of symptoms, but as many as 64% have limited improvement.[6]

RISK FACTORS

All individuals are potentially at risk for fatigue, regardless of age, gender, race, or ethnicity. Specific risk factors for chronic fatigue are linked to underlying causes of the condition.

Populations at Risk
Older Adults

The elderly are at greatest risk for experiencing fatigue due to physiological changes associated with aging and the fact that many elderly have underlying conditions contributing to fatigue. Middle-aged adults between ages 40 and 50 years are the most common group to experience chronic fatigue. Studies of secondary fatigue in cancer patients revealed that fatigue may be influenced more by developmental stage than by actual age. Although fatigue is reported by all age groups, researchers found that younger adults reported fatigue more frequently than older adults.[14] The researchers suggested that older adults may attribute the fatigue to other conditions they have or to their advanced age and thus may not view it as abnormal. Young adults, on the other hand, with heavy responsibilities of balancing career, marriage, and childbearing, may view this same fatigue as a significant change in their lifestyle.

Women

Women are more likely than men to experience fatigue; however, some researchers believe that data might be skewed because it is socially more acceptable for women to express unpleasant symptoms. Statistically, however, women have a greater risk than men to develop CFS, with 75% of patients diagnosed being female.[15]

Individual Risk Factors
Underlying Conditions

A large number of individuals experiencing fatigue have an underlying health condition. Fatigue is a common feature of many illnesses,

BOX 30-1   Centers for Disease Control and Prevention Criteria for Chronic Fatigue Syndrome

1. The individual has severe chronic fatigue for 6 or more consecutive months that is not due to ongoing exertion or other medical conditions associated with fatigue (these other conditions need to be ruled out by a doctor after diagnostic tests have been conducted).
2. The fatigue significantly interferes with daily activities and work.
3. The individual concurrently has 4 or more of the following 8 symptoms:
   - Postexertion malaise lasting more than 24 hours
   - Unrefreshing sleep
   - Significant impairment of short-term memory or concentration
   - Muscle pain
   - Multijoint pain without swelling or redness
   - Headaches of a new type, pattern, or severity
   - Tender cervical or axillary lymph nodes
   - Frequent or recurring sore throat

Source: From Centers for Disease Control and Prevention: Chronic fatigue syndrome: The 1994 case definition, 2012. Retrieved from http://www.cdc.gov/cfs/case-definition/1994.html.

such as anemia; depression; multiple sclerosis; eating disorders; autoimmune diseases (e.g., systemic lupus erythematosus); heart, liver, thyroid, or kidney disease; and many infections. A condition such as anemia, in which there is a loss or decreased production of red blood cells, represents an example of secondary fatigue. The resultant fatigue would be accentuated if the anemia occurred during a short period of time. Fatigue is highly correlated with mental health conditions. Fatigue is nearly always reported in people with depression, and depression is very high among those with CFS. The overlapping of depression and other psychological factors makes it difficult to determine causative factors. Sources estimate that medical or psychiatric diagnoses explain the fatigue in approximately two-thirds of patients.[6]

Treatment-Related Factors

Many cases of fatigue are attributable to medical treatments for other conditions. For example, β-blockers, a gold standard in the treatment of heart failure, have at times made patients' fatigue worsen. β-Blockers have been shown to increase free fatty acids and glycogenolysis, which lead to insufficient nutrient supply and thus increase fatigue.[16] Fatigue is a common side effect associated with many medications (e.g., sedative–hypnotics, antidepressants, muscle relaxants, opioids, antihypertensives, antihistamines, and many types of antibiotics). Psychoactive substances such as alcohol, nicotine, and caffeine can also result in fatigue, especially during periods of withdrawal. Therapy for cancer, such as radiation and chemotherapy, kills all fast-growing cells. This therapy can cause anemia, resulting in decreased tissue oxygenation and fatigue. Researchers studying fatigue have found that even those with minor surgery experience a 6- to 12-week period of fatigue during recovery.[6]

Nutritional Status

Proper nutrition is necessary to provide the body with essential nutrients for optional functioning. Individuals with nutritional deficiencies, particularly protein–calorie malnutrition, are at risk for experiencing fatigue due to inadequate energy sources. Because nutritional deficiencies accompany many chronic conditions, the fatigue symptoms may be attributed to both or either.

Lifestyle Choices

A person's lifestyle choices have a significant impact on fatigue. Physiological fatigue can be induced by exercising excessively, consuming a poor diet, excessive alcohol consumption, not sleeping, or working excessively. People with a history of working nights or rotating shifts are also at risk. A disruption of the circadian rhythm may make individuals feel tired when they need to be awake and/or interfere with sleeping, thus causing fatigue.[6]

ASSESSMENT

History

Because fatigue is a subjective experience, the best assessment should be focused on the patient's report about his or her fatigue experience. Use open-ended questions that encourage the patient to describe the fatigue in his or her own words. The patient's personal experience of fatigue must be understood so that an appropriate plan of care can be formulated. The following are components of a comprehensive history of fatigue:

- Personal description of the fatigue: Fatigue is a subjective experience, so it will be a different experience for each individual. Men and women often describe fatigue differently. Men will usually describe it as a feeling of being tired, whereas women might state that they feel depressed or anxious.[17] Most patients experiencing fatigue will describe their fatigue as the inability to complete specific activities because of a lack of energy or stamina. However, patients with depression describe their fatigue more globally and express that they are unable to do anything.[6]
- Onset and course: The nurse should ask the patient if the fatigue occurred suddenly or appeared more gradually. The nurse should also review the patient's medical history in order to evaluate if the patient has any potential risk factors that occurred at approximately the time of the onset of fatigue. Asking questions about the course of the fatigue will help the nurse determine if the fatigue has remained approximately the same, worsened, or improved.
- Duration and daily pattern: The nurse should ask the patient about the length of time he or she has experienced the fatigue. This will give the nurse information to determine if the problem is acute or chronic. Fatigue, as a symptom, is not a static entity and may change daily, so it is also important to determine the usual daily pattern of the fatigue. This will help the nurse to recognize the patient's usual fatigue pattern in order to identify when it worsens.
- Factors that alleviate or exacerbate: Finding out what makes the fatigue worse or better will help the nurse tailor patient-centered interventions. There may be other symptoms of other conditions that are contributing to the fatigue. For this reason, it is important to assess the existence of pain, sleep pattern disturbance, and poor nutrition. Assessing for interrelated concepts could help the nurse identify other contributing factors.
- Impact on daily life: The nurse should assess how the fatigue has impacted the patient's activities of daily living, such as his or her ability to work, socialize, participate in family activities, and libido. Once the nurse is aware of fatigue's impact, the nurse should assess what accommodations the patient/family has made to adjust.

Many self-report scales have been developed, but they often overlap with other symptoms and/or do not capture all the features of this multidimensional concept.[18] Table 30-1 presents reliable and valid instruments commonly used to measure the concept of fatigue. Studies of fatigue indicate that there is a strong positive correlation among

TABLE 30-1 Self-Report Instruments to Measure Fatigue

Instrument	Dimensions Assessed/ Target Population
Brief Fatigue Inventory (BFI)	Measures amount, activities affected by fatigue Cancer patients
Multidimensional Fatigue Inventory (MFI)	Measures general, physical, mental, reduced motivation, and reduced activity Various patient populations, including those with cancer, chronic fatigue syndrome, and COPD
Multidimensional Assessment of Fatigue (MAF)	Measures severity, distress, degree of interference in activities of daily living, timing (frequency of occurrence and changeability) Designed for arthritis patients; also used in cancer patients and those with chronic pulmonary disease
Fatigue Severity Scale (FSS)	Measures severity, how fatigue interferes with certain activities Developed for patients with multiple sclerosis and lupus

fatigue, depression, and perceived stress.[19] The nurse should ask questions about the patient's psychosocial status in order to rule out these disorders.

Examination Findings

The history can guide appropriate focused physical assessment and diagnostic tests to rule out underlying diseases. Recognition of secondary causes of fatigue is important so that the life-altering effects of fatigue can be diminished by appropriately treating this disease.

Inspection

The nurse should observe the individual's general appearance. Is the individual alert? Is he or she displaying any psychomotor agitation or impairment? Take note of the individual's personal grooming. Poor alertness, psychomotor impairment or agitation, and poor grooming could be evidence that the patient is experiencing a mood and affect disorder such as depression. If the patient's grooming appears unkempt, it could also indicate that the fatigue is affecting the patient's self-care. Look at the patient's posture. Does he or she appear slumped? Is the patient's gait appropriate? Observe the patient's skin.

Palpation and Auscultation

Palpation is indicated to assess for the presence of lymphadenopathy, thyroid nodules, or goiter. These findings could indicate the need to test further for cancer, thyroid disease, or infection. Examine muscle appearance, strength against resistance, deep tendon reflexes, and sensory and cranial nerve action to assess the neuromuscular system. Some neuromuscular diseases can decrease muscular bulk, tone, and strength, which increases the patient's risk for fatigue. Auscultation of the heart and lungs helps to identify underlying pulmonary or cardiac conditions that may be contributing factors.

Diagnostic Tests

There are no specific diagnostic markers for fatigue. Diagnostic testing is primarily completed to rule out underlying diseases.

Common laboratory tests include thyroid function tests, complete blood cell count with differential (to rule out anemia and infection), chemistry profile (to rule out electrolyte imbalances and alteration in glucose levels), tests of liver and renal function, HIV antibody, erythrocyte sedimentation rate (inflammatory disease), urinalysis (urinary infection and renal impairment), and a pregnancy test in women of childbearing age. Some health professionals use performance-based testing to determine if a patient experiences fatigue with difficult physical or cognitive activities. However, research indicates that measurement of motor or cognitive fatigue (reduction in power output over time) does not show significant correlations with perceived fatigue.[20]

CLINICAL MANAGEMENT

Primary Prevention

Primary prevention refers to purposeful activities to prevent disease. In the case of fatigue, basic primary prevention measures are associated with following a healthy lifestyle—meaning good nutrition, exercise, getting adequate sleep, and managing stress. In addition, the nurse can advocate for patients and families with fatigue risk so they can obtain resources needed to prevent fatigue. Patient teaching for individuals with risk factors, so they take measures to avoid fatigue, is another example of primary prevention. For example, women experiencing excessive menstrual flow can be advised to increase dietary intake of iron or iron supplements to avoid developing iron deficiency anemia, which is a common cause of fatigue.

Secondary Prevention (Screening)

Secondary prevention refers to screening efforts for early detection of disease. Because fatigue is a symptom associated with multiple health conditions, there are no population-wide screening efforts for fatigue. However, nurses can screen patients who are identified as being at risk for fatigue by asking additional questions during an interview or using a fatigue screening tool (see Table 30-1).

Collaborative Interventions

Collaborative interventions are geared toward assisting the patient who is experiencing fatigue to accomplish the activities of daily living, return to work, maintain interpersonal relationships, and perform some form of daily exercise. To accomplish these goals, the interprofessional team must first manage the fatigue associated with poor lifestyle choices or disease. The team can also utilize other treatment strategies, such as exercise/rest therapy, pharmacological treatment, and psychological care, to help the patient meet health goals.

Manage Physiological Fatigue

It is important for an individual to balance nutrition, sleep, stress, and psychological coping skills. For example, every individual should get an adequate amount of sleep. The amount of sleep considered adequate varies with different age groups, but it is usually 7 or 8 hours per night for adults, 9 hours for adolescents, and 11 or 12 hours for toddlers. When helping patients with sleep hygiene, discourage oversleeping because it will increase fatigue. Patient teaching in the areas of nutrition and stress management is another intervention geared toward minimizing contributory factors for fatigue.

Manage Secondary Fatigue

Because a large number of fatigue cases are caused by underlying health conditions, optimal management of the conditions helps to reduce fatigue. For example, teaching a patient with iron deficiency anemia about nutrition therapy could include taking iron supplements and eating iron-rich foods, such as lean meat, liver, shellfish, beans, and enriched cereal.

Exercise and Rest Therapy

Exercise can often help relieve the effects of fatigue, especially more short-lived, acute forms of fatigue. Usual exercise should include stretching and aerobic exercise such as walking for 30 minutes on a daily basis. Graded exercise therapy, a structured exercise regimen, may be more appropriate therapy for those who are more deconditioned.[21] Avoid overexertion because it can be detrimental to the body and add to the fatigue.[20] Yoga has been found to diminish fatigue in patients with cancer.[22]

Planned rest breaks throughout the day can also be a benefit to the patient. These naps should be short and limited to less than 1 hour. The best time for naps is early afternoon because fatigue in most patients worsens as the day progresses.[6] Energy conservation activities are also a valuable asset to avoid fatigue (Box 30-2).[23]

For CFS patients, exercise might make the fatigue worse. This is called "post-exertional malaise," and it occurs approximately 12–48 hours after exercise and remains for days or weeks. A carefully structured program of exercise that is balanced over time will help to build stamina and prevent increased fatigue.[24]

Pharmacological Agents

Agents aimed at treating underlying conditions. A number of pharmacologic agents may be used in the treatment of fatigue, with a focus on treating underlying diseases linked to the fatigue. For example, thyroxine may be administered to patients experiencing fatigue associated with hypothyroidism. Thyroxine, a synthetic hormone, will increase the basal metabolic rate to normal, resulting in a reduction of fatigue. As another example, antidepressants are often administered to those experiencing depression. Because fatigue often coexists with depression, an improvement in depression may alleviate the symptoms

of fatigue. If depression is not treated, then it is unlikely that the fatigue will respond to other therapies. These are but two examples of many pharmacological agents that improve fatigue through the treatment of the underlying condition.

Agents for treatment of fatigue. Several types of agents are utilized to specifically treat fatigue, but their exact mechanism of action to diminish fatigue is unknown. These medications are typically indicated for treatment of CFS. Amantadine and modafinil have a dopaminergic effect that increases alertness in those who are fatigued. For episodic situations requiring alertness, CNS stimulants such as methylphenidate (Ritalin), modafinil (Provigil), and caffeine can help. However, this group of drugs can cause headaches, restlessness, insomnia, and dry mouth. These drugs have been found to improve quality of life but do not return the patient back to his or her predisease state.[25] In fact, it has been found that the overuse of caffeine may actually make the fatigue worse.

Psychological Interventions

Most patients who experience chronic fatigue state that they believe their fatigue is misunderstood by health care professionals, and two-thirds of patients state that they are unsatisfied with their quality of medical care.[26] They believe that many caregivers doubt the fatigue's effects because of the inability to identify a physical or psychological cause. As health care providers, it is important to validate with patients that fatigue is a genuine problem and exists as they say it does. Nurses need to acknowledge that it is a subjective experience like pain and can significantly impact an individual's quality of life. Establishing a therapeutic relationship between the patient and the health care team could be instrumental in supporting the patient during this experience. Through this relationship, nurses can support the patient's feelings of control, which can help to lessen the patient's fatigue. Studies of cancer patients indicate that psychosocial support and individualized counseling have fatigue-reduction effects.[27] With chronic fatigue, cognitive–behavioral therapy (CBT) has been beneficial in treatment. CBT uses a series of sessions designed to help patients become aware of the stressors that make their symptoms worse and alter their beliefs and behaviors that might delay recovery.

INTERRELATED CONCEPTS

The concept of fatigue is closely interrelated with many concepts presented in this textbook (Figure 30-3). **Mood and Affect**, **Nutrition**, and **Pain** are shown as purple ovals with bidirectional arrows in Figure 30-3 because of the interrelated cause and effect on fatigue. With each of these concepts, fatigue is a prime symptom of many of their exemplars and can also increase the risk for fatigue. Depression is an example of this phenomenon. Fatigue is listed as one of the diagnostic criteria for depression,[28] an exemplar of mood and affect. In addition, fatigue can cause the individual to experience many losses, and this could lead to depression. **Gas Exchange**, **Perfusion**, **Cellular Regulation**, **Sleep**, and **Stress** (shown as pink ovals) are contributors to fatigue. Also, fatigue can significantly affect the concepts of **Mobility**, **Cognition**, and **Functional Ability**, shown as green ovals with an arrow pointing toward those concepts in Figure 30-3. If an individual is significantly exhausted, his or her ability to think, mobilize, and perform normal daily activities becomes impaired.

CLINICAL EXEMPLARS

Featured Exemplars

Many exemplars related to fatigue exist in the clinical arena and are seen in all areas of the population. The following featured exemplars

---

| BOX 30-2 | **Energy Conservation Strategies** |

- Assess height of work surfaces. Avoid working above head—better to keep items at waist level. Organize work centers so that equipment is within easy reach.
- Position equipment, furniture, or supplies for easy access; arrange household activities on one floor.
- Use adaptive equipment, gadgets, or energy-saving devices.
- Change body position during an activity. Use larger muscles, bend knees, and sit whenever possible.
- Eliminate part or all of an activity that is difficult.
- Delegate part or all of an activity to another person.
- Communicate needs for assistance to family members or others.
- Modify frequency or expected outcomes of an activity.
- Adjust priorities for energy expenditure.
- Simplify activities so they require less energy.
- Plan the day to balance work and rest times. Plan work around times of the day when fatigue is least.
- Change the time of day when an activity is done.
- Include rest periods in the day or rest at least an hour.
- Rest during fatiguing activities that take 30 minutes or longer.
- Organize ahead of time to avoid rushing.

Source: Adapted from Matuska K, Mathiowetz V, Finlayson M: Use and perceived effectiveness of energy conservation strategies for managing multiple sclerosis fatigue, *Am J Occup Ther* 61(1):62–29, 2007.

FIGURE 30-3 Fatigue and Interrelated Concepts

■■■ BOX 30-3   EXEMPLARS OF FATIGUE

Physiological
- Protein calorie malnutrition
- Excessive physical activity
- Sleep deprivation
- Excessive caffeine or alcohol use
- Pregnancy

Secondary
Acute Conditions Causing Fatigue
- Acute renal failure
- Mononucleosis
- Influenza
- Pneumonia
- Traumatic injury

Chronic Conditions Causing Fatigue
- Amyotrophic lateral sclerosis
- Anemia
- Cancer

- Chronic kidney disease
- Chronic obstructive pulmonary disease
- Depression
- Diabetes (type 1 and type 2)
- Fibromyalgia
- Heart failure
- HIV infection
- Hypothyroidism
- Multiple sclerosis

Treatment-Related Causes of Fatigue
- Chemotherapy
- Radiation therapy
- Surgery
- Side effects of medications

Unknown Etiology
- Idiopathic chronic fatigue
- Chronic fatigue syndrome

---

demonstrate conditions that can cause physiological, secondary, and unknown etiology fatigue. Box 30-3 presents additional common exemplars across the lifespan.

Cancer-Related Fatigue

The majority of cancer patients experience some level of fatigue during their course of treatment, and approximately one-third will have persistent fatigue for a number of years post treatment. [29] Prevalence rates for fatigue in cancer patients range from 78% to 96%, depending on the type of treatment and the stage of the cancer. For patients who undergo chemotherapy, the fatigue tends to be more cyclic. It is believed that these agents cause fatigue from direct CNS toxicity and indirectly through promoting menopause and poor mental health.

Diabetes

Diabetes is a condition in which abnormally high levels of sugar remain in the bloodstream instead of entering the body's cells, where it would be converted into energy. This results in the body tissues such as the muscles not receiving the needed nutrition to function appropriately despite the person having enough to eat. Without appropriate nutrition, the individual will experience fatigue. Fatigue is one of the presenting symptoms in both type 1 and type 2 diabetes.

Mononucleosis

Mononucleosis is characterized by the symptoms of fatigue, sore throat, fever, generalized lymphadenopathy, and splenomegaly. These symptoms vary greatly in type, severity, and duration. Patients will typically complain of difficulty maintaining their usual level of activity. The prognosis for recovery from the disease is good. The acute symptoms of the disease will last 7–10 days, and the fatigue will subside in approximately 1 month. In a few cases, the fatigue may extend for longer periods of 2 or 3 months.[30]

Pregnancy

Pregnancy is diagnosed by examining presumptive, probable, and positive indicators. One of the presumptive indicators of pregnancy is the subjective symptom of fatigue.[31] This symptom is particularly challenging during the first trimester, during which the pregnant woman will spend much time sleeping secondary to this increased fatigue. The exact cause of this fatigue is unknown, but it is believed that it might be caused by increasing levels of estrogen, progesterone, and hCG and the psychological/physical adaptations to the pregnancy.

Chronic Obstructive Pulmonary Disease

Chronic obstructive pulmonary disease (COPD) is a chronic condition associated with airway obstruction making it difficult to move air out of the lungs, leading to dyspnea and hypoxemia. A significant amount of energy is utilized by the patient just for the work of breathing. With COPD, a person has a decline in lung function, which can result in decreased exercise tolerance. Over time, patients may also experience decreased muscle strength from deconditioning. Although these patients are in the acute phase of the disease, they will need extensive help in meeting their activities of daily living.[32]

CASE STUDY

Source: Stockbyte/Thinkstock

Case Presentation

Helen Morris is a 55-year-old female who lives with her husband in a suburban community. She is the senior managing editor for a major newspaper. She presents to a health care clinic with the complaint of "getting the flu and cold" for the second time in 3 months and reports "feeling exhausted" and having to "drag herself into work." On the weekends, she describes spending most of her time resting so that she can go back to work on Monday. She adds, "The rest does not last long because by Wednesday I feel exhausted again. My life has become limited—all I can do is to go to work." She states that when she is at the office, by the afternoon she is exhausted and her muscles ache. She states that she has tried to eat better and stopped drinking anything with caffeine, but it has not seemed to make her fatigue any better. She describes the fatigue as starting approximately 6 months ago. The fatigue worsens with any activity. She expresses frustration at being unable to do the things she enjoys, and she wants to find the cause.

Her history reveals anemia with pregnancy, but otherwise she has had no health problems nor does she take any prescribed medications. She says she sleeps but does not feel rested when she wakes up. She denies weight loss or gain, polyuria, polydipsia, or cold intolerance. Her social history is negative for the use of alcohol, relationship problems, or situational stress. She denies having symptoms of depression.

On examination, the patient is alert and well groomed. Her skin is race appropriate, not pale or jaundiced. She is afebrile, and her vital signs are within normal limits. The heart, lung, musculoskeletal, and neurological exam yields normal results. She has no lymphadenopathy. She reports going through menopause and having no menstruation for 2 years. Her hemoglobin is 11.2 mg/dL, and total serum iron is 150 µg/L. Her thyroid-stimulating hormone, kidney, and liver enzymes are within normal limits.

Case Analysis

This case exemplifies the concept of fatigue. Helen is experiencing the exhaustion that is described typically by fatigue sufferers. The report of the fatigue lasting for nearly 6 months makes it chronic. Examining the history, physical, and diagnostic data, there are no underlying diseases that are causing the fatigue. Helen appears to have the classic symptoms of chronic fatigue syndrome as outlined by the Centers for Disease Control and Prevention.

ACCESS EXEMPLAR LINKS IN YOUR GIDDENS EBOOK

REFERENCES

1. Barroso J, Voss J: Fatigue in HIV and AIDS: An analysis of evidence. *J Assoc Nurses AIDS Care* 24:S5–S14, 2013.
2. Strauss S: Pharmacotherapy of chronic fatigue syndrome: Another gallant attempt. *JAMA* 292(10):1234–1235, 2004.
3. Multiple Sclerosis Council for Clinical Practice Guidelines: *Fatigue and multiple sclerosis: Evidence-based management strategies for fatigue in multiple sclerosis*, Washington, DC, 1998, Author.
4. Markowitz A, Rabow M: Palliative management of fatigue at the close of life: "It feels like my body is just worn out". *JAMA* 298(2):217, 2007.
5. Lee K, Hicks G, Nino-Murcia G: Validity and reliability of a scale to assess fatigue. *Psychiatry Res* 36(3):291–298, 1991.
6. Rosenthal T, Majeroni B, Pretorius R, et al: Fatigue: An overview. *Am Fam Physician* 78(10):1173–1179, 2008.
7. Centers for Disease Control and Prevention: Chronic fatigue syndrome: The 1994 case definition, 2012. Retrieved from: <http://www.cdc.gov/cfs/case-definition/1994.html>.
8. Barnett M: Fatigue. In Otto S, editor: *Oncology nursing*, ed 3, St Louis, 1997, Mosby.
9. Cella D: The Functional Assessment of Cancer Therapy—Anemia (FACT-An) scale: A new tool for the assessment of outcomes in cancer anemia and fatigue. *Semin Hematol* 3(Suppl 2):13–19, 1997.
10. Dantzer R, Heijnen CJ, Kavelaars A, et al: The neuroimmune basis of fatigue. *Trends Neurosci* 37(1):39–46, 2014.
11. Bower J, Ganz P, Aziz N, et al: T-cell homeostasis in breast cancer survivors with persistent fatigue. *J Natl Cancer Inst* 95:1165–1168, 2003.
12. Smith W, Noonan C, Buchwald D: Mortality in a cohort of chronically fatigued patients. *Psychol Med* 35:1301, 2006.
13. Joyce J, Hotopf M, Wessely S: The prognosis of chronic fatigue and chronic fatigue syndrome: A systematic review. *Q J Med* 90:223, 1997.
14. Ashbury F, Findlay H, Reynolds B, et al: A Canadian survey of cancer patients' experiences: Are their needs being met? *J Pain Symptom Manage* 15:298–306, 1998.
15. Prins J, van der Meer J, Bleijenberg G: Chronic fatigue syndrome. *Lancet* 367:346, 2006.
16. Kendall M: Do we need a new classification of beta-blockers? *J Hum Hypertens* 4:27–29, 1990.

17. Fahlen G, Knutsson A, Peter R, et al: Effort–reward imbalance, sleep disturbances and fatigue. *Int Arch Occup Environ Health* 79(5):371–378, 2006.

18. Lee K, Dziadkowiec O, Meek P: A systems science approach to fatigue management in research and health care. *Nurs Outlook* 62:313–321, 2014.

19. Lyon D, McCain N, Elswick R, et al: Biobehavioral examination of fatigue across populations: Report from a P30 Center of Excellence. *Nurs Outlook* 62:322–331, 2014.

20. Krupp L: Fatigue in multiple sclerosis: Definition, pathophysiology and treatment. *CNS Drugs* 14(4):225–234, 2003.

21. O'Connor P, Puetz T: Chronic physical activity and feelings of energy and fatigue. *Med Sci Sports Exerc* 37(2):299–305, 2005.

22. Mock V: Evidence-based treatment for cancer-related fatigue. *J Natl Cancer Inst Monogr* 32:112–118, 2004.

23. Matuska K, Mathiowetz V, Finlayson M: Use and perceived effectiveness of energy conservation strategies for managing multiple sclerosis fatigue. *Am J Occup Ther* 61(1):62–69, 2007.

24. Fulcher K, White P: A randomized control trial of grade exercise in patients with chronic fatigue syndrome. *Br Med J* 314:1647–1652, 1997.

25. Bruera E, Valero V, Driver L, et al: Patient controlled methylphenidate for cancer fatigue: A double-blind randomized, placebo-controlled trial. *J Clin Oncol* 24(13):2073–2078, 2006.

26. Deale A, Wessely S: Patients' perceptions of medical care in chronic fatigue syndrome. *Soc Sci Med* 52:1959, 2001.

27. Trijsburg R, van Knippengerg F, Rijpma S: Effects of psychological treatment on cancer patients: A comparison of strategies. *Psychosom Med* 54:489–517, 1992.

28. American Psychiatric Association: *Diagnostic and statistical manual of mental disorders*, ed 5, Arlington, VA, 2013, American Psychiatric Publishing.

29. Servaes P, Verfhagen S, Bleijenberg G: Determinants of chronic fatigue in disease free breast cancer patients: A cross-sectional study. *Ann Oncol* 13:589, 2002.

30. Hockenberry M, Wilson D: *Wong's nursing care of infants and children*, ed 9, St Louis, 2011, Mosby.

31. Lowdermilk D, Perry S, Cashion M, et al: *Maternity and women's health care*, ed 10, St Louis, 2012, Mosby.

32. Ignatavicius D, Workman M: *Medical–surgical nursing: Patient-centered collaborative care*, ed 7, St Louis, 2013, Saunders.

Stress

Lynne Buchanan

Stress is a common topic in society and is a frequently used term to express pressure or emotional strain. All people experience stress, a process involving cognitive appraisal and perception with physiological and psychological responses. Although early understandings viewed stress as unhealthy, contemporary views show stress as a mechanism of self-defense based on the individual's perceptions of the requirements of an event, demand, stressor, as well as the individual's pattern of response. Stress is a normal physiological process for regulation and homeostasis. How the individual perceives the stressor, the severity and duration of the stressor, and the individual's response to the stressor determine the outcome. Stress can have positive effects (referred to as eustress) associated with challenges and accomplishment. Stress can also be unhealthy (referred to as allostasis) when severe, sustained, and/or when the individual exhausts coping resources.

DEFINITION

The word "stress" has existed since the 14th century with a meaning of hardship, adversity, or affliction. In the early 20th century, Walter Cannon first described the stimulus and response (fight or flight) to the perception of a physical or emotional threat.[1] Hans Selye brought the concept of a general adaptation syndrome to popular society by proposing a reaction theory that stress is the sum of all the effects of factors that act on the body, with both pleasant and unpleasant stressors being equally important.[2,3] Although early experiments supported various species responding in a stereotypical reaction to events such as infection, trauma, nervous strain, heat, cold, or fatigue, continuing work demonstrated that there was not always a precise uniform response.[4] Later theorists proposed stress as a mediator between life events and the adaptation of stress as a process with a defined series of steps. The foundation for contemporary perspectives regarding stress evolved from this work.[5]

Throughout the years, stress has been characterized as a response, an interaction, and an outcome.[6] The stress response is a series of reactions to external and internal demands. The full reaction is determined by the duration, severity, resources, and coping skills. For example, a new father may appraise the birth of his newborn infant emotionally as a feeling of joy or as one of anxiety, depending on personal circumstances. This emotional feeling has an accompanying physiological response. The response may be a normal, short-term physiological process enabling regulation and homeostasis, or it may be of longer duration and severity when, for example, the response is driven by anxiety. The duration and severity of stress are determined by the perceived ability to manage the stressor within current environment, resources, and abilities—in other words, the perception that the stressor can or cannot be managed within the context of environment, available resources, and abilities.

For the purposes of this concept presentation, stress is defined as *an internal or external event or demand of life experienced by the individual that is perceived and appraised for scope and meaning on a continuum to determine whether resources and abilities for management are available, exceeded, or exhausted.* In nursing, stress has been proposed as a process with physical, psychological, and behavioral components in response to individuals' perception of the physical, environmental, or psychosocial demands placed on them.[7] Nursing has further conceptualized stress as a subjective experience involving cognitive appraisal, with potential for positive or negative effects on health and well-being.

SCOPE

The scope of stress as a concept ranges on a continuum from stress–neutral to challenge–manageable and threat–not manageable (Figure 31-1). Stress neutral is perceived as an event that is easy to manage and easy to mobilize resources. A challenge–manageable situation is perceived as requiring new ordinary resources that are currently available or can be easily accessed. Both of these conditions are associated with sustained homeostasis. Threat–not manageable with ordinary resources represents a situation perceived as requiring extraordinary resources, support, mobilization of resources that do not currently exist, or the exhaustion of existing resources and abilities. A situation perceived as a threat may be a new event or one that is prolonged in duration, severe in level, and viewed as extraordinary, overwhelming, and exhausting. Such a state triggers a stress response in order to manage the stressor.

Stress is also considered at the macro and individual or micro level context. An example of stress experience at the macro level is an environmental event such as a natural disaster or a large-scale terroristic attack. Although there are societal-level outcomes, each individual within the population involved will respond based on his or her own perception of the event and the personal impact it has for him or her.

FIGURE 31-1 Scope of Stress

Stress at the micro level focuses on the way a stressor affects an individual, specifically on the internal localized context (cells, organs, or body systems).

NORMAL PHYSIOLOGICAL PROCESS

In most cases, the day-to-day stress experienced by individuals is managed such that homeostasis and regulation are maintained with a minimal impact or interruption to the individual. The optimal stress response relies on intact, functioning body systems including the central nervous system, which processes information and makes meaning of events. When faced with a potential or actual stressor, the individual first appraises the situation. Perceived events or demands cause an anticipatory response beginning in the limbic system. If the stressor is perceived as minor, subtle physiological, psychological, and behavioral processes compensate for the stressor.

When a stressor is perceived as a more serious threat, a stress response is initiated by the nervous and endocrine systems, particularly the hypothalamus, sympathetic nervous system (SNS), the pituitary gland, and the adrenal gland. These systems synchronize a complex series of reactions leading to a coordinated response, directing energy for adaptation (Figure 31-2).

The hypothalamus secretes corticotropin-releasing factor (CRF), which activates the SNS, the anterior pituitary, and the posterior pituitary. Activation of the SNS causes the release of catecholamines (norepinephrine, epinephrine, and dopamine). Norepinephrine is released throughout the brain, triggering neural pathways for sensory information and stimulating arousal, vigilance, anxiety, and labile emotions.[8]

FIGURE 31-2 Physiology of Alarm Response Sympathetic Nervous System Effects

The physiological response (known as the *fight-or-flight response*) is due to the release of catecholamines epinephrine and norepinephrine. Specifically, these hormones lead to increased heart rate, blood pressure, and cardiac output; dilation of bronchial airways; pupil dilation; increased blood flow to the skeletal muscles; and increased blood glucose. There is a concomitant decrease in blood flow to nonessential organs (e.g., the digestive system).[8]

At the same time, CRF stimulates the anterior and posterior pituitary gland to release several hormones, including antidiuretic hormone, prolactin, growth hormone, and adrenocorticotropic hormone (ACTH). ACTH triggers the secretion of cortisol and aldosterone from the adrenal cortex. The activation of the adrenal cortex during the stress response leads to the secretion of cortisol, a glucocorticoid. Cortisol mobilizes cellular metabolism, particularly glucose and protein metabolism. The net effect is increased blood glucose (through gluconeogenesis and inhibition of glucose update and oxidation in selected body cells) and increasing amino acids (through catabolic effects of muscle). In elevated levels, cortisol also has a role in the immune response, including immunosuppressive and anti-inflammatory effects.

When the stressor or threat is eliminated or when the individual perceives the event as neutral or challenge (but manageable), the alarm response is halted. Sustained stress, however, has a negative impact on organs, body systems, and health and well-being. A prolonged or chronic situation involving a heightened stress response exhausts the ability to maintain homeostasis; physical, psychological, and behavioral manifestations lead to overt stress symptoms.[9]

Age-Related Differences

Because the stress response is based on a psychoneuro response, there are few discernable differences in the stress response across the lifespan. Age-related differences are primarily associated with cognitive appraisal of events that determine if a situation is a threat or not. Cognitive appraisal and coping strategies are associated with cognitive development and life experiences.

VARIATIONS AND CONTEXT

There are variations in stress seen across the lifespan, especially when stress is severe and/or prolonged.[9] For most individuals, stress is experienced in a similar way, and most individuals may not even be aware of the effects. Factors such as age, developmental level, maturation, environment, life experiences, and the individual's general mental and physical health status impact the response. The environment is important, especially if it is supportive of health and well-being and nurturing in developing skills and abilities to deal with life demands.

Sources of Stress
Physiological Stressors

Physiological stress refers to a stressor that originates as a physiological trigger and usually is specifically associated with an injury or illness (Box 31-1). Some acute physiological stressors are life-threatening states such as trauma, acute myocardial infarction, or acute renal failure. An acute stress response is immediate, often intense, and necessary for survival. Chronic physiological stress can lead to debilitating disease.

Psychological/Emotional Stressors

Psychological and emotional stressors are more common stressors encountered on a regular basis and generate a state of unpleasant arousal. Common stressors include occupational pressures, academic pressures, major life events (both positive and negative), financial

---

BOX 31-1 Examples of Stressors

Physiological Stressors
- Cancer
- Chronic obstructive pulmonary disease
- Dementia
- Diabetes
- Organ Failure (such as Heart, Renal, or Respiratory Failure)
- Myocardial infarction
- Acute and chronic pain
- Traumatic injury

Psychological/Emotional Stressors
- Birth of child
- Caregiving
- Change in health status
- Death of close family member or friend
- Diagnosis of terminal illness
- Divorce
- Environmental emergencies
- Failing an examination
- Loss of job
- Marriage
- Moral distress
- Moving
- Parenting
- Physical disability
- Relationship problems
- Social unrest
- Spiritual distress

---

stress, or bereavement (see Box 31-1). Psychological stress can be acute or chronic. An event in which danger is perceived (such as fleeing from a house fire or reacting to an automobile accident) or an emotionally traumatic event (such as the unexpected death of a close friend or family member) triggers an acute stress response. Chronic emotional stress is a long-term state associated with psychosocial stressors such as difficult relationships, ongoing occupational stress, or financial stress.

Types of Stress

In general, unhealthy stress is categorized as acute stress, episodic acute stress, and chronic stress.[8] The source of all three types of stress can be physiological or psychological/emotional (discussed previously):

- Acute stress: Acute stress is, by far, the most common type of stress and typically occurs for a short period of time. It usually occurs in reaction to a real or perceived demand, threat, or pressure. Resolution of the stressor leads to elimination of the stress response.
- Episodic acute stress: Episodic stress is often described as "self-inflicted" stress or in regular chaos and is common among type A personalities. This often occurs by taking on unrealistic assignments beyond what is typically or reasonably expected. These individuals may always be in a hurry and irritable. Constant worry is another form of episodic acute stress.
- Chronic stress: This type of stress represents a perpetual or sustained demand, threat, or pressure that is harmful to health because it wears on individuals continuously. It can stem from long-term stressors such as chronic occupational stress, relationship stress, and financial stress. Chronic stress is often associated with a loss of hope that the situation can improve.

CONSEQUENCES

Although stress is a normal physiological response, many consequences occur if stress is sustained over a long period of time or is severe. Chronic stress results in the continuous activation of the nervous system and eventually produces negative outcomes across multiple body systems:[8–12]

- Central nervous system: Chronic stress affects cognitive function, including headaches, nervousness, irritability, problems with decision making, insomnia, memory problems, confusion, anxiety disorders, and depression. Prolonged release of corticosteroids can also lead to stress-induced damage to the hippocampus, which can affect long-term memory.[8–11]

- Cardiovascular system: Chronic stress results in excessive activation of the SNS and in long-term exposure to catecholamines. This increases heart rate and blood pressure and can lead to cardiovascular disease such as hypertension, atherosclerosis, cardiac arrhythmias, myocardial infarction, or stroke.[8,13–16] Furthermore, individuals with preexisting cardiovascular disease are particularly at risk for exacerbation of the condition if exposed to prolonged stress.

- Immune system: Excessive and long-term exposure to cortisol has been shown to decrease white blood cells, leading to stress-induced immunosuppression placing the individual at greater risk for bacterial and viral infections.[17–19] There also appears to be a correlation between stress and immune-based conditions such as rheumatoid arthritis, multiple sclerosis, asthma, and cancer, although specific details of this relationship are unclear.

- Musculoskeletal system: The stress response is associated with muscle tension as a way to protect against injury. Chronic stress can result in an overly taut muscle over a long period of time, leading to pain and discomfort, particularly in the head, neck, and shoulders. Protracted muscle tension of both the head and the neck are two contributors to tension and migraine headaches.[8] Nervous tics may also develop with chronic stress because of muscle tension.

- Gastrointestinal system: Individuals under chronic stress may experience a number of gastrointestinal problems associated with excessive excretion of catecholamines and cortisol. Gastritis, ulcerative colitis, irritable colon, and diarrhea have been linked to chronic stress, as have obesity and eating disorders.[8,11,12]

- Integumentary system: The hair, skin, and nails may be affected by chronic stress. Elevated stress over time may cause excessive hair loss. There may be skin problems that are exacerbated by stress, including acne, eczema, and psoriasis. There may also be stress-related ulcers in the mouth from dry mouth and cold sores.[8]

- Sexuality and reproduction system: Chronic stress affects reproductive health in both men and women. In men, reduced sex drive, reduced testosterone production, reduced sperm production, maturation, erectile dysfunction, and impotence occur.[8] Among women, excessive stress may be associated with menstrual cycle disorders and dysmenorrhea, as well as exacerbation of menstrual symptoms (cramping, fluid retention and bloating, and irritability) or menopausal symptoms (irritability, mood swings, and hot flashes).[8,10,11]

RISK FACTORS

Populations at Risk

Individuals across all population groups are at risk for stress throughout the lifespan. Serious psychological distress is recognized in our society. According to the 2014 National Health Interview Survey, an estimated 3.1% of adults older than age 18 years experienced serious psychological distress in the previous 30 days; this was highest among middle-aged adults in the 45- to 64-year-old age group, Hispanics, and women.[20] The three populations that report the greatest level of general stress are lower-income Americans, young adults (particularly those with children), and women.[12]

Individual Risk Factors

One of the most common sources of stress is financial strain; this often leads to many other areas of stress, including stressful relationships, occupational stress, and strained family relationships. Individuals with health conditions or individuals in caregiving roles are also at risk for chronic stress. Medical conditions that are known to cause physiological stress are shown in Box 31-1. Individuals with brain disease or impaired cognition are at risk for negative outcome because of the inability to adequately appraise and process information related to stress and the environment. An appraisal assists with determining the meaning of the stressor (neutral, challenge, or threat); a full meaning of the stressor or event is gained through secondary appraisal. Information processing necessary to gain a full meaning of the scope of the event requires cognitive function, including long-term memory. Thus, any factor that impacts cognition and long-term memory will affect cognitive appraisal and outcome.[13] In a classic study, investigators found that the working memory in an adult is only able to hold seven items or elements of information at a time.[14] Therefore, adults who overload their working memory will also be at greater risk for disability or dysfunction.

ASSESSMENT

The priority of assessment should be evaluation of signs and symptoms of stress and the association to disease. Signs and symptoms can manifest in a variety of ways and may vary in severity. Stress can be evaluated using assessment tools that capture the physiological, cognitive, psychological/emotional, and behavioral signs and symptoms. Nurses should recognize individuals who are experiencing a challenging or threatening stress response (including psychological distress) so that appropriate interventions can be initiated.

History

When conducting a history, the nurse queries about the past and current state of health (past medical history, current conditions, and current medications), family history, psychosocial history, and stress symptoms associated with body systems. Clues about the presence of stress are often identified in the psychosocial component of the history. Specifically, the nurse should ask about mental health problems and past or current conditions or life events associated with psychological stress, such as a death, loss of job, or illness. Nurses should ask about demands and recent life events and the individual's perception of the event or demand, and nurses should consider physiological responses. The most common symptoms of stress include irritability, nervousness or anxiousness, fatigue, feeling overwhelmed, or feeling depressed or sad.[12] Also, nurses should ask about unexplained abdominal pain or indigestion, headaches, insomnia, fatigue, restlessness, lack of concentration, dizziness, excessive sweating, sweaty palms, back pain, tight shoulders or neck, skin eruptions, hair loss, hyperventilation, palpitations, and tightening of the chest.

A number of tools are available to further assist with assessment. Perhaps the most widely recognized tool is the Holmes Life Events Scale,[15] which can be easily administered and scored by nurses in clinic settings. Another stress assessment tool is the Ways of Coping Checklist, which helps to gain an understanding of how the patient responds to stressful situations.[16]

Examination

Examination findings associated with stress are usually consistent with sympathetic nervous system activation. In the acute phase, these signs may include elevated heart rate, irregular heart rate, elevated blood pressure, increased respiratory rate and depth, excessive sweating, dilated pupils, and muscle tension. Such findings may not be as evident when stress is chronic.

CLINICAL MANAGEMENT

Nurses in all areas of practice should be able to recognize stress and provide appropriate interventions. Figure 31-3 illustrates an organizing framework for the concept of stress that nurses can use in their practice, and Table 31-1 presents common interventions for the management of stress. In the framework, there are antecedents that include individual characteristics, family, community, and environment. The personal appraisal and reappraisal assist the individual to focus the scope of the experience and determine the magnitude of the

stressor. Psychological and physiological responses occur based on this appraisal, and clinical management strategies are identified.

Primary Prevention

The goal of clinical management and the treatment plan is to promote health and well-being. Primary care settings that focus on wellness, prevention of stress-related disease, and disability include the workplace, schools, senior centers, community wellness centers, primary health care clinics, and medical homes. Maintaining a positive attitude (e.g., feeling optimistic) contributes to health and well-being and serves as a foundation of primary prevention. Stress prevention also involves counseling, health education, nutrition counseling, exercise, and complementary/alternative strategies.[9] Health education for stress prevention is aimed at assisting the individual to understand the components of a healthy lifestyle and the relationship of chronic stress and disease.

Secondary Prevention (Screening)

A number of stress screening tools are available for use in clinical practice, and there are many screening inventory tools found online for consumers. There are currently no national recommendations for

FIGURE 31-3 Organizing Framework for the Stress and Nursing Practice

TABLE 31-1 **Clinical Management of Stress**

Stress Category	Signs and Symptoms	Examples of Intervention	Outcome
Psychological and emotional	Anxiety, anger, depression, irritability, frustration, overreaction, memory loss, lack of concentration	Cognitive–behavioral skills training Meditation Stress inoculation Time management	Reduced anxiety and anger Reduced depression Reduced strain
Physiological	Muscle tension, headache, stomachache, acid reflux, tachycardia, hyperventilation, elevated BP	Biofeedback Muscle relaxation Therapeutic touch/massage Exercise	Reduced somatization Reduced forehead muscle tension (EMG) Reduced BP Reduced level 0–10 scale Reduction in number and severity of stress warning signals Reduction in number and severity of stress signs and symptoms
Behavioral	Smoking, overeating, substance abuse	Health education Smoking cessation Counseling	Healthier lifestyle Improved health status

BP, blood pressure; EMG, electromyogram.

stress screening for general or designated populations, but the screening tools are useful for the assessment of stress.

Collaborative Interventions

Collaborative interventions are geared toward restoring the person to optimal function by initiating prompt interventions, follow-up, and education. There are four main categories of collaborative interventions for managing stress. Those that directly impact prevention or reduction of stress are therapeutic lifestyle change, relaxation/exercise therapy, pharmacologic agents, and complementary and alternative therapies.

Therapeutic Lifestyle Change

A therapeutic lifestyle change (TLC) collaborative intervention is aimed at promoting adaptation, coping, and support to promote positive changes that lead to checking of stress or of decreasing severity levels. The collaboration involves exercise, dietary, and counseling professionals who work with the nurse to develop a TLC treatment plan. Topics and skills include self-talk; muscle relaxation; exercise; and dietary approaches avoiding tobacco, alcohol, and drugs. Motivational interviewing is a useful strategy to motivate individuals to change.

Relaxation/Exercise Therapy

Relaxation and exercise are among the most effective measures for stress management. Specific plans are developed based on the individual's needs and underlying health conditions. The most common forms of relaxation activities include meditation, breathing, walking, stretching, and yoga.[17,18] Exercise therapy can be implemented in various settings, including a hospital, community center, or home. Exercise should be individualized but can include any cardiovascular–aerobic activity, including walking, running, swimming, and cycling. The benefits of exercise include relief of tension, reduction of stress, relaxation, and enhanced sense of well-being.[18,19]

Pharmacologic Agents

Although there are no medications used to prevent stress or treat stress directly, many types of medications are used in the management of stress, particularly conditions that coexist or are caused by stress. Drugs that act on the central and peripheral nervous systems, such as anxiolytics and hypnotics, antidepressants, antianxiety agents, psychotherapeutics, muscle relaxants, antimigraine agents, and narcotic pain medications, may be used. Selective serotonin reuptake

inhibitors and tricyclic antidepressants may be used for individuals with chronic stress and depression. Some of the most common drugs are for relief of muscle tension and pain associated with stress.[21] Stress often causes muscle tension and muscle spasm from prolonged contraction.

Complementary and Alternative Therapies

Another group of interventions effective for stress reduction includes complementary and alternative medicine strategies. Strategies listed as possibly effective for relieving stress include acupuncture, herbals/botanicals, aromatherapy, and massage. Relaxation techniques for stress reduction include a number of practices, such as progressive relaxation, guided imagery, biofeedback, self-hypnosis, and deep breathing exercises.[22]

INTERRELATED CONCEPTS

The concept of stress has multiple interrelated concepts featured in this textbook (Figure 31-4). The most closely aligned concepts are Coping and Anxiety. Coping represents how an individual perceives and responds to the stressor and is a determinant of the magnitude of response. Ineffective coping is associated with a challenged appraisal of stress, inadequate or inappropriate stress responses, and insufficient resources to resolve the stressor. Anxiety is also closely aligned with stress because this is a typical response to a stressor. Anxiety can be useful by mobilizing resources to cope with the stressor or can lead to overt mental health illnesses when the stressor is severe and/or sustained.

Functional Ability and Family Dynamics are shown as interrelated concepts because these are often associated with stressors. Many of life's most significant stressors are generated from problems managing life's events and challenges with relationships. Another key interrelated concept is the health and illness concept Cognition. Adequate cognitive skills are needed in order to perform a cognitive appraisal of an event because of the need to accurately process information. Chronic stress leads to cognitive impairment. For this reason, this is shown as a bidirectional arrow in Figure 31-4.

Many other consequences of chronic stress were mentioned previously in this chapter; they are represented by the concepts Mood and Affect, Perfusion, Sexuality, Sleep, and Immunity. Specifically, many stress-related illnesses result from sustained stress and are exacerbated by ineffective coping strategies.

FIGURE 31-4 Stress and Interrelated Concepts

CLINICAL EXEMPLARS

The clinical exemplars for this concept represent the most common or classic stress-related disorders (Box 31-2). These are disorders that result from or are exacerbated by chronic stress due to sustained exposure to catecholamines. A number of variables affect the onset and severity of the stress-related disorder and include the type of stressor, the perception of the stressor, copings skills, and length and severity of the stress. Stress-related illness is associated with chronic stress, and a brief discussion of selected exemplars is featured next. For detailed explanations and the nursing care exemplars, see medical–surgical, pediatric, and gerontology references.

Featured Exemplars

Anxiety Disorders

Anxiety is an adaptive response to stress that stretches on a continuum from mild anxiety to a panic disorder. Anxiety can be acute or chronic—consistent with the stressor involved. Anxiety affects individuals across the lifespan and represents the most common of mental health disorders among pediatric, adolescent, and adult populations. Individuals who develop anxiety disorders tend to have impairments in social, family, and occupational relationships.

Tension Headache

Tension headaches are the most common type of headache among adults and are associated with moderate to severe stress causing prolonged muscle tension. It is described as a bilateral, dull, bandlike or pressing pain that builds up gradually and has a prolonged duration. Tension headaches can occur periodically or for several days in a row, lasting from 30 minutes to days. This type of headache is worsened by noise and light. The severity of symptoms tends to be positively correlated with the frequency of occurrence.

Hypertension

Hypertension is a chronic elevation of blood pressure. This is one of the most common manifestations of stress related to catecholamine effect on the sympathetic nervous system. Catecholamines cause peripheral vasoconstriction and an increased rate and force of cardiac contraction, leading to the elevation of blood pressure. Hypertension

BOX 31-2 EXEMPLARS OF STRESS-RELATED DISORDERS

- Acne
- Anxiety disorders
- Autoimmune disorders
- Cardiac arrhythmias
- Coronary artery disease
- Depression
- Dysmenorrhea
- Dyspepsia
- Eating disorders
- Eczema
- Erectile dysfunction
- Fatigue
- Fibromyalgia
- Hypertension
- Immunodeficiency
- Insomnia
- Irritable bowel syndrome
- Low back pain
- Stroke
- Tension headaches

is most commonly diagnosed among adults, although hypertension among young adults and children is on the rise.

Insomnia

Insomnia represents a group of disorders associated with a disruption of sleep. Acute and chronic stress is one of the leading causes of insomnia. Insomnia is described as the inability to fall asleep or stay asleep. The effects include daytime sleepiness, generalized fatigue, irritability, and cognitive problems. Chronic insomnia is associated with multiple health-related conditions. Insomnia can affect individuals of all ages, but it is more commonly associated with adults and older adults.

Irritable Bowel Syndrome

Irritable bowel syndrome (IBS) refers to a group of symptoms associated with discomfort in the large intestine, including cramping pain, bloating, gas, diarrhea, and/or constipation. Because there is no identified pathology, IBS is not considered a disease but, rather, a functional syndrome with no known cause. However, stress has been identified as a common trigger of IBS. It affects an estimated 20% of the population at one or more times during their lifetime. IBS can occur at any age, but it most commonly affects adults and older adults and affects women more often than men.

Eczema

Eczema is a chronic condition associated with chronic inflammation of the skin. It presents as erythema, scaling, itching, and weeping sores. This condition is thought to be an autoimmune condition that is exacerbated by stress. In other words, eczema is not caused by stress, but the condition is made worse by stress. It occurs among individuals of all ages and affects men and women equally.

CASE STUDY

Source: MariaDubova/iStock/Thinkstock

Case Presentation

Jennifer Williams is a 43-year-old recently divorced female who has two teenage daughters aged 18 and 16 years. Her 16-year old daughter is 7 months pregnant. Jennifer's ex-husband is an alcoholic and is involved with her daughters but cannot be relied on for financial assistance. She lives in an older home in a low-income neighborhood. Her aging and widowed mother, who lives a few blocks away, is in the early stages of Alzheimer's disease and needs regular assistance. Ms. Williams is the main caregiver for her mother. She is employed full-time as an office assistant and regularly has difficulty making ends meet financially.

A number of recent events have been challenging for Jennifer. Her pregnant daughter recently broke up with her boyfriend and Jennifer knows she will be largely supporting and raising her grandchild. She also recently had an intense argument with her oldest daughter about attending college—something she supports but can't afford. In addition to all of these issues, Jennifer's mother fell and broke her arm. She is now trying to meet the increasing care her mother needs.

All these events have been weighing heavily on Jennifer's mind. She is feeling highly anxious and is experiencing difficulty sleeping. She has had intermittent diarrhea and has become highly irritable, leading to arguments at work with her coworkers. Jennifer also began experiencing headaches. Fearing she had something seriously wrong with her, she went to an urgent care clinic. After a brief visit focusing on her headache, she was told not to worry because she was "only experiencing a tension headache" and was a little hypertensive, and she was advised to see her primary care physician. Jennifer was relieved to learn she did not have a brain tumor, but she has no intention of seeing another physician for the headaches. She does not want to spend any more money on herself.

Case Analysis

This case exemplifies multiple psychological/emotional stressors and the physical effects of the stress. Because of the extensive demands on her time and limited income, Jennifer may not have extensive resources from which to draw. Unless she specifically shares these challenges with the health care professionals, it is unlikely that a comprehensive stress assessment and intervention will be developed. Unfortunately, many of these stressors will be ongoing and are likely to create even more demands on Jennifer, placing her at significant risk for stress-related disorders if she is unable to find appropriate coping mechanisms.

ACCESS EXEMPLAR LINKS IN YOUR GIDDENS EBOOK

REFERENCES

1. Cannon W: *Bodily changes in pain, hunger, fear and rage: An account of recent researches into the function of emotional excitement*, New York, 1915, Appleton.
2. Selye H: The general adaptation syndrome and the diseases of adaptation. *J Clin Endocrinol Metab* 6:117, 1946.
3. Selye H: Stress syndrome. *Am J Nurs* 65(3):97–99, 1965.
4. Selye H: Confusion and controversy in the stress field. *J Human Stress* 1:37–44, 1975.
5. Lazarus RS, Folkman S: *Stress, appraisal and coping*, New York, 1984, Springer.
6. Lazarus RS, Lazarus BN: *Passion and reason: Making sense of our emotions*, New York, 1994, Oxford University Press.
7. Mitchell P, Buchanan L: Physiologic adaptations during psychoemotional stress. In Underhill S, et al, editors: *Cardiac nursing*, ed 2, Philadelphia, 1989, Lippincott Williams & Wilkins, p 165.
8. Forshee BA, Clayton MF, McCance KL: Stress and disease. In McCance K, Huether S, Brashers V, et al, editors: *Pathophysiology: The biologic basis for disease in adults and children*, ed 6, St Louis, 2010, Mosby.
9. Horowitz JA: Stress management. In Edelman C, Kudzma E, Mandle C, editors: *Health promotion throughout the life span*, ed 8, St Louis, 2014, Elsevier.
10. Paradies Y: A theoretical view of psychosocial stress and health. In Barnes AB, Montefuscio JE, editors: *Role of stress in psychological disorders*, New York, 2011, Nova Science, pp 1–19.
11. Caplan RP: Stress, anxiety, and depression in hospital consultants, general practitioners, and senior health service managers. *BMJ* 309(6964):1261–1264, 1994.
12. American Psychological Association: Stress in America: Paying with our health, 2015. Retrieved from <http://apa.org/news/press/releases/stress/2014/stress-report.pdf>.
13. Sweller J, van Merrienboer J, Paas F: Cognitive architecture and instructional design. *Educ Psychol Rev* 10(3):251–296, 1998.
14. Miller GA: The magical number seven, plus or minus two: Some limits on our capacity for processing information. *Psychol Rev* 63:81–97, 1956.
15. Holmes TH, Rahe RH: Social readjustment rating scale. *J Psychosomat Res* 11:213–218, 1967.
16. Pearlin LI, Schooler C: The structure of coping. *J Health Soc Behav* 19(1):2–21, 1978.
17. Kim SD: Effects of yogic exercise on life stress and blood glucose levels in nursing students. *J Phys Ther Sci* 26(12):2003–2006, 2014.
18. Bruning NS, Frew DR: Effects of exercise, relaxation, and management skills training on physiological stress indicators: A field experiment. *J Appl Psychol* 72(4):515–521, 1987.
19. Sims J: The evaluation of stress management strategies in general practice: An evidence led approach. *Br J Gen Pract* 422:577–581, 1997.
20. Schiller J, Ward B, Freeman G, et al: National Health Interview Survey, Early Release Program. National Center for Health Statistics, 2014. Retrieved from <http://www.cdc.gov/nchs/nhis.htm>.
21. Karch AM: *Focus on nursing pharmacology*, ed 5, Philadelphia, 2011, Wolters Kluwer/Lippincott Williams & Wilkins, pp 299–512.
22. Kudzma E, Brunton J: Complementary and alternative strategies. In Edelman C, Kudzma E, Mandle C, editors: *Health promotion throughout the life span*, ed 8, St Louis, 2014, Elsevier.

Coping

Jean Giddens

When an individual experiences physiological or psychological stress, a response is needed to adapt or modify the impact of the stressor. Considering the large number and variety of stressors that humans experience throughout the lifespan, it should be no surprise that a wide variety of responses occur; some responses are helpful and some are not. Coping is a multifaceted concept involving human cognition, individual perception, and behavior. In nursing, understanding the concept of coping as a relationship between the person and the environment is an important component of care delivery.

DEFINITION

The definition of coping in nursing has not yet reached a consensus. Research in the area of coping has studied this concept from a number of perspectives. One of the classic definitions of coping is from Lazarus and Folkman, who described coping as *an ever-changing process involving both cognitive means and behavioral actions, in order to manage internal or external situations that are perceived as difficult and/or beyond the individual's current resources.*[1] This definition encompasses the relationship of the person and the environment. When the internal or external demands of the environment surpass current resources, the individual will attempt to maintain equilibrium by utilizing coping strategies. Ray and colleagues defined coping as *being action oriented toward a goal of changing a situation*—in other words, the conscious or unconscious behaviors of an individual to avoid harm and restore balance.[2] Keil further defined coping as *abstract thoughts based on past experiences to reduce stress.*[3]

It is apparent from the varying definitions that coping represents continual changes in behavior and cognition in order to modify or adapt the person–environmental relationship to reduce stress. This adaptation or modification requires conscious thought—a key differentiator from a physiological reflex or physiological defense mechanism.[4] Coping is based on individual perception, relationship to the environment, and evaluation of the environment as well as availability of resources. Furthermore, an individual's control over internal and external demands has an impact on coping and change.

SCOPE

The scope of the concept coping ranges from effective (or adaptive) coping to ineffective (or maladaptive) coping that result from constructive or destructive coping mechanisms (Figure 32-1). Coping behaviors result from a real or perceived stressor and are geared toward reduction or elimination of the stress. Constructive mechanisms occur when an individual treats the stressor as a warning and elects to resolve the problem.[5] Destructive mechanisms occur when an individual addresses the feeling associated with the stressor without resolving the problem. This continuum is not necessarily one or the other; some coping strategies may be partially effective or partially ineffective. Ineffective coping refers to the inability to assess the stressor and/or respond appropriately. When coping is ineffective, many problems can result, depending on the seriousness of the stressor event.

The scope of coping is also viewed from the perspective of an individual, family, or community. Individual coping links to the coping capacity of an individual/patient. Family coping refers the coping ability of family members when faced with challenges with one or more family members. On a community level, coping refers to the adaptive patterns and problem-solving capacity of a community when faced with challenges.[6] This concept presentation primarily focuses on individual coping.

NORMAL PHYSIOLOGICAL PROCESS

The coping process essentially involves an assessment of the stressor, an assessment of the available resources to deal with the stressor, and then engagement through the adoption of one or more coping strategies.[1] Outcomes are dependent on the effectiveness of the strategies selected. This is a complex, nonlinear process because of the multiple variables involved.[7]

Cognitive Assessment

Responding to stress begins with a cognitive assessment (or evaluation) of the situation in relation to the individual. This assessment represents the process of sorting out information to derive meaning and is the underlying factor in how an individual will respond.[4] There are two phases in cognitive assessment. The first involves *primary appraisal*, or an initial evaluation to understand the situation. The individual evaluates the potential for harm to self or to a loved one's well-being, self-esteem, or personal values and may determine how much personal control can be exercised over the situation. The second phase of cognitive assessment is *secondary appraisal*. Here, the individual evaluates the resources available to overcome, eliminate, or

FIGURE 32-1 Scope of Coping

reduce the stressor and determines to what extent the problem is controllable.

Therefore, primary and secondary appraisals require cognitive skills so that the stressor is accurately assessed and appropriate resources are identified. However, even with full cognitive capacity, there can be wide variability in how a stressor is perceived and the access, recognition, and application of appropriate resources.

Multiple variables influence perspectives for primary and secondary appraisals. One of the major influences is the characteristic and context of the stressful event, including perceived controllability. Key personal elements include level of education, past life experiences, current coping style, values, expectations, beliefs, self-efficacy, and worldviews. An individual's world is heavily influenced by his or her culture. A situation itself may or may not be perceived as stressful, depending on one's culture, and the response to an event is often culturally based—such as religious beliefs, social values, beliefs concerning the meaning or purpose an event, and the individual's beliefs concerning his or her own purpose in life. Cultural beliefs such as shame, discrimination, gender constraints, help-seeking activities, and stigma may affect how the individual copes in a situation.[8,9]

Engagement

The second process, which follows the cognitive assessment, refers to how the problem is addressed—or the individual's engagement with the problem. In other words, the primary and secondary appraisal drive the action an individual takes in attempts to cope with the stressor. After an individual takes action, a reappraisal process is done whereby the individual evaluates which coping mechanisms were effective and which ones were not, leading to the process of adaptation, or the incorporation of all coping processes to reach a new equilibrium or a return to the previous or normal state.

VARIATIONS AND CONTEXT

There is little agreement in the literature regarding the classification of coping strategies in stressful situations.[10] However, three predominate themes or common distinctions among the various strategies are problem-focused coping, emotion-focused coping, and meaning-focused coping (Figure 32-2):

- *Problem-focused coping* involves the cognitive process of evaluating the situation and then taking an action to manage or change the situation or circumstance associated with the stressor. The focus is usually geared toward eliminating or reducing the underlying cause of the stressor.[11]
- *Emotion-focused coping* emphasizes the regulation of emotional response that occurs in a given situation. No attempt is made to address the situation or stressor; rather, the focus is on controlling the emotional response as a result of the situation.[11]
- *Meaning-focused coping* involves a process whereby the individual draws on values, beliefs, and goals to modify the personal interpretation and response to a problem.[12]

Although individuals typically apply a combination of these strategies when attempting to cope with stress, research has shown that problem-focused approaches tend to be more effective than emotion-focused strategies, especially avoidance behaviors.[3] Some situations, however, are beyond the control of an individual; thus, problem-focused approaches are not always reasonable or indicated.

Inherent in these three categorical distinctions is the assumption that the individual is able to accurately appraise the situation and current resources and has the ability to determine an appropriate course of action that will produce change.[11,13] The types of coping strategies can change depending on the perceived outcomes of the stressor and the perceived availability of resources.[11] For example, when a role is threatened, the individual utilizes more of a problem-focused direct coping plan to relieve or eliminate the stressor.

A second major categorical distinction of coping is effective and maladaptive coping behaviors. Positive coping behaviors are those that address the underlying stressor and have a reasonable degree of success. Maladaptive coping behaviors are those that do not adequately address the underlying problem. These are addressed in more detail later.

CONSEQUENCES

Consequences of poor coping can result in multiple issues, particularly for the individual already in a stressful state. Specific consequences are difficult to describe because these are highly variable, depending on the type and number of stressors involved, the way the stressors are perceived, the length of time the stressor occurs, the type of coping mechanism (if any) implemented (and degree of effectiveness), and the resilience of the individual. In other words, two individuals faced with the same stressor often have very different outcomes because of the variables described. The consequences of poor coping can be physical, psychosocial, or both. Examples include a decline in physical health status; the development of mental health problems (e.g., depression and anxiety); a reduction in functional ability; a change in social status, financial status, or relationships; and alterations in family dynamics. Concept 31 (Stress) details the physiological and psychosocial consequences of unresolved stress.

The type of coping strategy or resource one uses can have an effect on the outcome. Maladaptive coping responses often lead to physical health problems. The use of alcohol or drugs to escape the stressor can lead to self-injury or long-term consequences such as addiction. Likewise, failure to adequately respond to a stressor can result in health consequences as a result of the stressor itself. An individual who uses avoidance or denial will have far less favorable outcomes associated with the stressful event.[11] In a study involving cardiac patients, Levine et al. found that patients in denial were less likely to follow discharge instructions (e.g., adding an exercise regimen). As a result, these patients had more re-hospitalizations 1 year following the cardiac event.[14] Avoidance, as a coping strategy,

FIGURE 32-2 Categories of Coping Strategies

can be somewhat useful in situations that are perceived as short term and uncontrollable.[15] However, avoiding the stressful event or feelings surrounding the stressful event can lead to increased emotional distress, longer recovery times, less effective problem solving, and maladaptive responses.

RISK FACTORS

All individuals use a variety of coping mechanism throughout life regardless of age, race, or gender. Although most individuals have effective coping mechanisms, there are risk factors associated with ineffective coping capacity. These depend on how the individual perceives the stressful event and the ability to identify and use resources. Any perceived threat to self or a loved one's well-being can be judged not only as a stressor but also as a situation in which one has little control. The ability to determine what resources are available and how those resources can be utilized is essential for coping. Therefore, risk factors for poor coping link to one or more of the following:

- Inability to accurately assess the stressor
- Denial or avoidance of the stressor
- An actual or perceived lack of control over the situation
- An actual or perceived lack of support
- No experience or poor past experiences handling stressful situations

Impaired Cognition

Limited cognitive functioning is a key risk factor for poor coping. How well an individual appraises the stressful event(s) and utilizes available resources is central to positive outcomes. Individuals with poor cognition may also have limited experience managing stressful events and thus may not take any action, either purposefully or as a form of denial.[12]

Limited Psychosocial Resources

Most researchers are in agreement that personality variables impact the perception of the stressor or stressful event, although there is controversy regarding how personality plays a role in coping.[16,17] Individuals who have poor self-esteem or those who feel depressed and lack motivation to respond to stressors are at risk for poor coping. Hardiness is the individual's sense of control over the stressful events, coupled with a commitment and challenge toward life events. Individuals who have a high degree of hardiness or resilience are generally better able to cope than those who have poor self-esteem.[18] Those with limited physical or financial resources are also at greater risk for poor coping because they may be less able to access appropriate interventions.

Age

Children

Research on children's perception of stressful events is based on age and developmental stages as well as the child's level of self-efficacy and self-control.[19] Self-efficacy and self-control are challenged by chaos and loss of autonomy.[20] Harsh experiences in childhood, including dysfunctional family dynamics, can lead to poor coping skills later in life. Studies have reported that younger children who are unexpectedly admitted to the hospital are usually at higher risk for poor coping. Also, children whose parents experience extreme amounts of stress also have shown poor coping behaviors.[21]

Adolescents

There is a well-established relationship between adolescent coping and high-risk behaviors. Adolescents who have poor or insufficient coping are at risk for drug use, high-risk sexual behaviors, psychological distress, and suicide. It is assumed that improving adolescent coping skills will result in changes in perception and reaction to stressors in different, more positive ways.[22] There is relatively little research related to the measurement of coping among adolescents; therefore, this is an area that requires additional exploration to further understand this concept.[22]

Older Adults

Older adults have unique risks for impaired coping compared to other age groups. Although they may have some advantage in coping experiences, many older adults may lack social supports or resources, may have less resilience because of health conditions, and may suffer from altered perceptions of stress events, particularly if cognitive function is impaired. There is a tendency for older adults with Alzheimer's disease to select escape mechanisms and emotional strategies as opposed to actually solving the underlying problem.[23] This underscores the importance of cognitive skills for adequate coping.

Changes in Health or Chronic Health Conditions

Individuals confronted with serious health issues are also vulnerable to poor coping styles. Franks and Roesch reported that individuals in a chronic state of disease who view their disease in a positive manner were more likely to use coping strategies.[24] However, individuals who viewed their disease negatively engaged in denial. Roesch and Weiner also reported that individuals who perceived their disease as uncontrollable were prone to denial and avoidance.[25]

ASSESSMENT

Nurses learn about an individual's perceived stressors and coping responses through a detailed history and examination. It is important to remember that coping is a way to manage a stressor. The assessment of coping should be kept separate from the outcome of the stressors. The individual may use maladaptive coping strategies to deal with the stressor, but this may or may not impact the outcome. Furthermore, the individual's background and culture may affect how the individual copes. In order to effectively help the individual, nurses should focus on the efficacy of the coping strategy rather than the final outcome of the given stressor. This information will guide the nurse in how to proceed with improving the individual's coping ability.

History

If an individual is experiencing a significant stressor, the history should provide data so the nurse can determine the individual's appraisal stage and determine coping strategies being used. It is also important to determine if the individual has used or is using problem-based or emotional-based coping strategies.

Perception of Threat

The assessment of the individual and how he or she will cope with a stressor may be a very delicate matter, depending on the given situation, the perceived threat, and the amount of control the individual has over the stressor. The nurse needs to understand the individual's perception of the event. This may be accomplished by asking the question, "What is the meaning of this event for you?" Recall that the meaning or perception is developed from several factors, including past experiences, internal needs, external needs, ability to acknowledge the problem, cognitive ability, values, expectations, culture, social supports, and perceived control over the situation. The nurse may want to also explore these areas with the individual in order to obtain a sense of how successfully the individual has coped in the past and if there are pertinent cultural beliefs that should be taken into consideration. This information will allow for the nurse to better understand the individual's coping ability as well as to aid the individual in finding more efficient ways to cope with the present stressor.

Past Coping Patterns

Ask how the individual has coped in the past. Did this person turn to alcohol use or seek a support person for help? It is also helpful to gain insight into the strengths and/or weaknesses of the individual's coping patterns. Did the alcohol use help the person relax to better deal with the stressors, or did the alcohol use become an additional problem? Did the person become withdrawn and isolative? Did the individual seek assistance from a support person? The individual himself or herself should serve as the primary source of this information. No one else can describe that individual's comprehensive internal perception attached to the given stressor or the effectiveness of past coping strategies.

Medical and Social History

As part of the interview, the nurse will want to understand the stressor event in the context of the individual's current and past health and social history. This is helpful to understand other health-related issues that can impact coping responses. Past social history may include questions concerning the individual's childhood caregivers, family history, and the family's coping strategies, as well as questions assessing how the individual navigated through difficult situations as a teenager. Relevant personal history also includes highest education level achieved, current and past occupations, social patterns, daily activities, sleeping patterns, eating patterns, and drug/alcohol use. The history also includes biographical data such as ethnicity, marital status and number of children, current living arrangements, and religious preference.

Examination

Observation of behavior is the key element associated with an examination of coping. This includes how the individual functions in the presence of the stressor and how the individual reacts when speaking of the stressor.[26] Because both primary and secondary appraisal require adequate cognitive functioning, a mental status assessment is essential. General observations such as personal appearance, grooming, facial expressions, and affect will aid the nurse in determining the extent to which the individual is reacting to the stressor, the individual's current cognitive ability, and the individual's current coping ability.[27] Assess the individual's thought process through conversation. This information may reveal coexisting mental health concerns such as mood disorders, anxiety, or impaired thinking.

Evidence of poor coping behaviors includes anger, anxiousness, sadness, or hopelessness. Evidence of adequate coping behavior includes insight and engagement with the primary appraisal and the development of a coping plan. Willingness to use coping strategies or problem-solving techniques is also consistent with positive coping. For example, perhaps the individual makes a written list of the advantages and disadvantages of the situation to determine if a threat actually exists, and then proceeds to make a list of support resources available to him or her.

The actual measurement of coping is very difficult because of the complexity of this concept. Many coping measurement instruments have been developed to quantify and measure coping. Several have been developed for specific age groups or situations. Box 32-1 presents examples of coping measurement instruments.

CLINICAL MANAGEMENT

The clinical management of coping can be very complex and challenging because coping is very personal and involves both internal and external needs. Once the individual's perception of the stressor, past coping experiences, and perceived control and support is understood, the nurse will be in a better position to guide the individual toward a positive coping experience.

Primary Prevention

Primary prevention strategies for coping are nonspecific and link to general strategies that optimize wellness. Maintaining good health and proper nutrition, exercising regularly, sustaining positive personal relationships and social support networks, and preserving positive self-esteem are all common mechanisms related to positive coping. Community-based support programs for situational stressors are described further in the Concept 31 Stress.

Collaborative Interventions

Clinical management of an individual with ineffective coping is directed toward the reduction of perceived threats and the reinforcement of perceived control over the stressor by adopting positive coping strategies. As mentioned previously, there are three general categories of coping strategies: problem-focused coping, emotion-focused coping, and meaning-focused coping.

- *Problem-focused coping strategies* are most commonly applied when stressors can be modified, changed, or controlled. These are strategies that attempt to find solutions or improvements to the underlying stressor. Examples of problem-focused coping strategies are a newly diagnosed patient attending a patient education seminar to learn about optimal disease management or a caregiver gaining support through the access of community resources.

- *Emotion-focused coping strategies* address the feelings one has as a result of the stressor. These strategies do not work toward a solution to the problem, but they can help create a feeling of well-being. Examples include performing physical activity to relieve stress associated with an overwhelming work schedule or attending a support group to discuss one's feelings.
- *Meaning-focused coping strategies* address an individual's personal values, beliefs, or goals and assumptions as a way to modify the personal interpretation and response to the stressor. Examples include a patient who is willing to change a personal goal as a way to cope with a stressor. For example, a patient who has lost functional ability following a stroke may change his or her personal expectation about walking without the use of assistive devices.

In many cases, a combination of problem-focused, emotion-focused, and/or meaning-focused coping strategies is utilized. It is important to emphasize that not all coping strategies are effective in all situations. Coping flexibility refers to the ability to change and adapt coping strategies over time based on changes in stressors and personal conditions.

Attempting to guide an individual toward enhanced coping abilities can be extremely challenging because there are numerous variables to consider. Once those variables have been identified, the nurse can more efficiently help the patient choose a clinical management strategy that will best support the individual's needs. Specific strategies include education, planning, accessing resources, and cognitive restructuring.

Education

Education regarding the situation and alternative coping measures is a powerful tool to increase self-efficacy and control. The cancer patient who is educated about treatment alternatives and is given a choice of treatment will feel more in control of the situation. Then, the nurse can help the individual select emotion-focused coping strategies. When emotion-focused and problem-focused coping strategies are combined, there is a greater sense of positive coping.

Developing an Action Plan

Another way to increase control and self-efficacy is to develop an action plan or coping plan with the individual. The nurse can assist the patient to consider various coping methods in various situations and develop an individualized plan. For example, the nurse might help the cancer patient identify several relaxation techniques or perhaps create a list of activities to complete when he or she is feeling better. The nurse may also help the individual to develop a list of tasks to accomplish while undergoing treatment, such as reading a book or learning to use a computer program—something that is interesting but not physically taxing.

Accessing Resources

Another important strategy is to identify and access supportive resources that can help the individual. Such resources can range from a support group to a mentor or a clinical service. Resources may also be beneficial for the individual to discuss problem-solving concerns or decision-making ideas.

Cognitive Restructuring

Another potential strategy involves a cognitive restructuring of the stressor—the primary strategy of mental-focused coping. This is referred to as positive reappraisal—that is, seeing the stressor from a more positive viewpoint.[12] When using this strategy, the nurse must understand and take into account the individual's worldview, which originates from the individual's values, beliefs, and culture. Positive appraisal has been shown to increase the individual's strategies for coping, sense of control, and perception of the stressor.[28] This change in the perception of the stressor can lead to changes in emotions, as well as behaviors toward the stressor, and can increase the individual's ability to cope. For example, an individual suffering from panic attacks attributable to an upcoming surgery may be asked to identify what aspect of the surgery he or she finds upsetting. The perception is likely negative; for example, a patient may fear not waking up from surgery. In this situation, the nurse could inform the patient about the surgery and the strengths of the surgeon, as well as the success rate of the procedure. The nurse has added doubt to the perception of, "I won't wake up from the surgery." The individual can then begin to turn the negative thinking into a more positive pattern of thought. This increased understanding can provide the patient with a greater sense of control and a much more positive perception of the upcoming surgery.

INTERRELATED CONCEPTS

The concept of coping is multifaceted and involves links to several interrelated concepts featured in this textbook. **Stress** is highly interrelated because coping is a stress response: Coping either is a positive response or is a cause of stress if it is maladaptive. Although stress is usually viewed as a negative event, it can also be perceived as a positive attribute with individual control. The terms stress and coping can be viewed as having an equal but different effect on an individual. Stress can be viewed as a situation requiring coping, or it can result from negative coping methods. Thus, coping is how the individual views and addresses the stressor.

A second interrelated concept is the health and illness concept **Cognition**. Adequate cognitive skills are essential for primary and secondary appraisal. Individuals with poor appraisal capabilities may fail to recognize or accurately perceive situations requiring attention, thereby exacerbating the situation.

Additional concepts also impact one's appraisal, including the attribute concepts **Culture**, **Spirituality**, and **Development**. Each of these concepts influences how an individual perceives or frames an event, shaped by the individual's development level and by the individual's value and belief system.

Functional Ability and **Family Dynamics** are additional concepts that link to coping strategies and can also be a reason for poor coping. The concepts **Addiction**, **Anxiety**, and **Mood and Affect** are interrelated because they can result from maladaptive coping, and they can also escalate poor coping strategies. These interrelated concepts are presented in Figure 32-3.

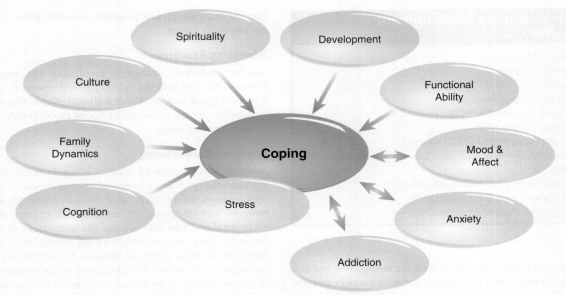

FIGURE 32-3 Coping and Interrelated Concepts

CLINICAL EXEMPLARS

Clinical exemplars of coping represent common coping behaviors from the context of positive and maladaptive. It is important to differentiate coping behaviors as exemplars as opposed to consequences of maladaptive coping. To help clarify this point, denial is an exemplar of an emotion-based maladaptive coping strategy, and the consequence could be increased anxiety. Substance use is a maladaptive coping strategy that could lead to addiction. Social isolation is a maladaptive coping strategy that could lead to depression. Although it is beyond the scope of this concept to list all examples, Box 32-2 presents common examples of both types of responses.

Featured Exemplars

Relaxation Techniques

One of the most common coping strategies is relaxation. Relaxation techniques reduce symptoms of stress by refocusing one's attention on something calming and increasing body awareness. There are many types of relaxation techniques, but most include one or more of the following four elements: autogenic relaxation (an internal process using visual and body awareness to reduce stress), progressive deep muscle relaxation (a focus on tension and relaxation of muscle groups), imagery (a cognitive strategy whereby calming, peaceful mental images are used to cope with a situation), and relaxed breathing (a process in which long, deep purposeful breaths are taken slowly over a period of several minutes).

Social Support

Social coping represents a group of strategies that involve gaining support from others. This can take the form of friends or family members, a community group, a spiritual group, and support groups organized by specific problems such as cancer survivors support groups. Social support has been shown to improve self-esteem or emotional well-being by moderating the impact of stress.[29] In addition to the improvement of emotional well-being, support groups usually help the individual make good decisions regarding actions to take in response to the problem. An exception to this is if the social support negatively influences behavior (e.g., codependency).

■■■ BOX 32-2 Exemplars of Coping

Positive Coping Behaviors
- Art therapy
- Counseling
- Distraction and diversion activities
- Education
- Massage
- Meditation
- Music therapy
- Physical activity
- Relaxation techniques
- Social support
- Spiritual resources

Maladaptive Coping Behaviors
- Avoidance coping
- Attacking or bullying
- Compartmentalizing
- Denial
- Dependency
- Displacement
- Dissociation
- Emotional outbursts
- Excessive eating
- Regression
- Rationalization
- Self-harm
- Sensitization
- Social isolation/withdrawal
- Substance use
- Violence

Reframing

Reframing refers to a positive coping strategy characterized by purposeful cognitive thoughts whereby the individual identifies positive aspects of the situation (finding "the silver lining") or makes a cognitive decision to make the best of the situation. In this case, the meaning or interpretation of the situation is reframed to a more positive state. For example, a pianist who is coping with functional loss of his hands may begin to reframe the loss as an opportunity for a new career path, such as music teacher or piano tuner.

Substance Use

A very common maladaptive coping strategy is the use of drugs or alcohol as a means to cope with a variety of stress, particularly job-related stress or relationship-based stress. Substance use is considered a short-term coping strategy because it provides a temporary relief, and it does not address the underlying problem. In many cases, this coping strategy can exacerbate the underlying problem if substance use escalates, creating an endless cycle of stress–use–relief–stress. If the substance use occurs over time, addiction can result.

Avoidance Coping

Avoidance coping is an emotion-focused maladaptive coping whereby the behavior response is based on attempting to avoid the thoughts and/or feeling associated with a situation. It can be demonstrated as doing things that are not helpful to a situation (e.g., washing dishes three times to address fear of food poisoning), failing to respond in a timely manner (e.g., delaying action to finish an unrelated task), or failure to do something (e.g., avoiding a conversation when one is necessary).

Regression

Regression is a maladaptive coping strategy whereby the individual reverts back to an earlier stage of development or a loss in functional status in an attempt to cope with situations that are uncomfortable or frightening. For example, an adolescent may demonstrate clingy childlike behaviors with a parent or other adult to cope with a significant disappointment, such as being rejected by a peer group. In response to an unexpected death of a spouse, an older adult may become dependent on others to carry out activates of daily living in which he or she is otherwise independent.

Dissociation

Dissociation is an extreme example of an ineffective emotion-based coping behavior in which an individual adopts another representation or perspective of his- or herself to cope with the situation. A person who dissociates may lose track of time and demonstrate a change in thought processes and behaviors. Dissociation results in the individual adopting a disconnected view of him- or herself in the individual's world. A person who dissociates "checks out" or "disconnects" from the reality of events in the real world and opts for a world in a different dimension free of thoughts, feelings, or memories that are unbearable.

CASE STUDY

Source: Josh Rinehults/iStock/
Thinkstock

Case Presentation

Carlie Wendell is a 10-year-old female who has recently been diagnosed with diabetes. She has no history of any major illnesses. Carlie lives with her single mother and four younger siblings in a small apartment. Her mother is unemployed, and the family has very limited resources. When the nurse meets with Carlie and her mother, Carlie's mother tells the nurse that her daughter did this to herself because she eats too much candy. Carlie appears withdrawn and tearful. The mother also mentions that she already knows how to "give the shots" because her own father had diabetes and was "in and out of the hospital a lot before he died." Carlie cries out in fear about having shots every day. Although Carlie's mother is present, she lacks full engagement in the discussion. She tells the nurse she cannot afford the medications needed to take care of Carlie's problem.

Case Analysis

This case represents a child with several known risk factors for ineffective coping. Carlie lacks the cognitive ability to fully grasp the situation, and she has a lack of control of her personal circumstances. She is upset with the diagnosis and perceives the treatments as a threat ("shots every day"); furthermore, she is blamed by her mother for the situation and lacks the capacity to draw on effective coping strategies. The situation is further complicated by her mother, who appears to have a limited understanding of Carlie's condition, is displaying avoidance coping, and does not perceive she has the resources to address the situation.

ACCESS EXEMPLAR LINKS IN YOUR GIDDENS EBOOK

REFERENCES

1. Lazarus RS, Folkman S: *Stress, appraisal, and coping*, New York, 1984, Springer.
2. Ray C, Lindop J, Gibson S: The concept of coping. *Psychol Med* 12(2):385–395, 1982.
3. Keil RMK: Coping and stress: A conceptual analysis. *J Adv Nurs* 45(6):659–665, 2004.
4. Mitrousi S, Travlos A, Koukia E, et al: Theoretical approaches to coping. *Int J Caring Sci* 6(2):131–137, 2013.
5. Stuart G: Stuart stress adaptation model of psychiatric nursing care. In Stuart GW, editor: *Principles and practice of psychiatric nursing*, ed 10, St Louis, 2013, Elsevier.
6. Ackley BJ, Ladwig GB: *Nursing diagnosis handbook: An evidence-based guide to planning care*, ed 8, St Louis, 2006, Mosby.
7. Yonhong Y, Jie H, Jimmy E, et al: Social support, coping strategies and health-related quality of life among primary caregivers of stroke survivors in China. *J Clin Nurs* 22:2160–2171, 2013.
8. Boss P: *Loss, trauma, and resilience: Therapeutic work with ambiguous loss*, New York, 2006, Norton.
9. Norris F, Alegria M: Mental health care for ethnic minority individuals and communities in the aftermath of disasters and mass violence. *CNS Spectr* 10(2):132–140, 2005.
10. Spivey J: *Coping with stress*, 2014. Retrieved from: <https://www.boundless.com/users/145830/textbooks/psychology-ed1f261f-c9c9-4c1e-855a-096bc90d7084/stress-and-health-psychology-17/improving-habits-and-managing-stress-89/coping-with-stress-337-12872>.

11. Folkman S, Lazarus R, Dunkel-Schetter C, et al: Dynamics of a stressful encounter: Cognitive appraisal, coping, and encounter outcomes. *J Personality Soc Psychol* 50(5):992–1003, 1986.

12. Folkman S, Moskowitz J: Coping: Pitfalls and promise. *Psychology* 55(1):745–774, 2004.

13. Clarke M: Stress and coping: Constructs for nursing. *J Adv Nurs* 9(1):3–13, 1984.

14. Levine J, Warrenburg S, Kerns R, et al: The role of denial in recovery from coronary heart disease. *Psychosomat Med* 49(2):109, 1987.

15. Suls J, Fletcher B: The relative efficacy of avoidant and nonavoidant coping strategies: A meta-analysis. *Health Psychol* 4(3):249–288, 1985.

16. Heth J, Somer E: Characterising stress tolerance: Controllability awareness and its relationship to perceived stress and reported health. *Personality Individ Diff* 33:883–895, 2002.

17. Tyson P, Pongruengphant R, Aggarwal B: Coping with organizational stress among hospital nurses in southern Ontario. *Int J Nurs Stud* 39(4):453–459, 2002.

18. Taylor S, Stanton A: Coping resources, coping processes, and mental health. *Clin Psychol* 3(1):377, 2007.

19. Zeitlin S, Williamson G: *Coping in young children: Early intervention practices to enhance adaptive behavior and resilience*, Baltimore, MD, 1994, Brookes.

20. Skinner E, Wellborn J: Children's coping in the academic domain. *Int J Behav Dev* 13:157–176, 1997.

21. Small L: Early predictors of poor coping outcomes in children following intensive care hospitalization and stressful medical encounters. *Pediatr Nurs* 28(4):393–401, 2002.

22. Garcia C: Conceptualization and measurement of coping during adolescence: A review of the literature. *J Nurs Schol* 42(2):166–185, 2010.

23. Nery de Souza-Talarioc J, Correâ Chaves E, Nitrini R, et al: Stress and coping in older people with Alzheimer's disease. *J Clin Nurs* 18:457–465, 2008.

24. Franks H, Roesch S: Appraisals and coping in people living with cancer: A meta-analysis. *Psycho-oncol* 15(12):1027–1037, 2006.

25. Roesch S, Weiner B: A meta-analytic review of coping with illness: Do causal attributions matter? *J Psychosomat Res* 50(4):205–219, 2001.

26. Edelman C, Mandle C: *Health promotion throughout the life span*, St Louis, 2010, Mosby.

27. Folkman S, Moskowitz J: Positive affect and the other side of coping. *Am Psychol* 55(6):647, 2000.

28. Moskowitz J, Folkman S, Collette L, et al: Coping and mood during AIDS-related caregiving and bereavement. *Ann Behav Med* 18(1):49–57, 1996.

29. Kim J, Han JY, Shaw B, et al: The roles of social support and coping strategies in predicting breast cancer patients' emotional well-being. *J Psychol* 15(4):543–552, 2011.

Mood and Affect

Robert Elgie

Mood and affect is a psychosocial concept that underlies all other concepts in the significant impact it has on health outcomes.[1] The purpose of this concept presentation is to enable the generalist practice nurse to have an understanding of mood and affect, develop an awareness of the expected variability or range of the mood spectrum, and recognize affective instability so that these patients can be managed safely and referred to advanced practitioners for evaluation and treatment of any possible mood spectrum disorders.

DEFINITION

The term *mood* is defined as *the way a person feels,* and the term *affect* is defined as *the observable response a person has to his or her own feelings.*[2] The term *euthymia* is used to describe normal, healthy fluctuations in mood. The *mood spectrum* is a continuum of all possible moods that any person may experience. *Mood spectrum disorders* disrupt the individual's ability to function normally, and individuals with mood spectrum disorders are at increased risk for many problems, such as health status impairment, addiction, and potential for violence.[1,3] Mood spectrum disorders must be diagnosed by physicians or other qualified advanced practitioners trained in making medical/psychiatric diagnoses; that is, the diagnosis of mood spectrum disorders is not within the scope of practice of the generalist nurse.

Because mood is a subjective experience of feelings, and affect is an objective reflection of feelings, the evaluation and description of mood is often done in terms of affect,[1] and generalist practice nurses are qualified and expected to assess affect. In particular, nurses must be able to recognize unstable affective states known as *affective instability.*[3] Signs of affective instability, such as crying, rage, euphoria, and blunting, indicate the need for further assessment because such individuals may have a mood disorder.[3] *Functional status* describes the individual's ability to perform activities of daily living and to realistically solve problems of daily living;[4] it is used as one indicator to determine the severity of a mood spectrum disorder.

SCOPE

From the simplest perspective, the scope of mood and affect can be thought of in terms of being low or depressive range, normal range,

and elevated range. There is considerable evidence to support a conceptual model of mood and affect in a single spectrum of possible affective states.[3] Normal mood, or euthymia, actually represents a *range* of expected mood cycles—normal happiness and normal sadness— and is shown in the middle of the spectrum in Figure 33-1; the curvy line illustrates normal euthymic mood cycling. The amplitude and frequency of euthymic mood cycles may be normally regular or irregular and vary from one person to another.[3]

The low end of the mood spectrum represents mild to moderate to severe melancholy. On the other end of the mood spectrum is mild to moderate to severe mania. As the mood cycles out of the euthymic range in either direction, the functional status decreases proportionally. In extreme mood states such as severe mania or severe melancholy, the individual may be completely disabled and experience symptoms of acute confusion such as hallucinations and/ or delusions. Figure 33-1 illustrates the full scope of the mood spectrum from extreme melancholy to extreme mania in language consistent with the current generalist nurse paradigm and scope of practice.

NORMAL PHYSIOLOGICAL PROCESS

Regulation of mood is complex and poorly understood, as it involves the integration of multiple brain functions and processes. Mood regulation depends on optimal function of neurons, neurotransmitters, and optimal coordination of several parts of the brain, including the prefrontal cortex, anterior cingulate cortex, and the limbic system. Changes to the function and/or coordination of any of these areas can dramatically impact mood regulation.

Neurotransmitters are chemicals that serve to transmit nerve signals from neuron to neuron and to different parts of the brain, such as the limbic system and prefrontal cortex. Neurotransmitters (especially dopamine, norepinephrine, and serotonin) have a powerful role in mood regulation by regulating appetite, sleep, thought, emotion, mood, learning, memory, motivation, and concentration. Excessive or insufficient levels of neurotransmitters are associated with mood disorders and other mental health conditions.

The prefrontal cortex and the anterior cingulate cortex are responsible for judgment, decision making, problem solving, feelings, and emotional responses.[3] The left half of the prefrontal cortex is involved with the establishment of positive feelings and the right half with

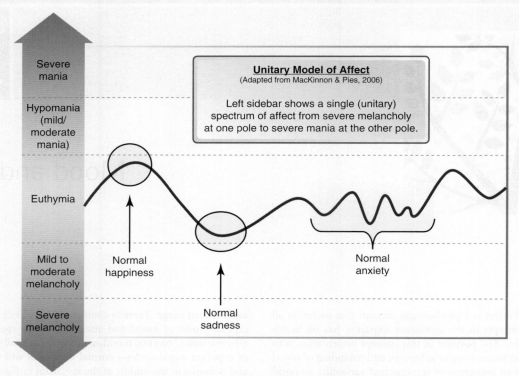

FIGURE 33-1 Unitary Model of Affect (shown here in euthymic range) The left sidebar shows the scope of affect in the generalist nurse paradigm from severe melancholy at one pole to severe mania at the other pole. The green line depicts normal mood as it cycles within the euthymic range from happiness to sadness and back to happiness. (Source: Adapted from MacKinnon DF, Pies R: Affective instability as rapid cycling: Theoretical and clinical implications for borderline personality and bipolar spectrum disorders, *Bipolar Disord* 8:1–14, 2006.)

negative feelings. The prefrontal cortex also has an indirect role in controlling mood by moderating feelings generated in the limbic structures and having an effect on neurotransmitter release. The limbic system is the area of the brain that is most directly involved in regulation of emotion, particularly the thalamus, amygdala, hippocampus, and cingulate gyrus. The amygdala is a limbic structure that is involved with memories, learning to fear events, and persistent negative thoughts. The hippocampus has a role in the creation and storage of new memories, and it also has a role in a major mood circuit known as the hypothalamic–pituitary–adrenal axis.[3]

Age-Related Differences in Emotional Regulation

Emotional regulation evolves throughout life and is closely linked with growth and development. This section briefly describes the evolution of emotional regulation.[3]

Infants and Children

There is a lack of agreement regarding at what point mood is experienced by infants. Mood can only be surmised based on what is observed. Initially, this is limited to facial expressions and behavior and is influenced by an increasing awareness of the environment. For example, infants initially smile beginning at approximately 6 weeks of age, often in response to a parent's smile; this response becomes more diverse as the child experiences positive feelings regarding things he or she sees and experiences. Thus an infant's expression of emotion is largely regulated by the degree of physical comfort and by cues from adults.

Emotional understanding emerges in toddlers as language, cognitive, and social development. Emotional regulation is thought to be associated with the child's ability to recognize the emotions of others and to mimic the behaviors he or she has observed and/or experienced. For example, toddlers will attempt to alleviate the distress of another by caressing or hugging. Preschool children continue to develop emotional regulation skills primarily based on observations of their parents or primary caregivers. An internalization of cultural norms regarding how they are expected to behave when they are feeling a certain way also becomes more developed.

The ability to self-regulate emotion becomes more evident during the middle childhood years. At this age, children understand the variety of verbal and nonverbal responses available for the expression of feelings. School-age children may be more willing to express feelings of sadness or anger toward a parent than toward a peer, and they develop an understanding of emotional states of others and the complexity of context in which they occur.

Adolescents

Adolescents typically have developed an array of skills to regulate their emotions and are highly aware of social circumstances related to emotional regulation. Evidence suggests that adolescents experience more variability in mood states and affect compared to adults. It is unclear if these differences are due to physiological changes such as hormonal imbalances or differences in emotional reactivity or emotional regulation.[5]

Older Adults

Mood regulation in older adults is generally physiologically consistent with what was previously described. However, despite the fact that older adults experience physical and cognitive decline, they often report higher levels of well-being (less negative affect and increased positive affect) and are more responsive to positive emotions compared to younger adults. It is thought that this difference can be explained by the fact that older adults activate emotional regulation processes to compensate for any negative stimuli they may experience.[6]

VARIATIONS AND CONTEXT

Conceptually, mood spectrum disorders occur when the mood cycles downward from the euthymic range into affective states seen as melancholy or when the mood cycles upward from the euthymic range into hypomania or severe mania. There are a large number of medical/psychiatric conditions with diagnostic criteria derived using medical reasoning in the fifth edition of the *Diagnostic and Statistical Manual of Mental Disorders (DSM-5)*.[7] In medical psychiatry, these conditions are grouped dichotomously as disorders in either the depressive spectrum or the manic spectrum. *Depression* and *mania* are medical/psychiatric diagnostic terms used to indicate the extreme poles of the mood disorders.[7] Although this dichotomous model is weakened by recent evidence supporting a unitary model of mood spectrum disorders,[3] it provides an excellent source for exemplars of the concept. There is a mixed state depression diagnosis that does not fit neatly in the depressive or the manic column because it contains features of both, and it provides useful borderline characteristics for concept analysis purposes. Suicide or suicidal behaviors in general may also be useful for analysis as exemplars.

Depressive Spectrum

Conceptually, depression is characterized by such overwhelming sadness and despair that one feels drained of energy. An individual suffering from depression may feel so sad and empty that he or she becomes incapacitated by a loss of the will to live, and suicidal thoughts may prevail. Caution should be exercised in the use of the word "depression" to avoid misunderstandings for two reasons. First, the word "depression" is commonly misused to describe normal euthymic sadness when there is little or no loss of functional status. Second, depression is a medical/psychiatric diagnostic term, and the clinical psychiatric use of the word "depression" has a variety of diagnostic applications. For clarity, the undiagnosed mood state characterized by sadness, despair, and loss of functional status is best referred to as *melancholy*.

Mania Spectrum

Individuals with *mania* are recognizable in the nursing paradigm by the presence of euphoric or agitated affective states, and they often suffer from varying degrees of *perceptual disturbances* as well, such as racing thoughts, grandiose delusions, difficulty concentrating, impulsivity, and lack of insight. Consequently, individuals with mania experience impaired functional status, and behavior associated with mania may be reckless and dangerous.

Another term used as a defining characteristic for some medical/psychiatric diagnoses is *hypomania*. Nurses are expected to be able to recognize hypomania as an unstable affective state. Hypomanic affective states are expansive or agitated and possibly euphoric but to a less severe degree than in mania and with less impairment. Although the individual with hypomania experiences racing thoughts and agitation or euphoria, perceptual disturbances are much less likely in hypomania. To facilitate the assessment of affective instability in the generalist nurse conceptual paradigm, the presence of perceptual disturbances is used to distinguish mania from hypomania.

CONSEQUENCES

The consequences of mood disturbances are significant from both a physical and a social perspective. Patients with mood spectrum disorders are high users of medical care, and the incidence of mood spectrum disorders is increased in general medical care patients.[8] Various neuroimaging studies of mood spectrum disorders demonstrate reduced blood flow and abnormal phosphorus metabolism in the cerebral cortex and especially the prefrontal cortex.[9] The activity of various neurotransmitters is also disturbed in mood spectrum disorders, particularly the levels of dopamine, norepinephrine, and serotonin. This is why medical interventions are aimed at restoring neurotransmitter balance.

Interpersonal relationships and productivity may be greatly limited by functional status impairment during mood spectrum disorders. Psychosocial variables such as negative life events, personality traits, and individual cognitive styles are associated with mood spectrum disorders.[3]

The most ominous consequence, of course, is the increased potential for suicide. Probably because of increased energy levels, patients on the manic or hypomanic pole of the mood spectrum are at a higher risk for suicide than are those with low energy at the melancholic pole.

RISK FACTORS

Fluctuations within the euthymic range occur normally and even daily among all populations and across the lifespan. However, although anyone may experience mood spectrum disorders, there are known risk factors. A landmark, broad-based assessment of mood spectrum disorders in the United States was the National Comorbidity Survey Replication (NCS-R) study conducted from 2001 to 2003; this study, based on 9282 interviews, provides a basis for understanding risk factors.[8]

Populations at Risk

According to the NCS-R, the 12-month prevalence of clinically significant depression in the general population was 6.6%, and the lifetime prevalence was 16.2%. The rate of depression among women is two or three times higher than that in men, and the first episode of depression for either gender usually occurs during adolescence or early adulthood. The incidence of depression peaks bimodally, occurring with the highest frequency during the late twenties/early thirties and again during the late sixties.

Individual Risk Factors

Individual risk factors for depression are stress, early trauma, neglect, abuse, family history, comorbid medical and psychiatric disorders, and personality disorders. Comorbid anxiety or substance-related disorders prevail in 75–80% of those with depression, and 22% of adults report comorbid substance dependence. Among those who reported no psychological distress, only 7% reported substance dependence.[8]

ASSESSMENT

Although generalist practice nurses are not qualified to diagnose mood spectrum disorders, they should be able to recognize affective instability as an outward manifestation of a possible mood spectrum disorder. Affective instability may present as any combination of agitation, sadness, elation, or blunting. Blunting is particularly difficult to recognize because it may not be noticeable immediately; blunting is an absence or diminished presence of any affect, and this should be considered a sign of affective instability. Speech may be monotone during blunting, and responses may be unusually brief. Blunting must not be overlooked because it may mask dangerously unstable affect.

The combined interaction between mood, energy, and cognition results in what is called affect;[3] therefore the recognition of affective instability is facilitated by an analysis of mood, thus energy, and cognition. The defining characteristics for the mood and affect concept in this analysis are derived from the diverse presentations of affective instability that result from the various problematic ways that mood, energy, and cognition interact. The defining characteristics are persistent mood disturbance, functional impairment, and disturbed vegetative functioning (sleep, appetite, and energy). To facilitate assessment, each of these characteristics is discussed individually.

Persistent Mood Disturbance

The assessment of mood is based on the patient's self-report. Occasionally, nurses will infer mood from affect, but this can be misleading because affect is not always congruous with mood. For example, individuals may laugh and cry simultaneously. In any case, persistent mood disturbance may include sadness, melancholy, irritability, lack of interest in normal activities (anhedonia), euphoria, elation, rage, or the lack of any ability to feel emotions at all. Moods should fluctuate normally in the full range of euthymia, but moods should not fluctuate so rapidly or to such extremes or for so long that functional status is disrupted.

The important point that underlies this defining characteristic is the idea of persistence. Anyone will normally experience sadness, irritability, and even euphoria or rage occasionally. However, daily, persistent melancholic feelings for longer than 2 weeks or persistent manic feelings for more than 4 days endorse a nursing assessment of persistent affective instability.[7] To illustrate useful reasoning in the recognition of persistent mania and hypomania by nurses, the fieldworkers who administered the face-to-face questionnaires during the NCS-R study were trained to ask the following:

Some people have periods lasting several days or longer when they feel much more excited and full of energy than usual. Their minds go too fast. They talk a lot. They are very restless or unable to sit still and they sometimes do things that are unusual for them, such as driving too fast or spending too much money. Have you ever had a period like this lasting several days or longer? … Or have you ever had a period lasting several days or longer when most of the time you were so irritable that you started arguments, shouted at people, or hit people?[10]

Functional Impairment

A useful way to assess functional impairment is to think of it as the inability to realistically solve ordinary problems of daily living.[4] Functional status may also be known as *functional ability*, although *functional ability* refers more specifically to the *capacity* of an individual to perform ADLs, whereas functional *status* refers to the individual's actual performance of the ADLs, which may not utilize his or her total functional capacity.[4] Functional impairment is closely linked to disturbed vegetative functioning.

Disturbed Vegetative Functioning

Vegetative functioning refers to the individual's appetite, sleep, and energy level. Some clinicians may evaluate sexual energy or changes in sexual desire (libido) as a separate measure of vegetative functioning. During a melancholic period, the patient typically exhibits reduced energy level, increased sleep, decreased appetite, and decreased interest in sex. Atypically, individuals with melancholy may overeat, may become more sexual, or may be too agitated to sleep—this is known as mixed state depression in the medical/psychiatric paradigm.[11]

Nurses may be confused to hear that the aforementioned increased appetite, hypersexuality, agitation, and insomnia present in the so-called mixed state depression diagnoses are also vegetative functioning characteristics in mania and/or hypomania. In fact, there is some debate in the medical/psychiatric paradigm regarding differentiation between mixed state depression diagnoses and the various bipolar diagnoses.[11] Although interesting, this debate is not very relevant in the nursing process, and nurses are advised to focus on assessing for the defining characteristics of mood and affect while avoiding speculation about possible medical/psychiatric diagnoses.

Mental Status Assessment

The mental status assessment is well within the nursing scope of practice and important in analyzing the defining characteristics for the mood and affect concept. In the same way that a nurse should generally be aware of any patient's pulse rate and character, respiratory rate and character, blood pressure, temperature, and pain, the nurse should also know the following elements of mental status assessment: general appearance, motor activity, mood, affect, speech, and alertness and orientation.[10]

The assessment and continuous monitoring of mental status enables the nurse to accurately assess cognitive status and functional status. Instruments such as the Mini-Mental State Exam, the Neecham Confusion Scale, and the Confusion Assessment Method Instrument permit the nurse to quantifiably measure mental status for particular situations, such as monitoring changes during or between shifts, day to day, or over the long term.[12] However, although these instruments can be very useful, they are not replacements for the continuous monitoring and documentation of the patient's mental status that makes it a sixth vital sign.

A complete discussion of the mental status examination is beyond the scope of this concept presentation, but sources are readily available that provide details of this part of the assessment. It is helpful to remember that the assessment of information processing lies at the heart of the mental status assessment. That is, assessing the patient's ability to process information is the purpose of the mental status assessment. Specifically, the following combine to form a clinical impression of the patient's total information processing ability and thereby form a basis for clinical management: the patient's appearance; motor functioning; speech and speech content; cognitive processes such as perception, judgment, insight, and memory; and alertness and orientation.

CLINICAL MANAGEMENT

An effective and easily remembered way for nurses to translate data from the mental status assessment to clinical management is by

FIGURE 33-2 Components of Affect Green line, mood; red line, energy; blue line, cognition. (Source: Adapted from MacKinnon DF, Pies R: Affective instability as rapid cycling: Theoretical and clinical implications for borderline personality and bipolar spectrum disorders, *Bipolar Disord* 8:1–14, 2006.)

analyzing it in the context of affect and the three main components of affect: mood, energy, and cognition. Figure 33-2 illustrates these components and the normal cycling of euthymia into an unstable melancholy and then back into euthymia. Note that during the unstable period illustrated in Figure 33-2, the individual displays a melancholic mood (green line) with reduced energy (red line) but increased cognition (blue line). Behaviorally, this individual would struggle with persistent sadness and low energy but agitated thoughts that disturbed his or her sleep. For individuals with affective instability, one or more of the three affective components will cycle out of euthymia in either direction, causing a variety of behavioral responses. By studying Figure 33-2, one can picture different affective (behavioral) manifestations. What makes the assessment of disorders associated with affective instability so challenging is that each affective component may cycle at different rates and extremes. Different combinations of affective components will have quite different manifestations. Also, when components occur simultaneously at the extremes, the disabling effects are increased.

Primary Prevention

Primary prevention measures for mood spectrum disorders are not well established, and efforts toward prevention focus on societal egalitarian interventions such as reduction in poverty, racism, violence, and stress.[2] According to systematic reviews,[2] programs that target prevention of mood disorders have been shown to reduce the severity of symptoms, but these programs tend to be early interventions rather than true prevention programs. Similar systematic reviews of universal prevention programs showed them to be ineffective.

Secondary Prevention (Screening)

Secondary prevention or screening efforts are aimed at early detection of mood spectrum disorders with the hope of preventing serious consequences, and there is compelling evidence to support mood disorder screening.[2] The U.S. Preventive Services Task Force (USPSTF) recommends the routine screening of adults for mood disorders in primary care.[13] The USPSTF further recommends that health care providers "remain alert" for mood spectrum disorders in children and adolescents, and that systems should be established to handle the diagnosis, treatment, and follow-up care for individuals who do screen positive for mood spectrum disorders. According to the USPSTF, the following two questions may be as effective as longer screening measures: "Over the past 2 weeks, have you ever felt down, depressed, or hopeless?" and "Have you felt little interest or pleasure in doing things?"[12]

Screening instruments do not diagnose mood spectrum disorders; instead, they measure the severity of associated symptoms.[13] By measuring the severity of symptoms associated with mood spectrum disorders, screening instruments assist clinicians to assess acuity and treatment effectiveness. There are numerous screening instruments validated for use at different times in the lifespan and appropriate for varying levels of cognition. Whatever instrument is used, it is important to realize that simple screening questions detect only approximately half of patients with mood spectrum disorders.[14] For this reason, it is recommended that nurses do not completely rely on screening instruments but, rather, use their assessment skills to detect affective instability followed by an assessment of functional status and potential for violence when indicated. It is noteworthy that diminished functional status may appear vaguely as somatic symptoms and vegetative complaints such as fatigue, sleep disturbance, pain, altered interest in sexual activity, or other persistent vague complaints.[12]

Collaborative Care

The generalist practice nurse who is proficient in the assessment of affective instability plays a key role in detecting mood spectrum disorders and providing patients with opportunities for preventing deterioration in functional status. The most extreme outcome the nurse may prevent is death or disability by suicide, and evidence supports the idea that when mood spectrum deterioration is prevented in an individual, he or she stands a good chance of living a long, happy, and productive life.

This point is illustrated in an ex post facto review of interviews with individuals prevented from jumping off the Golden Gate Bridge between 1937 and 1978.[15] During that period, 625 people are known to have died of suicide there, and perhaps another 200 possible deaths may have occurred unseen at night or in bad weather. Dr. Seiden carefully followed the 515 "attempters" who were restrained from leaping off the bridge. Of those who were prevented from suicide by jumping off the bridge, there were higher rates of violent death, but approximately 90% of those prevented from suicide did not die later by violent death. Other data from this study interpreted by Dr. Seiden enabled him to form the following conclusions:[15]

1. The chances are good that a person prevented from suicide will live a long and satisfying life. Ending one's life by suicide overlooks what might have happened—good feelings and good that could have been done.
2. Suicidal people should not be left to handle these emotions on their own. They should receive psychosocial help immediately, with at least 6 months of close support.
3. No matter how intense at the moment, the desire to die is temporary in almost all circumstances, negating the notion that "suicide is a choice."
4. Therapy, medication, relatives, friends, and groups all offer hope.

Individuals suffering from mood spectrum disorders are known to be lethargic in seeking treatment. Because the generalist nurse is quite likely to be the first clinician to detect the possibility of a mood spectrum disorder, it is imperative that the nurse is also able to discuss with the patient treatment options and reasonable expectations for treatment outcomes. In this way, the nurse may exert a substantial influence in convincing the patient to seek care. This influence is done most effectively with communication techniques called *motivational interviewing*.[16] Although additional training is helpful, motivational interviewing techniques lie within the generalist nurse scope of practice, and the effectiveness of motivational interviewing for mood spectrum disorders and suicidal ideation has been established.[16] Motivational interviewing was first developed to motivate individuals suffering from addictions to pursue change, and so it is further discussed in Concept 37 Addiction.

In addition to motivational interviewing, collaborative care for mood spectrum disorders consists of psychotherapy and/or pharmacotherapy and/or brain and vagus nerve stimulation therapies (e.g., electroconvulsive therapy). Collaborative care also includes managing emergent situations (potential for suicide and/or other violence) among individuals suffering from affective instability. Each of these areas of interventions is discussed next. The nursing role in collaborative care may include case management activities when functional status impairment persists.

Psychotherapy Options

There are many different types of psychotherapy, and no particular therapy has been found to be more effective than any other.[17] Compared to pharmacotherapy, there are fewer well-designed clinical trials of psychotherapy "because of the lack of a 'placebo therapy' condition."[17] However, there is sufficient evidence, including randomized controlled trials, to conclude that long-term outcomes of pharmacotherapy versus psychotherapy are similar.[17] Relapse rates appear to be lower in psychotherapy following termination of treatment. Psychotherapy has been found to take approximately 8 weeks for a 50% remission rate, 26 weeks for a 75% remission rate, and 52 weeks for an 80% remission rate.[18]

Because a person's thoughts and beliefs have been found to affect mood, cognitive therapy attempts to change thoughts and beliefs as needed to be more adaptive and healthy. In comparison, behavioral therapy is aimed at changing patterns of behavior that are repeated over time with the same negative results. Cognitive and behavioral therapy is a combined approach that has been found to be effective in numerous applications that share the characteristic of repetitive dysfunctional patterns.[18] Interpersonal therapy focuses on communication patterns and the way the patient relates to others. Grief issues respond well to interpersonal therapy, and the patient is provided the opportunity to learn ways to express such uncomfortable feelings. Variations of this modality have been demonstrated to be effective in managing bipolar spectrum disorders.[18] Family-focused therapy includes family members in a therapeutic process aimed at problem solving and managing conflict in ways that produce positive outcomes. All these therapeutic approaches are known to adapt well to the treatment of mood disorders in children and adolescents.[18]

Play therapy is an approach for children in which toys and games are used to establish rapport so that the child may better express him- or herself. Toys and games may also be used for children who lack the cognitive abilities of expression. Sand tray therapy is a variant of play therapy in which the child is encouraged to playfully make patterns in the sand. Other therapeutic modalities include light therapy, art therapy, and animal-assisted therapies, each with its own applications. Light therapy is used to treat seasonal affect disorder, a mood disorder that tends to occur during the winter months when there is less light. For some individuals, decreasing light is associated with melancholy. Animal therapies are often used in the recovery from psychological trauma, and art therapies may help with psychological self-healing.[18]

Pharmacotherapy for Mood Spectrum Disorders

The main drug categories used in the treatment of mood spectrum disorders are antidepressants and mood stabilizers; antianxiety agents (anxiolytics) are also used (see Box 33-1). In general, antidepressants are prescribed to treat patients diagnosed with depression and mood

---

BOX 33-1 Pharmacotherapy for Mood Spectrum Disorders

Antidepressants
- Selective serotonin reuptake inhibitors (SSRIs)
- Serotonin–norepinephrine reuptake inhibitors (SNRIs)
- Tricyclic antidepressants (TCAs)
- Norepinephrine–dopamine reuptake inhibiters (NDRIs)
- Monoamine oxidase inhibitors (MAOIs)

Mood Stabilizers
- Lithium
- Antiepileptic drugs (AEDs)
- Second-generation antipsychotic medications

stabilizers are used to treat diagnoses associated with mania and hypomania such as the various bipolar diagnoses.[7] Subcategories of antidepressants include the selective serotonin reuptake inhibitors (SSRIs), the norepinephrine–dopamine reuptake inhibiters (NDRIs), the tricyclic antidepressants (TCAs), the serotonin–norepinephrine reuptake inhibitors (SNRIs), and the monoamine oxidase inhibitors (MAOIs). The mood stabilizers are either lithium or antiepileptic drugs (AEDs), and numerous antipsychotic medications also have been approved as mood stabilizers.

Antidepressants. Many factors affect the choice of antidepressant medications, with remission or partial remission dependent on the particular neurochemical imbalance. The current first-line choice for the treatment of depression is the SSRI category because positive response rates are excellent and this category has the best rate of compliance as a result of its lower incidence of adverse effects.[17] SSRIs may be prescribed by primary care providers. If depression is complicated by anxiety, the anxiety may dissipate once the antidepressant medication takes effect, but this will take at least 3 weeks. During this period, anxiety may temporarily be treated with an anxiolytic, but persistent agitation may be treated with a mood stabilizer. Individual responses to any pharmacotherapy are highly variable. To achieve a positive response, the dose must often be increased after the initial 3 weeks; therefore it is not unusual for it to take 4–6 weeks to achieve a positive response.

The dual-action antidepressants known as SNRIs affect serotonin and norepinephrine levels, and these are also used in some cases of depression that does not respond to treatment, known as refractory depression.[17] For many years, the TCA antidepressants were the standard choice in the treatment of depression, and they are still used occasionally; however, because of their multiple adverse effects, TCAs are rarely or never used as first-line choices.[17] Overdose of TCA medications is lethally dangerous, so compliance and risk for suicide must be carefully evaluated before initiating medications from this category.

The MAOI antidepressants have also been demonstrated to be effective in the treatment of refractory depression, but they are never used as first-line treatment because of concerns about potentially fatal interactions (hypertensive crisis) between MAOI medications and foods containing tyramine. Tyramine occurs widely in foods, especially "spoiled" (fermented) or pickled foods. Foods to be avoided include many meats, chocolate, alcoholic beverages, cheese, tofu, beans, pineapples, plums, raspberries, figs, and nuts.

It is not unusual for patients to experience some mild side effects when SSRI medications are initiated or when the dosage is increased.[19] These side effects should subside within a few weeks and include insomnia, abdominal discomfort, and mild headaches. However, there is some potential for any antidepressant medication, including the safer SSRI category, to produce a dangerous condition known as *serotonin toxicity*.[19] Serotonin toxicity may occur abruptly, and initial presentation includes tachycardia, shivering, diaphoresis, dilated pupils, myoclonus (intermittent tremor or twitching), and hyperreflexia. Hyperthermia is common during serotonin toxicity, and temperatures may reach as dangerously high as 106°F (41°C). Serotonin toxicity is treated with serotonin blockade drugs such as chlorpromazine or cyproheptadine.

Patients should be instructed not to abruptly discontinue antidepressant medications because this may result in anticholinergic rebound symptoms known as SSRI withdrawal syndrome (also known as SSRI discontinuation syndrome). In SSRI withdrawal syndrome, the individual experiences flulike symptoms such as headache, diarrhea, nausea, vomiting, chills, dizziness, fatigue, insomnia, agitation, impaired concentration, and vivid dreams. Symptoms last from 1 to 7 weeks and may be dangerous if there is an increased presence of suicidal ideation.

Mood stabilizers. For many years, lithium and AEDs have been the two main types of pharmacologic agents used as mood stabilizers. In recent years, increasing numbers of later generation antipsychotic drugs have been approved and used for this purpose. The presumed action of lithium is through the regulation of the neurotransmitter glutamate. Kidney and thyroid function should be established before initiation of lithium therapy, and it is important to note that lithium has a very narrow therapeutic blood range of between 0.8 and 1.4 mEq/L. The toxic range begins at 1.5 mEq/L and may even overlap the therapeutic range, making dosage calculations difficult.

Patients taking lithium should be taught to recognize early signs of lithium toxicity, including diarrhea, vomiting, drowsiness, muscular weakness, and lack of coordination. Severe symptoms include ataxia (failure or irregularity of muscle action), giddiness, tinnitus (ringing in the ears), blurred vision, and a large output of dilute urine. Long-term side effects include thirst, frequent urination, tremors, diarrhea, weight gain, and edema. The cause of weight gain is not definitely known, and it may even be due to an increased consumption of caloric beverages for thirst.[19] Patients taking lithium should be instructed to maintain a steady fluid and electrolyte balance through dietary sources because lithium is lost during perspiration, affecting its narrow therapeutic range. Lithium should not be taken by pregnant or breast-feeding women. Antiepileptic medications such as carbamazepine, valproic acid/valproate, and lamotrigine are often used as mood stabilizers, but risk is substantial because AED overdose may be lethal.[19] Hepatic and renal functioning tests should be implemented prior to initiation of AED therapy and intermittently during treatment to detect and prevent long-term renal or hepatic damage.[19]

Brain Stimulation Therapy

The brain stimulation therapies are used primarily for treatment-resistant mood disorders that have failed to respond to other therapies.[18] During electroconvulsive therapy, the patient is sedated with a general anesthetic and a seizure lasting less than 1 minute is induced with electricity through electrodes placed at precise locations. It is not known exactly how brain stimulation works to relieve depression, but a general course of treatment is three sessions per week for 4 weeks. Common side effects include headaches, nausea, muscle aches, and occasional loss of memory. Magnetic pulses may be used instead of electricity in a brain stimulation therapy called repetitive transcranial magnetic stimulation.[18] Nursing management of patients who undergo brain stimulation therapies is identical to preoperative and postoperative nursing care of patients who are administered a general anesthetic. Nurses should perform teaching before the procedure so the patient will know what to expect. After the procedure, nurses should monitor the airway and mental status and assist the patient by orienting him or her to person, place, time, and situation as in any postoperative procedure.

Managing the Potential for Suicide and Other Violent Potential

The generalist nurse who suspects the possibility of a mood spectrum disorder should first assess for emergency situations. It should be considered an emergency when patients are at risk for suicide or violence; these patients should not be left alone. Any patient who presents with decreased functional status and affective instability should be evaluated for suicidal ideation. If there is any doubt regarding the severity of affective instability, functional status, or suicidal ideation, the nurse should order continuous observation and refer the patient for an

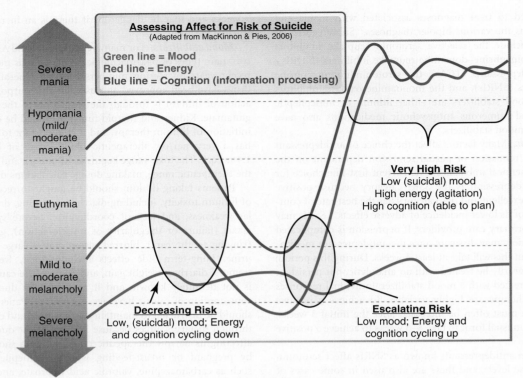

FIGURE 33-3 **Assessing Affect for Risk of Suicide** Green line, mood; red line, energy; blue line, cognition. (Source: Adapted from MacKinnon DF, Pies R: Affective instability as rapid cycling: Theoretical and clinical implications for borderline personality and bipolar spectrum disorders, *Bipolar Disord* 8:1–14, 2006.)

immediate, full evaluation. Figure 33-3 demonstrates affective states associated with varying levels of suicide risk and potential for violence. In this figure, the individual reflects a persistently low mood, as depicted by the green line. On the left side of the figure, cognition and energy are declining, so despite the low mood, he or she will tend to lack the energy and cognitive ability necessary to plan and carry out a suicidal act.

Comparatively, in the center of Figure 33-3, the individual's energy and cognition begin to cycle upward, increasing the risk of suicide. This condition may sometimes occur on initiation of antidepressant medications. On the far right side of the figure, the mood is very low, whereas energy and cognition are very high. The individual has a low, suicidal mood with sufficient energy and cognitive ability to plan and execute a suicidal act or other acts of violence. This person is unlikely to perceive reality accurately, and if mood were elevated here, then the individual would be manic and out of control—at risk for dangerous and reckless behaviors such as gambling, violence, and promiscuity. Such individuals are likely to have hallucinations and/or delusions.

Minimum standards of practice by the generalist nurse for managing the potential for suicide and other violence are not well established. In this concept, it is recommended that the minimum standard for the generalist nurse in any setting is to assess for violence potential, and when the potential for violence is endorsed, the patient should be assessed for acuity. This is done by asking the patient if he or she has been thinking about suicide or if he or she has any other thoughts of violence. The nurse should remember that talking about frightening thought content is known to provide relief for the patient.[20] It has been consistently demonstrated that talking about suicidal feelings does not increase the likelihood of acting on those feelings at any age.

The sudden appearance of unexplained euthymia in a person who has shown persistent affective instability may be an ominous sign of an impending suicidal act. In such cases, the appearance of euthymia results from the relief of making the decision to commit suicide. This decision may be accompanied by gift giving and acts of farewell. Not all suicides are predictable, especially impulsive suicide, but nurses who include assessment strategies discussed in this section will be more effective at recognizing possible mood spectrum disorders, initiating immediate interventions, and referring such patients to collaborative care. Other strategies include noting suicidal situations such as loss.[20] Loss may include the death of a loved one including pets, separation, illness, employment status, and self-esteem. Behavioral signals may warn of suicidal ideation, including writing or creating art about death; giving away prized possessions; and joking about death, dying, suicide, or leaving.[20]

INTERRELATED CONCEPTS

A number of concepts in this textbook are connected to mood and affect in some way. Three concepts are specifically worth mentioning and are shown in Figure 33-4. Like mood and affect, **Addiction** and **Cognition** share impairment in **Functional Ability** as a defining

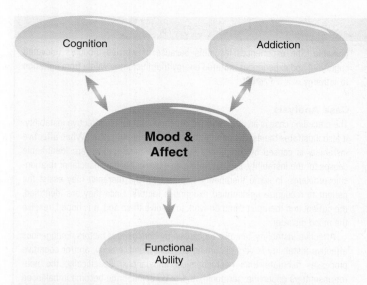

FIGURE 33-4 Interrelated Concepts of Mood and Affect Include Addiction, Cognition, and Functional Ability

characteristic. That is, any individual experiencing affective instability, addictions, or confusion will also experience functional status impairment. The affective disturbance may assume a variety of presentations, such as crying, rage, euphoria, or even flatness during loss of contact with reality, which is typical of confused states whether chronic or acute. Whatever the presentation, the standard of care should be to assess for any deficit in functional status and from that assessment proceed to establish a nursing diagnosis based on the presence or absence of other defining characteristics. For example, functional ability may be impaired by addiction, or it can be caused by confusion; it can also be caused by a mood spectrum disorder. Only by a thorough assessment can the nurse differentiate underlying etiologies.

CLINICAL EXEMPLARS

There are a large number of medical psychiatric conditions with diagnostic criteria (medical defining characteristics) derived using the medical reasoning in the *DSM-5*. These medically defined conditions provide useful exemplars for this concept. In medical psychiatry, these conditions are traditionally grouped dichotomously as disorders in either the depressive spectrum or the manic spectrum, but the unitary model of affect is more relevant to generalist nursing practice (Box 33-2).[21]

Featured Exemplars
Major Depressive Disorder

Major depressive disorder, one of the most common mental health conditions, is characterized by severe depressive mood symptoms that interfere with functional status, employment, and/or relationships that last for at least a 2-week period of time. This disorder can occur as a single episode, but more likely it occurs several times. This condition affects more than 6% of adults and 3% of adolescents in the United States each year. The average age of onset is 33 years; the populations at greatest risk are non-Hispanic whites and women.[8]

Persistent Depressive Disorder

Persistent depressive disorder (formerly known as dysthymic depressive disorder) differs from major depressive disorder in that the condition is chronic. Symptoms occur most of the day nearly every day for more than 2 years for adults or 1 year for children or adolescents. Symptom-free intervals last not longer than 2 months. Disqualifiers for use of this diagnosis include evidence of manic or hypomanic episodes during the first 2 years of symptoms, and the symptoms cannot be due to the direct use of substances (drugs and alcohol) or a medical condition.[8]

Disruptive Mood Dysregulation Disorder

As a new formal diagnosis to the *DSM-5*, disruptive mood dysregulation disorder is applied to children and adolescents who have a persistent or angry mood most of the day nearly every day with intermittent recurrent severe temper outbursts or episodes of explosive rage. The intensity and duration of the outbursts are out of proportion to the situation and must occur in at least two settings (e.g., home and school). The time of diagnosis should occur between ages 6 and 18 years, and the onset of symptoms must appear before age 10 years; not more than 3 months can pass without symptoms.[7]

Bipolar I Disorder

Bipolar I disorder is characterized by extreme mood swings—both lowering of mood and exaggerated elevation of mood. Although the cause is not well understood, bipolar I disorder is thought to be caused by an imbalance of neurotransmitters. There are several categories of this diagnosis, including manic, depressive, and mixed. Nearly 2.5 million adults in the United States have bipolar I disorder. The median age of onset is 18 years.[8]

Bipolar II Disorder

Like bipolar I, bipolar II disorder is also characterized by mood swings but is considered less severe. The main difference is a less exaggerated elevation of mood or "lesser mania" compared to bipolar I. This condition does not lead to life-threatening consequences, nor does psychosis occur. The median age of onset is 20 years, with a higher prevalence of bipolar II disorder among women.[8]

CASE STUDY

Source: Vico Images/Alin Dragulin/FogStock/Thinkstock

Case Presentation

Maya Rodgers is a 24-year-old college student whose mood is generally euthymic with stable affect. Her energy level, thinking, and mood fluctuate normally throughout the day. Ms. Rodgers has been struggling academically. She is informed by a course instructor that she must do well on an upcoming major exam or is at risk of failing the course. There is a lot riding on this exam, and Ms. Rodgers cannot stop thinking about the exam. Her vegetative functioning is affected, manifesting as insomnia at night and fatigue in the day. On the day of the exam, Ms. Rodgers has a bright affect, although her mood is anxious. Her energy and thinking are also elevated, although these fluctuations occur within the euthymic range.

The following day, Ms. Rodgers learns that she has failed the exam and may fail the course. Her mood begins to deteriorate through the euthymic range. Eventually, Ms. Rodgers feels melancholic and appears affectively unstable. She experiences insomnia because of worried thoughts (elevated cognition) and experiences agitated energy that fluctuates wildly from agitation to lethargy.

Case Analysis

The preceding case is an illustration of *exogenous* factors in affective instability. It also illustrates the assessment of the student's mental status. When affective instability is caused by exogenous factors, this means there are identifiable causes for the instability, such as failing an exam or having financial or relationship problems. In some therapeutic approaches, the therapist may assist the patient to recognize unidentified exogenous factors. Once they are identified, the patient and therapist can then work to resolve them and, it is hoped, resolve the mood disorder.

Affective instability can also be caused by *endogenous* factors. Endogenous affective instability is very disturbing because mood, energy, and/or cognitive processes fluctuate from neurochemical imbalances. Specifically, the neurotransmitters dopamine, serotonin, and/or norepinephrine become imbalanced for unknown reasons, as previously discussed. Neurotransmitters may also be affected by hormonal shifts. An individual with endogenous affective instability may, for example, suffer the same or worse agitation as an individual with exogenous instability, but with no externally known cause. This is very frightening and can become extreme, including perceptual disturbances and suicidal ideation.

ACCESS EXEMPLAR LINKS IN YOUR GIDDENS EBOOK

REFERENCES

1. Hofman SG, Sawyer AT, Fang A, et al: Emotion dysregulation model of mood and anxiety disorders. *Depress Anxiety* 29:409–416, 2012.
2. Venes D, editor: *Taber's cyclopedic medical dictionary*, Philadelphia, 2013, Davis.
3. Renaud SM, Zacchia C: Toward a definition of affective instability. *Harv Rev Psychiatry* 20(6):298–308, 2012.
4. Zisberg A, Shadmi E, Sinoff G, et al: Low mobility during hospitalization and functional decline in older adults. *J Am Geriatr Soc* 59(2):266–273, 2011.
5. Silvers JA, McRae K, Gabrieli JD, et al: Age-related differences n emotional reactivity, regulation, and rejection sensitivity in adolescence. *Emotion* 12(6):1235–1247, 2012.
6. Urry HL, Gross JJ: Emotion regulation in older adults. *Curr Directions Psychol Sci* 19(6):352–357, 2010.
7. American Psychiatric Association: *Diagnostic and statistical manual of mental disorders*, ed 5, Arlington, VA, 2013, American Psychiatric Publishing.
8. Kessler RC, Petukhova M, Sampson NA, et al: Twelve-month and lifetime prevalence and lifetime morbid risk of anxiety and mood disorders in the United States. *Int J Methods Psychiatr Res* 21(3):169–184, 2012.
9. Harper DG, Jensen JE, Ravichandran C, et al: Tissue-specific differences in brain phosphodiesters in late-life major depression. *Am J Geriatr Psychiatry* 22(5):499–509, 2014.
10. National Institute of Mental Health: *Symptoms of depression and mania*, 2010. Retrieved from <http://www.nimh.nih.gov/health/publications/men-and-depression/symptoms-of-depression-and-mania.shtml>.
11. Angst J, Cui L, Swendsen J, et al: Major depressive disorder with subthreshold bipolarity in the National Comorbidity Survey Replication. *Am J Psychiatry* 167(10):1194–1201, 2010.
12. Registered Nurses Association of Ontario: *Screening for delirium, dementia and depression in older adults 2010 supplement*, Toronto, Ontario, Canada, 2010, Author.
13. O'Connor EA, Whitlock EP, Gaynes B, et al: *Screening for depression in adults and older adults in primary care: An updated systematic review*, Evidence Syntheses No. 75, Rockville, MD, 2009, U.S. Agency for Healthcare Research and Quality. Retrieved from <http://www.ncbi.nlm.nih.gov/books/NBK36406>.
14. National Institute of Mental Health: *Real men. Real depression. Men and depression: Screening and treatment in primary care settings*, 2010. Retrieved from <http://www.nimh.nih.gov/health/topics/depression/men-and-depression/healthprovider_may1_34671.pdf>.
15. Seiden R: Where are they now? A follow-up study of suicide attempters from the Golden Gate Bridge. *Suicide Life Threat Behav* 8(4):203–216, 1978.
16. Berger BA, Villaume WA: *Motivational interviewing for healthcare professionals*, Washington, DC, 2013, American Pharmaceutical Association.
17. Pigott HE, Leventhal AM, Alter GS, et al: Efficacy and effectiveness of antidepressants: Current status of research. *Psychother Psychosom* 79(5):267–279, 2010.
18. National Institute of Mental Health: *Psychotherapies*, 2010. Retrieved from <http://www.nimh.nih.gov/health/topics/brain-stimulation-therapies/brain-stimulation-therapies.shtml>.
19. Taylor DL: Psychopharmacology. In Stuart GW, editor: *Principles and practice of psychiatric nursing*, ed 10, St Louis, 2014, Mosby, pp 523–559.
20. Stuart GW: Self-protective responses and suicidal behavior. In Stuart GW, editor: *Principles and practice of psychiatric nursing*, ed 10, St Louis, 2014, Mosby, pp 523–559.
21. MacKinnon DF, Pies R: Affective instability as rapid cycling: Theoretical and clinical implications for borderline personality and bipolar spectrum disorders. *Bipolar Disord* 8:1–14, 2006.

Anxiety

Sean Convoy

Anxiety is an adaptive response to stress that is ubiquitous across the lifespan. Anxiety is a subjective experience that can be measured objectively through physiological and psychological dimensions. As an adaptive response, anxiety has and continues to serve an evolutionary purpose. Early man spent most of his time hunting, gathering, and maintaining shelter. Survival was predicated on the ability to address basic needs and simultaneously remain vigilant to potential threat. Upon exposure to threat, humans relied on their evolutionary ability to rapidly translate sensory information into a cascade of internal biochemical responses that heightened awareness and generated the necessary energy to either fight or retreat. Although modern humans have fewer threats to contend with, their biochemical temperament has not appreciably changed. The excrescence of the human's prehistoric brain in present-day society can be conceptualized as anxiety.

Anxiety can be episodic or chronic, mild or severe, adaptive or functionally impairing, a symptom or a disorder. The nurse who understands the concept of anxiety is in a unique position to assess and meaningfully deliver care that has the potential to reduce illness, promote wellness, and instill self-efficacy.

DEFINITION

Several definitions of anxiety are found within the literature. While studying animals under stress, Cannon conceptualized the "fight-or-flight response" or the physiological reaction that occurs in response to perceived threat.[1] This observation influenced many of the definitions of anxiety that followed. Peplau defined anxiety as a "response to a psychic threat" and codified it along a continuum that is discernable through the lenses of *observation*, *focus*, and *learning ability*.[2] Freud initially conceptualized anxiety as a "physiologic buildup of libidinal energy" but later redefined it as a "feeling of impeding danger that can be based on objective, neurotic or moral threats."[3,p61] Barlow and Cerney defined anxiety as a "diffuse state characterized by an unpleasant affective experience marked by a significant degree of apprehension about the potential appearance of future aversive or harmful events."[4,p1] Beck proposed that anxiety is the product of "biased information processing of stimuli, which results in a systematic distortion of the person's thinking and construction of his or her experiences."[5,pxvi] A psychobiological definition of anxiety would invariably involve a complex interaction of anatomical activation coupled with neurotransmitter activation and

sensitivity that manifests above a clinical threshold as a constellation of symptoms. Each definition shares common themes involving both the perception of threat and a subsequent reaction. For the purpose of this concept presentation, anxiety is defined as *a subjectively distressful experience activated by the perception of threat, which has both a potential psychological and physiological etiology and expression*.

SCOPE

Simply conceptualized, anxiety exists along a continuum (Figure 34-1) comparable to Peplau's model ranging from mild anxiety to moderate anxiety, severe anxiety, and panic.[2] This is considered a continuum because the level of anxiety any individual experiences at any given time fluctuates. It is widely accepted that in the mild to moderate form, anxiety can actually be beneficial because it promotes learning, motivation, and heightens awareness. In more severe or chronic forms, anxiety can be debilitating because it restricts cognitive capability and degrades functioning (Table 34-1). In that regard, anxiety is analogous to rainfall because it is needed regularly to promote growth but not so often that one risks drowning.

NORMAL PHYSIOLOGICAL PROCESS

Anxiety is the product of a number of complex physiological and psychological processes best presented through the flight-or-flight response, the general adaptation syndrome, and neurophysiology.

Fight-or-Flight Response

During the "fight-or-flight response," the sympathetic division of its autonomic nervous system interacts with the adrenal cortex to release adrenalin, which causes the heart to speed up and circulate blood faster, the lungs to dilate to increase the oxygen-carrying capacity of the blood, the liver to release stored glucose for a quick infusion of energy, the pupils to dilate for improved visual acuity, and the stomach to inhibit peristalsis as a means to conserve energy.[1] Secondary to these organ system changes, there are observable signs of the fight-or-flight response that include tachycardia, disambiguation, bladder relaxation, tremors, blushing, xerostomia, delayed digestion, and hyperacusis. If the experience is both infrequent and of short duration, the human body has the endogenous capacity to downregulate and return to homeostasis.

FIGURE 34-1 Scope of Anxiety

TABLE 34-1	Peplau's Four Levels of Anxiety		
Mild Anxiety	**Moderate Anxiety**	**Severe Anxiety**	**Panic Anxiety**
• Sharp senses	• Narrowed perceptional field	• Concentration progressively narrowed	• Complete lack of focus
• Increased motivation	• Less alert	• Severe impairment of attention	• Tendency to misperceive environment
• Heightened awareness	• Decreased concentration	• Severe cognitive impairment	• Marked change in baseline behavior
• Enhanced learning	• Decreased problem solving	• Physical symptoms	• Marked functional impairment
• Optimal functioning	• Muscular tension	• Emotional symptoms	• Emotional and behavioral dysregulation
	• Restlessness		

General Adaptation Syndrome

Building on Cannon's research, Hans Selye's general adaptation syndrome is relevant to our conceptual discussion of anxiety.[6,7] The *general adaptation syndrome* model establishes that an event (or *stressor*) that threatens an organism's well-being leads to a predictably staged process of bodily response:

Stage 1—Alarm: Upon perceiving the stressor, the body reacts with an autonomic response that activates the sympathetic nervous system (see Fight-or-Flight Response), thus mobilizing the body's resources to respond to the stressor.

Stage 2—Resistance: The parasympathetic nervous system attenuates the reaction, returning many physiological functions to homeostasis while other functions remain hyperactive, ensuring that the body remains alert and ready to respond.

Stage 3—Exhaustion: If the nature of the stressor is sufficiently intense or of a protracted nature, it may exceed the body's capacity to compensate, thus exposing susceptibility to disease and death.

Brain Structure and Neurochemistry

A variable that is relevant to a discussion of brain structure and neurochemistry involves individual genotype (or genetic makeup). As an individual blueprint for development, one's genotype drives the division of every cell that splits and diversifies within one's body. The development of vital neuroanatomy, neural circuits, and neurotransmitter systems within the brain is genotypically directed. Changes in genotypic expression set the stage for potential vulnerability to stress and anxiety. Although there is no one single gene complicit, the evidence suggests a number of possible gene variations may explain the range of vulnerability that is seen. Changes in genomic expression represent the antecedent element of vulnerability. Genotype cannot be underestimated because it contextualizes why some appear to be more or less vulnerable or resilient than others.

Although the field of neuroscience is not yet so advanced to declaratively implicate all of the brain structures, neural circuits, and neurotransmitter systems associated with anxiety, it has made considerable progress. Critical structures within the limbic system, such as the thalamus, hypothalamus, cingulate gyrus, amygdala, hippocampus, and basal ganglia appear to play a central role in anxiety. Likewise, critical neurotransmitters and hormones such as serotonin, norepinephrine,

γ-amino butyric acid (GABA), dopamine, and thyroid hormone are also central to anxiety.

The state of the science is able to trace certain symptoms of anxiety back to certain neural circuits and neurotransmitter systems. For example, anxiety-based symptoms such as panic and phobia are linked to a malfunction within the amygdala-centered neural circuit that integrates the amygdala, orbitofrontal cortex and anterior cingulate cortex, and a number of different neurotransmitters systems (e.g., serotonin, norepinephrine, GABA, glutamate, and corticotropin-releasing factors).[8] Similarly, the symptom of worry can be traced back to a malfunction within a neural circuit incorporating the cortico-striatal-thalamo-cortical circuit and its unique constellation of neurotransmitter systems (e.g., serotonin, GABA, dopamine, norepinephrine, and glutamate).[8]

Age-Related Differences

The evidence assessing age-related differences in anxiety is mixed. The symptom of worry appears to play a less prominent role in the presentation of anxiety, suggesting older adults experience anxiety differently than younger adults.[9] A reasonable argument can be made that, although anxiety occurs across the lifespan, critical windows of vulnerability for certain expressions of anxiety exist. Likewise, an argument can also be made to suggest that the perceptual experience of anxiety changes over the lifespan.

VARIATIONS AND CONTEXT

The concept of anxiety can be symptomatically expressed a number of ways as shown in Figure 34-2 . Figure 34-3 is a contextual representation of anxiety based on symptom duration, intensity, and functional impairment. Anxiety must be of a sufficient intensity, duration, and degree of functional impairment to be recognizable. That point of observable recognition is defined as the *clinical threshold*. *Clinical perception* is defined as the nurse's ability to recognize anxiety-based symptoms. The novice or advanced beginner nurse may possess a sufficient understanding of anxiety to recognize overt symptoms of anxiety such as a panic attack or an obsessive compulsion. Through experience, the proficient nurse is potentially able to widen his or her clinical perception to recognize other, more subtle, symptoms of anxiety. The expert nurse understands the concept of anxiety and its

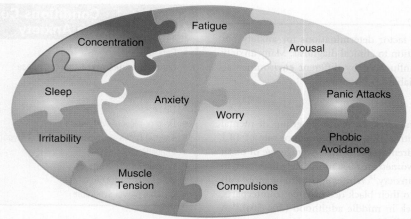

FIGURE 34-2 Symptomatic Expressions of Anxiety (Source: Redrawn from Stahl SM: *Stahl's essential psychopharmacology:* ed 4, Cambridge, UK, 2013, Cambridge University Press.)

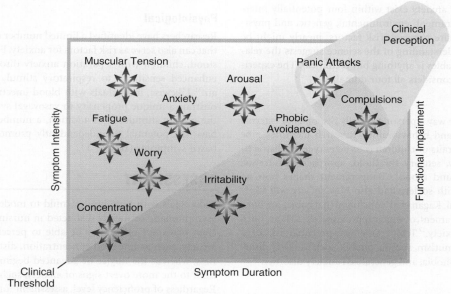

FIGURE 34-3 Anxiety Symptoms Based on Intensity and Duration

symptomatic expression so well that he or she is sometimes able to perceive anxiety below the clinical threshold.

The clinical opportunity for the nurse lies in the ability to understand anxiety and all of its symptomatic manifestations, overt and subtle. Being able to recognize the earlier, subtler symptoms can create new opportunities that exist below the clinical threshold. Such opportunities can dramatically influence the trajectory of care, health, and wellness.

CONSEQUENCES

If the physiological consequences of anxiety are dependent on symptom duration, symptom intensity, and degree of functional impairment, one can reasonably conclude that the physiological consequences of anxiety are variable. The general adaptation syndrome establishes that certain stressors are powerful enough to result in exhaustion and subsequent physiological consequence. The physiological realization of

alarm, resistance, and exhaustion is varied. This variation is influenced by endogenous (or genotype), exogenous (or environment), and the dynamic interaction between endogenous and exogenous (or epigenetic) sources.

Physiological consequences of anxiety link back to the deleterious effect of chronic sympathetic activation on renal, cardiovascular, endocrine, gastrointestinal, immune, neurologic, and psychiatric systems. Recent research has provided additional evidence associating anxiety disorders with future projected risk for medical morbidity, specifically cerebrovascular, atherosclerosis, ischemic heart, gastrointestinal, hypertensive, respiratory, and genitourinary system diseases.[10-11]

Advances in psychoneuroimmunology (or the study of interactions between psychological, neurologic, and immune systems) have established that the mind and body have equal potential to both influence and be influenced by the other. The symptomatic manifestations and potential consequences of anxiety are both psychological and physiological in nature.

RISK FACTORS

Research associated with risk factor determinations for anxiety has largely been performed in relation to clinical diagnosis. Many anxiety disorders appear to also be influenced by different environmental, temperament, and genetic variables.[12]

Populations at Risk

Anxiety disorders represent the most prevalent subgroup of mental illness in the United States, with a 12-month prevalence rate of 18.1 and 25.1% for adults and children, respectively.[13] Average age of onset is 11 years. Demographically, women are 60% more likely than men to manifest clinically significant anxiety.[12] Whites appear to be more vulnerable to anxiety compared to their black or Hispanic counterparts. Age prevalence appears to peek in middle adulthood (30s–50s).[14] A systematic review of research linking socioeconomic status (SES) among youth with anxiety reveals that lower SES is associated with higher rates of depressed mood and anxiety.[15]

Individual Risk Factors

Individual risk factors for anxiety exist within four potentially interrelated domains of temperament, environmental, genetic, and physiological. Although the desire to weigh risk factors linearly might be enticing, our evolving understanding of the science suggests the relationship among these variables is anything but rectilinear. The experienced nurse dynamically considers all four domains.

Temperament

Temperament refers to the way a person typically responds to external events both emotionally and behaviorally.[16] Research identifies nine different temperamental traits of children (i.e., activity level, distractibility, intensity, regularity, sensory threshold, approach/withdrawal, adaptability, persistence, and mood). Temperament shapes how an individual will interact with society and also how society will likely interact with the individual. Kagan et al. concluded that babies are born with an established temperament, of which approximately 20% are born with a predisposition to anxiety.[17] Temperament is a potential risk factor for anxiety with selective mutism, specific phobia, social anxiety disorder, panic disorder, agoraphobia, and generalized anxiety disorder.[15]

Environmental

Environmental factors are linked to certain clinical manifestations of anxiety. For example, separation anxiety disorder centers on a stress event defined by loss, death, or profound change. Parental social inhibition may serve as a role model for selective mutism among children. A number of environmental factors appear to influence the development of phobias, including parental overprotectiveness, parental loss or separation, and physical or sexual abuse. Childhood maltreatment and adversity during childhood appear to be risk factors for social anxiety disorder. Physical and sexual abuse appear to be more common among those with panic disorder than other anxiety disorders. Stressful life events during early childhood appear to be a risk factor for agoraphobia.[14]

Genetics

Heritable evidence associated with anxiety continues to evolve. Separation anxiety disorder research established a 73% heritability rate among a sample of 6-year-old twins.[14] There is some early evidence demonstrating genetic susceptibility to zoophobia among patients with first-degree relatives who possess the same condition.[14] Those traits that predispose individuals to social anxiety disorder (e.g., behavioral inhibition) are strongly influenced by genetics. A number of gene

variations have been implicated in increasing the vulnerability to panic attacks and panic disorder.[18,19] Agoraphobia has the strongest and most specific genetic linkage and a heritability rate of 61%.[20]

Physiological

Researchers have identified a limited number of physiological variables that can also serve as risk factors for anxiety. For reasons not yet understood, children with separation anxiety disorder display particularly enhanced sensitivity to respiratory stimulation with CO_2-enriched air.[21] Likewise, individuals with blood injection injury phobias demonstrate a unique propensity to vasovagal syncope in the presence of the phobic stimulus.[22] In addition, a number of medical conditions have the potential to independently promote anxiety and anxiety-based symptoms (Box 34-1).

ASSESSMENT

Individuals with time-limited, mild to moderate anxiety may appear asymptomatic or merely distracted in nursing assessment. The proficient or expert nurse may be able to perceive more subtle signs of anxiety, such as impaired concentration, distractibility, and talkativeness, whereas the novice or advanced beginner is usually only sensitized to the more overt signs of anxiety, such as panic or compulsion. Regardless of proficiency level, assessment for anxiety requires the collection of a history, physical assessment, and mental status examination (Box 34-2).

History

Prior to collecting a history, meaningful effort must be put into establishing a therapeutic rapport. Perfunctorily asking a list of rote questions involving extraordinarily sensitive medical history without building rapport is at best ill-advised and at worst unprofessional. The goal of the history is to obtain vital and time-sensitive health information that has the potential to immediately and significantly influence the trajectory of care.

When collecting history, be advised that not every individual understands or even acknowledges terms such as "anxiety" or "panic." Although some individuals may have experienced clinically significant and functionally impairing symptoms for years, they will not necessarily understand or convey the symptom experience the way the nurse does so. Consequently, the nurse is advised to strip away psychological terminology when communicating with patients. As opposed to asking, "Do you experience anxiety?" the nurse should ask, "Do you find yourself worrying a lot and feel unable to control it?" Instead of asking, "Do you ruminate?" the nurse should ask, "Do you find it hard to shut

---

BOX 34-1 Conditions Commonly Associated with Anxiety

- Cancer
- Chronic obstructive pulmonary disease
- Asthma
- Heart Disease
- Diabetes
- Drug or alcohol withdrawal
- Thyroid Disease (Hyperthyroidism or Hypothyroidism)
- Pheochromocytoma
- Chronic Infections
- Vestibular dysfunction
- Irritable bowel syndrome

BOX 34-2 Nursing Assessment of Anxiety

Medical History
- Risk factor identification
- Mental health history
- Substance use history
- Current medical problems
- Familial medical history
- Trauma exposure

Physical Examination
- Vital signs
- Auscultation of heart and lungs
- Palpation of thyroid
- Cranial nerve assessment
- Blood and urine studies

Mental Status Examination
- Appearance
- Attitude
- Behavior
- Mood and affect
- Speech
- Thought process
- Thought content
- Perceptions
- Cognition
- Insight
- Judgment

off your mind from overthinking?" A good exercise prior to assessing a patient for anxiety is to review the symptomatic expressions of anxiety (see Figure 34-2) and develop more user-friendly, nonclinical terms for the identified symptoms. Somatic symptoms often require a systematic measure of assessment to improve reliability. For this reason, employing scaled questions such as "On a scale of 1 to 10, with 1 being no distress and 10 being severe distress, how is your anxiety today?" becomes a way to operationalize subjective data in a meaningful way.

Physical Assessment

Understanding human physiology, the competent nurse can reasonably anticipate many of the physical manifestations of anxiety. Autonomic activation can manifest in hypertension, tachycardia, tachypnea, diaphoresis, ataxia, tremulousness, gastrointestinal distress, and muscular tension. Although many of these physical findings are sensitive to anxiety, they are by no means specific to anxiety. Making a determination of anxiety should never be done until other high-risk medical explanations (e.g., myocardial infarction, embolism, and stroke) have been ruled out. Serial evaluation of physical symptoms is vital to determine both functioning and response to treatment.

A well-executed mental status examination (MSE) is another objective data point that can meaningfully quantify anxiety. As established in Box 34-2, the MSE systematically evaluates a number of variables (e.g., distractibility, psychomotor agitation, tremulousness, rapid rate of speech, confusion, perseverated thought, and impaired short-term memory) that are potentially sensitive to anxiety.

Diagnostic Tests and Screening Measures

There is no specific test or study that can definitively rule anxiety in or out. However, there are a number of studies worthy of discussion. Laboratory studies (complete blood count, comprehensive metabolic profile, arterial blood gas, thyroid function test, spinal fluid analysis, urinalysis, and urine drug screen), radiologic studies (computerized tomography), or procedural studies (electrocardiogram, stress test, or electroencephalogram) often provide vital findings that contextualize suspected anxiety-based symptoms. Sometimes the only way to rule in anxiety is to first rule out all other medical explanations.

Evidence-based screening tools are also available to assess for anxiety across the lifespan. The fifth edition of the *Diagnostic and Statistical Manual of Mental Disorders* (*DSM-5*) has implemented a cross cutting symptoms measure, for both children and adults, that also has general value as a crude psychiatric assessment.[14] The Beck Anxiety Inventory for Youth (BYI),[23] Spence Children's Anxiety Scale

(SCAS),[24] and Revised Children's Manifest Anxiety Scale (RCMAS-2)[24] are all well-established screening tools for children and adolescents. The Hamilton Anxiety Scale,[25] Beck Anxiety Inventory (BAI),[26] Generalized Anxiety Disorder–7 Item (GAD-7),[27] and PTSD Checklist (PCL-5)[28] are all well-researched tools for adults.

CLINICAL MANAGEMENT

Primary Prevention

Primary prevention seeks to deter injury or illness via risk reduction. This is done by education, altering risk behaviors, decreasing exposure, and enhancing resistance to those agents that promote anxiety. Prevention measures used to target anxiety-based disorders are growing in both frequency and scope.[29-32] Our developing understanding of neuroscience suggests that the psychobiological damage of mental illness commonly precedes symptomatic expression. Consequently, prevention measures are vital.

Primary prevention targeting anxiety theoretically begins during pregnancy by promoting the health, wellness, and functioning of the pregnant mother and associated family support system. Mental health-focused well visits across the lifespan conducted by informed health care professionals are integral to risk recognition. Therein, a thorough family history that quantifies mental illness is critical. Resources and investment into strengthening family functioning and stability can serve as a protective measure against anxiety.

Secondary Prevention

Secondary prevention involves screening for the early detection of an illness. There are no population-based screening recommendations for anxiety, although screening tools (previously discussed) are available to use if symptoms have been recognized. Maintaining an awareness of and monitoring for symptoms and functional impairment allows for early identification and treatment.

Collaborative Management

Anxiety is commonly recognized as one of the most treatable psychiatric conditions. Because psychiatric illness is etiologically multifactorial and requires multimodal responses, it is uncommon that one treatment approach alone effectively and definitively treats anxiety. More often, a combination of therapies is associated with the best results. It is also important to distinguish between treatment and symptom management. Psychotropic interventions have great potential to manage symptoms, and psychotherapeutic interventions have the greatest potential to resolve the disorder.

Pharmacotherapy

Dating back to the mid-1950s, anti-anxiety agents such as meprobamate, otherwise known as "mother's little helper," quickly found a lucrative market in American society, with an estimated 36 million prescriptions filled in the first decade of its existence. In the 1960s, benzodiazepines became the prescribed drug of choice for anxiety. Although benzodiazepines continue to dominate the pharmaceutical market, a number of other agents have expanded treatment options during the past three decades.

β-adrenergic receptor antagonists. Considering Figure 34-3, some individuals only episodically or situationally experience anxiety above the clinical threshold. In those instances, there may be an indication for a psychotropic agent that can be used *pro re nata* (PRN). β-Adrenergic antagonists or β-blockers (e.g., propranolol, metoprolol, clonidine, and atenolol) have been used to treat varied expressions of anxiety (e.g., performance anxiety, traumatic nightmares, and extrapyramidal side effects of antipsychotic medications) for decades.[33,34]

β-Blockers work by binding the β-adrenergic receptor and subsequently blocking the effects of epinephrine and norepinephrine, consequently (and temporarily) blocking the physiological manifestations of anxiety. Although β-blockers are generally well tolerated, they can commonly result in postural hypotension, dizziness, and bradycardia.[35]

Benzodiazepines. Benzodiazepines (BZAs) are a commonly used anti-anxiety agent prescribed on a scheduled and as-needed basis. BZAs (e.g., lorazepam, alprazolam, clonazepam, and diazepam) enhance the effect of the neurotransmitter GABA, which is known to inhibit or calm nerve activity, and are exceptionally effective for the short-term management of anxiety symptoms. Unfortunately, BZAs are also highly addictive agents that pose serious risk for complicated, potentially life-threatening withdrawal. They also pose risk for central nervous system sedation and rebound anxiety. It is for these reasons that long-term scheduled use of a BZA is ill-advised.

Non-benzodiazepine anti-anxiety agents. Buspirone is a serotonin 1A partial agonist that diminishes serotonin activity postsynaptically, consequently delivering anxiolytic actions with less central nervous system sedation. Hydroxyzine is an antihistaminergic agent that blocks histamine 1 receptors, consequently prompting sedation. Each agent may be able to provide some degree of symptomatic relief of anxiety but will likely be of less utility if the patient has already been sensitized to the effects of a benzodiazepine.

Antidepressant agents. Although antidepressant agents have historically been used to treat symptoms of depression, a commonality between depression and anxiety is serotonin and norepinephrine dysregulation. Consequently, there are now a number of antidepressants on the market that hold a U.S. Food and Drug Administration (FDA) indication for the treatment of anxiety:

- *Tricyclic antidepressants (TCAs)*: TCAs influence a number of different neurotransmitter receptors potentially relevant to anxiety. Doxepin is the only drug in this group that has an FDA indication for the treatment of anxiety. Although effective, this is considered third- and fourth-tier treatment choice due to significant side effects and potential for suicidal thinking and suicidality.
- *Monoamine oxidase inhibitors (MAOIs)*: MAOIs (e.g., isocarboxazid, phenelzine sulfate, tranylcypromine sulfate, and selegiline) inhibit the activity of monoamine oxidase enzymes, obstructing the breakdown of monoamine neurotransmitters and hence increasing monoamine availability. Phenelzine sulfate is effective in treating symptoms associated with social anxiety,[36,37] but it is considered a second- or third-tier choice compared to the newer agents with fewer side effects.
- Selective serotonin reuptake inhibitors (SSRIs): SSRIs (e.g., fluoxetine, paroxetine, sertraline, citalopram, and escitalopram) inhibit the reuptake of the neurotransmitter serotonin presynaptically, thus increasing the availability of serotonin postsynaptically. SSRIs indicated for anxiety disorders include fluoxetine, paroxetine, sertraline, and escitalopram. SSRIs are generally well-tolerated agents but demonstrate an increased risk for a life-threatening condition (serotonin syndrome) when combined with other serotonin agonists. Abrupt discontinuation of SSRIs can lead to discontinuation syndrome.
- Serotonin–norepinephrine reuptake inhibitors (SNRIs): Like their SSRI counterparts, SNRIs (e.g., venlafaxine, duloxetine, and desvenlafaxine) block the presynaptic reuptake of both serotonin and norepinephrine, thus increasing the availability of both neurotransmitters postsynaptically. The SNRIs indicated for anxiety include venlafaxine (for panic disorder, social anxiety disorder, and GAD) and duloxetine (for GAD). Like SSRIs, abrupt discontinuation of SNRIs can lead to discontinuation syndrome.

Psychotherapy

A number of different psychotherapeutic modalities have demonstrated efficacy in treating clinically significant anxiety.

Psychoeducation. Psychoeducation is a modality of care that provides patients and their support systems with basic instruction on a wide array of topics, including diagnosis, treatment, risk management, health promotion, illness prevention, and anticipatory guidance. A meta-analysis published in 2009 established that brief passive psychoeducational interventions can reduce symptoms.[38] Although not as stimulating as other forms of therapy, psychoeducation is a foundational resource that is vital to all treatment, especially anxiety.

Cognitive–behavioral therapy. Of all the recognized psychotherapies, cognitive–behavioral therapy (CBT) has the largest evidentiary base supporting its utility for the treatment of anxiety. CBT is based on the notion that how one perceives and processes sensory stimuli has a direct bearing on the reaction one has to that situation. CBT employs a systematic process of Socratic questioning to expose cognitive distortions and core beliefs. Once identified, the therapist and patient collaborate in a process of initially recognizing and neutralizing and later modifying those cognitive distortions and core beliefs. The result of this process is the alleviation of anxiety symptoms.

Prolonged exposure therapy. Prolonged exposure (PE) is a specialized form of psychotherapy that targets anxiety born of trauma by systematically exposing patients to their own trauma via a structured process of education, breathing retraining, and real-world (or *in vivo*) and imaginal exposure. Conceptually, the goal of PE is to take patients back to their index trauma and systematically expose them to those sensory aspects of the trauma, thereby changing the subsequent reaction to the sensory trigger henceforth.

Cognitive processing therapy. Cognitive processing therapy (CPT) is a manualized form of cognitive therapy that also targets anxiety born of trauma.[39–43] CPT (1) provides psychoeducation about trauma symptoms and its etiology, (2) heightens awareness of one's own thoughts and feeling associated with trauma, and (3) teaches skills for managing distressing thoughts and feelings. It ultimately aspires to understand how beliefs associated with safety, trust, control, self-esteem, other people, and relationships have changed.

Mindfulness-based cognitive therapy. Whereas traditional CBT teaches the patient to challenge his or her own cognitive distortions, mindfulness-based cognitive behavioral therapy (MBCT) teaches the patient to reconceptualize cognitive distortions as a transient experience that is a predictable part of the human experience. MBCT has established efficacy with numerous anxiety disorders.[44–48] MBCT aspires to teach the patient how to develop the skill of nonjudgmental awareness of his or her own thoughts and feelings because doing so delimits the symptomatic experience that commonly follows.

Eye movement desensitization and reprocessing. Eye movement desensitization and reprocessing psychotherapy is a fairly new nontraditional manualized form of psychotherapy that aspires to process traumatic memories while simultaneously focusing on other sensory stimuli (e.g., sounds, hand taps, and/or eye movements). Although the therapeutic mechanism of action still eludes researchers, the evidence of its benefit has steadily grown.[49,50]

Other therapies. A number of other therapies (e.g., animal-assisted therapy, lifestyle modification, and complementary and alternative medicine) have shown evidence of benefit for a number of anxiety-based conditions. Animal-assisted therapy is building an evidentiary base as a complimentary treatment for trauma.[51–53] Likewise, a number of complementary and alternative medicine methods (e.g., supplements, botanical remedies, meditation and spiritual practices, acupuncture, and dietary practices) appear to also demonstrate benefit in

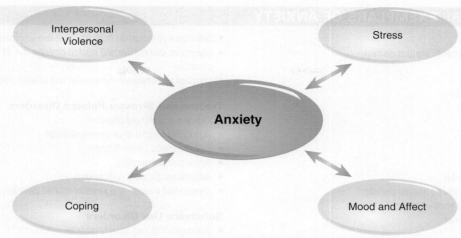

FIGURE 34-4 Anxiety and Interrelated Concepts

the treatment of anxiety-based disorders.[54–57] Although there are a number of supplements (e.g., kava kava, valerian root, and St. John's wort) on the market that boast efficacy in treating anxiety, these agents are not subject to the rigorous scrutiny of a governing body such as the FDA to ensure quality control. Likewise, there are demonstrated risks associated with combining supplements with psychotropic medications.

INTERRELATED CONCEPTS

There are several interrelated concepts that potentially demonstrate a linkage with anxiety (Figure 34-4), including Stress, Coping, Mood and Affect, and Interpersonal Violence. Individuals with clinically significant anxiety are by definition in **Stress** overload. It logically follows that if stress can exacerbate anxiety, so too can anxiety make one more vulnerable to stress. **Coping** is the response to stress and is linked to anxiety particularly if coping skills are ineffective to resolve the stress. **Mood and Affect** comprise the subjective (mood) and objective (affect) manifestation of stress, coping, and anxiety. Lastly, **Interpersonal Violence** is defined as a set of overt behaviors that have the potential to place both the patient and others at risk. Therein, we can establish interpersonal violence as one of many potential excrescences of stress, coping, and anxiety.

CLINICAL EXEMPLARS

There are a number of exemplars of anxiety that represent established medical diagnoses (Box 34-3). It is beyond the scope of this text to provide detailed information on each of these exemplars, but a brief explanation of some of the most important exemplars is presented in the section that follows. For detailed information and nursing care for each of these exemplars, consult a nursing psychiatric, mental health textbook.

Featured Exemplars

Simple Phobia

A simple phobia is characterized as an intense fearful reaction to an object or situation. The reaction is disproportionate and excessive and goes against rational thinking. Examples of common simple phobia "triggers" include fear of insects, heights, water, or closed spaces. When exposed to the object or situation, the individual typically has a panic-like experience and a subsequent strong urge to avoid or eliminate the situation. Some individuals develop simple phobias as a result of a

physical or psychological traumatic exposure, such as being bitten by a dog prompting cynophobia or being trapped in a closed space prompting cleithrophobia.

Social Phobia

Social phobia refers to a type of anxiety characterized by extreme fear of situations involving social interactions in public settings. Examples include attending social events, eating in public, speaking in public, and using public bathrooms. An individual with social phobia often seeks ways to avoid social situations. When faced with an event, the individual will often experience anxiety nearing panic leading up, during, and after a social situation.

Panic Disorder

A panic disorder occurs when an individual experiences a constellation of anxiety-based symptoms that approximate panic two or three times a day, with each episode lasting 10–20 minutes. Panic triggers include a fear of an impending disaster or fear of losing control in the absence of an actual threat. These recurrent panic events can interfere with one's life to the point that they become disabling. Common physical symptoms include a racing or pounding heart, chest pain, difficulty breathing, sweating, weakness, and dizziness. Panic disorders affect approximately 6 million Americans, occur twice as often in females as in males, and most often develop in adolescents or adults.

Generalized Anxiety Disorder

A generalized anxiety disorder is described as generalized worry (and often an inability to control worry) accompanied by uncomfortable symptoms of anxiety that can near the level of panic. The nature of the worry typically involves varied aspects of the individual's life and would be considered disproportionate or excessive by other people's standards. Examples include worries related to completing tasks on time, worrying about performance, and worrying about family members.

Obsessive–Compulsive Disorder

Obsessive–compulsive disorder (OCD) is a psychological state characterized by obsessive thoughts that manifest as compulsive behavior. Common examples include a need to repeatedly wash hands, check things, repeat an action, count things, a preoccupation with symmetry, and hoarding. The inability to fulfill the ritual is commonly associated with profound anxiety. An individual with OCD spends 1 hour or more per day engaged in the repetitive thoughts or behaviors, which interfere with the individual's daily life.

■■■ BOX 34-3   EXEMPLARS OF ANXIETY

Depressive Disorders
- Major depressive disorder with anxious distress

Anxiety Disorders
- Separation anxiety disorder
- Selective mutism
- Specific phobia
- Social anxiety disorder
- Panic disorder
- Agoraphobia
- Generalized anxiety disorder
- Substance-/medication-induced anxiety disorder
- Anxiety disorder due to a another medical condition
- Unspecified anxiety disorder

Obsessive–Compulsive and Related Disorders
- Obsessive–compulsive disorder
- Body dysmorphic disorder
- Hoarding disorder
- Trichotillomania
- Excoriation disorder

- Substance-/medication-induced obsessive–compulsive and related disorder
- Obsessive–compulsive and related disorder due to another medical condition
- Unspecified obsessive–compulsive and related disorder

Trauma and Stressor-Related Disorders
- Reactive attachment disorder
- Disinhibited social engagement disorder
- Post-traumatic stress disorder
- Acute stress disorder
- Adjustment disorder with anxiety
- Unspecified trauma- and stressor-related disorder

Substance Use Disorders
- Substance-induced anxiety disorder

Personality Disorders (Cluster C)
- Avoidant personality disorder
- Dependent personality disorder
- Obsessive–compulsive personality disorder

CASE STUDY

Source: Shelly Perry/iStock/ Thinkstock

Case Presentation

Roger is a Reserve Army Sergeant with 11 years of military service and three operational deployments (2005 for 6 months to Kuwait City, Kuwait; 2007 for 18 months to Baghdad, Iraq; 2010 for 7 months to Kabul, Afghanistan). Roger has significant family history for both anxiety and alcohol dependence. Roger's first deployment was unremarkable because he saw no direct combat and reported only limited stress associated with geographical separation from his family. His second deployment to Baghdad was markedly different because he participated in more than 100 supply runs between Baghdad and Mosul during the peak period of the war. During this deployment, he incurred three improvised explosive device (IED) attacks, two small arms fire exchanges with the enemy resulting in two confirmed kills, and perpetual risk of mortar attack. In his second IED event, two of his close friends died of injuries, with one dying in his arms (this event represents the index trauma). In the months that followed his return from the second deployment, Roger avoided all reminders of his experiences in Baghdad, and began to consume excessive amounts of alcohol to facilitate sleep. His marriage disintegrated, he alienated his support system, and his work performance declined, resulting in missed opportunities for promotion. His third deployment to Kabul was more intense than that to Baghdad. He began to experience intrusive recollections of the deaths of his friends (index trauma) from Baghdad with flashbacks and nightmares. Each time he put on his Kevlar in anticipation of going outside the safe zone, he would experience disabling panic. His ability to avoid triggers of his trauma at home was impossible to continue in the combat zone. While at home, he used avoidance and alcohol to tolerate his symptoms. Absent either option in theater, he developed a plan to kill himself by leaving the safe zone without support with the intent to kill as many insurgents as he could before they killed him. After informing his chaplain of his plans, Roger was medically evacuated out of theater.

Case Analysis

Roger's trauma experiences reflect severe anxiety and panic. The stress he was exposed to was of a sufficient intensity, duration, and frequency to eclipse his internal ability to resist, thus leading to exhaustion. His exposure to trauma has indelibly influenced his ability to tolerate stress absent clinically significant and functionally impairing anxiety. His ability to compensate with social avoidance and alcohol at home reflected his attempt to control his trauma symptoms. Consistent with Figure 34-3, the combination of symptom intensity, symptom duration, and functional impairment crossed over the clinical threshold during his third deployment to Afghanistan.

ACCESS EXEMPLAR LINKS IN YOUR GIDDENS EBOOK

REFERENCES

1. Cannon W: *Bodily changes in pain, hunger, fear and rage*, New York, 1929, Appleton-Century-Crofts.
2. Peplau HE: *Interpersonal relations in nursing, a conceptual frame of reference for psychodynamic nursing*, New York, 1952, Putnam.
3. Hall CS: *A primer of Freudian psychology*, Cleveland, OH, 1954, World Publishing.
4. Barlow DH, Cerny JA: *Psychological treatment of panic*, New York, 1988, Guilford Press.
5. Beck AT, Emery G, Greenberg RL: *Anxiety disorders and phobias: A cognitive perspective*, 15th anniversary ed, Cambridge, MA, 2005, Basic Books.
6. Selye H: *Stress in health and disease*, Boston, 1976, Butterworths.
7. Selye H: *The stress of life*, rev ed, New York, 1978, McGraw-Hill.

8. Stahl SM: *Stahl's essential psychopharmacology: The prescriber's guide*, ed 5, Cambridge, UK, 2014, Cambridge University Press.

9. Brenes GA: Age differences in the presentation of anxiety. *Aging Ment Health* 10(3):298–302, 2006.

10. Bowen RC, Senthilselvan A, Barale A: Physical illness as an outcome of chronic anxiety disorders. *Can J Psychiatry* 45(5):459–464, 2000.

11. Harter MC, Conway KP, Merikangas KR: Associations between anxiety disorders and physical illness. *Eur Arch Psychiatry Clin Neurosci* 253(6):313–320, 2003.

12. American Psychiatric Association: *Diagnostic and statistical manual of mental disorders*, ed 5, Arlington, VA, 2013, American Psychiatric Publishing.

13. Stucky KJ, Kirkwood MW, Donders J: *Clinical neuropsychology study guide and board review*, Oxford, UK, 2014, Oxford University Press.

14. The National Institute of Mental Health: *Anxiety disorders*, 2014. Retrieved from: <http://www.nimh.nih.gov/health/publications/anxiety-disorders/index.shtml?rf=57640>.

15. Lemstra M, Neudorf C, D'Arcy C, et al: A systematic review of depressed mood and anxiety by SES in youth aged 10–15 years. *Can J Public Health* 99(2):125–129, 2008.

16. Medina JJ: The genetics of temperament: An update, *Psychiatric Times* 2010. Retrieved from: <http://www.psychiatrictimes.com/articles/genetics-temperament%E2%80%94-update>.

17. Kagan J, Snidman N, Kahn V, et al: The preservation of two infant temperaments into adolescence. *Monogr Soc Res Child Dev* 72(2):1–91, 2007.

18. Domschke K, Tidow N, Schrempf M, et al: Epigenetic signature of panic disorder: A role of glutamate decarboxylase 1 (GAD1) DNA hypomethylation? *Prog Neuropsychopharmacol Biol Psychiatry* 46:189–196, 2013.

19. Judd FK, Burrows GD, Hay DA: Panic disorder: Evidence for genetic vulnerability. *Aust N Z J Psychiatry* 21(2):197–208, 1987.

20. Kendler KS, Karkowski LM, Prescott CA: Fears and phobias: Reliability and heritability. *Psychol Med* 29(3):539–553, 1999.

21. Pine DS, Klein RG, Coplan JD, et al: Differential carbon dioxide sensitivity in childhood anxiety disorders and nonill comparison group. *Arch Gen Psychiatry* 57(10):960–967, 2000.

22. Sarlo M, Buodo G, Munafo M, et al: Cardiovascular dynamics in blood phobia: Evidence for a key role of sympathetic activity in vulnerability to syncope. *Psychophysiology* 45(6):1038–1045, 2008.

23. Steer RA, Kumar G, Ranieri WF, et al: Use of the Beck Anxiety Inventory with adolescent psychiatric outpatients. *Psychol Rep* 76(2):459–465, 1995.

24. Essau CA, Muris P, Ederer EM: Reliability and validity of the Spence Children's Anxiety Scale and the Screen for Child Anxiety Related Emotional Disorders in German children. *J Behav Ther Exp Psychiatry* 33(1):1–18, 2002.

25. Maier W, Buller R, Philipp M, et al: The Hamilton Anxiety Scale: Reliability, validity and sensitivity to change in anxiety and depressive disorders. *J Affect Disord* 14(1):61–68, 1988.

26. Osman A, Kopper BA, Barrios FX, et al: The Beck Anxiety Inventory: Reexamination of factor structure and psychometric properties. *J Clin Psychol* 53(1):7–14, 1997.

27. Beard C, Bjorgvinsson T: Beyond generalized anxiety disorder: Psychometric properties of the GAD-7 in a heterogeneous psychiatric sample. *J Anxiety Disord* 28(6):547–552, 2014.

28. Demirchyan A, Goenjian AK, Khachadourian V: Factor structure and psychometric properties of the posttraumatic stress disorder (PTSD) checklist and DSM-5 PTSD symptom set in a long-term postearthquake cohort in Armenia. *Assessment* 2014. [Epub ahead of print].

29. Christensen H, Batterham P, Mackinnon A, et al: Prevention of generalized anxiety disorder using a web intervention, iChill: Randomized controlled trial. *J Med Internet Res* 16(9):e199, 2014.

30. Corrieri S, Heider D, Conrad I, et al: School-based prevention programs for depression and anxiety in adolescence: A systematic review. *Health Promot Int* 29(3):427–441, 2014.

31. Johnstone J, Rooney RM, Hassan S, et al: Prevention of depression and anxiety symptoms in adolescents: 42 and 54 months follow-up of the Aussie Optimism Program–Positive Thinking Skills. *Front Psychol* 5:364, 2014.

32. Stallard P, Taylor G, Anderson R, et al: The prevention of anxiety in children through school-based interventions: Study protocol for a 24-month follow-up of the PACES project. *Trials* 15:77, 2014.

33. Bachmann S, Muller-Werdan U, Huber M, et al: Positive impact of the beta-blocker celiprolol on panic, anxiety, and cardiovascular parameters in patients with mitral valve prolapse syndrome. *J Clin Psychopharmacol* 31(6):783–785, 2011.

34. Chaturvedi SK: Metoprolol, a new selective beta-blocker in anxiety neurosis. *Psychopharmacology (Berl)* 85(4):488, 1985.

35. Epocrates I: *Drug search*, 2014. Available at: <https://online.epocrates.com/noFrame>.

36. Aarre TF: Phenelzine efficacy in refractory social anxiety disorder: A case series. *Nord J Psychiatry* 57(4):313–315, 2003.

37. Blanco C, Heimberg RG, Schneier FR, et al: A placebo-controlled trial of phenelzine, cognitive behavioral group therapy, and their combination for social anxiety disorder. *Arch Gen Psychiatry* 67(3):286–295, 2010.

38. Donker T, Griffiths KM, Cuijpers P, et al: Psychoeducation for depression, anxiety and psychological distress: A meta-analysis. *BMC Med* 7:79, 2009.

39. Holliday R, Link-Malcolm J, Morris EE, et al: Effects of cognitive processing therapy on PTSD-related negative cognitions in veterans with military sexual trauma. *Mil Med* 179(10):1077–1082, 2014.

40. Morland LA, Mackintosh MA, Greene CJ, et al: Cognitive processing therapy for posttraumatic stress disorder delivered to rural veterans via telemental health: A randomized noninferiority clinical trial. *J Clin Psychiatry* 75(5):470–476, 2014.

41. Mullen K, Holliday R, Morris E, et al: Cognitive processing therapy for male veterans with military sexual trauma-related posttraumatic stress disorder. *J Anxiety Disord* 28(8):761–764, 2014.

42. Nixon RD: Cognitive processing therapy versus supportive counseling for acute stress disorder following assault: A randomized pilot trial. *Behav Ther* 43(4):825–836, 2012.

43. Walter KH, Varkovitzky RL, Owens GP, et al: Cognitive processing therapy for veterans with posttraumatic stress disorder: A comparison between outpatient and residential treatment. *J Consult Clin Psychol* 82(4):551–561, 2014.

44. Hofmann SG, Sawyer AT, Witt AA, et al: The effect of mindfulness-based therapy on anxiety and depression: A meta-analytic review. *J Consult Clin Psychol* 78(2):169–183, 2010.

45. McManus F, Surawy C, Muse K, et al: A randomized clinical trial of mindfulness-based cognitive therapy versus unrestricted services for health anxiety (hypochondriasis). *J Consult Clin Psychol* 80(5):817–828, 2012.

46. Rapgay L, Bystritsky A, Dafter RE, et al: New strategies for combining mindfulness with integrative cognitive behavioral therapy for the treatment of generalized anxiety disorder. *J Ration Emot Cogn Behav Ther* 29(2):92–119, 2011.

47. Sharma MP, Mao A, Sudhir PM: Mindfulness-based cognitive behavior therapy in patients with anxiety disorders: A case series. *Indian J Psychol Med* 34(3):263–269, 2012.

48. Wong SY, Mak WW, Cheung EY, et al: A randomized, controlled clinical trial: The effect of mindfulness-based cognitive therapy on generalized anxiety disorder among Chinese community patients—Protocol for a randomized trial. *BMC Psychiatry* 11:187, 2011.

49. Chen YR, Hung KW, Tsai JC, et al: Efficacy of eye-movement desensitization and reprocessing for patients with posttraumatic-stress disorder: A meta-analysis of randomized controlled trials. *PLoS One* 9(8):e103676, 2014.

50. McGuire TM, Lee CW, Drummond PD: Potential of eye movement desensitization and reprocessing therapy in the treatment of post-traumatic stress disorder. *Psychol Res Behav Manag* 7:273–283, 2014.

51. Beck CE, Gonzales F, Jr, Sells CH, et al: The effects of animal-assisted therapy on wounded warriors in an occupational therapy life skills program. *US Army Med Dep J* 38–45:2012.

52. Berget B, Braastad BO: Animal-assisted therapy with farm animals for persons with psychiatric disorders. *Ann Ist Super Sanita* 47(4):384–390, 2011.

53. Rossetti J, King C: Use of animal-assisted therapy with psychiatric patients. *J Psychosoc Nurs Ment Health Serv* 48(11):44–48, 2010.

54. Bazzan AJ, Zabrecky G, Monti DA, et al: Current evidence regarding the management of mood and anxiety disorders using complementary and alternative medicine. *Expert Rev Neurother* 14(4):411–423, 2014.

55. Bystritsky A, Hovav S, Sherbourne C, et al: Use of complementary and alternative medicine in a large sample of anxiety patients. *Psychosomatics* 53(3):266–272, 2012.

56. Ekor M, Adeyemi OS, Otuechere CA: Management of anxiety and sleep disorders: Role of complementary and alternative medicine and challenges of integration with conventional orthodox care. *Chin J Integr Med* 19(1):5–14, 2013.

57. McPherson F, McGraw L: Treating generalized anxiety disorder using complementary and alternative medicine. *Altern Ther Health Med* 19(5):45–50, 2013.

Cognition

Jean Giddens

The ability to think has long been considered a defining characteristic of what it means to be human. Attesting to this are the words of the French philosopher Rene Descartes, who said "Cogito, ergo sum," which translates to "I think, therefore I am." Thus the understanding of cognition, a term derived from the Latin verb "to think," is essential to understanding human behavior in health and in disease.

The study of cognition is multidisciplinary in scope with involvement and contributions from psychologists, philosophers, linguists, artificial intelligence scientists, and neuroscientists.[1] Two fields exclusively dedicated to the study of cognition are cognitive psychology and cognitive neuroscience. Cognitive psychology is committed to the study of cognition from an information processing perspective.[1] Cognitive neuroscience is the combined study of the mind and brain.[2]

DEFINITION

Cognition is a comprehensive term used to refer to all the processes involved in human thought.[1] These processes relate to the reception of sensory input, its processing, its storage, its retrieval, and its use.[2] For the purposes of this concept presentation, cognition is defined as *the mental action or process of acquiring knowledge and understanding through thought, experience, and the senses.*[3] Six domains of cognitive function include perceptual motor function, language, learning and memory, social cognition, complex attention, and executive function.[4] Three related terms—perception, memory, and executive function—are also described here for further clarification. *Perception* is the interpretation of the environment and is dependent on the acuity of sensory input. A related construct is awareness or consciousness, which refers to the ability to perceive or be sensitive to stimuli in the environment and respond to them. Attention is a focus on a particular area of conscious content. It implies selection as well as the ability to direct cognitive effort.[2]

Memory broadly refers to the retention and recall of past experiences and learning. It is not a single, unified mental ability but, rather, a series of different neural subsystems, each of which has a unique localization in the brain. These different subsystems support different types of memory—namely declarative episodic memory, declarative semantic memory, immediate memory, working memory, and procedural memory. Declarative memory refers to the ability to consciously learn and recall information. When the information relates to specific events, the terminology used is declarative episodic memory. This is distinct from declarative semantic memory, which refers to

memory of knowledge, words, and facts.[5] Declarative memory provides for long-term storage of large amounts of information. Immediate memory or "attention span" allows memory of very small amounts of information, such as a series of six or seven digits, for a very short time.[5] Working memory allows a small amount of information (approximately four chunks or meaningful units) to be actively maintained and manipulated for a short period of time. Procedural memory refers to the retention and retrieval of motor skills. It requires extensive training and provides for long-term storage of a moderate amount of information. Related to memory is visuospatial cognition, which is the capacity to comprehend, retain, and use visual representations and their spatial relationships.[6]

Executive function refers to the higher thinking processes that allow for flexibility, adaptability, and goal directedness. Executive function determines the contents of consciousness, supervises voluntary activity, and is future oriented.[2]

SCOPE

At the most basic level, cognition may be described as intact or impaired. Intact cognition means that an individual exhibits cognitive behaviors that are considered to be within the range of normal for age and culture. Impaired cognition signifies an observable or measurable disturbance in one or more of the cognitive processes resulting from an abnormality within the brain or a factor interfering with normal brain function (Figure 35-1). Cognition represents a continuum because the level of cognition is not a matter of "all or none"; it can change over time, and the degree of impairment can be mild to severe.

Among individuals with impaired cognition, there is variability related to the degree of impairment because of a number of influencing variables. In addition to considering the degree of impairment, cognitive changes can also be considered from a time perspective—that is, a temporary state or a chronic (permanent) state. Depending on the underlying cause, chronic states of impaired cognition can remain stable or can be associated with steady decline over time.

NORMAL PHYSIOLOGICAL PROCESS

One of the most distinctive features of humans, compared to other forms of life, is advanced cognitive abilities. In the absence of injury or disease, cognitive development occurs throughout life, with the

FIGURE 35-1 Scope of Cognition Ranges from Cognitive Impairment to Higher Order Cognitive Functioning

most significant changes from infancy through adolescence. Less dramatic development and maintenance of cognition occurs during adulthood.

There are four major units of the human brain: cerebrum, diencephalon, brain stem, and cerebellum (Figure 35-2A). The brain is responsible for multiple processes, including those that involve purposeful thought and responses and those that are automated and occur without purposeful thought (e.g., breathing, heart rate, reflexes, hormonal control, temperature regulation, and sensory regulation).

Most cognitive tasks occur in the cerebrum, which is divided into two hemispheres (right and left); each hemisphere has four lobes (frontal lobe, parietal lobe, temporal lobe, and occipital lobe) (see Figure 35-2B). Another key area of the brain that supports cognitive processing is the limbic system, which is a structure that overlaps the cerebrum and diencephalon. The ability to reason, function intellectually, express personality, and purposefully interact with the external environment is a result of a highly advanced brain. The cerebral cortex is primarily responsible for carrying out such functions, in which highly sophisticated neurons and neurotransmitters deliver information through complex networks. The brain is continually involved in receiving internal and external data signals. These signals are integrated and interpreted, which then triggers a sensory or motor response. This process is continuous and automatic.

Cognitive thought requires the ability to take in data signals and actively think about (integrate) and act on the information. Data signals that represent important information are transferred to memory. The hippocampus (a part of the limbic system) plays a significant role in committing information to long-term memory. Anatomic areas that have been identified as playing a key role in specific cognitive functions are presented in Table 35-1.[2,7] Optimal brain function depends on the continuous perfusion of oxygenated and nutrient-rich blood. Decreases in oxygen and glucose supply as well as electrolyte and acid–base imbalances significantly impair cognitive function.

Age-Related Differences
Infants and Children
Significant cognitive development occurs during infancy and childhood. Although the brain stem and spinal cord are fully developed (and needed to sustain extrauterine life), the limbic system and cerebral cortex are in undeveloped states at birth. Thus newborn infant

FIGURE 35-2 **Brain Structures** A, Four main areas of the brain. B, Lobes of the cerebrum. (Source: Modified from Herlihy B: The human body in health and illness, ed 5, St Louis, 2014, Saunders.)

TABLE 35-1   Cognitive Function and Associated Anatomic Location in the Brain

Cognitive Function	Anatomic Location
Memory	
Declarative episodic memory	Hippocampus, medial thalamus
Declarative semantic memory	Temporoparietal association cortices
Immediate memory/attention	Primary auditory or visual cortex
Working memory	Lateral frontal cortex
Procedural memory	Basal ganglia, association neocortices
Language	
Receptive language function	Auditory association areas: posterior superior temporoparietal supramarginal gyrus
Expressive language function	Lateral inferior posterior frontal lobes
Visuospatial Cognition	
	Occipital lobe, inferior temporal and posterior parietal lobes
Executive Function	
	Network of brain regions anchored by prefrontal and anterior lobe neocortex

FIGURE 35-3 Categories of Cognitive Impairment

behavior (e.g., sleeping, crying, feeding, sucking, kicking, and other reflexive behaviors) is controlled by the lower brain. The process of cognitive development from infancy throughout childhood has been described by many—perhaps most notable is Piaget.[8] According to Piaget, cognitive development is an orderly and sequential process that occurs in four stages: sensorimotor (birth to age 2 years), preoperational (ages 2–7 years), concrete operational (ages 7–11 years), and formal operational (age 11 years and older). (Piaget's theory of cognitive development is presented in Concept 1 Development.)

From a physiological perspective, three primary changes occur that influence the developing brain: increase in brain mass, neuronal–synaptic connections, and myelination. The growth of the brain and development of cognitive processing occur throughout infancy and childhood. The brain itself triples in weight during the first year, representing the single greatest change in brain size after birth. Along with an increase in brain mass, the number of neurons in the brain increases until approximately age 2 years. A massive explosion of neuronal–synaptic connections develops after birth and continues throughout childhood and adolescence, fueling the progression of cognitive developmental milestones. The connections occur in different regions of the cerebral cortex (e.g., sensory cortex, temporal lobes, and frontal lobes) during this time, which explains the various milestone achievements typically seen at different stages of development. Another physiological change is myelination of the neurons. Myelination occurs with the formation of a myelin sheath around nerve fibers needed for efficient neurotransmission of signals between neurons within the brain. This has a direct impact on cognitive development. Although infants are born with very little myelination, the process of myelination occurs throughout childhood and continues well into young adulthood, allowing for more complex or advanced thought with aging.

Older Adults

The size and weight of the brain and number of neurons decrease with aging. The reduction in and atrophy of neurons results in less efficient neurotransmission and a slowing of neural responses. However, these normal physiological changes with aging are not necessarily associated with a loss of cognitive function. In other words, cognitive impairment or intellectual loss is not a part of normal aging; rather, it is indicative of disease.[7] Throughout life, humans have the ability to continue to learn. The ability to retain cognitive function is often associated with brain "exercise"—meaning that regular purposeful thought is correlated to cognitive function, particularly among the oldest of older adults. A decline in memory is associated with aging, but the extent and degree are highly variable. Committing new information (particularly complex information) to memory is less efficient in older adults, but the majority of memory functioning remains intact.[9] This is especially true when older adults are in familiar situations and doing things they have done before.

VARIATIONS AND CONTEXT

Cognitive impairment refers to deficits in intellectual functioning. It is estimated that more than 16 million people in the United States have some degree of cognitive impairment.[10] A wide range of categories for cognitive impairment exists. For the purposes of this concept presentation, the following categories are used: delirium, neurocognitive disorders (NCDs), cognitive impairment not dementia, focal cognitive disorders, intellectual disabilities, and learning disabilities (Figure 35-3).

Delirium

Delirium is a state of disturbed consciousness and altered cognition with a rapid onset occurring over hours or a few days. During a delirious state, the individual experiences a dulled awareness of the environment and a reduced ability to focus, sustain, and shift attention. Memory and judgment are impaired, and disorientation may occur. Speech is rapid, rambling, and/or incoherent. Sudden, intense emotional swings, hallucinations, vivid dreams, and delusions may also occur. Restlessness is common, although in some cases activity may be reduced.

Delirium is the most frequent complication of hospitalization in the elderly population. A number of underlying conditions can lead to delirium such as dehydration, electrolyte imbalances, fever, hypoxia, sleep deprivation, adverse effect of medications, and illicit drug use to name a few. It may also be the initial symptom of life-threatening problems such as pneumonia, urosepsis, or myocardial infarction. Delirium is usually reversible with prompt treatment of the underlying problem and management of related predisposing factors.[11,12]

Neurocognitive Disorders

Neurocognitive disorders (NCDs) refer to a group of disorders better known as dementia. The commonality within these disorders is an acquired and progressive deterioration of all cognitive functions (with little or no disturbance of consciousness or perception), including impairment in memory, judgment, calculation ability, attention span, and abstract thinking. These impairments develop over a period of months to years. Primary dementia is irreversible and not secondary to another disease. Secondary dementia occurs as a result of another disease process.[12]

There are many types of dementia that are classified as etiologic subtypes of NCDs.[4] These subtypes include Alzheimer's disease, Parkinson's disease, HIV infection, frontotemporal, Lewy body type, traumatic brain injury, vascular, substance induced, Huntington's disease, prion disease, and other medical conditions. Each of these subtypes is classified as major or minor, depending on the degree of cognitive decline and functional ability.[4]

Cognitive Impairment, Not Dementia

Individuals with mild cognitive impairment, also known as cognitive impairment, not dementia (CIND), demonstrate a greater reduction of cognitive function than expected for an individual's age and education, but it does not interfere with functional ability. This is in itself not a medical diagnosis but, rather, a recognized state between normal cognitive function and true cognitive impairment. Individuals with mild cognitive impairment are at higher risk of progressing to dementia compared to the general population.[13,14]

Focal Cognitive Disorders

Focal cognitive disorders, unlike delirium and dementia, affect a single area of cognitive function. The area involved may be memory, language, visuospatial ability, or executive function.[7] These disorders may be associated with a neurocognitive disorder or may be seen independently. For example, one focal cognitive disorder involving memory is an amnestic disorder characterized by a significant decline in the ability to learn and recall new information and to recall previously learned material. This leads to impaired social and occupational function.[12]

Intellectual Disability

Intellectual disability refers to limitations of cognitive functioning and below-average intelligence (IQ score <70), in addition to limitations in conceptual skills, social skills, and activities of daily living.[15] Intellectual disability differs from neurocognitive disorders in that the cognitive processing never fully develops and the symptoms are identified before age 18 years. Intellectual disability is described as mild (IQ scores of 55–70, representing 85% of the population with intellectual disability), moderate (IQ scores of 40–55, representing 10% of the population with intellectual disability), severe (IQ scores of 25–40), or profound (IQ scores <25).[16] Common intellectual disabilities include chromosomal abnormalities (e.g., Down syndrome), genetic/inherited conditions (e.g., fragile X syndrome and Tay–Sachs), and other conditions that damage the developing brain (e.g., exposure to toxins, malnourishment, and cerebral anoxia).

Learning Disability

Learning disabilities represent another category of impaired cognition. Often identified during childhood, there exists a challenge in taking data signals in and then processing the information received. Learning disorders occur among individuals having average or

above-average intelligence, which is an important distinction compared to intellectual disability. Like intellectual disabilities, the severity of impairment ranges from mild to profound and can involve one or more areas of learning, including speaking, listening, reading (skills and comprehension), writing, and mathematics (calculation and reasoning).[16]

CONSEQUENCES

The consequences of cognitive impairment can be devastating for the affected person and for family and friends. Cognitive impairment places an individual at significant risk for a number of adverse physical, psychological, and social outcomes. Individuals with cognitive impairment are at higher risk for injury due to falls (particularly those with dementia) and other injuries within the environment due to the lack of accurate perceptions, risk recognition, and/or lack of capacity for an appropriate response to dangerous situations. Impaired cognition also complicates disease management, making optimal health management a challenge.[12] Cognitive impairment is associated with a higher incidence of hospitalization and long-term care. Advanced forms of cognitive impairment affect functional ability, the patient's capacity for independent living, and normal social interaction. The need for assistive services can range from help with some of the instrumental activities of daily living to constant supervision and complete care. Financial hardship and caregiver burden can result.

RISK FACTORS

Preventative interventions aimed at modifiable risk factors and risk recognition are an essential strategy with cognitively impaired patients. Early identification of cognitive impairment is also essential. There are many different types of cognitive impairment and many causes of each, with a wide array of risk factors, not all of which apply to every case.

Populations at Risk

Individuals across all population groups are potentially at risk for developing cognitive impairment. Results of several studies indicate that a primary risk factor for cognitive impairment is advancing age.[13] Moreover, the primary age group at risk is the elderly population.[17] No differences in impairment have been found across populations based on race, ethnicity, or gender; however, correlated risk factors among women and men differ. Significant risk factors found for women are overall poor health status, dependency, lack of social support, and insomnia. Risk factors specific to men include a history of stroke or diabetes.[13]

Individual Risk Factors

Many individual risk factors are associated with impaired cognition. The most common factors are personal behaviors, environmental exposures, congenital or genetic conditions, and other health-related conditions.

Personal Behaviors

Personal behaviors that predispose to impaired cognition are those related to chemical exposure and risk of traumatic injury to the brain. Specific examples of high-risk behaviors include substance abuse (e.g., alcohol, amphetamines, cannabis, cocaine, hallucinogens, inhalants, opioids, phencyclidine, sedatives, hypnotics, and anxiolytics); participation in high-risk activities that could result in traumatic brain injury; and omission of basic safety measures, such as wearing a helmet (e.g., skiing, cycling, motorcycle riding, and rock climbing) or wearing a seat belt (or seat restraint for children) when riding in vehicles. Accidental injuries associated with work, recreation, or violence in the absence of high-risk behaviors can also lead to brain injury and cognitive impairment.

Environmental Exposures

Environmental exposures to toxic substances can negatively impair cognitive function. Despite changes in environmental regulations, lead exposure continues to be a problem due to the presence of lead in the soil and dust, as well as old lead-based paint. Lead exposure among young children is particularly concerning because the developing brain is especially vulnerable. Other chemical agents, such as pesticides, can also negatively impair cognitive function.[18]

Congenital and Genetic Conditions

The term congenital means "present at birth"; genetic conditions differ in that the genetic problem exists at birth, but the condition may or may not be present at birth, manifesting later in life. Many congenital and genetic conditions are associated with impaired cognition. Some are related to maternal conditions (e.g., fetal alcohol syndrome or cocaine or methamphetamine exposure), and some are caused by birth injuries (e.g., cerebral palsy). Cognitive impairment also results from many chromosomal abnormalities (e.g., Down syndrome or fragile X syndrome) or other genetic conditions evident in infancy (e.g., phenylketonuria and galactosemia)[19] or those that emerge later in life (e.g., Huntington's disease, in which mental deterioration begins typically in the fourth decade of life).

Physical Disability and Reduced Mobility

There appears to be a relationship between physical disability and a decline in cognitive function. In a study of older adults, Rajan and colleagues found that cognitive function declines faster following disability in basic and instrumental activities of daily living.[20] In fact, slow gait is considered a predictor of cognitive decline.[21,22]

Health Conditions

Many health conditions can lead to temporary or long-term impairments in cognition. Fluid and electrolyte imbalance, systemic or intracranial infection, fever, pain, hypoglycemia, and anoxia can cause delirium that is reversible with treatment of the precipitating cause. Stroke and intracranial tumor can cause irreversible long-term amnestic and other cognitive impairments. Many chronic conditions, such as cardiovascular disease,[23] chronic pulmonary disease, and depression, have also been found to be significant risk factors for cognitive impairment in both men and women. Individuals with type 2 diabetes have been shown to have cognitive impairment due to poor disease management.[24]

Changes in cognition may occur as an adverse effect of medical treatments and medications. This is a particular risk among the elderly population because of decreased physiological reserve, decline in hepatic and renal function, altered metabolism, the presence of chronic disease, and multiple drug regimens. Psychoactive drugs are particularly notorious—these agents can cause delirium or cognitive decline. Examples include sedative–hypnotics (especially the long-acting benzodiazepines flurazepam and diazepam), narcotics (especially meperidine), anticholinergics (e.g., antihistamines, antispasmodics, heterocyclic antidepressants, neuroleptics, and antiparkinsonians), digitalis glycosides, antidysrhythmics (e.g., quinine and procainamide), and antihypertensives such as β-blockers. H_2-antagonists, nonsteroidal anti-inflammatory drugs, corticosteroids, and anticonvulsants as well as over-the-counter sleep aids, cold and sinus medications, and anti-nausea and acid reflux preparations can also lead to changes in cognition. Chemotherapy, used to kill cancer cells, has been shown to impair normal brain function—a long-term consequence referred to as chemo-brain.[25]

ASSESSMENT

Characteristics of normal cognitive status vary with the individual's stage of development. In infants and young children, expected cognitive development is indicated by achievement of developmental milestones and tasks, with specialized age-appropriate tests of development used when indicated to determine developmental delays (see Concept 1 Development). During the remaining lifespan, identification of new problems with cognition relies primarily on routine observations by health care providers, patient self-report, and report of family or others.

History
Adults

Assessment of cognitive functioning occurs as part of the health history. It begins with assessment of consciousness because unless the patient is fully aware of self and the environment, other cognitive assessments may not be valid. The nurse observes the patient for wakefulness, alertness, and appropriate responses to introductions and to the environment as the health history interview is begun. The patient's speech pattern and content are noted, and memory, logic, and judgment are assessed while the interview progresses.[26] Questions related to cognition included in the interview relate to history of intracranial disease or trauma; substance abuse; use of medications that can impair cognition; environmental or occupational exposure to hazards such as lead or insecticides; the presence of symptoms such as difficulty in forming words or saying what is meant, headache, behavior changes, or seizures suggestive of a brain disorder; unexplained emotional or behavioral changes; and any noticed change in memory or mental function. If any abnormalities are noted, a more specific cognitive assessment is performed. A family member who can assist with the history helps to provide greater understanding of the patient's cognitive level prior to hospitalization.[27]

Infants and Children

Parents should be asked about prenatal and birth history, in addition to a three-generation family health history (to establish familial syndromes).[28] Intellectual disability may have an association with the pregnancy or birth process. Having an understanding of developmental tasks met and those not met provide helpful clues regarding impairment.

Examination

A mental status assessment forms the basis for cognitive assessment and includes general appearance, behavior, and cognitive functions.

General Appearance

Observation of general appearance often provides initial clues to an individual's cognitive functioning. The posture and body movements should be relaxed, coordinated, and smooth. Slumped posture, slow movements while walking, and dragging feet may be indicative of dementia. Observe the patient's dress and overall hygiene, and consider if it is appropriate for the weather, setting, gender, and age. Individuals with cognitive impairment may present with inappropriate dress and/or poor hygiene.

Behavior

Assess the level of consciousness. The expected finding is an individual who is awake, alert, and aware of the environment. Abnormal findings include lethargic, obtunded, stupor, or confusion.

Facial expressions should be appropriate and consistent with the situation. Flat expressions could be associated with dementia. Note the quality of speech. Expected findings include effortless conversation that is fluent, articulate, and of moderate pace. Individuals with impaired cognition may have trouble recalling words, blocking, distorted speech, disconnected sentences, or loose associations. Confabulation (the fabrication of events to fill in memory gaps) may also be demonstrated.

Assessment of Cognitive Function

Formal assessment of cognition goes further to include a test of orientation to person, place, and time and also attention, memory, judgment, insight, spatial perception, calculation, abstract reasoning, thought process, and content. Orientation is usually established during the course of the interview by asking the patient to state his or her name, provide date of birth, state, address, etc. Typically, a patient is considered orientated if he or she is aware of the date, time, and location. The Mini-Mental State Exam (MMSE) is one of the most common standardized cognitive assessment tools used across care settings to screen for dementia and delirium, to detect cognitive impairment occurring during illness, and to monitor response to treatment. The test consists of 11 cognitive tasks that cover the categories of time orientation, place orientation, immediate recall, short-term memory recall, serial 7's, reading, writing, drawing, and verbal/motor comprehension. The test takes 5–10 minutes, and is simple to administer. The lower the score (out of a total of 30), the more severe the impairment. Individuals who score below 27 should be referred for further evaluation.[29] Another simple cognitive assessment tool for memory impairment involves recall of three words written down by the patient followed by three shapes drawn by the patient, termed the Three Words Three Shapes test. Kiral and colleagues found that use of the MMSE and Three Words Three Shapes test was effective for early detection of memory impairment among individuals in a community-based setting.[30] For delirium, a short screening test called the Confusion Assessment Method (CAM) (CAM-ICU for patients who are unable to speak as a result of intubation) is used.

Several assessment tools are available for use in clinical practice that assess various aspects of cognitive skills; some of these are listed in Box 35-1. Regardless of the tests used, adults should be able to evaluate and respond appropriately in situations requiring judgment; demonstrate a realistic insight into self; state the abstract meaning of a metaphor appropriate to their culture; and exhibit logical, coherent, and goal-directed thought processes based on reality.[31] Adults with normal cognition have an attention span and calculation ability adequate to complete a task such as counting backwards from 100 by subtracting 7 each time. Short-term memory allows functions such as repeating a list of three words after 5 minutes of another conversation. Long-term memory allows for correctly responding to questions about events occurring 24 hours or more in the past.

Adults with intact cognitive processes also exhibit spatial perception sufficient to allow copying of a simple shape without difficulty and identify right and left sides of the body. Observable behaviors associated with altered cognition have been well documented, named, and defined. Terms used to describe abnormal cognitive findings are

---

BOX 35-1 Common Cognitive Assessment Tools

Global Cognitive Performance

- *Mini-Mental State Examination (MMSE)*: A 30-item, 10-minute questionnaire to measure cognitive impairment and progression of disease.
- *Severe Impairment Battery (SIB)*: Used with significantly cognitively impaired patients to assess lower levels of cognitive function; in other words, provides differentiating clarity among individuals who score less than 12 on the MMSE.

Executive Functioning

- *Controlled Oral Word Association Test (COWAT)*: Assesses ability to generate a list of as many words starting with a designated letter as possible in 1 minute. Tests attention, thought process, judgment, aphasia and memory, ability to adhere to a set of rules to assess attention, thought process, and judgment.
- *Behavioral Dyscontrol Scale (BDS)*: Nine-item screening test to evaluate the capacity of an older adult related to independent functioning. The tool evaluates motor control processes and insight regarding accuracy of performance.

Motor Speed

- *Hand Tapping Test*: Used to evaluate motor speed and involves tapping the hands. Slowed tapping speed is associated with cognitive impairment.

Episodic Memory

- *Three Words Three Shapes Test*: Measures memory, recall, and recognition using verbal and nonverbal information.
- *Fuld Object Memory Evaluation*: Tests for recognition, memory, and learning in older adults. Ten objects in a bag are presented to individuals who are asked to identify the objects by touch (stereognosis) and then allowed to see if they were correct. After a few minutes, they are asked to recall the things in the bag.

Cognitive Impairment

- *Global Deterioration Rating Scale (GDRS)*: Behavioral rating scale assessment for three phases of cognitive impairment: forgetfulness, confusion, and dementia.

---

presented in Table 35-2.[2,6] Cognitive assessment of infants and children also includes behavioral, cognitive, and psychosocial development. This is presented in Concept 1 Development.

Diagnostic Tests

There are no laboratory tests that diagnose cognitive impairment, although laboratory tests are critical in determining the presence of associated disease or contributing factors. Brain imaging techniques such as magnetic resonance imaging and positron emission tomography scans can identify some brain abnormalities such as intracranial tumors, infarcts associated with vascular dementia, and frontotemporal lobe atrophy. However, their usefulness is limited in the majority of cases of cognitive impairment. Formal neuropsychometric testing by a neuropsychologist is needed for the identification of mild cases of cognitive impairment. Such testing uses more detailed standardized tests of memory and advanced methods of determining visuospatial function, which can identify impairments missed by standard clinical evaluation tests.[6]

TABLE 35-2 Common Cognitive Functional Abnormalities and Definitions

Cognitive Area	Abnormality	Definition
Memory	Anterograde amnesia	Loss of ability to learn and recall new information on an ongoing basis
	Retrograde amnesia	Impaired ability to retrieve information from the past
Language	Aphasia	Language impairment at the conceptual level; may have difficulty with production or comprehension of language or both
	Wernicke's aphasia	Impaired comprehension of both written and verbal language, even understanding single words; speech fluent and person is unaware that words used are incorrect
	Broca's aphasia	Impaired language expression characterized by nonfluent, labored speech; comprehension of language intact
	Global aphasia	Both language reception and expression impaired
	Anomia	Impaired ability to name places or objects; may have difficulty with sentence repetition, although comprehension and expression abilities are basically intact
Visuospatial	Alexia	Impaired reading ability
	Agraphia	Inability to write
	Agnosia	Impaired ability to recognize objects or persons through sensory stimuli; may be visual, tactile, auditory, olfactory, or gustatory
	Object agnosia	Impaired ability to recognize visual forms
	Prosopagnosia	Impaired ability to recognize faces
	Simultanagnosia	Impaired ability to integrate complex visual scenes
	Apraxia	Inability to perform purposeful movements or manipulate objects, although sensory and motor ability is intact
	Constructional apraxia	Inability to reproduce figures on paper
	Ideomotor apraxia	Inability to translate an idea into action
	Hemispatial (unilateral) neglect	Inability to process and perceive stimuli on one side of the body or the environment despite intact senses; results in a deficit in attention and awareness to the affected side
Calculation	Dyscalculia	Inability to perform calculations correctly
Abstract reasoning	Conceptual concreteness	Inability to describe in abstractions, generalize, or apply principles
Thought process and content	Flight of ideas	Topic of speech changes within a sentence
	Confabulation	Making up answers without regard to facts
	Circumstantiality	Indirect speech characterized by countless details and explanations with resultant prolonged time to reach point
	Echolalia	Involuntary repetition of a word or sentence spoken by someone else
	Clanging	Use of meaningless, rhyming words
	Blocking	Unconscious interruption in the train of thought manifested as a sudden obstruction to the spontaneous flow of speech
	Pressured speech	Frantic, energetic, jumbled speech; speech trying to keep up with thoughts
	Word salad	Meaningless mixture of words or phrases

CLINICAL MANAGEMENT

Nursing practice has four major dimensions of concern relative to an individual's cognitive status: recognition of risk for impaired cognition, cognitive assessment, the planning and delivery of individualized care appropriate to level of cognitive ability, and evaluation of outcomes.

Primary Prevention

Promoting a healthy lifestyle—including optimal nutrition, exercise, social activity, regular medical care to prevent and/or manage chronic diseases, avoidance of substance abuse (especially during pregnancy), and other high-risk behaviors—through teaching and community programs is basic to prevention across the spectrum of cognitive impairment. It is essential for healthy pregnancies, growth and development into adulthood, healthy aging, and decreasing vulnerability to delirium and vascular dementia.

Genetic counseling is another primary prevention strategy related to risk for disorders characterized by impaired cognition. This ranges from pregnancy risks associated with advanced maternal age (e.g., Down syndrome) to available genetic testing for inherited disorders (e.g., Huntington's disease) that could affect decisions about having children.

Primary prevention specific to delirium involves educating health care providers about changes in practice that can decrease vulnerability to the disorder. Practices that constitute risk factors for delirium, such as use of sleeping medications, use of urinary bladder catheters, and immobilization, need to be identified along with alternative methods of care.

Secondary Prevention (Screening)

Secondary prevention, or screening, refers to periodic assessment of specified population groups to detect early onset of a condition. Several screening tests to assess cognitive function were presented in the Assessment Section and Box 35-1. According to the U.S. Preventive Services Task Force,[32] the current evidence is insufficient to recommend for or against routine screening of cognitive impairment in older adults. Addressing dementias, including Alzheimer's disease, is part of the national Healthy People 2020 policy effort, although no specific screening recommendations are made.[33] Likewise, no routine screening tests are recommended for early detection of intellectual disability.

Collaborative Interventions

Cognition is a consideration in virtually all areas of health care and for all members of the health care team. It is a critical element in communicating with the patient and in the determination of care.[12] It is also critical to discharge planning from acute care facilities and is one determinant of need for home care services or placement in a long-term care facility.

The focus of treatment varies, depending on the underlying cause of the cognitive impairment. Clearly, the management of a child with intellectual disability differs from the focus of care for an older adult with dementia. In some cases, the treatment of a precipitating trauma or disease is possible, but in many cases of cognitive impairment, the disease process is not well understood and no treatments or only treatments with limited effectiveness are available. However, several underlying principles apply to all individuals with intellectual impairment. For example, regardless of the cause, management of the patient with cognitive impairment involves a multidisciplinary effort. Depending on the type and cause of the impairment, one or more of the following services may be required: nursing, medicine, physical therapy, occupational therapy, psychological intervention, individual and/or family counseling, nutritional consulting, speech and language services, audiology services, home health or homemaker assistance community services such as day care, caregiver support groups, and assistive technologies.

General Management Strategies

Promoting adequate rest, sleep, fluid intake, nutrition, elimination, pain control, and comfort are essential elements of care for persons with cognitive impairment. Also of great importance is ensuring an appropriate level of environmental stimulation because excessive stimulation can create agitation and confusion, whereas a lack of stimulation can result in sensory deprivation effects and withdrawal. If behavior is a problem, attempts should be made to identify and manage environmental triggers while avoiding the use of physical and pharmacologic restraints.[12]

Virtually all patients with cognitive impairment benefit from predictable routines, consistent caregivers, simple instructions, eye contact, and the presence of familiar people and objects. If needed, sensory aids such as eyeglasses and hearing aids should be used consistently to maximize accurate sensory input. To the extent possible, patients should be involved in self-care and decision making even if the latter is limited to deciding which of two shirts to wear or whether to drink milk or juice. Verbal reorientation to time and place should be provided if needed, and a clock and calendar should be within easy vision. For patients with delirium or who are otherwise agitated, a private room, soft music, relaxation tapes, or massage can be helpful.

Safety is a priority concern for all patients with cognitive impairment. Precise interventions needed vary with the person's age, developmental status, and degree of impairment. Patients should not drive, use machinery, or handle firearms, and the environment should be kept free of potential hazards. Supervision is generally needed with activities such as cooking or taking medications. If the patient wanders, an identification tag or bracelet should be worn or, if appropriate, a wander guard device should be used.

Pharmacologic Agents

In the management of patients with cognitive impairment, pharmacologic agents primarily treat associated diseases and control behavioral alterations such as sleeplessness, anxiety, agitation, and depression.[34] In the management of Alzheimer's disease (AD), however, pharmacologic therapy is aimed at maintaining cognitive function and slowing disease progression by regulating neurotransmitters in the brain. The two classes of drugs used in the treatment of AD are the cholinesterase inhibitors and a glutamate receptor antagonist. The three cholinesterase inhibitors approved by the U.S. Food and Drug Administration for the treatment of AD are donepezil (Aricept), rivastigmine (Exelon), and galantamine (Razadyne). All three of these drugs have been shown to help maintain memory, thinking, and speaking skills for a few months to a few years in *some* patients with mild to moderate AD; donepezil also is used in severe AD. The glutamate receptor antagonist memantine (Namenda) has been shown to delay functional decline in moderate to severe disease.[34]

Family and Caregiver Support

Engaging family members or significant others in goal setting and care planning also is essential. Advanced planning should be encouraged, and caregiver needs for education and support should be recognized and addressed. Information should be provided about support groups, respite options, day care, and other community services. Parents of a child born with intellectual disability require a great deal of support, particularly when they learn their child will have lifelong special needs. Caregivers of individuals with intellectual disability and dementia should be referred to support groups and other community resources.

INTERRELATED CONCEPTS

Because cognition depends on the interplay of multiple elements within the physical, psychological, and social dimensions, and because it allows for purposeful interaction with the environment, a multitude of concepts can be identified as influencing and/or being influenced by it. Figure 35-4 depicts the most prominent of these interrelationships. The physiologically focused concepts of Glucose Regulation, Mobility, Nutrition, Gas Exchange, Perfusion, Fluid and Electrolytes, and Acid–Base Balance have a clearly reciprocal relationship with cognition. These concepts are represented in Figure 35-4 by the ovals surrounding the upper half of the cognition conception and double-headed arrows because of their mutual interaction with it. The concepts of Functional Ability and Development are shown at the very bottom of the figure with arrows pointing from cognition to them because of the primarily unidirectional relationship of these concepts.

CLINICAL EXEMPLARS

Exemplars of impaired cognition are classified into categories described previously in this chapter and include delirium, neurocognitive disorders, focal cognitive disorders, intellectual disability, and learning disability; these are presented in Box 35-2. Although it is beyond the scope of this textbook to present each of these exemplars in detail, brief descriptions of the most important exemplars are featured here. Refer to other resources, particularly a pediatric and geriatric textbook, for a more comprehensive presentation of these conditions.

Featured Exemplars

Delirium

Delirium is a state of disturbed consciousness and altered cognition. Three categories of delirium exist: hyperactive delirium, hypoactive delirium, and mixed. Delirium is caused by a number of variables.

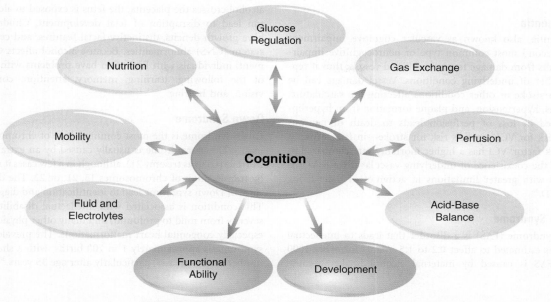

FIGURE 35-4 Cognition and Interrelated Concepts

■■■ BOX 35-2   EXEMPLARS OF IMPAIRED COGNITION

Neurocognitive Disorders (NCDs)
- Alzheimer disease
- Vascular NCD
- Frontotemporal NCD
- Lewy body dementia
- Parkinson's disease
- HIV-associated NCD
- Huntington's disease
- Prion disease
- Traumatic brain injury
- Substance-induced NCD
- NCD due to other medical conditions

Cognitive Impairment, Not Dementia
- Mild cognitive disorder
- Post-concussion syndrome

Focal Cognitive Disorders
- Amnesia
- Aphasia

Intellectual Disability
- Down syndrome
- Fragile X syndrome
- Prader–Willi syndrome
- Galactosemia
- Hunter's syndrome
- Phenylketonuria
- Rett syndrome
- Tay–Sachs disease
- Fetal alcohol syndrome
- Congenital hypothyroidism

Learning Disability
- Dyslexia
- Dyscalculia
- Dysgraphia
- Dyspraxia

Some of the most common causes include pharmacologic agents (particularly when four or more pharmacologic agents are given in combination), metabolic dysfunction, dehydration, electrolyte imbalance, hypoglycemia, renal impairment, urinary retention, fecal impaction, hypoxia, acute illness, infection, and trauma.[27]

Alzheimer's Disease

Alzheimer's disease is the most common form of dementia among individuals older than age 65 years, and it is the sixth leading cause of death among adults aged 18 years or older. Estimates vary, but experts suggest that up to 5 million Americans aged 65 years or older have AD, and this number is expected to double by 2050.[35] It is thought that AD is caused by a combination of Tau protein clumps that form inside neurons and amyloid plaques that form in spaces between brain cells, leading to neuronal dysfunction and death. Symptoms include a combination of deficits, including loss of memory, language skills, visual perception, focus, attention, reasoning skills, and functional ability.[4]

Lewy Body Dementia

Dementia with Lewy bodies (DLB) is a type of synucleinopathy characterized by the formation of balloon-like protein structures inside the neurons. This represents the third most common form of dementia. Early symptoms, which can appear as long as a decade before dementia occurs, include loss of smell, visual hallucinations, and difficulty sleeping; these symptoms are often attributed to other causes. Once dementia occurs, symptoms of DLB are similar to those of AD, and parkinsonian signs and symptoms are often noted.

Vascular Dementia

Vascular dementia, also known as vascular cognitive impairment (VCI), is the second most common type of neurocognitive impairment. VCI results from damage to cerebral blood vessels; thus it represents a number of underlying conditions. Vessel damage can be associated with stroke or other conditions affecting the vasculature, such as diabetes, hypertension, and plaque formation from hyperlipidemia. Reduced or loss of perfusion leads to death of neurons affected. The risk for VCI parallels risk for stroke—in fact, stroke is the greatest risk factor. VCI has a higher mortality rate compared to AD because of the coexistence of underlying vascular disease; VCI is also associated with greater limitations in activities of daily living compared to AD.[36]

Fetal Alcohol Syndrome

Fetal alcohol syndrome (FAS) is a disorder that leads to intellectual disability and is estimated to affect 0.2 to 1.5 infants for every 1000 live births.[37] FAS is caused by maternal alcohol intake; because alcohol crosses the placenta, the fetus is exposed to alcohol and this can lead to disruption of fetal development. Children with FAS have growth deficits, distinctive facial features, and central nervous system (CNS) abnormalities. Because alcohol affects CNS development, individuals with FAS often have problems with one or more of the following: learning, memory, attention, communication, vision, and hearing.

Down Syndrome

Down syndrome is the most common type of chromosomal abnormality. Down syndrome is usually caused by an extra chromosome 21 (referred to as trisomy 21), although in a few cases it may be caused by translocation of chromosomes 15, 21, or 22. The distinctive features of Down syndrome lead to identification and diagnosis at birth. This condition is associated with intellectual disability (ranging in severity from mild to profound) and many other physical conditions, especially congenital heart malformations. The prevalence of Down syndrome is approximately 1 in 700 births; with a sharp rise as the mother's age increases, particularly after age 35 years.[38]

CASE STUDY

Source: BakiBG/iStock/Thinkstock

Case Presentation

As part of a community health awareness event, a community health nurse has presented a program on problems associated with aging and their management; the nurse is available for meetings with individuals who have questions or concerns. One of the persons requesting a meeting was a middle-aged woman named Karen, who expressed concern regarding her mother's condition and asked for guidance. Karen explained that her mother, Ruby Long, is 79 years old and has no known medical conditions. Ruby lives with Karen and has become increasingly difficult to manage during the past 8–10 months. Karen states that her mother has become lax in her hygiene, is very forgetful of details of recent events, seems to be only focused on herself and unconcerned with anyone else's needs, is unwilling to try new things or go new places, and has lost interest in activities that she formally enjoyed. Karen also tells the nurse that her mother sometimes makes what appear to be poor decisions, has trouble managing money, and becomes very upset if any mistakes are mentioned. Upon further questioning, the nurse learns that Ruby Long wears eyeglasses (last eye exam 2 years ago) and has difficulty hearing (but does not use a hearing aid). Ruby has a family physician; her last visit was approximately 1 year ago. Karen tells the nurse that her grandparents and two aunts on her mother's side had dementia, although she is not exactly sure exactly what caused dementia in her relatives.

The nurse encourages Karen to arrange for Ruby to have a complete physical examination to rule out a physical cause of the behaviors and to determine the presence of any comorbidities, including a hearing and vision examination (to determine if the observed problems are resulting from changes in sensory perception). The nurse stresses the importance of maintaining a safe environment for Ruby. The nurse also discusses with Karen the possibility that she will need to plan for management of life affairs, such as power of attorney and advance directives. Finally, the nurse refers Karen to a local community resource for further education and support for caregivers.

Case Analysis

The behaviors described on the part of the mother are consistent with signs of cognitive impairment. There are two major risk factors present for dementia: advanced age and family history. Current sensory status is uncertain: Vision has not been recently checked, hearing has not been tested, and both age and history suggest a possibility of impairment. Sensory input is a determinant of cognition. Physical disease could be responsible for the behaviors; no physical examination has been done in more than 1 year. There is a clear potential for caregiver role strain implicit in the situation and in the daughter's words "increasingly difficult to manage."

ACCESS EXEMPLAR LINKS IN YOUR GIDDENS EBOOK

REFERENCES

1. Wiley J, Jee BD: Cognition: Overview and recent trends. In Aukrust VG, editor: *Learning and cognition in education*, New York, 2011, Academic Press.

2. Baars BJ, Gage NM: *Cognition, brain and consciousness: Introduction to cognitive neuroscience*, ed 2, New York, 2010, Academic Press.

3. Oxford Dictionaries: Cognition, 2015. Retrieved from: <http://www.oxforddictionaries.com/us/definition/american_english/cognition>.

4. American Psychiatric Association: *Diagnostic and statistical manual of mental disorders*, ed 5, Arlington, VA, 2013, American Psychiatric Publishing.

5. Magnussen S, Brennan T: Memory. In Baars BJ, Gage NM, editors: *Cognition, brain and consciousness. Introduction to cognitive neuroscience*, ed 2, New York, 2010, Academic Press.

6. Aminoff MJ: Regional cerebral dysfunction: Higher mental functions. In Goldman L, Ausiello D, editors: *Cecil medicine*, ed 23, Philadelphia, 2008, Saunders, pp 2262–2266.

7. Goldman L, Schafer M, editors: *Cecil medicine*, ed 24, Philadelphia, 2012, Saunders.

8. Piget J: *The theory of stages in cognitive development*, New York, 1969, McGraw-Hill.

9. Perrot A, Bherer L, Messier J: Preserved special memory for reaching to remembered three-dimensional targets in aging. *Exp Aging Res* 38(5):511–536, 2012.

10. Centers for Disease Control and Prevention: Cognitive impairment: A call for action, now! 2011. Retrieved from: <http://www.cdc.gov/aging/pdf/cognitive_impairment/cogImp_poilicy_final.pdf>.

11. Inouye SK: Delirium and other mental status problems in the older patient. In Goldman L, Schafer M, editors: *Cecil medicine*, ed 24, Philadelphia, 2012, Saunders.

12. Halter MJ: *Varcarolis' foundations of psychiatric mental health nursing: A clinical approach*, ed 4, Philadelphia, 2014, Saunders.

13. Plassman B, Langa K, McCammon R, et al: Incidence of dementia and cognitive impairment, not dementia in the United States. *Ann Neurol* 70(3):418–426, 2011.

14. Group Health: Dementia and cognitive impairment diagnosis and treatment guideline, 2012. Retrieved from: <http://www.ghc.org/all-sites/guidelines/dementia.pdf>.

15. Mefford HC, Batshaw ML, Hoffman EP: Genomics, intellectual disability and autism. *N Engl J Med* 366(8):733–743, 2012.

16. Tynan WD: Cognitive deficits, 2014. Retrieved from: <http://www.emedicine.medscape.com/article/91729-overview>.

17. Davey A, Dai T, Woodard J: Profiles of cognitive function in a population-based sample of centenarians using factor mixed analysis. *Exp Aging Res* 39:125–144, 2013.

18. Brooks M: Long-term pesticide exposure linked to cognitive decline, *Medscape News Today*, 2010. Retrieved from: <http://www.medscape.com/viewarticle/734960>.

19. Hockenberry MJ, Wilson DW: *Wong's essentials of pediatric nursing*, ed 9, St Louis, 2013, Mosby.

20. Rajan KB, Hebert LE, Scherr PA, et al: Disability in basic and instrumental activities of daily living is associated with faster rate of decline in cognitive function of older adults. *J Gerontol Ser Biol Sci Med Sci* 68(5):624–630, 2013.

21. Mielke M, Roberts R, Savica R, et al: Assessing the temporal relationship between cognition and gait: Slow gait predicts cognitive decline in the Mayo Clinic study of aging. *J Gerontol A Biol Sci Med Sci* 68(8):929–937, 2013.

22. Holtzer R, Wang C, Lipton R, et al: The protective effects of executive functions and episodic memory on gait speed decline in aging defined in the context of cognitive reserve. *J Am Geriatr Soc* 60(11):2093–2098, 2012.

23. Ganguli M, Fu B, Snitz BE, et al: Mild cognitive impairment: Incidence and vascular risk factors in a population-based cohort. *Neurology* 80(23):2112–2120, 2013.

24. Tran D, Baxter J, Hamman RF, et al: Impairment of executive cognitive control in type 2 diabetes, and its effects on health-related behavior and use of health services. *J Behav Med* 37:414–422, 2014.

25. Mayo Clinic: Chemo brain, (n.d.). Retrieved from: <http://www.mayoclinic.org/diseases-conditions/chemo-brain/basics/definition/con-20033864>.

26. Wilson S, Giddens J: *Health assessment for nursing practice*, ed 5, St Louis, 2013, Mosby.

27. Gillis AJ, MacDonald B: Unmasking delirium. *Can Nurse* 102(9):19–24, 2006.

28. Habela CW, Hamosh A: Genetic testing for intellectual disability: A role in diagnostic evaluation. *Contemp Pediatr* 30(6):21–30, 2013.

29. Alzheimer's Society: The Mini Mental State Examination (MMSE), (n.d.). Retrieved from: <http://www.alzheimers.org.uk/site/scripts/documents_info.php?documentID=121>.

30. Kiral K, Ozge A, Sungur M, et al: Detection of memory impairment in a community-based system: A collaborative Study. *Health Soc Work* 38(2):89–96, 2013.

31. Lin J, O'Connor E, Rossom R, et al: Screening for cognitive impairment in older adults: A systematic review for the U.S. Preventative Services Task Force. *Ann Intern Med* 159(9):601–612, 2013.

32. U.S. Preventive Services Task Force: Cognitive impairment in older adults: Screening, 2014. Retrieved from: <http://www.uspreventiveservicestaskforce.org/Page/Topic/recommendation-summary/cognitive-impairment-in-older-adults-screening?ds=1&s=>.

33. Healthy People 2020: Dementias, including Alzheimer's disease, 2015. Retrieved from: <https://www.healthypeople.gov/2020/topics-objectives/topic/dementias-including-alzheimers-disease>.

34. Staurt GW: *Principles and practice of psychiatric nursing*, ed 10, St Louis, 2012, Mosby.

35. National Institutes of Health: The dementias: Hope through research, NIH Publication No. 13-2252, 2013. Retrieved from: <http://www.ninds.nih.gov/disorders/dementias/the-dementias.pdf>.

36. Gure TR, Kabeto MU, Plassman BL, et al: Differences in functional impairment across subtypes of dementia. *J Gerontol A Biol Sci Med Sci* 65A(4):434–441, 2010.

37. Centers for Disease Control and Prevention: Fetal alcohol spectrum disorders, 2015. Retrieved from: <http://www.cdc.gov/ncbddd/fasd/index.html>.

38. Centers for Disease Control and Prevention: Down syndrome: Data and statistics, 2015. Retrieved from: <http://www.cdc.gov/ncbddd/birthdefects/downsyndrome/data.html>.

Psychosis

Sean Convoy

Much like many other psychiatric experiences, psychosis has been misjudged, misunderstood, and mislabeled for centuries. Society's relative lack of understanding of psychosis produces rich soil from which stigma and social injustice have traditionally flourished. The purpose of this concept presentation is to present basic elements of psychosis for application into nursing practice, with a secondary intent to strip away commonly held misperceptions and illuminate the evidence so that the nurse is better able to understand psychosis and those it affects.

DEFINITION

Although psychosis has not appreciably changed over the centuries, human understanding and subsequent definition of it have changed considerably. One of the oldest medical references published in 1500 BC, the Egyptian Ebers Papyrus, spoke generally to what would later be referred to as psychosis in a chapter titled "The Book of Hearts," crudely defining it as a "madness" born of "poison, demons, fecal matter and blood trouble."[1] During the Middle Ages, the treatment of those with psychosis was undistinguished from that of criminals, commonly involving physical punishment and torture. When torture did not "cure" the psychosis, witchcraft was then conveniently suspected.[2]

The term *psychosis* was formally coined in 1845 and was synonymously linked with terms such as mental handicap and psychopathy.[3] Although present-day understanding and tolerance of psychosis have unquestionably improved, society's persisting fear and misunderstanding of it continue to complicate an already complex condition.

The *Diagnostic and Statistical Manual of Mental Disorders*, fifth edition (*DSM-5*), currently defines psychosis as abnormalities in five different symptomatic domains: delusions, hallucinations, disorganized thought, disorganized or abnormal motor behavior, and negative symptoms.[4] A psychobiological definition of psychosis would implicate dysregulation of dopamine transport systems between the limbic system and prefrontal cortex. Stephen Stahl defines psychosis as a syndrome associated with many different disorders in which a "person's mental capacity, affective response, and capacity to recognize reality, communicate, and relate to others is impaired."[5] Each definition provides a unique but arguably incomplete description of a complex state. For the purpose of this concept presentation, *psychosis* is defined as *a syndrome of neurocognitive symptoms that impairs cognitive capacity leading to deficits of perception, functioning, and social relatedness.*

SCOPE

The scope of psychosis exists along a continuum ranging from absence of psychosis to severe psychosis (Figure 36-1). Between the extremes there exists a line of demarcation where the symptoms are of a sufficient intensity, duration, and degree of functional impairment to be considered clinically significant. Symptoms that exist below this threshold are consequently referred to as subclinical. Like most health states, psychosis is not static. Rather, psychosis is best conceptualized in the form of a distinct episode of clinically significant symptoms. The frequency of psychotic episodes is contingent upon the etiology of the psychosis. Psychosis can be acute in onset and relatively short in duration, as can be seen with a delirium or substance-induced psychotic episode. Likewise, psychosis can be chronic, as can be seen with schizophrenia or schizoaffective disorder.

NORMAL PHYSIOLOGICAL PROCESS

Under no circumstances should the symptoms associated with psychosis be considered "normal" or acceptable. Regardless of etiology, the duration of untreated psychosis is associated with poor outcomes.[6]

Normal physiology is defined by the absence (or reduced number) of vulnerability gene mutations that influence the development of critical neural pathways in the brain. In other words, in the absence of critical gene variations, development and maturation of critical neural circuits in the brain occur. Thus the brain is better able to regulate dopamine, leading to optimal dopaminergic neurotransmission between critical neural circuits that span the distance between the limbic system and prefrontal cortex.[7] The absence of psychosis would reflect normal regulation of dopamine within each of the four pathways (mesocortical, mesolimbic, nigrostriatal, and tuberoinfundibular) and the subsequent absence of psychosis.

VARIATIONS AND CONTEXT
Etiologies of Psychosis

Psychosis can manifest from varied etiologies and can be categorized as either primary or secondary in origin.[8] *Primary* psychosis has a

FIGURE 36-1 Scope of Concept The concept of psychosis ranges from an absence of psychosis to severe psychosis.

psychiatric etiology, as can be seen in schizophrenia, schizoaffective disorder, and, in some instances, other psychiatric illnesses. *Secondary psychosis* has an organic etiology, as can be seen in acute substance intoxication, delirium, or dementia. Primary and secondary forms of psychosis are not mutually exclusive; not only do they coexist but also in some instances they potentiate the other. Absent a primary source of psychosis, individuals that manifest secondary psychosis have greater potential to recover from a psychotic episode without clinically significant sequelae. Those with a primary etiology of psychosis are more likely to manifest subsequent episodes of psychosis due to the predisposing genomic variation and subsequent neural circuit compromises.

Primary Psychosis

Schizophrenia spectrum and other psychotic disorders. Within the Schizophrenia Spectrum and Other Psychotic Disorders classification, psychosis is the principal symptom(s) of interest. Clinical disorders in this category include delusional disorder, brief psychotic disorder, schizophreniform disorder, schizophrenia, schizoaffective disorder, and catatonia.[4] As a primary etiology of psychosis, the schizophrenia spectrum and other psychotic disorders reflect greater potential for long-term disability due to their genomic and neurodevelopmental etiology. Schizophrenia is a diagnosis of exclusion in that all other possible (typically medical) explanations must be first ruled out.

Other psychiatric illnesses. Other psychiatric illnesses can also manifest psychotic symptoms or episodes. Disorders such as bipolar I disorder and major depressive disorder have the potential to manifest psychosis.[4] More than half of those diagnosed with bipolar disorder will experience psychosis at some time in their life.[9] Psychosis associated with bipolar disorder is commonly an acute presentation that has potential to subside but is associated with poor outcomes.[10] Among the depressive disorders, psychosis is exclusively associated with the most severe expressions of clinical depression and occurs in 14–20% of those who are clinically depressed.[11] Psychotic episodes that manifest in the context of a depressive disorder are more commonly acute in presentation and typically have high rates of recovery with treatment.

Psychotic symptoms are not explicitly seen within the personality disorders. However, personality disorders can be comorbid with a number of conditions that have the potential to manifest psychosis. For example, personality disorders have a 13.4% comorbidity rate with major depressive disorders, 8.1% with bipolar spectrum disorders, 10.9% with alcohol use disorder, and 5.6% with substance use disorders.[12] Consequently, the presentation of psychosis (e.g., acute or chronic) is typically dependent on the comorbid condition and not the personality disorder.

Secondary Psychosis

Toxic psychosis. Toxic psychosis is the product of an underlying and untreated medical issue. Delirium is an example of toxic psychosis. Psychosis associated with delirium is typically rapid in onset and defined by a hallmark sign of dramatic fluctuations in mental status. Between 10% and 30% of medically ill inpatients and 80% of terminally ill patients exhibit delirium.[7] Medically treating a secondary source of psychosis as one would a primary source of psychosis will not resolve the psychosis and actually increases the relative risk that the underlying medical illness will further deteriorate. Provided the health care team isolates and treats the underlying medical issue, there is a reasonable expectation of complete resolution of psychosis.

Dementia. Dementia is one of many neurocognitive disorders that have potential to manifest psychosis. Dementia can be the product of multiple etiologies, including Alzheimer's, Lewy bodies, vascular, HIV, prion, Parkinson's, traumatic brain injury, and Huntington's disease.[4] A slow but progressive manifestation of psychotic symptoms within the context of a suspected neurocognitive disorder is more consistent with a demanding condition and requires specialty consultation.

Medical illness. Numerous medical conditions can, given the right circumstances, manifest symptoms of psychosis. Patients can manifest psychosis secondary to endocrinopathies (e.g., adrenal or thyroid disorders), metabolic disorders (e.g., porphyria and Wilson's disease), nutritional and vitamin deficiencies (e.g., vitamin A, D, and B_{12}, magnesium, and zinc deficiency), central nervous system disorders (e.g., cerebral vascular accident, epilepsy, and hydrocephalus), degenerative disorders (e.g., Friedriech's ataxia), autoimmune disorders (e.g., multiple sclerosis and paraneoplastic syndrome), infections (e.g., encephalitis, neurosyphilis, Lyme disease, and sarcoidosis), space-occupying lesions (e.g., congenital vascular malformations and tuberous sclerosis), and chromosomal abnormalities (e.g., Klienfelter's and fragile X syndrome).[8] When recognized, this secondary source of psychosis will commonly be classified as a Psychotic Disorder Due to Another Medical Condition. Due to the diverse etiologies, the presentation of psychosis is varied in expression but more commonly resolves in accordance with the concurrent illness state.

Toxins, drugs, and medications. Psychosis can also be a product of numerous toxins, drugs, and medications. This form of psychotic expression is typically most challenging to causally identify. When recognized, this secondary source of psychosis will commonly be classified as a Substance-/Medication-Induced Psychotic Disorder.[4] Toxins known to potentially induce psychosis include but are not limited to carbon monoxide, organophosphates, and heavy metals such as arsenic, magnesium, mercury, and thallium.[8] Possible drugs that can induce psychosis include synthetic cannabis (or Spice), synthetic cathinones (or bath salts), alcohol, cocaine, methamphetamine (or crystal meth), psychotomimetic (or LSD), cannabis (or marijuana), and anabolic steroids. Likewise, certain prescribed medications also demonstrate an elevated risk for psychosis as a side effect, including sedative–hypnotic agents, amphetamines, anticholinergic agents, antiseizure agents, corticosteroids, and mefloquine. Depending on the substance used, psychosis can potentially go unrecognized and consequently insufficiently treated. Unless the patient has a preexisting psychotic condition, psychosis that manifests within the context of a toxin or substance will typically be acute in onset with a high rate of recovery after the substance is eliminated from the system.

BOX 36-1   Symptomatic Domains of Psychosis

- *Delusions*: Fixed beliefs that are not amenable to change in light of conflicting evidence
- *Hallucinations*: Perception-like experiences that occur without an external stimulus
- *Disorganized thinking*: Most commonly inferred from speech, defined by derailment, loose associations, tangentially, and incoherence
- *Disorganized/abnormal motor behavior*: Markedly abnormal behavior ranging from agitation to catatonia that is commonly situationally incongruent
- *Negative symptoms*: Alogia, affective blunting, asociality, anhedonia, and avolition

TABLE 36-1   Physiological Sequelae of Psychosis and Treatment

Pharmacotherapy Related	Behaviorally Related
• Extrapyramidal side effects	• Activity intolerance
• Hyperglycemia	• Obesity
• Dyslipidemia	• Substance use
• Hypertension	• Violence-related risk
• Hepatotoxicity	• Infectious disease exposure
• Immune compromise	• Vitamin deficiency
• Lens opacities (cataracts)	

Source: Data from Keks NA, Hope J: Long-term management of people with psychotic disorders in the community, *Australian Prescriber, An Indepedent Review* 30(2):44–46, 2007.

Symptomatic Variations of Psychosis

The presence of psychosis suggests progressively compromised neural circuits. Psychiatric (or primary) etiologies of psychosis typically reflect epigenetically mediated neural circuit compromise long before symptoms reach the clinical threshold. Some secondary causes of psychosis (e.g., those caused by drugs, toxins, and medical illness) are not necessarily associated with a progressive neural circuit compromise, hence variations in symptoms.

A number of symptoms can be expressed in a state of psychosis. Classic symptoms are described in Box 36-1. A conceptual representation of symptomatic expression of psychosis is presented in Figure 36-2. Symptoms must be of a sufficient intensity, duration, and degree of functional impairment to be recognizable as such. That point of observable recognition is defined as the *clinical threshold*.

CONSEQUENCES

Physiological Consequences

Regardless of the underlying cause, untreated psychosis is associated with poor outcomes.[6] Untreated, psychosis reflects a persisting

neurotoxic state that has the potential to further degrade neural pathways over time,[13] which may explain why dementia occurs twice as often among those diagnosed with schizophrenia.[14] The physiological consequences of psychosis are largely dependent on etiology and those variables that influence symptom duration, symptom intensity, and functional impairment.

Untreated psychosis has the potential to cause dementia; thus a determination of consequences follows the trajectory of both the etiology and symptoms. Much like how a compromised nuclear power plant is unable to control its core reactor temperature, the consequence of unregulated neural circuits is the release of inflammatory markers that further degrades the circuit.[15] Consequently, early and decisive treatment of psychosis is critical.

Although neural circuit degradation is the primary consequence of psychosis, there are also a number of secondary consequences worth mentioning (Table 36-1). Ironically, many of the secondary consequences are associated with treatment. Although the use of antipsychotic medications has revolutionized the treatment of psychosis, antipsychotic agents are not without risk. Long-term use of antipsychotic medications is associated with elevated risk of drug-induced movement disorders; metabolic syndrome; and cardiovascular, hepatic, and immune system problems.

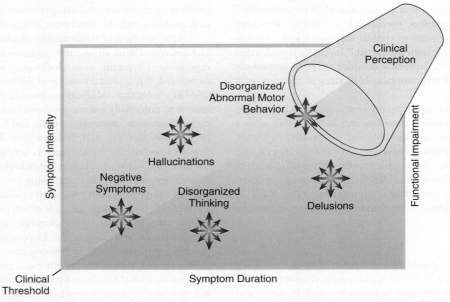

FIGURE 36-2 Symptomatic Expressions of Psychosis below and above the Clinical Threshold

Psychosocial Consequences

Behaviorally related consequences are influenced by both the symptomatic expression of psychosis and its treatment. Psychotic symptoms, coupled with the sedating effects of many of the antipsychotic agents, can commonly lead to decreased activity and weight gain.[16,17] The comorbidity of psychosis and substance abuse is well documented; nearly half of those diagnosed with a schizophrenia spectrum disorder have either alcohol or illicit substance dependence, and more than 70% are nicotine dependent.[18] Also concerning, individuals with persisting psychosis typically shun and are shunned by society. This reality brings with it major implications in terms of employment, housing, and one's ability to attend to basic needs. The seriously mentally ill (SMI) population is subsequently more vulnerable to violence, infectious disease, and malnutrition.[19]

RISK FACTORS

All individuals are potentially susceptible to psychosis regardless of age, gender, race, and/or ethnicity. There are no conclusive factors for psychosis in general; however, family history for psychosis, past psychotic episodes, substance use, stress intolerance, ineffective coping skills, and preexisting psychiatric illness are common variables among those who manifest psychosis. A large body of research exists on risk factors associated with schizophrenia; for this reason, discussion of risk factors is presented from this perspective. Risk factor determination reflects both genetic and environmental influences.

Populations at Risk

Schulz et al. identified that children with a premorbid IQ in the learning disability range demonstrate a statistically significant risk for schizophrenia.[20] Likewise, Werner et al. determined that lower individual- and community-level socioeconomic status at the time of birth are associated with an increased risk for schizophrenia.[21] Interestingly, the prevalence of schizophrenia has also been correlated with population density in cities with populations exceeding 1 million.[7]

Individual Risk Factors

Individual risk factors for psychosis exist within four potentially interrelated domains of temperament, environment, genetics, and physiology.

Temperament

Research has established that those with a preexisting personality disorder appear to be more vulnerable to brief psychotic disorder. An increased risk of schizophrenia may also be associated with asociality.[22]

Environmental

Environmental risk factors for schizophrenia spectrum disorder are clustered temporally by early life (e.g., obstetric complication, season of birth, prenatal/postnatal infection, maternal malnutrition, and maternal stress), childhood (e.g., adverse childrearing, child abuse, and head injury), and later life (e.g., drug abuse, migration/ethnicity, urbanization, social adversity, and life events).[23]

Genetic

The research suggests that schizophrenia currently has the strongest demonstrated genetic linkage among the known psychiatric disorders. Gene variants increase the relative risk for the development of psychosis through the subsequent degradation of key neural pathways in the brain over time. Although psychosis is not defined by a single gene variant, there is evidence that both the number of gene variations and the temporal sequence of those variations in relation to environmental stress can increase the relative risk for psychosis. Recent research has established that specific gene mutations associated with chromosomes 1, 6, 8, 12, 13, and 22 demonstrate an increased vulnerability to psychotic disorders.[5] The concordance rate for a schizophrenia spectrum disorder is 48% among monozygotic twins, 17% among fraternal twins, 9% among siblings, and 6% among parents.[24]

Physiological

In terms of potential biomarkers, some research establishes that decreased cortical gray matter may also be associated with increased risk for schizophrenia spectrum disorder.[25] Currently, there is active research on many fronts seeking to establish reliable biomarkers for schizophrenia. There is also strong evidence that sleep deprivation has the potential to induce psychotic states.[26]

ASSESSMENT

Assessment for psychosis requires the systematic collection of a history, physical assessment, mental status examination, and diagnostic testing (Box 36-2). As mentioned previously, psychosis is associated with progressively compromised neural circuits; for this reason,

---

BOX 36-2 Nursing Assessment of Psychosis

History
- Risk factors
- Personal medical history
- Mental health history
- Substance use
- Perinatal trauma
- Developmental history
- Family history
- Trauma exposure
- Culture and beliefs

Physical Examination
- Vital signs
- Cranial nerve assessment
- Mental status examination
  - Appearance
  - Attitude
  - Behavior
  - Mood and affect
  - Speech
  - Thought process
  - Thought content
  - Perceptions
  - Cognition
  - Insight
  - Judgment

Diagnostic Tests
- Laboratory tests
- Imaging

the symptoms are progressive and evolve over time. Many subclinical symptoms occur before the patient is overtly psychotic (see Figure 36-2); thus early recognition requires a critical eye. To the casual observer, individuals with subclinical symptoms of psychosis may appear odd, socially awkward, or easily distracted. The proficient or expert nurse is better able to perceive subtle signs of psychosis, such as hallucinations and negative symptoms, whereas the novice or advanced beginner is usually only sensitized to the more overt signs of psychosis, such as delusional and disorganized behavior.[27] The expert nurse understands the concept of psychosis and its symptomatic expression so well that he or she is sometimes able to perceive psychosis below the clinical threshold.

History

The goal of the history is to obtain vital and time-sensitive health information that has the potential to immediately and significantly influence the trajectory of care. Cognitive impairment and diminished reality testing commonly complicate history taking with a psychotic patient. Thus obtaining collateral information from friends, family, coworkers, and past health care professionals is vital. A complete health history includes subjective data from the patient and (when available) a collateral source. Questions should be straightforward, concrete, and open-ended. The nurse should afford the patient with suspected psychotic symptoms additional time to answer questions. Psychotic patients commonly experience paranoia, which makes rapport building very important.

Patients who are experiencing psychosis often lack self-awareness of their own medical condition or disability. Consequently, using clinical terms such as *hallucination*, *delusion*, *paranoia*, and *catatonia* with a suspected psychotic patient is contraindicated. Develop questions using non-clinical terms as part of the interview. For example as opposed to asking, "Are you experiencing hallucinations?" ask, "Do you ever see or hear things that other people can't see or hear?" Instead of asking, "Are you delusional?" nonjudgmentally ask a patient about those beliefs he or she feels strongly about and assess the nature of those beliefs in relation to reality. As opposed to asking, "Do you feel paranoid a lot?" ask, "Are you influenced strongly by the beliefs of others?"

Physical Assessment

Physical manifestations of psychosis follow etiology. If the etiology of psychosis is medically or chemically induced, any number of physical symptoms may be present. For example, a psychotic patient under the influence of a psychoactive stimulant would also demonstrate those symptoms associated with psychoactive stimulant intoxication or withdrawal (e.g., mydriasis, bruxism, nonintentional tremor, elevated blood pressure, tachypnea, and hyperthermia). Alternatively, a psychotic patient with a comorbid history of dementia would also manifest symptoms associated with dementia (e.g., memory loss, impaired judgment, impaired abstract reasoning, impaired communication skills, and disorientation). Regardless of etiology, a mental status examination is used to assess symptoms.

Diagnostic Tests

Although there currently are no diagnostic tests that definitively rule in or out psychosis, a number of tests are available that can aid the nurse in differentiating between the primary and secondary etiologies of psychosis. Laboratory studies such as a complete blood count, chemistry panel (Chem18), thyroid function test, rapid plasma reagin, dexamethasone suppression test, HIV test, heavy metals panel, urinalysis, urine drug screen, urine culture and sensitivity, computerized tomography, and magnetic resonance imaging can rule out a number of potential organic etiologies.[7]

CLINICAL MANAGEMENT

Clinical management of psychosis is principally dependent on etiology. If the nature of the psychosis is secondary, the health care team must treat the underlying cause of the psychosis while simultaneously managing the symptoms of psychosis. In instances in which psychosis does not have a secondary cause, a number of treatment options are available to manage psychosis. For the purposes of this section, clinical management focuses on the primary etiology of psychosis.

Primary Prevention

Understanding that psychosis is born of both genomic and environmental variables, primary prevention targeting the genomic influence would focus on prepregnancy genetic counseling. Alternatively, primary prevention targeting the environmental influence requires a reconsideration of previously discussed environmental risk factors (e.g., obstetric complication, maternal health, malnutrition and stress, stable parenting, and injury prevention).

Secondary Prevention (Screening)

The focus of secondary prevention as it relates to psychosis involves screening individuals with a family history and monitoring for subclinical symptoms. A number of evidence-based screening instruments may aid in diagnosis, including the Brief Psychiatric Rating Scale (BRPS),[28] the Positive and Negative Syndrome Scale (PANSS),[29] the Minnesota Multiphasic Personality Inventory–2 (MMPI-2),[30] and the *DSM-V*'s Level I Cross-Cutting Symptoms Measure.[4]

Available evidence indicates that early intervention within the prodromal phase (the period in which subtle symptoms of psychosis begin to rise to the level of clinical significance) is associated with the best possible outcome. In that regard, the proficient or expert nurse who is able to discern symptoms at or below the clinical threshold is in a particularly unique position to positively influence the trajectory of care.

Collaborative Interventions

The clinical management of psychosis is subdivided into four classifications of pharmacologic (Box 36-3), nonpharmacologic, lifestyle modification, and community integration. Although nearly half of those with a schizophrenia spectrum disorder do not receive care, those who do typically do not receive comprehensive care. The National Institute of Mental Health funded the Schizophrenia Patient Outcomes Research Team (PORT) to develop and disseminate evidence-based recommendations for the treatment of schizophrenia.[31] The results of the PORT study recommended an individualized, multimodal approach to care involving interventions from all four classifications.

Pharmacotherapy

First-generation antipsychotics. Most first-generation antipsychotics are no longer considered first-tier choices for the treatment of psychosis; however, they are still seen in community-based and forensic settings throughout the country. First-generation antipsychotics (see Box 36-3) reduce the transmission of dopamine at the D_2 receptor site of four key dopaminergic pathways in the brain. Their ability to target the positive symptoms associated with a schizophrenia spectrum disorder is well-established. However, they are known for significant side effects including anticholinergic side effects, high-risk extrapyramidal side effects (EPS), and sedation that has historically led to medication adherence problems.

Second-generation antipsychotics. Second-generation antipsychotic agents (see Box 36-3) also target positive symptoms of psychosis with their D_2 antagonism; in addition, they target negative symptoms with their 5-HT_{2a} antagonism and (for certain agents) 5-HT_{1a} agonism.[32]

BOX 36-3 Pharmacologic Agents for the Treatment of Psychosis

First-generation antipsychotics
- Haloperidol (Haldol)
- Fluphenazine (Prolixin)
- Thiothixene (Navane)
- Trifluoperazine (Stelazine)
- Perphenazine (Trilofon)
- Chlorpromazine (Thorazine)
- Thioridazine (Mellaril)
- Loxapine (Loxitane)

Second-generation antipsychotics
- Clozapine (Clozaril)
- Olanzapine (Zyprexa)
- Risperidone (Risperdal)
- Quetiapine (Seroquel)
- Aripipazaole (Abilify)
- Paliperidone (Invega)
- Ziprasidone (Geodon)
- Asenapine (Saphris)

Anticholinergic agents
- Cogentin
- Parlodel
- Artane
- Benadryl

Their tendency to more loosely bind to targeted receptor sites, consequently resulting in a lower risk for EPS. Although the second-generation antipsychotics are considered first-line choices for the treatment of psychosis and have a lower risk for EPS, they have a marked increased risk for metabolic disorders such as dyslipidemia, diabetes, and weight gain if used for long periods of time.

Anticholinergic agents. Anticholinergic agents (see Box 36-3) are used to treat EPS resulting from antipsychotic medication use. EPS can occur because of excessive D_2 binding within the nigrostriatal pathway. Because certain forms of EPS are considered medical emergencies (e.g., acute pharyngeal dystonia) and potentially permanent (e.g., tardive dyskinesia), anticholinergic agents can be delivered both orally and intramuscularly to target EPS.

Nonpharmacologic Therapies

Social skills training. Psychosis, by its very definition, has the potential to slowly and progressively dissolve interpersonal relational skills. Social skills acquisition and maintenance can be seen as a bridge to long-term symptom management. Social skills training (SST) is typically done in a homogeneous group format and teaches individuals about verbal, nonverbal, and paraverbal communication.[33] Assertiveness training is also an element of SST, as is social cue interpretation.

Family focused therapy. Tailored to a family influenced by schizophrenia spectrum disorder, family focused therapy (FFT) educates the family on the nature of psychosis, its symptoms, and common management strategies. Research has established that FFT improves medication adherence, reduces the rate of relapse, and reduces psychiatric readmission rates.[34–36]

Cognitive–behavioral therapy for psychosis. Cognitive–behavioral therapy is premised upon the notion that how one perceives and interprets sensory stimuli has a direct bearing on the reaction one has to that situation. Upon initial consideration, this form of therapy would seem contraindicated for an individual struggling with psychosis. It is important to note that an individual with a schizophrenia spectrum disorder is not perpetually psychotic and can go months, if not years, without psychotic symptoms. Evidence suggests that cognitive–behavioral therapy for psychosis can improve medication adherence, insight, and social functioning.[37–39]

Cognitive enhancement therapy. Cognitive enhancement therapy employs elements of cognitive–behavioral therapy with social skills training for symptomatically stable individuals with severe mental illness. Delivered via computer-based training and group-based activities, cognitive enhancement therapy focuses on improving mental stamina, active information processing, and learning how to negotiate unrehearsed social challenges.[40]

Electroconvulsive therapy. Electroconvulsive therapy (ECT) is a medical procedure in which electrical currents are passed through the brain with the intent to trigger seizure activity, which has the potential to cause changes in brain chemistry and subsequently influence psychotic symptoms. ECT has great efficacy in treating catatonia but poses a risk for cognitive and memory side effects.[41] Depending on the severity of symptoms, 6–12 rounds of ECT commonly demonstrate target symptom improvement, with the potential for longitudinal maintenance sessions thereafter.

Lifestyle Modification

Lifestyle modification addresses behaviors that have the potential to either improve or worsen ones' health state. Most second-generation antipsychotics have an increased risk for weight gain and impaired glucose tolerance.[42] For this reason, lifestyle modification approaches are a critical element to the long-term management of psychotic disorders and, if implemented in a group-based format, can also reinforce social skills development.[43]

Serial health monitoring. Second-generation antipsychotic agents have greatly improved the management of positive and negative symptoms. Research suggests that a second-generation antipsychotic metabolic monitoring process that serially assesses abdominal obesity, triglycerides, high-density lipoprotein cholesterol, blood pressure, and fasting glucose has the potential to mitigate some degree of the risk associated with the long-term use of these agents.[44]

Case management. Case management employs a team of health care workers to serve as a liaison between the patient and the community to maximize patient autonomy without compromising patient health and well-being. Assertive community treatment (ACT) is a popular model that includes a team consisting of a case manager, primary care provider, mental health provider, and nurse and in which care is decentralized away from the traditional brick-and-mortar environment and accessible 24 hours a day. ACT has proven to be both clinically and fiscally efficacious.[45–47]

Vocational therapy. Vocational therapy is a process that individualizes resources for those with functional, psychological, developmental, or cognitive impairments to overcome barriers to accessing, maintaining, or returning to employment. In individuals with a schizophrenia spectrum disorder, vocational therapy has been proven to improve cognitive and negative symptoms,[48] clinical outcomes,[49] and social functioning.[50]

INTERRELATED CONCEPTS

Multiple concepts are clearly interrelated to the concept of psychosis (Figure 36-3). Incorporating several key psychosocial concepts and professional nursing concepts is essential to improving healthy outcomes when caring for psychotic patients. Health Policy is important in the context of regulations that oversee the delivery of mental health care in the United States. The concepts of Ethics and Health Care Law relate to ensuring appropriate use of restrictive treatment interventions (i.e., seclusion, sedation, and restraints). In terms of psychiatric commitment, the legal concepts of habeas corpus and justification for involuntary treatment must be respected. Communication is a key concept because this represents an important skill needed to establish therapeutic relationships with psychotic patients. The concept of Patient Education links to the instructional treatment of protocols, disease process, and pharmacologic interventions. Collaboration is essential for effective treatment and includes

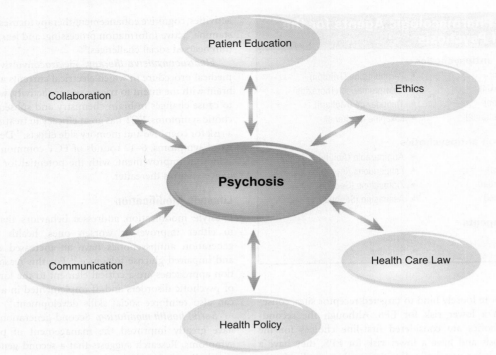

FIGURE 36-3 Psychosis and Interrelated Concepts

the interprofessional team to optimize specialty-related patient outcomes.

CLINICAL EXEMPLARS

As already established, psychosis can manifest from multiple etiologies. Box 36-4 presents common exemplars associated with psychosis. A comprehensive description and explanation of each exemplar is beyond the scope of this text; here, however, some of the most common exemplars are featured with a short description. Refer to psychiatric/mental health references for detailed information about each of these conditions.

Featured Exemplars
Schizophrenia

Schizophrenia is an SMI defined by a constellation of positive symptoms (e.g., hallucinations, delusions, disorganized speech and behavior, catatonia, and agitation), which commonly distance society from the patient, and negative symptoms (e.g., alogia, affective blunting, asociality, anhedonia, and avolition), which frequently distance the patient from society. Schizophrenia commonly manifests insidiously during early adulthood with a prodromal phase and requires lifelong management to control psychotic episodes. In addition to psychotherapy, treatment typically involves the use of antipsychotic agents.

Major Depressive Disorder, Severe with Psychotic Features

Major Depressive Disorder, Severe with Psychotic Features is defined by a primary constellation of major depressive symptoms with a symptomatic overlay of psychotic features. Psychosis seen within the context of this condition is episodic in nature but nonetheless a poor prognostic indicator. In addition to psychotherapy, treatment for major depressive disorder, severe with psychotic features requires antidepressant and antipsychotic agents to control target symptoms.

Delirium

Delirium is defined by rapid changes in brain function and cognitive capacity that occur within the context of a co-occurring physical condition. Symptoms can manifest as disturbance in attention, cognition, and behavior.[4] Consequently, psychosis or psychotic behavior can result from a delirium state. A cardinal symptom of delirium is defined by a waxing and waning of mental status. Delirium is considered a medical emergency. Common sources of delirium can be substance withdrawal, severe electrolyte abnormality, systemic infection, poor nutrition or dehydration, multiple co-occurring medical problems, and polypharmacy. Treatment follows the underlying etiology of the delirium state.

Major Neurocognitive Disorder

Major neurocognitive disorder is defined by a demonstrable cognitive decline from a previous level of performance as seen within different cognitive domains.[4] Consequently, psychosis or psychotic behavior can also result from a progressing neurocognitive disorder. The onset of symptoms with a major neurocognitive disorder is slow and progressive and not defined by a waxing and waning of mental status. Most etiologies of a major neurocognitive disorder are not typically reversible but can be slowed with different forms of pharmacotherapy and rehabilitation.

Substance-/Medication-Induced Psychotic Disorder

Substance-/medication-induced psychotic disorder is a time-limited manifestation of psychotic symptoms triggered by the ingestion of a substance or medication known to promote psychosis. Psychotic symptoms typically have a rapid onset with no evidence of prodrome and commonly dissipate after the substance has sufficiently degraded within the body. Long-term use of some agents (e.g., marijuana, cocaine, methamphetamine) can lead to an increased risk for chronic psychosis.[51-54]

■■■ BOX 36-4 EXEMPLARS OF IMPAIRED PSYCHOSIS

Schizophrenia Spectrum and Other Psychotic Disorders
- Schizotypal personality disorder
- Delusional disorder
- Brief psychotic disorder
- Schizophreniform disorder
- Schizophrenia
- Schizoaffective disorder
- Substance-/medication-induced psychotic disorder
- Psychotic disorder due to a general medical condition
- Catatonia associated with another mental condition
- Catatonic disorder due to another medical condition
- Unspecified catatonia
- Other specified schizophrenia spectrum disorder and other psychotic disorder
- Unspecified schizophrenia spectrum and other psychotic disorder

Bipolar and Related Disorders
- Bipolar I disorder with psychotic features

- Substance-/medication-induced bipolar and related disorder
- Bipolar and related disorder due to another medical condition

Depressive Disorders
- Major depressive disorder with psychotic features
- Substance-/medication-induced depressive disorder
- Depressive disorder due to another medical condition

Substance-Induced Disorders
- Substance intoxication and withdrawal

Neurocognitive Disorders
- Delirium
- Major neurocognitive disorder
- Substance-/medication-induced major disorder

Personality Disorders
- Cluster A personality disorders

CASE STUDY

Source: veronica89/iStock/Thinkstock

Case Presentation

Ethan is a 21-year-old unemployed, homeless male readmitted to the state hospital after a serious suicidal gesture when he attempted to walk into oncoming traffic on the highway. Prior to this most recent admission, Ethan's established diagnosis was *schizophrenia, first episode, currently in partial remission*, and *nicotine dependence*. Ethan has a significant family history of psychosis, with both his biological brother and father diagnosed with schizophrenia prior to the age of 20 years. His father completed suicide at age 30 years, and his brother is currently incarcerated. Ethan's mother is alcohol dependent and has historically been an unreliable support system. Ethan's first break of psychosis occurred at age 18 years during his first 6 months at college. His prodromal period was more prominent for negative symptoms (e.g., alogia, affective blunting, asociality, anhedonia, and avolition), with positive symptoms (e.g., audio–visual hallucinations and disorganized speech and behavior) surfacing much later and remitting much quicker with treatment. Ethan was initially prescribed Risperdal and achieved remission of all positive symptoms and some portion of his negative symptoms after 3 months of treatment with two hospitalizations and an eventual transition to a

long-acting injection form of Risperdal (Consta). A review of his outpatient record indicates that his negative symptoms have fluctuated around the clinical threshold during the past 3 years and he has been struggling with suicidal thoughts for the better part of the past 6 months. The persisting nature of his depressive symptoms prompts a diagnostic reconsideration of *schizoaffective disorder, multiple episodes, in acute episode*. During this hospitalization, Ethan's positive symptoms again quickly resolved, but his negative symptoms persisted, prompting the decision to add an antidepressant (Prozac) to his medication plan. Upon stabilization, Ethan was transferred to a partial hospitalization program, where cognitive enhancement therapy, art therapy, nutritional counseling, case management, and vocational rehabilitation was provided. With this augmented plan of care, Ethan was able to get remarkably better control of his negative symptoms and is now currently working part-time in a bookstore and is considering re-enrolling in a local community college.

Case Analysis

Ethan's case exemplifies how genomic vulnerability (e.g., familial history for schizophrenia) coupled with environmental stress (e.g., paternal suicide, unstable parental support, and stress of matriculating to college) expose vulnerable neural circuits, which over time manifest as psychosis. Positive symptoms of psychosis are more commonly targeted for treatment than are negative symptoms. Ethan's readmission is reflective of the high rate of psychiatric readmission seen with this population. Ethan's comprehensive remission of both positive and negative symptoms resulted from a medication plan that targeted both positive and negative symptoms augmented by a number of psychotherapeutic resources.

ACCESS EXEMPLAR LINKS IN YOUR GIDDENS EBOOK

REFERENCES

1. Juhas D: Throughout history, defining schizophrenia has remained a challenge. *Sci Am* 24(1):2013.
2. Mandal A: *Psychosis history*. Retrieved from: <http://www.news-medical.net>, 2014.
3. Beer MD: Psychosis: A history of the concept. *Compr Psychiatry* 37(4):273–291, 1996.
4. American Psychiatric Association: *Diagnostic and statistical manual of mental disorders*, ed 5, Arlington, VA, 2013, American Psychiatric Publishing.

5. Stahl SM: *Stahl's essential psychopharmacology: The prescriber's guide*, ed 5, Cambridge, UK, 2014, Cambridge University Press.
6. Penttila M, Jaaskelainen E, Hirvonen N, et al: Duration of untreated psychosis as predictor of long-term outcome in schizophrenia: Systematic review and meta-analysis. *Br J Psychiatry* 205(2):88–94, 2014.
7. Sadock BJ, Sadock VA, Ruiz P: *Kaplan & Sadock's synopsis of psychiatry: Behavioral sciences/clinical psychiatry*, ed 11, Philadelphia, 2014, Wolters Kluwer.
8. Freudenreich O: Differential diagnosis of psychotic symptoms: Medical "mimics." *Psychiatric Times* 2012.
9. Keck PE, Jr, McElroy SL, Havens JR, et al: Psychosis in bipolar disorder: Phenomenology and impact on morbidity and course of illness. *Compr Psychiatry* 44(4):263–269, 2003.

10. Harrow M, Grossman LS, Herbener ES, et al: Ten-year outcome: Patients with schizoaffective disorders, schizophrenia, affective disorders and mood-incongruent psychotic symptoms. *Br J Psychiatry* 177:421–426, 2000.

11. Meyers BS: Psychotic depression: Underrecognized, undertreated—and dangerous. *Psychiatric Times* 2014.

12. Lenzenweger MF, Lane MC, Loranger AW, et al: *DSM-IV* personality disorders in the National Comorbidity Survey Replication. *Biol Psychiatry* 62(6):553–564, 2007.

13. McGlashan TH: Schizophrenia in translation: Is active psychosis neurotoxic? *Schizophr Bull* 32(4):609–613, 2006.

14. Hendrie HC, Tu W, Tabbey R, et al: Health outcomes and cost of care among older adults with schizophrenia: A 10-year study using medical records across the continuum of care. *Am J Geriatr Psychiatry* 22(5):427–436, 2014.

15. Fillman SG, Cloonan N, Catts VS, et al: Increased inflammatory markers identified in the dorsolateral prefrontal cortex of individuals with schizophrenia. *Mol Psychiatry* 18(2):206–214, 2013.

16. Bonfioli E, Berti L, Goss C, et al: Health promotion lifestyle interventions for weight management in psychosis: A systematic review and meta-analysis of randomised controlled trials. *BMC Psychiatry* 12:78, 2012.

17. Faulkner G, Cohn TA: Pharmacologic and nonpharmacologic strategies for weight gain and metabolic disturbance in patients treated with antipsychotic medications. *Can J Psychiatry* 51(8):502–511, 2006.

18. Winklbaur B, Ebner N, Sachs G, et al: Substance abuse in patients with schizophrenia. *Dialogues Clin Neurosci* 8(1):37–43, 2006.

19. Foster A, Gable J, Buckley J: Homelessness in schizophrenia. *Psychiatr Clin North Am* 35(3):717–734, 2012.

20. Schulz J, Sundin J, Leask S, et al: Risk of adult schizophrenia and its relationship to childhood IQ in the 1958 British birth cohort. *Schizophr Bull* 40(1):143–151, 2014.

21. Werner S, Malaspina D, Rabinowitz J: Socioeconomic status at birth is associated with risk of schizophrenia: Population-based multilevel study. *Schizophr Bull* 33(6):1373–1378, 2007.

22. Smith MJ, Cloninger CR, Harms MP, et al: Temperament and character as schizophrenia-related endophenotypes in non-psychotic siblings. *Schizophr Res* 104(1–3):198–205, 2009.

23. Dean K, Murray RM: Environmental risk factors for psychosis. *Dialogues Clin Neurosci* 7(1):69–80, 2005.

24. Heckers S: 2009: Who is at risk for a psychotic disorder? *Schizophr Bull* 35(5):847–850, 2005.

25. National Alliance on Mental Illness: *First episodes of psychosis.* Retrieved from: <http://www.nami.org/Template.cfm?Section=First_Episode>, 2014.

26. Petrovsky N, Ettinger U, Hill A, et al: Sleep deprivation disrupts prepulse inhibition and induces psychosis-like symptoms in healthy humans. *J Neurosci* 34(27):9134–9140, 2014.

27. Benner PE: *From novice to expert: Excellence and power in clinical nursing practice*, Menlo Park, CA, 1984, Addison-Wesley.

28. McGorry PD, Goodwin RJ, Stuart GW: The development, use, and reliability of the brief psychiatric rating scale (nursing modification)—An assessment procedure for the nursing team in clinical and research settings. *Compr Psychiatry* 29(6):575–587, 1988.

29. Kay SR, Fiszbein A, Opler LA: The Positive and Negative Syndrome Scale (PANSS) for schizophrenia. *Schizophr Bull* 13(2):261–276, 1987.

30. Butcher JN: *MMPI-2: Minnesota Multiphasic Personality Inventory-2: Manual for administration, scoring, and interpretation*, rev ed, Minneapolis, MN, 2001, University of Minnesota Press.

31. Kreyenbuhl J, Buchanan RW, Dickerson FB, et al: Schizophrenia Patient Outcomes Research Team: The Schizophrenia Patient Outcomes Research Team (PORT): Updated treatment recommendations 2009. *Schizophr Bull* 36(1):94–103, 2010.

32. Stahl SM: *Stahl's essential psychopharmacology: Neuroscientific basis and practical application*, ed 4, Cambridge, UK, 2013, Cambridge University Press.

33. Hofmann SG, Tompson MC: *Treating chronic and severe mental disorders: A handbook of empirically supported interventions*, New York, 2002, Guilford.

34. Bressi C, Manenti S, Frongia P, et al: Systemic family therapy in schizophrenia: A randomized clinical trial of effectiveness. *Psychother Psychosom* 77(1):43–49, 2008.

35. O'Brien MP, Miklowitz DJ, Candan KA, et al: A randomized trial of family focused therapy with populations at clinical high risk for psychosis: Effects on interactional behavior. *J Consult Clin Psychol* 82(1):90–101, 2014.

36. Simon GE: Family focused psychoeducational therapy decreases relapse and rehospitalisation in people with a manic episode and bipolar disorder. *Evid Based Ment Health* 6(4):114, 2003.

37. Eack SM, Hogarty SS, Greenwald DP, et al: Cognitive enhancement therapy in substance misusing schizophrenia: Results of an 18-month feasibility trial. *Schizophr Res* 161(2–3):478–483, 2015.

38. Li Z, Guo Z, Wang N, et al: Cognitive–behavioural therapy for patients with schizophrenia: A multicentre randomized controlled trial in Beijing, China. *Psychol Med* 45(9):1893–1905, 2015.

39. Velligan DI, Tai S, Roberts DL, et al: A randomized controlled trial comparing cognitive behavior therapy, cognitive adaptation training, their combination and treatment as usual in chronic schizophrenia. *Schizophr Bull* 41(3):597–603, 2015.

40. Hogarty GE, Flesher S, Ulrich R, et al: Cognitive enhancement therapy for schizophrenia: Effects of a 2-year randomized trial on cognition and behavior. *Arch Gen Psychiatry* 61(9):866–876, 2004.

41. Kellner CH: ECT and catatonia: Out of the shadows. *Psychiatric Times* 2013.

42. Fontaine KR, Heo M, Harrigan EP, et al: Estimating the consequences of anti-psychotic induced weight gain on health and mortality rate. *Psychiatry Res* 101(3):277–288, 2001.

43. Rosenbaum S, Watkins A, Teasdale S, et al: Aerobic exercise capacity: An important correlate of psychosocial function in first episode psychosis. *Acta Psychiatr Scand* 131(3):234, 2015.

44. Grundmann M, Kacirova I, Urinovska R: Therapeutic drug monitoring of atypical antipsychotic drugs. *Acta Pharm* 64(4):387–401, 2014.

45. Karow A, Reimer J, Konig HH, et al: Cost-effectiveness of 12-month therapeutic assertive community treatment as part of integrated care versus standard care in patients with schizophrenia treated with quetiapine immediate release (ACCESS trial). *J Clin Psychiatry* 73(3):e402–e408, 2012.

46. Lambert M, Bock T, Schottle D, et al: Assertive community treatment as part of integrated care versus standard care: A 12-month trial in patients with first- and multiple-episode schizophrenia spectrum disorders treated with quetiapine immediate release (ACCESS trial). *J Clin Psychiatry* 71(10):1313–1323, 2010.

47. Schottle D, Schimmelmann BG, Karow A, et al: Effectiveness of integrated care including therapeutic assertive community treatment in severe schizophrenia spectrum and bipolar I disorders: The 24-month follow-up ACCESS II study. *J Clin Psychiatry* 75(12):1371–1379, 2014.

48. Bio DS, Gattaz WF: Vocational rehabilitation improves cognition and negative symptoms in schizophrenia. *Schizophr Res* 126(1–3):265–269, 2011.

49. Kilian R, Lauber C, Kalkan R, et al: The relationships between employment, clinical status, and psychiatric hospitalisation in patients with schizophrenia receiving either IPS or a conventional vocational rehabilitation programme. *Soc Psychiatry Psychiatr Epidemiol* 47(9):1381–1389, 2012.

50. Suresh Kumar PN: Impact of vocational rehabilitation on social functioning, cognitive functioning, and psychopathology in patients with chronic schizophrenia. *Indian J Psychiatry* 50(4):257–261, 2008.

51. Glasner-Edwards S, Mooney LJ: Methamphetamine psychosis: Epidemiology and management. *CNS Drugs* 28(12):1115–1126, 2014.

52. Roncero C, Daigre C, Gonzalvo B, et al: Risk factors for cocaine-induced psychosis in cocaine-dependent patients. *Eur Psychiatry* 28(3):141–146, 2013.

53. Roncero C, Daigre C, Grau-Lopez L, et al: Cocaine-induced psychosis and impulsivity in cocaine-dependent patients. *J Addict Dis* 32(3):263–273, 2013.

54. In brief: Study strengthens evidence that early marijuana use increases risk of psychosis. *Harv Ment Health Lett* 27(11):7, 2011.

Addiction

Robert Elgie

The financial cost of addiction is staggering. It is estimated that addiction costs nearly $1000 a year for every man, woman, and child in the United States,[1] but financial loss does not account for the terrible grief suffered by families as a result of addiction. The purpose of this concept presentation is to develop a generalist nurse conceptual paradigm for the recognition and assessment of addiction on individual, family, and community levels. A conceptual understanding of addiction will enable nurses to analyze patient data for the planning and implementation of interventions necessary to ensure patient safety during emergency management and to motivate patients toward successful recovery from addiction during nonemergency management.

DEFINITION

Terminology related to the concept of addiction is controversial and subject to debate. For the purpose of this concept presentation, the term addiction is defined as *"a compulsive, abnormal dependence on a substance (such as alcohol, cocaine, opiates, or tobacco) or on a behavior (such as gambling, Internet, or pornography). The dependence typically has adverse psychological, physical, economic, social, or legal ramifications."*[2] The American Psychiatric Association (APA) defines a wide range of mental disorders in the *Diagnostic and Statistical Manual of Mental Disorders* (*DSM*); the terms *substance-induced disorders* and *substance use disorders* are used as diagnostic categories.[3] Substance-induced disorders refer to direct effects of the substance, and substance use disorders include cognitive, behavioral, and physiological symptoms associated with long-term use.[4] These distinctions are clarified further in the sections that follow. The term *intoxication* is used to describe behavioral and/or physical symptoms that result from substance use. *Craving*, in the context of this concept, is used to describe a desire to use a substance and is a symptom associated with substance use disorder. *Tolerance*, another symptom indicating substance use disorder, is defined as an increasing need for the substance to achieve its reward. A lack of reward from the same dose as previously taken would also be considered tolerance. *Withdrawal* refers to a syndrome of symptoms that occurs from a sudden cessation of taking the substance.[3]

SCOPE

This concept presentation examines addiction from the perspective of two broad categories—the substance addictions and the behavioral addictions (Figure 37-1). There is some controversy regarding whether behavioral addictions exist, but as new developments occur in understanding brain neurochemistry, it is becoming more evident that substance addictions and behavioral addictions are the result of similar neurochemical processes.[4]

NORMAL PHYSIOLOGICAL PROCESS

Unlike most concepts presented in this book, the concept of addiction does not have a "normal" physiological process because addiction is never considered normal. However, there is an expected physiological process associated with addiction. Discussions of addiction physiology focus either on the exogenous signs and symptoms of substance abuse (shown later in Box 37-1) or on the endogenous neurochemistry underlying these signs and symptoms. The neurochemical relationship between addictive behaviors or substances and various neurotransmitters in the brain depends on complex models now being explored on the frontiers of addiction science.[5]

It is believed that neurochemical interactions related to addiction originate in the caudate nucleus, the nucleus accumbens, and the ventral tegmental areas of the brain—otherwise known as the reward centers. The reward centers are affected in different ways depending on which neurotransmitters and other brain areas are involved in various reward pathways. It is evident that the neurotransmitter dopamine plays a key role in many or all addictive processes, whether chemical addiction[5] or behavioral addictions.[4] Dopamine is directly associated with the euphoric reward known as being "high," and other neurotransmitters are associated with dopamine regulation. Examples of other neurotransmitters identified as involved in reward pathways include the endogenous opioids γ-aminobutyric acid, glutamate, acetylcholine, norepinephrine, and serotonin.

VARIATIONS AND CONTEXT

As mentioned previously, the scope of this concept is represented by two broad categories: substance addictions and behavioral addictions.

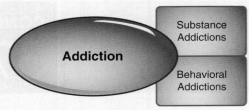

FIGURE 37-1 Scope of Addiction

Substance Addictions

There are two major categories of problems stemming from substance addictions: substance-induced and substance use disorders.

Substance-Induced Disorders

Substance-induced disorders are temporary and reversible, caused by the immediate use of a substance (intoxication) and the immediate effect that occurs when the substance use is discontinued (withdrawal). The substance affects the central nervous system, causing physiological, psychological, and/or behavioral effects; the symptoms of intoxication or withdrawal are related to the specific substance or substances used. Thus these disorders can include not only the intoxication/withdrawal but also other conditions associated with intoxication and withdrawal, such as depression, anxiety, or psychosis.[5]

Substance Use Disorders

Substance use disorders result from continued, frequent use of a substance; the consequences occur over time as a cumulative effect as the addiction progresses. Substance use disorder combines abuse and dependence into a single diagnostic category with mild, moderate, and severe subclassifications. Although each substance is its own disorder (i.e., alcohol use disorder, heroin use disorder, opioid use disorder, etc.), the same overarching criteria for diagnostic purposes are used. According to the *DSM-5*, meeting 2 of 11 criteria within a 12-month period is indicative of substance use disorder. The severity is based on the number of criteria met (2 for mild, 4 for moderate, and 6 or more for severe).[3]

Behavioral Addictions

Although less clearly defined, there are many examples of behavioral addictions found in the literature. Like substance addictions, there are several behaviors that produce a reward response similar to the neurochemical processes previously described. An alternative perspective is that behavioral addictions actually represent impulse control disorders. This perspective has given rise to significant debate regarding the legitimacy of formally recognizing behavioral addictions. Although only one behavioral addiction (gambling disorder) was included in the *DSM-5* diagnostic criteria,[3] a less restrictive view is used for this concept presentation. Other behavioral addictions found in the literature (e.g., Internet addiction, gaming addiction, food addiction, and sex addiction) are included.

CONSEQUENCES

Depending on the individual and the particular addiction, the consequences of addiction are highly variable. However, an understanding of particular neurochemical processes known as *habituation* and *adaptation* forms a conceptual foundation for understanding all addictions. Habituation begins when neurons that receive a repetitive stimulus chemically inhibit their own receptors to restrict the stimulus. Habituation permits the organism to tolerate primal suffering such as hunger pain during a famine, but habituation also facilitates higher order functioning. For example, it allows students to study in the presence of background noise. As a result of habituation, city dwellers are able to sleep in the presence of city sounds such as traffic noise or sirens.

If a repetitive stimulus persists, then neurons will permanently restrict a sufficient number of their own receptors to permit functioning of the organism in the presence of the stimulus; this is called *adaptation*. In evolutionary terms, adaptation began as a survival mechanism allowing the organism to establish a new equilibrium in the presence of an unceasing, long-term stimulus. Once adaptation to a repetitive stimulus occurs, the stimulus must be increased to overcome the adaptation for there to be perception of the same stimulus. A user of cocaine who has adapted to a particular dose, for example, will no longer perceive a high on the same dose; therefore the dose of cocaine must be increased to get high. In turn, the brain neurochemically adapts to the increasing doses of cocaine in an addictive cycle known as *tolerance*. That is, habituation and adaptation cause tolerance.

Any behavioral reward, such as pleasure, is in fact a neurochemical process mediated by neurotransmitters; therefore the brain will habituate and adapt neurochemically to repetitive behaviors such as gambling in the same way as it will adapt to ingested substances such as cocaine. Gamblers have to gamble more often for higher stakes to overcome the brain's adaptation to the gambling high. All the neurochemical consequences of substance use—whether alcohol, tobacco, cocaine, amphetamines, opiates, or others—apply to non-substance addictions such as money, power, relationships, sex, pornography, computer games, television, work, exercise, sports, and even addictive thought patterns such as worry or rumination.[4]

The processes of habituation, adaptation, tolerance, and withdrawal are well illustrated by an individual who is too anxious to sleep. The anxiety triggers the release of adrenaline as part of the fight-or-flight response, and insomnia results from the adrenaline. The brain recognizes the importance of sleep and will eventually block the anxiety stimulus so that sleep will occur. Some motor vehicle drivers have experienced this mechanism—the brain chemically overwhelms the alertness necessary to stay awake and accidents occur when drivers fall asleep at the wheel.

Tolerance and withdrawal enter the picture if a sedative is taken to artificially overwhelm the stimulus of anxiety to achieve sleep. In this case, instead of blocking the anxiety stimulus, the brain will block the sedative by signaling the release of more adrenaline. The need for increasing doses of the sedative to overcome the increasing level of adrenaline is tolerance. If the sedative is abruptly discontinued, the brain does not immediately stop signaling the release of adrenaline, and therefore the opposite effect of the sedative occurs in the form of restlessness and insomnia even if the original stimulus for anxiety is resolved. This restlessness and insomnia are called the rebound effects of withdrawing the sedative. After one or two nights, the neurons will readjust and these rebound effects will cease, but if the sedative is continued to artificially counter the rebound effects, then adaptation will take place and there will be addiction to the sedative.

RISK FACTORS

Examples of predisposing risk factors associated with addiction include family history of addiction, burnout, mood disorders, and stress.[5] Homelessness is also a significant risk factor for addiction.[6] Other risk

BOX 37-1 **Symptoms and Behaviors of Addiction**

- Fatigue
- Insomnia
- Headaches
- Seizure disorder
- Changes in mood
- Anorexia, weight loss
- Vague physical complaints
- Overabundant use of mouthwash or toiletries
- Appearing older than stated age, unkempt appearance
- Leisure activities that involve alcohol and/or other drugs
- Sexual dysfunction, decreased libido, erectile dysfunction
- Trauma secondary to falls, auto accidents, fights, or burns
- Driving while intoxicated (more than one citation suggests dependence)
- Failure of standard doses of sedatives to have a therapeutic effect
- Financial problems, including those related to spending for substances
- Frequent reference to alcohol or alcohol use indicating preoccupation with and importance of alcohol in the person's life
- Problems in areas of life function (e.g., frequent job changes; marital conflict, separation, and/or divorce; work-related accidents, tardiness, absenteeism; legal problems, including arrest; social isolation; and estrangement from friends and/or family)

Source: Modified from Lewis SL, Dirksen SR, Heitkemper MM et al: *Medical-surgical nursing: assessment and management of clinical problems*, ed 9, St Louis, 2014, Mosby.

factors identified by the National Institute on Drug Abuse (NIDA) include early aggressive behavior, lack of parental supervision, drug availability, and poverty.[7] Individuals with previous histories of dependence on opiates are at much higher risk for becoming addicted to opioid analgesics.[8] Use of illicit drugs, tobacco, and alcohol is much higher among adults with co-occurring severe psychological distress.[9] The unique challenges faced by those with co-occurring disorders are discussed in the Clinical Management section of this concept presentation.

Prevalence

The National Survey on Drug Use and Health (NSDUH) analyzes data from interviews of more than 67,000 persons; it contains the most recent and extensive information on substance use in the United States.[10] According to NSDUH, the most prevalent abuse of addictive substances used in the United States is alcohol abuse, followed in decreasing order by abuse of tobacco products, marijuana, non-medical use of psychotherapeutics, cocaine, hallucinogens, inhalants, and heroin.[10] Because they are less studied, the prevalence of behavioral addictions is not well-established. The more commonly recognized behavioral addictions are gambling, shopping, Internet use, video games, exercise, food addictions, and several subtypes of sex addiction.[4]

More than 50% of all Americans surveyed in NSDUH reported that they drink alcohol, and more than 20% reported binge drinking. Binge drinking is defined by NSDUH as five or more drinks on one occasion in the 30 days preceding the survey. Heavy drinking is defined as binge drinking on at least 5 days during the 30 days preceding the survey, and 1.2% reported heavy drinking. Among underage persons (defined as ages 12–20 years), 6.2% reported binge drinking and 6% reported heavy drinking.

NSDUH defines illicit drug use as the unlawful use of a drug within 1 month before the interview. According to NSDUH, the national rate for illicit drug use in 2013 was 9.4% of the total population. Almost 9% (8.8%) of individuals between the ages of 11 and 18 years used illicit drugs in 2007.

ASSESSMENT

The first priority of nursing assessment for persons experiencing addictions is aimed at identifying those in need of emergency management so they can be referred immediately for stabilization. Nonemergency priorities of the assessment are aimed at identifying possible addictions by interview and screening so that treatment options for recovery can be explored. Screening tools are used during the history and examination; these are discussed under Secondary Prevention in the Clinical Management section.

History

There are a number of general symptoms an individual with substance use or induced disorders may mention while taking a patient history (Box 37-1). The patient history also includes exploring the use of prescription and over-the-counter drugs, herbal and homeopathic products, caffeine, tobacco products, alcohol, and recreational drug use. However, the patient may consider the disclosure of addictions to be risky, so it is important to reassure the patient that the information is confidential. Even so, because of the presence of deception in addictive processes, patients are unlikely to disclose addictions accurately.[11] For this reason, it is recommended that the nurse build trust and rapport by using a therapeutic communication technique called motivational interviewing.

The use of motivational interviewing is discussed further (in the Clinical Management section) because it has been demonstrated to improve recovery significantly.[12] However, it is also recommended that the nurse use motivational interviewing methods during the assessment to identify the following defining characteristics for addiction: (1) tolerance and withdrawal, (2) deception of the self and others, and (3) relapse processes (loss of willpower). This interview technique allows the nurse to explore the defining characteristics as they arise without loss of rapport. The following discussion of the defining characteristics of addiction is provided to facilitate the assessment.

Tolerance and Withdrawal

Tolerance and withdrawal are the result of the neurochemical processes already discussed: habituation and adaptation. The nurse can identify tolerance when the patient acknowledges the need for increasingly more of the stimulus to achieve reward. Withdrawal symptoms occur when sufficient quantities are not obtained to achieve reward because of tolerance or because of reducing consumption. There are two categories of withdrawal symptoms: the stress reaction symptoms and the rebound symptoms. Stress reaction symptoms are mediated by the autonomic nervous system and result from the stress of stopping the addictive behavior. Stress reaction symptoms range from mild uneasiness and irritability to extreme agitation, rapid pulse rate, tremors, and panic.

Rebound symptoms occur when adaptive changes in the brain that counter the effects of the addiction continue despite cessation of the addictive substance or behavior. Therefore the effects of the rebound symptoms are the exact opposite of the effects of the addiction. If the addiction is stimulating, then rebound symptoms will be sedating and manifest as lethargy. If the addiction is sedating, then the rebound symptoms will manifest as agitation. This explains why stimulant addicts experience a "crashing" of mood and energy as a rebound symptom but also have anxiety as a stress reaction symptom. Agitation will be a rebound symptom to stopping the use of substances that are sedating, such as alcohol or benzodiazepines, and the agitation may be compounded as a reaction to the stress of stopping the substance.

Deception of the Self and Others (Denial)

Deception of the self and others may be loosely referred to as denial. Sometimes addicts deliberately deceive others to hide their addiction, but they may also deceive themselves. The need to fulfill the addiction is so great that good people will do bad things in pursuit of their addictions. Addicts may commit crimes to pay for the addiction or use sex to obtain assistance in maintaining the addiction. Deception underlies much pain and suffering experienced by the families of addicts and explains why addiction is sometimes known as a "family disease."[13]

Relapse (Loss of Willpower)

Relapse processes are invariably linked to addiction, and they are addressed in the Clinical Management section because they are directly related to recovery.

Physical Examination

A routine physical exam may disclose evidence of addiction. Long-term use of toxic substances may harm the liver and result in symptoms of liver failure, such as jaundice, fatigue, abdominal discomfort, or ascites. Intravenous drug users may have damaged veins and be at risk for coronary complications that include endocarditis. Opiates and stimulants reduce appetite, so users of these substances tend to develop an undernourished, emaciated appearance. Physical signs typical of a withdrawal stress reaction should be noted, such as anxiety, palpitations, shakiness, increased heart rate, and diaphoresis. Other physical exam findings are listed in Box 37-1.

Diagnostic Tests

Diagnostic tests detect the presence of drug and alcohol metabolites in the blood and urine. Tests may also be ordered to detect addiction-related disorders, such as evidence of hepatitis, liver disease, and smoking-related disease.

CLINICAL MANAGEMENT

Primary Prevention

To prevent addiction, nurses need to understand the individual and social contexts in which addiction occurs. This section examines primary prevention from the community perspective and from the individual perspective.

Community Health

Successful models for the prevention of addiction promote healthy families in healthy communities.[14,15] Examples of large-scale community treatment programs shown to be effective in preventing addiction have been implemented in Australia[15] and Vancouver, British Columbia.[16] In the United States, NIDA has established recommendations to support research-based community prevention.[7] NIDA suggests that a well-constructed community plan first identifies the specific drug problems in the community and then builds on existing resources to develop short-term goals and projects that include the assessment of outcomes.[7] Numerous examples of educational and community-based programs are offered at HealthyPeople.gov[17] and on the NIDA website.[7]

Individual Positive Coping Strategies

Individual prevention strategies are well illustrated by a general discussion of positive coping strategies aimed at preventing addiction among nurses. The impairment of nurses by substance abuse is documented as long ago as during Florence Nightingale's time in the 19th century.[18] The American Nurses Association (ANA) officially addressed the problem of impaired nurses in 1984 and estimates that 6–8% of nurses are impaired by substance abuse. The ANA reports that 68% of state board disciplinary actions are related to substance-related impairment, and one descriptive study found that only 3% of nurses in substance abuse recovery had been reported to their respective state nursing boards.[18]

Because stress and burnout have been suggested as risk factors for addiction, it may be presumed that effectively managing stress and burnout will reduce the incidence of addiction, but more research is needed to confirm this.[18] Work overload, lack of support, and unreasonable expectations are factors that may lead to burnout. Short-term personal coping strategies that may help mitigate these stressors include participating in simple self-care activities such as exercise, meditation, and journaling; pursuing a personal spiritual orientation; maintaining a sense of humor with positive attitude; and enjoying recreational activities.[18] Long-term personal coping strategies include developing a nursing care philosophy; setting limits at work by saying "no" to unreasonable expectations; debriefing stress through supportive professional relationships; and developing rituals for coping with loss, grief, and death. It is recommended that all nurses reflect upon and further explore ideas for the positive management of stress so that they can experience long and rewarding careers free from addiction.

Secondary Prevention (Screening)

The United States Preventative Services Task Force recommends screening all adults over age 18 for alcohol misuse.[19] Some evidence endorses the use of the National Institute on Alcohol Abuse and Alcoholism (NIAAA) Quantity and Frequency Questionnaire and the CAGE questionnaire by generalist nurses.[20] Box 37-2 presents these instruments with recommendations for their use to detect possible addictions by nurses. The CAGE questionnaire is easily adapted for screening of other substances and behaviors.[20] Initially developed by Ewing in 1984 to screen for alcohol addiction, the reliability and validity of the CAGE questionnaire have been established.[21] It does not distinguish between past and present problems, but it is an expedient and nonthreatening approach to assessing patients for the defining characteristics of any addiction.[20]

Collaborative Interventions

The clinical management of addictions and consequences of addictions by the generalist practice nurse consists of emergency management measures to stabilize life-threatening complications and nonemergency measures to facilitate the recovery from substance abuse.

Emergency Management

Generalist practice nurses are likely to encounter many different emergency scenarios related to adverse drug reactions and/or overdose. The primary goal of emergency management is to prevent life-threatening complications that occur as a result of substance consumption or that result as the substance clears the system.[22] Agency-specific protocols should be followed when indicated.

BOX 37-2   Alcohol Screening

NIAAA Quantity and Frequency Questions
1. On average, how many days per week do you drink alcohol?
2. On a typical day when you drink, how many drinks do you have?
3. What is the maximum number of drinks you had on any given occasion during the last month?

CAGE Questions
In the Last 12 Months:
1. Have you ever felt like you should **C**ut down on your drinking?
2. Have people **A**nnoyed you by criticizing your drinking?
3. Have you ever felt bad or **G**uilty about your drinking?
4. Have you ever had a drink first thing in the morning to "steady your nerves" or get rid of a hangover (**E**ye opener)?

Screen Positive If:
A positive response on one or more questions from CAGE and/or consumption:
Men >14 drinks/week or >4 drinks/occasion
Women >7 drinks/week or >3 drinks/occasion
Over 65 years old >7 drinks/week or >3 drinks/occasion

Source: From National Institute on Alcohol Abuse and Alcoholism. Helping patients who drink too much: a clinician's guide. NIH Publication No. 07-3769. Retrieved from: http://pubs.niaaa.nih.gov/publications/practitioner/CliniciansGuide2005/guide.pdf

Presenting signs and symptoms depend on the doses of substance or substance combinations that may have been taken, and the nurse should institute basic life-support measures as needed until toxicology findings are confirmed and resuscitation efforts are directed by advanced practice personnel. Many agents impact the respiratory system, and respiratory management includes monitoring (rate, depth, and oxygen saturation) and support (oxygen administration, ventilation, and medication administration). Cardiovascular support includes monitoring (heart rate, blood pressure, and electrocardiograph) and support (intravenous fluids, medications, and/or resuscitation).

Opiate Overdose. Opiate overdose risks respiratory arrest, and naloxone is a rapid-acting drug that restores respiratory function by blocking opiate receptors almost immediately. Nurses who administer naloxone should be aware of the potential for violence by the patient attributable to panic and fear as consciousness is restored.

Acute alcohol withdrawal syndrome. Acute alcohol withdrawal syndrome is a life-threatening condition that may occur unexpectedly whenever long-term, daily alcohol consumption is abruptly discontinued. This may occur in any setting—for example, on admission to the hospital for some other reason. Such patients may deny alcohol use for fear of legal implications or because of shame. Consequently, the nurse may be unprepared for the sudden onset of acute alcohol withdrawal syndrome (also known as delirium tremens).

When it occurs, the onset of alcohol withdrawal syndrome is highly variable, usually beginning within 6 to 9 hours of the last drink.[22] Signs that may lead the nurse to suspect the onset of alcohol withdrawal syndrome are alterations in mental status, tremors, seizures, tachycardia, and hypertension. Late signs such as bradycardia or hypotension are indicative of cardiovascular collapse and the impending need for resuscitation. Other signs of possible alcohol withdrawal syndrome are irritability, depressed mood, impaired

concentration, dizziness, hyperreflexia, ataxia, pyrexia, anorexia, and insomnia.[22]

Wernicke's encephalopathy and Korsakoff's syndrome. Wernicke's encephalopathy and Korsakoff's syndrome are two stages of the same emergency problem: Heavy alcohol use leads to poor nutritional intake and also inhibits B vitamin absorption (especially vitamin B_1 [thiamine]). This leads to alcohol neuropathy from irreversible brain damage with manifestations of psychosis, ataxia, abnormal eye movements, and death. Therefore standard treatment for alcohol withdrawal for all patients should also include daily injections of B-complex vitamins.

Substance Abuse Recovery: The Nonemergency Management of Addictions

During substance abuse recovery, the individual struggles to achieve sufficient willpower to maintain long-term sobriety from addiction. The essence of this struggle is known as the relapse process, and an understanding of the relapse process is essential to understanding addiction. For some, addiction recovery may only involve attendance to group support meetings, whereas others may have much more complicated rehabilitation needs. Rehabilitation refers generally to a broad spectrum of treatment options that may be inpatient or outpatient and may include initial detox treatment, group therapy, individual therapy, mental health treatment, psychosocial rehabilitation, and others such as comprehensive community support services.[23]

The term *recovery* is used to depict an individual who is sober from an addiction and getting the help needed to maintain sobriety.[24] In successful recovery, craving is recognized as part of the relapse process, and therefore coping strategies are planned in advance to prevent use of the substance or behavior in response to craving. This process is an ongoing struggle as the individual moves through early sobriety from 1 month to 1 year, sustained sobriety from 1 to 5 years, and stable sobriety that begins at approximately 5 years.[24]

It is a common misunderstanding among many patients and even some clinicians that recovery means simply the absence of addictive behavior, as depicted by line A in Figure 37-2. Unfortunately, recovery is complicated by a distinct split between the will for freedom and the will of addiction. Consequently, the recovery from addiction is rarely or never a straight line to freedom, as depicted in line A of Figure 37-2. Rather, as soon as anyone suffering from addiction begins to pursue freedom from it, the will of the addiction begins to draw him or her back into it. Therefore recovery is better demonstrated by lines B and C in Figure 37-2 because these lines depict

Line A

Line B

Line C

FIGURE 37-2 Recovery and the Relapse Process

the two opposing forces of will that pull in one direction down toward addiction and in the other direction up toward freedom. It is important for the person in recovery to understand that this process is normal so that his or her self-esteem can withstand any feelings of failure that may result from the inevitable relapse into craving. The idea is that relapse is recognized on the emotional level as craving *before use reccurs,* and therefore use can be prevented by implementing the positive coping strategies as planned. Success in doing this enhances self-esteem and strengthens recovery, whereas failure to understand this can damage self-esteem and undermine recovery.

Often, it is said that an individual who has been struggling with addiction "has entered rehab." What this means clinically is that to a certain extent the individual has overcome his or her resistance to changing an addictive behavior and is motivated to commit to a treatment program. The overarching goal of any rehabilitation program is to establish and maintain sobriety by helping the patient manage the relapse challenges that will certainly arise. Rehabilitation may also include advanced practice care to manage any mood spectrum problems that emerge as addictive coping subsides. This specialized area of addiction care, which is known as the care for co-occurring disorders or dual diagnosis, is discussed in more detail later.

Motivational interviewing. It is well-known that in modern health care, individual patient outcomes are greatly influenced by the patient's motivation to change lifestyle behaviors.[12] There are hundreds of ran-domized, controlled trials of the motivational interviewing method in health care that endorse this simple truth: *Efforts to persuade patients to change increase their resistance to change.* Clearly, nurses become more effective by "asking patients why they would want to make a change and how they might do it rather than telling them that they should."[12,p9]

It has been reliably demonstrated that whatever approach is selected in the treatment of addiction, the most significant factor is the motivation of the patient. Motivational interviewing is especially useful in the management of addictions.[25] The underlying "spirit of motivational interviewing"[12,p6] does not involve convincing the patient to do something he or she does not want to do. Rather, it is a collaborative effort that honors the autonomy of the patient to make informed decisions about his or her behavior. In motivational interviewing, the nurse should listen more than talk. The patient will almost certainly have ambivalent feelings about his or her problem behaviors, and it is important to understand the ambivalence. In particular, the *benefits* of the addiction should be well understood for any plan of change to be effective.

A homeless woman addicted to amphetamines provides a poignant example of the benefits of addiction. In this example, the woman's addiction to amphetamines began when she was sleeping in parks and shelters, where her motivation to use the drugs emerged from a need to stay vigilant at night to avoid being raped, as had happened previously. In addition to the benefit of surviving the night, amphetamines were beneficial in providing her with a temporarily enhanced mood in an otherwise bleak and hopeless setting. Amphetamines provided her with temporary relief from symptoms of rape trauma syndrome. Once the individual's ambivalent situation is understood in this way, the patient and nurse can then collaborate to resolve the motivations underlying the addiction with a personal plan for recovery that antici-pates relapse processes.

To enhance their abilities to do this, nurses are encouraged to par-ticipate in motivational interviewing workshops. As a brief overview, when patients are committed to change, the nurse is able help them to determine the best course of action, but most patients are not initially interested in change or they are ambivalent about changing. When the patient is not interested in changing, it is recommended that the nurse remain empathetic but raise doubt, provide information with permis-sion, and let the patient know that he or she may return if an interest in change develops.[12]

When patients are ambivalent about changing addictive behaviors, the nurse should consider ways to tip the balance toward change without arguing. Arguing with an ambivalent person will put the person in a defensive position in which he or she is resistant to change. One way already discussed to tip the balance toward change is by analyzing the benefits of the addiction so that ideas for meeting the benefits by healthier means can be planned. Another technique is to develop a discrepancy between the patient's current behavior and important goals.

There are compassionate, respectful ways to point out discrepan-cies, and it is important that the nurse is authentic in his or her style of communication. In the example of the homeless woman who is addicted to amphetamines, lecturing her on the harm of amphet-amines is likely only to alienate her and make her defensive. As an alternative, the nurse might ask this patient how she would like her life to be in 2 years. Chances are she would like to have a nice home and a job, providing the nurse with a point of leverage because there is a discrepancy between having a nice home and job while addicted to amphetamines.

The nurse should determine how motivated the woman is to achieve these goals and perhaps chat about how nice it would be to have her own apartment and a job. Patient motivation can be reported on a scale of 1 to 10. This opens the door to establish a discrepancy between amphetamine addiction and having a nice apartment and job. For example, the nurse might state, "Gosh, it would be really hard to hold down a job and pay rent while supporting an amphetamine addiction, wouldn't it?" Once the discrepancies are established, then resources for relapse prevention and support services can be arranged collaboratively.

Pharmacotherapy in substance abuse recovery. Relapse preven-tion is improved by reducing craving and withdrawal symptoms. This is the aim of pharmacotherapy in recovery.[23] A complete dis-cussion of the full scope of pharmacotherapy in the routine treat-ment of addictions is beyond the scope of this concept, and there are numerous text sources available for information on this subject.[23] The following is a brief overview to provide the nurse with a frame-work for deeper research:

- *Methadone*: Medications to treat opiate withdrawal either are sub-stitutes for street opiates or are aimed at reducing the symptoms of withdrawal.[23] Methadone is a long-acting opiate that may be pre-scribed as a replacement; methadone can be gradually tapered once the withdrawal is stabilized.
- *Buprenorphine*: Buprenorphine may be prescribed rather than methadone; buprenorphine is a partial opioid agonist and, as such, higher doses can be administered with fewer side effects.[23]
- *Suboxone*: Buprenorphine may also be prescribed in a combined preparation with naloxone called Suboxone. Suboxone is taken sub-lingually, and the addition of the opiate antagonist naloxone in this preparation reduces the potential for abuse of buprenorphine alone by eliminating the opioid euphoria.
- *Clonidine*: The antihypertensive clonidine may also be prescribed for symptomatic relief of opiate withdrawal.
- *Nicotine*: Nicotine gum and nicotine patches may be prescribed to deliver nicotine into the body during withdrawal from tobacco products. These products are intended to alleviate withdrawal

symptoms while tapering the dose of nicotine to zero. There are also nasal sprays and inhalers that serve the same purpose, but they are less popular.[23]

- *Bupropion*: Bupropion may also be prescribed for nicotine withdrawal; it is a non-nicotine replacement medication that reduces craving.
- *Naltrexone, nalmefene, and acamprosate*: Besides the emergency management for acute alcohol withdrawal, a number of pharmacologic approaches may be taken to facilitate the recovery from alcohol addiction. Naltrexone, nalmefene, and acamprosate are all used to reduce cravings for alcohol.
- *Disulfiram*: Disulfiram may be prescribed as aversion therapy for alcohol addiction meant to prevent impulsive drinking.[23] The intent of aversion therapy is to extinguish a negative behavior by pairing it with an unpleasant stimulus. Disulfiram works by disrupting the metabolism of alcohol so that toxic blood levels of alcohol metabolites occur in the bloodstream, causing severe headache, nausea, vomiting, palpitations, flushing, tachycardia, chest pain, and dizziness. Severe reactions that include convulsions and death may also occur, but these are rare. Taking disulfiram usually requires written consent to ensure that the patient is fully informed of the risks and aware that he or she must not consume anything containing alcohol. Therefore patient teaching is of critical importance. Such food items as vanilla extract and over-the-counter preparations of cough medicine and mouthwash often contain alcohol and are likely to induce the side effects of disulfiram and alcohol incompatibility. No form of alcohol should be consumed for at least 2 weeks after discontinuation of disulfiram.[23]

Co-occurring Disorders

Also known as dual diagnosis, co-occurring disorders refer to the unique challenges faced by individuals who are chemically dependent and have serious psychological distress (SPD). There are two broad etiologies of co-occurring disorders. Persons with mental illness may turn to substance abuse to self-medicate the SPD, or the substance use may cause SPD. In either case, motivational interviewing is recommended as part of a comprehensive treatment approach to unravel the motivations that underlie the problem.[26]

Safe detoxification from the substances of abuse is usually the first step, but ongoing therapeutic communication skills such as active listening and affirmation will help establish trust so that the etiologies can be understood to avoid years of "revolving door" treatment for these individuals, sometimes labeled as "frequent flyers." By doing so, case management can be established to intervene in the underlying causes of the disorder. For example, there are likely to be logical benefits for the use of illicit drugs and alcohol for individuals with SPD.[26] Street drugs may alleviate symptoms of anxiety and psychosis. Intoxication may facilitate social interactions and mask psychosis as substance induced—among the users of street drugs, substance-induced psychosis is socially acceptable, whereas psychosis from "being mental" is not. An understanding of all the logical reasons *not* to stop taking street drugs will facilitate the development of treatment plans that are more likely to result in long-term remission by addressing these needs as logical within the patient's social ecology.

There are some contraindications for the use of motivational interviewing in dual diagnosis. The patient might be too psychotic to benefit from motivational interviewing.[26] If so, the psychosis will have to be stabilized before motivational interviewing can be of any significant value. These patients may also be too dangerous for motivational interviewing.[26] Dangerousness necessitates the removal of freedom, and this contradicts the principle of autonomy in motivational interviewing.

For patients who have a degree of orientation to reality despite their confusion or psychosis, the generalist nurse may modify his or her motivational interviewing method by frequently paraphrasing what the patient says to help maintain an organized dialogue. Nurses should try to keep motivational change talk very concrete and target compliance with medications and other treatments. To avoid escalating anxiety, nurses should avoid exploring despair and instead explore the patient's motivation for using street drugs. As in the ordinary motivational interviewing method, once the motivation is understood, then discrepancy can be established between the drug use and the patient's goals.[26]

INTERRELATED CONCEPTS

Addiction as a concept does not exist in isolation, and there are many other interrelated concepts, depending on the specific context of the patient situation. Three common interrelated concepts are Coping, Family Dynamics, and Cognition. When coping, family dynamics, or cognition become ineffective, the individuals within these systems are at risk for addiction. Mood and Affect also overlaps with a risk for addiction. Nurses will benefit by mentally applying the defining characteristics of addiction to these related concepts in their own analyses (Figure 37-3).

CLINICAL EXEMPLARS

There are numerous exemplars of addiction, representing both substance addictions and behavioral addictions; some of the most common are presented in Box 37-3. This list is brought to life by the story of a student in an addictions' concept class discussion who mentioned that her boyfriend was addicted to pornography. Inspired to change by the harm his addiction was causing their relationship, he drove to a distant city where he discarded his entire pornography collection in a dumpster. Evidently, it became clear to him that he was unable to defeat the will of his addiction without help when he found himself in that same dumpster at 3:00 AM rummaging for remnants of his precious pornography collection.

Stories such as this clearly illustrate tolerance, withdrawal, deception, loss of willpower, and relapse, but interrelated concepts are also clear. The boyfriend's will for freedom was motivated by the harm his addiction had on his family dynamics, mood, and cognition, but his coping abilities were not adequate to withstand the will of addiction. The nurse's role in this story is to recognize how these concepts interrelate so that the boyfriend's motivation to cope can be strengthened with a collaborative plan that will vary, depending on the local resources and the individual's sense of what will work for him.

Featured Exemplars
Tobacco Use Disorder and Tobacco Withdrawal

Tobacco use is the most common addictive disorder and the leading cause of preventable disease, disability, and death. Nicotine, a stimulant substance found in tobacco, increases arousal and alertness; increases heart rate, blood pressure, and cardiac output; and decreases appetite. Cigarette smoking is the most predominate form of tobacco use. It is estimated that 85% of smokers who try to quit on their own relapse within 1 week because of the withdrawal symptoms that include irritability, craving, depression, anxiety,

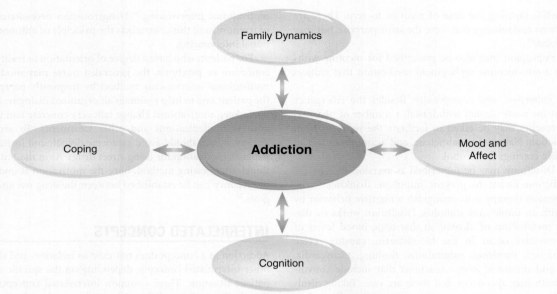

FIGURE 37-3 Addiction and Interrelated Concepts

BOX 37-3 EXEMPLARS OF ADDICTION

Substance-Induced Disorders

- Alcohol-induced disorders
- Cocaine-induced disorders
- Heroin-induced disorders
- Inhalant-induced disorders
- Marijuana-induced disorders
- Methamphetamine-induced disorders
- Opioid-induced disorders
- Tobacco-induced disorders

Substance Use Disorders

- Alcohol use disorder
- Cocaine use disorder

- Heroin use disorder
- Inhalant use disorder
- Marijuana use disorder
- Methamphetamine use disorders
- Opioid use disorder
- Tobacco use disorder

Behavioral Addictions

- Food addiction
- Gambling addiction
- Gaming addiction
- Internet addiction
- Sex addiction
- Shopping addiction

---

cognitive and attention deficits, sleep disturbances, and increased appetite.[27]

Alcohol Intoxication

Alcohol intoxication is one of the most common substance-induced disorders. It occurs when alcohol is ingested faster than the liver can metabolize it. Physiological effects of alcohol intoxication are related to the dose. Euphoria, reduced social inhibitions, and flushed skin are associated with lower levels of alcohol intake. Drowsiness and progressive impairments in balance, coordination, judgment, and erratic or sometimes violent behavior occur with greater levels of alcohol intake. Sufficiently high levels of intake lead to nausea, vomiting, and potentially lethal depression of the central nervous system.

Alcohol Use Disorder

Alcohol use disorder (AUD) is one of the most prevalent of the substance use disorders. It is estimated that 17 million adults (older than age 18 years)[28] and more than 850,000 adolescents between ages 12 and 17 years[29] had an AUD in 2012. AUD results from long-term excessive alcohol use and is characterized by the inability to cut down or stop drinking, craving, interference with family or job, alcohol tolerance, withdrawal, deception of the self and others, and relapse processes (loss of willpower).

Opioid Use Disorder

Opioid use disorder involves the misuse of a wide range of drugs from multiple sources, including prescription pain medications (e.g., codeine, morphine, and oxycodone), street drugs (e.g., heroin), and drugs to treat addictions (e.g., methadone). Opioids cause central nervous system depression, leading to analgesia, euphoria, drowsiness, relaxation, and detachment from the environment and impaired decision making. The annual rate of chronic non-medical use of opioid analgesics in people age 12 years or older is estimated to be 3.8%, with males and individuals between the ages of 18 and 50 years the major users.[30]

Gambling Disorder

Compulsive gambling, a behavioral addiction, involves an uncontrollable urge to gamble despite social consequences. Gambling disorder is characterized by gaining a thrill from gambling risk; preoccupation with gambling; taking increasingly larger gambling risks; and using the behavior as a means to cope with problems, guilt, or depression. Gambling disorder closely resembles substance use disorders in the physiological response but also social consequences, including relationships, economic, and occupational. It is estimated that of the 80% of adults who have gambled, 2% or 3% have experienced a gambling problem —representing more than 1 million individuals with gambling disorders.[31]

CASE STUDY

Source: NADOFOTOS/iStock/Thinkstock

Case Presentation

Jim Wright is a 45-year-old white male. He is married to Darla and has two children: 16-year-old Ryan and 9-year-old Jenny. The interview with Jim stemmed from a family therapy meeting to plan Jim's care in a substance treatment program. Jim is charming, funny, and talkative. His interview began with the CAGE questionnaire, and Jim affirmatively acknowledged all four CAGE questions. Jim further acknowledged more than two decades of heavy alcohol and substance use. He says he has tried Narcotics Anonymous and Alcoholics Anonymous meetings, "but they didn't help much." He says that after such meetings, he and other addicts would go out to drink and use drugs together.

Jim says tearfully that he has tried family therapy as well, "because of me our whole family is screwed up." As a youth, Jim was involved in gang activity; at age 16 years, he served time in the youth detention system for assault and battery and making threats with a deadly weapon. Jim has been arrested and incarcerated numerous times for reasons related to drug and alcohol use. While in jail, Jim would drink a fermented jailhouse concoction called "pruno" and use drugs with other inmates.

Jim has recently been released from jail and Darla has told him she does not want him around until he can stop drinking and using drugs. He plans ways to manipulate Darla into taking him back. His current plan is to be kind and generous with her at first, and he thinks he "might even have to get a job for a while." Knowing rules of confidentiality, Jim admitted that coming in for this interview was part of manipulating Darla.

"Alcoholism runs in the family," Jim says. Like others in his family, Jim has gone through alcohol withdrawal several times. "Withdrawal sucks," he says. "It can last a couple days or more. … Your skin's all a-crawlin,' your heart's a-pounding, and you want that drink so bad … you get all shaky and once in jail I almost died from a seizure. See, you should take some Valium for that, but I was in jail and they didn't care. Sometimes you see things. … I once saw a six foot rabbit and another time I thought snakes were crawling on me."

Case Analysis

This case illustrates several aspects of this concept. Alcohol use and alcohol-induced disorders are clearly described in this case. The substance use is creating challenges within Jim's relationships, particularly with his family. He has two significant risk factors (family history of addiction and early aggressive behavior). The fact that he mentions support groups without success is evidence of recurrence in his disease management.

ACCESS EXEMPLAR LINKS IN YOUR GIDDENS EBOOK

REFERENCES

1. National Institute on Drug Abuse: *Drug abuse costs the United States economy hundreds of billions of dollars in increased health care costs, crime, and lost productivity*, 2008. Retrieved from: <http://www.drugabuse.gov/publications/addiction-science-molecules-to-managed-care/introduction/drug-abuse-costs-united-states-economy-hundreds-billions-dollars-in-increased-health>.
2. Venes D, editor: *Taber's cyclopedic medical dictionary*, Philadelphia, 2013, Davis.
3. American Psychiatric Association: *Diagnostic and statistical manual of mental disorders*, ed 5, Arlington, VA, 2013, American Psychiatric Publishing.
4. Holden C: Psychiatry: Behavioral addictions debut in proposed *DSM-V*. *Science* 327:935, 2010.
5. National Institute on Drug Abuse: *Drugs, brains and behavior: The science of addiction*, Bethesda, MD, 2010, U.S. Department of Health and Human Services, National Institutes of Health. Available at: <http://www.drugabuse.gov/sites/default/files/sciofaddiction.pdf>.
6. National Coalition for the Homeless: *Addiction disorders and homelessness*, 2009. Retrieved from: <http://www.nationalhomeless.org/factsheets/addiction.pdf>.
7. National Institute on Drug Abuse: *Preventing drug abuse among children and adolescents*, 2010. Available at: <www.nida.nih.gov/prevention/risk.html>.
8. Federation of State Medical Boards: *Model policy on the use of opioid analgesics in the treatment of chronic pain*, Washington, DC, 2013, Author. Retrieved from: <http://www.fsmb.org/Media/Default/PDF/FSMB/Advocacy/pain_policy_july2013.pdf>.

9. Ruiz MA, Douglas KS, Edens JF, et al: Co-occurring mental health and substance use problems in offenders: Implications for risk assessment. *Psychol Assess* 24(1):77–87, 2012.
10. U.S. Department of Health and Human Services: Substance use and mental health estimates from the 2013 national survey on drug use and health: Overview of findings. *The NSDUH Report* 2014. Retrieved from: <http://store.samhsa.gov/shin/content//NSDUH14-0904/NSDUH14-0904.pdf>.
11. Boniface S: How is alcohol consumption affected if we account for under-reporting? A hypothetical scenario. *Eur J Public Health* 23(6):1101–1262, 2013.
12. Rollnick S, Miller WR, Butler CC: *Motivational interviewing in health care: Helping patients change behavior*, New York, 2008, Guilford.
13. Carpenito L: *Nursing diagnosis: Application to clinical practice*, ed 13, Philadelphia, 2010, Lippincott.
14. Liddle HA: Adapting and implementing an evidence-based treatment with justice-involved adolescents: The example of multidimensional family therapy. *Fam Process* 53(3):516–528, 2014.
15. Stafford J, Allsop S, Daube M: From evidence to action: Health promotion and alcohol. *Health Promotion J Austr* 25(1):8–13, 2014.
16. Vancouver Coastal Health: *2011 Health watch*, 2011. Retrieved from: <http://www.vch.ca/media/HealthWatchNOV2011.pdf>.
17. U.S. Department of Health and Human Services: *Healthy People 2020: Educational and community based programs*, 2011. Retrieved from: <http://healthypeople.gov/2020/topicsobjectives2020/overview.aspx?topicid=11>.
18. Fearon C, Nicol M: Strategies to assist prevention of burnout in nursing staff. *Nurs Stand* 26(14):35–39, 2011.
19. United States Preventative Services Task Force: *Alcohol Misuse: Screening and Behavioral Counseling Interventions in Primary Care*, 2015. Retrieved from: <http://www.uspreventiveservicestaskforce.org/Page/Document/UpdateSummaryFinal/alcohol-misuse-screening-and-behavioral

-counseling-interventions-in-primary-care?ds=1&s=Alcohol%20 screening>.

20. Connors GJ, DiClemente CC, Velasquez MM, et al: *Substance abuse treatment and the stages of change: Selecting and planning interventions*, New York, 2013, Guilford.

21. Meneses-Gaya C, Zuardi AW, Loureiro SR, et al: Is the full version of the AUDIT really necessary? Study of the validity and internal construct of its abbreviated versions. *Alcoholism Clin Exp Res* 34(8):1417–1424, 2010.

22. Kumar CN, Andrade CA, Murphy PM: A randomized, double-blind comparison of lorazepam and chlordiazepoxide in patients with uncomplicated alcohol withdrawal. *J Stud Alcohol Drugs* 70:467–474, 2009.

23. Taylor DL, Stuart GW: Chemically mediated responses and substance-related disorders. In Stuart GW, editor: *Principles and practice of psychiatric nursing*, ed 9, St Louis, 2009, Mosby.

24. Buddy T: *What exactly is recovery? It's more than just being sober, panel says*, 2014. Retrieved from: <http://alcoholism.about.com/od/faq/a/recovery.htm>.

25. Butler Center for Research: *Research update: Project MATCH: A study of alcoholism treatment approaches*, 2010, Hazelden Foundation. Retrieved from: <www.hazelden.org/web/public/document/bcrup_0600.pdf>.

26. Martino S, Moyers TB: Motivational interviewing with dually diagnosed patients. In Arkowitz H, Westra HA, Miller WR, et al, editors: *Motivational interviewing in the treatment of psychological problems*, New York, 2008, Guilford, pp 277–303.

27. National Institutes of Health, National Institute on Drug Abuse: *Tobacco/nicotine: Is nicotine addictive?* 2012. Retrieved from: <http://www.drugabuse.gov/publications/research-reports/tobacco/nicotine-addictive>.

28. Substance Abuse and Mental Health Services Administration: *2012 National Survey on Drug Use and Health (NSDUH), Table 5.8A— Substance Dependence or Abuse in the Past Year among Persons Aged 18 or Older, by Demographic Characteristics: Numbers in Thousands*, 2011 and 2012. Available at: <http://www.samhsa.gov/data/sites/default/files/NSDUH-DetTabs2012/NSDUH-DetTabs2012/HTML/NSDUH-DetTabsSect5peTabs1to56-2012.htm#Tab5>.

29. Substance Abuse and Mental Health Services Administration: *2012 National Survey on Drug Use and Health (NSDUH), Table 5.5A— Substance Dependence or Abuse in the Past Year among Persons Aged 12 to 17, by Demographic Characteristics: Numbers in Thousands*, 2011 and 2012. Available at: <http://www.samhsa.gov/data/sites/default/files/NSDUH-DetTabs2012/NSDUH-DetTabs2012/HTML/NSDUH-DetTabsSect5peTabs1to56-2012.htm#Tab5.5A>.

30. U.S. Department of Health and Human Services, Behavioral Health Committee: *Addressing prescription drug abuse in the United States*. 2013. Retrieved from: <http://www.cdc.gov/HomeandRecreationalSafety/pdf/HHS_Prescription_Drug_Abuse_Report_09.2013.pdf>.

31. GamblingRecovery.Org: *Prevalence of problem gambling*, 2015. Retrieved from: <http://www.gamblingrecovery.org/prevalence-of-problem-gambling.php>.

Interpersonal Violence

Pam Schultz

Violence is pervasive and common. It occurs among all people of all ages. There are many facts, relationships, associations, risk factors, and theories about violence. It is a multifaceted problem. Perhaps it is part of the human condition. At the very least, it is a destructive behavior. We have legal and moral rules, cultural traditions, political beliefs, and religious ramifications surrounding violence. It is a quality of humanity. The more we try to understand it, the more complicated it becomes. Perhaps we give it more power in the lives of people by compartmentalizing it. However, interpersonal violence is a health concept as well as an elusive human concept. The purpose of this concept presentation is to introduce the concept, including how to recognize it and the role of the nurse as related to interpersonal violence.

DEFINITION

The World Health Organization (WHO) has defined *violence* as *the intentional use of physical force or power, threatened or actual, against oneself, another person, or against a group or community that either results in or has a high likelihood of resulting in injury, death, psychologic harm, maldevelopment, or deprivation.* Furthermore, it has categorized violence into three subtypes: self-directed violence, collective violence, and interpersonal violence.[1] Interpersonal violence refers to violence between individuals. When violence is defined in part as the use of power, then other concepts come into play, such as intimidation and bullying. The WHO definition also encompasses the nature of interpersonal violence—for instance, physical, psychological, sexual, and neglect and/or deprivation. Intimate partner violence (IPV) is recognized as a public health problem, but it is also a crime. Assault, battery, homicide, weapon use, kidnapping, and unlawful imprisonment are frequent crimes of domestic violence.[2] This concept does not discuss abuse or violence by strangers, street crime, gang warfare, or military conflict.

SCOPE

Interpersonal violence is a complex concept seen in many forms across the lifespan. In order to fully understand this concept, one must not restrict oneself to the *recipient* of the violence but consider the *perpetrator* as well, who is also part of the public health problem. When considering interpersonal violence, one must also consider the *nature* of the violence, the *environment* in which the violence occurs, the *relationship* between the perpetrator and the recipient of the violence, and possibly the *motivation* of the violence (Figure 38-1).

In 1995, Johnson proposed a model of IPV that separated the violence into two types: *patriarchal terrorism* and *situational violence*.[3] The first category included cases in which the male partner attempted to dominate and assume control over his partner. The second category included cases in which a situation produced an escalation of conflict and the partner initiated physical aggression based in the situational conflict. The first category was considered the most physically violent. Other studies have shown that as physical violence increases, danger of death also increases.[4,5] When considering the nature of the violence, there can be an overlap among the physical, sexual, and psychological components, and in children neglect is also often a part of the pattern of violence.

When considering interpersonal violence as a concept to be understood, the etiology of violence becomes an area of interest. Violence is closely related to criminality because most violence is criminal in nature. Through the 20th century, the dominant model for understanding violence and criminality had been a sociological model. Raine has proposed that violence and criminality may have a biological basis.[6]

VARIATIONS AND CONTEXT

There are many categories of interpersonal violence that is seen across the lifespan. Many of these categories overlap and include child abuse/neglect, elderly abuse/neglect, youth violence, bullying, IPV, sexual abuse, and psychological/emotional maltreatment (Figure 38-2).

Child Abuse and Neglect

Child abuse and neglect encompasses a wide variety of forms of child maltreatment, including physical abuse, sexual abuse, and neglect. The Federal Child Abuse Prevention and Treatment Act (CAPTA), which was amended by the Keeping Children and Families Safe Act of 2003, defined child abuse and neglect as occurring when there is any recent act or failure to act on the part of a parent or caretaker that results in death, serious physical or emotional harm, sexual abuse, or exploitation, or when there is any act or failure to act that presents an imminent risk of serious harm.[7]

FIGURE 38-1 Scope of Interpersonal Violence

Elder Abuse and Neglect

Elder abuse refers to abuse to an older person by the older person's family members or caregivers. National estimates indicate that 1 in 10 older adults experience elder abuse.[8] Individuals who are older than 75 years, African-American, and of low socioeconomic status are at greater risk of elder abuse. According to the National Center on Elder Abuse, females are more likely to be abused than males. Ninety percent of abusers are family members. In 2010, one study reported that 47% of participants with dementia had experienced abuse from their caregivers.[9] Other possible risk factors have been identified as cognitive and physical function impairment. In the elderly, emotional abuse is significantly associated with higher levels of psychological distress compared to physical abuse.[10] There is no consensus regarding the definition of elder abuse.[11] The age range of the "older person" is not consistent across studies. Abuse can consist of omission or commission, and it can be physical, psychological, sexual, financial, or other forms of maltreatment such as neglect. Like child maltreatment, elder maltreatment can have an element of neglect. Maltreatment by individuals to elders can occur in homes or institutions. Family members who maltreat their elders can continue to maltreat them when they are transferred to an institution. The institution can be abusive and/or neglectful, and/or the employees of the institution can be abusive. The elder is restricted in his or her response to abuse by his or her physical and cognitive abilities. Elder abuse situations tend to be more complex than those experienced by intimate partners and children. Elder abuse often concerns multiple forms of abuse and multiple parties, including the victim, the perpetrator, neighbors, other family members, and service providers such as nurses, social workers, attorneys, adult protective workers, and physicians.[11,12] Elders can become prisoners to their caregivers, and death is often the end result of the abusive cycle.

Youth Violence

Youth violence refers to harmful behaviors (e.g., slapping, hitting, or other forms of physical assault with or without weapons) that can start early and continue into young adulthood. The young person can be a victim, an offender, or a witness to the violence. Patterns of behavior change over developmental stages. During teen and young adult years, violence seems to be most prevalent.

Bullying

Bullying consists of intimidation or domination toward an individual who is perceived as weak. Often, the perpetrator does this as a way to establish perceived superiority over another or to get something through coercion or force. Bullying tactics can be physical, verbal, or emotional—often through social and cyber-bullying approaches. Although most prevalent in school-age children and adolescents, adult bullying also exists and is reported in the workplace.

As a result of school shootings in the United States, professionals have turned their attention to school bullying.[13] Bullying is considered to be the most prevalent form of violence perpetrated by youth. The Surgeon General's Task Force on Youth Violence found that 30–40% of males commit a serious violent offense by age 17 years.[14]

Intimate Partner Violence

IPV refers to any behavior within an intimate relationship that results in physical, psychological, or sexual harm, such as physical aggression, psychological abuse (which could include intimidation and humiliation), forced sexual coercion, and other behaviors designed to control the recipient of the violence.

Sexual Violence

Sexual violence is defined by WHO as any sexual act, attempt to obtain a sexual act, unwanted sexual comments or advances, or acts to traffic (or otherwise direct) a person's sexuality using coercion. It can be committed by any person regardless of his or her relationship to the victim and in any setting, including, but not limited to, home and work. Rape involves any penetration of the vulva or anus with any other body part or object. Rape of a person is considered gang rape if there are two or more perpetrators.[15]

Psychological/Emotional Maltreatment

It is difficult to define psychological maltreatment and therefore little research has been done to understand the consequences of this form of maltreatment. However, in 1995, the American Professional Society on the Abuse of Children (APSAC) published *Guidelines for Psychosocial Evaluation of Suspected Psychological Maltreatment of Children and Adolescents*,[16] which defined six subtypes of psychological maltreatment: spurning; terrorizing; isolating; exploiting/corrupting; denying emotional responsiveness; and mental health, medical, and educational neglect.

Spurning includes verbal and nonverbal acts that reject and degrade a child. Terrorizing is behavior that threatens or is likely to physically hurt, kill, or abandon in dangerous situations. Isolating acts confine the child or place unreasonable limitations on the child's freedom to move or communicate with others. Exploiting/corrupting includes acts that promote inappropriate behaviors from the child, such as criminal, antisocial, or deviant behaviors. Denying emotional responses includes showing no emotion in interactions with the child.

CONSEQUENCES

Physical Consequences

Physical consequences of interpersonal violence include traumatic injury and physiological symptoms associated with stress and anxiety

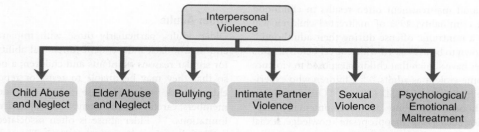

FIGURE 38-2 Categories of Interpersonal Violence across the Lifespan

caused by IPV. Common patterns of injury and related symptoms that have been identified in the literature include headaches, back pain, choking sensations, hyperventilation, gastrointestinal symptoms, chest pain, facial fractures, and other head and neck injuries.[17–21] It has been reported that 83% of fractures experienced by victims of assault involved the face, and 69% of patients with violence-related injuries had involvement of the craniofacial region. Others have reported that the dominant cause of facial fractures in North America is interpersonal violence.[22] In a study of more than 2000 patients with craniofacial fractures, Lee reported that patients whose fractures were caused by IPV were more likely to need surgery.[23] The nature of IPV fractures tends to be different in that the fracture is caused by a punch or kick to the face and prominent points are targeted, such as the cheek, the angle of the jaw, and the nose. Other studies have found an increase in chronic health problems during midlife when previously exposed to IPV.[24]

Sexual violence can occur in the context of child abuse and/or IPV, or it can occur as an isolated incident. The health consequences depend on the age of the victim, the relationship between the victim and the perpetrator, the circumstances of the environment, and the severity and/or types of other violence accompanying the incident.

Unintended pregnancy and gynecologic complications—such as bleeding, infection, pain during intercourse, chronic pelvic pain, sexually transmitted diseases, HIV transmission, and urinary tract infections—are associated with sexual violence.[25–27] Violence that occurs during pregnancy can have detrimental effects not only on the mother but also on the fetus. In the United States, estimates of abuse during pregnancy range from 3% to 38%, and there is increased risk of miscarriage, stillbirth, premature labor and delivery, fetal injury, and low birth weight. There is also an increased risk of maternal mortality.[26]

Mental Health Consequences

Post-traumatic stress disorder (PTSD) is one of the most common mental health consequences of exposure to interpersonal violence, particularly IPV.[28–31] The incidence of PTSD among those exposed to IPV varies by study from 33% to 84%. The nature of the violence is predictive of the severity of the symptoms of PTSD. For instance, the use of a weapon and sexual abuse result in more severe symptoms. The characteristic symptoms of PTSD are threefold. *Re-experiencing* includes intrusive and recurrent thoughts, images, and flashbacks of the violence; *avoidance* and *numbing* include feelings of detachment and persistent avoidance of memories that relate to the violence; and *increased arousal* can include insomnia, difficulty focusing, and hypervigilance.[32] Rape by an intimate partner results in PTSD in many circumstances and is usually associated with greater severity of violence.

Depression is also a common reaction to IPV.[24,29,33] Depression inhibits the ability of abused individuals from formulating a plan to deal with the abuse. This inertia prevents the victim from taking proactive steps to leave the abusive situation. Humphreys and Lee reported that the presence of social support mitigates the depressive effects of IPV.[24] When an individual experiences depression, there is an increased risk of suicide, and there are increased suicide attempts in women experiencing IPV.[26]

Studies have shown a link between mental disorders and violence[29] in that there is a high rate of lifetime victimization among psychiatric patients. However, there does appear to be evidence that suggests that mental illness is exacerbated by exposure to violence, and it may also contribute to interpersonal violence. Many of the physical sequelae are associated with mental health disturbances, such as gastrointestinal disorders, headaches, choking sensations, hyperventilation, and other somatic complaints commonly associated with increased physical stress.

Consequences of Bullying

A great deal of research has investigated the consequences of bullying; it has been shown that bullying behaviors in childhood and adolescence have ramifications in adulthood. There is strong evidence that childhood bullies are at risk of developing antisocial behaviors as adults.[13] In addition, adult childhood bullies are likely to have more criminal convictions and traffic violations than their less aggressive peers. The victims of bullying often view themselves as outcasts and failures. Victims often display signs of anxiety and depression in conjunction with isolationism, school absenteeism, loneliness, and suicidal ideation.[13]

Costello reported that bullying predicts poorer functioning up to 40 years from the bullying incident(s).[34] Poorer functioning includes psychological distress, depression, poor physical health, and poorer cognitive functioning.[35,36] Others have found higher incidences of agoraphobia, generalized anxiety, and panic disorder.[37] It has been reported that individuals who have been bullied at school were three times more likely to have suicidal ideation in adulthood.[38]

In a study of 2833 adults, individuals were categorized as those who experienced bullying and those who did not experience bullying in childhood.[36] After adjusting for demographics, the effect of bullying was significantly associated with poorer levels of mental health. In another study of adult men, those who had experienced bullying in childhood had a significantly higher frequency of depression.[39]

In an effort to understand the consequences of violence, it should be obvious that violence can be an initiating event that produces consequences on the offender as well as the victim. Depending on age and/or criminality, the violence can be considered bullying, child abuse, IPV, elder abuse, or youth violence.

Consequences of IPV Experienced by Infants and Children

As with adults, physical sequelae of childhood abuse are determined by the type of violence done to the child. In some cases, the social and emotional consequences are severe.

A history of childhood maltreatment often results in childhood delinquency and adult criminality; 49% of maltreated children will have been arrested for a nontraffic offense during their adulthood.[40] Aggression has been shown to be associated with neglect before 2 years of age.[41] Multiple studies have shown that children exposed to violence are more likely to become violent as adults.[42–45] Children who experience sexual abuse have high rates of PTSD (>34%).[46] Other common consequences of childhood sexual abuse are developmentally inappropriate sexual behavior, such as age-inappropriate knowledge, sexual preoccupation, and excessive masturbation.[47]

Neglected children have learning problems, developmental delays, passivity, low self-esteem, and juvenile delinquency. Multiple emotional problems and social competency problems are associated with psychological maltreatment during childhood, such as anxiety, depression, low self-esteem, suicidal ideation, impulse control problems, substance abuse, eating disorders, isolating behavior, social phobia, aggression, and violent behavior.[48] Exposure to intrafamily violence also often leads to behavioral problems such as anxiety, depression, and aggression.[49] Children experience many fears and worries that are developmentally inappropriate such as PTSD, which is often more detrimental than the violence itself.[50,51] Guilt is highly correlated with the severity of PTSD, and resolving guilt is difficult because of the child's inability to accept that the violence was beyond his or her control.[51]

Long-term health consequences of childhood abuse are often related to specific behavioral risk factors such as smoking, alcohol abuse, poor diet, and lack of exercise linking to many illnesses in adulthood, including ischemic heart disease, cancer, chronic lung disease, irritable bowel syndrome, and fibromyalgia.[26]

In a study of 595 individuals, participants were divided into those who had experienced childhood trauma and those who had not.[40] It was reported that those who had experienced a childhood traumatic experience demonstrated more aggressive behavior in later life and they were at greater risk of paranoid hostility. This study emphasized the lifetime effects of childhood trauma.

RISK FACTORS

As mentioned previously, interpersonal violence involves all age groups and all races and ethnicities, it is not restricted to any one special interest group or any socioeconomic group, and it can involve all genders. Literally, all individuals have potential risk of experiencing interpersonal violence—either as a recipient or as a perpetrator of violence. Violence has many complex linkages. Some factors are relative to one type of interpersonal violence, but in many cases there are commonalities in that violence can share multiple and identical risk factors.

Populations at Risk
Infants and Children
Infants and children are at risk for abuse because of the power differential that exists with adolescents and adults. They are unable to resist the abuse and unable to report it. The ages for child abuse most often reported were among infants from birth to 1 year of age, with the rate decreasing with increasing age.[52] Children and adolescents who are killed by their parents are battered to death (32.9%), physically assaulted (28%), drowned (4.3%), burned (2.3%), stabbed (2.1%), or shot (3.0%).[6] The peak age at which a child will most likely be killed by the mother or father is within the first few months of life. A child is 100 times more likely to be killed by a stepparent than by a genetically related parent. Compared to genetic parents, stepparents are six times more likely to abuse their genetically unrelated child younger than the age of 2 years.[6]

Older Adults
Older adults, particularly those with impaired cognitive function and/or who lack independent functional ability, are at risk for abuse for similar reasons as infants and children; a power differential exists so that they may be unable to resist or report. Factors that place elders at risk for sexual abuse include dependence on others (family members, caretakers, and agency staff), physical frailty, and cognitive limitations.[53–56] Elder abuse is often associated with physical frailty and/or alterations in mental status.[57] These dependency factors are barriers to detecting elder sexual abuse and can provide for increased risk of abuse with continued low rates of reporting.[58] Ageism is the stigmatization of older people and is likely an element of the etiology of elder abuse. Negative attitudes toward aging and the glorification of youth may contribute to elder abuse.

Gender
The overwhelming incidence of IPV is perpetrated by men to women. In the United States, approximately one in three homicides of females is committed by an intimate partner, whereas approximately 5% of male homicide victims are killed by intimate partners.[8–10]

Studies from developed countries have reported a higher incidence of elder abuse among males.[59] In consideration of child abuse, higher reports of maltreatment occurred for boys versus girls (51% vs. 48.3%, respectively), and 56% of the perpetrators were women.[60]

Individual Risk Factors
Substance Use
A common underlying factor associated with interpersonal violence involves the use/misuse of alcohol. Alcohol has been reported to be a risk factor in IPV, child abuse, youth violence, and elder abuse.[61]

Mental Health Conditions
Factors that have been identified as risk factors for a man abusing his intimate partner include young age, depression, personality disorders, and low academic achievement.[61,62]

Exposure to Violence in Childhood
In homes in which IPV occurs, children are exposed to that violence at the very least and often become additional recipients of that violence. IPV usually predates abuse of the child.[63] Individuals who were witness to and/or the victim of interpersonal violence during childhood are at greater risk of becoming perpetrators as adults; this is especially notable with IPV and child abuse.[61]

Sociocultural Factors
In North America, a sociocultural view of the etiology of IPV is rooted in the family and society in the form of a historical legacy of oppression and colonization. From the beginning of the colonization of the Americas, there has been a stratified caste system based on race, ethnicity, religion, and sexuality.[64] Europeans were privileged over non-Europeans and men over women. Therefore the patriarchy was racialized. At an interpersonal and intrafamilial level, power leads to a culture that breeds violence. Studies have suggested that migration, acculturation, underemployment, undereducation, and economic stress contribute to domestic violence, including IPV, child abuse, and elder abuse.[64] A high socioeconomic status has generally been considered to be protective against IPV but not necessarily; generally, women living in poverty are disproportionately affected.[61]

Factors influencing the likelihood of youth violence are low intelligence; low levels of achievement; poor parental supervision; harsh physical punishment of children; a large number of siblings; low socio-economic status; income inequality; racism; or the presence of gangs, guns, and drugs in the environment.[14]

ASSESSMENT

All health professionals should maintain continuous vigilance for evidence of interpersonal violence with all health care encounters. It is often difficult to differentiate injuries caused by violence from those caused accidentally. Clues are usually present, but only if the astute nurse is keeping an open mind to the presence of signs and symptoms.

History

There are certain elements in the medical history that raise concern for physical abuse. Perpetrators may provide a history of events that is incomplete or inconsistent with injuries seen. Many individuals who experience interpersonal violence are unable or afraid to provide an accurate account of events. Specific examples include a history of trauma that is inconsistent or implausible with the physical examination, a history of no trauma with evidence of injury, a history of self-inflicted trauma that is developmentally unlikely, and serious injuries blamed on siblings or playmates.[65]

One study reported that older adults are exposed to far more abuse than they are willing to admit.[66] Elders were much more likely to report physical and sexual abuse and less likely to report other types of abuse. This creates a serious situation in that direct questioning of elders may not be the best way to determine incidence of abuse. Much more work needs to be done to better understand the pervasiveness of elder abuse and the way it impacts quality of life.

Examination Findings

Examination findings for interpersonal violence range from subtle to obvious. Some may manifest as old or new injuries that may seem mild to more significant (e.g., cuts, bruises, burns, or fractures) and may not raise concern. For this reason, it is critical to consider the history in relation to injuries seen. The nurse should also maintain a high degree of awareness for injuries that are not typically seen in the context of day-to-day living, such as unusual patterns of bruising or burn marks. In some cases, specific physical injuries are common. Traumatic brain injury usually occurs in infants younger than 1 year of age. Shaken baby syndrome is also common in infants and young children. Studies have shown that 15–25% of these injuries are fatal, and 80–90% of the survivors are left with varying degrees of compromise, including learning disabilities, blindness, seizures, and paralysis.[65] Abdominal injuries caused by punching or kicking, which lead to internal bleeding, are the second most common cause of death in child abuse. Burns are a common injury associated with abuse; in fact, it is believed that 10% of all physical abuse cases involve burns, usually with scalding water.[65] Burns with a stocking pattern or circular burn marks always should raise suspicion.

CLINICAL MANAGEMENT

Primary Prevention

The prevention of interpersonal violence is considered a key public health priority. The lead federal organization for violence prevention, established by the Centers for Disease Control and Prevention, is the National Center for Injury Prevention and Control (NCIPC). One of three divisions of the NCIPC is the Division of Violence Prevention (DVP). The strategic directions established by the DVP include reducing rates of various forms of violence (including child maltreatment, IPV, sexual violence, and youth violence) through individual, community, and societal change. A comprehensive discussion of the national strategic direction for DVP is beyond the scope of this concept analysis, but it is important for nurses to know these directions exist and are readily available on the CDC website (http://www.cdc.gov/injury/index.html)

Secondary Prevention (Screening)

A large number of screening tools have been developed to screen for various types of interpersonal violence in a number of health care settings. Nurses should be aware of appropriate tools to use in various settings, such as emergency departments, school-based clinics, inpatient settings, or community-based clinics. A useful resource for screening tools is the *Intimate Partner Violence and Sexual Violence Victimization Assessment Instruments for Use in Healthcare Settings* published by the Centers for Disease Control and Prevention.[67] This resource presents a variety of screening tools that have been tested and validated for multiple types of interpersonal violence and among various population groups (age and ethnic/cultural). It is beyond the scope of this concept analysis to describe each screening tool, but nurses are encouraged to become aware of the most appropriate screening tools used in their particular practice settings.

Collaborative Interventions

When interpersonal violence is suspected or identified, the priority intervention is to protect the infant, child, adult, or elder from further abuse. It is the legal and ethical duty of nurses and all health professionals to report suspected abuse. All states have laws for mandatory reporting of child abuse and other forms of violence. When the victim is a child or compromised elderly individual, referrals are made to the state agency child or human welfare departments for a formal investigation; based on these findings, the child or elderly person may be left in the home or removed and placed in another setting. Adult victims of IPV may need a referral to a "safe house" such as a battered women's shelter and/or may need a referral to seek a legal restraining order.[68]

Emotional support and appropriate referrals are also needed for the patient and family. A focus on minimizing the physiological consequences is needed, particularly helping those who have suffered emotionally to experience and establish positive relationships. Education and counseling are often needed to ensure adequate coping strategies. Nurses can also help patients and families gain access to appropriate community agencies and support groups as available.

During the past decade, much research has been done to draw attention to the problem of IPV. Many studies have shown the serious consequences of IPV. However, there is still an underreporting of IPV; hence, there is a lack of formal help-seeking behaviors, which may be a result of sociocultural barriers.[17] Bauer et al. suggested that sociocultural barriers included cultural stigma of abuse, dedication to the family unit, social isolation, and language barriers.[69] When nurses are able to view diversity as an indication of resilience instead of weakness, perhaps help-seeking behaviors will increase.[29] Compared to women with no lifetime exposure to interpersonal violence, it was reported that women who have experienced IPV were more likely to be unemployed, to have lower incomes, and to be married. It was also found that they had fewer individuals in their support systems.[19]

INTERRELATED CONCEPTS

Many of the sequelae of interpersonal violence result in other health and illness concepts. For instance, interpersonal violence could

FIGURE 38-3 Interpersonal Violence and Interrelated Concepts

conceivably involve almost all health and illness concepts depending on the physical and psychological effects of the violence. In fact, interpersonal violence sequelae are cumulative and long-lasting beyond the violence events.[19] Figure 38-3 features important interrelationships to consider. Common psychological consequences of interpersonal violence include Anxiety, Stress, and Mood and Affect. Individuals who experience interpersonal violence rely on Coping strategies as part of the response to such events. Interrelationships with several professional nursing concepts also are important to note. Nurses have a *legal* (Health Care Law) and *ethical* (Ethics) obligation to report abuses. Because of widespread prevalence, Health Policy initiatives have resulted in national strategies to address interpersonal violence.

CLINICAL EXEMPLARS

There are many examples of interpersonal violence, many of which have been described throughout this concept analysis. It is important to remember that this occurs across the lifespan and it can happen to any individual. Box 38-1 presents common examples of interpersonal violence.

Featured Exemplars

Child Abuse

It is difficult to know the actual figures of child maltreatment. Much of it is unreported. In 2008, the national rate of reports of child maltreatment was 10.3 per 1000 children.[48] The U.S. Department of Health and Human Services reported that 71% of these children experienced neglect, 16% were physically abused, 9% were sexually abused, and 12% experienced other forms of abuse.[14] An estimated rate of physical abuse of 49 per 1000 children was obtained when the following behaviors were included: hitting the child with an object, hitting the child somewhere other than the buttocks, kicking the child, beating the child, and threatening the child with a weapon.[60]

Neglect

Neglect is parental failure to meet a child's basic needs[11] or a caregiver's failure to meet a dependent adult's needs. Five subtypes of child neglect are physical neglect, psychological or emotional neglect (these parents typically ignore their child's desire for comfort), medical neglect (not providing medical treatment), mental health neglect, and educational neglect.[47] It is difficult to differentiate neglect from abuse. Most believe neglect is a form of abuse. The legal definition of child neglect is "the failure of a parent or other person with responsibility for the child to

> ### BOX 38-1 EXEMPLARS OF INTERPERSONAL VIOLENCE
>
> **Child Abuse**
> - Physical abuse
> - Sexual abuse
> - Emotional abuse
> - Neglect
>
> **Bullying**
>
> **Youth Violence**
>
> **Intimate Partner Violence**
> - Physical violence
> - Sexual violence
> - Emotional abuse
>
> **Elder Abuse**
> - Physical abuse
> - Sexual abuse
> - Emotional abuse
> - Neglect
> - Abandonment
> - Financial abuse

Source: From Centers for Disease Control and Prevention: Injury Prevention and Control, Division of Violence Prevention, 2015. Retrieved from: http://www.cdc.gov/violenceprevention.

provide needed food, clothing, shelter, medical care, or supervision to the degree that the child's health, safety, and well-being are threatened with harm."[11,70]

Bullying

Bullying is a serious concern, and the prevalence is on the rise. Most bullying occurs during childhood and adolescent years, with a peak among middle school children. In most cases, bullying occurs while at school, but this can also occur outside the school grounds, such as on the way to and from school or during extramural youth activities. It is estimated that between 15% and 25% of students are bullied frequently, and nearly 20% reported bullying others often. There is a direct relationship between being a bully or being bullied and other types of violence (including youth violence).[27]

Youth Violence

Youth violence is a serious worldwide problem, and the common quality is that both the perpetrators and the recipients of violence are youths. Worldwide, the highest rates of youth homicide are from Latin America (36.4/100,000 youths), and in the United States this rate is 11/100,000 youths.[71] According to the Centers for Disease Control and Prevention, youth violence is the second leading cause of death among young people between ages 10 and 24 years (see http://www.cdc.gov/violenceprevention/pdf/YV-FactSheet-a.pdf).

Intimate Partner Violence

According to 48 population-based studies from several countries, 10–69% of women reported being victims of IPV during their lifetime.[19] In the United States, the prevalence of IPV in minority women is higher than that in white women, with Hispanic women reporting a greater frequency of rapes and Native American women reporting more violent victimization.[71] It has been reported that IPV exposure causes more severe health consequences than other types of trauma.[64]

Sexual Violence

Sexual violence occurs across the lifespan. The U.S. Department of Health and Human Services reported that 9% of children were sexually abused.[11] Older adults also are subjected to sexual abuse within their own homes, nursing homes, or community. In a study evaluating 284 elders who experienced sexual assault, the mean age was 78.8 years; the age of offenders ranged from 13 to 90 years, and the large majority of victims were female.

Elder Abuse

There are no national data on the prevalence or incidence of elder abuse. Pillemer and Finklehor reported an overall prevalence rate of 3.2% and a 1 in 14 reporting rate.[66] In a later study by Pillemer, it was reported that at least 36% of nursing home personnel witnessed physical abuse within the previous year and 40% admitted to committing an act of psychological abuse within the preceding year.[55] In a study of 730 hospitalized elder patients in Israel, 6% reported that they had experienced elder abuse of varying types. Of those reporting abuse, 25% reported 1 type, and the remaining patients reported 2–10 types of abuse.[72]

CASE STUDY

Source: Cameron Whitman/iStock/Thinkstock

Case Presentation

Amanda Soto, a 22-year-old female, presents to an outpatient clinic with a chief complaint of headaches and problems sleeping. Yvonne Sanchez, the nurse at the clinic, remembers seeing Amanda in the clinic not long ago. She reviews Amanda's medical record before seeing her and notes that Amanda has been in the clinic four times in the past 5 months, each time with vague symptoms, and each time she was sent home with a nonspecific diagnosis. The nurse reviews her social history and sees that Amanda is married and has two children, ages 2 and 4 years and works as a receptionist. Amanda has no medical conditions and takes no medications other than oral contraceptives.

When Yvonne enters the examination room, she observes Amanda sitting on the examination table with her knees held tightly against her torso and rocking back and forth. Yvonne asks Amanda to describe the symptoms she has been experiencing. Amanda states her headaches have been occurring off and on for a while, and she describes them as "intense" and often keeping her awake at night. As she talks, Yvonne notes a flat affect in Amanda's communication pattern. She also notices bruising to her neck, just above the clavicle, and on her upper arms. When Yvonne asks Amanda when was the last time she experienced the headache, she tells Yvonne she cannot remember exactly, but perhaps 1 or 2 weeks ago.

Yvonne suspects Amanda may be experiencing violence. She pulls out the Partner Violence Screening tool, available at her office, and asks Amanda the following three questions:

1. Have you been hit, kicked, punched, or otherwise hurt by someone within the past year? If so, by whom?
2. Do you feel safe in your current relationship?
3. Is there a partner from a previous relationship who is making you feel unsafe now?

Amanda begins to cry and acknowledges she is in trouble. She states her husband has a drinking problem and every couple of weeks he gets drunk and becomes violent. He always feels badly after he becomes sober, but she has become frightened at what he will do to her or the children. She states that he has never hurt the children, but they see him regularly hit her. Amanda tells Yvonne she has contemplated leaving, but she does not think she can. She explains that her husband controls all of the money, and she has nowhere to go. She is sure she does not earn enough money to support herself and her children, and she is worried that he will track her down anyway. Amanda feels completely trapped and unable to remove herself from the situation.

Case Analysis

This case exemplifies interpersonal violence, specifically intimate partner violence. Individuals are often reluctant to report this violence; thus the nurse must maintain a keen awareness of the possibility when interacting with every patient. Yvonne first noticed a pattern of frequent clinic visits; she also noted Amanda's flat affect and body posturing, as well as the bruises to the neck and arms. Alone, any one of these findings might not seem significant, but together these are indeed concerning. Yvonne used a common screening tool for domestic violence and positively identified this problem.

As a nurse, Yvonne's next steps are to ask Amanda if she would like to speak to a law enforcement officer, to provide her with resources for emotional support, and to direct Amada to community agencies that can assist her to extricate herself and her children from her abuser. Because of her fear of retaliation, it is unlikely that Amanda will want to press charges against her husband.

ACCESS EXEMPLAR LINKS IN YOUR GIDDENS EBOOK

REFERENCES

1. Dahlberg L, Krug E: Violence—A global public health problem. In Krug E, Dahlberg L, Mercy J, et al, editors: *World report on violence and health*, Geneva, 2002, World Health Organization.
2. Schaffer B: Male veteran interpersonal partner violence (IPV) and associated problems. *J Aggress Matr Trauma* 19:414, 2010.
3. Johnson M: Patriarchal terrorism and common couple violence: Two forms of violence against women. *J Marriage Fam* 57:283, 1995.
4. Wilkinson D: Violent youths' responses to high levels of exposure to community violence: What violent events reveal about youth violence. *J Commun Psychol* 36:1026, 2008.
5. Windom C, Maxfield M: *An update on the "Cycle of Violence,"* 2001, National Institute of Justice Research Brief, U.S. Department of Justice, Office of Justice Programs. Available at: <https://www.ncjrs.gov/pdffiles1//nij/184894.pdf>.
6. Raine A: *The anatomy of violence*, New York, 2013, Pantheon.
7. Giardino A, Lyn M, Giardino E: Introduction: Child abuse and neglect. In Giardino A, Lyn M, Giardino E, editors: *A practical guide to the evaluation of child physical abuse and neglect*, New York, 2010, Springer.
8. Dong X: Elder abuse: Research, practice, and health policy. *Gerontologist* 54:153, 2012.
9. Wiglesworth A, Mosqueda L, Mulnard R, et al: Screening for abuse and neglect of people with dementia. *J Am Geriatr Soc* 58:493, 2010.
10. Pico-Alfonso M, Garcia-Linares M, Celda-Navarro N, et al: The impact of physical, psychological, and sexual intimate male partner violence on women's mental health: Depressive symptoms, posttraumatic stress disorder, state anxiety, and suicide. *J Womens Health* 15:599, 2006.
11. Child Welfare Information Gateway: *Definitions of child abuse and neglect*, Washington, DC, 2014, U.S. Department of Health and Human Services, Children's Bureau.
12. Nerenberg L: Communities respond to elder abuse. *J Gerontol Soc Work* 46(3–4):5–33, 2006.
13. Smokowski P, Kopasz K: Bullying in school: An overview of types, effects, family characteristics, and intervention strategies. *Children & Schools* 17:101, 2005.
14. U.S. Department of Health and Human Services: *Youth violence: A report of the Surgeon General*, Rockville, MD, 2001, Author.
15. Jewkes R, Sen P, Garcia-Moreno C: Sexual violence. In Krug E, Dahlberg L, Mercy J, et al, editors: *World report on violence and health*, Geneva, 2002, World Health Organization.
16. American Professional Society on the Abuse of Children: *Guidelines for psychosocial evaluation of suspected psychological maltreatment of children and adolescents*, Chicago, 1995, Author.
17. Federal Bureau of Investigation: *Crime in the United States*, Washington, DC, 2007, U.S. Department of Justice.
18. Centers for Disease Control and Prevention: Surveillance for violent deaths—National violent death reporting system, 16 states 2007. *Morbid Mortal Weekly Rep* 59:SS4, 2010.
19. Hien D, Ruglass L: Interpersonal partner violence and women in the United States: An overview of prevalence rates, psychiatric correlates and consequences and barriers to help seeking. *Int J Law Psychiatr* 32:48, 2009.
20. Schumacher A, Jaramillo D, Uribe T, et al: The relationship of two types of trauma exposure to current physical and psychological symptom distress in a community sample of Colombian women: Why interpersonal violence deserves more attention. *Health Care Women Int* 31:946, 2010.
21. Giardet R, Giardino A: Evaluation of physical abuse and neglect. In Giardino A, Lyn M, Giardino E, editors: *A practical guide to the evaluation of child physical abuse and neglect*, New York, 2010, Springer.
22. Alvi A, Doherty T, Lewen G: Facial fractures and concomitant injuries in trauma patients. *Laryngoscope* 113:102, 2003.
23. Lee K: Interpersonal violence and facial fractures. *J Oral Maxillofac Surg* 67(9):1878–1883, 2009.
24. Humphreys J, Lee K: Interpersonal violence is associated with depression and chronic physical health problems in midlife women. *Issues Ment Health Nurs* 30:206, 2009.
25. Pallito C, O'Campo P: The relationship between intimate partner violence and unintended pregnancy. *Int Fam Plan Perspect* 30:165, 2004.
26. Stark E, Flitcraft A: *Women at risk: Domestic violence and women's health*, Thousand Oaks, CA, 1996, Sage.
27. National Center for Educational Statistics and Bureau of Justice Statistics: *Indicators of school crime and safety*. Available at: <http://nces.ed.gov/pubs2010/2010012.pdf>, 2009.
28. Meuleners L, Lee A, Hendrie D: Effects of demographic variables on mental illness admission for victims of interpersonal violence. *J Public Health* 31:162, 2008.
29. Astin M, Lawrence K, Foy D: Posttraumatic stress disorder among battered women: Risk and resiliency factors. *Violence Victims* 8:17, 1993.
30. Golding J: Intimate partner violence as a risk factor for mental disorders: A meta-analysis. *J Fam Violence* 14:99, 1999.
31. Jones L, Hughes M, Unterstaller U: Post-traumatic stress disorder (PTSD) in victims of domestic violence: A review of the research. *Trauma Violence Abuse* 2:99, 2001.
32. Hegadoren K, Lasiuk G, Coupland N: Posttraumatic stress disorder. Part III: Health effects of interpersonal violence among women. *Perspect Psychiatr Care* 42:163, 2006.
33. Campbell J: Health consequences of intimate partner violence. *Lancet* 359:1331, 2002.
34. Costello E: Adult outcomes of childhood bullying victimization. *Am J Psychiatry* 171:709, 2014.
35. Takizawa R, Maughan B, Arseneault L: Adult health outcomes of childhood bullying victimization: Evidence from a five-decade longitudinal British birth cohort. *Am J Psychiatry* 171:777, 2014.
36. Allison S, Roeger L, Reinfeld-Kirkman N: Does school bullying affect adult health? Population survey of health-related quality of life and past victimization. *Aust N Z J Psychiatry* 43:1163, 2009.
37. Copeland W, Dieter W, Angold A, et al: Adult psychiatric outcomes of bullying and being bullied by peers in childhood and adolescence. *JAMA Psychiatry* 70:419, 2013.
38. Roeger L, Allison S, Korossy-Horwood R, et al: Is a history of school bullying victimization associated with adult suicidal ideation? *J Nerv Ment Dis* 198:728, 2010.
39. Lund R, Nielsen K, Hansen D, et al: Exposure to bullying at school and depression in adulthood: A study of Danish men born in 1953. *Eur J Public Health* 19:111, 2008.
40. Dragioti E, Damigos D, Mavreas V, et al: Effects of childhood trauma on hostility, family environment and narcissism of adult individuals. *Int J Care Science* 5:137, 2012.
41. Runyan D, Wattam C, Ikeda R, et al: Child abuse and neglect by parents and other caregivers. In Krug E, Dahlberg L, Mercy J, editors: *World report on violence and health*, Geneva, 2002, World Health Organization.
42. Mercy J, Butchart A, Farrington D, et al: Youth violence. In Krug E, Dahlberg L, Mercy J, et al, editors: *World report on violence and health*, Geneva, 2002, World Health Organization.
43. Slovak K, Carlson K, Helm L: The influence of family violence on youth attitudes. *Child Adolesc Social Work J* 24:77, 2007.
44. Weaver C, Borkowski J, Whitman T: Violence breeds violence: Childhood exposure and adolescent conduct problems. *J Commun Psychol* 36:96, 2008.
45. Legge S: Youth and violence: Phenomena and international data. *New Directions Youth Dev* 119:17, 2008.
46. Berliner L: Child sexual abuse: Definitions, prevalence, and consequences. In Myers J, editor: *The APSAC handbook on child maltreatment*, Los Angeles, 2011, Sage.
47. Erickson M, Egeland B: Child neglect. In Myers J, editor: *The APSAC handbook on child maltreatment*, Los Angeles, 2011, Sage.
48. Hart S, Brassard M, Davidson H, et al: Psychological maltreatment. In Myers J, editor: *The APSAC handbook on child maltreatment*, Los Angeles, 2011, Sage.

49. Lemmey D, Malecha A, McFarlane J, et al: Severity of violence against women correlates with behavioral problems in their children. *Pediatr Nurs* 27:265, 2001.

50. Graham-Berman S, Howell K: Child maltreatment in the context of intimate partner violence. In Myers J, editor: *The APSAC handbook on child maltreatment*, Los Angeles, 2011, Sage.

51. Kletter H, Weems C, Carrion V: Guilt and posttraumatic stress symptoms in child victims of interpersonal violence. *Clin Child Psychol Psychiatr* 14:71, 2009.

52. DePanfils D: Child protection system. In Myers J, editor: *The APSAC handbook on child maltreatment*, Los Angeles, 2011, Sage.

53. Wyandt MA: A review of elder abuse literature: An age old problem brought to light. *Californian J Health Promot* 2(3):40–52, 2004.

54. Swagerty DL, Takahashi PY, Evans JM: Elder mistreatment. *Am Fam Phys* 59(10):2804–2808, 1999.

55. Pillemer K, Moore D: Highlights from a study of abuses of patients in nursing homes. *J Elder Abuse Neglect* 2:5, 1990.

56. Anetzberger G: Elder abuse. In Bonder B, Dal Bello-Haas V, Wagner M, editors: *Functional performance in older adults*, Philadelphia, 2009, Davis.

57. Anetzberger G: Elder abuse. In Bonder B, Dal Bello-Haas V, Wagner M, editors: *Functional performance in older adults*, Philadelphia, 2009, Davis.

58. Marshall CE, Benton D, Brazier JM: Primary care—Elder abuse: Using clinical tools to identify clues of mistreatment. *Geriatrics* 55(2):42–44, 47–50, 2000.

59. Cohen M, Levin S, Gagin R, et al: Elder abuse: Disparities between older people's disclosure of abuse, evident signs of abuse, and high risk of abuse. *J Am Geriatr Soc* 55:1224, 2007.

60. U.S. Department of Health and Human Services: *Child maltreatment 2007*, Washington, DC, 2007, U.S. Government Printing Office.

61. Xue Y, Zimmerman M, Cunningham R: Relationship between alcohol use and violent behavior among urban African American youths from adolescence to emerging adulthood: A longitudinal study. *Am J Pub Health* 99:2041, 2009.

62. Taft C, Murphy C, King L, et al: Posttraumatic stress disorder symptomatology among partners of men in treatment relationship abuse. *J Abnorm Psychol* 114:259, 2005.

63. Amar A, Bess R, Stockbridge J: Lessons from families and communities about interpersonal violence, victimization, and seeking help. *J Forensic Nurs* 6:110, 2010.

64. Heise L, Garcia-Moreno C: Violence by intimate partners. In Krug E, Dahlberg L, Mercy J, et al, editors: *World report on violence and health*, Geneva, 2002, World Health Organization.

65. Reece R: Medical evaluation of physical abuse. In Myers J, editor: *The APSAC handbook on child maltreatment*, Los Angeles, 2011, Sage.

66. Pillemer K, Finklehor D: The prevalence of elder abuse: A random sample survey. *Gerontologist* 28:51, 1988.

67. Basile KC, Hertz MF, Back SE: *Intimate partner violence and sexual violence victimization assessment instruments for use in healthcare settings: Version 1*, Atlanta, GA, 2007, Centers for Disease Control and Prevention, National Center for Injury Prevention and Control. Available at: <http://www.cdc.gov/violenceprevention/pdf/ipv/ipvandsvscreening.pdf>.

68. Gist JH, McFarlane J, Malecha A, et al: Women in danger: Intimate partner violence experienced by women who qualify and do not qualify for a protective order. *Behav Sci Law* 19:637, 2001.

69. Bauer H, Rodriques M, Quiroga S, et al: Barriers to health care for abused Latina and Asian immigrant women. *J Health Care Poor Underserved* 11:33, 2000.

70. Greenbaum J, Dubowitz H, Lutzker J, et al: *Practice guidelines: Challenges in the evaluation of child neglect*, Elmhurst, IL, 2008, American Professional Society on the Abuse of Children.

71. Flores-Ortiz Y: Domestic violence in Chicana/o families. In Velasquez R, Arellano L, McNeill B, editors: *The handbook of Chicana/o psychology and mental health*, New York, 2004, Erlbaum.

72. Wolf R, Daichman L, Bennett G: Abuse of the elderly. In Krug E, Dahlberg L, Mercy J, et al, editors: *World report on violence and health*, Geneva, 2002, World Health Organization.

Professional Nursing and Health Care Concepts

I n the not-too-distant past, health care was delivered in a disease-centered model whereby health care providers controlled and directed care, with little input from patients regarding their desires or their concerns about the impact of the treatment plan on their lives. Patients were apprised of the plan as opposed to discussing options for disease management.

The first theme is ***Attributes/Roles of a Professional Nurse***. Concepts within this theme represent roles nurses play within health care delivery and the attributes or characteristics desired of professional nurses; these are the behaviors nurses incorporate into all patient care encounters. Specific concepts represented include *Professional Identity, Clinical Judgment, Leadership, Ethics, Patient Education,* and *Health Promotion.*

The second theme is ***Care Competencies***. The term *competency* refers to being competent or well qualified to complete a skill or task. In the context of nursing and health care, competencies are identified knowledge, skills, and attitudes deemed important for safe and effective care. Specific concepts include *Communication, Collaboration, Safety, Technology and Informatics, Evidence,* and *Health Care Quality.* Although the concepts featured within this theme are not intended to be comprehensive of all competencies, some of the most common to all nurses, regardless of area of practice, are included.

The third theme is **Health Care Delivery**. These concepts represent the context of the application and care delivery situations or models. There are literally thousands of health care delivery models; those included are some of the most important to be aware of and include *Care Coordination, Caregiving, Palliative Care,* and *Health Disparities.*

The final theme is **Health Care Infrastructures**. These concepts are foundational to health care delivery and the practice of nursing. *Health Care Organizations, Health Care Economics, Health Policy,* and *Health Care Law* represent specific concepts within this theme.

Professional Identity

Nelda Godfrey and Nancy Crigger

Professional identity is an attribute of a nurse professional that is initially acquired during one's nursing education. As a novice member of a professional group, the student nurse uses multiple experiences and reflections to embrace the characteristics, norms, and values of the nursing discipline and begins to think, act, and feel like a nurse.[1,2] The process of gaining this understanding is called professional identity formation, which together with professional identity encompass what is sometimes referred to as professionalism. Professional identity is formed as a person transitions from layperson to a nurse professional during the educational process,[3] and it is fostered throughout the nurse's career as professional identity is challenged and matures through experiences within the profession.[4]

DEFINITION

Based on earlier work from medical colleagues,[1,2] professional identity in nursing is defined as *a sense of oneself that is influenced by characteristics, norms, and values of the nursing discipline, resulting in an individual thinking, acting, and feeling like a nurse.* Professional identity is part of the larger notion of identity, "an umbrella term used throughout the social sciences to describe an individual's comprehension of him- or herself as a discrete, separate entity."[5,p119] Within the concept of identity one would find personal identity, with professional identity as a subset of personal identity (Figure 39-1).[6]

SCOPE

Novice professionals in any discipline begin to form a sense of professional identity as their education and training begin. Professional identity is developed in many ways, although real and simulated experiences, reflection, and role modeling by professional colleagues seem to be the most meaningful strategies.[1,7–24] Nursing incorporates many, if not most, of these strategies in "clinicals," a highly valued[25,26] opportunity for experiential learning in clinical sites under the guidance of a preceptor or faculty member. In some schools, these experiences progress to apprenticeship opportunities[3] in which a student works the shift of a nurse in practice to better learn the knowledge, skills, and attitudes needed in that practice environment.

Today, *professional identity* and *professional identity formation* are replacing nursing terminology such as *professional role* and *professionalism*, largely because of important work from colleagues in academic medicine. More than a decade ago, medical faculty determined that students needed to understand the nature of professionalism and internalize the value system of the medical profession.[1] Teaching and assessment efforts ensued, but faculty discovered that only part of what made up professionalism was addressed with these methods. Jarvis-Selinger et al. argue that focusing on role (a social construct) and competencies (behaviors), and assuming that the process of becoming a professional is a linear, learning-related developmental process, is inadequate.[16] Instead, a broader focus should acknowledge the crisis nature of identity formation and that with every adoption of a new identity, an old identity has to be deconstructed that leads to discontinuity and crisis. Jarvis-Selinger et al. suggest a model in which role, competencies, and identities more equally explain the realities of professional identity formation (Figure 39-2).[16]

ATTRIBUTES AND CRITERIA

Professional identity is composed of five subcategories or attributes: doing, being, acting ethically, flourishing, and changing identities.

Doing

"Doing," or the consensus or sociological perspective, incorporates the societal and professional codes and standards that are part of the nursing discipline. It also includes a skill orientation, or a "doing" component.[27] Because of its sociological origins, *role*—how one functions as a part of a group—is central to understanding the "doing" part of professional identity, and it is seen in functionalistic approaches to accomplishing goals.[16,28] In the early stages of any new role, there is usually a strong focus on external expectations and tasks—the "doing."[16] An example is diploma nursing education of the 1950s, when each nurse or nursing student had a specific role or duty and needed to fulfill that role to be deemed successful. The "doing" orientation remains a part of professional identity formation in nursing today, but it does not entirely explain how laypersons become nurse professionals.[3,27,29]

FIGURE 39-1 The Concept of Professional Identity as a Subset of Identity and Personal Identity

Being

"Being," or the personal or psychological view of the nurse professional, explains what it means to do the right thing even when no one is looking.[27] Decisions and actions come from within, from a desire to do what is good. This attribute is about "being" a professional and about adopting attitudes and behaviors that reflect the value of how a professional thinks, feels, and acts. This perspective may incorporate rules and principles, but it is beyond the laws, codes, and standards within the discipline or society. It is more a personal sense of being a nurse and functioning within the norms and values that are characteristic of nursing as a discipline.[27]

Acting Ethically

Doing the right thing, or acting ethically, is a critical component of professional identity and professional identity formation. According to Socrates, "The really important thing is not to live, but to live well. And to live well [means] … to live according to your principles." Living well means being attentive to what is considered right and good from both a societal and a professional perspective. For instance, it is not right to accept a date from a patient who is in your care in the hospital. Nor is it ethical to tell your family member details about a patient's condition.

FIGURE 39-2 Scope of Concept Professional identity formation involves roles, competencies, and identities. (Source: Data from Jarvis-Selinger S, Pratt D, Regehr G: Competency is not enough: Integrating identity formation into the medical education discourse, *Acad Med* 87(9):1185–1190, 2012.)

Flourishing

Not only is it necessary to better understand the doing and being of the discipline of nursing but also one must do so with a sense of positive and transformational growth. A transformational or human flourishing perspective is necessary for professional identity to move past the initial phases of formation. Not all professionals move to the expert stage of development; some opt to be experienced non-experts who choose not to deepen their understanding of their profession.[30] Box 39-1 shows the five key qualities for sustainable, life-long growth as a professional. This perspective can also be found in Magnet Recognition Program materials, in which excellence and the effort to strive for excellence is a core value. These ideas are as old as the ancient Greeks, who believed that each person's life has a purpose and that the function of one's life is to attain that purpose. Flourishing is an important component of both forming and fostering professional identity.[27]

Changing Identities

From adolescence on, each time a new identity emerges, a reworking of the person's identity occurs in order to resolve this new developmental issue.[31] However, because each person has multiple identities (i.e., son, daughter, student, employee, grandchild, or parent) at any one time, identity formation for persons preparing for the professions looks more like disequilibrium and subsequent assimilation than a developmental transition.[1,16,31] Recognition of changing identities is the final attribute of professional identity and the process of professional identity formation.

THEORETICAL LINKS

The research base for professional identity formation is underdeveloped,[23] and no unified theoretical framework for understanding the process of professional identity formation exists.[15] However, a number of other theories strongly influence the current understanding of professional identity.

Marcia and Josselson note that identity issues first arise in late adolescence when society and adolescents expect beliefs and vision for future career goals will start to form.[31] For the adolescent and growing young adult, this occurs within an environment of exploration and commitment. It is manifested through four identity statuses: identity diffusion, foreclosure, moratorium, and identity achieved. *Identity diffusion* is characterized by a lack of interest in commitment, and even in exploration. The catchphrase for this would be "whatever seems good at the moment." The second identity status is *foreclosure*, in which the person keeps talking about changing those around him or her and conspicuously not about making change him- or herself. *Moratorium*, the third identity status, is

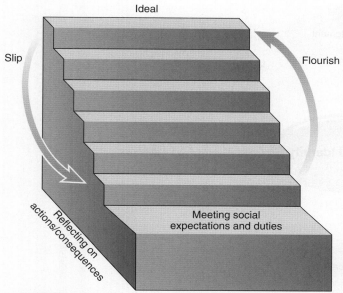

FIGURE 39-3 Stairstep Model of Professional Transformation (Source: Redrawn from Crigger N, Godfrey N: *The making of nurse professionals: A transformational, ethical approach*, Burlington, MA, 2011, Jones & Bartlett Learning, www.jblearning.com. Reprinted with permission.)

BOX 39-2   Professional Identity Statement for Nurses

At the University of Kansas Hospital, we strive to create a dynamic culture of professional behavior that requires personal and team accountability, self-reflection, integrity and respect. A nurse at the University of Kansas Hospital has a professional obligation to provide the highest quality of care that is reflective of the culture and to adhere to organizational policies and best practices. This culture is actualized through image, attitudes and behavior.

Source: From The University of Kansas Hospital Department of Nursing. Retrieved from http://www.kumed.com/careers/career-profiles/nursing.

characterized by overwhelming anxiety that is "hard to sit through" with someone. The fourth status, *identity achieved*, means that the person is reasonably self-aware, has a sense of self, and can manage overwhelming anxiety should it occur.[31]

Crigger and Godfrey's work with a stairstep model of professional transformation for nursing (Figure 39-3) visually represents the dynamism in professional identity formation.[27] The main ethical traditions are represented in the model, along with the transformational nature of nursing with the reality of slips and progress (flourishing) that occur throughout the trajectory of one's career. Finally, the progress toward the ideal is a function of individual and group efforts, with influences from many experiences.[27]

From an intervention standpoint, Bandura's social learning theory, in which learning occurs through observations of others, and Mezirow's transformational learning theory, in which growth and development are outcomes of transformational learning when sufficient levels of cognitive functioning are present, form part of the theoretical basis for professional identity and professional identity formation interventions.[32,33]

CONTEXT TO NURSING AND HEALTH CARE

Three illustrations of the connection between professional identity with nursing and health care follow: (1) forming and fostering professional identity, (2) an interprofessional perspective on professional identity and professional identity formation, and (3) interventions to achieve professional identity formation.

Forming and Fostering Professional Identity

Forming a professional identity in beginning pre-licensure nursing education is a challenge. First, the amount of empirical work in this

area is limited, although it is growing. Second, it seems that a variety of terms have been used to describe the same phenomenon, making comparisons difficult. However, a small set of studies indicate that faculty incivility can be a barrier to the development of professional identity[34]; observing the behaviors of registered nurses positively impacts students' development of their own sense of professional identity[17,35]; and, for students, the greatest barrier to growing a professional identity was the "unanticipated expectations" of the professional and academic nursing role. Students found that they needed to relinquish preconceptions and acclimate to their academic and professional climate in order to develop a sense of professional identity and to be successful.[36]

Even less is known about the impact of professional identity in nursing practice. Some data suggest that a robust professional identity can inoculate the nurse to bullying and incivility activity in the workplace. An example of an academic health center's professional identity statement for nurses is shown in Box 39-2.

An Interprofessional Perspective

Much of what is known about nursing and professional identity derives from interprofessional education and practice research. The Core Competencies for Interprofessional Collaborative Practice (IPEC) have set a clear standard for interprofessional collaboration in education and practice settings. With an eye on behavior change in the early stages of professional education, interprofessional education efforts are evident in nearly every nursing program nationally.[37]

Early interprofessional education research findings indicate that novice learners may marginalize other professionals based on their group affiliation, and this may result from lack of knowledge and oversimplification.[38] Interprofessional education opportunities can address this issue in more focused ways and strategize about ways to diminish this behavior. Findings show that the stronger the perceived professional identity of the learner, the more confidence one has with interprofessional collaboration,[39] making the case for ensuring adequate professional identity formation efforts. Furthermore, medical students' early attachment with the nursing profession engenders more respect for it,[40] and nurses' greater levels of education (i.e., master's degree) yield higher scores on the Readiness for Interprofessional Learning Scale (RIPLS) and on the professional identity subscale,[41] indicating that higher levels of education may enhance interprofessional learning. Professional identity was greatest in students with cognitive flexibility (able to structure knowledge), previous work experience in these environments, better understanding of team work, and a greater knowledge of their own profession.[42]

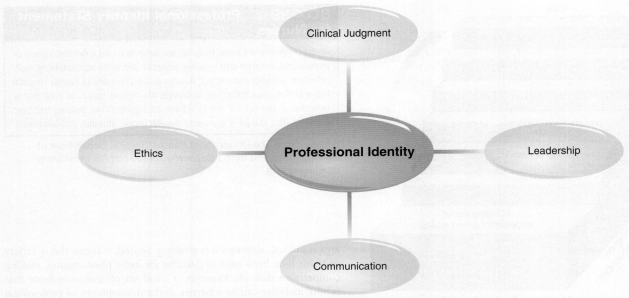

FIGURE 39-4 Professional Identity and Interrelated Concepts

Interventions to Achieve Professional Identity Formation

The following interventions will be helpful for students in building a professional identity:

- *Hear expectations clearly.* Most nursing education programs are highly complex and may seem difficult to understand. Listen carefully to expectations and advice for success.
- *Value debriefing and feedback from role models.* Studies have shown that role modeling is critically important in learning a profession. One study describes the most important component of the educational process as the "supportive yet challenging relationship" the learner has with the faculty member or mentor.[35] Recognize that these relationships are not only important in the future but also a valuable part of the student's learning in the nursing program in the present.
- *Engage in reflection.* Reflection has been increasingly shown to positively influence student learning.[43] Sometimes the reflection will be guided, through assignments in and outside of class; other times, reflection will be expected to be spontaneous, such as in post conferences following clinical. Reflection is a time to internalize what is occurring with the patient and family and also what is happening and changing one's own perspective.
- *Actively adopt a professional identity.* There is increasing evidence that labeling what nurses do as part of nursing's standards and codes is an important step in building language within the discipline.[15,28,44] Adopting a clear sense of professional identity that includes growing understanding of how integrity, compassion, courage, humility, advocacy, and human flourishing fit within the identity of nursing will in turn clarify the nurse's purposes as he or she relates to patients, families, and health care colleagues.[45]
- *Understand your own responsibilities for learning and be accountable for them.* People's beliefs in their ability to influence events that

affect their lives is known as self-efficacy.[46] Your ability to recognize your potential to grow and flourish will help propel you to greater personal and professional levels of self-efficacy.
- *Build relationships with those around you.* Building relationships is about understanding the importance to engage in the learning environment and following through so that these relationships become stronger and more meaningful. Relationship building and engaging with others is an important part of identity formation. In their integrative review of professional identity formation in higher education, Trede et al. reported that students need authentic experiences on which to reflect and active engagement that employs collaborative learning from practice environments.[23]
- *Develop personal self-care habits.* The American Nurses Association (ANA) Code for Nurses addresses the importance of nurses' self-care as part of nurses' ethical code. Caring for oneself is a key component of solidly developing a professional identity—in any field.
- *Embrace any opportunity for experiences with patients.* Holden et al. report that both real and simulated unique experiences with patients are valuable in forming professional identity.[15] Early experiences with patients or simulations are also important in this component of professional identity development.

INTERRELATED CONCEPTS

The concept of professional identity is interrelated with four professional nursing and health care concepts (Figure 39-4). **Clinical Judgment** depends on a deep and meaningful understanding of the professional identity of the nurse, incorporating health and illness concepts along with the norms and values that characterize the nurse as a designer, manager, and coordinator of care and as a member of a profession.[1,25] Principles of **Leadership** and **Ethics** govern the nurse's social contract with patients and families in his or her care, affirming that advocacy for the patient and family is a primary consideration for all decisions made within the health care environment.[30] **Communication** is fundamental to the nursing discipline and as such constitutes a substantial part of what actually happens in moment-to-moment nursing practice.

CLINICAL EXEMPLARS

There are many examples of professional identity in nursing practice. Box 39-3 presents some of the most common situations or examples seen in clinical practice, including language choice, attire (assurance), interaction, being "present," interacting in a professional way with the family, and acting as an agent for healing. It is beyond the scope of this text to provide details on all exemplars, but some are featured here.

Featured Exemplars
Integrity
Considered a fundamental character trait, integrity is evident in nearly every nursing action. If one has integrity, she does what she says she will do and acts with consistency and purpose. Integrity is often the basis for trust—for families and patients and for coworkers. A breach of integrity can erode one's trust in another, making this exemplar a critical consideration when providing care to vulnerable patients and their families.[27]

Compassion
Not to be confused with sympathy or empathy, compassion is feeling what another is feeling and responding to it with the intent of doing something to help.[47] Compassion is akin to caring, although they are difficult to separate in concept analysis. Caring and the ethic of care are intricately intertwined with the notion of compassion, and together they constitute a sense of response and accompanying action with those in need.[27]

Courage
In the context of professional identity, courage has two meanings: (1) to affect change and (2) "to stand in opposition for moral rightness."[27,p125] Courage can also be categorized as physical or moral.[27] The nurse who put herself between the patient and falling debris from a tornado demonstrated physical courage. The nurse who escalated a patient care situation by consulting higher ranking members of the medical staff exhibited moral courage.

Humility
Sometimes misunderstood, humility is "like a buoy that rides the waves of disappointments and accomplishments."[27,p121] When a person demonstrates humility, he or she views the world with equanimity, taking neither an overstated amount of credit nor blame for a particular situation.[27] Such an approach encourages a realistic view of circumstances, events, and the actions of others.

Advocacy
In situations in which nurse professionals employ advocacy, nurses and patients alike view this action as the "last line of defense" on behalf of the patient. This normative conception of the nurse as patient advocate is an example of a "signature image" of professional identity among nursing and other professions.[30]

BOX 39-3　EXEMPLARS OF PROFESSIONAL IDENTITY

Integrity
- Following through with pain medication
- Calling the physician when the patient asks you to
- Checking the Code Cart by the prescribed time
- Giving medications within the 30-minute window

Compassion
- Taking time to talk with a troubled family member
- Responding to a patient's call light with genuine interest
- Comforting a colleague who has just had a death in his or her family
- Using eye contact to apologize for a misstep with a colleague

Courage
- Speaking up when a colleague did not wash his or her hands before entering a patient room
- Conveying the details of the conversation a dying patient had with you to other members of the health care team
- Taking practice issues to the practice council to positively change practice on your nursing unit
- Speaking out about bullying occurring on the nursing unit

Humility
- Realistically viewing family members' ability to cope with a crisis
- Being nonjudgmental as staff deal with a unit-based crisis
- Clearly identifying your part in an error and not accepting more blame than is yours
- Seeing the larger picture when issues arise with patients, families, and coworkers

Advocacy
- Sharing with family members the details of a conversation you had with their loved one previously in the day
- Listening carefully to help family members carry out their wishes, and working with the hospital to do what you can to help that happen
- Communicating with the family about their loved one's surgery schedule, course of events, and expected finish time
- Working to get prescriptions filled before a homeless person leaves the hospital

Human Flourishing
- Encouraging patients in their difficult times
- Seeking additional resources for patients with limited discharge planning issues
- Encouraging coworkers to seek employee assistance options for difficulties they are having
- Creating a positive, encouraging environment for patients and families

---

Human Flourishing
The notion of human flourishing arises in conversation when virtues or normative views of a discipline are discussed. Grounded in the writings and beliefs of the ancient Greeks, the purpose of *being human* is to flourish. As nurses and fellow humans, we have a duty to do what is possible to foster outcomes that lead to human flourishing. Similar normative language is found in the ANA Code for Ethics for Nurses.[48]

CASE STUDY 1

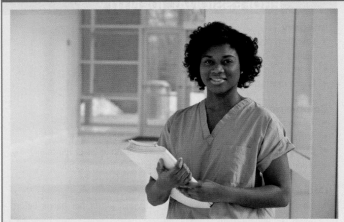

Source: Huntstock/Thinkstock

Case Presentation

Jane King is a 22-year-old female who has just begun her BSN nursing program. She is in her first clinical experience, and although she has been taught about giving bed baths, she is not sure that she is at all comfortable doing so. Her patient today is a 78-year-old male renal failure patient with limited mobility. Within her 8-hour assignment, Jane will need to complete all of her patient's personal care.

Although Jane has cared for young children in baby-sitting jobs since she was 11 years old, she has no experience caring for adults. She is particularly concerned about perineal care. Jane has had instruction—but what about the actual experience of doing peri care? This is new to Jane, and she does not know what to do.

Case Analysis

This is a time when the learning experience is not solely about Jane. As she tries on her new identity, she has not had any of these experiences and does not know what to do. Because this is her first semester in her nursing program, she has not had much time to "feel, think, and act" like a nurse professional. However, this patient is in a difficult situation in which he needs her care.

Compassion and engaged role modeling from Jane's clinical instructor will help her take the next step in her own professional identity formation. As one takes on a new identity, there can be some sadness in "letting go" of the person's previous perception of him- or herself. The clinical instructor needs to be aware that just as the student is constructing a new sense of professional identity in nursing, this often occurs in crisis (as in this situation), and often "deconstruction"—grieving the loss of the previous identity—occurs as the person takes on this new understanding of self. This example illustrates how such a situation reaches beyond role or job title. This student is experiencing a formative moment, and it is likely that she will be able to re-tell the story years from now. This is precisely why positive, insightful role modeling is needed by the clinical instructor. The student needs to see what the instructor does, how she treats the patient and the student, and what it means to provide professional nursing care in difficult situations. Furthermore, the instructor needs to ask the student to reflect on this experience within the next few days, and together they should discuss the student's thoughts and reactions. Role modeling, reflection, feedback, and encouragement are important strategies to help students as they incorporate additional identities into their own sense of professional identity.

CASE STUDY 2

Source: michaeljung/iStock/Thinkstock

Case Presentation

Jackie Wilson is a junior nursing student who was assigned on Tuesday to her first day of operating room (OR) observation. The OR staff was excited that Jackie was able to see one of the transplants on a day when several transplants were performed. Later that evening, Jackie shared with her family how interesting it was to see the transplant and to see the staff work so well together and function as a high-performing team. She also shared many details about the surgery because, of course, the staff had been sharing these details with her.

Three days later, the academic health center released a press briefing to media outlets in the region reporting that Tuesday had been a record day for transplants at the academic health center. That morning at work, Jackie's father told his colleagues that his daughter had been in the OR for one of these transplants, and he proceeded to communicate many of the details that Jackie had shared at the family dinner table.

Case Analysis

One of the lapses in professional identity that appears in the research literature is that of breach of confidentiality. That is certainly the main problem in this case. However, there are other influences that more fully tell the story—the inclusive approach that health care providers had for a new learner, the enthusiasm that faculty have for what students are learning, and the genuine interest in being part of something so intriguing. What is difficult to understand is where and how to draw the line in a situation such as this—for the student, for the OR staff, and even for the faculty. Students hear clinical examples in class and discuss specific details of their patients' circumstances in clinical conferences. Of course, all students sign confidentiality agreements—but do they really understand?

This is a situation in which a rule-based approach is probably not as helpful as helping the students build their own understanding of professional identity as it relates to confidentiality. Being more reflective and conversational with the students would probably yield better outcomes in the long term. A combination of specific examples of what *not* to do along with conversation about other possible scenarios would better prepare novice professionals for the complex system expectations that exist in health care today.

CASE STUDY 3

Source: Photodisc/Thinkstock

Case Presentation

John Roberts is a pre-licensure nursing student who has been asked to be part of an interprofessional education activity at his school. His school has students doing clinical at many hospitals in the area, and he also works in a local hospital as a nurse tech. He loves the clinical environment and is quite competent in his nurse tech role.

This interprofessional education activity includes students in occupational therapy, physical therapy, respiratory therapy, pharmacy, and nursing. In his work experience, John has worked (although minimally) with people who are in each of these fields, but he is sure that they do not have the "real picture" of what patients experience—particularly because he has often floated the hospital as he has worked his shift as a tech.

The small group portion of this interprofessional educational activity includes John, two occupational therapy students, and one physical therapy student. Going into the exercise, John is sure that he is the one who will have more knowledge and understanding than any of the other students.

Case Analysis

Findings indicate that novice learners often marginalize other novice learner abilities. In fact, minimizing others' knowledge is actually a rhetorical strategy. Although it is unlikely that a novice student would intentionally diminish a student from another profession, such initial thinking is not unusual, especially when one is inexperienced. Interprofessional education learning opportunities are excellent opportunities to change behaviors and promote colleagueship among various professional groups. John needs to be aware of this documented tendency among novice professionals and do what he can to foster an environment of teamwork and collaboration with fellow students. Such actions will encourage reflection for John and provide feedback for other members of the interprofessional team.

ACCESS EXEMPLAR LINKS IN YOUR GIDDENS EBOOK

REFERENCES

1. Cruess RL, Cruess SR, Boudreau JD, et al: Reframing medical education to support professional identity formation. *Acad Med* 89(11):1446–1451, 2014.
2. Merton RK: Some preliminaries to a sociology of medical education. In Merton RK, Reader LG, Kendall PL, editors: *The student physician: Introductory studies in the sociology of medical education*, Cambridge, MA, 1957, Harvard University Press, pp 3–79.
3. Benner P, Sutphen M, Leonard V, et al: *Educating nurses: A call for radical transformation*, Stanford, CA, 2010, The Carnegie Foundation for the Advancement of Teaching.
4. Godfrey N, Crigger N: Ethics and professional conduct: Striving for a professional ideal. *J Prof Regul* 3(1):32–37, 2012.
5. Sharma S, Sharma M: Self, social identity and psychological well-being. *Psychol Stud* 55(2):118–136, 2010.
6. Tsang SKM, Hui EK, Law BCM: Positive identity as a positive youth development construct: A conceptual view. *Sci World J* 2012:Article ID 529691, 2012.
7. Baldwin A, Mills J, Birks M, et al: Role modeling in undergraduate nursing education: An integrative literature review. *Nurse Educ Today* 34:e18–e26, 2014.
8. Boudreau JD, MacDonald ME, Steinert Y: Affirming professional identities through an apprenticeship: Insights from a four-year longitudinal case study. *Acad Med* 89(7):1038–1045, 2014.
9. Brown J, Stevens J, Kermode S: Supporting student nurse professionalization: The role of the clinical teacher. *Nurse Educ Today* 32:606–610, 2012.
10. Curran C, Fitzpatrick T: *Claiming the corner office: Executive leadership lessons for nurses*, Indianapolis, IN, 2013, STT.
11. Finn G, Garner J, Sawdon M: "You're judged all the time" Students' view on professionalism: A multicenter study. *Med Educ* 44:814–825, 2010.
12. Gazzola N, De Stefano J, Audet C, et al: Professional identity among counseling psychology doctoral students: A qualitative investigation. *Couns Psychol Q* 24(4):257–275, 2011.
13. Goldie J: The formation of professional identity in medical students: Considerations for educators. *Med Teach* 34:e641–e648, 2012.
14. Hendelman W, Byszewski A: Formation of medical student professional identity: Categorizing lapses of professionalism, and the learning environment. *BMC Med Educ* 14:139, 2014.
15. Holden M, Buck E, Clark M, et al: Professional identity formation in medical education: The convergence of multiple domains. *HEC Forum* 24:245–255, 2012.
16. Jarvis-Selinger S, Pratt D, Regehr G: Competency is not enough: Integrating identity formation into the medical education discourse. *Acad Med* 87(9):1185–1190, 2012.
17. Keeling J, Templeman J: An exploratory study: Student nurses' perceptions of professionalism. *Nurse Educ Pract* 13:18–22, 2013.
18. Lim FA: Nursing as a virtue: Strategies for value education. *Medsurg Nurs* 22(4):10, 2013.
19. MacIntosh J: Reworking professional nursing identity. *West J Nurs Res* 25(6):725–741, 2003.
20. Noble C, Coombes I, Shaw PN, et al: Becoming a pharmacist: The role of curriculum in professional identity formation. *Pharm Pract (Granada)* 12(1):380, 2014.
21. Ohlen J, Segesten K: The professional identity of the nurse: Concept analysis and development. *J Adv Nurs* 28(4):720–727, 1998.
22. Thompson JL, Mallet-Boucher M, McCloskey C, et al: Educating nurses for the twenty-first century abilities based outcomes and assessing student learning in the context of democratic professionalism. *Int J Nurs Educ Scholarsh* 10(1):219–226, 2013.
23. Trede F, Macklin R, Bridges D: Professional identity development: A review of higher education literature. *Stud High Educ* 37(3):365–384, 2012.
24. Wong A, Trollope-Kumar K: Reflections: An inquiry into medical students' professional identity formation. *Med Educ* 48:489–501, 2014.
25. American Association of Colleges of Nursing: *Baccalaureate essentials for professional nursing practice*, Washington, DC, 2008, Author.
26. American Association of Colleges of Nursing: *Expectations for practice experiences in the RN to baccalaureate curriculum*, Washington, DC, 2012, Author.
27. Crigger N, Godfrey N: *The making of nurse professionals: A transformational, ethical approach*, Sudbury, MA, 2011, Jones & Bartlett.
28. Khalili H, Hall J, DeLuca S: Historical analysis of professionalism in Western societies: Implications for interprofessional education and collaborative practice. *J Interprof Care* 28(2):92–97, 2014.
29. Benner P: Formation in professional education: An examination of the relationship between theories of meaning and theories of the self. *J Med Philos* 36:342–353, 2011.

30. Colby A, Sullivan WD: Formation of professionalism and purpose: Perspectives from the preparation for the professions program. *Univ St Thomas Law J* 5(2):404–426, 2008.

31. Marcia J, Josselson R: Eriksonian personality research and its implications for psychotherapy. *J Pers* 81(6):617–629, 2013.

32. Bandura A: *Social learning theory*, New York, 1971, General Learning Press.

33. Merriam SB: The role of cognitive development in Mezirow's transformational learning theory. *Adult Educ Q* 55(1):60–68, 2004.

34. Del Prato D: Student voices: The lived experience of faculty incivility as a barrier to professional formation in associate degree nursing education. *Nurse Educ Today* 33(3):286–290, 2013.

35. Severinsson E, Sand A: Evaluation of the clinical supervision and professional development of student nurses. *J Nurs Manag* 18:669–677, 2010.

36. Goodolf D: *Growing a professional identity: A grounded theory of the educational experience of baccalaureate nursing students*, dissertation abstract. Chester, PA, 2013, Widener University.

37. American Association of Colleges of Nursing, American Association of Colleges of Osteopathic Medicine, American Association of Colleges of Pharmacy, American Dental Education Association, Association of American Medical Colleges, Association of Schools of Public Health: *The core competencies for interprofessional collaborative practice*, Washington, DC, 2011, Interprofessional Education Collaborative.

38. Lingard L, Resnick R, Espin S: Forming professional identities on the health care team: Discursive constructions of the "other" in the operating room. *Med Educ* 36(8):728–734, 2002.

39. Jakobsen F, Hanson TB, Eika B: Knowing more about the other professions clarified my own profession. *J Interprof Care* 25(6):441–446, 2011.

40. Helmich E, Derksen E, Prevoo M, et al: Medical students' professional identity development in an early nursing attachment. *Med Educ* 44(7):674–682, 2010.

41. Williams C: *Factors that relate to registered nurse readiness for interprofessional learning in the context of continuing professional development*, dissertation abstract. Berrien Springs, MI, 2014, Andrews University.

42. Adams K, Hean S, Sturgis P, et al: Investigating the factors influencing professional identity of first year health and social care students. *Learning Health Social Care* 5(2):55–68, 2006.

43. Horton-Deutsch S, Sherwood G: Reflection: An educational strategy to develop emotionally competent nurse leaders. *J Nurs Manag* 16(8):946–954, 2008.

44. Fitzpatrick JJ: Educating our students regarding the standards of professional practice and professional performance. *Nurs Educ Perspect* 35(3):143, 2014.

45. Crigger N, Godfrey N: From the inside out: A new approach to teaching professional identity formation and professional ethics. *J Prof Nurs* 30:376–382, 2014.

46. Bandura A: Self-efficacy. In *Corsini encyclopedia of psychology*, New York, 2010, Wiley.

47. Pellegrino ED, Thomasma DC: *The virtues in medical practice*, New York, 1993, Oxford University Press US.

48. American Nurses Association: *Code of ethics for nurses with interpretive statements*, Washington, DC, 2015, American Nurses Publishing.

Clinical Judgment

Ann Nielsen and Kathie Lasater

The delivery of health care in general and the practice of nursing have become very complex. Larger numbers of patients with complicated medical conditions and health care financing and reimbursement have become major determinants of health care practices and policies; thus patients with interrelated comorbidities are now admitted to acute care settings for shorter periods of time, and sicker patients are cared for in community-based settings, such as home health and long-term care.[1] There is increasing evidence that acute deterioration in patients goes unrecognized by nurses and therefore nursing responses and/or referrals are delayed, putting patient safety at risk.[2,3] More than simple knowledge acquisition is needed to support increased recognition and appropriate responses.[2]

The increased complexity requires nurses to provide care in situations in which patients' conditions may be changing rapidly. Ebright concluded that nurses in acute care medical–surgical settings must prioritize or "restack" patient care tasks multiple times throughout a shift.[4] This restacking involves a myriad of unexpected events that necessitate reorganizing tasks, such as changes to patient schedules, changing patient conditions, multiple discharges and admissions, and patient care staffing issues. Between the restacked tasks, nurses engage in a thinking process that results in crucial decisions about patient care, often with little time to think about or plan for the next steps. The foundation of safe and effective nursing practice is the ability to consistently make good clinical judgments. Clinical judgment as a concept is presented from a theoretical perspective to help the student gain an understanding of the complexities of this process.

DEFINITION

The concept of clinical judgment in general refers to interpretations and inferences that influence actions in clinical practice. The most recent nursing literature uses the term *clinical judgment* as an inference or interpretation made in a caregiving setting,[5–10] a process resulting in such an inference or interpretation,[7–17] or the capacity for making inferences or interpretations about patient care.[6,7,12,15,17,18] The definition of clinical judgment used for this concept presentation is "*an interpretation or conclusion about a patient's needs, concerns, or health problems, and/or the decision to take action (or not), use or modify standard approaches, or improvise new ones as deemed appropriate by the patient's response.*"[9,p204]

Two other terms, clinical reasoning and critical thinking, are often used interchangeably in the literature with the term clinical judgment; thus differentiation is needed. *Clinical reasoning* is the thinking process by which a nurse reaches a clinical judgment.[10,19] It is defined as "an iterative process of noticing, interpreting, and responding—reasoning in transition with a fine attunement to the patient and how the patient responds to the nurse's actions."[12,p230] Encompassed in clinical reasoning is the ability to perceive the relevance of scientific evidence and its fit with the specific patient situation.[20]

Herein lies the complexity of nursing: Clinical judgments require that the nurse recognize the unique situation of the patient, originating from deep knowledge of a variety of interrelated physiologic and psychosocial concepts resulting in a profound understanding of the clinical situation. In other words, clinical judgment requires the nurse to apply knowledge, both tacit and explicit, to the unique patient situation to make sense of it and respond appropriately in the specific context of care.

SCOPE

Standards-Based Approach

Early research behind clinical judgment focused on trying to understand all the factors involved in clinical judgments about patient care, making them explicit. This resulted in a rules-based or standards-based approach that located the nurse and the individual needs of the patient outside the caregiving situation rather than situating the specific patient issue in a context of care. Decision making from this perspective involves selection from options of mutually exclusive possibilities, implying that there is one right decision. This approach often involves use of algorithms, decision trees, and patient care guidelines. These tools provide clear-cut guidance that standardize approaches to patient care within an institution based on best practices for a typical patient population and are important to general patient care quality. Algorithms direct care in emergent situations, such as a cardiopulmonary arrest, that involve multiple personnel from several disciplines. These standardized tools can be very useful to support safe patient care, especially for the beginning clinician who lacks knowledge and/or experience. However, their use may or may not result in the best possible care for a particular patient in a given situation. They also may limit options and creative solutions.

A principle that relates decision-making tools to clinical judgment is that if there is a rule that covers the situation, clinical judgment is not required. Also, clinical judgment may be required in decision making about whether or not a given standard is applicable or appropriate in a given patient care situation.[20] In fact, research has shown that although standards or guidelines may be useful beginning points, expert nurses rarely use them alone.[9,20] This is because the expert nurse nuances his or her understanding of the individual patient situation along with knowledge of standards to employ a much more interpretivist approach.

Evidence-Based Practice and Clinical Judgment

All clinicians are expected to use the best evidence to inform practice. Use of evidence-based guidelines, informed by research, improves patient outcomes.[21] It is important to note that clinical judgment is an integral aspect of safe implementation of evidence-based practice (EBP). EBP is defined by the Agency for Healthcare Quality and Research as "applying the best available research results (evidence) when making decisions about health care. Health care professionals who perform evidence-based practice use research evidence along with clinical expertise and patient preferences."[22]

As implied in the definition, EBP is implemented with clinical judgment. Safe and effective nursing care requires scientific knowledge, as well as practical experience, to understand when particular research evidence is relevant.[2,20] The nurse must accurately assess the patient and care context and then apply EBPs that are most appropriate in a given situation. Clinical judgment also guides nurses to question current practices and consider when guidelines need to be updated.[20]

Interpretivist Perspective

Interpretivist approaches originate from the belief that life experiences are culturally bound, that individuals interpret these experiences on the basis of their encounters within a given culture,[23] and that one circumscribed approach is often not appropriate for a large number of patients.[9] The nature of nursing care is not linear, and in fact, in numerous situations there are many unknowns; therefore, approaches that consider multiple factors in clinical reasoning are often more appropriate.[9] Because there are often no clear-cut answers about nursing care or because of the influence of the individual patient circumstances and context of care, clinical judgments by nurses become very specific to a given patient care situation. Interpretivist approaches situate the nurse squarely in the context of care and account for what the nurse personally contributes to the caring encounter, including previous experiences, values, and emotions.[12] The creation or construction of understanding the patient and caregiving situation using empirical knowledge, knowledge of the patient, and knowledge of the clinical environment facilitates decisions about care, thereby setting the stage for what the nurse notices and how the nurse interprets and responds.[9,12,24]

Reasoning in interpretivist approaches may involve "rule of thumb" methods and be intuitive. It involves understood knowledge,[25] is often inductive in nature, and is referred to by some authors as engaged, practical reasoning.[9,12,15,26] In contrast, rules-based approaches tend to rely heavily on analytic reasoning that requires systematically dividing a situation into parts, examining alternatives, and weighing options.[9] One example of the analytic approach is diagnostic reasoning—considering the evidence that supports each diagnosis.[27]

ATTRIBUTES AND CRITERIA

Using the interpretivist perspective of clinical judgment and clinical reasoning from the nursing literature, clinical judgment has three significant defining attributes that are useful to understand the concept:

- *Holistic view of the patient situation*: Clinical judgment is inherently complex and influenced by many factors related to the particular patient and caregiving situation, and it therefore requires a holistic view.[12,14,15,25] Making excellent clinical judgments requires a willingness to consider all factors involved in patient care, including certain characteristics of the nurse, and is much more than simply a combination of the individual aspects.[9,14]

- *Process orientation*: Clinical judgment is circular, interactive, and moves fluidly between and among all of the aspects of the process.[8,9,12,15] To make clinical judgments, the nurse employs a deep understanding of the individual patient situation and his or her own background, experience, and values. Patients and nurses are unique and bring different backgrounds to the caregiving situation. The nurse notices salient (or relevant) features of a situation based on these factors and intervenes. While the nurse observes the patient response, he or she determines what the next steps are going to be. After the caregiving situation, the nurse connects the patient outcomes in a way that enhances further understanding of future patients' care, utilizing reflection.[9,11,16,24,28] These aspects do not have a linear relationship but, rather, continuously influence each other in complex ways.

- *Reasoning and interpretation*: Clinical judgment involves reasoning and interpretation. As described previously, reasoning is the process that leads to clinical judgments. At least three types of reasoning are used: analytic, intuitive, and narrative.[9] The type of reasoning used depends on the caregiving situation and the nurse's previous experience. When a situation is unfamiliar, the nurse (expert and novice alike) tends to rely on analytic reasoning processes, consider the possibilities, and deduce the solution. At other times, the expert nurse may recognize a situation immediately and act intuitively and tacitly. Nurses may also process their reasoning in narrative form— that is, recognizing the significance of the situation at hand to the patient's experience with illness and engaging in interventions based on this understanding.

THEORETICAL LINKS

The model of clinical judgment is a comprehensive approach to clinical judgment that was developed based on three decades of clinical judgment research and through an extensive review of research done primarily with expert nurses in practice.[9] The model (Figure 40-1) rests on assumptions about complexities in the environment of care and the interplay of multiple factors that affect nurses' clinical thinking. In the model, four aspects of clinical judgments are described. Influenced by background and contextual factors, the nurse *notices* various things about the caregiving situation, such as clinical assessment findings, lab work, data, patient demeanor, and family situation. Through clinical reasoning patterns, collecting additional clinical data as needed, and conferring with colleagues, the nurse develops an understanding of the particular clinical situation—a process called *interpreting*. Based on the interpretation of the situation, the nurse determines appropriate actions, which is termed *responding* in the model. The nurse observes the patient's reaction to the nursing action and decides if the action has addressed the primary concerns, if the action needs some refinement to adjust for

FIGURE 40-1 Tanner's Model of Clinical Judgment Source: Adapted from Tanner CA: Thinking like a nurse: A research-based model of clinical judgment, *J Nurs Educ* 45(6):204–211, 2006. Reprinted with permission from SLACK Incorporated.

the particular patient, or if a completely different response is required. This is referred to as *reflection-in-action*. Nursing reflection after the fact, *reflection-on-action*, helps the nurse to connect patient responses with outcomes in a way that contributes to the nurse's further understanding of patient care.[9] Despite the fact that these aspects are described in separate sections, they do not have a linear relationship but, rather, continuously influence each other in a complex manner. Thus the consideration of them as separate aspects may be artificial but is offered here as an in-depth means to better understand the concept.

Noticing

Noticing is most often the impetus for clinical reasoning and is critical to making an effective judgment to address a patient issue. Several important factors impact what the nurse notices. In fact, Tanner asserts that the factors behind the nurse's eyes are as important as what is in front.[9] These include the background of the nurse (including intrapersonal characteristics, ethical grounding for what is right, previous experiences, and theoretical knowledge), the nurse's relationship with the patient, and the context of care (for more detail about these precursors to noticing, see Box 40-1). Influenced by these factors, the nurse develops expectations about potential patient needs that set the stage for *noticing*. Expectations derived from the nurse's experiences with similar patients allow the nurse to anticipate the patient's appearance and needs, both currently and in the next hours and days. Without these experiences, the nurse uses theoretical, decontextualized knowledge.

The nurse enters the care situation and collects pertinent information and patient data. Broad knowledge based on experience and theoretical understanding as well as understanding a particular context allows nurses to notice what factors are the most salient in terms of caring for a particular patient. Nurses select from a very broad set of data and patient assessment findings, searching for patterns that are consistent with previous experiences and using that information to guide care in the current situation. Less experienced nurses may have

BOX 40-1 Factors that Influence Noticing

Intrapersonal Characteristics of the Nurse
- Ethical grounding and personal sense of importance
- Trustworthiness—asking questions/seeking help when unsure
- Developmental maturity in thought and knowing processes; formulates opinions and values relative to the context of learning
- Skill in using various ways of knowing—empirical, experiential, and ethical

Theoretical and Experiential Knowledge of the Nurse
- Novice and less experienced nurses use deductive reasoning, rules, and comparisons of the patient with the textbook in a systematic analysis of the situation.
- Expert nurses look at the whole picture and use pattern recognition and intuition derived from their experiences to make judgments.

Knowing the Patient
- Knowing the range of patient's pattern of responses
- Knowing the patient as a person, including preferences and desires

Context or Environment of Care
- Setting in which the nurse interacts with the patient
- Unique aspects of nursing practice/patient care needs in a given setting

difficulty extracting the most important patient data and findings in a particular situation.[12,29]

Knowing the patient (whether it is knowing a given type of patient or knowing a specific patient) in a particular context influences what a nurse notices. For example, a home health nurse who has made visits to an older adult patient in his home over several months has a different level of "knowing the patient" than a nurse who sees a patient in an acute care setting. Knowing the older adult allows the home health nurse to know the patient's baseline mental status and to notice subtle changes in cognition or affect. The nurse assuming care for this same patient in an acute care setting might not realize that medication-related confusion demonstrated by the patient postoperatively is not typical for this patient and might make the assumption that the patient has dementia or other cognitive impairment.

Based on what is noticed, the nurse may have an immediate grasp of the situation—recognition of a pattern or cluster of cues that signals one concern. On other occasions, the nurse, despite extensive experience, may have noticed that the situation is not as expected but does not quite have a clear grasp. Depending on this initial understanding, various reasoning patterns may be triggered. Once an issue is noticed, the nurse immediately gathers additional information and draws on his or her background, including theoretical knowledge, past experiences with similar patients as well as his or her relationship and knowledge of this particular patient within the specific context of care, and ethical beliefs about what is right in this situation. Because each individual nurse and patient and the context of care are different, what happens next is also very unique; in many situations, there is no one correct way.

Interpreting

Using the particular patient data as well as germane theoretical and experiential knowledge, the nurse begins to assemble all the information to make sense of it. For the expert nurse, certain data carry more weight than others with respect to the patient. For example, in the long-term care setting, a patient's age and kidney function may well impact the nurse's clinical judgment about using ibuprofen for pain relief even though the drug may be ordered. The nurse uses reasoning to make that determination.

According to Tanner, expert nurses draw on a variety of reasoning patterns (analytic, intuitive, and narrative) to interpret the meaning of what has been noticed.[9] The types of reasoning used seem to vary with the experience of the nurse.[12] For example, students and novice nurses, or more experienced nurses encountering unfamiliar situations, tend to rely on analytic reasoning based on theoretical knowledge. The nurse makes a hypothesis or best guess about the patient care situation and then tests the hypothesis. Sometimes this reasoning is not situation specific but, rather, based on generalizations. Expert nurses often use intuitive reasoning based on unstated but understood knowledge about the patient, the caregiving context, and their previous experiences.[12,30] A third type of reasoning, narrative reasoning, is a way of making sense of a situation through telling and interpreting stories.[9,31] Narrative reasoning supports deep understanding of caregiving situations.[9,12] Nurses hear patients' stories of their experiences with illness, how they understand their symptoms, what meaning they attribute to their illness, how they cope with it, and what they hope for resolution. This type of reasoning helps nurses understand the specific patient experience, setting the stage for individualizing care.[9] Nurses may also use narrative reasoning in their own reflections about patient care.

Responding

Once the patient data have been sorted and interpreted, the nurse uses his or her interpretation to respond to the particular patient issue through one or more nursing interventions. Depending on the level of expertise, the nurse may or may not be able to judge the effectiveness of the intervention before initiating it. For example, the nurse knows that the ordered pain medication is likely to help the newly admitted postoperative patient with a pain level of 8 out of 10. What the nurse may not know is what dose will be effective or the level to which it will reduce the patient's pain. The nurse's past experience with and knowledge about the effects of the pain medication will initially direct the

dosage the nurse chooses. As the nurse comes to understand the particular patient's response to the medication and dosage required, the reasoning process moves from primarily analytic to more intuitive/narrative.

Reflecting

Many theorists have described reflective thinking and its usefulness. In fact, an early 20th-century educator made the bold statement that "reflective thinking alone is educative."[32,p2] Other theorists consider that reflection and the ability to learn from one's actions are marks of a professional.[33] The clinical judgment model includes two types of reflection: reflection-*in*-action and reflection-*on*-action. Both have significant bearing on clinical judgment.

Reflection-in-Action

Reflection-in-action refers to the nurse's understanding of patient responses to nursing actions while care is occurring.[9] In observations and interactions with the patient, the nurse determines patient status and adjusts care accordingly. It is the thinking that happens in "real time" during patient care. Because of the ambiguous and complex nature of clinical judgments and the particular needs of each patient, reflecting is a critical step in evaluating the patient's reaction to the intervention. To continue the example of the postoperative patient, the nurse chooses a pain medication dose based on many factors; while administering the medication intravenously, the nurse is continually assessing and reflecting on the patient's response to medication. This is an example of reflecting-in-action. If the desired response is not achieved, the nurse may need to return to interpreting the data in order to respond with a different intervention.

Reflection-on-Action

Reflection-on-action is consideration of the situation after the patient care occurs. In reflection-on-action, the nurse contemplates a situation and considers what was successful and what was unsuccessful. Reflection-on-action is critical for development of knowledge and improvement in reasoning. It is how learning from practice is incorporated into personal experience for consideration in future patient care situations.[34] In the previous example, the nurse may take some time at the end of his or her shift to analyze why he or she intervened in a specific way for this particular patient and to consider whether the intervention was successful. Reflection-on-action is when significant learning from practice occurs and is important to the development of increasing skillfulness as a nurse.[31,34,35] Often, nurses spend more time reflecting on negative results, but it is equally important to consider successful interventions in order to improve practice.

Nurses may use verbal narrative to engage in reflection-on-action, to make sense of their own experiences and to process thinking. Listen to nurses in clinical settings when they talk; they often tell stories about their patients, especially if some aspect of care is perplexing. Telling stories is often a way of problem solving or learning from the experiences of others.

CONTEXT TO NURSING AND HEALTH CARE

All Nurses, All Settings

Clinical judgment is an integral aspect of nursing care of all patients and patient populations. Nurses in all specialty areas and practice settings—whether in public health nursing, community-based nursing, long-term care, or acute care—exercise clinical judgment; thus it is considered an essential skill of the professional nurse.[30] Clinical judgment, however, is not required for every patient care activity or intervention. Some nursing actions are obvious. For example, a postanesthesia recovery nurse knows that it is appropriate to take an immediate postoperative patient's vital signs quite frequently in the first few hours in order to recognize early signs of a problem. This is based on the nurse's knowledge that patients can sometimes have breathing or circulatory difficulties following administration of a general anesthetic and surgical interventions. The nurse also knows that the earlier such a sign or symptom is identified, the better the outcome for the patient.

Environmental Context

As mentioned previously, the context or setting of care influences what a nurse notices. The specific environment of care also has a significant influence on care. Demanding environments of care can add increasing burden to making clinical judgments[4,8,9,24] and can actually interfere with competent clinical judgment.[36] On the other hand, context may also be a boon for easing the burden of clinical judgments. For example, consider the case of a patient experiencing a myocardial infarction in the emergency department, where a wide range of medications, including oxygen, are readily available. Monitoring devices are already on the patient and, in fact, may have signaled an impending life-threatening dysrhythmia. Nurses in this context are trained to respond quickly and confidently; because of the setting, they are anticipating emergent situations. By contrast, consider the nurse who encounters a person experiencing a myocardial infarction in a public setting, such as a park or a church. Very different actions must be employed, including making a decision about what to do first, who should call for help, who should be involved in the resuscitation process, and how long resuscitation should be continued.

Experience, Theoretical Knowledge, and Expertise

Clinical judgment, or thinking like a nurse, requires deep clinical knowledge and several types of thinking. Not surprisingly, deep clinical knowledge provides the nurse with the background needed to recognize patterns and therefore differences when they occur in patients, signaling the need for nursing care. As nurses become more experienced, clinical judgments become more intuitive, with nurses instantly recognizing patterns and grasping the meaning of situations they have previously encountered to immediately know what their response to the situation should be. As such, it may appear that experienced nurses have not engaged in all aspects of clinical judgment, but, in fact, all aspects may occur almost simultaneously and subconsciously.[9] Inexperienced nurses (novices) tend to treat all pieces of information with similar importance. They have difficulty identifying the most important aspects of a given situation. Early in practice, it is more challenging to individualize and contextualize patient care. Expert nurses look at the whole picture and use pattern recognition and intuition derived from their experiences to make judgments, whereas those with less experience most often use deductive reasoning, rules, and comparisons of the patient with the textbook in a systematic analysis of the situation.[9,12,26,27,37,38]

Consider the experienced nurse in a clinic-based setting, such as an internal medicine clinic. Through honing his or her cardiopulmonary assessment skills over a number of years, the nurse has become familiar with the early signs of impending acute congestive heart failure. A nurse new to that clinic may not as readily recognize the pattern of breathing correlated with patient color, including the nuanced blue tinge of oral mucous membranes, and complaints of increased fatigue with activities of daily living. The outcome of such experience may well be faster initiation of treatment for this patient, thereby preventing a hospitalization.

This concept has introduced the idea that students and novice nurses rely on theoretical knowledge and analytic reasoning to make clinical judgments. That theoretical grounding is very important to student nurse practice and beyond. Understanding the principles of nursing care, communication, altered states of health, patient teaching, and other aspects of care is fundamental to becoming a nurse. As students and novice nurses acquire more experience, thinking, and clinical judgment, they use previous experiences, along with an understanding of this particular patient, the current context, and the best available, relevant evidence to ground their thinking about patient care. In fact, one study found that preceptors believed that new graduate nurses were ready for independent practice when they were able to integrate multiple sources of knowing and individualize care to the patient.[15] Recent evidence suggests that certain strategies promote development of clinical judgment.[5] With that in mind, the next section explores ways to facilitate clinical judgment development.

Developing Clinical Judgment

Acquisition of clinical judgment is a developmental process.[39] Novice nurses and nursing students often admire nurses who possess high-level clinical judgment skills. Taking advantage of a wide range of clinical learning opportunities and working closely with experienced nurses foster clinical judgment. Analyzing situations in which appropriate nursing actions are not obvious or clear-cut can enhance development of clinical judgment. Search for factors that impact the judgments that are made—nursing values, theoretical knowledge, previous experiences, knowing the patient, and the patient care environment. Consider how these factors influence the situation. Simulation is commonly used in nursing programs to supplement learning in clinical situations. Learning in simulation can contribute to clinical judgment skills,[40,41] including skill in care of patients with acute deterioration in patient status.[3,42]

Knowledge or Deep Understanding

Knowing how to respond to a patient issue requires a deep knowledge of the complex interconnected factors that impact the issue.[43] This includes theoretical knowledge about the patient population, relevant physiology and pathophysiology, and potential nursing interventions.[20,44] For example, in maternal–newborn nursing, a deep understanding of the birthing process is essential. However, knowledge of interconnected concepts—such as the normal and problematic signs of impending delivery, the physiological transition of hormonal influences in the immediate postdelivery phase (both physical and psychological), and also the potential impact of a new member on the family's dynamics—will facilitate the nurse's clinical judgments in that context of care. In this example, the nurse will need specialty-specific knowledge about lab findings, subtle signs of depression, and community resources/supports that are available for new mothers. Deep knowledge provides a basis for focused assessments, including salient factors, and for interpreting findings that lead to appropriate clinical judgments, specific to the patient's needs.

Learning to Recognize Patterns

Pattern recognition of specific conditions is a significant aspect of noticing and interpreting patient care needs and leads to a deeper understanding of patient issues.[45] For instance, a patient with septic shock will likely display a pattern of elevated heart rate, poor perfusion, decreased oxygen saturation, low blood pressure, and a left shift on the white blood cell count differential. Knowing this pattern alerts the student or nurse to note what signs or symptoms may be present or absent in order to determine an appropriate response. As students and nurses gain more experience, patterns related to nursing care become more apparent.

Apply Concepts to Nursing Practice

Search for opportunities to learn about patient care concepts; then compare and contrast how the concepts present in various patients in order to see patterns.[45] For example, consider how a particular patient with sepsis matches the pattern of sepsis just described as well as what signs or symptoms are different.[46] Then consider how the context (caregiving situation, your own values, knowing the patient and his or her specific personal qualities and needs, and your own past nursing and personal experiences with the concept) impacts the particular caregiving situation. This may help you to recognize how the specific situation influences the nursing response to the individual patient with sepsis.

Another opportunity to do this might occur on a pediatric rotation. In this rotation, you may care for a patient with respiratory problems that require oxygen, perhaps a patient with asthma. Consider why your patient is receiving supplemental oxygen and other factors (physical, developmental, and pathophysiological) that impact oxygenation and oxygen administration to your patient. Then visit another student's patient who is also administered oxygen, perhaps a patient with pneumonia. Consider the same questions for your classmate's patient. Compare and contrast the two patients. What are the similarities? What are the differences? What learning will you apply to future situations?

Skillful Responding

An important aspect of responding involves setting priorities and modifying them as the situation changes. Pay attention to how RN preceptors prioritize patient care. Consider the factors they use to make decisions about planning and replanning their shift. Discuss prioritization of care as a part of your daily routine in clinical. Identify the resources in the clinical setting that support skill-related decision making and performance, such as procedure references. Think about what you might expect the patient response to the intervention might be, and then observe the actual response.[46,47]

Reflective Practice

Reflection is a learning activity included in many nursing programs and with good reason. Reflecting helps students to process and consolidate learning about caregiving situations.[31,35] Reflection on clinical experiences can support application of theoretical knowledge to clinical situations and improve prioritization of future nursing care.[34,48] As a student and as a practicing nurse, it is important to reflect on both successful and unsuccessful interventions during a caregiving experience. Nursing students are often acutely aware of their knowledge deficits as well as their shortcomings in performing a particular nursing skill. Although recognizing the need for improvement and analyzing how that will happen are critically significant parts of nursing practice, it is important to reinforce in one's mind those things that you did well.

Telling stories about practice is often a part of clinical post-conference and journaling and is integral to reflective learning.[48] By being an active part of this important learning opportunity and considering carefully the patients described by classmates, students multiply their exposure to different patient issues and gain deeper understanding of nursing practice.[34,40,49] Questioning each other and expressing different possibilities can help students broaden their thinking about nursing care options. Fostering personal habits of reflection during nursing school, whether individually in writing or in group discussions, provides a strong foundation for continued learning through reflection when one enters practice.

INTERRELATED CONCEPTS

Several concepts in this textbook are interrelated to the concept of clinical judgment—in fact, all concepts related to patient care activities have this link. Featured in Figure 40-2 are seven concepts that are especially closely related to clinical judgment.

Clinical judgment is integral to the **Safety** of patients. Consider the situation of an older adult postoperative patient getting up to walk postoperatively for the first time. The nurse may know that particular

FIGURE 40-2 Clinical Judgment and Interrelated Concepts

caution should be exercised because falls are very common in the hospital context, and there may be unit guidelines regarding fall prevention. From theoretical knowledge, the nurse knows that although falling is a danger when ambulating, there are significant dangers associated with immobility and staying in bed. In making the decision to get the patient up, the nurse considers many factors, including the patient's level of consciousness, strength, pain control status, motivation, and environmental context. The nurse's previous experiences with ambulating older adult patients will significantly inform his or her decisions.

The nurse who is committed to high-quality patient care is alert to patterns that may indicate that there are concerns for **Health Care Quality** in a given hospital unit or agency. For example, if medications consistently arrive from pharmacy in mid-morning rather than early in the shift, some nurses become involved in other caregiving activities and then forget to administer the medications once they arrive on the unit. Based on theoretical knowledge, the nurse recognizes this as a systems problem. Experiential knowledge of unit culture and organization informs how the nurse takes action to communicate with the unit manager and the pharmacy in order to get medications to the unit on time.

Leadership choices are almost always fraught with multiple competing factors. For example, the charge nurse of an adult medical–surgical unit may have to consider the mix of nursing staff needed for a shift, given the patients' acuity. What staffing combination will best serve the needs of the patients on the unit at any given moment? The charge nurse may need to respond by asking for help at a higher level if the staffing mix is inadequate. On the same unit, an individual nurse may delegate certain aspects of more stable patients' care to a certified nursing assistant, allowing greater focus on those more seriously ill. These kinds of leadership choices are dependent on knowing the patient(s) as well as the backgrounds of the nursing staff.

Determining when and how much **Patient Education** a patient and/or family needs frequently requires clinical judgment. A patient newly diagnosed with diabetes needs to know about diet, medication, exercise, and foot care, how to perform blood glucose monitoring, and medication administration. Because it is impossible for a patient to learn everything in one visit, the home health nurse must assess the patient's knowledge and prioritize information. Depending on the patient's ability and ease of learning, the nurse may need to use clinical judgment to refine her teaching to best address the patient's needs. Clinical judgment is exercised throughout the entire learning process—noticing how much the patient remembers from the last visit and assessing learning outcomes.

In making clinical judgments, nurses consider a variety of **Evidence** from research studies, clinical guidelines, and standards of care. The nurse may also use evidence from past experiences with "what works" for patient care within a particular unit culture, as well as practice experiences with a given patient ("knowing the patient") or understanding other contextual factors that impact a caregiving situation. The best available evidence may well impact how the nurse interprets a patient situation and responds to it, but other factors impact nursing actions as well. Using clinical judgment, values regarding individualizing patient care, and knowledge of the patient, the nurse identifies additional needs and resources and then advocates for the patient in order to meet the unique needs.

Clinical judgment is applied in situations in which the nurse relies on **Professional Identity** in interactions with patients and/or their families. Consider the patient who is newly diagnosed with late-stage lung cancer. The nurse caring for this patient will need to notice the patient's mood and level of interest to determine when the patient needs information about hospice care. The nurse may also have firsthand experience with a family member who had a similar diagnosis. Is there an appropriate opportunity for the nurse to relate to and encourage this patient's family, based on that experience, or is it better with this particular family to focus only on their experience? This situation requires careful noticing and interpretation.

Clinical judgment is used in **Care Coordination** situations to help the patient achieve optimal health care outcomes. When planning an older adult patient's discharge after a motor vehicle accident resulting in multiple fractures, the nurse may uncover information that is critical for coordinating the patient's care—information about a patient's home situation that will impact the older adult's recovery. Based on previous experiences with complicated patients, the nurse may request a case conference with members of the health care team, patient, and family in order to foster the transition for a quality outcome.

CLINICAL EXEMPLARS

Clinical judgment is applied in all areas of nursing practice; thus there are multiple examples. Box 40-2 presents five general areas in which nurses potentially apply clinical judgment within practice: application of clinical skills, recognizing and responding to urgent/emergent situations, communication, medication management, and management of care.

BOX 40-2 EXEMPLARS OF CLINICAL JUDGMENT

Clinical Skills
- Decisions about urinary or intravenous catheter placement, such as determination regarding size and type of urinary or intravenous catheter or whether placement is needed
- Decisions about timing and extent of bathing and personal care
- Assessment of a wound and determining next steps
- Selection of an appropriate dressing

Urgent/Emergent Situations
- Detection of subtle signs of sepsis
- Early treatment of patient hemorrhage
- Starting oxygen to respond to decreased saturation levels
- Early recognition of anaphylaxis

Communication
- Content and depth of patient teaching at discharge, pre- and postoperatively
- Advocacy for patient at care coordination conferences
- Communication with distraught or fearful patient or family
- Defusing potentially confrontational interactions

Medication Management
- Selection of dose when a range is ordered
- PRN decisions
- Holding a medication
- Early recognition of adverse reaction or side effect from medication

Management of Care and Nursing Leadership
- Delegation to ancillary nursing personnel
- Prioritization of care among patients
- Calling a physician
- Referral to another health professional (e.g., wound care specialist, dietitian)
- Decisions about patient assignments

Featured Exemplars
Clinical Skills: Determining Type of Catheter

A nurse caring for an older adult postoperative patient with anesthesia-associated urinary retention needs to make a decision about whether to catheterize the patient, and if so if a straight catheterization procedure or placing a Foley (retention) catheter would be best. The nurse considers the evidence, unit policy for catheter placement, and his knowledge of his patient, including mobility, cognitive status, and preferences. From clinical experience, he estimates how long the typical older adult might experience anesthesia-related urinary retention. Contextual knowledge may include the time of day; for example, placement of a Foley catheter may allow the patient to rest through the night.

Management of Care: Patient Assignments

On a busy day in an adult surgical unit, the charge nurse must decide to whom a newly admitted patient should be assigned. She uses her background knowledge of general patient care on the unit and unit policy regarding nurse/patient ratios and the current context of care involved in the patients on the unit. She also uses her knowledge of the nursing staff. Does someone have particularly strong organizational skills or knowledge about the anticipated care needs of the patient to be admitted? The experienced nurse leader realizes that safe patient assignment goes well beyond abiding by the unit guidelines for patient/nurse ratios.

Urgent/Emergent Situation: Child with Sepsis

The nurse caring for a 4-year-old being treated for leukemia notices a blood pressure (BP) of 70/40. To interpret this reading, the nurse uses background and theoretical knowledge (normal BP for 4-year-olds and knowledge of this patient's usual BP trends over time). He considers contextual factors, including therapies the child is receiving that may lower blood pressure. Prompted by theoretical knowledge of presenting signs of sepsis, his previous experiences with septic patients, and awareness of the patient's risk factors, additional data are collected to determine if the patient's symptoms resemble sepsis. With these additional data, the nurse contacts the physician to discuss the next steps in the care.

Clinical Skills: Community-Based Client

A volunteer nurse at a free clinic sees a client just released from jail and living in a single-room occupancy hotel. The client has an open wound on his left hip. The client lives alone and has no family or close friends nearby who can assist. The nurse must use her background knowledge to select an appropriate dressing from a wide range of available materials and her knowledge of the patient to help the patient change the dressing. Safe patient care includes ensuring that patients can manage their own care, sometimes in challenging circumstances.

CASE STUDY

Source: metin Kiyak/iStock/Thinkstock

Case Presentation

Leon Rowen is a growing premature infant whose 32-year-old mother, Cassandra Rowen, is described by the nurses in the unit as "difficult." The baby is nearing discharge, but Cassandra is reported to be "resistant" to learning about how to feed and care for her infant. She has other children at home, but none of them were premature. A nursing care priority for the day is parental teaching about safe feeding of her premature baby.

Ruth, the nurse assigned to care for Leon, has worked in this unit for 10 years. She observes the entire caregiving situation and sees that Leon's condition is stable. Ruth meets Cassandra and notices she is quiet and sullen. Rather than beginning by explaining how to feed the baby, Ruth asks about Cassandra's other children and shares a little bit about the challenges of parenting her own children who are of similar ages as Cassandra's other children. Cassandra smiles

and agrees. As time passes, Cassandra begins to talk about what a frightening experience having a premature baby has been. Ruth acknowledges those feelings. Cassandra smiles and begins to ask questions about how to care for Leon. Ruth answers those questions in a way that is tailored to what the mother has revealed about her family. Cassandra demonstrates feeding Leon in a developmentally appropriate way (side-lying position to prevent aspiration) based on Ruth's teaching. At the end of the shift, Ruth believes Cassandra has made significant progress toward competence in meeting her baby's unique needs. On the drive home, Ruth considers the experience. She realizes that prioritizing getting to know the mother and building a relationship by sharing a bit about herself as a parent helped to create emotional safety and trust so that Cassandra could talk about her apprehension as a first-time mother of a premature baby and then focus on learning infant care.

Case Analysis

In this case study, Ruth's previous encounters with mothers of premature infants and her knowledge of the family experience inform her nursing actions. Experienced nurses incorporate much information simultaneously. Notice that Ruth determines that the baby's physiologic condition is stable while she is beginning to interact with the mother. In this action, she is prioritizing patient safety. While she interacts with the mother, Ruth may interpret Cassandra's behavior as a pattern sometimes displayed by mothers in the neonatal intensive care unit. She understands how frightening it is to have a hospitalized newborn and knows from experience that fear can take on many faces. This may be evidence of Ruth's intrapersonal characteristics that value empathy and consider the patient experience. Rather than focusing on Cassandra's negative response to her, Ruth focuses on relationship building before moving on to teaching. This action opens the door to effective teaching. Notice that Ruth takes some time afterward to consider what went well in this challenging situation. This will inform future interactions with mothers of patients.

REFERENCES

1. Institute of Medicine: *The future of nursing*, Washington, DC, 2010, Author.
2. Rattray JE, Lauder W, Ludwick R, et al: Indicators of acute deterioration in adult patients nursed in acute wards: A factorial survey. *J Clin Nurs* 20(5–6):723–732, 2011.
3. Lindsey PL, Jenkins S: Nursing students' clinical judgment regarding rapid response: The influence of a clinical simulation education intervention. *Nurs Forum* 8(1):61–70, 2013.
4. Ebright PR: The complex work of RNs: Implications for healthy work environments. *OJIN Online J Issues Nurs* 15(1):Manuscript 4, 2010.
5. Capelletti A, Engel J, Prentice D: Systematic review of clinical judgment and reasoning in nursing. *J Nurs Educ* 53(8):453–458, 2014.
6. Lasater K: Clinical judgment development: Using simulation to create an assessment rubric. *J Nurs Educ* 46(11):496–503, 2007.
7. Rhodes ML, Curran C: Use of the human patient simulator to teach clinical judgment skills in a baccalaureate nursing program. *Comput Inform Nurs* 23(5):256–262, 2005.
8. Samuels JG, Fetzer S: Pain management documentation quality as a reflection of nurses' clinical judgment. *J Nurs Care Qual* 24(3):223–231, 2009.
9. Tanner CA: Thinking like a nurse: A research-based model of clinical judgment in nursing. *J Nurs Educ* 45(6):204–211, 2006.
10. Victor-Chmil J: Critical thinking versus clinical reasoning versus clinical judgment: Differential diagnosis. *Nurse Educ* 38(1):34–36, 2013.
11. Becker D, Kaplow R, Muenzen PM, et al: Activities performed by acute and critical care advanced practice nurses: American Association of Critical-Care Nurses study of practice. *Am J Crit Care* 15(2):130–148, 2006.
12. Benner P, Tanner C, Chesla C: *Expertise in nursing practice: Caring, clinical judgment and ethics*, ed 2, New York, 2009, Springer.
13. del Bueno D: A crisis in critical thinking. *Nurs Educ Perspect* 26(5):278–282, 2005.
14. Di Vito-Thomas P: Nursing student stories on learning how to think like a nurse. *Nurs Educ* 30(3):133–136, 2005.
15. McNiesh S: Demonstrating holistic clinical judgment: Preceptors perceptions of new graduate nurses. *Holist Nurs Pract* 21(2):72–78, 2007.
16. Pesut DJ: Education: Clinical judgment—Foreground/background. *J Prof Nurs* 17(5):215, 2001.
17. Roberts K, Lockhart R, Sportsman S: A competency transcript to assess and personalize new graduate competency. *J Nurs Adm* 39(1):19–25, 2009.
18. Bambini D, Washburn J, Perkins R: Outcomes of clinical simulation for novice nursing students: Communication, confidence, and clinical judgment. *Nurs Educ Perspect* 30(2):79–82, 2009.
19. Simmons B: Clinical reasoning: Concept analysis. *J Adv Nurs* 66(5):1151–1158, 2010.
20. Benner P, Hughes RG, Sutphen M: Clinical reasoning, decision making, and action: Thinking critically and clinically. In Hughes RG, editor: *Patient safety and quality: An evidence-based handbook for nurses*, Rockville, MD, 2008, Agency for Healthcare Research and Quality, pp 1–23.
21. Agency for Healthcare Research and Quality: *Evidence-based decision making*, 2015. Retrieved from <http://www.ahrq.gov/professionals/prevention-chronic-care/decision/index.html>.
22. Agency for Healthcare Research and Quality: *Glossary of terms*, (n.d.). Retrieved from <http://effectivehealthcare.ahrq.gov/index.cfm/glossary-of-terms/?pageaction=showterm&termid=24>.
23. Crotty M: *The foundations of social research: Meaning and perspective in the research process*, London, 1998, Sage.
24. Kaplow R, Reed K: The AACN synergy model for patient care: A nursing model as a force of magnetism. *Nurs Econ* 26(1):17–25, 2008.
25. Braude HD: Clinical intuition versus statistics: Different modes of tacit knowledge in clinical epidemiology and evidence-based medicine. *Theor Med Bioeth* 30(3):181–198, 2009.
26. Wolf AW: Comment: Can clinical judgment hold its own against scientific knowledge? *Psychotherapy* 46(1):11–14, 2009.
27. Croskerry P: A universal model of diagnostic reasoning. *Acad Med* 84(8):1022–1028, 2009.
28. Redding DA: The development of critical thinking among students in baccalaureate nursing education. *Holist Nurs Pract* 15(4):57–64, 2001.
29. Benner P: *From novice to expert: Excellence and power in clinical nursing practice* [commemorative edition], Upper Saddle River, NJ, 2001, Prentice Hall.
30. Coles C: Developing professional judgment. *J Contin Educ Health Prof* 22:3–10, 2002.
31. Bruner J: *The culture of education*, Cambridge, MA, 1996, Harvard University Press.
32. Dewey J: *How we think: A restatement of the relation of reflective thinking to the educative process*, Chicago, 1933, Regnery.
33. Schön D: *Educating the reflective practitioner: Toward a new design for teaching and learning in the professions*, San Francisco, 1987, Jossey–Bass.
34. Glynn D: Clinical judgment development using structured classroom reflective practice: A qualitative study. *J Nurs Educ* 51(3):134–139, 2012.
35. Schön D: *The reflective practitioner: How professionals think in action*, New York, 1983, Basic Books.
36. Dillard N, Sideras S, Ryan M, et al: A collaborative project to apply and evaluate the clinical judgment model through simulation. *Nurs Educ Perspect* 30(2):99–104, 2009.
37. Burritt J, Steckel C: Supporting the learning curve for contemporary nursing practice. *J Nurs Adm* 39(11):479–484, 2009.
38. Busch F, Schmidt-Hellerau C: How can we know what we need to know? Reflections on clinical judgment formation. *J Am Psychoanal Assoc* 52(3):689–707, 2004.
39. Ashley J, Stamp K: Learning to think like a nurse: The development of clinical judgment in nursing students. *J Nurs Educ* 53(9):519–525, 2014.
40. Kelly M, Hager P, Gallagher R: What matters most? Students' rankings of simulation components that contribute to clinical judgment. *J Nurs Educ* 53(2):97–101, 2014.
41. Lasater K, Johnson E, Ravert P, et al: Role modeling clinical judgment for an unfolding older adult simulation. *J Nurs Educ* 53(5):257–264, 2014.
42. Fisher D, King L: An integrative literature review on preparing nursing students though simulation to recognize and respond to the deteriorating patient. *J Adv Nurs* 69(11):2375–2388, 2013.
43. Benner P, Sutphen M, Leonard V, et al: *Educating nurses: A call for radical transformation*, San Francisco, 2010, Jossey–Bass.
44. Modic MB: Tanner's model of clinical judgment applied to preceptorship: Part 1. *J Nurs Prof Dev* 29(5):274–275, 2013.
45. Modic MB: Tanner's model of clinical judgment applied to preceptorship: Part 2. *J Nurs Prof Dev* 29(6):335–337, 2013.
46. Modic MB: Developing skills in interpretation. *J Nurs Prof Dev* 30(1):274–275, 2014.
47. Modic MB: Clinical judgment: Developing the skill of responding. *J Nurs Prof Dev* 30(2):105–106, 2014.
48. Modic MB: Clinical judgment: Developing skills in reflection. *J Nurs Prof Dev* 30(3):157–158, 2014.
49. Lavoie P, Pepin J, Boyer L: Reflective debriefing to promote novice nurses' clinical judgment after high-fidelity simulation: A pilot test. *Dynamics* 24(4):36–41, 2013.

Leadership

Nancy Hoffart

Leadership is an old concept that applies to all aspects of life—from close to home, such as leading a family, to more distant situations, such as leading an international organization. Most people can name leaders in their experiences at school, work, and recreational and volunteer activities. Practical familiarity with the concept of leadership is gained through such experiences.

This concept presentation focuses on leadership as an essential aspect of the role of the registered nurse (RN). Registered nurses are summoned to be leaders as part of their daily work, and most RN competencies delineate leadership as an important capability for professional nurses. Nurses are expected to exhibit leadership when delivering patient care and when working with others to address issues that affect the practice of nursing.[1] Nurses also have been called on to play a leadership role in health policy and in shaping the health care system of the future.[2,3] This concept presentation introduces the general principles of leadership and their application in nursing and health care.

DEFINITION

Although there is a vast body of literature on leadership in work settings, a universally accepted definition of the term does not exist. For the purposes of this concept analysis, leadership is defined as *"an interactive process that provides needed guidance and direction."*[4,p820] Leadership involves three dynamic elements: a leader, a follower, and a situation. The leader provides guidance to followers, directing them toward a vision or goal and giving support to enable their success in the particular situation or setting.

SCOPE

The scope of leadership encompasses formal leadership and informal leadership (Figure 41-1). Individuals who occupy designated administrative or management positions in an organization are considered to hold formal leadership positions. Chief executive officer, chief nurse executive, vice president for patient services, and nurse manager are common examples of formal leadership positions in health care. Depending on the location of the institution and type of setting, titles may vary. For example, in some settings, titles such as

head nurse and nursing supervisor are still used. Another type of formal leadership position is an elected or appointed position in professional nursing associations, such as president or committee chairperson.

Informal leadership by individuals who do not occupy a designated administrative or management position also occurs in organizations. Individuals are perceived as informal leaders by their supervisors and peers because of their capabilities and actions. An example is experienced staff nurses who are recognized as clinical leaders because of their expertise, their willingness to be spokespersons for other staff, or their involvement in important issues for patient care and nurses. Individuals who are perceived as informal leaders sometimes, but not always, move into formal leadership positions.

ATTRIBUTES AND CRITERIA

The following six attributes must be present for effective leadership to occur: followers, vision, communication, decision making, change, and social power. These attributes are presented in Figure 41-2 and are described in the following sections.

Followers

There are no leaders without followers and no followers without leaders. In fact, most employees spend a large part of their work life as followers. Even leaders are followers in some settings, activities, and situations. Because followers and leaders are interdependent, each can influence the effectiveness of the other. Leaders, as discussed in the Featured Exemplars section, use different approaches to motivate, support, and reward their followers. How followers interact with leaders can be viewed on a continuum, with responses ranging from resistance to passivity and active participation in organizational activities. Consequently, success of an organization is closely tied to the interactions between leaders and followers.[5]

Figure 41-2 uses a broken line to show a boundary between leaders and followers. The strength and permeability of the boundary between a leader and followers will depend on the leader's style. Autocratic leaders will maintain more distance from followers, interacting with them less than a leader who employs a democratic style. Transformational leaders also will have high interaction with followers.

FIGURE 41-1 Leadership Scope

Vision

A vision is a leader's ideological statement of a desired, long-term future for an organization. It is the future that a leader wants to create; thus it is something to be worked toward over a period of time. The aim of leadership, as indicated by its definition, is to guide and direct followers toward the organization's vision or toward goals instrumental for attaining the vision. The importance leaders place on vision will depend on their leadership style. Articulating a clear vision is an essential component of transformational leadership, whereas in transactional leadership the leader is focused on performance goals for followers. To move followers toward a vision, a leader will use several processes. Three commonly used processes are communication, decision making, and change.

Communication

Communication is an essential function of effective leadership. In fact, leadership has been referred to as an ongoing conversation between a leader and followers. Leaders communicate with their followers, other leaders, the organization's clients, and people outside the organization to give and receive information. Figure 41-2 depicts communication between the leader and followers as a process that spans the boundary between parties. The way in which a leader communicates with followers will depend on the leader's style. Laissez-faire leaders will have little communication with their followers. Authentic leaders will use open communication and transparency to build trust with their followers.

Decision Making

All leaders make decisions that affect others and their organization's success. Good decisions are among the most critical features of good leadership, but good decisions are also among leaders' most invisible actions. Like communication, decision making occurs at the boundary between a leader and followers (Figure 41-2) and varies depending on the leader's style. Democratic leaders will use a participatory style of decision making. Autocratic leaders are more likely to make decisions without follower input. Laissez-faire leaders generally allow followers to make independent decisions except in a crisis.

Change

Change is the transition process from an old state to a new state. Leaders guide the change process by working with their followers to move the organization or department toward the established vision and goals. A leader's change management skills are vital in the change process. Aspects of leadership that influence change are using effective communication skills, understanding the organizational culture, considering alternate paths to achieve a goal, identifying and dealing with differences among followers, and creating leverage to motivate followers toward the vision.

Social Power

Social power is the potential influence of one individual over another. Leaders derive their social power from a variety of sources, as outlined by French and Raven's bases of power model (Table 41-1).[6] A leader's style influences how he or she will use power. For example, formal

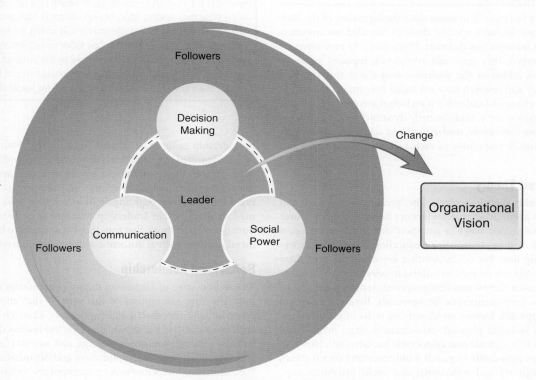

FIGURE 41-2 Attributes of Leadership

TABLE 41-1 Bases of Social Power

Type of Power	Description
Coercive	Uses threat of punishment to get followers to respond. Followers expect to be punished by their leader if they fail to conform to leader's influence. Leader must monitor followers' work in order to allocate punishment. Followers who like their leader are more likely to respond to leader's threats than are followers who do not like their leader. Research also has shown that women are more responsive to coercive power than men.
Legitimate	Recognition that formal leaders have power over their followers because of the position they hold. A legitimate power relationship between two individuals can also be based on reciprocity (i.e., "You did 'X' for me, so I should do 'Y' for you"), equity (i.e., "I have done 'X' for you, so I have a right to ask you to do 'Y' for me"), and dependence (i.e., "I have an obligation to help others who cannot help themselves"). Internalized values dictate the extent to which individuals will respond to legitimate power.
Referent	Results when followers identify with or aspire to be like their leader. It does not require a direct relationship between leader and followers, or action on the part of the leader. Referent power is positive when followers voluntarily mold themselves to the leader. Referent power is negative when followers do not like or want to be like their leader.
Reward	Ability of one person to reward another for compliance with expectations. Leader must monitor the follower in order to give the reward. Like coercive power, reward power is stronger when followers like their leader, and women are more responsive to reward power than men.
Expert	Results when followers respond to their leader's directions because they perceive that the leader knows best. The range of expert power is limited to the leader's area of expertise. For example, one may have expert power as a registered nurse but not as an engineer. Like referent power, there is a negative variation on expert power. In this case, followers recognize the expertise of the leader but assume the leader will act in his or her own best interests rather than the followers' interests.
Informational	Based on the leader's ability to influence followers to act by using clear logic, rational argument, and information. Leader may present the information to followers directly or indirectly (e.g., through hints and suggestions). Use of indirect informational power is more effective than direct informational power when followers are trying to influence their leader.

Source: Data from Raven BH: The bases of power: Origins and recent developments, *J Social Issues* 49:227, 1993.

leaders' power is derived, in part, from the position they hold; transactional leaders use reward power, and authentic leaders use information power.

THEORETICAL LINKS

Leadership theory has evolved in waves since the beginning of the 20th century. Each wave includes specific theories founded on common assumptions and incorporates different dimensions. As new waves of theory have emerged, they have not completely replaced previous waves but instead added to the understanding about this complex concept. As theory and research have advanced over time, the concept of leadership has changed. Leadership is no longer seen as a set of traits; it is now understood as a multifaceted, dynamic process. Today's leaders must know themselves, understand and relate effectively with their followers, and be responsive to varied situational dynamics and needs.

Great Man/Trait Theory

The oldest leadership theories illustrate the "great man" approach and are based on the assumption that leaders are born, not made. These theories hypothesize that when a situation demands leadership, a leader emerges to assume control; prior education or special preparation for leadership does not occur. Another key assumption of these theories is that traits can be used as criteria to select effective leaders. When the great man theory was first proposed, leaders were almost exclusively males from aristocratic backgrounds. Research based on the great man approach focuses on identifying traits of great leaders. Historically, this included physical characteristics (e.g., height) and demographic traits (e.g., male and aristocratic background). Now this research addresses personality (e.g., self-confidence and decisiveness), intellect (e.g., high IQ and reflection), and social attributes (e.g., friendliness and sense of humor). Gradually, the great man approach

BOX 41-1 An Example of the "Great Man" Theory in Nursing

Florence Nightingale is internationally recognized as the founder of modern nursing and is well-known for her work in Scutari during the Crimean War, when she led an effort to provide better health care for British soldiers. Like many great man leaders, Miss Nightingale came from an aristocratic background, and although female, she and her only sibling, a sister, were educated and received encouragement from their father to read and study the texts that served as the educational core for men during the Victorian era.[8] Nightingale has been the subject of innumerable biographies, many of which attempt to identify the traits and attributes that made her the leader she became.

to leadership came to be termed "trait theory." Four attributes commonly identified by respondents throughout the world who were asked what qualities they look for and admire in leaders are (in rank order) honesty, forward looking, inspiring, and competent.[7] The many biographies of Florence Nightingale illustrate how trait theory has been used to describe her leadership characteristics (Box 41-1).[8] Recent nursing research shows that trait theory continues to be used to recommend qualities such as authenticity for today's nursing leaders.[9]

Behavioral Leadership

The second wave of leadership theory concentrates on leader behaviors. The core assumption of this wave is that effective leaders use different behaviors than ineffective leaders. Research using behavioral leadership theories has shown that effective leaders demonstrate high concern for employee needs, feelings, and morale (i.e., consideration) and also address task accomplishment and organizational productivity (i.e., initiating structure). A contemporary behavioral leadership theory popular in nursing is emotional intelligence.[10] Emotional intelligence (EI) is composed of five components: self-awareness, self-regulation, motivation, empathy, and social skill. The theory hypothesizes that to improve their effectiveness, leaders must develop their capabilities in all five components. Emotional intelligence has been used by nurse researchers to study the impact of nursing leadership styles on patient outcomes[11] and nurses' responses to hospital restructuring.[12] EI highlights the importance of knowing one's self, reflection, openness to feedback, and continuous learning in the leadership role.

Situational and Contingency Theory

The third wave of leadership theory, situational and contingency theory, aims to explain why some leadership approaches are effective in one situation and not in another. This wave takes into consideration the subtle and complex ways in which a leader's traits and behaviors, followers' needs and values, and situational parameters interact. It challenges the assumption that there is "one best way" to lead. Education and training to enhance leader effectiveness gained importance during this wave.

Two leadership development programs were designed to provide formal nurse leaders at the frontlines of care delivery with skills specific to situations they encounter. The Nursing Leadership Institute was a year-long program that included a 4-day workshop, mentoring, organizational support, and online networking for frontline leaders in British Columbia. When interviewed at the end of the program, participants reported that nursing-focused leadership content helped them more in their practice than general leadership content because of its specificity, and that leadership style changes achieved throughout the year helped them meet situational needs on the job.[13] The second leadership program, offered for charge nurses employed by one Florida health care system, was designed to address communication difficulties, conflict management, and supervision and delegation. Anecdotal feedback was positive, but the charge nurses reported needing specific training for managing different types of conflict situations—for example, with physicians, patients and their families, and among nurses.[14]

Charismatic and Transformational Leadership

The fourth wave of leadership theory is referred to as charismatic and transformational leadership. The underlying assumption is that leaders inspire, intellectually stimulate, and recognize the contributions of their followers. Charismatic leaders influence followers through their personality and charm; they develop an emotional relationship that inspires and motivates followers. Transformational leaders possess similar characteristics and, in addition, convey high expectations to their followers, challenging their assumptions about what can be attained and building their commitment to an organizational vision. Transformational leaders rouse followers to achieve something of significance. They positively affect individual initiative and accomplishment, and they encourage trust and performance within workgroups.[15] Many have advocated for the use of transformational leadership in nursing.[16-18] Studies of charismatic and transformational nursing leadership have shown that they are associated with high nurse satisfaction, low nurse turnover, empowerment, and high productivity and effectiveness.[19]

Complexity Leadership

The complexity leadership approach is derived from complexity science, a relatively new theory that reflects the dynamism and knowledge-based nature of the world in the 21st century. Using complexity science as a framework produces markedly different approaches to leadership than the theories presented previously. Complexity science assumes interconnectedness among the parts of a system and between the system and its external environment. Interaction among the interconnected parts can affect the entire system, often in substantial ways. Another assumption of complexity science is nonlinearity. Throughout the decades, organizational theory has been based on the assumption of predictability—that organizations are designed to work "like a well-oiled machine." Complexity science, however, recognizes that organizational processes are often nonlinear and unpredictable. Through the dynamic interplay of negative and positive feedback, an organization is able to make changes to keep abreast of the environmental context. Self-organization is another assumption of complexity science. Employees at the frontlines will self-organize to enable the organization to adapt to change, innovate, and create new capabilities.[20-22]

Leaders who apply complexity science will not direct or control the process of solving organizational problems. Instead, they invite workers to connect with each other to create a solution. The complexity leader will provide resources to them, such as data and information about the problem; help them recognize their ability to find a solution, including innovations that already may have been implemented at the frontlines; set parameters for action and boundaries for the solution; and remove organizational barriers so that the solution can emerge from the workers most affected by the problem. Complexity science is beginning to appear in the nursing literature. In one report, the use of complexity science approaches helped newly licensed RNs manage patient care dilemmas that threatened the quality of patient care.[23] An investigation of care for nursing home residents showed that interaction strategies aligned with complexity science increased the staff's ability to deliver better care.[24]

CONTEXT TO NURSING AND HEALTH CARE

An expected role and competency of all RNs is leadership; thus it is a characteristic of all nurses in all settings. The application of leadership begins in nursing school (with role formation) and continues throughout one's career. Three categories of nursing leadership are formal leadership, clinical leadership, and interprofessional leadership.

Formal Nursing Leadership

The increasing complexity and rapid change in health care demand effective leadership. The aims of nursing leadership are to ensure quality patient care and to create supportive practice environments for nurses. Nurses who hold executive-level leadership positions, such as chief nursing officer or vice president for patient care services, partner with other executives to establish the organizational vision and then align the goals and operations of the nursing department with the organizational vision. Nurses in lower level leadership positions, such as directors and nurse managers, report to the nurse executive. Their focus is to ensure that day-to-day patient care operations meet established standards, to empower staff to participate in improving patient care, and to create work environments that foster professional practice and nurse satisfaction.

The size and structure of the nursing leadership team depend on the size of the health care agency. For example, a small rural hospital may have only one formal nursing leader—a director who supervises all nursing staff. Home health and public health agencies that have offices in several communities may have designated nurse leaders for each site who report to an executive nurse leader at a central location. Urban quaternary medical centers may have four or five levels of nursing leadership, creating a hierarchy with considerable distance between the nurse executive and nurses who provide direct patient care.

Preparation for Formal Leadership

Jennings and colleagues reviewed 5 years of writing about leadership and management to identify the top categories of competencies

BOX 41-2 Recommended Competencies for Nursing Leaders

- Personal qualities
- Interpersonal skills
- Thinking skills
- Setting the vision
- Communicating
- Initiating change
- Developing people
- Health care knowledge (clinical, technical, as a business)
- Management skills (e.g., planning, organizing)
- Business skills (e.g., finance, marketing)

Source: Adapted from Jennings BM, Scalzi CC, Rodgers JD III, et al.: Differentiating nursing leadership and management competencies, *Nurs Outlook* 55:169, 2007.

recommended for nursing leaders.[25] These are presented in Box 41-2. Education and training are needed to cultivate these competencies. Academic education is the foundation for nurses who aspire to leadership positions. The position of the Council on Graduate Education for Administration in Nursing is that nurse managers should be minimally prepared at the bachelor's degree level but preferably at the master's in nursing level. Nurses seeking executive-level positions should hold a doctorate degree.[26]

Although some individuals have natural leadership tendencies, the most effective leaders are those who have participated in leadership training. Leadership development is essential for all levels of leadership. It is not a single event but, rather, an ongoing and interactive process that enables the leader to learn, apply, and receive feedback that guides further learning. Studies have shown that nurses' participation in leadership development programs can bring significant and sustained improvements in leadership skills and competencies.[17,18,27]

Many leadership development options are available, including self-study, seminars, workshops, experiential learning, and mentorship from experienced leaders. Programs generally incorporate several components and extend over a period of time. Hospitals, community health agencies, and professional nursing associations offer leadership development workshops for new and aspiring leaders. Several well-established national programs sponsored by universities, professional associations, and health foundations enable executive nurses to broaden and deepen their leadership knowledge and competencies.[3] Local programs such as that described by Schwarzkopf and colleagues have been designed to address the developmental needs of leaders at the unit level.[14] The program's aims were to enhance charge nurses' interpersonal and team management skills, give them tools to improve nurse–physician collaboration, and reduce charge nurse turnover. Evaluation of a 12-month transformational leadership training program for unit-level managers in a Belgian hospital showed that the program improved manager communication with staff, which in turn improved job clarity for nurses and increased their sense of empowerment.[28]

The Impact of Leadership on Outcomes

Several researchers have conducted studies to determine if there is a relationship between formal nursing leadership and RN outcomes. Investigations have shown that nursing leadership based on consideration for followers and leader visibility in the clinical setting is positively related to feelings of empowerment and autonomy, work commitment, as well as staff nurse job satisfaction and retention.[19,29]

Authentic leadership by nurse managers also has been shown to have a positive effect on RN job satisfaction and performance.[30] Nursing leadership based on emotional intelligence is positively associated with work environment characteristics that support professional nursing practice, such as more opportunities for staff development, good teamwork between nurses and physicians, positive work culture, and greater use of research in practice.[12,19,31]

The relationship between nurse leadership and patient outcomes has also been examined. An investigation of the impact of nurse leader tenure showed that when a nursing home's director of nursing had less than 1 year of experience at the facility, there were four times as many deficiencies in care compared to nursing homes whose director had 15 or more years of experience at the facility.[32] A systematic review of 20 studies showed that positive nurse leader practices were associated with fewer adverse patient events, particularly medication errors, decreased patient mortality, and higher patient satisfaction. The authors suggested that effective nurse leaders create practice environments that have sufficient nurse staffing, resources, and care delivery processes.[33]

Clinical Leadership

Clinical leadership has been defined as

> *staff nurse behaviors that provide direction and support to clients and the health care team in the delivery of patient care. A clinical leader is a registered nurse who influences and coordinates patients, families, and health care team colleagues for the purpose of integrating the care they provide to achieve positive patient outcomes.*[34,p450]

Clinical leadership also has been defined as "a professional competency demonstrated in clinical care that galvanizes the nurse to influence others to continuously improve the care they provide."[35,p269] Clinical leaders do not hold formal management positions; instead, they are informal nurse leaders whose colleagues perceive them to be leaders.

Characteristics of Clinical Leaders

An integrative research review identified three categories of clinical leader characteristics.[36] The first category is clinical characteristics: practice skills (e.g., advanced nursing care and coordination); expert knowledge (clinical, leadership, and management); use of evidence-based rationale; and systematic, critical circumspect, and rapid thinking skills. The second category is follower/team: effective communication skills, role modeling, behaviors that support colleagues, and team empowerment. The final category is personal qualities: positive attitudes toward the nursing profession; reflective practice; leadership of change; and individual attributes such as dynamism, integrity, and consistency.[36] Clinical leaders' influence with colleagues is based on referent, expert, and informational power. In addition, a study of nearly 500 Canadian nurses showed that staff nurse clinical leadership was affected positively when their nurse managers created an empowering unit work environment.[34]

Developing Clinical Leadership Skills

Every RN has the potential to be a clinical leader. A study of 32 nursing students and 21 RNs at different career stages was conducted to identify how students and nurses learn and practice clinical leadership.[35] A five-stage model emerged. The first stage is "I am aware of clinical leadership in nursing," and it was described, primarily by students, as being able to discriminate between a positive and a negative nurse leader. Stage 2 was "integration of clinical leadership in my actions." In this stage, students and new nurses identify their personal strengths and weaknesses and identify a role model. Stage 3, described by senior students and new nurses, was "active leadership with patient/family, sometimes with colleagues." Patient/family successes inspire them to continue to develop, and they begin identifying their own leadership style and competencies. Stage 4 is "active leadership with the team" and includes mobilizing intra- and interprofessional teams, acting as a resource, and adapting leadership style to the context. Expert nurses described stage 5 as "embedded clinical leadership extended to organizational level and beyond." These clinical leaders take part in organizational decision making, propose changes that depart from the status quo, anticipate problems, manage conflicts, and act as mentors.[35]

Learning to be a clinical leader starts in the academic setting through coursework and guided experience.[37] After entering the practice setting, RNs can seek clinical leadership development opportunities offered by their employer, continuing education providers, and professional associations. Active and experiential learning are particularly important to enable aspiring clinical leaders to link theoretical knowledge with clinical practice. Mentorship from experienced clinical leaders, reflection on leadership actions, and feedback on leadership progress are important components of clinical leadership development programs.[38] Frequent and meaningful contact between leaders and the staff they lead also provides opportunities for aspiring leaders to observe and role model effective leadership behaviors and become more self-aware of their own style.[31] Clinical leaders are encouraged to develop their presentation and professional writing skills and to learn how to maintain a professional portfolio.[39]

Research on clinical nursing leadership is in its infancy, and to date it has focused on understanding the attributes and characteristics of clinical leaders, as reported previously in this concept presentation. A few studies have been conducted to assess the outcomes of clinical leadership development programs. For example, one comprehensive development program designed to prepare staff nurses for shared clinical leadership showed improvements in self-reported leadership behaviors such as accountability for clinical problem solving, confidence, negotiation skills, and interprofessional team skills. In turn, program participants reported that they were better able to meet patient needs and promote their recovery and thereby positively influence patient satisfaction.[38]

Interprofessional Leadership

Today's health care system requires leadership that goes beyond a specific discipline or health profession. In many health care agencies and health sector businesses, nurses have interprofessional leadership responsibilities. For example, countless nurses in executive-level leadership positions in hospitals and home health agencies carry titles such as vice president for patient care services and, in addition to nursing, are responsible for other patient care departments, such as pharmacy, physical therapy, and chaplaincy. Nurses also move into formal leadership positions in areas such as clinical informatics and quality management. In these roles, nurses draw on their knowledge and experience as clinicians, their understanding of the health care system, and their leadership training to ensure safe and effective patient care.

Nurse leaders at all levels of the organization, formal and informal, are called on to become full partners in the interprofessional care environment.[3,40] Interprofessional collaboration reduces the use of redundant services and develops more creative solutions to complex patient care problems. In particular, patients with chronic conditions, patients who are critically ill, and the elderly population benefit from coordinated interprofessional care. Research also has shown that interprofessional collaboration can improve quality of care and patient outcomes.[41–43] Nurses are typically the health care providers who have the most frequent and sustained interaction with patients and their families. Thus, it is incumbent on nurse leaders to position the nursing staff to use their close relationships with patients and families as the vantage point for strengthening interprofessional collaboration and, in turn, the quality of health care services.

INTERRELATED CONCEPTS

Several concepts within this textbook are interrelated to the concept of leadership. These are presented in Figure 41-3 and described here.

Health Care Organizations are the setting in which most nurse leaders work. Formal nurse leaders play an important role in the operations of health care organizations. Clinical nurse leaders usually emerge at the front lines of the organization where patient care is delivered.

FIGURE 41-3 Leadership and Interrelated Concepts

Nursing is a practice discipline geared toward the delivery of health care, and the coordination of safe and effective patient care falls on the shoulders of leaders. As mentioned previously, there are multiple levels of leadership; thus, some leaders are further removed from direct patient care than others. Nonetheless, the efforts of nursing leaders ultimately link to the coordination of patient care. **Care Coordination** refers to the process of connecting health care services and resources to patients and is one of the distinctive contributions that clinical nurse leaders make in patient care.

Because **Communication** is an attribute of effective leaders (described previously), it is a key interrelated concept. Clear communication is central to effective leadership. Leaders who communicate unambiguous and consistent messages in a timely manner help followers understand the organization's direction, decision-making processes, and changes that may be underway. Listening is an essential aspect of communication. Only by listening to peers, followers, patients, and others will the leader understand all dimensions of a problem or opportunity. Effective leaders also provide mechanisms to foster clear communication throughout the organization.

Effective **Collaboration** within and among organizations, and within and across disciplines, is essential to efficient organizations. Skilled nurse leaders encourage and role model this behavior. Collaboration enhances communication and delivery of care.

Nurse leaders help ensure that the actions of the organization, unit, and individuals contribute to **Health Care Quality**. Formal and clinical nurse leaders are attuned to the standards and processes that an organization uses to provide high-quality care. They are involved in improvement initiatives and other change processes to meet the quality goals of their organization. Often, nurse leaders collaborate with others through professional organizations and regulatory bodies to establish the quality standards for nursing and health care.

Use of **Evidence** is important for effective leadership. Formal leaders use evidence about different leadership and management approaches to create organizational processes and work environments that contribute to satisfaction, productivity, and retention of nursing staff. Clinical leaders use research-based evidence and best practices to ensure health care quality and often guide other nurses in evidence-based practice.

Ethics is also important for effective leadership. Ethical integrity is a core element of all types of leadership. Formal leaders practice and role model high ethical standards. Clinical and interprofessional leaders rely on their knowledge of ethical principles and decision-making models to protect and advocate for patients in all aspects of patient care.

CLINICAL EXEMPLARS

Every hospital, community health department, and long-term care facility is likely to have a variety of leadership positions. Box 41-3 presents common examples of formal, clinical, and interprofessional leaders.

Leaders are made, not born. Leadership in health care is not an act reserved only for designated administrators and managers. Clinical leaders are needed in every setting to ensure that quality patient care is delivered and that new evidence and research findings are adopted to improve patient care. It is incumbent on nurses who aspire to be leaders, as well as those who are leaders, to embrace opportunities to continue to develop their leadership skills. Research investigating the relationship between nursing leadership and nurse outcomes shows that people-oriented leadership approaches are positively associated with nurse satisfaction and retention and supportive work

---

■■■ BOX 41-3 EXEMPLARS OF LEADERSHIP

Leadership Roles
Formal Nurse Leader
- Chief nursing officer
- Nursing director/assistant director
- Nurse manager
- Charge nurse/team leader
- Dean
- Associate dean
- State board of nursing executive director

Clinical Nurse Leader
- Experienced staff nurse
- Clinical nurse educator
- Experienced advanced practice nurse

Interprofessional Leader
- Director of clinical service line (e.g., primary care services)
- Associate director of infection control department
- Chairperson, quality improvement committee (e.g., ER)
- Chairperson, reaccreditation steering committee

Leadership Styles
- Autocratic
- Democratic
- Laissez-faire
- Transactional
- Transformational
- Authentic
- Shared

---

environments. An increasing number of studies also show that effective nurse leaders can positively influence patient satisfaction with care and other indicators of health care quality.

Featured Exemplars

Nurses experience situations in which different leadership styles are portrayed. The exemplars presented here are those most likely to be encountered.

Autocratic Leaders

Autocratic leaders make all decisions and are generally most concerned with the tasks to be accomplished. They maintain distance from their followers, motivating them through the threat of punishment and offer of rewards as incentives. Traditionally, autocratic leadership was thought to be effective for leading new employees and large groups and for controlling work that needs to be coordinated among many departments. It is often used when a decision needs to be made quickly, such as in emergencies.

Democratic Leaders

Democratic leaders involve followers in the decision-making process by using a participatory leadership style. They show more concern about followers than do autocratic leaders. Democratic leadership is useful when the followers are experienced workers, particularly when they have professional education and socialization. It is effective when organizational success requires that followers are committed to the goal. Democratic leaders help followers develop technical and emotional maturity.

Laissez-Faire Leaders

Laissez-faire leaders do not interfere with employees and their work. They stand at a distance, giving followers freedom to make decisions and accomplish their work. They provide minimal information to followers and have little communication with them about their work. Typically, laissez-faire leaders wait until a crisis develops to make decisions. This leadership style works best when followers are highly experienced in their work, but it often results in employee apathy, inefficiency, and chaos.

Transactional Leaders

Transactional leaders focus on the daily operations of an organization and develop an exchange relationship with their followers. The transaction entails rewarding followers when they perform and correcting them when necessary. Transactional leaders focus on getting things done and satisfying their own and their followers' self-interests.

Transformational Leaders

Transformational leaders use approaches that change or transform individuals. They inspire and intellectually stimulate followers and recognize their contributions. Expectations are high and often challenge followers' assumptions about what can be attained. They communicate an organizational vision to their followers, moving them to accomplish more than expected. Their focus is long term and involves developing people and organizations.

Authentic Leaders

Authentic leaders are transparent and ethical in their dealings with followers. They are genuine, empathic, reliable, and believable. They are perceived by others to be open, optimistic, warm, and respectful. They focus on establishing relationships that embody trust and show commitment to the development of their followers.

Shared Leadership

A type of leadership associated with work teams is shared leadership, an approach in which employees are empowered to distribute leadership responsibilities broadly within a group. They lead one another to achieve a goal. Shared leadership is effective with professionals and with project-focused workgroups. It is highly interactive and enables employees to develop their skills and professionalism.

CASE STUDY

Source: Fuse/Thinkstock

The case study is a clinical nurse leader who applied all three types of clinical leadership characteristics (clinical, follower/team, and personal qualities) to address a difficult patient/family situation.

Case Presentation

We had a very long-term patient in our medical/surgical ICU who was with us from early October until January 1 when he died. He had amyotrophic lateral sclerosis and a very aggressive, untreatable cancer, but he and his family were not willing to accept his diagnosis, thus kept him as a Full Code. His mind was intact until the last few days when he developed renal failure.

His wife was very difficult, constantly criticizing our care, constantly "checking him over," looking for a sheet crease or something to pin his deterioration on. She was so difficult, that most nurses gave up trying to even talk to her.

I spoke with my manager, who challenged me to understand her and to have her understand us and his prognosis. I remember telling my manager that I didn't need any more challenges, but I ended up taking it on! I spoke with all his doctors (even those who had "checked off" the case to understand their position[s]), used the Social Services and Case Management teams of nurses/social workers. I finally spoke with him alone to see what his end of life decision[s] were and then I spoke with her alone. He and she both wanted to maintain the Full Code status, so then we discussed his probable course. It took many conferences with her but she came to trust me and eventually called me "his favorite nurse." It taught me that patience is crucial and that was nothing I thought I had in my arsenal!

His room had a small window, but he hadn't been outside in many months other than his transfer from the ambulance from his rehab center to our hospital in October. The respiratory therapist and I decided to take him outside for some sun. We cleared it with the doctors, the charge nurse, and finally with the patient. He was terrified and I explained we'd bag him while he was outside and then he could see the life outside. He agreed. It was a major undertaking, but he smiled in the slightly overcast day. We bundled him in warm blankets and he was out there for about 15 minutes, with the wind blowing his hair and he beamed. His wife was thrilled and asked if we could do it again, so we repeated the adventure the following day with her. That day was sunny, so we stayed out longer. We had four to five trips outside over the next 2 weeks.

His deterioration was substantial after Christmas; his code status was changed to No Code and she asked for a priest to come to give him a final blessing. Eventually, she agreed, on January 1, to take him outside, off the ventilator and allow him to go in peace in the sun where he had enjoyed some last pleasant days. It was a rainy day, but the sun came out for an hour and a half. He breathed for 45 minutes and had his family (real family and hospital family of RNs and "his" respiratory therapist, who had been with me on our first venture outside) around him when he finally passed away. It was one of the most beautiful experiences of my life and one I've learned a lot from!

Case Analysis

This RN showed her leadership in the following ways: She was a visible role model who demonstrated clinical competence and knowledge. She was an effective communicator, engaging other members of the interprofessional team, the patient, and the patient's family in making decisions about his care. Her care for the patient illustrated her professional values and use of ethical principles, particularly related to patient autonomy and dignity. Her actions illustrate how she functioned as a care coordinator and empowered, motivated, and opened others to new possibilities in caring for a difficult patient. In writing about this experience, she used reflection. This case also illustrates how a nurse manager can empower a staff nurse to become a clinical leader.

Source: Reprinted with permission from National Council of State Boards of Nursing: *Report of findings from the post-entry competence study*, research brief, vol 38, p. 18, Chicago, 2009, Author.

ACCESS EXEMPLAR LINKS IN YOUR GIDDENS EBOOK

REFERENCES

1. American Association of Colleges of Nursing: *Essentials of baccalaureate education for professional nursing practice,* 2008. Retrieved from <http://www.aacn.nche.edu/education-resources/BaccEssentials08.pdf>.
2. Holm AL, Severinsson E: The role of the mental health nursing leadership. *J Nurs Manag* 18:463, 2010.
3. Institute of Medicine: *Transforming leadership.* In *The future of nursing: Leading change, advancing health,* Washington, DC, 2011, National Academies Press. Retrieved from <http://www.iom.edu/Reports/2010/The-Future-of-Nursing-Leading-Change-Advancing-Health.aspx>.
4. Goethals GR, Sorenson GJ, Burn JM, editors: *Encyclopedia of leadership,* Thousand Oaks, CA, 2004, Sage.
5. Kean S, Haycock-Stuart E, Baggaley S, et al: Followers and the co-construction of leadership. *J Nurs Manag* 19:507, 2011.
6. Raven BH: The bases of power: Origins and recent developments. *J Social Issues* 49:227, 1993.
7. Kouzes JM, Posner BZ: *The leadership challenge,* ed 4, San Francisco, 2007, Wiley.
8. Gill G: *Nightingales: The extraordinary upbringing and curious life of Miss Florence Nightingale,* New York, 2004, Ballantine.
9. Waite J, McKinney N, Smith-Glasgow ME, et al: The embodiment of authentic leadership. *J Prof Nurs* 30:282, 2014.
10. Akerjordet K, Severinsson E: The state of the science of emotional intelligence related to nursing leadership: An integrative review. *J Nurs Manag* 18:363, 2010.
11. Cummings GG, Midodzi WK, Wong CA, et al: The contribution of hospital nursing leadership styles to 30-day patient mortality. *Nurs Res* 59:331, 2010.
12. Cummings G, Hayduk L, Estabrooks C: Mitigating the impact of hospital restructuring on nurses: The responsibility of emotionally intelligent leadership. *Nurs Res* 54:2, 2005.
13. MacPhee M, Skelton-Green J, Bouthillette F, et al: An empowerment framework for nursing leadership development: Supporting evidence. *J Adv Nurs* 68:159, 2011.
14. Schwarzkopf R, Sherman RO, Kiger AJ: Taking charge: Front-line nurse leadership development. *J Cont Ed Nurs* 43:154, 2012.
15. Wang X-H, Howell JM: Exploring the dual-level effects of transformational leadership on followers. *J Appl Psychol* 95:1134, 2010.
16. Clavelle JT, Drenkard K, Tullai-McGuinness S, et al: Transformational leadership practices of chief nursing officers in Magnet organizations. *J Nurs Admin* 42:195, 2012.
17. Martin JS, McCormack B, Fitzsimons D, et al: Evaluation of a clinical leadership programme for nurse leaders. *J Nurs Manag* 20:72, 2012.
18. Kelly LA, Wicker TL, Gerkin RD: The relationship of training and education to leadership practices in frontline nurse leaders. *J Nurs Admin* 44:158, 2014.
19. Cummings GG, MacGregor T, Davey M, et al: Leadership styles and outcome patterns for the nursing workforce and work environment: A systematic review. *Int J Nurs Stud* 47:363, 2010.
20. Holden LM: Complex adaptive systems: Concept analysis. *J Adv Nurs* 52:651, 2005.
21. Avolio BJ, Walumbwa FO, Weber TJ: Leadership: Current theories, research, and future directions. *Annu Rev Psychol* 60:421, 2009.
22. Weberg D: Complexity leadership: A healthcare imperative. *Nurs Forum* 47:268, 2012.
23. Kramer M, Brewer BB, Halfer D, et al: Changing our lens: Seeing the chaos of professional practice as complexity. *J Nurs Manag* 21:690, 2013.
24. Anderson RA, Toles MP, Corazzini K, et al: Local interaction strategies and capacity for better care in nursing homes: A multiple case study. *BMC Health Svc Res* 14:244, 2014.
25. Jennings BM, Scalzi CC, Rodgers JD, III, et al: Differentiating nursing leadership and management competencies. *Nurs Outlook* 55:169, 2007.
26. Council on Graduate Education for Administration in Nursing: *Position statement on the educational preparation of nurse executives and nurse managers,* 2011. Retrieved from <http://www.cgean.org/assets/docs/cgean_positon_on_educational_preparation.pdf>.
27. Chappell KK, Willis L: The Cockcroft difference: An analysis of the impact of a nursing leadership development programme. *J Nurs Manag* 21:396, 2013.
28. de Casterlé BD, Willemse A, Verschueren M, et al: Impact of clinical leadership development on the clinical leader, nursing team and care-giving process: A case study. *J Nurs Manag* 16:753, 2008.
29. Germain PB, Cummings GG: The influence of nursing leadership on nurse performance: A systematic literature review. *J Nurs Manag* 18:425, 2010.
30. Wong CA, Laschinger HKS: Authentic leadership, performance, and job satisfaction: The mediating role of empowerment. *J Adv Nurs* 69:947, 2012.
31. Cummings GG, Olson K, Hayduk L, et al: The relationship between nursing leadership and nurses' job satisfaction in Canadian oncology work environments. *J Nurs Manag* 16:508, 2008.
32. Lerner NB, Trinkoff A, Storr CL, et al: Nursing home leadership tenure and resident care outcomes. *J Nurs Regul* 5:48, 2014.
33. Wong CA, Cummings GG, Ducharme L: The relationship between nursing leadership and patient outcomes: A systematic review update. *J Nurs Manag* 21:709, 2013.
34. Patrick A, Laschinger HKS, Wong C, et al: Developing and testing a new measure of staff nurse clinical leadership: The clinical leadership survey. *J Nurs Manag* 19:449, 2011.
35. Pepin J, Dubois S, Girard R, et al: A cognitive learning model of clinical nursing leadership. *Nurs Ed Today* 31:268, 2011.
36. Mannix J, Wilkes L, Daly J: Attributes of clinical leadership in contemporary nursing: An integrative review. *Contemp Nurs* 45:10, 2013.
37. Kling VG: Clinical leadership project. *J Nurs Educ* 49:640, 2010.
38. George V, Burke LJ, Rodgers B, et al: Developing staff nurse shared leadership behavior in professional nursing practice. *Nurs Adm Q* 26(3):44, 2002.
39. Lannon SL: Leadership skills beyond the bedside: Professional development classes for the staff nurse. *J Contin Educ Nurs* 38:17, 2007.
40. Sorensen R, Iedema R, Severinsson E: Beyond profession: Nursing leadership in contemporary healthcare. *J Nurs Manag* 16:535, 2008.
41. Reeves S, Zwarenstein M, Goldman J, et al: Interprofessional education: effects on professional practice and health care outcomes. *Cochrane Database of Systematic Rev* Art. No. CD002213, 2008.
42. Martin JS, Ummenhofer W, Manser T, et al: Interprofessional collaboration among nurses and physicians: Making a difference in patient outcome. *Swiss Med Wkly* 140:w13062, 2010. doi: 10.4414/smw.2010.13062.
43. Hutchinson RW: Treating diabetes in underserved populations using an interprofessional care team. *J Interprof Care* 28:568, 2014.

Ethics

Deb Bennett-Woods

A m I ever justified in withholding the truth from a patient? Should I respect the wishes of the family or the wishes of the patient? Is there a point at which the treatment I am providing causes more harm than good? What do I do when I suspect my best friend is caring for patients while under the influence of alcohol? When short-staffed, how do I divide my time between too many patients? Is there a limit to how many scarce resources I should provide to any one patient?

These are difficult questions, and not everyone will agree on the answers. On one level, these are practical problems and decisions that need to be made in order to do a job. However, on a deeper level, they are moral and ethical choices that speak to more than just our formal training and job description. They cannot be answered with simple logic or by referring to a policy or procedure manual. Rather, how you respond to such questions is a reflection of the core values, beliefs, and character that make you the person that you are and, ultimately, the professional that you become. The actions you take in response to ethically challenging situations often require great courage, compassion, or commitment. At the same time, failure to act or respond ethically can lead to serious and even dangerous errors, personal stress, and professional burnout.

Very few of us start our day wondering, "How can I harm someone today?" or "What unethical action should I take first?"[1] In fact, most of us would like to end the day feeling as though we made a positive difference in the world and satisfied that we did our best. We want the respect of our colleagues and patients. Most important, we want to feel at home in our own skin. We want a sense of personal and professional integrity—the feeling of wholeness we experience when our actions are consistent with our core beliefs and values. Technical proficiency in nursing is important but not enough, in and of itself, to guarantee this sense of integrity. To achieve the ideal of professional integrity, one also needs the skills and abilities of ethical practice, including moral sensitivity, ethical reflection, ethical analysis, and ethical decision making.

DEFINITION

Morality is a broad term without a single commonly recognized definition. Generally, the term *morality* is used to refer broadly to an accepted set of social standards or morals that guide behavior. Ethics and its

various approaches deal more specifically with concepts of right and wrong. Although the terms ethics and morality, and the descriptors ethical and moral, are often used interchangeably, it is helpful to think of the various approaches to ethics as a foundation for morality and moral behavior. Thus a simple working definition of ethics is *the study or examination of morality through a variety of different approaches.*[2] To understand morality, an understanding of underlying concepts, assumptions, and methods of the various approaches to ethics is needed.

Ethics is also a process involving critical thought and action. *Ethical sensitivity* helps us recognize when there is an ethical problem or dilemma, *ethical reflection and analysis* enable us to think critically to rank our ethical obligations and priorities, and *ethical decision making* is a method for ensuring that the action we take is well reasoned and can be justified. Finally, *moral courage* enables us to act on our decisions even under the most challenging circumstances.

Each individual has his or her own moral comfort zone, or personal morality, within which ethical reflection and analysis occur. This comfort zone is both influenced by societal concepts of morality and unique to the individual and his or her own ethical foundations. Most of us do not give much thought to our ethical comfort zone. We think of ourselves as being ethical without entirely understanding how we act ethically in practice or why we so often falter ethically when confronted with difficult choices. Knowing and understanding who you are as a moral being, how you think ethically, and why you make certain decisions are critical to ethical practice as a nurse.

The various approaches to ethics begin with *metaethics*, the branch of philosophy that considers fundamental questions about the nature, source, and meaning of concepts such as good and bad or right and wrong. Rather than making judgments about right and wrong, metaethics provides a foundation for how to think about right and wrong or good and bad, and it provides a common language to use when considering the ethical or moral dimensions of a situation.[1]

Normative ethics, on the other hand, deals with very specific judgments about right and wrong in everyday actions. Normative ethics uses the language of ethics, along with factual information, prior experience, commonly held values and beliefs, and acceptable standards of behavior, to make everyday judgments.[1]

Finally, when faced with a moral choice, *applied ethics* refers to the process of applying ethical theory and reasoning to daily life. Applied ethics is sometimes also referred to as *practical ethics*,[2] and it provides the justification for specific actions based on ethical reflection and reasoning.

SCOPE

The scope of ethics is broad, encompassing many different dimensions of our lives. For example, we all live and work within larger systems, each of which has its own moral and ethical dimensions. We are all members of a larger society, we work in organizational settings, and we function within the parameters of a particular profession. To fully understand the scope of ethics, one must consider how each of these dimensions interacts with us, as individuals, in shaping our ethical foundation and behavior (Figure 42-1).

Societal Ethics

At the top, there are societal ethics that serve the larger community. Society provides a strong normative basis for ethical behavior through the legal and regulatory systems. Law is a minimum standard of behavior to which all members of society are held and that, generally, serves the interests of society as a whole. Laws prohibiting fraud and abuse or unauthorized release of medical information are examples of behaviors that society has deemed immoral and unethical. Legal standards such as the clinical standard of care, liability, negligence, and malpractice are based on legal and ethical obligations owed to patients. Other areas of our professional lives are guided by regulatory parameters such as the practice act that defines educational requirements and your scope of practice as a nurse or the accreditation standards that determine how a health care facility must operate. Compliance with these minimum standards for practice is expected of all health care professionals and the organizations within which they practice.[3] Following the law is the most basic ethical standard required for the privilege of working as a licensed professional in health care. However, even as a minimum standard, law can create moral conflict for nurses, which is evident in issues such as abortion and physician-assisted suicide, on which there remains broad disagreement within society.

Organizational Ethics

Organizational ethics involves a set of formal and informal principles and values that guide the behavior, decisions, and actions taken by members of an organization as well as the organizational structures, systems, practices, policies, and procedures developed to ensure ethical operation. The billions of dollars spent annually as a result of health care fraud and abuse is an example of ethical failures at the level of the organization.[4] Ideally, organizational ethics directs all aspects of an organization from its mission and values to how it treats both its customers and its employees, its financial practices, and how it responds to the needs of the larger community and the environment.[5]

Professional Ethics

Professional ethics refers to the ethical standards and expectations of a particular profession. Because professions have held a privileged role in society, their members are often held to a higher standard in terms of ethics. Therefore ethics becomes a fundamental element of one's professional identity and character as a nurse. As stated by Crigger and Godfrey, "The relationship between the patient and the nurse is, first and foremost, an ethical one."[6,p33] Ethical standards and expectations of practice are often expressed in a code of ethics or code of conduct that embodies the unique demands and philosophies of a particular profession. Unlike the minimum standard of the law, professional codes of ethics tend to offer general guidelines that are aimed at the highest ideals of practice. The Code of Ethics for Nurses of the American Nurses Association (ANA) establishes clear priorities in the ethical practice of nursing, such as compassion, respect, and primary commitment to the patient as well as advocacy for patient rights.[7] For example, the first principle in the ANA's Code of Ethics for Nurses states the following:

> *The nurse, in all professional relationships, practices with compassion and respect for the inherent dignity, worth and uniqueness of every individual, unrestricted by considerations of social or economic status, personal attributes, or the nature of health problems.*

Although this is an admirable ideal, how many of us can say that we live our lives or practice our professions in ways that *always* treat others with perfect compassion and respect, valuing every individual equally, and without any form of bias? Instead, it is the responsibility of the individual nurse to interpret this statement in terms of what it means in each unique situation and how well or poorly it is being demonstrated in his or her professional practice.

Bioethics and Clinical Ethics

Bioethics and its subcategory of clinical ethics are closely related to professional ethics. *Bioethics* deals broadly with ethical questions surrounding the biological sciences, emerging health care technologies, and health policy. *Clinical ethics* is involved primarily with decision making at the bedside and other patient-specific issues. *Research ethics* is a specialized field within bioethics that examines the ethical conduct of research using human subjects and animals.

Personal Ethics

Finally, and perhaps most important, personal ethics describes an individual's own ethical foundations and practice. Our personal ethics continuously intersects with these other categories of ethics; however, they do not perfectly overlap, so there is much potential for conflict. In addition, the sources of our ethics change over time just as we continue to change with time.

ATTRIBUTES AND CRITERIA

The attributes of ethical nursing practice begin with the sources of ethics and involve skills and abilities needed to identify and distinguish ethical problems and dilemmas and then apply a disciplined approach to analysis and action.

Ethics

Societal Ethics
Organizational Ethics
Bioethics/Clinical Ethics
Professional Ethics
Personal Ethics

FIGURE 42-1 Scope of Ethics

Family
Peers
Religion
Culture
Society
Profession
Personal
Experiences

FIGURE 42-2 Sources of Ethics

Sources of Ethics

The beliefs, values, and methods that define ethical practice are influenced by a variety of sources. Natural intersections and places of agreement exist between the various sources; however, they can also conflict with each other, creating competing beliefs and inconsistency in the way we approach ethical issues (Figure 42-2).

Family initially forms the most powerful influence on ethics, providing many of our earliest lessons about "right and wrong." A similar influence is the culture in which we are raised, including cultural practices related to our ethnicity, geographic area, socioeconomic status, and faith tradition. Peers become a source of ethical awareness and practice, especially as we move into adolescence, begin to look outside the family for direction, and are exposed to new experiences in the larger world. Education introduces new ways of thinking about difficult issues. Professional education, in particular, is charged with both your technical training and your awareness of the ethical practice of the profession. Once in the workplace, your colleagues and the organization where you work may further alter your views and your behaviors.

Ethical Problems and Dilemmas

An *ethical problem* is simply a problem with an ethical dimension. Most ethical problems have a reasonably clear solution, whereas others can be quite complex or involve competing ethical priorities. An *ethical dilemma* involves a problem for which in order to do something right you have to do something wrong. For example, in order to be loyal to one friend, you have to be disloyal to another. An example in patient care is determining whether aggressive treatment at the end of life will cause more harm than benefit. In other words, it is not possible to meet all of the ethical requirements in the situation. Instead, you must be sensitive to the ethical dimensions of the situation, able to use ethical concepts to analyze and reflect on the ethical conflicts within the dilemma, determine an ethically justifiable solution, and take action.

Ethical Analysis and Decision Making

When faced with an ethical problem or dilemma, it is helpful to apply a systematic approach of ethical analysis to the process of making a decision. There are many different methods for ethical analysis.[8] A practical approach is to use some form of decision model, and there are a number of different decision models from which you might select.[9]

One popular model for clinical decision making is the four topics method of Jonsen et al.[10] The four topics are medical indications, patient preferences, quality of life, and contextual features. Within each topic, questions are posed that clarify factual aspects of the case with an emphasis on common ethical principles. Answering the various questions provides a framework within which different options for action can be considered.

Any approach to ethical analysis will depend heavily on one's ability to ask good questions. Asking the wrong question or failing to ask an important question will generally result in a wrong or incomplete answer. An *ethical question* is a question that challenges you to consider a particular ethical concept, principle, or perspective in your analysis. The following are examples of ethical questions:

- Do I have a duty to tell the truth?
- What is the greater harm?
- To whom is my primary loyalty?
- What are the best interests of my patient?

Framing good ethical questions is the key to strong ethical analysis, and the ability to use a variety of ethical concepts and theories naturally expands the range and quality of questions.

THEORETICAL LINKS

The study of ethics can be traced back to philosophers in the ancient world such as Aristotle in the West and Confucius in the East. In medicine, the Hippocratic Oath, although probably not written by Hippocrates himself, is dated to sometime near the fourth century BC.[11] The body of theory in ethics is vast, reflecting the diversity of human thought and action.

Think of each theory or principle as a camera lens. Different lenses have different magnifications and filters that allow us to view exactly the same scene but from a different angle or in a slightly different light. This body of ethical theory provides the "language of ethics" and allows us to explore situations from many different perspectives and points of view. The perspectives can be quite diverse; therefore most of us feel more strongly about some principles and are drawn toward one or two theories at most. We may have a very difficult time even trying to think in the language of other theories. Ethical conflict occurs between parties when this language fails and each party simply cannot understand the other party's reasoning or point of view.

Ethical Principles

An ethical principle is a general guide, basic truth, or assumption that can be used with judgment to help determine a course of action.[12] Principles have long been used in bioethics and clinical ethics to describe the most common ethical concerns one must consider in most cases. Although all of the principles are important, they can conflict with each other in certain situations. The four principles most often cited are respect for persons, nonmaleficence, beneficence, and justice.[12] Less often mentioned, but equally important, is the principle of fidelity.

Respect for Persons

Respect for persons simply maintains that human beings have an unconditional moral worth that requires us to treat each individual person with great value, dignity, and respect.[13] The ethical principle of *autonomy* is an important extension of this principle and suggests that patients must be treated in a way that respects their self-determination by expressing their wishes and making informed choices about their treatment.[13] Another ethical principle closely related to autonomy is *veracity* or the principle of truth telling. A patient is not able to make an informed choice about treatment unless he or she has received the truth about his or her condition and the proposed treatment, and in a manner that is understandable to the patient.[13]

Nonmaleficence

Nonmaleficence directs us to act in ways that avoid harm to others, including even the risk of harm.[13] In health care, the primary focus is on harms such as pain, disability, or death; however, harm is difficult to define, and both patients and providers may be concerned about a wide range of perceived harms.[12] Another challenge in health care is that we are often required to inflict some harm and risk in order to benefit the patient and avoid a greater harm. However, these harms are not avoidable if we are to properly treat the patient, so we are required to carry out such treatments in ways that are unlikely to cause undue risk or needless harm.

Beneficence

Beneficence is an obligation to do good by acting in ways that promote the welfare and best interests of others.[12] Patients can reasonably expect that you, as a nurse, will promote their health and well-being. However, much like harm, the concept of good is difficult to define. A patient may define his or her best interests very differently than the nurse or other health care professional.[13]

Justice

The concept of *justice* is particularly complex, and there are no universally accepted definitions of what constitutes justice. However, at a minimum, the principle of justice is concerned with treating people equitably, fairly, and appropriately.[12] This means we owe our patients care and treatment that do not arbitrarily discriminate against them as an individual or as a member of a class of individuals. Returning to the ANA's Code of Ethics for Nurses, justice is the underlying principle that prohibits a nurse from treating patients differently based on their social or economic status, their personal attributes, or the nature of their health problems.[7] Each patient is entitled to the same level of care and consideration. Also of concern is the concept of distributive justice and the allocation of scarce health care resources. For example, should patients receive health care resources based on an equal share, what they need, or what they deserve based on contribution or effort? Related concepts include compensatory justice, such as occurs in a malpractice settlement, and procedural justice, which requires a system of fair treatment such as the system for allocating organs to people on the waiting list.[13]

Fidelity

Fidelity is the principle that requires us to act in ways that are loyal. In the role of a nurse, such action includes keeping your promises, doing what is expected of you, performing your duties, and being trustworthy.[13] Fidelity sounds easy enough, but it is probably the most frequent source of conflict for health care professionals because they owe loyalty to so many parties. In any particular situation, nurses may find themselves at odds between what they believe is right and what is in their own self-interest, what the patient or family wants, what other members of the health care team expect, what organizational policy dictates, or what the profession or the law requires.

Ethical Theories

There are many ethical theories, and we can only highlight a few major approaches in very simplified terms. Each theoretical approach offers a very different view of the same situation—views that may or may not lead to similar conclusions about an ethical problem or dilemma.

For example, most of us have a preference for either the consistency of rule-based approaches or the flexibility of consequence-based approaches. Likewise, some of us will be more comfortable with the highly contextual and emotionally engaged approach of relational ethics, whereas others are more comfortable with a highly rational and detached approach to ethical analysis.

Ethics of Duty

An ethics of duty is based on the ethical approach of deontology, in which moral duties are seen as self-evident, needing no further justification. Moral action is then based on acting according to a specific duty simply because it is the right thing to do.[13] Although the consequences of our actions are important, they are a secondary consideration to duty and our intention to do the right thing. The ethical question posed is, "What is my duty?" For example, if a nurse becomes aware that a friend and colleague has been diverting narcotics because she has developed an addiction, and the nurse reports her friend to her supervisor because that is what the organizational policy requires, she is complying with her ethical duty to report.

Ethics of Consequences

An ethic of consequences is based on a teleological view that moral actions are defined entirely on the basis of the outcomes or consequences of an action. Reaching a particular goal is what defines the ethical justification of an act regardless of your sense of duty or moral intent.[13] Consequence-based theories often weigh the advantages and disadvantages, or the harms and benefits, of different actions in the same situation. Utilitarianism, a common teleological theory, assumes that a moral action is one that results in the greatest good for the greatest number. The basic ethical question posed is, "What action will promote the greatest good with the least harm?" For example, if the nurse mentioned previously reports her friend because she is concerned that some patients are being harmed when their pain medications are diverted and all patients are at risk if her friend is practicing under the influence, then her actions are primarily based on a consideration of consequences. Her goal is to protect as many patients as possible rather than following a particular rule as a matter of duty. In fact, she might act outside of the policy if she believed reporting would not result in appropriate action by her supervisor.

Ethics of Character

Theories that emphasize character are classified under the general category of virtue ethics. Unlike the ethics of duty or consequences, which use external principles and rules to guide actions, virtue ethics relies on the character of the individual as the primary source of moral action.[13] Character develops over time based on life experiences and our willingness to reflect on our actions and motives. Virtues are character traits that predispose a person with good intentions to act with practical wisdom. Moral virtues include respect, honesty, sympathy, charity, kindness, loyalty, and fairness, whereas practical virtues include intelligence, patience, prudence, and shrewdness.[14] In general, a moral act must both promote good and intend good based on the moral predispositions of our character. The basic ethical question might be, "What is the wise action to take?"

Crigger and Godfrey argue strongly for virtue theory to be the core of nursing ethics, with an emphasis on the virtues of compassion, integrity, humility, and courage.[6] In particular, the virtue of courage lies at the heart of ethical practice. It is one thing to know what one's intention should be and another to have the courage to act on that intention. The concept of virtue has been central to the definitions of professional, professionalism, and professional identity.[6] Common criticisms of virtue ethics are that character varies between individuals, leading to ethical inconsistency, and our choices may change over time with additional experience and character development. However, a strength of a virtue-based approach to nursing ethics is that it assumes character must be continually developed and refined in practice throughout a nurse's career. Ethics is a dynamic element of practice that cannot be reduced to simple habits of following rules or weighing outcomes. In the case of our nurse with the impaired colleague, a character-based approach would lead her to act based on a combination of her own good intentions to protect her friend, the patients, and the organization while also seeking the best possible outcome for all. She would be guided primarily by some combination of her own moral and practical virtues, and on the basis of her professional sense of identity, rather than by the externally dictated rules and consequences.

Ethics of Relationship

Ethical theories that emphasize relationship are focused on the nature and obligations inherent in human relationships and community. With some roots in feminist thought, the ethic of care approaches difficult ethical situations in a context-specific manner that searches for solutions in the particular details of the situation. Universal principles are used only to the extent they can be applied based on the unique circumstances of each situation. Primary attention is paid to preserving relationships, improving communication, enhancing cooperation, and minimizing harm to everyone involved while promoting an ideal of caring.[15] The basic ethical question in the ethic of care might be, "What is the caring response?"

Such an approach is very different from the highly abstract, rational, unemotional, and rule-oriented approach of most Western ethical traditions. Although duty-based, consequence-based, and, to a lesser extent, character-based approaches have dominated the fields of bioethics, clinical ethics, and medical ethics (physicians), nursing has long embraced an ethic of care and other relational approaches. Returning once more to our nurse with the impaired colleague, the ethic of care will direct her first toward gaining a full and empathetic understanding of the context of the situation, including the various relationships that must be protected and preserved if possible. She will seek open communication and a collaborative approach that emphasizes caring and minimizes harm to all parties. For example, she might first approach her friend and offer to accompany her to speak with the appropriate party in the organization to arrange for treatment and address the legal implications of her actions.

CONTEXT TO NURSING AND HEALTH CARE

Applied ethics addresses the process of ethical analysis and decision making in actual cases or with respect to specific topics. Although the range and complexity of ethical theory can be daunting, applied ethics is fairly straightforward insofar as you have a specific decision that needs to be made and you are free to incorporate any ethical concepts you consider relevant to making that decision.

Ethical Decision Making in Practice

There will be times when you must assess a situation and make a difficult ethical decision on your own. However, health care decisions are generally not made in a vacuum, and the nurse is often participating in ethical decision making as a member of an interprofessional patient care team or an administrative team. Although there is likely to be some conflict when people with different perspectives are involved, such conflict can be used to enhance the depth and breadth of the analysis by forcing everyone to consider the situation from various viewpoints. Therefore group or team decision making can often result in a more refined solution.

When conflict within the team or between the team and the patient or patient's family cannot be resolved, an organizational ethics committee can be consulted to assist with mediating the conflict. Most acute care hospitals and some extended care facilities have an ethics committee onsite or they have access to one. An ethics committee does not make clinical decisions; however, the assigned consult team or the full committee can guide the discussion and act as mediator when there is conflict among the parties.

For organizational issues such as adherence to regulations, safety standards, quality of care, conflict of interest, or billing fraud and abuse, most organizations have a compliance committee or compliance officer, and they may even offer a compliance hotline for reporting of suspected violations. When the dilemma involves other professional issues, state and local chapters of professional associations may have similar ethics committees or experts with whom one can consult.

Ethical Issues in Nursing

A large study by Fry and Riley examined (1) the ethical issues encountered by registered nurses (RNs) in their practice, (2) the frequency that ethical issues occur in practice, (3) the degree to which RNs are concerned by these issues, (4) the way RNs handle ethical issues, and (5) the types of ethics education topics and resources that RNs perceive as helpful in practicing ethically.[16]

According to study findings, the following are the most frequent ethical issues experienced by RNs:
- Protecting patients' rights and human dignity
- Respecting/not respecting informed consent to treatment
- Providing care with possible risk to the nurse's health
- Using/not using physical or chemical restraints
- Working with staffing patterns that limit patient access to nursing care

Issues that RNs find most disturbing include the following:
- Coping with staffing patterns that limit patient access to nursing care
- Prolonging the living/dying process with inappropriate measures
- Not considering the quality of a patient's life
- Implementing managed care policies that threaten quality of care
- Working with unethical/impaired colleagues

More than 30% of the respondents reported encountering ethical issues in their practice one to four times per week or daily. In handling their most recently experienced ethical issue, more than 83% reported that they discussed the issue with nursing peers, whereas more than 66% discussed the issue with nursing leadership. On the other hand, more than 5% of the nurses reported that they did not deal with the ethical issue at all.[16]

Moral Distress

There has been much research on moral distress, with evidence of moral distress within all health care disciplines.[17–23] *Moral distress* occurs when you are unable to act upon what you believe is the morally appropriate action to take or when you otherwise act in a manner contrary to your personal and professional values.[24] In other words, you know what to do but believe you cannot do it due to internal or external barriers. Self-doubt, lack of assertiveness, and the perception

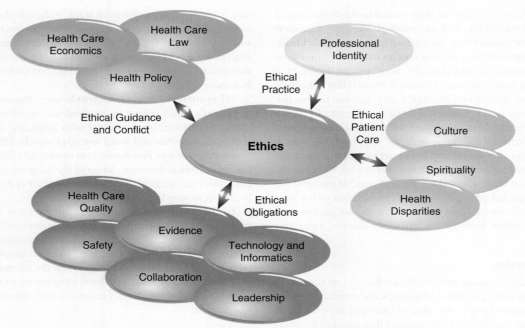

FIGURE 42-3 Ethics and Interrelated Concepts

of powerlessness are examples of internal barriers. External barriers include inadequate staffing, lack of organizational support, poor relationships with colleagues, and policies that conflict with the care needs of patients.[17]

Situations that have been shown to cause moral distress are very similar to the common ethical issues noted previously. Many of them occur in end-of-life situations and involve what is perceived to be overly aggressive treatment and inappropriate use of resources. Working with other physicians and nurses who one considers incompetent is another common situation that has been shown to result in moral distress.[25]

The impact of moral distress occurs in two parts.[17] When the situation first occurs, moral distress can result in frustration, anger, guilt, anxiety, withdrawal, self-blame, and other stress-related symptoms. The second part of moral distress is referred to as *reactive distress* or *moral residue*, and it is characterized by lingering feelings that can accumulate over time with each subsequent experience of moral distress. At least three patterns of response to moral residue have been described. In the first pattern, a heightened response leads health care professionals to engage in activities of conscientious objection, such as voicing opposition to a plan of care or refusing to follow orders. In the second pattern, they experience a desensitization with a tendency to be passive or to simply withdraw from situations in which they feel ethically challenged. The third pattern is characterized by strong, ongoing physical and psychological stresses that often lead to burnout and leaving the profession.[17] In all cases, the health care professional's core values, integrity, and professional identity have been undermined.

Because of the strong negative impact of unresolved moral distress on the job satisfaction and retention of nurses and other health care professionals, leaders in health care organizations are becoming aware of the need to create an organizational climate in which ethical issues can be openly discussed and resolved.[26] Interventions have included ethics debriefings, more support for ethics committees, and better access to ethics education and other resources.

INTERRELATED CONCEPTS

As evident in Figure 42-3, ethics is closely intertwined with many other concepts related to nursing. Health Policy, Health Care Law, and Health Care Economics can all be the source of both ethical guidance and ethical conflict. For example, legal requirements may provide guidance in most situations but may create conflict in a specific situation that does not quite fit the context for which the legal requirement was intended. Professional Identity is contingent upon a conception of ethical practice.

The concepts Health Care Quality, Safety, Evidence, Collaboration, and Technology and Informatics are all grounded in ethical obligations such as preventing needless harm, acting in a patient's best interest, ensuring the best outcomes for the most patients, and serving as a good steward of scarce health care resources. The concept of Leadership has additional ethical obligations, such as balancing loyalties and the interests of patients, employees, the organization, and the community.

Patient care and the process of nursing are fraught with ethical problems and dilemmas. For example, the ethical practice of nursing requires that the nurse treat each patient with respect, recognizing and responding to each patient's unique experience of illness and injury; however, ethical challenges can arise at the intersections of patient care, Culture, and Spirituality, as well as in the face of Health Disparities.

CLINICAL EXEMPLARS

The scope of ethical issues in nursing can be generally examined across the broad categories of clinical, organizational, and health policy issues, with many issues falling into more than one category. Clinical issues can be further subdivided into those at the beginning of life, across the lifespan, and at the end of life. Box 42-1 provides an expanded list of examples of potential ethical issues faced in nursing practice. It is beyond the scope of this text to describe all of these exemplars; however, a few are featured here.

■■■ BOX 42-1 EXEMPLARS OF ETHICS

Clinical Ethics and Bioethics
Beginning of Life
- Abortion
- Assisted reproduction
- Child abuse
- Complications of pregnancy
- Emergency contraception
- Genetic enhancement
- Minor consent to or refusal of treatment
- Prenatal genetic selection
- Prenatal genetic testing
- Severely impaired newborns

Lifespan
- Confidentiality
- Cultural conflicts
- Decisional capacity
- Domestic and elder abuse
- Genetic testing
- Informed consent
- Pain management and addiction
- Patient noncompliance
- Patients as research subjects
- Protecting patient rights

End of Life
- Advance directives
- CPR orders
- Chronically critically ill
- Nonbeneficial treatment
- Organ allocation

- Organ procurement
- Patients without a proxy decision maker
- Proxy decision making
- Terminal sedation
- Withholding or withdrawal of life support

Organizational Ethics
- Allocation of scarce resources
- Conflict of interest
- Conscience policies
- Disclosure of medical errors
- Fraud and abuse
- Impaired providers
- Inadequate staffing levels
- Patient safety
- Uncompensated care
- Use of restraints

Health Policy Ethics
- Abortion
- Provider-assisted suicide
- Allocation of research funding
- Medical marijuana
- Health care for the uninsured
- Health care for undocumented immigrants
- Access to experimental treatment
- Privacy of health information
- Rural access to health care
- Drug shortages
- Tort reform (malpractice)

Featured Exemplars
Genetic Enhancement

Advances in genetics continue to pose numerous ethical issues in practice, particularly at the beginning of life. Preimplantation and prenatal genetic screening not only allow for parents to select embryos free of genetic diseases or predispositions but also are now used to select nonmedical traits such as gender. Soon, parents will be able to select for a range of nonmedical traits and genetic enhancements, such as eye and hair color, height, and perhaps even intelligence, raising basic questions of respect for persons, parental autonomy, needless harm, and justice.

Confidentiality

Confidentiality is an issue that can arise across the lifespan in many situations. A particularly complex dilemma involves mandatory reporting of potential domestic or elder abuse. The legal duty to report may be very much at odds with the patient's wishes and may result in unwanted intervention and disruption in the patient's life.

Advance Directives

Advance directives for health care pose many dilemmas at the end of life. A patient's autonomous wishes, or what we think the patient

wanted based on the directive, may be strongly opposed by the family or the health care team. Even patients often change their minds when faced with the reality of their directive.

Uncompensated Care

Organizations face numerous ethical challenges. A common source of ethical conflict for health care organizations and their employees is ensuring high-quality and cost-effective operations while also maintaining safe levels of staffing, purchasing current technologies, and continuing to deliver necessary but unreimbursed care to uninsured or underinsured patients.

Conflict of Interest

Many ethical dilemmas at the bedside begin at the level of health care policy. For example, medical marijuana is now legal in nearly half of the United States; however, federal drug laws directly conflict with the ability of pharmacists and health care organizations to dispense it. In addition, there is a lack of strong evidence-based research for or against its use, particularly in children, posing ethical questions for both individual providers and organizations when treatment with the drug is requested by patients or parents.

CASE STUDY

Source: Thomas Northcut/Digital Vision/Thinkstock

Case Presentation

Josh is a pleasant and intelligent 17-year-old male who was diagnosed with an aggressive bone cancer and underwent amputation of his left leg; however, his cancer has now metastasized to his chest, skull, and lungs. Josh and your son have been friends at school for years, and you knew him before his illness. Since then, you have been his nurse on occasion and he has talked to you about his disease. He has told you that talking about it upsets his parents and makes his friends uncomfortable, so it is nice to have someone with whom he can be honest. You have always been impressed with the maturity and insight he demonstrates.

Josh has been readmitted, his prognosis is grim, and he is experiencing a great deal of pain. Although you have not been assigned to care for him, you are aware that members of the clinical team have struggled with an ongoing request by Josh's parents that the health care personnel limit the information they share with him. Despite the many questions he asks, Josh has not been told the extent of the metastases or that he will likely die within a few weeks. Members of the care team have frequently omitted information and even lied to Josh at the insistence of his parents and with the reluctant agreement of his attending physician. Members of the care team have questioned the unit director several times; however, she continues to instruct them to respect the wishes of the parents to avoid any legal problems. Joshua's parents also insist that he continue to receive every possible intervention, and another clinical trial is being considered.

One evening, Josh notices you in the hall and calls you into his room. He confronts you and tells you he knows he is not being told everything. He says he believes he is dying and, although it frightens him, he is ready to die. He has not been able to attend school for several months, his friends no longer come to see him, he knows his younger brother and sister get very little attention because of him, and he is in nearly constant pain. He is tired of pretending to be "strong and brave." He has tried to talk to his parents, but they refuse to even listen to him. He says, "I trust you to tell me exactly what's happening and what I need to do to stop treatment, even if it is against my parents' wishes."

Case Analysis

This case presents you with a true ethical dilemma as you are faced with the practical problem of how to respond to his request to be told the truth of his condition and how to discontinue treatment. Numerous ethical questions and assumptions can be raised, and there is no one correct solution to the dilemma. You will need to consider Josh's autonomy and that of his parents, whether he is being needlessly harmed both by withholding information and by aggressive treatment, and how to define his best interest. Issues of veracity, fidelity, and justice can also be identified. Each ethical theory will pose a somewhat different approach to the case, providing you with many different points of view. Unfortunately, Josh is sitting in front of you expecting an answer now, which is why ongoing practice with ethical reflection and analysis is so important to your practice. You will not always have the luxury of time to explore your options, so you need to be able to quickly and effectively assess the ethical dimensions of a situation. How would you respond to Josh?

ACCESS EXEMPLAR LINKS IN YOUR GIDDENS EBOOK

REFERENCES

1. Bennett-Woods D: *Nanotechnology: Ethics and society,* Boca Raton, FL, 2008, CRC Press.
2. Tubbs JB: *A handbook of bioethics terms,* Washington, DC, 2009, Georgetown University Press.
3. Darr K: *Ethics in health services management,* Baltimore, 2005, Health Professions Press.
4. U.S. Department of Health and Human Services and U.S. Department of Justice: *Health care fraud and abuse control program: Annual report for fiscal year 2013, February 2014.* Retrieved from <http://oig.hhs.gov/publications/docs/hcfac/FY2013-hcfac.pdf>.
5. Boyle PJ, DuBose ER, Ellingson SJ, et al: *Organizational ethics in health care: Principles, cases and practical solutions,* San Francisco, 2001, Jossey–Bass.
6. Crigger N, Godfrey N: *The making of nurse professionals: A transformational approach,* Sudbury, MA, 2011, Jones & Bartlett.
7. American Nurses Association: *Code of ethics for nurses,* 2001. Retrieved from <http://nursingworld.org/MainMenuCategories/ThePracticeofProfessionalNursing/EthicsStandards/CodeofEthics.aspx>.
8. Sulmasy DP, Sugarman J: The many methods of medical ethics (or, thirteen ways of looking at a blackbird). In Sugarman J, Sulmasy DP, editors: *Methods in medical ethics,* ed 2, Washington, DC, 2010, Georgetown University Press.
9. Johnson C: *Meeting the ethical shadows of leadership,* ed 4, Los Angeles, 2011, Sage.
10. Jonsen A, Siegler M, Winslade W: *A practical approach to ethical decisions in clinical medicine,* ed 7, New York, 2010, McGraw-Hill.
11. Devettere R: *Practical decision making in health care ethics,* ed 3, Washington, DC, 2010, Georgetown University Press.
12. Beauchamp TL, Childress JF: *Principles of biomedical ethics,* ed 6, New York, 2008, Oxford University Press.
13. Bennett-Woods D: *Ethics at a glance,* Denver, CO, 2005, Regis University, Center for Ethics and Leadership in the Health Professions. Retrieved from <http://rhchp.regis.edu/HCE/EthicsAtAGlance/index.html>.
14. Munson R: *Intervention and reflection: Basic issues in medical ethics,* ed 9, Belmont, CA, 2011, Wadsworth.
15. Noddings N: *Caring: A feminine approach to ethics and moral education,* Berkley, CA, 1984, University of California Press.
16. Fry ST, Riley JM: *Ethical issues in clinical practice: A multi-state study of practicing registered nurses,* Boston, 2002, Nursing Ethics Network. Retrieved from <http://jmrileyrn.tripod.com/nen/research.html#anchor195458>.
17. Epstein EG, Hamric AB: Moral distress, moral residue and the crescendo effect. *J Clin Ethics* 20(4):330–342, 2009.
18. Forde R, Aasland OG: Moral distress among Norwegian doctors. *J Med Ethics* 34:521–525, 2008.

19. Hamric AB, Blackhall LJ: Nurse–physician perspectives on the care of dying patients in intensive care units: Collaboration, moral distress, and ethical climate. *Crit Care Med* 35(2):422–429, 2007.

20. Schwenzer KJ, Wang L: Assessing moral distress in respiratory care practitioners. *Crit Care Med* 34(12):2967–2973, 2006.

21. Carpenter C: Moral distress in physician therapy practice. *Physiother Theory Pract* 26(2):69–78, 2010.

22. Kalvemark Sporrong S, Hoglund AT, Arnets B: Measuring moral distress in pharmacy and clinical practice. *Nurs Ethics* 13(4):416–427, 2006.

23. Austin W, Rankel M, Kagan L, et al: To stay or to go, to speak or to stay silent, to act or not to act: Moral distress as experienced by psychologists. *Ethics Behav* 15(3):197–212, 2005.

24. American Association of Critical Care Nurses: *Moral distress [Position statement]*, 2008. Retrieved from <www.aacn.org/WD/Practice/Docs/Moral_Distress.pdf>.

25. Zuzelo PR: Exploring the moral distress of registered nurses. *Nurs Ethics* 14(3):344–359, 2007.

26. Bell J, Breslin JM: Healthcare provider moral distress as a leadership challenge. *Healthcare Law Ethics Regul* 10(4):94–97, 2008.

CONCEPT
43

Patient Education

Barbara Carranti

ducation empowers. Patient education is no exception. Effective patient education allows patients and their families the opportunity to control their own health, reduce risk for illness, improve longevity, and enhance overall wellness. Specifically, the goals of patient education are to learn and adapt by forming connections and associations that will facilitate changes in behavior, resulting in enhanced health and well-being or improved treatment of illness.[1] Lamiani and Furey note that the emphasis of patient education frequently focuses on the disease as opposed to the patient, and they stress the importance of incorporating exploration of the patient's illness experience into the educational plan to ensure high-quality care.[2]

The importance of patient education is supported by *Healthy People 2020*. This science-based program, in existence for more than 30 years, has used evidence to establish objectives to improve the health of Americans. Patient education is the key to achievement of the overarching goals of *Healthy People*, specifically increasing the quality and years of healthy life and eliminating health disparities.[3]

DEFINITION

For the purposes of this concept presentation, patient education is defined as "*a process of assisting people to learn health-related behaviors so that they can incorporate these behaviors into everyday life.*"[4,p11] This is a purposeful process whereby the patient is learning health-related information to support healthy lifestyle or behavior change. A similar term, *patient teaching*, is used interchangeably. The role of the nurse in patient education is to assist the patient in forming goals; assess patient need, motivation, and ability; plan educational interventions to achieve goals; and evaluate patient outcomes toward goal attainment. In short, nurses empower patients. This empowerment is accomplished by providing information to enhance wellness, reducing the risk for illness, and encouraging autonomy by enhancing self-care skills while maintaining a patient-centered approach.

SCOPE

As a concept, patient education can include provision of information in a wide range of formats and can be described from two perspectives: the delivery approach and educational domains. The process varies depending on multiple variables, including the intended outcome and the characteristics of the learner. For example, is the educational intervention intended to teach the patient a skill or impart knowledge related to a known health problem, increase the probability of successful treatment, prepare for discharge, or to promote a healthy lifestyle and enhance well-being? Thoughtful consideration of intended outcomes will enhance the patient's learning by matching an approach to intended goals. The nurse must ask, "What change in the patient is the desired outcome of this activity?" The type of education offered will require that the nurse match the approach, method, and evaluation to this desired outcome.[5]

Educational Approaches

Patient educational approaches can range from formal educational programming such as group lecture settings to informal, individualized one-on-one teaching and to self-directed learning by the patient that is facilitated by the nurse.[1] Formal patient education courses or classes are useful to address needs common to a group of patients or as individual teaching sessions. Formal courses are often taught using a curriculum/course plan with standardized content. In contrast, informal teaching often occurs in one-on-one sessions with the patient and/or family. Informal sessions may be planned or spontaneous, but they do not follow a specified formalized plan. An informal approach represents a large portion of patient education done by nurses. In fact, the majority of critical education occurs with each patient encounter when medications, diet, or treatment is explained or simply when answering questions about the patient's issues or concerns. Individual or self-directed education results when a patient or family obtains and/or completes an educational activity independent from the nurse or other health care providers. With the influence of consumerism and the availability of information, a great deal of education can occur through self-directed learning employing written material or media (e.g., Internet and video) designed to assist the patient with information about health topics, a particular disease, treatments, or a specific skill (Figure 43-1).[1]

Because of the increasing dependence on technology in all aspects of life, the use of Internet resources for patient education cannot be ignored. A majority of adults in America use the Internet to find information on many aspects of life, including health, healthy lifestyles, and treatment options.[5] This use of technology expands the role of the nurse in patient education to include teaching on evaluation of

FIGURE 43-1 Scope of Patient Education Concept

Internet sources. Patients should be encouraged to search for information sources that list authors and their credentials and contact information. The source of information should also be listed, and any photographs, charts, graphs, or other graphics should contain helpful understandable information. Any links associated with the site should be functional, active links. It is also important that patients be taught to search for government (.gov), educational (.edu), and nonprofit (.org) sites because they are considered to be the most credible sources of information. Finally, sites chosen for use in gathering information should clearly identify how consumers can contact a site administrator and should be secure sites.[6]

For this discussion of approaches to patient education to be complete, the educated and motivated consumer should be considered. Many patients will be active consumers of health information and use self-directed approaches to education. Patients may present the nurse with articles, computer printouts, and other materials gathered in an attempt to learn about health promotion, symptoms, diagnoses, and treatments. These materials can be incorporated into the nurse's assessment of the patient and the educational plan. The tendency to pursue learning opportunities addresses motivation and presents the nurse with an opportunity to ask the patient to discuss what has been learned. This also gives the nurse the opportunity to teach the patient evaluative skills, looking at sources and content of the material for credibility and reliability.[7]

Learning Domains

Patient education can also be conceptualized from the perspective of learning domains—in other words, in terms of the type of learning a patient will need. The three main domains are cognitive, psychomotor, and affective (Figure 43-2).[1] Education intended to increase a patient's knowledge of a subject, for example, is cognitive in nature, and using methods such as written material, lecture, and discussion is appropriate. Skill teaching or psychomotor teaching requires that the patient have opportunities to touch and manipulate equipment and practice skills. A patient who must learn to change a dressing over a wound is an example. Education that is intended to change attitudes, such as viewing the lifestyle modifications associated with the treatment of coronary artery disease as a positive change rather than a burden, is known as the affective domain in education.[5]

FIGURE 43-2 Learning Domains

To illustrate this, consider an example of a patient with a new diagnosis of a degenerative neurologic disorder that will require the patient to self-catheterize. The nurse will need to teach the patient the complex *psychomotor* skill of self-catheterization, and the teaching will be successful when the patient is able to competently demonstrate this skill. Part of this teaching will include physiological information designed to enhance the patient's understanding of the necessity of this procedure (*cognitive* learning) as well as assistance with lifestyle alterations and coping to help the patient to adapt and continue to live fully (*affective* domain).[1]

ATTRIBUTES AND CRITERIA

For patient education to occur, there must be an identified need for learning. Although this need may be identified by the nurse, learning will not occur without readiness on the part of the learner. Ultimately, it is patient motivation that determines when, how, and if patient education will occur.[1] In addition to an identified need, the following are other major attributes of patient education:
1. Planning is involved.
2. The outcomes are goal oriented.
3. The patient is motivated to learn.

Like any other teaching-learning process, patient education requires that the teacher (nurse) know the intended audience and plan appropriately. This is a process that must be in place even in the most routine patient encounters. There must also be a goal, which is usually a change in behavior or attitude of some sort. The learners (patient and/or significant other) not only should be identified as the target of the teaching plan but also should be motivated by the outcome of the behavioral or attitudinal change. The nurse then develops the plan and evaluation to be consistent with the patient needs.

The nurse must determine the overall appropriateness of patient education. This requires asking, "Is the timing right, are the involved parties ready, and are the goals clear?" Only after these answers are determined can true education of the patient occur.

THEORETICAL LINKS

The goal of all patient education is to produce change. It is helpful to examine theories of behavior and learning in addition to nursing theory to understand patient need and motivation to change.

Theories of Health Behavior

The health belief model was developed by Rosenstock in the mid-20th century to help explain individual decisions to use health screening opportunities. It has been adapted many times to explain compliance and behavior as they relate to health.[8] According to the health belief model, individual perceptions of susceptibility to and severity of disease are the primary motivators for making attempts to change health behavior. These motivators are modified by demographic, social, psychological, and structural variables that may heighten or dampen motivation. The primary motivation of patient perception then allows the patient to be open to cues to act, which of course leads to patient education opportunities.[8]

For example, a patient who is aware that her risk for breast cancer is high because of genetics may be likely to participate in some form of education about risk for the disease. This education can enhance the patient's knowledge level to produce lifestyle changes that reduce risk.

Simply stated, the health belief model states that for an individual to change behavior related to health and wellness, there first must be a belief that illness can be avoided and that taking a particular action can reduce risk. Furthermore, the individual must believe that he or she is capable of making the needed change.

Nola Pender's health promotion model (HPM), developed in 1987 and revised in the late 1990s, is "an attempt to depict the multidimensional nature of persons interacting with their interpersonal and physical environment as they pursue health."[9,p44] The HPM is based on the health belief model that was expanded by Pender to include factors that can influence the patient's motivation to change behavior, such as previous experience with behavior changes to address the problem, and the patient's perception of success in these attempts. This model also expands the view of patient motivation by including social supports and competing priorities as factors to consider.

Pender's model is focused on achieving optimum wellness rather than avoiding disease, which Rosenstock's original model stressed as the primary motivator for changing behaviors. Pender points out, for example, that consideration of the patient's prior experience with attempting to change health behaviors is a key factor for the nurse when planning strategy, including educational strategy. An obese patient with comorbidities of coronary artery disease and type 2 diabetes will likely be told to lose weight to avoid serious complications. The HPM dictates that part of the nursing assessment would be to ask the patient about prior attempts at weight reduction and perceived success of these efforts. The patient response to these inquiries will assist the nurse in development of educational interventions to address patient need. Pender also emphasizes that how the patient views the benefits and barriers to behavior change as well as the patient's own perception of ability to succeed will impact the nurse's plan for education.[9]

Nursing Theory

There are many theories that can be used as a basis for formulating patient education plans. Dorothea Orem's self-care deficit theory is based on optimizing the patient's ability to assume responsibility for his or her own care and that motivation is based on the anticipation of resuming this responsibility. Orem defines self-care as a regulatory function that is "a deliberate action to supply or ensure the supply of necessary materials needed for continued life, growth, development and maintenance of human integrity."[10,p134] Orem addresses the role of family and others in the patient's social support system as assuming the responsibility of the patient's care when the patient is unable. Utilization of Orem's theory can assist the nurse to determine if teaching materials are consistent with factors discovered during the assessment process so that selection can move the patient toward meeting self-care demands.[11]

CONTEXT TO NURSING AND HEALTH CARE

Education of patients is integral to professional nursing practice; this fact is illustrated in multiple documents, including the American Nurses Association's *Nursing: Scope and Standards of Practice*,[12] each state's Nurse Practice Act, the Institute of Medicine's *Future of Nursing* report,[13] and the *Quality and Safety Education in Nursing* competencies.[14] Nursing practice has been defined as "the protection, promotion, and optimization of health and abilities, prevention of illness and injury, alleviation of suffering through the diagnosis and treatment of human response, and advocacy in the care of patients, families, communities, and populations."[12,p1] These positive patient outcomes are often achieved through education.

Numerous agencies require that patients and families be provided with information required to make decisions about health care and treatment of illness.[15] Modifications in health care in terms of delivery style and financer expectations have also changed the role of the

patient in participating in his or her own care. This new level of patient engagement in health care requires that patient education be a priority for the registered nurse in the provision of patient care.[16]

Consumerism has also made more individuals want to take control of their own health and wellness and is promoting more individuals to seek health education opportunities in many venues. Patient education, however, is a cornerstone of nursing practice and is one of the ways in which members of care teams collaborate to achieve quality patient care outcomes. Quality patient education requires appropriate assessment, planning, implementation, and evaluation of this often-complex process.

The educational process and the nursing process are essentially the same[4] and include learner assessment, planning, implementation, evaluation, and documentation. Each of these steps is discussed in detail.

Learner Assessment

Learner assessment begins with a comprehensive assessment of the patient's learning needs. This may include a formalized written assessment, may be incorporated as part of the health assessment interview, or certainly may be a stated need from the patient. The assessment should include patient resources (education level, literacy level, social support, and financial resources), educational resources, and nursing resources. Assessment data should be used to develop a teaching plan that is appropriate for the patient but also one that will meet the desired goal. To fully individualize the educational plan for a patient, the nurse will consider the age, stage of development, and motivation to change behavior.

Psychosocial Development

Educational interventions must attend to the patient's achievement of developmental tasks. Erikson's theory of development is based on an eight-stage process in which each stage requires the achievement of a particular task. Completion of each stage forms the foundation of the next stage.[17] An understanding of Erikson's theory of development assists the nurse in patient education by understanding approaches necessary to accomplish the goal. For example, the educational approach taken by the nurse in teaching a patient how to use a metered dose inhaler for delivery of steroids will be different for a school-age child than for a middle-aged adult. Using play-type activities to teach the procedure and identifying a celebrity or other role model who may need a similar treatment will appeal to the school-age patient. The middle-aged adult is more concerned with fitting this treatment into his or her normal life patterns. Finally, it is critical for the nurse to incorporate the patient's own culture to make the teaching process meaningful.

Pedagogy Versus Androgogy

An appropriate next step to follow when utilizing Erikson's theory of development is to ensure that the type of educational method used is appropriate to the individual stage of development. Pedagogy is the methodology used to assist children to learn, or the strategies of traditional teaching. Androgogy conversely describes adult learning.[5] This implies that the strategies used with great success for teaching children in classrooms may not translate to successful outcomes for the nurse teaching adults. The nurse should attend to the developmental level of the individual and tailor learning activities to account for these differences. In general, learning in the adult is focused on an immediate need to address a personal issue or to solve a problem. The nurse is viewed as one who can facilitate that goal rather than simply impart knowledge. All learning activity should be directed toward meeting the learning goals of the adult patient. It is also important to note that most adults enter any learning situation with a rich history of experiences that can be, and should be, drawn on by the nurse to enhance present learning.[1] Adults tend to learn best when there is a perceived need to learn the information (internal motivation) and the information perceived is pertinent to address an immediate problem or need, when learning is self-directed using learner-centered strategies with application, and when learning draws on the past experiences of the learner. The nurse further enhances learning in the role of a facilitator and by providing timely feedback.

Hierarchy of Needs

Maslow's hierarchy of needs theory is based on a simple premise that for higher level needs to be addressed, lower level needs must be met. Maslow, a humanist, concluded that if environmental conditions are appropriate to meet basic needs, then individuals will be able to learn and self-actualize.[18] This is an important concept in all types of teaching and is clear in all levels of education. A school-age child has limited ability to concentrate if the child is hungry. A college student has limited ability to concentrate and learn after an all-night study session. Of course, this extends to patients as well. For example, inadequate oxygenation, safety deficits, and food, water, and elimination needs must be addressed before the patient can adequately learn. A patient who needs to learn a complex skill must have the needs of pain management and comfort met before he or she attempts to meet learning needs. The motivation for patient education may also be linked to survival, representing a much more basic level of need. For example, a patient learning to self-administer insulin for the first time may feel a great sense of accomplishment at mastering this complex task, but the ability to self-administer this drug is truly a matter of survival for the diabetic patient.

Generational Differences

Generational differences are also a consideration when approaching patient education. Much has been reported about differences in the learning styles between generations, relating not only to the age of the patient but also to the era in which the individual was raised, as well as the social and political experiences of a group.[19] Educational approaches may need to differ for those born before 1946; members of this age group usually are self-motivated and do not seek feedback for their performance. On the other hand, members of Generation Y are dependent on technology and desire immediate feedback.[20] This generational factor, perhaps more than any other, will dictate how the nurse approaches patient education.

Literacy Level

The ability to read and understand the written word is, of course, critical if the educational process is to include any written material. Based on the 2003 National Assessment of Adult Literacy, 43% of adults in the United States had literacy skills at the basic or below basic level.[21] It is also important to consider the patient's ability to understand and interpret health-related information and instructions —the individual's level of health literacy.[4] Although assessment of literacy levels can be very difficult in adult patients because of the stigma and shame often associated with limited reading ability, patients may give cues to limited literacy, such as avoiding reading materials provided (the patient may state "I forgot my glasses") or demonstrating repeated inability to follow written instructions. If there is a suspicion that the patient may not be able to read written material or that the information is written at a level that the patient cannot understand, the nurse must use alternate methods of instruction to ensure patient understanding. Although beyond the scope of this text, several methods exist for the nurse to quickly evaluate written material for readability for those with limited reading skills.

Barriers

There are a number of barriers to learning that must be considered as part of learner assessment. The lack of available social support systems, which may impair the patient's motivation to learn or ability to participate in classes or programs, is one common barrier. Lack of support may also limit the patient's ability to practice new skills. Additional patient-related barriers include cultural differences, lack of financial resources or time, and frequent interruptions. It may be within the patient's or the nurse's ability to control or remove these barriers to enhance patient learning and outcomes.

Barriers on the part of the nurse to participate in patient education include lack of time and multiple competing demands. The teaching role of the professional nurse is often not prioritized because of issues with staffing, payment, and perception of effectiveness of educational efforts. Furthermore, the nurse's professional motivation and confidence in education skills may pose a barrier to patient education. Again, assessing the nurse's attitudes can assist in identification of these professional barriers and development of interventions to overcome them.[1]

Planning

Planning is the determination of what methods will be used to meet the educational need. This includes deciding if the outcome is a cognitive (knowledge) change, a psychomotor (performance of a skill) change, or an affective (feeling or attitude) change. Determining the type of outcome dictates the approach as well as the goal. For example, a patient diagnosed with type 1 diabetes may need to learn about the overall pathophysiology of the disease so that he or she can appreciate the physical and lifestyle impact. However, the patient also needs to develop practical psychomotor skills (e.g., injection and testing) to cope with this disease. The nurse must plan not only to describe what diabetes is but also to demonstrate blood glucose testing and self-injection of insulin, allowing for practice and re-demonstration from the patient and perhaps significant others as well. The teaching methodology used should match the domain of learning.

Implementation of Educational Plan

Implementation or carrying out the plan is an area in which flexibility is key. The nurse will need to determine the length of educational sessions, content to be covered, and methodology for teaching. These plans may be influenced by numerous unpredictable factors, such as patient condition and competing priorities. The nurse must adjust the teaching session to accommodate the priorities of the patient.

Evaluation

Evaluation of learning outcomes should be consistent with the domain of learning as well. Psychomotor skills, for example, require that the patient be able to *do* something, such as perform a skill. Using a survey or other measurement tool to evaluate a skill will not adequately measure this outcome. Surveys and questionnaires can be used to measure affective behavior change as well as patient satisfaction with the teaching experience. Because the goal of patient education is behavior change, the evaluation of the process may need to be conducted over time and be dependent on multiple sources of data.

Returning to the example of teaching a patient diagnosed with type 1 diabetes, the nurse will likely include cognitive information about disease pathology to appropriately manage the condition. This patient will probably need to master the psychomotor skill of blood glucose monitoring and insulin injection. The nurse will also be concerned with the affective dimension of the diagnosis of chronic disease. Evaluation of all of these dimensions will require that the nurse observe the skills for level of mastery, discuss the "why" of diet and exercise with the patient on multiple occasions, evaluate the impact of the patient's daily decisions on disease management, and use repeated assessment of the patient's acceptance of the condition to fully evaluate behavior change.

No discussion of patient education would be complete without consideration of patient adherence. There are many factors that block patient adherence, such as lack of understanding, literacy, financial problems, lack of environmental or interpersonal support, previous experiences with treatment or self-management, and motivation.[3] These issues should be included in the assessment process and addressed in the educational plan for the patient in an attempt to enhance compliance.

Documentation

To ensure consistency in care, documentation of patient education is included in the patient record. This documentation should be comprehensive and include not only a description of the information that the patient was taught but also an assessment of the patient's motivation, ability to learn (any physical or cognitive issues that may inhibit the process), developmental level, and resources (personal and financial, if appropriate). A detailed plan should be included in the documentation so that other professionals can reinforce the process if education is to be continued across care settings. This should include goals and progress toward them. Finally, the patient response to the educational plan and adjustments to accommodate changes in patient condition or other factors should be included to ensure consistent, successful patient education outcomes.

INTERRELATED CONCEPTS

Patient education as a concept is central to the role of the nurse in the delivery of quality patient care (Figure 43-3). The professional roles and attributes of **Collaboration** and **Communication** are essential in

the development, planning, and delivery of patient education, whereas the nurse's role as an educator is central to his or her **Professional Identity**. The nurse works not only with the patient but also with teams of providers in determining care needs, and quality patient education is one of the results of this skilled collaborative effort. To accomplish this, the nurse's knowledge of **Technology and Informatics** along with the ability to teach patients and families the use of health care technology are critical when transitioning care from the acute care facility into the home. The result of current changes in health care requires the nurse to engage **Leadership** skills not only to assist patients and families but also to prepare the consumer for this evolution of health care.

The role of the nurse in **Health Promotion**, an area in which nurses generally take the lead, is also a critical professional dimension that is related to patient education. The nurse's knowledge and skill in recognizing opportunities to improve wellness, health, and function through lifestyle modification are used in all patient encounters and are a critical professional role in the education of patients.

Patient education incorporates the patient's attributes and resources. The nurse approaches each patient encounter as an opportunity to educate. This involves a determination of the patient's developmental level (**Development**) as well as an analysis of the dynamics of relationships (**Family Dynamics**) to assist in determination of supports and stressors. The patient's cultural background (**Culture**) and prior experiences with **Adherence** to prescribed regimens are also concepts that have a direct relationship to patient education and in fact form the foundation of the assessment and planning process.

CLINICAL EXEMPLARS

Examples of patient education exist in many formats for a broad range of topics, intended for use in a variety of ways. Box 43-1 represents some of the most common examples. Grouped by the primary focus as well as how the teaching/learning may be accomplished, Box 43-1 also highlights the numerous types, venues, and media types that can be considered in patient education.

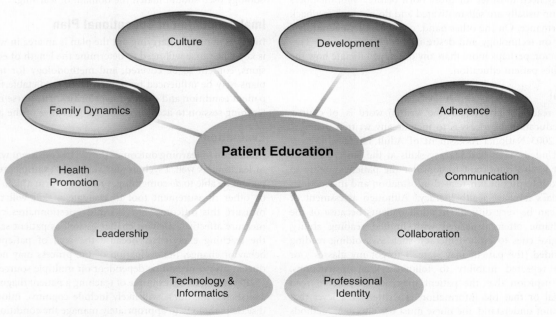

FIGURE 43-3 Patient Education and Interrelated Concepts Professional nursing concepts are represented in blue; health care recipient concepts are represented in red.

BOX 43-1   EXEMPLARS OF PATIENT EDUCATION

Illness Related
Formal Patient Education Programming
- Cancer support groups
- Cardiac education
- Coumadin classes
- Diabetes education
- Group preoperative teaching
- Ostomy support group

Informal Patient–Nurse Encounters
- Discharge teaching
- Disease-specific diet teaching
- High-tech home care teaching
- Medication teaching
- Symptom control
- Targeted written materials
- Wound care

Self-Directed Patient Education Activities
- Common literature (e.g., magazines, journals, newspapers)
- Instructional videos specific to condition or treatment
- Internet resources (e.g., American Cancer Society, American Heart Association)
- Self-help books (e.g., diet plans, herbal remedies, alternative and complementary treatment, coping with addiction)

Health Promotion
Formal Patient Education Programming
- Childbirth classes
- Complementary and alternative therapy
- Drug abuse avoidance
- Elder care classes
- Parenting classes
- Risk reduction activities
- Smoking cessation programs
- Strength/endurance building
- Weight reduction classes
- Wellness education programs

Informal Patient–Nurse Encounters
- Advanced care planning
- Age-specific screening needs
- Breast-feeding
- Counseling
- Genetic screening
- Health counseling
- Immunization teaching
- Preventing sexually transmitted diseases

Self-Directed Patient Education Activities
- Common literature (e.g., magazines, journals, newspapers)
- Exercise videos (e.g., aerobics, yoga, Pilates)
- Instructional videos specific to health-related topic
- Internet resources (e.g., WebMD, Real Age)
- Self-help books (e.g., diet plans, herbal remedies, alternative and complementary treatment, coping with addiction)
- Television (e.g., health-related programming, FIT TV)

Featured Exemplars

Although a discussion of all the exemplars presented in Box 43-1 is beyond the scope of this concept presentation, brief descriptions of a few of the most common and important exemplars are presented next. Refer to other resources for detailed information about these and any of the other exemplars.

Diabetes Education

Diabetes patient education is aimed at increasing the patient's ability to self-manage this endocrine disorder. Diabetes education programs can take many forms, including group classes and one-to-one teaching. Typical topics included in diabetes education programs are the physiological alterations present in this disease, diet and medication management, monitoring of blood glucose, and risk reduction. Also critical to address in a comprehensive education plan is the psychosocial impact of this condition. If patients are unable to self-manage, family members and other support people can be educated to assist in the care.[22]

Genetic Screening (Testing) Education

Although nurses are an excellent source of general information regarding genetic testing and screening, it is important to advise patients to consult with a genetics counselor if they are considering genetic testing. This professional can provide the most accurate information about cost, confidentiality of results, and the risks and benefits of testing. General information that can be provided to patients involves the information that can be gleaned from genetic testing as it relates to risk of developing a particular disease and passing that risk on to offspring.[22]

Internet Resources

Many patients have the ability to actively research symptoms, diagnoses, and treatment options through use of the Internet. Although often an excellent resource, the nurse remains an active partner in the education of the patient and family by answering questions, reviewing material and websites for accuracy, and assisting the patient and family to locate high-quality health information. It is also important to note that use of Internet resources requires access to a computer or mobile device and some comfort with technology.[22]

Complementary and Alternative Therapy

Inquiry into the use of complementary and alternative therapies should be part of a complete health assessment. This information is incorporated into a teaching plan for the patient. Teaching should include information about the specific type of complementary or alternative therapy (e.g., herbal supplements and meditation, acupuncture, or chiropractic intervention) and how these therapies may relate to more conventional treatments. For example, patients using herbal remedies should be instructed about the storage and use of these remedies and any potential medication or food interactions and also about potential complications of use in the perioperative period.[22]

Smoking Cessation Programs

Smoking cessation programs are designed to assist smokers to stop their use of cigarettes and other forms of tobacco. These programs provide education on the dangers and risks of tobacco use, but they are more focused on methods of stopping habitual use. Interventions may vary depending on the type or sponsor of the smoking cessation program, but they may include nicotine replacement, behavior modification, counseling, support, and relapse prevention. Education plans may also include non-nicotine drugs that may assist the patient to quit, such as some antidepressant medications.[22]

Cardiac Education

Information covered in cardiac education can include medication and treatment options as well as risk reduction. The following are all important topics to include in prevention programs as well as post-diagnosis education programs: alterations in lifestyle such as diet modification, weight loss, and control of diabetes; interpretation of common laboratory values (lipid profile); and sleep patterns and stress reduction. Concerns related to return to work, sexual activity, and exercise should be included in a comprehensive education plan. This information can be covered in group classes, which offer the benefit of support of others, or one-to-one teaching.[22]

CASE STUDY

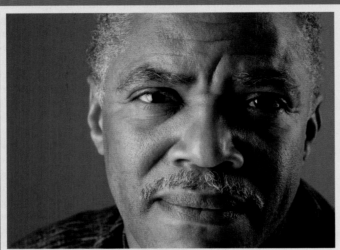

Source: Fuse/Thinkstock

Case Presentation

Mr. Jacobs is a 55-year-old college-educated male recently diagnosed with colon cancer. He is scheduled for surgery with formation of a colostomy. Prior to meeting the patient, the nurse reviews the health record and notes that Mr. Jacobs is able to read English, has family support, and is currently not working. Mr. Jacobs' wife works in retail.

Mr. Jacobs is very health conscious, and his goals are to return to "normal" life. The nurse notes a comment made by Mr. Jacobs that "a colostomy is the one thing I said I would never live with." Based on the information gathered, the nurse develops a teaching plan for Mr. Jacobs. The plan includes the provision of written material about colon cancer, anatomy and physiology of the gastrointestinal tract, and alterations presented by having a stoma. Options for care of the stoma are also provided in writing. A second visit to demonstrate how the ostomy appliance is fitted, emptied, and changed is planned. A manikin abdomen will be used to demonstrate and practice stoma care with the patient.

Mr. Jacobs is in the developmental stage of *generativity versus stagnation.*[12] When planning for his learning needs, the nurse uses multiple sources of information to teach Mr. Jacobs according to his level of education but also attends to the fact that psychomotor learning is required. To evaluate the outcome of the educational intervention conducted, the nurse follows-up with Mr. Jacobs to determine his competency (both actual and perceived) in performing the necessary skills of care and Mr. Jacobs' emotional and attitudinal changes related to the ostomy and his illness. Plans are changed and adjusted according to Mr. Jacobs' progress toward his goals, incorporating family members while Mr. Jacobs becomes ready for this step.

Case Analysis

In this case, the nurse attended carefully to assessment before beginning the educational process. Because the patient was well educated, the nurse could rely on multiple forms of education, including written materials. The nurse used hands-on practice to incorporate psychomotor skill. By asking about goals and listening to Mr. Jacobs' as he discussed his feelings about living with an ostomy before initiating the educational plan, the nurse gathers valuable information about perceptions and attitudes. With this information, the nurse is able to incorporate strategies for addressing the affective domain that will be most effective. Including the family members before the patient is ready may hamper education efforts by limiting trust in the nurse–patient relationship.

The patient's desire to return to his normal life indicates to the nurse that this patient, in Erickson's stage of generativity versus stagnation, wants to resume a productive life as soon as possible, lending to motivation to learn. This could have been further enhanced by incorporating frank discussions about the impact on Mr. Jacobs' sexuality into the teaching plan.

Failing to attend to the patient during assessment would have resulted in failure of the patient's educational experience. For example, if the nurse assumed that the patient would want his wife included from the beginning and arranged the educational sessions with Mrs. Jacobs rather than the patient alone, the nurse would have limited the patient's ability to express his own needs in the educational encounter.

ACCESS EXEMPLAR LINKS IN YOUR GIDDENS EBOOK

REFERENCES

1. Bastable SB, Gramet P, Jacobs K, et al: *Health professional as educator: Principles of teaching and learning,* Boston, 2011, Jones & Bartlett.
2. Lamiani G, Furey A: Teaching nurses how to teach: An evaluation of a workshop on patient education. *Patient Educ Couns* 75(2):270–273, 2009.
3. U.S. Department of Health and Human Services: *Healthy People 2020,* 2015. Retrieved from <http://www.healthypeople.gov>.
4. Bastable SB: *Essentials of patient education,* Boston, 2006, Jones & Bartlett.
5. Clark DR: *Dick and Carey instructional design model,* 2014. Retrieved from <http://nwlink.com/~donclark/history_isd/carey.html>.
6. Anderson AS, Klemm P: The Internet: Friend or foe when providing patient education? *Clin J Oncol Nurs* 12(1):55–63, 2008.

7. Bradley SM: The Internet: Can patients link to credible sources? *Medsurg Nurs* 17(4):229–236, 2008.
8. Richards E: Compliance, Motivation, and Health Behaviors of the Learner. In Bastable SB, editor: *The nurse as educator: Principles of teaching and learning for nursing practice,* ed 3, Boston, 2013, Jones & Bartlett.
9. Pender NJ, Murdaugh CL, Parsons MA: *Health promotion in nursing practice,* ed 6, Upper Saddle River, NJ, 2011, Pearson Prentice Hall.
10. McEwen M, Wills EM: *Theoretical basis for nursing,* ed 3, Philadelphia, 2011, Lippincott Williams & Wilkins.
11. Wilson FL, Wood DW, Risk J, et al: Evaluation of education materials using Orem's self-care deficit theory. *Nurs Sci Q* 16(1):68–76, 2003.
12. American Nurses Association: *Nursing: Scope and standards of practice,* Silver Spring, MD, 2010, Author.
13. Institute of Medicine: *The future of nursing: Leading change, advancing health,* Washington, DC, 2010, National Academies Press. Retrieved from <http://books.nap.edu/openbook.php?record_id=12956&page=23>.

14. QSEN Institute: *Quality and safety education in nursing.* Retrieved from <http://qsen.org/competencies/pre-licensure-ksas>.
15. Nelson MJ: Ethical, Legal, and Economic Foundations of the Education Process. In Bastable SB, editor: *Essentials of patient education*, Boston, 2006, Jones & Bartlett.
16. Gruman J, Rovner MH, French ME, et al: From patient education to patient engagement: Implications for the field of patient education. *Patient Educ Couns* 78:350, 2010.
17. Edelman CL, Mandle CL: *Health promotion throughout the lifespan*, ed 8, Philadelphia, 2014, Elsevier.
18. Braungart M, Braungart RG, Gramet R: Applying Learning Theories to Health Care Practice. In Bastable SB, editor: *Nurse as educator: Principles of teaching and learning for nursing practice*, ed 4, Burlington, MA, 2014, Jones & Bartlett.
19. Zalenski RJ, Raspa R: Maslow's hierarchy of needs: A framework for achieving human potential in hospice. *J Palliat Med* 9(5):1120–1127, 2006.
20. Moreno-Walton L, Brunett P, Akhtar S, et al: Teaching across the generation gap: Consensus from the Council of Emergency Medicine Residency Directors 2009 Academic Assembly. *Acad Emerg Med* 16(12, Suppl 2):S19–S24, 2009.
21. National Center for Education Statistics: *National assessment of adult literacy (NAAL)*, 2003. Retrieved from <http://nces.ed.gov/naal/kf_demographics.asp>.
22. Lewis SL, Dirksen SR, Heirkemper MM, et al: *Medical–surgical nursing: Assessment and management of clinical problems*, ed 9, St Louis, 2014, Mosby.

Health Promotion

Jean Giddens

During the past century, technological advancements have resulted in dramatic changes in nearly every aspect of our daily lives—particularly in the areas of transportation, communication, food production, and food acquisition. Technological advances have afforded humans with many conveniences incomprehensible 100 years ago. Along with these advances, there have been many consequences. Over time, the lifestyles of people worldwide have changed, resulting in a largely sedentary society with epidemic rates of obesity and many other related chronic diseases. According to the U.S. Department of Health and Human Services (USDHHS), unhealthy lifestyles and unhealthy environments are responsible for a large percentage of morbidity and mortality in the United States.[1]

Early technological advances in medicine fueled an initial interest in developing improved methods for the diagnosis and treatment of disease. As societal changes occurred, it became clear that a focus on health prevention was also necessary. Thus during the past several decades there has been a significant shift in national attention from the treatment of illness to the promotion of health.

Health promotion is a national health priority and foundational to the provision of care for people of all ages; it also influences health policy, economics, and distribution of resources. As the largest group of health care providers, nurses are central to meeting national health promotion goals through interactions with individuals, families, and communities. Not surprisingly, health promotion is a standard of professional nursing practice specifically identified by the American Nurses Association.[2] The purpose of this concept presentation is to introduce health promotion and describe how this concept is applied within nursing practice.

DEFINITION

Initially, the concept of health promotion may seem simple—that is, a focus on improvement of health and prevention of disease. This concept, however, is actually very complex, involving multiple dimensions. For the purposes of this concept presentation, the World Health Organization's definition is proposed: *Health promotion is the process of enabling people to increase control over, and to improve, their health.*[3] Health promotion requires the adoption of healthy living practices and often necessitates a change in behavior. For this reason, long-term success of health promotion efforts is largely dependent on adaptation

to change. Disease prevention (also referred to as health protection) is considered a component of health promotion and refers to behaviors motivated by a desire to avoid illness, detect illness early, and manage illnesses when they occur.

To fully understand health promotion, one must have an understanding of various dimensions underlying this concept. Health promotion encompasses health, wellness, disease, and illness. First, what is meant by *health*? The World Health Organization defines *health* as "a state of complete physical, mental, and social well-being and not merely the absence of disease and infirmity."[4] Despite the fact that this definition is nearly 60 years old, it remains the most popular definition of health worldwide.[5] A similar term is *wellness*, but unlike health, there is no universally accepted definition. Wellness refers to a positive state of health of an individual, family, or community. It is multidimensional, encompassing several dimensions, including physical, mental, spiritual, social, occupational, environmental, intellectual, and financial. Wellness is seen as a continually changing state ranging from high-level to low-level wellness. *Disease* is a functional or structural disturbance that results when a person's adaptive mechanisms to counteract stimuli and stresses fail.[6] Although similar to disease, *illness* is seen as the physical manifestations and the subjective experience of the individual. Illness can be present in the absence of disease, and it is possible to have no illness when a disease is present. Likewise, many individuals experience wellness in the presence of an illness. For example, a person who has type 2 diabetes (a chronic illness) can experience high-level wellness. Low-level wellness is seen as an unfavorable state in which illness may result. Throughout the years, there has been ongoing debate about the relationship between health and illness—as paired entities at opposite ends of a single continuum or as separate entities.[7-9] The complex interrelationship of health, wellness, illness, and disease as components of health promotion would suggest the latter is a more realistic view.

SCOPE

Health promotion is viewed broadly as behaviors that promote optimal health across the lifespan within an individual, family, community, population, and environment. The scope of health promotion is represented through levels of prevention, first defined by Leavell and Clark: primary, secondary, and tertiary prevention (Figure 44-1).[6]

FIGURE 44-1 Scope of health promotion includes three levels (primary, secondary, and tertiary) applied across the lifespan with an individual, family, community, population, and environmental focus.

Specific recommendations vary according to the level of prevention and the unique characteristics of an individual (e.g., age, gender or race, family history, or medical history), a community, or a population. Health promotion recommendations for population groups often are presented in the context of age groups, including infants, toddlers, school-age children, adolescents, adults, and older adults.

Community is a collective group of people identified by geography, common interests, concerns, characteristics, or values.[10] Thus, community may be a localized area or may involve groups of people without geographic boundaries. It is also important to recognize the entire world as a global community—meaning that events rarely occur in isolation of one country or region so a very broad perspective of potential impact must be considered.

Primary Prevention

Primary prevention refers to strategies aimed at optimizing health and disease prevention. The focus is on health education for optimal nutrition, exercise, immunizations, safe living and work environments, hygiene and sanitation, protection from environmental hazards, avoidance of harmful substances (e.g., allergens, toxins, and carcinogens), protection from accidents, and effective stress management. Specific health promotion strategies are not linked to a single disease entity. For example, avoiding smoking helps to promote health and reduce the individual's risk for pulmonary, cardiovascular, and immunologic disease. Also, it is important to understand that a combination of strategies is usually advised for the prevention of specific conditions. For example, there are many known strategies that prevent or reduce one's risk for developing cardiovascular disease, including implementing a healthy diet, exercising regularly, and avoiding smoking; additional measures may be advised based on other personal risk factors.

Secondary Prevention (Screening)

The goal of secondary prevention is to identify individuals in an early state of a disease process so that prompt treatment can be initiated. Early treatment provides an opportunity to cure, limit disability, or delay consequences of advanced disease. Secondary prevention measures typically involve screening tests. Screenings are typically indicated and recommended if they are safe, cost-effective, and accurate and if the effort makes a substantial difference in the morbidity and/or mortality of conditions. Screenings are recommended for an individual, family, population, or community based on known risk factors.

To be considered accurate, a screening method must have a high degree of reliability and validity. A screening instrument, test, or method is considered reliable if the approach produces the same results when different individuals (with a similar skill set) perform the test. Validity reflects the ability of the test to accurately detect disease.

Ideally, a screening measure will accurately differentiate individuals who have a condition from those who do not have a condition 100% of the time. *Sensitivity* is a measure related to the proportion of those with a condition who are correctly identified. A test with poor sensitivity fails to identify disease in people who actually have a condition—known as a false-negative result. *Specificity* refers to the ability to currently identify those who do not have a condition. If a screening measure has poor specificity, many people who are disease free will have a false-positive test result.

Tertiary Prevention

Tertiary prevention involves minimizing the effects of disease and disability; the focus of tertiary prevention is restorative through collaborative disease management. The aim is to optimize the management of a condition and minimize complications so that the individual can achieve the highest level of health possible. Specific strategies include rehabilitative efforts to increase adherence to medication, nutrition, physical activity, and other disease management strategies. Many strategies used as primary prevention strategies are also used for tertiary prevention. The difference is not the strategy itself but, rather, the intent, goal, and context of the strategy. For example, aerobic exercise is used as a primary prevention strategy to maintain health, but it may be a specific weight loss intervention for the obese patient or a rehabilitation strategy following an acute myocardial infarction.

ATTRIBUTES AND CRITERIA

Attributes are qualities, characteristics, or elements that validate parameters of the concept. Health promotion is characterized by four elements:

- *Optimization of health*: The focus on optimizing health includes measures to maintain high-level wellness, measures to prevent illness, and strategies for early detection and management of disease when it occurs.
- *Evidence*: Health promotion guidelines are based on evidence; for this reason, recommendations are periodically updated to reflect new knowledge generated through research efforts. The recommendations are usually disseminated through practice guidelines for health professionals and via consumer-targeted media for the general public. In many cases, recommendations are presented as a matter of priority based on the level of evidence. For example, the U.S. Preventive Services Task Force (USPSTF) has five levels of evidence; each recommendation statement is accompanied by a recommendation grade that ranges from A to D or grade I (Box 44-1). As applied to two examples of cancer screening, USPSTF recommends biennial mammography screening for women aged 50–74 years (grade B recommendation)[11] and recommends against

routine screening for bladder cancer in adults (grade D recommendation).[12]

- *Patient/community centered*: Incorporation of health promotion measures must be valued and desired by the individuals impacted. On an individual level, personal motivation to incorporate the strategies is required. On a community level, leadership from individuals within the community is needed for successful implementation. It is critical that the wishes and desires of the targeted individual(s) are considered and understood. A patient/family/community assessment must be done in order to gain an understanding of the wishes and desires of the individual(s) impacted.[5]

- *Enculturation*: Designing and implementing health promotion require cultural competence and sensitivity to differences among cultures. Nurses must be willing to listen to and learn from patients and communities so that interventions are provided within appropriate languages and within the context of health belief practices.[13] Often, health care providers make recommendations for actions from their own perspective of what is appropriate and expected behavior—an ethnocentric perspective based on their own set of values and beliefs. Enculturation refers to the full internalization of values of a culture group. To be successful, health promotion plans incorporate the beliefs, attitudes, values, behaviors, and interpersonal dynamics into the planning, implementation, and evaluation of health promotion activities.

THEORETICAL LINKS

Numerous models and theories of health, health behavior, and health promotion have evolved during the past 30 years as the science and evidence of health promotion have expanded. Two areas of health promotion models include those focusing on the individual as a patient and those focusing on the community.

TABLE 44-1 Models of Health Promotion Targeting the Individual

Model Name and Theorist	Brief Description
Health promotion model (Pender)	This model shows that healthy behaviors (behavioral outcomes) are influenced by integration of unique characteristics and experiences of an individual (prior behavior and personal factors) and by influences of behavior (perceived benefit and barriers to action, perceived self-efficacy, activity-related affect, and interpersonal and situational influences).
Transtheoretical model (Prochaska and DiClemente)	This model proposes that health-related behavior progresses through six stages of behavior change on a continuum from motivational readiness to change of a problem behavior. The six stages are precontemplation, contemplation, preparation for action, action, maintenance, and termination. These changes occur regardless of specific behavior change and have been observed both among individuals adopting healthy behaviors and among those stopping an unhealthy behavior (e.g., smoking).
Theory of reasoned action and planned behavior (Ajzen and Fishbein)	This theory is built on an understanding of attitudes and subjective norms and the influence these have on changes in behavior. According to the model, the intention to change is driven by the attitude toward the behavior and the subjective norm for the behavior.
Social cognitive theory (Bandura)	This is a social cognitive theory used to design individual behavioral change. Self-belief influences behavior; self-beliefs are formed through self-observation and self-reflection. The major concepts within this theory are self-direction, self-regulation, and self-efficacy.
Health belief model (Stretcher and Rosenstock)	This model explores behaviors of individuals who take actions to avoid illness and those who fail to take preventive actions and thus has been used to predict which individuals would or would not use preventive measures.

Individual-Focused Models

Models that focus on the individual typically share common themes, including cognition, decision making, motivation, behavior, and environment. Although it is beyond the scope of this concept presentation to detail all the models and theories associated with health promotion, some of the most prominent, contemporary models are presented in Table 44-1.

Community-Focused Models

True community interventions focus on the community as a whole or the majority of the population within a community; this is in contrast to the application of interventions to individuals within a community. Community-focused models share common attributes, including (1) a focus on community values and norms, (2) legitimization of desirable behaviors and environmental changes, (3) participation of

TABLE 44-2 Models of Health Promotion Targeting the Community

Model Name and Theorist	Brief Description
Social ecology models	These are models that emphasize social and cultural contexts of people within an environment—and recognition of multiple variables that influence health behaviors. Consideration for health promotion interventions includes an integration of environmental resources and lifestyles of individuals within that environment.
PRECEDE-PROCEED model (Green)	This is a nine-stage model designed to guide the planning to health programs by identifying the most appropriate intervention strategies. PRECEDE stands for *p*redisposing, *r*einforcing, *e*nabling constructs in *e*cosystem, *d*iagnosis, and *e*valuation. PROCEED recognizes forces outside the control of individuals and stands for *p*olicy, *r*egulation, *o*rganizational constructs in *e*ducation, and *e*nvironmental *d*evelopment.
Diffusion of innovations model (Rogers)	This is a model that emphasizes dissemination of health behavior interventions. Rogers' model identifies four steps of diffusion: (1) the innovation, (2) communication channels (spreading the word), (3) time, and (4) social systems. The underlying assumption of adoption is the perceived value placed on the new behavior or innovation.
Social marketing models	Social marketing models influence behavior change by influencing adoption of an idea by the general public. Foundational to social marketing models are product, price, place, and promotion. When applied to health promotion, the "product" is the desired application, the "price" is the cost (social and economic) to the community as a result of adoption, "place" refers to the location where the program(s) is available, and "promotion" refers to strategies used to entice individuals to accept the change through adoption.

BOX 44-2 Overarching Goals for *Healthy People 2020*

1. Attain high-quality, longer lives free of preventable disease, disability, injury, and premature death.
2. Achieve health equity, eliminate disparities, and improve the health of all groups.
3. Create social and physical environments that promote good health for all.
4. Promote quality of life, healthy development, and healthy behaviors across all life stages.

Source: From U.S. Department of Health and Human Services: *Healthy People 2020.* Accessed at www.healthypeople.gov/2020/about/default.aspx.

fact, nurses have a significant responsibility for enhancing the health of individuals across the lifespan; this occurs in the context of a therapeutic relationship and requires skillful commination by the nurse.

National Health Care Agenda and Health Care Economics

Health promotion is a central focus of health care delivery that has been shown to add quality years of life and to decrease health care costs.[5] National goals and objectives for improving the health of Americans have been outlined in a series of reports beginning in 1979 with the publication of the first of the *Healthy People* series—*Healthy People: The Surgeon General's Report on Health Promotion and Disease Prevention*—and a companion document published in 1980—*Promoting Health/Preventing Disease: Objectives for the Nation.* Since that time, the USDHHS has published three additional reports (in 1990, 2000, and 2010) outlining goals and objectives for the upcoming decade. The most current document, *Healthy People 2020*, outlines four national goals for the nation to achieve by 2020; these goals are presented in Box 44-2. The four goals link to 42 topic areas, each with a set of objectives and target indicators to measure progress.[15]

The support for health promotion and illness prevention services is also demonstrated through the changes in coverage for such interventions by third-party payers. The impact of providing such services is continually evaluated; to maintain support, the cost of providing such services (including to those who are uninsured or underinsured) must outweigh the consequences of the absence of such services, particularly in the face of rising health care expenditures. Such issues have been central to health policy debate.

Vulnerable Populations and Health Disparities

Vulnerable populations refer to groups of individuals who are at greatest risk for poor health outcomes. These people are more likely to develop health-related problems and experience significantly worse outcomes when they occur. Health disparities is a term (and a concept presented in this textbook) that refers to inequities in heath within vulnerable population groups. Vulnerable populations are often politically marginalized in society; they experience discrimination and intolerance and may not have basic human needs met. The most consistent predictor of life expectancy, morbidity, mortality, and nearly all indicators of health status is low socioeconomic status,[16,17] although race/ethnicity, education, and occupation are also powerful indicators. Thus, two of the most highly vulnerable populations

community leadership, and (4) a planned change in which community members have control.[14] A number of community-focused models exist for planning and dissemination of health promotion agendas; a few of these are presented in Table 44-2.

CONTEXT TO NURSING AND HEALTH CARE

Nurses have involvement in health promotion on a number of levels, including working with an individual or family to enhance health, working with communities and organizations to enhance health, and participating in the development and implementation of health policy. The most common roles of nurses include the assessment, planning, and implementation of interventions and the evaluation of health promotion strategies for individuals. In are persons with low socioeconomic status and persons who are members of ethnic and racial minorities. Health policy to eliminate health disparities aims to increase accessible health services, requiring community involvement. Cultural competence is especially important to the elimination of health disparities because it facilitates integration of culturally appropriate interventions based on the values and beliefs of the targeted group. Thus, before working with vulnerable populations, nurses must be committed to developing skills in cultural competence.[18]

Assessment

Health assessment is the foundation for establishing a health promotion plan and the basis for application of health promotion into practice. Assessment can target an individual, family, or community.

Individual Assessment

The primary components of assessment for individuals include a comprehensive assessment of health status, health behaviors, and risk. Advances in genetic research have enhanced the ability to assess risk; thus, family history is a critical component of health assessment. In addition, assessment includes gaining an understanding of personal factors such as health preferences, values, and social relationships. The assessment of health is performed by nurses in nearly all settings and includes conducting a history and physical examination. Effective communication skills are essential to obtain necessary information for a successful health promotion process. The nurse–patient relationship is truly the context of care; the nurse must be sensitive to each person's goals and values.

Family Assessment

A family assessment is necessary to promote health within families. Family assessment includes gaining an understanding of health promotion and disease prevention activities within the family (including risk factors), family strengths, and the relationships among family members—how family members influence behaviors and decision making of others. A genogram is a useful method to understand family members across multiple generations.[19]

Community Assessment

Community assessment is a necessary component of assessment when developing community-based health promotion strategies—usually in the context of community health nursing and public health nursing. Community assessment is conducted in participation with community representatives and through community data collection strategies including observation, interviews from community residents, and data collection using instruments that quantify data. Additional information about a community typically incorporated into an assessment includes the structure of a community; census; population/demographic statistics; morbidity rates; mortality rates; epidemiologic data; environmental data (e.g., pollution indices); and community resources such as health care services, government services (fire, police, and other emergency services), schools, and other local government agencies. These data can be collected from a variety of sources, including the Internet and city/government offices.

Health Promotion Interventions

Health promotion interventions are planned and initiated on the basis of data gained from assessment. Guidelines for health promotion interventions based on age or other risk factors are readily available for health professionals; nurses should know how to access and interpret the guidelines so these can be incorporated into patient care. The

interventions described here are broadly applied to all levels of health promotion (primary, secondary, and tertiary) and can be applied to all targeted groups (individual, family, and community).

Education

Education is a cornerstone for health promotion; this is also one of the most important contributions of nursing. Education intersects with each area of health promotion—as a primary, secondary, and tertiary health promotion strategy. Education is applied to individuals (patient education), families, and communities. Nurses have an opportunity to assist individuals to optimize their health by educating individuals and families about healthy lifestyle choices and encouraging appropriate screening and management of disease when necessary. Teaching involves not only providing information but also helping to align resources and access so health services can be provided. This is especially important among individuals from vulnerable populations.

Vaccinations

Edward Jenner is credited with being the father of immunology because he was the first person to successfully develop a vaccination in 1798. Smallpox vaccination was a new and innovative way to prevent disease and provided the foundation for the science of immunology. Since that time, vaccinations have become one of the most effective primary prevention interventions; development and research efforts for new immunizations are ongoing. Nurses are commonly involved in this area of health promotion by providing patient education regarding immunizations, allaying fears of immunization, identifying those who are in need of immunization, and administering vaccines. Vaccinations are recommended for individuals across the entire lifespan from infancy through geriatric populations. Although it is beyond the scope of this concept analysis to describe all vaccinations, nurses should know where to find and interpret current immunization guidelines. The Centers for Disease Control and Prevention (CDC) website (http://www.cdc.gov) is a reliable resource to find current immunization guidelines for all age groups.

Screening

Screening is a secondary prevention strategy; the goal is for disease detection in the early stages of the disease process. Screening usually involves testing that has high reliability and validity—and screens for important conditions in which early detection is paramount. The benefits must outweigh the consequences and must be feasible from an economic and resource perspective. Specific routine screening guidelines have been developed for individuals across the lifespan. The USPSTF offers reliable screening recommendations, as do many other government agencies and organizations such as the CDC, the American Cancer Society, the American Heart Association, and the American Academy of Pediatrics. Screening is also done based on an individual's risk. Genetic screening, for example, is not routinely performed on all individuals, but it is indicated in cases in which the history supports the need.

Nutritional Health

It is estimated that more than 60% of all deaths are associated with chronic diseases such as obesity, cardiovascular disease, cancer, and diabetes; a large percentage of these diseases are caused or exacerbated by poor or unhealthy nutritional behaviors.[20] According to the National Center for Health Statistics,[21] 18.1% of children between ages 12 and 19 years and 19.6% of children between ages 6 and 11 years are overweight. Children who are overweight or obese are at significant risk for many health-related problems as adults. For these reasons, one of the most important health promotion interventions is nutrition counseling.

The *Dietary Guidelines for Americans 2015* provides the basis for dietary recommendations and guides state and federal policies related to nutrition.[22] A consumer-friendly translation of the *Dietary Guidelines*, known as *MyPlate*, serves as a useful tool for dietary teaching and planning and can be found at the following website: http://www.choosemyplate.gov.

The promotion of an adequate diet is included in nearly all health promotion plans—either as a primary or as a tertiary prevention focus. For example, a healthy individual whose weight is within normal range may set a goal to increase the servings of fruits and vegetables consumed each day to meet the dietary recommendations found in *MyPlate*. Another individual who is obese and has cardiovascular disease may reduce saturated fats and calorie consumption as a treatment measure with a goal to reduce weight and decrease levels of serum lipids. In addition to improving dietary intake, other topics related to nutrition include dietary supplements, food safety, and nutritional screening.[6]

Physical Activity

The human body was designed to move; therefore, it should be no surprise that regular physical activity is an essential component of maintaining optimal physical and psychologic health. Physical activity encompasses any bodily movement involving skeletal muscles and energy expenditure. Physical activity occurs as part of routine daily activities, occupational activities, and recreational activities. Exercise training (purposeful bodily movement with the intention to improve physical fitness) is recommended for individuals across the lifespan and also is an important component to maintaining a healthy weight.

The benefits of physical activity are well documented for individuals across the lifespan. According to the USDHHS, there is strong evidence that regular physical activity among children and adolescents resulted in improved bone health, improved cardiorespiratory and muscular fitness, improved cardiovascular and metabolic health

biomarkers, and increased favorable body composition.[21] For adults and older adults, there is strong evidence that regular physical activity lowers the risk for multiple conditions, including coronary heart disease, stroke, hypertension, elevated lipids, type 2 diabetes, metabolic syndrome, breast and colon cancers, weight gain, and depression.[23] There is also a reduced risk for falls and improved cognitive function. In addition to being a primary prevention strategy, physical activity and exercise are also common tertiary health promotion interventions. Examples include physical activity as part of cardiac rehabilitation or following a stroke and physical therapy following joint replacement surgery.

Pharmacologic Agents

In addition to immunizations, many pharmacologic agents are useful for health promotion efforts. Details of drugs are primarily discussed in specific concept chapters, but two common examples are provided here.

Drugs used for smoking cessation. Several U.S. Food and Drug Administration (FDA)-approved medications are available to assist smoking cessation. Most of these drugs are nicotine replacement therapy for short-term use to reduce nicotine craving and provide relief of symptoms from nicotine withdrawal. These are available in the form of patches, gums, or lozenges.[24]

Drugs used for weight loss. There are four FDA-approved medications for weight loss. Three of these (phentermine, diethylpropion, and phendimetrazine) are for short-term use (up to 3 months) in adults as appetite suppressors. The fourth (orlistat) is a lipase inhibitor that blocks the ability of the body to absorb fat. This is recommended for long-term use (up to 1 year) for adults and children older than age 12 years.[25]

INTERRELATED CONCEPTS

Several important concepts interrelated to health promotion are presented in Figure 44-2. Health promotion actually is linked to every

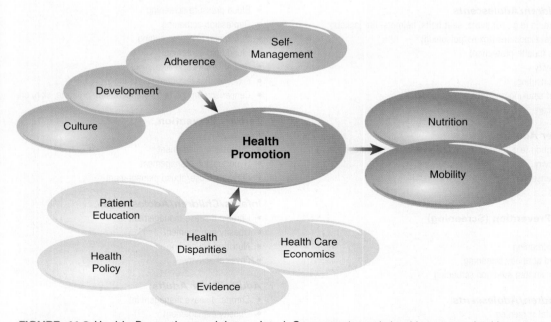

FIGURE 44-2 Health Promotion and Interrelated Concepts Interrelationships among health care recipient concepts (in blue), health and illness concepts (in purple), and professional nursing concepts (in yellow).

health and illness concept within this book as a matter of prevention, screening, or tertiary care. Interrelationships with the health and illness concepts Nutrition and Mobility are especially important based on the health promotion interventions discussed in the previous section. Health care recipient concepts Development, Culture, Adherence, and Self-Management are interrelated and form a concept cluster; these impact the type of health promotion interventions and approaches offered, as well as factors that influence the success of behavior change. Self-management and adherence are particularly important in the area of disease management.

Patient Education, a professional nursing concept, is based on patient attributes and significantly influences the success of health promotion interventions. Recommended health promotion guidelines are based on Evidence, and the effectiveness of health promotion recommendations is evaluated. Because of evidence, health promotion guidelines are implemented through Health Policy. A significant amount of evidence exists showing the connection between Health Disparities among vulnerable populations, thus underscoring the need for measures to enhance health promotion access and practices. These concepts form a natural concept cluster (see Figure 44-2). Health promotion is also interrelated to Health Care Economics. The delivery of health promotion interventions must be financed, and these interventions should be cost-effective.

CLINICAL EXEMPLARS

Considering the recommendations across the lifespan, there are literally thousands of exemplars for health promotion. Box 44-3 presents some of the most common exemplars of health promotion for individuals. Major exemplars for the promotion of health for individuals are often considered in terms of primary prevention, secondary prevention, and tertiary prevention. Box 44-3 is not comprehensive and does not include community or environmental health promotion strategies. Specific details for all exemplars presented can be found in multiple textbooks and on many websites devoted to health promotion.

Featured Exemplars
Vaccination
Vaccination represents standard health promotion measures for individuals of all ages. Vaccines provide immunity, or the ability to resist infection from many dangerous communicable diseases. The specific vaccines given to an individual is dependent on age, previous vaccinations, health status, medical history, lifestyle, type of employment, and travel history. Immunization schedules are available from the CDC's website for various age groups, including infants and children, adolescents, and adults.

■■■ BOX 44-3   EXEMPLARS OF HEALTH PROMOTION

Primary Prevention
Prenatal
- General prenatal care
- Folic acid supplementation
- Vaccinations (e.g., rubella, hepatitis B)
- Abstinence from smoking, alcohol, and other drugs
- Nutrition counseling
- Genetic counseling

Infants/Children/Adolescents
- Injury prevention (e.g., car seats, seat belts, helmets, life jackets)
- Environmental exposures (toxins/poisoning)
- Vaccinations (health protection)
- Physical activity
- Nutrition counseling
- Avoidance of smoking and other substance use
- Dental/oral care

Adults/Older Adults
- Injury prevention (e.g., safety belts, fall prevention measures)
- Physical activity
- Nutrition counseling
- Vaccinations

Secondary Prevention (Screening)
Prenatal
- Ultrasound screening
- Rh factor and antibody screening
- Sexually transmitted infection screening

Infants/Children/Adolescents
- Developmental screening
- Hearing screening
- Vision screening
- Body mass index screening
- Blood pressure screening
- Depression screening
- Substance abuse screening

Adults/Older Adults
- Hearing screening
- Vision screening
- Body mass index screening
- Blood pressure screening
- Depression screening
- Substance abuse screening
- Blood lipid screening
- Cognitive function screening
- Functional assessment screening
- Cancer screenings (e.g., breast, colon, prostate, skin, oral)

Tertiary Prevention
Prenatal
- Diabetes management
- Hypertension management
- Substance use/abuse management

Infants/Children/Adolescents
- Chronic disease management
- Obesity management
- Nutrition counseling
- Physical activity

Adults/Older Adults
- Chronic disease management
- Obesity management
- Nutrition counseling
- Physical activity

Oral Hygiene

Oral hygiene is an important health promotion measure for people of all ages and includes brushing teeth, flossing, drinking fluoridated water, dental sealants, and regular visits to a dental care professional. Oral hygiene prevents dental caries (considered the most common chronic condition in childhood) and periodontal disease (which affects an estimated 47% of adults older than age 30 years).[26]

Nutrition Counseling

Patient education regarding optimal dietary intake is one of the most common forms of health promotion and includes both primary prevention and tertiary prevention (disease management). Although most individuals as early as childhood are aware of the importance of eating a healthy diet, many children, adolescents, adults, and older adults have diets that are not optimal for a variety of reasons, including access to healthy foods; poor food choices; or conditions interfering with appetite, intake, digestion, or elimination.

Physical Activity

Physical activity is a fundamental health promotion measure for all individuals. Physical activity helps to control weight and improves cardiovascular health, musculoskeletal strength and agility, sleep, and mental health. Common activities include walking, running, cycling, swimming, and weight training. School-based, community-based, and employer-based programs to increase physical activity are examples of the greater awareness of physical activity as an important health promotion activity.

Blood Pressure Screening

Screening for hypertension involves regular blood pressure assessment. This is one of the most common health screenings because of its relative ease and cost-effectiveness. Although the USPSTF recommends blood pressure screening every 2 years after age 20 years,[27] other agencies recommend routine blood pressure screening for children age 3 years or older.[28,29]

Breast Cancer Screening

Screening measures to detect breast cancer depend on an individual's age and risk factors. A clinical breast exam, conducted by a health care professional, involves palpation of the breasts and axilla for the presence of lumps. A mammography is a radiographic test that detects tumors in the breast tissue that are too small to feel. Magnetic resonance imaging is used among women with high-risk factors for breast cancer.

Colorectal Cancer Screening

Colorectal cancer screening efforts focus on detecting and removing precancerous polyps in the colon and early detection of colorectal cancer. Screening measures include high-sensitivity fecal occult blood testing, sigmoidoscopy, or colonoscopy. Routine screening is recommended for all adults beginning at age 50 years (with regular screening intervals based on an individual's risk factors) through age 75 years.[30]

CASE STUDY

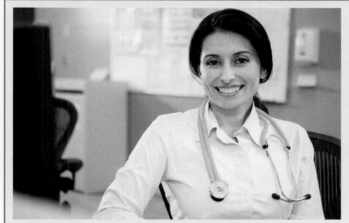

Source: monkeybusinessimages/iStock/Thinkstock

Case Presentation

Natalie Jemez, DNP, a pediatric nurse practitioner, works for a community-based health center. After hearing about the death of a 12-year-old boy who suffered head trauma at the local skateboard park, Natalie and her colleagues at the community center decided to initiate an injury reduction program targeting local youth and their families. Specifically, they were interested in raising awareness regarding traumatic brain injury and providing a mechanism to increase helmet use among children skateboarding and riding bicycles at the city park. Natalie wrote a grant in partnership with the local school district to secure state funds for a 3-year project that would achieve the following four goals: (1) development of informational brochures to be mailed to the families of children attending the local schools, (2) development of an age-appropriate information video "Helmet Heads" to be shown to children within the school system, (3) providing a mechanism for parents to purchase helmets at a significant discount from a local retailer, and (4) purchasing a large number of helmets for free use (by checking the helmets out at the local park service center) while children and their families are at the park.

Natalie was awarded grant funding for a 3-year project. As the program was implemented, other community stakeholders (including the local hospital, the orthopedic physician group, and the neurosurgeon physician group) became interested and provided additional funds to purchase additional protective equipment and to track data regarding use of equipment and number and types of reported injuries.

Case Analysis

This case is an example of a community-based health promotion project targeting a specific focus and population group. Traumatic injuries are among the most common cause of death and disability in children. Helmets can reduce head injury associated with bicycle accidents as much as 85%, but they are effective only if children wear them. Two significant barriers include lack of education and access to properly fitting helmets. The project specifically included education for parents and children and access to helmets to address these known barriers. Natalie's plan also illustrates the benefit of collaborating with multiple community stakeholders (school system, hospital, and physician groups) to gain widespread support.

ACCESS EXEMPLAR LINKS IN YOUR GIDDENS EBOOK

REFERENCES

1. U.S. Department of Health and Human Services: *Healthy People 2010*, Washington, DC, 2000, U.S. Government Printing Office.
2. American Nurses Association: *Nursing: Scope and standards of practice*, Silver Spring, MD, 2010, Author.
3. World Health Organization: *Ottawa charter for health promotion*, Geneva, 1986, Author.
4. World Health Organization: *Constitution of the World Health Organization*, 2006. Retrieved from <http://www.who.int/governance/eb/who_constitution_en.pdf>.
5. Pender NJ, Murdough CL, Parsons MA: *Health promotion in nursing practice*, ed 7, Upper Saddle River, NJ, 2015, Pearson.
6. Edelman CL, Mandle CL: *Health promotion throughout the life span*, ed 7, St Louis, 2010, Elsevier.
7. Oelbaum CH: Hallmarks of adult wellness. *Am J Nurs* 74:1623, 1974.
8. Sullivan M: The new subjective medicine: Taking the patient's point of view on health care and health. *Social Sci Med* 56:1595–1604, 2003.
9. Dunn HL: *High level wellness*, Thorofare, NJ, 1980, Charles B. Slack.
10. World Health Organization: *Community health nursing: Report of a WHO expert committee*, report No. 559, Geneva, 1974, Author.
11. U.S. Preventive Services Task Force: *Screening for breast cancer*, 2009. Retrieved from <www.uspreventiveservicestaskforce.org/uspstf/uspsbrca.htm>.
12. U.S. Preventive Services Task Force: *Screening for bladder cancer in adults*, 2004. Retrieved from <www.uspreventiveservicestaskforce.org/uspstf/uspsblad.htm>.
13. Chinn JL: Culturally competent care. *Pub Health Rep* 115:25–33, 2000.
14. Minkler M, Wallerstein N, Wilson S: Improving health through community organization and community building. In Glanz K, Rimer BK, Lewis FM, editors: *Health behavior and health education theory, research, and practice*, ed 4, San Francisco, 2008, Jossey–Bass, pp 287–312.
15. U.S. Department of Health and Human Services: *Healthy People 2020: Improving the health of Americans*, Washington, DC, 2010, Author. Retrieved from <https://www.healthypeople.gov/2020>.
16. Braverman PA, Cubbin C, Egerter S, et al: Socioeconomic disparities in health in the United States: What the patterns tell us. *Am J Public Health* 100:S186–S196, 2010.
17. Braverman PA, Egerter SA, Mockenahaupt RE: Broadening the focus: The need to address the social determinants of health. *Am J Prev Med* 40:S4–S18, 2011.
18. Giger J, Davidhizar RE, Poole VL: Health promotion among ethnic minorities: The importance of cultural phenomena. *Rehabil Nurs* 22(6):303–307, 1997.
19. Wilson S, Giddens J: *Health assessment for nursing practice*, ed 4, St Louis, 2009, Elsevier.
20. World Health Organization: *The world health report 2002: Reducing risks, promising healthy life*, Geneva, 2002, Author.
21. Ogden C, Carroll M: *National Center for Health Statistics Health E-Stat: Prevalence of obesity among children and adolescents: United States, trends 1963–1965 through 2007–2008, 2010*. Retrieved from <www.cdc.gov/nchs/data/hestat/obesity_child_07_08/obesity_child_07_08.pdf>.
22. U.S. Department of Agriculture and U.S. Department of Health and Human Services: *Dietary guidelines for Americans*, 2015. Retrieved from <http://health.gov/dietaryguidelines>.
23. U.S. Department of Health and Human Services: *Physical activity guidelines for Americans*, 2008. Retrieved from <http://www.health.gov/paguidelines>.
24. U.S. Department of Health and Human Services: *FDA 101: Smoking cessation products*, 2015. Retrieved from <http://www.fda.gov/forconsumers/consumerupdates/ucm198176.htm>.
25. National Institutes of Health: *Weight control information network: Prescription medications for the treatment of obesity*, (n.d.). Retrieved from <http://win.niddk.nih.gov/Publications/prescription.htm>.
26. Eke P, Dye B, Wei L, et al: Prevalence of periodontitis in adults in the United States: 2009–2010. *J Dent Res* 91(10):914–920, 2012.
27. U.S. Preventive Services Task Force: *Blood pressure in adults (hypertension) screening*, 2007. Retrieved from <http://www.uspreventiveservicestaskforce.org>.
28. National Institutes of Health: *The seventh report of the Joint National Committee on Prevention, Detection, Evaluation, and Treatment of High Blood Pressure*, 2004. Retrieved from <http://www.nhlbi.nih.gov/files/docs/guidelines/jnc7full.pdf>.
29. National Institutes of Health: *Expert Panel on Integrated Guidelines for Cardiovascular Health and Risk Reduction in Children and Adolescents*, 2012. Retrieved from <https://www.nhlbi.nih.gov/files/docs/peds_guidelines_sum.pdf>.
30. U.S. Preventive Services Task Force: *Colorectal cancer screening*, 2008. Retrieved from <http://www.uspreventiveservicestaskforce.org>.

Communication

Lorraine Buchanan and Nelda Godfrey

Communication is an essential form of human behavior—so fundamental to human social systems that our world would be barely recognizable without it. As a fundamental behavior, communication is so pervasive that the profound impact on our ability to engage with our world cannot be underestimated. Communication is unavoidable within the context of social life.[1] Human social interaction is accomplished through the relationships that develop between people, and these relationships are mediated by communication. These relationships vary from the intimacy of family to the more distant or more formal relationships between members of a community or nation. However, all of these relationships are dependent on communication for the creation and coordination of social interaction through the exchange of messages between participants. This exchange of information allows for the creation and coordination of social action, the integration of disparate individuals into social groups, and the subsequent formation of social relationships. Therefore communication is the essential process that ties people together, whether the ties create a family, an organization, a culture, or a nation.

DEFINITION

There are many definitions of communication in the literature, and these really only vary slightly. A synthesized definition would need to include the use of symbols to convey meaning through an interactive process. Because there is no way to directly communicate mind-to-mind with others, people must communicate through the use of symbols.[2] These symbols are used to create a message that is transmitted to others, usually through spoken or written language but also through gestures, facial expressions, or body movements.[3] Symbolic interaction between people becomes an expression of mind states and a means to transmit ideas. Thus, for the purposes of this concept presentation, communication is defined as *a process of interaction between people in which symbols are used to create, exchange, and interpret messages about ideas, emotions, and mind states.*

SCOPE

Communication encompasses all means by which people exchange messages with each other. The scope of the communication concept ranges from effective communication to no communication.

Ineffective communication lies within this continuum. Three primary categories of communication are linguistic, paralinguistic, and metacommunication (Figure 45-1).

The most obvious form of communication is *linguistic*—the verbal exchange of messages through spoken words and written symbols. Conversing face-to-face, reading newspapers and books, and even cell phone texting are all common forms of linguistic communication. In addition to overt verbal messages, more subtle forms of communication are included in this category. Silence can be a form of communication in the sense that some messages may be eloquently expressed when one or more persons in the communication exchange choose either to withhold messages or to avoid the interaction. Omission and/or avoidance in communication may also relay a message, depending on the circumstances of the exchange.

Communication also includes the nonverbal exchange of symbols —*paralinguistics*. Paralinguistics include less recognizable, though important, means of transmitting messages. These include the use of gestures, eye contact, and facial expressions. Paralinguistics are necessary for a complete understanding of the message sent because nonverbal gestures and facial expressions provide important cues about emotions, moods, and/or psychological states. Nonverbal messages are also conveyed through the use of color, artwork and graphic design, and dress. Uniforms, for example, provide information about the wearer's social role in a given context.

Metacommunication consists of the factors that comprise the context of the message. Because the ultimate goal of communication is to create meaning, the particular context or situation in which the communication act is occurring will have an effect on the meaning derived from the message.[2] Metacommunication factors that affect how messages are received and interpreted include internal personal states (e.g., disturbances in mood), environmental stimuli related to the setting of the communication, and contextual variables (e.g., the relationship between the people in the communication episode).

ATTRIBUTES AND CRITERIA

As defined, communication simply describes the transmission of ideas between people. However, the concept of communication becomes very complex when studied in-depth and is therefore a major field of study for academics and professionals in specialized fields such as

FIGURE 45-1 Categories of Communication

speech therapy and linguistics. There are three attributes of communication that form the basis of study in the nursing sciences: a process of complementary exchange, context, and learned skill.[4]

Process of Complementary Exchange

The process of complementary exchange occurs between people. In the exchange, each participant is, in turn, either a sender or a receiver. In the act of communication, the reception and transmission of messages between participants is iterative, where sustained dialogue serves to support the creation of shared meaning. The sender encodes a message using symbols (both verbal and nonverbal) and transmits the created message to the receiver. As each transmission is completed, the receiver perceives the message, interprets the symbols, and then responds with another act of encoding and transmission of a response to the sender. The implication is that the meaning created for participants during the communication act is negotiated during the exchange while messages are perceived, decoded, and interpreted.[5] Because meaning results from negotiation, effective communication depends on mutual engagement and on the authenticity of each participant's contributions during an exchange. The interpretation of meaning explains why communication by nurses to patients is subject to distortion or misinterpretation when the patient is ill, anxious, or distracted by pain. Communication messages and responses between nurse managers and staff nurses can be misread or negatively perceived if the nurses distrust the manager's intentions or the manager lacks credibility.

Context

The context of communication is relevant because communication cannot occur in a vacuum.[5] The metacommunication aspect, or context of communication, is important to the quality of meaning derived by participants during the process of complementary exchange. Contextual factors are those characteristics of the environment in which the communication occurs that affect perception and subsequent interpretation of messages by participants. Context can include factors such as the relationship between participants, internal mood states, mental and physical condition, experience and education, and external noise emitted from the environment.

Communication between people is both subject to and a reflection of relationships.[4] The relationship could be relatively distant, such as between shopkeepers and customers, or more intimate, as are the relationships between family members. Relationships always affect the communication process.[5] Hierarchical relationships, such as between parents and children or between managers and workers, involve power and status and thus affect the communication between these different types of participants. Children might fear upsetting their parents with some kinds of information because of the consequences of parental reactions. The same holds true with management/staff communication in the workplace. The effect of power and status on communications can be significant, especially if the result is a distortion of meaning that leads to a misunderstanding or a failure to fully appreciate the message being sent.

Learned Skill

Communication is a learned skill that develops over time and through interactions with others. Furthermore, these interactions constitute a complex learning experience that includes the need to understand the meaning of a diverse array of linguistic and paralinguistic symbols. Studies of language acquisition among infants and toddlers indicate that infants receive cues about meaning from the facial expressions of their caregivers during verbal interactions.[6] These verbal and nonverbal cues to children while they learn to communicate are an essential part of growth and development, especially for children with developmental disabilities.[1,7,8]

People continuously learn new ways to communicate throughout their lifetime. For some, this might mean the acquisition of a new language, either a spoken language or perhaps a specialized language, such as sign language or the vocabulary specific to a profession. Health care workers use a specific language developed for the purpose of communicating information among members of the group. This specialized language features words and terms that carry specific meanings related to the work for members working in the profession. Learning professional languages integrates people into the specialized social network of health care and helps to create group cohesion while facilitating the coordination of care. Professional nursing has a language that developed over time and is used to express and transmit the concepts and ideas relevant to the profession. An example of a term with particular relevance to nursing is *caring*. For nurses, this term is loaded with an array of meanings, some of which are specific to particular patient situations or conditions. Other examples of professional nursing language are the use of a nomenclature for body systems, medications and treatments, and terms that describe patient care practices. Learning this nomenclature is a necessary part of the education of nursing students, just as is learning how to communicate in therapeutic relationships. The term *therapeutic communication* probably has little meaning to a layperson, but it is so fundamental to the professional nursing role that it is a major component of nursing education.

THEORETICAL LINKS

The most basic theory of communication is a linear process model that describes a *sender* transmitting a *message* to a *receiver* (Figure 45-2).[1] The process starts with a sender encoding a message, either verbally or nonverbally, and sending it to the receiver through some medium, such as voice or print. Upon perceiving the message, the receiver decodes and interprets the message, creating meaning from the symbols.

This simplistic representation fails to convey the true richness of the communication exchange as a means to create shared meaning among participants. As noted previously, there are a great many factors that affect the perception and interpretation of messages. In addition, a simple model such as this does not reflect the iterative complexity of communication acts in which messages are passing back and forth between participants in the exchange.[9] Actual communication episodes involve multiple acts of perception and interpretation, in addition to the creation of a mutually negotiated meaning. A more accurate representation is shown in the complex model of communication (Figure 45-3), in which the interactive process depicts the influence of multiple factors on the meaning created during the interaction between participants.

To be effective, communication needs to have clarity, be goal directed, and possess vigor. In other words, effective communication is vivid and memorable.[10] The negotiation of shared meaning in the communication act is impaired if the purpose of the communication

FIGURE 45-2 Basic Communication Theory

is unclear or the symbols used for expression of ideas are inappropriate. A poorly worded memo can create much confusion or consternation among members of a workgroup because the true meaning of the message is questionable. Course syllabi that fail to provide clear direction because of incomplete information or errors will result in uncertainty for students. For nonnative speakers, the colloquialisms common to any foreign language can be inexplicable and the source of error and embarrassment. In all these cases, the clarity and goals of the message transmitted are lost, and the ultimate meaning of the message is distorted.

CONTEXT TO NURSING AND HEALTH CARE

Health care is a major social activity established for the purpose of helping people with their health concerns. It encompasses a variety of social structures that reflect the myriad of specialized relationships necessary for supporting the delivery of health care services. Nurses can expect to engage in multiple acts of communication daily in their work environments, perhaps even more so than in their personal lives. For nurses, effective communication is critically important. The professional role requires that nurses develop and practice a variety of communication skills that will ensure successful role function as well as the delivery of quality patient care. Because health care is relationship based, communication competence is highly valued for nurses, whether that communication is with patients or with other members of the health care services environment. Patient safety and health care quality, the electronic health record, and advocacy are also key elements of communication in today's health care environment.

Communication Competence

Communication competence in nursing means that communication is both *effective* and *appropriate*. Effectiveness is achieved when the goals of the communication are met. Appropriate means the communication has been adapted to the people and situation involved in the act of communication.[1] Because communication is a learned skill, instruction begins early in nursing education related to a variety of behaviors and attitudes that produce the framework for communication competence in the nurse. Communication competence among nurses continues to evolve with experience and professional development throughout a nursing career. Professional nurses can expect to be tasked with the need to communicate as a caregiver and as a member of a health care profession, both of which require skill in interpersonal communication. As a caregiver, nurses are expected to effectively and appropriately communicate with patients and families and with members of the health care team. As members of the profession, nurses are expected to competently voice the concerns of patients, families, and communities to others both within the profession and in the larger health services' sector. Achieving communication competence in nursing is important for optimizing safety and quality in health care and for creating the voice and authority needed to advocate for better systems and safer workplaces.

Patient Safety and Health Care Quality

The Institute of Medicine (IOM) captured national attention in 2001 with the report, *To Err Is Human: Building a Safer Health Care System*.[11]

In this report, the IOM noted that an estimated 98,000 medical errors each year were leading to unnecessary injury and even death for patients in the U.S. health care system. IOM reports since then have critically evaluated the safety and quality problems inherent to our health care systems, especially how these problems are related to the actions of health care professionals, including nurses.[12,13] Communication is a frequently cited cause of errors in the delivery of health care,[14] including being the leading cause of *sentinel events*, defined as unusually serious, unexpected events that occur during episodes of care. Sentinel events—such as wrong-site surgery, adverse drug events, or patient falls—not only result in harm to the patient but also lead to increased health care costs. Consequently, communication competence has become a critical skill that promotes quality of care and patient safety.

One recommendation by the IOM is to educate health professionals to use practices and tools that support effective communication. One tool that supports consistent and accurate communication between professionals is the ISBARR communication technique. ISBARR stands for *i*dentify self, *s*ituation, *b*ackground, *a*ssessment, *r*ecommendations, and *r*ead back orders.[15] This tool is a structured routine for passing information between team members, most notably between nurses and other health care providers such as physicians and nurse practitioners. When using this tool, the nurse will *identify self*, describe the patient *situation*, explain the *background information relevant to the situation*, provide an *assessment*, provide *recommendations* for action, and *read back orders*.[15]

This structured approach to communicating patient care information provides the health care provider with the information necessary to make decisions about proposed interventions while also respecting the nurse's status as a member of the care team.[16]

Electronic Health Record

Another fundamental communication skill for nurses is accurate and timely documentation in the patient record. The patient's health care record is a communication tool for documenting progress, treatments, interventions, and patient responses to care. Because many members of the health care team document their care interventions in the health care record, it is an important source of information and a major means of communication between members of the team. The health care record is also considered to be a legal document that records the actions of health care providers and is subject to legal review to determine if standards of care were met. Therefore, clear and accurate documentation of health care provider actions and observation of the patient's response not only is important but also might be the best available evidence that a provider's actions were appropriate and effective.

With the advent of the electronic health record (EHR), the potential for improving communication among health care providers in a variety of settings is enhanced. A digital record of a person's health history facilitates the timely transmission of complete and accurate information between providers. For example, the EHR provides the means by which emergency personnel can access prior history and medical condition for patients who are too ill or too injured to provide a complete medical history. However, the speed of digital transmission and the potential for widespread dissemination of electronic records also create increased concerns related to accuracy and confidentiality.

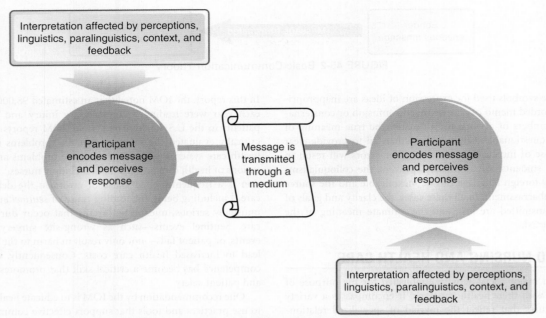

FIGURE 45-3 Complex Model of Communication Theory

Documentation errors or omissions in the EHR can jeopardize patient safety and the quality of care provided because multiple providers access these records and then make health care decisions based on inaccurate or faulty information. The potential also exists for personal health care information to be accessed by others who do not have a right to access or a need to know the information. Nurses working with an EHR need to be cognizant of these potential threats to the quality of care and patient safety. Access to an EHR has the potential to greatly enhance the delivery of efficient, timely, and patient-centered care, but it also increases the requisite for diligence in documentation of that care as well as the need to strictly maintain the confidentiality of the patient's health record.

Advocacy

Communication competence is a necessary component for nurses to effectively function in the role of advocate. Advocacy is the act of speaking for others to assist them to meet needs, and it is an expectation for all who assume the role of professional nurse. The advocacy might be in the form of interceding with members of the health care team on behalf of patients or families, advocacy on behalf of these same members of the health care team, or even advocacy on behalf of the profession. The ability to speak out assertively, credibly, and authoritatively is a highly valued communication skill critical to effective advocacy. Principles of assertive communication are routinely taught in basic nursing education courses with continued refinement of the skill through professional development and graduate education.

INTERRELATED CONCEPTS

Communication is the exchange of information between participants that leads to a negotiated, mutual understanding of a situation or phenomenon. As such, there are related concepts that are closely associated with communication (Figure 45-4).

Communication is the structure that supports social interaction. Social interaction is the primary means for **Collaboration** and **Care Coordination**. Nurses collaborate with patients and families in the development of a plan of care. Nurses also collaborate with members of the health care team, often functioning as the link between the patient and the rest of the team. As the link, nurses routinely coordinate care to ensure that the care is appropriately and safely delivered and that it is beneficial to patients. The importance of effective collaboration and care coordination to quality care and patient safety cannot be overemphasized. It is crucial that communication between the patient and the health care team as well as communication between the members of the health care team be clear, accurate, and timely. Errors, omissions, and gaps in communication can lead to dangerous and costly errors in care.

Culture and communication exist in a symbiotic relationship. Cultures develop on the basis of an infrastructure of communications. Communications, especially the symbols used in language, dress, and patterns of behavior, are expressions of culture. Behavioral expectations and norms, values and traditions, the way relationships are built and maintained, the definition of personal space as dictated by cultural norms, and even the significance of words and gestures are possible because people are able to transmit ideas, values, emotions, and needs through communication acts. The relationship between culture and communication has important implications for nurses. As a profession that interacts with people from all cultures, nurses will frequently encounter different, culturally based communication practices. Nurses need a fundamental appreciation of cultural differences and the potential effect of these differences on care. By recognizing these differences, nurses are able to proactively address potential misperceptions and misunderstandings that might arise during the implementation and evaluation of care.

The appreciation of cultural differences extends beyond the need to think about the language and culture of patients and their families. Organizational cultures have a strong impact on nursing practice

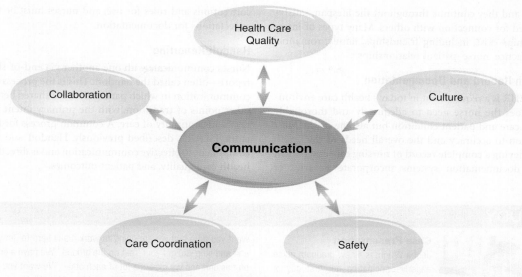

FIGURE 45-4 Communication and Interrelated Concepts

because most nurses work in some kind of organization, whether a hospital, community health agency, school, hospice, or some other kind of health care unit. Organizational cultures also have norms and values; expectations for appropriate behavior and language; and rituals, symbols, and artifacts.

Communications in organizations are both affected by the prevailing culture and also serve to help mold the organizational culture. This is particularly important in health care because of the links between communication, organizational culture, Safety, and Health Care Quality. Communications and systems for communications must allow for clear, timely, and accurate communications between professionals working together in order to deliver quality patient care, unimpeded by contextual factors such as power and status. Lessons learned from aviation safety programs indicate that effective communication is fundamental to safe systems, leading to the adoption of improved communication strategies by health care organizations to ensure quality care.[17,18]

CLINICAL EXEMPLARS

Communication for nurses encompasses a wide range of practices, most of which support effective interactions with others. Exemplars of communication represent situations within the context of professional nursing practice. A list of exemplars is presented in Box 45-1. Some of these exemplars are featured next.

Featured Exemplars

Assertive Communication

Assertive communication refers to a process in which positive and negative ideas and feeling are expressed in an open and direct way. Intentionally using assertive communication helps the nurse to advocate for the patient with other health care professionals. Many personal factors can play a role in a nurse's communication with others. Some of the influencing factors on communication are culture, gender, personality type, and level of self-confidence.[19] Assertive communication respects the rights of all involved while allowing the sender to stand up for his or her beliefs.

BOX 45-1 EXEMPLARS OF COMMUNICATION

- Assertive communication
- Therapeutic communication
- Intrapersonal communication (self-talk)
- Interpersonal communication
- Interprofessional communication
- Handoff/reporting
- Documentation—Electronic health record

Therapeutic Communication

Therapeutic communication is defined as "an interactive process between the nurse and the client that helps the client overcome temporary stress, to get along with other people, to adjust the unalterable, and to overcome psychological blocks which stand in the way of self-realizations."[19,p2164] Therapeutic communication becomes an important part of the healing process for patients and families. This type of communication promotes understanding and builds relationships that lead to positive patient outcomes.

Intrapersonal Communication

Part of an internal perspective, intrapersonal communication takes place within the individual. Often called self-talk, it can be positive and helpful to the person, or it can be negative and self-destructive.[9,20] Positive self-talk can be part of an overall mental hygiene regime or part of formalized psychological therapy. A nurse should be aware of intrapersonal communication and the impact it could have on one's way of thinking, behavior, and, in turn, on nursing practice.

Interpersonal Communication

Embedded in relationships, interpersonal communication is the verbal and nonverbal interaction that occurs among human beings.[20] This interaction can be one-to-one or occur within groups. Interpersonal communication and the resulting relationships begin at birth with the infant and parent, and they continue throughout the lifespan, satisfying the human need for connection with others. Many types of interpersonal relationships exist, including friendships, family, romantic, and, in nursing practice, nurse–patient relationships.

Electronic Health Record and Documentation

Skill in using the EHR is a requirement in today's health care environment. Not only does the nurse need to adequately and thoroughly document patient care and patient condition but also he or she must do so with attention to accuracy and the overall needs of the health care system in retrieving a complete record of nursing care and patient condition. Most documentation systems incorporate a series of conventions and rules for use, and nurses must be fully aware of the expectations for documentation.

Handoff/Reporting

Nurses communicate with one another via end-of-shift or end-of-day report—often called the handoff. This is the process of nurse-to-nurse communication in which patient data are shared between shifts and at other points of transition, with the primary intent of ensuring accuracy and continuity of care. A common process for handoff reporting is the ISBARR, described previously. Handoff and reporting is a key component to effective communication and is directly related to safety, health care quality, and patient outcomes.[15]

CASE STUDY

Source: monkeybusinessimages/ iStock/Thinkstock

Case Presentation

Jenna Wright is a new graduate nurse eagerly anticipating her first day of work. She has been hired as a nurse in the surgical intensive care unit (ICU) of a large hospital and was selected for a 6-month residency program for new nurses offered by the hospital.

Jenna reports to her new nursing unit early on her first day. She waits at the nurses' station for her assigned preceptor, Diane Miller, who has 20 years of nursing practice experience. Diane was chosen by the unit manager to be Jenna's preceptor because of her communication skills and effective mentorship. Diane is familiar with the "first-day jitters" common with new nurses, so she also arrives slightly early and meets Jenna at the nurses' station. Diane walks directly to Jenna, smiles, and greets her: "Hi, you must be Jenna. I'm Diane and I will be your preceptor during your residency. I have worked on this unit for the last 5 years and find I really enjoy the challenge of the surgical ICU." Jenna smiles shyly and nods her head, "I am so excited to be here…. It's great to finally be starting out, no longer a student." Diane laughs and nods her head, "Oh yes, I know. Students are fun to have on the unit but I also know there are limits on what they can do. Getting to spread your wings and learn this new role can be very exciting and we want you to be excited. We want you here and we are going to work really hard to get you oriented to the unit and help you get your 'feet on the ground.' We have a great team of nurses on this unit and we expect a lot of each other. We want you to be a part of that team and to learn and grow in the position. After all, that helps all of us, right? So let's find a place for your things and then we will go to report. You know, I think there is another new nurse working in the medical intensive care unit. Let's see if we can arrange to have lunch with her and her preceptor."

Case Analysis

In this small conversation, Diane demonstrates different attributes of effective communication. From her experience, she knows that new nurses are uncertain about themselves and their place in a new workplace. By approaching Jenna directly, Diane creates the first contact needed to begin the acculturation process for new members to the unit. She indicates acceptance of Jenna's uncertainty and uses inclusive language with Jenna, stating that she and the other nurses on the unit welcome a new member. Diane also acknowledges that Jenna is at a legitimate professional transition point, from student to nurse, and she provides Jenna with some information about unit culture and expectations. Diane is also thinking about Jenna's further needs, such as introductions to other staff members, especially another new nurse who might become a social support for Jenna in the future. Diane uses verbal and nonverbal communication strategies (inclusive language, smiling, and head nodding) to indicate to Jenna that she is hearing Jenna's message, accepts her as a new member of the team, and is willing to support Jenna while she learns a new culture and grows into professional practice. In addressing the cultural expectations of teamwork and collaboration, Diane is communicating to Jenna the cultural norms for behavior and attitude that will be the foundation of her successful transition to the surgical ICU.

ACCESS EXEMPLAR LINKS IN YOUR GIDDENS EBOOK

REFERENCES

1. Wood J: *Interpersonal communication: Everyday encounters*, ed 6, Boston, 2010, Wadsworth.
2. Samovar L, Porter R, McDaniel E: *Communication between cultures*, Boston, 2010, Wadsworth.
3. Arnold E: Theoretical perspectives and contemporary dynamics. In Arnold E, Boggs K, editors: *Interpersonal relationships: Professional communication skills for nurses*, St Louis, 2011, Elsevier, pp 1–23.
4. Finkelman A: *Leadership and management in nursing*, Upper Saddle River, NJ, 2006, Prentice-Hall.
5. Worley D, Worley D, Soldner L: *Communication counts: Getting it right in college and life*, Boston, 2007, Allyn & Bacon.
6. Green J: Lip movement exaggerations during infant-directed speech. *J Speech Language Hearing Res* 53:1529–1543, 2010.
7. Adamson L, Romski M, Bakeman R, et al: Augmented language intervention and the emergence of symbol-infused joint engagement. *J Speech Language Hearing Res* 53:1769–1774, 2010.
8. McDuffie A, Yoder P: Types of parent verbal responsiveness that predict language in young children with autism spectrum disorder. *J Speech Language Hearing Res* 53:1026–1040, 2010.
9. Arnold E: Self-concept in the nurse–client relationships. In Arnold E, Boggs K, editors: *Interpersonal relationships: Professional communication skills for nurses*, St Louis, 2011, Elsevier, pp 62–82.
10. Hattersley M, McJanet L: *Management communications: Principles and practice*, ed 3, Boston, 2007, McGraw-Hill/Irwin.
11. Institute of Medicine: *To err is human: Building a safer health care system*, Washington, DC, 2000, National Academies Press.
12. Institute of Medicine: *Crossing the quality chasm: A new health care system for the 21st century*, Washington, DC, 2001, National Academies Press.

13. Institute of Medicine: *Keeping patients safe: Transforming the work environment of nurses*, Washington, DC, 2004, National Academies Press.

14. Joint Commission Center for Transforming Health Care: *Hand-off communications*, (n.d.). Retrieved from <http://www .centerfortransforminghealthcare.org/news/press/handoff.aspx>.

15. Shanks LC, Enlow M, Guhde J: Student's ability to communicate a critical situation after implementation of ISBARR in an undergraduate nursing curriculum. *Int J Innovation Educ Res* 1-02:1–6, 2013.

16. Kowalski K: Building teams through communication and partnerships. In Yoder-Wise P, editor: *Leading and managing in nursing*, ed 5, St Louis, 2011, Elsevier, pp 345–371.

17. Weinstock M: Can your nurses stop a surgeon? *Health Hospital Networks* September:39–46, 2007.

18. Pronovost P, Berenholtz S, Goeschel C, et al: Creating high reliability in health care organizations. *Health Services Res* 41(Pt 2):1599–1617, 2006.

19. North Carolina Concept-Based Learning Editorial Board: Communication. In *Nursing: A concept-based approach to learning*, vol 2, New York, 2011, Pearson, pp 2147–2203.

20. Burger J: Communication. In Potter PA, Perry AG, Stockert PA, et al, editors: *Fundamentals of nursing*, ed 8, St Louis, 2013, Mosby, pp 309–327.

Collaboration

Judy Liesveld

When thinking about the profession and practice of nursing, the words "collaboration" and "nursing" seem inseparable. Nurses work with patients, families, communities, and other professionals in a multitude of settings from state-of-the-art hospitals to remote rural home settings and clinics. Collaboration involves building models of health care using the best ideas of our patients and our partners in the health care setting. Understanding collaboration is perhaps the key component for reducing errors in patient care. Unfortunately, collaboration remains an unclear concept with varying meanings and perspectives among health professionals. Exploration of the concept of collaboration will help to crystallize its meaning and its potential for advancing the nursing profession and for improving the health outcomes of our patients.

DEFINITION

The word *collaborate* is derived from the Latin word *collaborare*, meaning to labor together. Collaboration usually has the connotation of working with others in an intellectual endeavor. Nurses labor with patients, families, and health care workers such as physicians, pharmacists, social workers, physical therapists, medical assistants, and other lay health workers using knowledge, reasoning, and critical thinking skills to promote or restore health. For the purposes of this concept presentation, collaboration in nursing is the *development of partnerships to achieve best possible outcomes that reflect the particular needs of the patient, family, or community, requiring an understanding of what others have to offer.* Collaboration also involves a joint responsibility for patient outcomes.[1]

SCOPE

The scope of collaboration spans four overarching categories, each based on collaboration with the nurse: nurse–patient, nurse–nurse, interprofessional, and interorganizational collaboration (Figure 46-1).

Nurse–Patient Collaboration

Nurses are inherent collaborators. The American Nurses Association identifies six standards for nursing practice known as the nursing process: assessment, diagnosis, outcomes identification, planning, implementation, and evaluation.[2] Opportunity for nurse–patient collaboration exists at each level of the process. Nurses particularly collaborate with patients as fully functional members of the health care team in making health care decisions.[3] For example, nurses collaborate with patients regarding health promotion and disease prevention behaviors, treatment strategies and options, lifestyle changes, and end-of-life decision making.

The historical context for nurse–patient collaboration is rich and extensive. Florence Nightingale encouraged collaboration with the patient, assessing what is needed or wanted.[4] In an early use of nurse–patient collaboration, Hildegard Peplau described a component of the working phase of her nursing theory as the patient participating with and being interdependent with the nurse.[5] Also, in her human-to-human relationship model of nursing, Joyce Travelbee defined nursing as an interpersonal process whereby the nurse assists an individual, family, or community to prevent or cope with the experience of illness and suffering and, if needed, to find meaning in these experiences.[6] Throughout the years, many other nurse theorists have examined and defined the nurse–patient relationship with elements of nurse–patient collaboration existing in many of the theories.

Nurse–Nurse Collaboration

Nurse–nurse collaboration, or intraprofessional collaboration, is also important to consider. How do nurses collaborate together? Nurses develop nursing teams on hospital units, in clinics, and in community settings that provide collaboration and support in patient caregiving. Nurses from various specialty areas also collaborate: nurse managers, nurse researchers, nurse educators, advanced practice nurses, as well as novice nurses with expert nurses.[7]

Mentoring

Mentoring is a special type of collaboration, or creative partnership, typically between a novice nurse and an expert nurse, that has been recognized as beneficial to the development of professional nurses.[8] Mentoring is described as purposeful activities that facilitate the career development, personal growth, caring, empowerment, and nurturance that are important to nursing practice and leadership.[9] The purpose of mentoring is to enable a smooth transition from novice nurse to a knowledgeable practitioner who is self-reflective and self-confident and who is able to negotiate both professional and patient relationships.[10] Despite the valuable benefits of mentoring, challenges to successful and constructive mentorships exist. Ketola stated that mentoring needs to go beyond the acquisition of knowledge and skills

Nurse-Patient

Nurse-Nurse (Intraprofessional)

Collaboration

Interorganizational

Interprofessional

FIGURE 46-1 Scope of Collaboration

and include the socialization of a nurse transmitting the values, norms, and accepted modes of behavior for the professional nurse.[11] Jakubik also encouraged mentoring to progress from the traditional approach of fostering support, competency, and job retention to a more modern approach of promoting career development and advancement, similar to mentoring in the business world.[12]

Shared Governance

Shared governance is another type of collaboration found in nursing. Shared governance is a nursing practice model that fosters a decentralized style of management that creates an environment of empowerment.[13] Shared governance is seen as an important component of professional practice and pursuit of Magnet designation from the American Nurses Credentialing Center.[14] The goal of shared governance is to transition from a traditional hierarchical management style to one in which nursing staff are more involved in decision-making processes and managers are facilitative rather than controlling.[15] Nurses practicing in a shared governance environment truly labor together and collectively develop collaborative relationships. Collaborating in the shared governance model, nurses can help to improve quality of care and clinical effectiveness, facilitate the development of knowledge and skills, and increase professionalism and accountability.[15] Shared decision making, the cornerstone of shared governance, is an essential element to improve the health care system of the future.[14]

Interprofessional Collaboration

The true essence of collaboration involves working across professional roles. With interprofessional collaboration, individual areas of expertise are represented along with diverse perspectives influenced by professional orientation, experience, age, gender, education, and socioeconomic status.[16] The goal of interprofessional collaboration is the formation of a partnership between a team of health providers and a patient in a participatory, collaborative, and coordinated approach to share in decision making of health and social issues.[17] The scope of interprofessional collaboration is vast and could include professionals from nursing, medicine, pharmacy, occupational therapy, physical therapy, dentistry, social work, education, law, or many others interacting with the patient and family.

Not surprisingly, different professions perceive collaboration in different ways. For example, nurses typically perceive a greater need for collaboration than do physicians;[18,19] however, physicians perceive a higher occurrence of collaboration.[20] In a study by Matziou and colleagues, more than 60% of nurses reported that physicians did not collaborate during the therapeutic or decision-making process nor did they accept nurses' opinions. Contrarily, more than 90% of the physicians in the study stated that they respected nurses' work and accepted the nurses' responsibility in patients' care. An important barrier that was identified by the physicians was that they did not recognize the nurses' professional role.[21] Makary and colleagues observed that nurses in the operating room setting described collaboration as shared decision making, whereas physicians described it as having their needs

anticipated and their directions followed.[22] Interprofessional collaboration involves navigating different professional cultures and specialized languages and understanding different viewpoints and goals, including various measures of success.[16]

A growing trend in professional health care curricula is to offer interprofessional courses as a means of facilitating mutual respect, understanding, and commitment to common goals; joint problem solving; mutual give and take; shared accountability; and collegial communication.[17] Best practices to deliver interprofessional education are being researched and developed. General opinion in interprofessional education is that students benefit from learning to collaborate in an academic setting before they are expected to practice together in a care delivery setting. One study shows little change in medical student attitudes about communication and collaboration before and after interprofessional education experiences compared to nursing student attitudes.[23] However, other studies have shown positive changes in medical students' attitudes toward their nurse colleagues when introduced to the diverse roles on interprofessional teams. Pfaff and colleagues found that new graduate nurses were more confident in interprofessional collaboration if their unit educator and manager had close proximity and were easily accessible, if different health care disciplines were worked with daily, and if satisfaction with the team existed.[24] New graduate nurses in acute care settings had more confidence in interprofessional collaboration than did community or long-term care new graduates.[25]

Interorganizational Collaboration

Consideration of interorganizational collaboration is important in today's health care environment. Pooling of resources and information between organizations can benefit patients and communities at regional, national, or international levels. Interorganizational collaboration often takes place in the form of coalitions or consortiums. For example, nurses have been involved in coalitions addressing health care disparities, diabetes prevention, teen pregnancy, immunization rates, and health care for the homeless. Health care consortiums often exist in communities or regions to ensure integrated care delivery, information, and networking among health care deliverers.

ATTRIBUTES AND CRITERIA

The Interprofessional Education Collaborative Expert Panel (a panel representing the nursing, pharmacy, medical, osteopathic, public health, and dental professions) identified four competencies or attributes necessary for effective interprofessional collaboration.[1] These attributes are transferable to intraprofessional collaboration, and they represent the ingredients (attributes) needed for successful collaboration. They are (1) values/ethics, (2) roles/responsibilities, (3) communication, and (4) teamwork/team-based practice. These are further described with several specific competencies mentioned for each attribute.

Values/Ethics

Values and ethics, undergirded with mutual respect and trust, are an important component in creating a professional and interprofessional identity. These values and ethics are imbedded in patient-centeredness and strive for safer, more efficient, and more effective systems of care. Demonstration of interprofessional values would be evidenced by professionals working together and applying principles of altruism, excellence, caring, ethics, respect, communication, and accountability to achieve high-level health and wellness in individuals and communities.[1] The ethical principles considering health care as a right and balance in the distribution of resources are also important. Respect for diversity that is found in the individual expertise each profession contributes to care delivery is also considered. Ten competencies were identified for the attribute of values/ethics. The following four are highly pertinent for collaborative practice:

- Embrace the cultural diversity and individual differences that characterize patients, populations, and the health care team.
- Respect the unique cultures, values, roles/responsibilities, and expertise of other health professions.
- Work in cooperation with those who receive care, those who provide care, and others who contribute to or support the delivery of disease prevention and health services.
- Demonstrate high standards of ethical conduct and quality of care in one's contributions to team-based care.

Roles/Responsibilities

Collaboration requires an understanding of how professional roles and responsibilities support patient-centered care. Clearly articulating one's professional role and responsibilities to other professions and conversely understanding other professions' roles is a key element for effective collaboration. Recognizing legal boundaries and limits of professional expertise is also needed. Understanding that roles and responsibilities might change based on a specific care situation is important. The following three competencies are representative of roles and responsibilities in collaboration:

- Engage diverse health care professionals who complement one's own professional expertise, as well as associated resources, to develop strategies to meet specific patient care needs.
- Use the full scope of knowledge, skills, and abilities of available health professionals and health care workers to provide care that is safe, timely, efficient, effective, and equitable.
- Communicate with team members to clarify each member's responsibility in executing components of a treatment plan or public health intervention.

Communication

Communication has been defined as a core aspect of collaborative practice. Health professionals communicate a readiness to collaborate by being available in place and time, as well as being receptive through displaying interest, engaging in active listening, conveying openness, and being willing to discuss.[26] A common language for team communication that avoids professional jargon is considered a key to safe and effective communication. Dismantling professional hierarchies created by demographic and professional differences is also valued in interprofessional communication. All professions and team members are equally empowered to speak up in firm, respectful ways regarding patient care issues. Finally, consideration of health literacy and effective use of communication technologies are viewed as important components of interprofessional communication. The following three competencies are shared as examples of collaborative communication:

- Organize and communicate information with patients, families, and health care team members in a form that is understandable, avoiding discipline-specific terminology when possible.
- Listen actively, and encourage ideas and opinions of other team members.
- Recognize how one's own uniqueness, including experience level, expertise, culture, power, and hierarchy within the health care team, contributes to effective communication, conflict resolution, and positive interprofessional working relationships.

Teams and Teamwork

Learning to be a good team player is an important component of collaboration. Teamwork behaviors involve collaboration in the patient-centered delivery of care and also in coordinating care with other health professionals so that gaps, redundancies, and errors are avoided. Teamwork also involves shared accountability, shared problem solving, and shared decision making. The process of teamwork can occur in microsystems such as hospital units or with increasing complexity between organizations and communities. The following three competencies are representative for collaborative teamwork:

- Describe the process of team development and the roles and practices of effective teams.
- Engage other health professionals—appropriate to the specific care situation—in shared patient-centered problem solving.
- Apply leadership practices that support collaborative practice and team effectiveness.

THEORETICAL LINKS

Theory of Collaborative Decision Making in Nursing Practice

Kim's theory of collaborative decision making in nursing practice offers a solid framework for the concept of collaboration.[27,28] Kim developed her theory in the early 1980s following society's renewed interest in human rights and demand for informed consent. Kim recognized that many different types of nursing care decisions are made for patients that influence their health in various ways and that patients have the resources required to be active participants in making health care decisions affecting the outcomes of nursing care.[27] Collaboration was defined as a process in which two or more individuals work together for the attainment of a goal—a process by which a joint influence on an action is produced. Kim's theoretical framework included the initial context of participant, both the patient and the nurse and their accompanying role expectations and attitudes, knowledge, personal traits, and definition of the situation. This initial context then influenced the context of the situation, including organizational components of decision making and the nursing care decision type, such as immediate- or long-term effects. Next, the primary outcomes of the decision-making process, the level of collaboration, and the nature of the decision were assessed. Kim stated that collaborative decision making could be assessed on a continuum in which the lowest level of collaboration is expressed as complete domination of decision making by the nurse and the highest level of collaboration is expressed as an equally influencing joint decision making.[27] Finally, the patient outcomes, the result of the primary outcomes, were determined: goal attainment, feelings of autonomy and control, satisfaction, health status, and recovery.

Kim's model specifically addresses collaboration between the patient and the nurse but could extend to collaboration with other family members or health professionals at the context of participant level, such as patient, caregiver, and nurse. Kim proposed several research questions to develop a knowledge base for the theory of collaboration in nursing.[27] These questions continue to hold relevancy for collaboration with patients, nurses, and other health professionals. The following is a list of some of these questions:

- Are there opportunities for patients to collaborate in making nursing care decisions?
- Do nurses believe in the value of patients' collaboration in making nursing care decisions?
- What are the relationships between the patients' collaboration in making nursing care decisions and patient outcomes?
- What are the consequences to nurses of patients' collaborations in making nursing care decisions?

Interprofessional Education Collaborative Model

The Interprofessional Education Collaborative developed a model that incorporates the four attributes of collaboration as previously

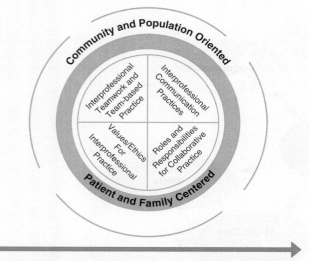

The Learning Continuum pre-licensure through practice trajectory

FIGURE 46-2 Interprofessional Collaborative Practice Domains (Source: From Interprofessional Education Collaborative Expert Panel: *Core competencies for interprofessional collaborative practice: Report of an expert panel*, Washington, DC, 2011, Interprofessional Education Collaborative.)

described.[1] The model was derived from social theories of learning and complexity theory.[29] These theories recognize the social and experiential nature of interprofessional collaboration and the complex health care environment in which it occurs. The attributes of communication, roles and responsibilities, values/ethics, and teamwork and team-based practice are equally distributed in a fluid circle surrounded by patient- and family-centered care (Figure 46-2). A final outer layer including the importance of community- and population-oriented care is included. A straight arrow representing the learning continuum from prelicensure through practice trajectory is situated at the bottom of the circle in Figure 46-2.

CONTEXT TO NURSING AND HEALTH CARE

The implications for collaboration and the nursing profession are expansive. The American Nurses Association's *Code of Ethics for Nurses* specifically addresses the importance of collaboration.[30] The code addresses the complexity of health care delivery systems, requiring a multidisciplinary approach with the strong support and active participation of all health professions. The code states that within the context of collaboration, nursing's unique contribution, scope of practice, and relationship with other health professionals needs to be clearly articulated, represented, and preserved. Nurses are encouraged to work together to ensure all relevant parties have a voice in informed decision making and patient care issues. Nurses are also encouraged to promote collaborative planning to ensure the availability and accessibility of quality health services. The code also addresses the importance of intraprofessional collaboration—that is, collaboration of practice nurses with educators, researchers, and administrators—because effective care is accomplished through the interdependence of nurses in differing roles.

The Quality and Safety Education for Nurses (QSEN) initiative anticipates that collaboration will have a major impact on positive patient outcomes and improve quality of care.[31] To date, conclusive results from research have been difficult to determine because of various definitions of collaboration, difficulty in measuring levels of collaboration, and small sample sizes.

There are hundreds of published narratives and reports involving interprofessional collaboration, but only a few studies have evaluated the effects of practice-based interventions occurring as a result of interprofessional collaboration.[32] Daily interprofessional rounds in inpatient medical wards in an acute care hospital had a positive impact on length of stay and total charges but had no impact on length of stay in a community hospital telemetry ward.[33,34] In another study, monthly multidisciplinary team meetings improved prescribing of psychotropic drugs for nursing home patients.[35] Videoconferencing, compared to audioconferencing, of multidisciplinary case conferences was found to decrease the number of case conferences per patient and to shorten the length of treatment in another study.[36] Cheater and colleagues reported that multidisciplinary meetings led by an external facilitator, who used strategies to encourage collaborative working practices, had teams using beneficial auditing that improved patient outcomes.[37]

Collaboration also has great potential to benefit nursing and other health professionals. A strong team work culture has been found to promote job retention and to decrease resignation rates.[38] Collaborative practice environments favorable to nursing have shown improved perceptions of registered nurse–physician communication, which was predictive of registered nurse job satisfaction.[39] Other benefits that have been observed include improved communication skills, greater leader satisfaction, improved problem-solving skills,[40] high levels of group cohesion, and increased satisfaction with patient care decisions.[41]

Collaboration has also been shown to benefit health care at the organizational level. A study led by Cowan compared traditional management of general medicine patients with nurse practitioner/hospitalist/multidisciplinary team-based planning. Results showed that length of stay was reduced (5 vs. 6 days) and profit to the hospital was higher ($1591 vs. $639) when multidisciplinary collaboration was used to manage patients.[42]

INTERRELATED CONCEPTS

Because there are many closely related concepts, collaboration is at times a fluid concept. Figure 46-3 presents these interrelationships. Professional Identity involves use of nursing's full scope of knowledge, skills, and abilities while clearly articulating the role of nursing in collaboration and respecting the boundaries of diverse professions. Ethics involves nurses' ethical comportment when working in cooperation with various professions, patients, and families. Altruism, excellence, caring, respect, and accountability are important considerations. Communication is also an important ingredient of collaboration because individuals from diverse backgrounds and professions need openness and clear communication skills and strategies for collaboration to occur.

The concept of Care Coordination is closely aligned and intertwined with collaboration; it is not possible to achieve highly efficient coordination of care without clearly effective collaboration among health care professionals and resources. Care coordination involves ensuring appropriate delivery of services and information as well as coordination of resources to ensure optimal health and care across settings and time. These efforts occur while nurses, patients, and interprofessional teams collaborate to resolve a specific caregiving situation.

The outcomes of collaboration include health care quality and safety. Health Care Quality is a desired outcome when collaboration occurs. Serious quality problems continue to plague the health care industry despite highly trained and technically skilled professionals. Error prevention, specifically reducing sentinel events and near-miss events, requires a whole systems' approach that seeks to understand

FIGURE 46-3 Collaboration and Interrelated Concepts

the parts and their interactions as well as the broader context in which they are embedded. Questions involving the expectations, assumptions, habits, behaviors, history, and tradition that influenced an adverse situation must be asked. A better understanding of the whole is needed for intelligent leadership and quality results in today's health care organizations. Collaboration with diverse professionals and patient-centeredness can make this happen. Safety is also a concept that is influenced by collaboration. Multiple threats to patient safety and errors occur at all levels of health care delivery. The Institute of Medicine (IOM), along with the QSEN initiative, has changed from an emphasis on errors to widespread system change to ensure safety. A culture of safety is being promoted. The IOM encourages training programs for effective communication and collaboration including transitions and handoffs. Collaboration is at the heart of resolving safety issues and creating a culture of safety in nursing and health care.

CLINICAL EXEMPLARS

The concept of collaboration with patients, nurses, and other professionals clearly has the potential to improve the safety and quality of health care delivery. Nurses must continue to find ways to clearly articulate the nursing component of health care in collaborative arenas. Involvement of nurses in the development of models of collaboration and development of collaborative interventions is needed. These collaborative strategies will continue to benefit patients, nursing, other professions, and health care organizations. There are many examples of collaboration within nursing and health care. These are presented as exemplars in Box 46-1 using the categories previously discussed.

Featured Exemplars
Patient Care Handoffs
Handoffs using communication tools such as SBAR (*s*ituation, *b*ackground, *a*ssessment, and *r*ecommendation) offer opportunity for collaboration in many situations. Collaborative handoffs can occur between nurses during shift change, between nurses when transferring patients to different units or facilities, between nurses and providers when receiving orders on patients, or between nurses and other health care workers when communicating critical information about patients. Many entities, such as the Joint Commission, the Institute for Health

---

■■□ BOX 46-1   EXEMPLARS OF COLLABORATION

Nurse–Patient Collaboration
- Collaboration on plan of care
- Collaboration from time of assessment to discharge plan
- Home care models
- Community partnerships
- Community-based participatory research

Nurse–Nurse Collaboration
- Quality improvement project
- Mentoring programs
- Dedicated information exchange: meetings, memos, e-mail
- Shared governance
- Patient care handoff
- Student nurse collaborative learning

Interprofessional Collaboration
- Rapid response teams
- Ethics committees
- Specialty care teams
- Patient rounding
- Team meetings for information exchange
- Quality improvement committee to discuss near-miss or sentinel events
- Patient care handoff
- Disaster preparedness teams
- Interprofessional education
- Interprofessional practice

Interorganizational Collaboration
- Regional, national, or international coalitions
- Health care consortiums

Improvement, and nursing's QSEN initiative, recognize collaborative handoffs as an important strategy for the safety of patients.

Interprofessional Education

Participation in interprofessional education (IPE) events in educating nurses, medical students, pharmacy students, and many other health care professions is an outcome goal in almost every health care college or university. Students are exposed to many different disciplines and their role in caring for patients. Students collaborate with each other on a variety of interprofessional projects, including quality and safety initiatives, community health projects, disaster preparedness, collaborative care in clinical settings, and many other interprofessional opportunities. IPE is recognized as an important educational component as students enter the workforce and collaborate for the best outcomes for patients, families, and communities.

Community Partnerships

Health care professionals from many disciplines come together to work on a common initiative important to their community, such as a collaborative initiative on child abuse and neglect. In such an example, the collaborative collectively works on goals and strategies to ameliorate this identified community problem. Other examples of community collaboratives include homelessness, access to health care, nutrition in schools, and care of the elderly. The potential for positive health care outcomes for local, national, and international communities is endless with individuals and communities working toward a common goal.

Patient Rounding

Patient rounding refers to the process of purposeful rounds to see each patient in each room or area on a regular basis. Patient rounding is often done by interprofessional teams to monitor progress and clearly communicate goals and a plan for each patient. Patient rounds are frequently mentioned as a means for collaboration, but reviews are mixed with regard to whether this is an effective strategy for collaboration.[33,34] Patient rounding may also be done by a nursing staff with the goal to check on patients on a predetermined basis (e.g., hourly) to determine if they have any needs, such as addressing pain level and assisting them with basic needs.

Specialty Care Team

A specialty care team is an interprofessional team of health care professionals who work together around a specific type of patient or population need. Specialty team members represent various disciplines (medicine, nursing, pharmacology, physical therapy, occupational therapy, nutrition, social work, etc.) and contribute to the team by sharing their area of expertise, thus providing the best collective thinking for patient care. Examples of specialty care teams include pediatric, geriatric, pain, wound care, pulmonology, oncology, cardiac, and palliative care teams.

CASE STUDY

Source: monkeybusinessimages/iStock/Thinkstock

Case Presentation

Melanie is a 4-year-old girl with cystic fibrosis and developmental delays. She is from a small rural community. Melanie is currently hospitalized at a large tertiary care center for a "tune-up" consisting of vigorous chest physiotherapy and antibiotics. Kayla is an experienced registered nurse mentoring Janelle, a new graduate nurse who has not worked with patients with cystic fibrosis. Together they are working with Melanie's parents on a nursing plan of care during the hospitalization. The Child Life program has also been included in Melanie's plan of care to ensure developmental appropriateness for Melanie's hospital experience.

The pediatric pulmonary team (consisting of the pulmonologist, social worker, nutritionist, nurse practitioner, and nurse educator) meets with Melanie's parents and the pediatric unit nursing staff to discuss the need for a gastrostomy tube because of Melanie's poor weight gain and past aspiration episodes. Via telehealth modalities, Melanie's primary care provider, a pediatric nurse practitioner from Melanie's home town, joins the team conference. Kayla has also linked Melanie's family with a parent advocacy group and has invited a representative to be present at the meeting to ensure understanding of the presented information. Melanie's parents ask many questions regarding the gastrostomy tube placement. The questions are met with open, honest answers using evidence-based information as appropriate. Joint decision making occurs with agreement to have the surgery scheduled. At the end of their shift, Kayla and Janelle handoff information to the oncoming nurse at Melanie's bedside. The parents are present to hear and contribute to the report and plans for Melanie's care. Kayla and Janelle leave work feeling a sense of joy and accomplishment.

Case Analysis

The model case exemplifies many opportunities for collaboration: nurse–patient–family collaboration, intraprofessional collaboration (Kayla mentors Janelle), and also interprofessional collaboration (the interprofessional team meets with Melanie's family). Interorganizational collaboration also occurs when the parent advocacy organization participates with the hospital team and Melanie's family.

The attributes of collaboration are embedded in the case and are the foundation for this hospital unit and for the interprofessional team that meets with Melanie's parents. Values and ethics are displayed in the patient-centered care and in the respect, trust, and accountability that the nurses and team display. The nurses and team appear to truly work in cooperation with one another.

The attribute of roles and responsibilities is particularly exemplified by the nurses when they involve the family and Child Life workers in Melanie's plan of care. The nurses mobilize resources for the family, ensuring that the primary care provider, as well as the parent advocacy worker, participates in the team meeting. Ensuring that the essential health care professionals were present for the team meeting took time and coordination. This is an important component of collaboration and promotes the most efficient and effective care.

The attribute of communication is apparent in the case. An openness and willingness to discuss and ask questions is evident. Inviting the parent advocate helped to level the field of professional hierarchy and perhaps acted to avoid the use of professional jargon. The use of telehealth was also an effective means to involve and communicate with Melanie's primary care provider. The handoff of shift information at Melanie's bedside was a safe and effective way to provide information for the oncoming nurse and for Melanie's parents. Teamwork was exemplified as diverse professions, the parent advocate, and Melanie's parents problem solved regarding Melanie's need for a gastrostomy tube.

ACCESS EXEMPLAR LINKS IN YOUR GIDDENS EBOOK

REFERENCES

1. Interprofessional Education Collaborative Expert Panel: *Core competencies for interprofessional collaborative practice: Report of an expert panel*, Washington, DC, 2011, Interprofessional Education Collaborative.

2. American Nurses Association: *Nursing: Scope and standards of practice*, Washington, DC, 2004, Author.

3. The Joint Commission: *The Joint Commission: Advancing effective communication, cultural competence, and patient- and family-centered care: A roadmap for hospitals*, Oakbrook Terrace, IL, 2010, Author.

4. Nightingale FN: *Notes on nursing: What it is and what it is not (Com ed)*, Philadelphia, 1992, Lippincott (original work published 1859).

5. Peplau HE: *Interpersonal relations in nursing*, New York, 1988, Springer (original work published 1952, New York, Putnam's Sons).

6. Travelbee J: *Interpersonal aspects of nursing*, ed 2, Philadelphia, 1971, Davis.

7. Benner P: *From novice to expert: Excellence and power in clinical nursing practice*, Menlo Park, CA, 1984, Addison-Wesley.

8. Metcalfe S: Educational innovation: Collaborative mentoring for future nurse leaders. *Creat Nurs* 16(4):167–170, 2010.

9. Wroten S, Waite R: A call to action: Mentoring within the nursing profession—A wonderful gift to give and share. *ABNF J* 20(4):106–108, 2009.

10. Santucci J: Facilitating the transition into nursing practice: Concepts and strategies for mentoring new graduates. *J Nurses Staff Dev* 20(6):274–284, 2004.

11. Ketola J: An analysis of a mentoring program for baccalaureate nursing students: Does the past still influence the present? *Nurs Forum* 44(4): 245–255, 2009.

12. Jakubik L: Mentoring beyond the first year: Predictors of mentoring benefits for pediatric staff nurse protégés. *J Pediatr Nurs* 23(4):269–281, 2008.

13. Doherty C, Hope W: Shared governance—Nurses making a difference. *J Nurs Manag* 8(2):77–81, 2000.

14. Porter-O'Grady T: Is shared governance still relevant? *J Nurs Adm* 31(10):468–473, 2001.

15. Ballard N: Factors associated with success and breakdown of shared governance. *J Nurs Adm* 40(10):411–416, 2010.

16. Disch J: Teamwork and collaboration competency resource paper. *Quality Saf Educ Nurs* 2010.

17. Canadian Interprofessional Health Collaborative: *A national interprofessional competency framework*, Vancouver, British Columbia, Canada, 2010, Author.

18. Sterchi L: Perceptions that affect physician–nurse collaboration in the perioperative setting. *AORN J* 86(1):45–57, 2007.

19. Thompson S: Nurse–physician collaboration: A comparison of the attitudes of nurses and physicians in the medical–surgical patient care setting. *Medsurg Nurs* 16(2):87–104, 2007.

20. Hamric A, Blackhall L: Nurse–physician perspectives on the care of the dying patients in intensive care units: Collaboration, moral distress, and ethical climate. *Crit Care Med* 35(2):422–429, 2007.

21. Matziou V, Vlahioti E, Perdikaris P, et al: Physician and nursing perceptions concerning interprofessional communication and collaboration. *J Interprof Care* 28(6):526–533, 2014.

22. Makary M, Sexton J, Freischlag J, et al: Operating room teamwork among physicians and nurses: Teamwork in the eye of the beholder. *J Am Coll Surg* 202(5):746–752, 2006.

23. Delunas L, Rouse S: Nursing and medical student attitudes about communication and collaboration before and after an interprofessional education experience. *Nurs Educ Perspect* 35(2):100–105, 2014.

24. Pfaff K, Baxter P, Jack S, et al: Exploring new graduate nurse confidence in interprofessional collaboration: A mixed methods study. *Int J Nurs Stud* 51:1142–1152, 2014.

25. Mathastein N, Klingenberg M: Students working with nurses. *Med Educ* 44:1138–1139, 2010.

26. Baggs J, Schmitt M: Nurses' and resident physicians' perceptions of the process of collaboration in the MICU. *Res Nurs Health* 20:71–80, 1997.

27. Kim H: Collaborative decision-making in nursing practice: A theoretical framework. In Chinn P, editor: *Advances in nursing theory development*, Rockville, MD, 1983, Aspen, pp 271–283.

28. Kim H: Collaborative decision-making with clients. In Hannah KJ, editor: *Clinical judgment and decision-making: The future with nursing diagnosis*, New York, 1987, Wiley, pp 58–62.

29. Sargeant J: Theories to aid understanding and implementation of interprofessional education. *J Contin Educ Health Prof* 29(3):178–184, 2009.

30. American Nurses Association: *Code of ethics for nurses with interpretive statements*, Washington, DC, 2001, Author.

31. Cronenwett L, Sherwood G, Barnsteiner J, et al: Quality and safety education for nurses. *Nurs Outlook* 55:122–131, 2007.

32. Zwarenstein MG: Interprofessional collaboration: Effects of practice-based interventions on professional practice and healthcare outcomes. *Cochrane Database Syst Rev* (3):CD000072, 2009.

33. Curley C, McEachern J, Speroff T: A firm trial of interdisciplinary rounds on the inpatient medical wards. *Med Care* 36(Suppl):AS4–AS12, 1998.

34. Wild D, Nawaz H, Chan W, et al: Effects of interdisciplinary rounds on length of stay in a telemetry unit. *J Public Health Manag Pract* 10(1): 63–69, 2004.

35. Schmidt I, Claesson C, Westerholm B: The impact of regular multidisciplinary team interventions on psychotropic prescribing in Swedish nursing homes. *J Am Gerontol Soc* 46(1):77–82, 1998.

36. Wilson S, Marks R, Collins N, et al: Benefits of multidisciplinary case conferencing using audiovisual compared with telephone communication: A randomized control trial. *J Telemed Telecare* 10:351–354, 2004.

37. Cheater F, Hearnshaw H, Baker R, et al: Can a facilitated programme promote effective multidisciplinary audit in secondary care teams? An exploratory trial. *Int J Nurs Stud* 42:779–791, 2005.

38. Mohr D, Burgess J, Young G: The influence of teamwork culture on physician and nurse resignation rates in hospitals. *Health Serv Manage Res* 21(1):23–31, 2008.

39. Manojlovich M: Linking the practice environment to nurses' job satisfaction through nurse–physician communication. *J Nurs Scholarsh* 37(4):367–373, 2005.

40. Boyle D, Kochinda C: Enhancing collaborative communication of nurse and physician leadership in two intensive care units. *J Nurs Adm* 34(2):60–70, 2004.

41. Messmer P: Enhancing nurse–physician collaboration using pediatric simulation. *J Contin Educ Nurs* 39(7):319–327, 2008.

42. Cowan M, Shapiro M, Hays R, et al: The effect of multidisciplinary hospitalist physician and advanced practice nurse collaboration on hospital costs. *J Nurs Adm* 36(2):79–85, 2006.

Safety

Gail Armstrong and Gwen Sherwood

Patient safety has always been fundamental to the delivery of responsible health care, but recently new knowledge, skills, and attitudes have redefined how it is understood and operationalized. New theories and frameworks inform current applications of safety science that describe how errors and near misses are recognized and reported, ways to manage the myriad of human factors that impact safe care delivery, and competencies required for health professionals to work in cultures of safety. These undergird an emerging approach to safety first developed in other high-performance industries and are being adapted to health care systems. Important shifts in these advances focus not only on considering personal responsibility and accountability in the delivery of safe care but also on how to direct efforts to system changes to mitigate the possibility of errors. Nursing has historically focused on maintaining patient safety and integrating new concepts of keeping patients safe. Safety science now calls for new knowledge, skills, and attitudes to achieve practice changes identified in national reports from the Institute of Medicine (IOM), which are addressed next. The new focus extends personal responsibility and accountability to incorporate safety from a systems perspective so that analysis of events includes system changes to prevent future occurrences.

DEFINITION

Many of the safety concepts in the health care literature originate from the IOM's groundbreaking work in patient safety. Beginning with the 2000 publication *To Err Is Human*, the IOM alerted the health care industry and the public to the problem of deaths from preventable errors. In this report, the IOM offers a definition of safety as "freedom from accidental injury."[1] An expanded definition of patient safety is offered in this report's appendix: "Freedom from accidental injury; ensuring patient safety involves the establishment of operational systems and processes that minimize the likelihood of errors and maximizes the likelihood of intercepting them when they occur."[1,p11] In *Crossing the Quality Chasm* (2001), the IOM defines safe care as "avoiding injuries to patients from the care that is intended to help them."[2,p5] An important emphasis in this IOM report is the expectation of consistent safety in our health care systems:

The health care environment should be safe for all patients, in all of its processes, all of the time. This standard of safety implies that organizations should not have different, lower standards of care on nights and weekends or during time of organizational change.[2,p45]

In a third report in this series, *Keeping Patients Safe* (2004), the IOM defines safe care as care that maintains a focus on using evidence in clinical decisions so to maximize the health outcomes, while also reducing the potential for harm. In its exploration of safe care, this IOM report addresses errors of commission as well as errors of omission.[3]

The National Patient Safety Foundation (NPSF) is an independent, not-for-profit organization with a mission to improve the safety of care for all patients. NPSF defines patient safety as the "prevention of health care errors, and the elimination or mitigation of patient injury caused by healthcare errors."[4] To further clarify this definition, NPSF defines health care errors as unintended health care outcomes caused by a defect in the delivery of care to a patient. Health care errors may be errors of commission (doing the wrong thing), omission (not doing the right thing), or execution (doing the right thing incorrectly). Errors may be made by any member of the health care team in any health care setting.[4]

A 2014 NPSF report, *Safety Is Personal: Partnering with Patients and Families for the Safest Care*, expands the concept of patient safety to reflect recent research. The report emphasizes how collaboration with patients and families through ongoing engagement can transform safety outcomes. Specific action items are clearly identified to enable health leaders, clinicians, and policymakers to accentuate the overlap of engagement and patient safety as interrelated phenomena. A key component is how providers work with the patient and family as a safety ally; they can be invited to observe and report gaps or omissions in care to help avoid errors and near misses.[5]

The work of defining safety and safe care by the IOM is relevant for all health care professionals and emphasizes safety from the patient's perspective. In nursing, a Robert Wood Johnson Foundation–funded national initiative, Quality and Safety for Nurses (QSEN), builds on IOM's work and defines safety as "minimizing risk of harm to patients and providers through both system effectiveness and individual performance."[6] This competency definition is further explicated by the necessary knowledge, skill, and attitude elements

FIGURE 47-1 Scope of Safety

to demonstrate safety in one's practice and can be found on QSEN's website (http://qsen.org).

Levels of errors are important definitions to understand. The IOM offers definitions of an adverse event and a near miss[3] and The Joint Commission[7] offers a definition of a sentinel event as follows:

- *Adverse event*: An event that results in unintended harm to the patient by an act of commission or omission rather than by the underlying disease or condition of the patient.[7]
- *Near miss*: An error of commission (did not provide care correctly) or omission (did not provide care) that could have harmed the patient, but serious harm did not occur as a result of chance (e.g., the patient received a contraindicated drug but did not experience an adverse drug reaction), prevention (e.g., a potentially lethal overdose was prescribed, but a nurse identified the error before administering the medication), or mitigation (e.g., a lethal dose was administered but discovered early and countered with an antidote).[7]
- *Sentinel event*: A sentinel event is an unexpected occurrence involving death or serious physical or psychological injury, or the risk thereof. Serious injury specifically includes loss of limb or function. The phrase "or the risk thereof" includes any process variation for which a recurrence would carry a significant chance of a serious adverse outcome. Such events are called "sentinel" because they signal the need for immediate investigation and response.[7]

SCOPE

The concept of safety is broad and encompasses the ideal of keeping all patients safe to the unfortunate reality that errors can lead to injury or death (Figure 47-1). Several key elements associated with this perspective include gaining an understanding of the types of errors, placement of errors, and ways of building a culture of safety.

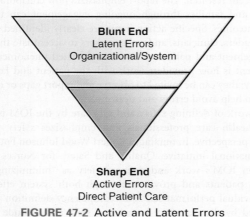

FIGURE 47-2 Active and Latent Errors

Types of Errors

In nursing, safety has focused on the safe execution of specific procedures and tasks. However, recent safety work has emphasized the variety of errors that compromise patient safety and the range of variables that impact the occurrence of errors in health care. Understanding types of errors in health care is a vital element in addressing individual practice and improving health care systems. In its early report, the IOM cites a pioneer in the field of patient safety, Lucian Leape, who identified four types of errors:[8]

1. Diagnostic errors are the result of a delay in diagnosis, failure to employ indicated tests, use of outmoded tests, or failure to act on results of monitoring or testing.
2. Treatment errors occur in the performance of an operation, procedure, or test; in administering a treatment; in the dose or method of administering a drug; or in avoidable delay in treatment or in responding to an abnormal test.
3. Preventive errors occur when there are failures to provide prophylactic treatment and inadequate monitoring or follow-up of treatment.
4. Communication failure (meaning a lack of communication or a lack of clarity in communication) can lead to many types of errors.

By employing a standardized system for classifying different types of errors, best practices can be developed to address safety compromises in health care systems.

Placement of Errors

Along with types of error, the placement of errors may be described as active or latent. This distinction is important in further understanding the etiology of health care errors and appropriate improvements. In health care, active errors are made by those providers (e.g., nurses, physicians, and technicians) who are providing patient care, responding to patient needs at the "sharp end," which is at the point of care (Figure 47-2).[9,10] Latent conditions are the potential contributing factors that are hidden and lie inactive in the health care delivery system, originating at more remote aspects of the health care system, far removed from the active end.[11] Latent errors—more organizational, contextual, and diffuse in nature or design-related—are called errors occurring at the "blunt end."[9] A latent failure is a flaw in a system that does not immediately lead to an accident but establishes a situation in which a triggering event may lead to an error.[12] Identifying errors as either active or latent in origin allows the exact system that needs improvement to be more accurately identified and corrected. Most bedside nurse clinicians operate at the sharp end of health care and are involved with active errors or inherit latent errors that can be manifest as active errors. For example, a nurse who administers the incorrect medication because of a failure to check the medication order is involved in an active error. However, a medication error can occur where a latent error can lead to an active error. For example, a latent error can lead to an active error if a Pyxis (or other medication administration system) is incorrectly stocked with a look-alike, sound-alike medication that a nurse mistakenly administers based on what should have been stocked in a certain Pyxis compartment. As nurses learn about differences between active and latent errors, they can more accurately identify and contribute to processes or systems for improvement.

Culture of Safety

The IOM's work in the past decade has facilitated a clearer focus on patient outcomes for health care clinicians and facilities. Historically, a culture of blame has been pervasive in health care. When an error occurred, the focus was often on identifying the clinician at fault and meting out discipline.[13] With greater focus on patient outcomes, health care teams now investigate what went wrong rather than just blaming the individual clinician who executed the error. Balancing the historical emphasis on blame within the broader context of a culture of safety is vital to effectively addressing error occurrence. A commonly cited definition of safety culture derives from the Health and Safety Commission of Great Britain and is utilized by the Agency for Healthcare Research and Quality (AHRQ): "The safety culture of an organization is the product of individual and group values, attitudes, perceptions, competencies, and patterns of behavior that determine the commitment to, and the style and proficiency of, an organization's health and safety management."[14] Organizations with a positive safety culture are characterized by communication guided by mutual trust, shared perceptions of the importance of safety, and confidence that error-preventing strategies will work.[15]

From an organizational context, a culture of safety acknowledges the influence of complex systems and human factors that influence safety. In a culture of safety, the focus is on teamwork to accomplish the goal of safe, high-quality care. When errors or near misses occur, the focus is on what went wrong rather than on who committed the error. The focus shifts from identifying fault to establish blame and determine discipline to acknowledging and reporting errors and near misses to improve the system. Accountability is a critical aspect of a culture of safety; recognizing and acknowledging one's actions is a trademark of professional behavior.

A 2003 study surveying trends in how hospitals report errors to patients revealed significant variability in the way hospitals disclose errors and share information with patients.[16] Although hospitals are increasingly reporting serious injury to patients, hospitals in the survey that were concerned about malpractice implications or disclosure were less likely to disclose incidents of preventable harm to patients.[16]

A recent extensive review of safety culture literature identified seven aspects of the concept that contribute to a culture of safety in a health care organization: Leadership, teamwork, an evidence base, communication, learning, a just culture, and patient-centered care.[17] Safety culture is a complex phenomenon that requires support from the leadership level, the policy level, and the bedside clinician level.[17] Empowering staff to participate in an error-reporting system without fear of punitive action is an important aspect of creating a culture of safety. In surveying nurses and physicians, a barrier to reporting medication errors and near-miss events is the fear of professional or personal punishment.[18–20] As the largest segment of the health care workforce, nurses are central to creating and maintaining a culture of safety in any health care setting. From the bedside to the administrative suite, nurses can contribute to all aspects of a culture of safety.

ATTRIBUTES AND CRITERIA

What knowledge, skills, and attitudes are required for nurses to effectively contribute to safety in health care? The QSEN project has been the national leader in defining the competency for safety by specifying the knowledge, skill, and attitude objectives for prelicensure students. A national expert panel of thought leaders in each competency used an iterative process to reach consensus on the essential knowledge, skill, and attitude objectives that all nurses need to contribute to emerging systems of safety in health care.

Knowledge

Historically, the emphasis in nursing has been on the safe execution of discrete skills. However, contemporary nurses need to be knowledgeable in examining human factors and other basic safety design principles as well as make the distinction with commonly used unsafe practices (e.g., workarounds and dangerous abbreviations). Nurses need to be able to describe the benefits and limitations of selected safety-enhancing technologies (e.g., barcodes, computerized provider order entry, medication pumps, and automatic alerts/alarms). Educating nurses in effective strategies to reduce reliance on memory (e.g., checklists) encourages nurses to understand safety as an individual as well as a systems phenomenon. As nurses become more knowledgeable about safety at the systems level, they can delineate general categories of errors and hazards in care (e.g., active vs. latent and diagnostic, treatment, and preventive errors). Nurses need to be able to describe factors that create a culture of safety (e.g., open communication strategies and organizational error-reporting systems). Nurses must understand the processes used in understanding the cause of error and allocation of responsibility and accountability through such processes as root cause analysis (RCA) and failure mode effects analysis. An important facet of nurses' knowledge is their appreciation of the potential and actual impact of national patient safety resources, initiatives, and regulations to effectively use and contribute to these important facets of standardized safe practices.

Skills

Nurses need skills to utilize tools that contribute to safer systems. For example, nurses must develop skills in the effective use of technology and standardized practices that support safety and quality as well as effectively use strategies to reduce risk of harm to self or others. Communication failures are the leading cause of inadvertent patient harm.[21] A vital skill set for nurses is to communicate observations or concerns related to hazards and errors to patients, families, and the health care team. Nurses have the responsibility to use organizational error-reporting systems for near miss and error reporting and to participate in analyzing errors and designing system improvements (e.g., RCAs). Nurses are responsible for their own individual practices while also contributing to the development of safer systems. Applying the national patient safety resources to his or her professional development will also enhance the capacity to focus attention on safety in care settings.

Attitudes

Nurses' personal and professional attitudes are instrumental in shaping their nursing practice and recognizing the cognitive and physical limits of human performance. Safety systems utilize principles of standardization and reliability as part of error prevention strategies. Professionals value their own role in preventing errors and realize the difference that one person can make in prevention, even for one patient and family. Developing an attitude of collaboration across the health care team to ensure safe coordination of care contributes to safe care. It is the collective and shared environmental scanning and vigilance by all team members (e.g., patients, families, and all disciplines and staff) that prevents errors. As nurse clinicians perceive their own local practices as components of the broader national safety initiatives, patient outcomes can be incrementally improved at the local and national levels.

THEORETICAL LINKS

Theoretical links that further explicate safety include human factors, crew resource management, and high reliability organizations.

Human Factors

Human factors are adapted from engineering and expanded to address processes in health care by studying the interrelationship between people, technology, and the environment in which they work.[22] Human factors consider the ability or inability to perform exacting tasks while attending to multiple things at once. Human factors offer a systematic approach to studying process and outcome effectiveness for greater error prevention and greater efficiency. Within human factors health care research, attention is paid to all levels of care provision: external environment, management, physical environment, human–system interfaces, organizational/social environments, the nature of the work being done, and individual characteristics and aspects of performance.[11]

In employing a human factors framework to health care, the emphasis is on both supporting health care professionals' performance and eliminating hazards. Supporting health care professionals' performance in systems design includes physical performance, cognitive performance, and social/behavioral performance.[23] Simultaneously, consideration should be given to designing systems that avoid hazards. A hazard is anything that increases the probability of errors or patient/employee injury.[23] The dual consideration of supporting health care professionals and eliminating hazards is a qualitative shift to the development of systems that do not respond reactively to error occurrence but instead work proactively to avoid errors in an anticipatory way through the purposeful design of safer systems. A culture of safety requires organizational leadership that gives attention to human factors such as managing workload fluctuations, seeking strategies to minimize interruptions in work, and attending to communication and coordination across disciplines including power gradients and excessive professional courtesy.

Applying a human factors framework to guide research in appreciating and quantifying processes that lead to error will increase our understanding of the complexity of nurses' work in the acute care environment. Ebright and colleagues identify eight patterns that relate to complexity of nursing work in the acute care environment:[12]

- Disjointed supply sources
- Missing or nonfunctioning supplies and equipment
- Repetitive travel
- Interruptions
- Waiting for systems/processes
- Difficulty in accessing resources to continue care
- Breakdown in communication
- Communication media

Using a human factors paradigm to guide research highlights how work complexity can threaten patient care continuity and contribute to medical error.[12] Nurses are challenged by numerous human factors that impact safety, such as multitasking, distractions, complacent attitudes, fatigue, task fixation that limits environmental scanning, and failure to follow up or follow protocol. Helping nurses understand human factors can inform their understanding of safety and further facilitate nursing's contributions toward the development of safer health care delivery systems.

Crew Resource Management

Crew resource management (CRM) training was developed in the aviation industry to standardize procedures, standardize communication, decrease errors, and increase efficiency. Within aviation, crew resource management has been defined as a set of instructional strategies designed to improve teamwork by applying well-tested training tools (e.g., performance measures, exercises, and feedback mechanisms) and appropriate training methods (e.g., simulators, lectures, and videos) targeted at specific content (i.e., teamwork knowledge, skills, and attitudes).[24] CRM emphasizes the role of human factors in high-stress, high-risk work environments. The work environments of health care and aviation share the characteristics of high stress, complexity, the need for highly functioning teams, the importance of accurate and precise communication, and the high cost of system failures.[25]

CRM has been used to improve team functioning in operating rooms, emergency departments, for labor and delivery teams, and for perioperative teams. CRM programs are tailored to an individual organization to consider specific human factors that contribute to errors and near misses in that particular environment.[26] Critical reviews of CRM training programs in health care indicate the need for further study to validate effectiveness[24] to determine the transfer of the learned behavior to provision of care.

Application of CRM principles to guide improvement work in health care settings is becoming more common. A 2013 unit-based project applied sterile cockpit principles to protect nurses from distractions during medication administration through the use of "Do Not Disturb" signs and donning of orange vests by nurses administering medications.[27] In tracking the type and frequency of distractions, there was a decrease in the number of distractions over time as well as a decrease in medication error rates. The generalizability and sustainability of CRM interventions is a common question because unit culture and staff buy-in can vary dramatically between agencies.

High Reliability Organizations

High reliability organizations (HROs) manage work that involves hazardous environments (e.g., nuclear power plants and air traffic control agencies) in which the consequence of errors is high but the occurrence of error is low.[28] AHRQ offers resources for hospitals or other organizations to adapt and apply the principles and characteristics of HROs.[29] Five characteristics describe the mindset of HROs:

- HROs exhibit sensitivity to operations. Beyond policies and manuals, there is a "situational awareness" among HROs in which process anomalies and outliers are quickly identified. Sensitivity to operations both reduces the number of errors and facilitates prompt recognition to avoid larger consequences from errors.
- HROs are preoccupied with failure and focused on predicting and eliminating errors rather than being in the position of reacting to errors. HROs view near misses as opportunities to improve current systems by examining strengths and weaknesses and addressing gaps.
- HROs have a reluctance to simplify. These high-functioning organizations accept the complexity inherent in their work and do not accept simplistic solutions for challenges intrinsic to complex systems. In complex work environments, different team members may have information at different times.
- Effective HROs exhibit deference to expertise and cultivate a culture in which team members and organizational leaders defer to the person with the most knowledge of the current issue or concern. The team member with the most information may not be the individual with the highest rank, deemphasizing hierarchy.
- HROs exhibit a commitment to reliance. HROs pay close attention to their ability to quickly contain errors and return to functioning despite setbacks.[29]

HROs share power and standardized communication. Especially in the acute care setting, nurses are often the most informed bedside clinicians to an emerging error and have an obligation to speak up to share critical information. HROs have an explicit value of safety at the organizational level. Organizational leadership helps align safety goals with mission and vision so that safety is valued throughout all areas and levels of the system. A hospital is a system, a set of interdependent components that interact to achieve a common goal. Hospitals are composed of interdependent components such as service lines, nursing care units, ancillary care departments, and outpatient care clinics that interact to achieve a common goal of care delivery. The way in which these separate but united system components interact and work together is a significant factor in delivering high-quality safe care, and the more that clinicians understand the interrelationships, the more effectively they can coordinate care. HROs have a multilevel focus on safety; it is pervasive in the culture, and all employees must have mindfulness to observe where the next error may occur and implement prevention strategies.

CONTEXT TO NURSING AND HEALTH CARE

Just Culture

Data about errors have not always been accessible to health care professionals or to health care consumers. To create a culture of safety, adverse events must be reported so they can be analyzed for lessons learned and new procedures drafted to improve the system. "Just culture" refers to a system's explicit value of reporting errors without punishment. A just culture is one in which people can report mistakes or errors without reprisal or personal risk.[29] Just culture does not mean individuals are not accountable for their actions or practice, but it does mean that people are not punished for flawed systems. A just culture promotes sharing and disclosure among stakeholders.[29]

A just culture seeks to balance the need to learn from mistakes and the need to implement disciplinary action.[3] The IOM recommends that in most cases front-line workers should be protected from disciplinary action when they report injuries, errors, and near misses, even if they were personally involved, to encourage transparency in the system. These recommendations are based on literature review of other high-risk industries such as aviation safety, nuclear power, and high-reliability military operations. Without such protections, injury-reporting rates may drop and thus impede the ability to prevent future injuries. The IOM provides exceptions to such protection, however, if an error involves criminal behavior, active malfeasance, or cases in which an injury is not reported in a timely manner.[3]

Consequences for errors in a just culture are commonly addressed by a model proposed by David Marx. Marx differentiates *human error* from *at-risk* behavior and reckless behavior. Human error is inadvertent action: a slip or lapse. At-risk behavior is behavioral choice that increases risk when risk is not recognized or is mistakenly believed to be justified. Reckless behavior is a behavior choice to consciously disregard a substantial risk. Each level of error involves differing responses from leadership. Human error is best remedied by training, redesigning the system, and improving procedures. At-risk behavior is best mitigated by creating incentives for healthy behaviors, increasing situational awareness, and providing education. Marx suggests remedial or punitive action in instances of reckless behavior.[30]

Transparency in Health Care

The IOM recommends new rules to redesign and improve care by increasing transparency in health care.[2] The health care system should make information available to patients and families that allows them to make informed decisions about where and from whom to receive their care. This information should include information on a system's performance on safety, evidence-based practice, and patient satisfaction. The Hospital Compare website, operated by the U.S. Department of Health and Human Services (http://www.hospitalcompare.hhs.gov), makes Health Care Quality Information from the Consumer Perspective (HCAHPS) available to consumers.

More than just making quality information available to consumers, transparency is also defined as open communication and information sharing with patients and their families about their care, including adverse and sentinel events. Timely, open, honest communication with patients and families about adverse events helps restore trust. Professionals trained in the principles and practice of transparency, usually risk management staff, communicate with the patient and family as soon as an adverse event is recognized and the patient is ready physically and psychologically to receive this information, usually within 24 hours. There are specific recommendations to help health care professionals understand how transparency can be operationalized in a health care system and fit within the framework of just culture. Patients should be told what happened, and those involved should take responsibility, apologize, and explain how the organization will respond and what will be done to prevent future events.[31]

Transparency and disclosure are interrelated experiences. Rick Boothman and colleagues have developed a standardized model around transparency and disclosure (often referred to as the Michigan model) that focuses on compensating patients quickly and fairly when inappropriate care causes injury, supporting clinical staff when the care was reasonable, and reducing patient injuries by learning from patients' experiences. This transparent disclosure model has demonstrated a decrease in rate of new claims, a decline in lawsuits, and decreased overall compensation costs.[32]

INTERRELATED CONCEPTS

Safety is a multidimensional term as applied in health care with several interrelated concepts. The concepts featured in this text that are most closely interrelated with safety are shown in Figure 47-3.

Health Care Quality is very closely interrelated to safety—so much so that they really overlap. Health care quality is defined as identifying the gap that occurs between ideal care and actual care delivered. Quality improvement is an approach to practice that measures the variance in ideal and actual care and implements strategies to close the gap. Quality measures include benchmarks from other areas of the same institution or from peer institutions across the health care industry, such as comparisons of the National Database of Nursing Quality Indicators (NDNQI), led by the American Nurses Association.[33]

How well health care professionals work together accounts for as much as 70% of health care errors.[1] For this reason, Communication, Collaboration, and Care Coordination are closely related to safety. Standardized communication can ensure safe handoffs between providers or between settings, provide clear direction in seeking and sharing information between providers, and instill collaborative behaviors for speaking up to prevent errors from occurring. Ineffective communication, hierarchy, and disruptive behavior are challenges to patient safety. Care coordination requires cross-disciplinary communication, knowing scope of responsibility, and organizational support for speaking up when safety is compromised. Collaboration begins with self-development based on emotional intelligence to monitor appropriate reactions and responses to team members. Nurses need

FIGURE 47-3 Safety and Interrelated Concepts

BOX 47-1 EXEMPLARS OF SAFETY

Point of Care
- Prevention of decubitus ulcers
- Medication administration
- Fall prevention
- Invasive procedures
- Diagnostic workup
- Recognition of/action on adverse effects
- Communication with patients/families
- Communication with other health care providers

Systems Level
- Care coordination
- Documentation/electronic records
- Team systems
- Work processes
- Communication process
- Environmental systems
- Error reporting/analysis
- Regulatory systems
- National quality benchmarks

---

skills in problem solving, conflict resolution, and negotiation to be able to coordinate safe care across interprofessional teams. Shared leadership based on the provider most expert in the situation is consistent with HROs.

CLINICAL EXEMPLARS

Because multiple exemplars exist for safety and injury prevention within health care, it is not possible to list them all. Box 47-1 presents the most common safety issues at the point of care and the systems level. A few of the most important exemplars are briefly described here.

Featured Exemplars
Fall Prevention
Prevention of falls is a safety concern in all living environments, especially for older adults. The American Geriatrics Society (http://www .americangeriatrics.org) offers evidence-based clinical practice guidelines for older adults living independently, in assisted living, in long-term care facilities, and for those being cared for in the acute care environment. These guidelines address recommended screening, elements of a focused history, physical examination, and functional assessment. In addition, the guidelines synthesize common fall prevention interventions and tailor them for various living situations: adaptation of the environment; minimization of psychoactive medications; attention to postural hypotension; management of foot problems and footwear; and exercises that emphasize balance, strength, and gait training.

Medication Administration
Medication administration is an essential aspect of nurses' work, especially in the acute care setting. Medication errors are the most common errors in the hospital setting, and they usually involve the frontline nurse clinician. From 26% to 32% of medication errors occur at the administration stage and involve nurses.[34] Interventions to decrease medication administration errors often focus on technology such as bar code medication administration or computer physician order entry, standardization of medication administration practices, or alterations to the nurses' environment to decrease distractions or interruptions.

Care Coordination
Poorly coordinated care systems contribute to safety compromises in the delivery of care. Integrated care systems are an effective method to address such system gaps. The development of care coordination models has grown out of the need to address fragmented service delivery, cost inefficiencies, and poor health outcomes. Care coordination can be defined as a set of activities purposefully organized by a team of personnel that includes the patient to facilitate the appropriate delivery of the necessary services and information to support optimal health care across settings and over time.

Team Systems
Health care professionals provide care on teams. Safety outcomes are often closely tied to effective team functioning. Understanding team systems in health care is complex because of the high degree of variability in settings, microsystem culture, care delivery, and members of the care team. Effective team systems in health care contribute to safe, patient-centered outcomes. Evidence suggests that high-functioning teams in health care are related to clear role definition, timely information about a patient's changing health status, mutual respect among team members, consistent feedback, and participation of patient or family on team, when desired.[35]

Error Reporting

Adverse outcomes in health care can only be addressed when reported; thus error reporting is essential to error prevention. A reluctance to report errors may be attributed to a perceived lack of impact of the error on the patient or a patient outcome, a fear of a punitive response by leadership or a system, or a personal sense of embarrassment about the error.[36] There is also wide variation in how errors are defined, which information should be reported, and the best approaches to mitigating the effects of errors.[36] Addressing reluctance to error reporting at the unit culture level through implementation of just culture concepts is one evidence-based approach to this complex issue.[37]

CASE STUDY

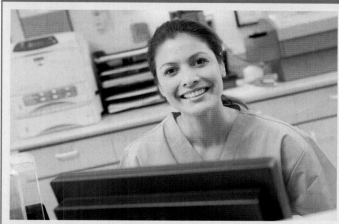

Source: monkeybusinessimages/iStock/Thinkstock

Case Presentation

Gloria considers herself an expert nurse on her medical/surgical unit. She has been a registered nurse (RN) on this unit for 12 years and has seen some important changes in how care is provided. Keeping up with these changes is an important part of Gloria's practice, and many RNs look to Gloria for guidance in understanding the latest evidence.

Lately, Gloria has been concerned about the occurrence of decubitus ulcers on her unit. She knows that there are several strategies that must be employed to effectively address this deleterious patient outcome.[38] When caring for Mr. Brown, a postoperative spinal stenosis patient, Gloria knows that at the individual practice level it is important that she establish a schedule of turning this patient every 2 hours. Evidence supports the impact of this nursing intervention at the individual clinician level in preventing decubitus ulcers.[39]

As Gloria goes off shift after caring for Mr. Brown, she thinks about the importance of clear communication with the rest of the health care team about decubitus ulcer prevention for Mr. Brown. Therefore, to address safety at the health care team level, Gloria posts a reminder above his bed for all health care team members to turn Mr. Brown every 2 hours.

While Gloria cares for Mr. Brown for consecutive shifts, she thinks about the variety of ways that nurses can work with other members of the health care team to prevent decubitus ulcers. On his second postoperative day, Mr. Brown's surgeon mentions to Gloria that because he has been prescribed steroids, he is at especially high risk for developing decubitus ulcers. Gloria decides to address this safety concern for Mr. Brown at the unit level, and she seeks input on his care from the physical therapist to learn about skin protection products and from the dietitian to address nutritional strategies to help prevent decubitus ulcers in Mr. Brown.

When speaking with the physical therapist and dietitian about decubitus ulcer prevention for Mr. Brown, both colleagues mention the increase in occurrence of decubitus ulcers on this medical/surgical unit. Gloria works with her manager and the quality improvement department to track the decubitus ulcer rate on her medical/surgical unit for the previous 6 months and plans to compare this rate with state and national quality benchmarks for decubitus ulcer prevention. She is also aware that many studies have been published by the Institute for Healthcare Improvement (http://www.ihi.org) on best practices for decubitus ulcer prevention. Once Gloria has retrieved the data from her own unit to compare to other benchmarks, she will collaborate with her manager and RN colleagues to identify some systematic strategies that can be adopted on her unit. Gloria understands that safety needs to be addressed at the individual clinician level as well as at the systems level.

Case Analysis

Any source of potential injury to patients can be examined on a continuum from an individual practice perspective to a safe systems perspective. The case provides several levels of instruction to improve patient safety outcomes. Safety is a multilevel phenomenon. However, in nursing, safety has been traditionally understood as primarily the responsibility of the individual nurse clinician. Until recently, safety was considered only the individual nurse's responsibility to prevent medication errors, to prevent a patient from falling, or to prevent decubitus ulcers. Applying principles from safety science to health care systems offers a broader understanding of safety with several levels of implementation. Gloria's decisions in her own nursing practice to prevent the development of a decubitus ulcer for Mr. Brown exemplify individual clinician strategies that are important and effective. In addition, Gloria's work in collaborating with other members of the health care team and comparing unit-level data to system, state, and national data represent valuable strategies in addressing patient safety from a larger perspective. To improve patient safety outcomes, compromises to safety need to be addressed on many levels simultaneously.

ACCESS EXEMPLAR LINKS IN YOUR GIDDENS EBOOK

REFERENCES

1. Institute of Medicine: *To err is human: Building a safer health system*, Washington, DC, 2000, National Academies Press.
2. Institute of Medicine: *Crossing the quality chasm*, Washington, DC, 2001, National Academies Press.
3. Institute of Medicine: *Keeping patients safe: Transforming the work environment of nurses*, Washington, DC, 2004, National Academies Press.
4. National Patient Safety Foundation: *Our definitions*, (n.d.). Retrieved from <http://s197607105.onlinehome.us/au/mission_definitions.php>.
5. National Patient Safety Foundation's Lucian Leape Institute: *Safety is personal: Partnering with patients and families for the safest care*, 2014. Retrieved from <http://www.npsf.org/?page=safetyispersonal>.
6. Cronenwett L, Sherwood G, Barnsteiner J, et al: Quality and safety education for nurses. *Nurs Outlook* 55(3):122–131, 2007.
7. The Joint Commission: *Sentinel events*, 2011. Retrieved from <http://www.jointcommission.org/assets/1/6/2011_CAMBHC_SE.pdf>.
8. Leape L, Lawther AG, Brennan TA, et al: Preventing medical injury. *Qual Rev Bull* 19(5):144–149, 1993.

9. Cook R, Woods D: Operating at the sharp end: The complexity of human error. In Bogner M, editor: *Human error in medicine*, Hillsdale, NJ, 1994, Erlbaum, pp 255–310.

10. Reason J: *Managing the risks of organizational accidents*, Burlington, VT, 1997, Ashgate.

11. Henrickson K, Dayton E, Keyes MA, et al: Understanding adverse events: A human factors framework. In Hughes RG, editor: *Patient safety and quality: An evidence-based handbook for nurses*, Publication No. 08-0043, Rockville, MD, 2008, Agency for Healthcare Research and Quality, pp 1-67–1-85.

12. Ebright PR, Patterson ES, Chalko BA, et al: Understanding the complexity of registered nurse work in acute care settings. *J Nurs Admin* 33(12):630–638, 2003.

13. Barnsteiner JH: *Safety competency resource paper*, Washington, DC, 2010, American Association of Colleges of Nursing QSEN Education Center.

14. Health and Safety Commission Advisory Committee on the Safety of Nuclear Installations: *Organizing for safety: Third report of the ACSNI study group on human factors*, Sudbury, UK, 1993, HSE Books.

15. Gadd S, Collins AM: *Safety culture: A review of the literature, definition of "safety culture" as suggested by ACSNO, HSE*, 2002. Retrieved from <http://www.hse.gov.uk/research/hsl_pdf/2002/hsl02-25.pdf>.

16. Lamb RM, Studdert DM, Bohmer RM, et al: Hospital disclosure practices: Results of a national survey. *Health Aff (Millwood)* 22(2):73–83, 2003.

17. Sammer C, Lynken K, Singh K, et al: What is patient safety culture? A review of the literature. *J Nurs Schol* 42:156–165, 2010.

18. Cohoon BD: Learning from near misses through reflection: A new risk management strategy. *J Healthcare Risk Manage* 23(2):19–25, 2003.

19. Schmidt CE, Bottoni T: Improving medication safety and patient care in the emergency department. *J Emerg Nurs* 29(1):12–16, 2003.

20. Bullock LM: Transform into a culture of safety. *Risk Management* 42(7):14–15, 2011.

21. Leonard M, Graham S, Bonacum D: The human factor: The critical importance of effective teamwork and communication in providing safe care. *Qual Saf Health Care* 13:i85–i90, 2004.

22. Karsh BT, Holden RJ, Alper SJ, et al: A human factors engineering paradigm for patient safety: Designing to support the performance of the healthcare professional. *Qual Saf Health Care* 15(Suppl 1):i59–i65, 2006.

23. Salas E, Prince C, Bowers C, et al: A methodology for enhancing crew resource management training. *Hum Factors* 41:161–172, 1999.

24. Rivers RM, Swain D, Nixon WR: Using aviation safety measures to enhance patient outcomes. *J Ass Operating Room Nurses* 77(1):158–162, 2003.

25. Oriol MD: Crew resource management. *J Nurs Admin* 36(9):402–406, 2006.

26. Salas E, Wilson KA, Burke CS, et al: Does crew resource management training work? An update, an extension and some critical needs. *Hum Factors* 48(2):392–412, 2006.

27. Fore AM, Sculli GL, Albee D, et al: Improving patient safety using the sterile cockpit principle during medication administration: A collaborative, unit-based project. *J Nurs Manage* 21:106–111, 2013.

28. Baker DP, Day R, Salas E: Teamwork as an essential component of high-reliability organizations. *Health Services Res* 41(4):1576–1598, 2006.

29. Agency for Healthcare Research and Quality: *Becoming a high reliability organization: Operational advice for hospital leaders*, Rockville, MD, 2008, U.S. Department of Health and Human Services. Retrieved from <http://archive.ahrq.gov/professionals/quality-patient-safety/quality-resources/tools/hroadvice/hroadvice.pdf>.

30. Marx D: *Patient safety and the "just culture": A primer for health care executives*, New York, 2001, Columbia University.

31. Harvard Hospitals: *When things go wrong: Responding to adverse events*, Burlington, MA, 2006, Massachusetts Coalition for the Prevention of Medical Errors.

32. Boothman RC, Imhoff SJ, Campbell DA: Nursing a culture of patient safety and achieving lower malpractice risk through disclosure: Lessons learned and future directions. *Front Health Services Manage* 28(3):13–28, 2012.

33. American Nurses Association: *The National Center for Nursing quality indicators*, (n.d.). Retrieved from <http://www.nursingworld.org/ncnq>.

34. Hughes RG: Nurses at the "sharp end" of patient care. In Hughes RG, editor: *Patient safety and quality: An evidence-based handbook for nurses*, Publication No. 08-0043, Rockville, MD, 2008, Agency for Healthcare Research and Quality. Retrieved from <http://www.ncbi.nlm.nih.gov/books/NBK2672>.

35. Sevin C, Moore G, Shepherd J, et al: Transforming care teams to provide the best possible patient-centered, collaborative care. *J Ambulatory Care Manager* 32(1):24–31, 2009.

36. Wolf ZR, Hughes R: Error reporting and disclosure. In Hughes RG, editor: *Patient safety and quality: An evidence-based handbook for nurses*, Publication No. 08-0043, Rockville, MD, 2008, Agency for Healthcare Research and Quality, pp 2-333–2-379.

37. Boysen PG: Just culture: A foundation for balanced accountability for patient safety. *Ochsner J* 13:400–406, 2013.

38. Soban LM, Hempel S, Munjas BA, et al: Preventing pressure ulcers in hospitals: A systematic review of nurse-focused quality improvement interventions. *Jt Comm J Quality Patient Saf* 37(6):245–252, 2011.

39. Lyder CH, Ayello EA: Pressure ulcers: A patient safety issue. In Hughes RG, editor: *Patient safety and quality: An evidence-based handbook for nurses*, Publication No. 08-0043, Rockville, MD, 2008, Agency for Healthcare Research and Quality.

Technology and Informatics

Diane Skiba and Helen Connors

Health care providers have always gathered patient data and information to provide the best care possible. What has changed over time is the use of technology to gather, process, and manage data and information. With the advent of new technologies in health care, health information technology (IT) has become essential to providing safe, effective, efficient, and quality care and with it, a new discipline of informatics has emerged. Health care professionals with expertise in specialty areas or practice, along with a background in computer and information science, became focused on furthering and broadening their specialty area of practice with informatics. The field of health IT and informatics is rapidly advancing and must include a workforce prepared to meaningfully use these evolving technologies. There is a growing requirement for practicing nurses, nurse educators, nurse researchers, and nurse administrators to ensure that expected competencies in informatics are met. Despite widespread use of the term informatics, few seem to understand exactly what it means.

DEFINITION

Technology describes the knowledge and use of tools, machines, materials, and processes to help solve human problems. It can be applied to a specific discipline such as education technologies, medical technologies, or health technologies. Technology is the product of creative human action, and it is sustained by human action.[1] For the purpose of this concept presentation, the focus is on *health information technology (health IT)* as the essential antecedents for health informatics. In today's world, you cannot have health informatics without health IT.

Health IT provides the umbrella framework to describe the comprehensive management of health information and its secure exchange between consumers, providers, government and quality entities, and insurers. Health IT is generally viewed as the most promising tool for improving the overall quality, safety, and efficiency of the health delivery system.[2-4] The efficacy and effectiveness of health IT tools are also being examined in terms of their engagement of patients, the families, and caregivers in their health care decisions.

Informatics, like technology, also is a broad term and is derived from the French word *informatique*—it is the science that encompasses information science and computer science to study the process, management, and retrieval of information.[5] In this concept, the focus is on health informatics.

Health informatics is a discipline in which health data are stored, analyzed, and disseminated through the application of information and communication technology (Box 48-1). It involves the use of technology and information systems to support the health care industry. Today, the term informatics as it relates to health care is ubiquitous and ambiguous because of the many health professions and related disciplines that use health data. Health informatics encompasses the interprofessional study of the design, development, adoption, and application of IT-based innovations in health care services delivery, management, and planning.[6] The American Medical Informatics Association noted "the term health informatics to refer to applied research and practice of informatics across the clinical and public health domains."[7] As a broad term, health informatics includes the discipline of informatics as applied to clinical care and public health.

SCOPE

The scope of this concept is represented by the idea that health IT and health informatics intersect with the science of health to provide powerful tools and processes for advancing health practices and serve as an infrastructure to support and promote a continuously learning health care system (Figure 48-1).[8]

The tools are used by various groups and serve as part of the infrastructure of a health care delivery system. These groups include consumers, patients and their families, caregivers, health care professionals, administrators, and any personnel supporting the delivery of health care. One such tool is the electronic health record (EHR), which is a central component of the health IT infrastructure. An EHR is an individual's official, digital health record and is shared among multiple facilities and agencies. Other tools include the electronic medical record (EMR), which is an individual's health record within a health care provider's facility, and decision support tools to guide practice and decision making. Tools for patients, their families, and caregivers as well as consumers consist of mobile health tools such as wellness monitoring devices (physical activity monitors such as FitBit), personal health records, patient portals, and physiologic monitoring (pulse oximetry, digital stethoscope, and glucose monitors) and sensors. In addition, there are infrastructure health information technologies such as health information exchanges (HIEs) that support the sharing of health data across health care institutions, data warehouses that are repositories of stored data, and communication networks. The plethora of health IT and informatics tools provide the opportunity for engaging consumers in health care and creating a connected health system.

ATTRIBUTES AND CRITERIA

Health IT is a precursor or antecedent to health informatics and is summarized in Table 48-1. The defining characteristics and consequences of health IT are reflected in the analysis of health informatics. The results of the health IT and informatics concept analysis suggest the following attributes: hardware and software, data standards and terminology, policies and procedures, privacy and security, informatics workforce, and organizational skills.

Hardware and Software

Health IT is the application of information processing involving computer hardware, computer software, communications, and networking technologies that enables the storage, retrieval, sharing, and use of health care data, information, knowledge, and wisdom for communication and decision making.[9] Certified *clinical information systems*

(CIS) offer the best set of tools for achieving quality outcomes and are at the heart of health care IT and informatics. CIS consist of information technology that is applied at the point of clinical care. They include electronic health records, clinical data repositories, decision support programs, handheld and mobile devices for collecting data and viewing reference material, imaging modalities, and communication tools such as electronic messaging systems and patient portals. Increasingly, care is provided in multiple settings, thus creating a need for clinicians to share data with providers at other locations. Advances in computer networking, broadband, and wireless communication technologies have now made it possible for clinicians to access these data from any location—whether in the office, the hospital, at home, or even when traveling out of town.

An increasing number of digital tools are being used as part of health information technologies and used by patients and their families, caregivers, and consumers. These digital tools include patient portals including secure messaging that are available on numerous devices (tablets, smart phones, and desktop computers) and mobile applications software that collects and shares patient-generated health data (daily glucose readings, physical activities measures, etc.) with other consumers or their health care providers. The mobile applications can also be used to connect patients or consumers with social network groups. The use of these digital tools in the connected health

---

BOX 48-1 **Informatics Definitions**

- *Technology* is the knowledge and use of tools, machines, materials, and processes to help solve human problems.
- *Health information technology (health IT)* is the application of information processing involving both computer hardware and computer software that deals with the storage, retrieval, sharing, and use of health care data, information, and knowledge for communication and decision making.
- *Informatics* is derived from the French word *informatique*. Simply stated, informatics is the science that encompasses information science and computer science to study the process, management, and retrieval of information.
- *Health informatics* is a discipline in which health data are stored, analyzed, and disseminated through the application of information and communication technology.
- *Informatician* is a person who works in the field of informatics, sometimes called an informaticist.
- *Information science* is an interprofessional science primarily concerned with the analysis, collection, classification, manipulation, storage, retrieval, and dissemination of information.
- *Computer science* is a branch of engineering that studies computation and computer technology, hardware, and software as well as the theoretical foundations of information and computation techniques.

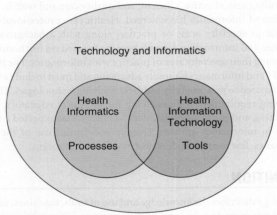

FIGURE 48-1 Scope of Technology and Informatics

TABLE 48-1 **Health Information Technology Summary**

Antecedent	Defining Characteristics	Outcomes
Need for a tool, machine, materials, and/or processes to improve health care	Technology (hardware and software) that supports discipline of health informatics (e.g., EHR)	Improves health provider's workflow
Information science	Clinical point-of-care tools	Improves health care quality
Computer science	Interoperable and connected	Prevents medical errors
Health discipline science (e.g., nursing, medicine)	Evolutionary and updated to provide new functionality	Reduces health care costs
Information technology specialist	Interoperable systems and tools	Increases administrative efficiencies
Informed patients, families, and caregivers	Technology-competent and engaged patients, families, and caregivers	Decreases paperwork
		Improves disease tracking
		Creates cultural, social, organizational, and intellectual change
		May be used in unintended ways
		Serves as an infrastructure for a learning health system
		Promotes and supports patient and family engagement in health decisions
		Connected Health

world helps patients and families, caregivers, and consumers manage their health, wellness, and health conditions, especially chronic illnesses such as heart disease, stroke, and diabetes. Digital tools that collect patient-generated health data may be used for personal management and may or may not be shared with providers. Health care providers also may use remote monitoring tools and sensor technologies to monitor patients in their homes.

Standardized Information Systems and Terminology

The proliferation of clinical information systems has created a pressing need for standardization of patient information systems and terminology. Standardized terminology within the EHR is critical for communicating care to the interprofessional team and exchanging health information. The universal requirement for quality patient care, efficiency, and cost containment makes it imperative to express data, information, and knowledge in a meaningful way that can be shared across disciplines and care settings.[10] EHRs must use consistent, codified terminology to eliminate ambiguity and confusion and to ensure interoperability. The many different ways of organizing data, information, and knowledge are built on taxonomies and nomenclature developed over decades using a clear coding scheme. The terminologies recognized by the American Nurses Association (ANA) are listed in Table 48-2.

Policies

Responsibility for developing an overall policy infrastructure that supports health IT and HIEs primarily lies with the Office of the National Coordinator for Health IT (ONC). ONC has worked closely with the Centers for Medicare & Medicaid Services (CMS) to assist in establishing policies related to Medicare and Medicaid payment for "meaningful use" of EHRs. ONC rules specify the standards, implementation specifications, and other criteria for EHR systems and technologies to be certified, whereas CMS rules specify how hospitals, physicians, and other eligible professionals must demonstrate their meaningful use of these technologies in order to receive Medicare and Medicaid payment incentives.[11]

In addition to meaningful use criteria and certification standards, the ONC health IT policy committee has issued recommendations regarding health information extension centers, workforce training, and privacy and security. Once the policies are established at the federal level, states, professional organizations, and institutions adopt and adapt these fundamental practices at the local level to reduce barriers to health information exchange.

Privacy and Security

A major concern with health care information, as with other highly sensitive personal data, involves privacy and security. The privacy and security rules issued under the Health Insurance Portability and Accountability Act (HIPAA) of 1996 along with multiple state laws create a complex network of laws and regulations that address patient privacy and consent for the use of identifiable personal health information. In 2013, HIPAA rules were modified to reflect new technologies and to enhance personalization and the quality of health care.[12] Building and maintaining the public's trust in health IT requires comprehensive privacy and security protections that establish clear rules on how patient data can be accessed, used, and disclosed.

TABLE 48-2   ANA-Recognized Terminologies

Terminology	Terminology URL	Nursing Process Within Terminology	Date Recognized by ANA	Integrated Within Other Terminologies
CCC: Clinical Care Classification	http://www.sabacare.com	Diagnoses, interventions, and outcomes	1992	NLN-UMLSSNOMED CT
ICNP: International Classification of Nursing Practice	http://www.icn.ch/icnp.htm	Diagnoses, interventions, and outcomes	2004	NLN-UMLSSNOMED CT
NANDA: NANDA International	http://www.nanda.org	Nursing diagnoses	1992	NLM-UMLSSNOMED CTPNDSHL7
NIC: Nursing Interventions Classification	http://www.nursing.uiowa.edu/center-for-nursing-classification-and-clinical-effectiveness	Interventions	1992	NLN-UMLSSNOMED CTHL7
NOC: Nursing Outcomes Classification	http://www.nursing.uiowa.edu/center-for-nursing-classification-and-clinical-effectiveness	Outcome indicators	1998	NLM-UMLSSNOMED CTHL7
Omaha System	http://www.omahasystem.org	Problem classification scheme Intervention scheme Problem rating scale for outcomes	1992	NLM-UMLSSNOMED CTHL7LOINC
PNDS: Perioperative Nursing Data Set	http://www.aorn.org/PNDS	Diagnoses, interventions, and outcomes	1999	NLM-UMLSSNOMED CTHL7
SNOMED CT: Systematic Nomenclature of Medicine Clinical Terms	https://www.nlm.nih.gov/research/umls/Snomed/snomed_main.htm	Assessment concepts, diagnoses, interventions, and outcomes	2002	NLM-UMLS

Informatics Workforce

An informatics workforce with the right skill set is critical to the advancement of health IT and informatics. During the past decade, a great deal of work has been done in nursing and other disciplines to define informatics competencies; however, currently there is no single consolidated list of competencies. Several professional organizations are working toward identifying informatics competencies, such as the American Medical Informatics Association (AMIA) and the Health Information Management Systems Society (HIMSS). In nursing, the ANA has defined the scope and standards for an informatics nurse and an informatics nurse specialist.[13] In addition, the Technology and Informatics Guiding Education Reform (TIGER) initiative in 2006 advocated that all nurses need informatics knowledge and skills to practice in a technology-intensive health care environment. In addition, the Quality and Safety Education for Nurses (QSEN) initiative and American Association of Colleges of Nursing's documents have determined informatics competencies for nurses being prepared at the prelicensure and graduate levels. As a result of the various initiatives, informatics competencies have been developed for all levels of nursing as well as competencies for specialization as an informatics nurse and an informatics nurse specialist. Certification as an informatics nurse is available through the American Nurses Credentialing Center (ANCC).

Informaticians are informatics specialists with advanced education and training who collaborate with other health care professionals and IT specialists to enhance and support patient-centered quality health care. Informaticians use their knowledge of patient care (e.g., nursing and medicine) combined with their understanding of informatics concepts, methods, and tools to analyze, design, implement, and evaluate information and communication systems that enhance individual and population health as well as provide efficient administrative services.[14] The hallmark of nursing informatics practice is its cross-disciplinary nature, with nurse informaticians often leading the team to create practical informatics solutions for use by many disciplines.[13] In 2013, clinical informatics was recognized as a board-certified subspecialty. Physicians take the Clinical Informatics Certification Exam to become board certified. Nurses can become certified in nursing informatics through the ANCC.

Peopleware and Organizational Skills

Informatics is not limited to the hardware and software; it includes people and organizational skills. When talking about widespread use of health IT and informatics, technical skills alone are not sufficient for implementation success. Peopleware, a key component of successful implementation, is a term used to refer to anything that has to do with the role of people in the development and use of computer hardware and software systems. Peopleware involves the sociologic side of informatics implementations and includes issues such as productivity, teamwork, group dynamics, project management, organizational factors, human interface design, and human–machine interaction. When introducing new technologies into an organization, the peopleware issues become as important and at times more important than the technological issues. Learning to manage people is crucial to managing technological change.[15] Table 48-3 summarizes the concept analysis of health informatics and its impact on nursing practice and consumer/patient health.

THEORETICAL LINKS

Classic theories that underpin the concept of informatics are from information science and computer science. Other sciences that play a role in the implementation of informatics are cognitive science and organizational science. Discipline-specific science, such as nursing science or medical science, is what differentiates informatics in the specialty areas of practice or domains of informatics and provides the fundamental building blocks for knowledge and wisdom.[13,16]

Information Science

Information science is a branch of applied mathematics and electrical engineering that involves the quantification of information. It is a collection of mathematical theories, based on statistics, concerned with methods of coding, transmitting, storing, retrieving, and decoding information. Its application includes the design of systems, such as clinical information systems, that are involved with data transmission, encryption, compression, and other information processing techniques. Recent advances in health information technologies and health information exchange have resulted in an enormous increase in health care data requiring large storage capacities, powerful computing resources, and accurate data analysis algorithms. Every clinical decision is based on this availability of the information that is transmitted. If the exchange of information works well, clinical care is solidly based on best evidence, whereas poor transmission of clinical data can lead to poorly informed decisions.[16]

Computer Science

Computer science is the study of the theoretical foundations of information and computation as these techniques relate to implementation and application of computer systems. It is frequently described as the systematic study of algorithmic processes that create, describe, and transform information. Computer science is a broad field of study that focuses on computation, algorithms and data structures, programming methodology and languages, and computer elements (hardware, software, and networks) and architecture. It also includes fields such as software engineering, artificial intelligence, computer networking and communications, database systems, and human–computer interaction.[17]

Cognitive Science

Cognitive science is the interprofessional study of mind, intelligence, and behavior from an information processing perspective. It encompasses how people think, understand, remember, synthesize, access, and respond to stored information and knowledge. Cognitive science provides the scaffolding for the analysis and modeling of complex human performance in technology-mediated settings. Theories from cognitive science inform and shape design, development, implementation, and assessment of health information systems. The mind is frequently compared to a computer, and experts in cognitive science try to model human thinking using the artificial networks of the computer.[16]

Organizational Science

Organizational science is an emerging field that focuses on behavior of organizations and includes a wide variety of topics, such as individual, group, and organizational decision making; the management of human resources; and the design of organizations and interorganizational networks. Understanding an organization and particularly understanding how culture, behavior, and social change impact an organization are essential requirements for successful implementation of health IT and health informatics within and among organizations.[18] Health care has been determined to be a complex adaptive system and as such involves patients, providers, and policymakers alike to ensure that every health care decision is guided by timely, accurate, and

TABLE 48-3 Health Informatics Summary[a]

Antecedents	Defining Characteristics	Nurse Outcomes	Patient Outcomes
Certified health IT hardware and software (CIS and computer applications)	Interoperable EHR and tools that allow for formal representation of data/information/knowledge	Clinical decision support tools at point of care Reduces duplication of services Evidence-based practice Opportunity for shared learning environment	Consumers adopt personal health record Decreased cost of health care Patient-centered, personalized health care and user-generated data
Standard terminology for data collection and electronic exchange of health information	Data structure that allows for uniform input and retrieval of health data Algorithms that support evidence-based clinical decision making and provide safety checks	Mechanism to determine costs of nursing and other health care services Accurate, timely, and up-to-date information at point of care	Better understanding of health care benefits and services Improved quality of health care and reduced medial errors
Policies for data transmission and use	Policy framework for development and adoption of health IT infrastructure and information exchange	Ensures security and privacy of health information and exchange	Confidentiality of health data
Broadband capacity for widespread electronic data transmission and download	Sufficient bandwidth requirement to achieve full functionality of health IT applications	Ability to transfer health data among providers and across health care systems	Health data available at point of care
Persons with specialized education in informatics Persons with technical knowledge and skill	Informatics specialist as team member Health information management and health IT professionals as team members	Maximize use of clinical information system	
End users with basic informatics competencies and discipline-specific knowledge and wisdom	Clinicians (nurses) with knowledge of phenomena of nursing in their area of practice as a team member	Broad-based team approach to patient care to support clinical judgment and meaningful use	
Patient, families, and caregivers informed about health and healthcare decisions	Patient, families, and caregivers central to the health care team		Improved patient engagement
Organizational culture that supports a learning health care system	Dynamic interprofessional team-oriented digital culture focused on peopleware and organizational skills	Use of data to inform clinical care and support research and knowledge development	Improved patient education, self-management, and health literacy

[a]Working definition: *Health informatics* is a discipline that sorts, enhances, processes, operates on, organizes, makes usable, and retrieves information related to human health and illness through the application of technology for the purpose of sharing information, knowledge, and wisdom among health providers, among consumers, and across organizations.

comprehensive health information to guarantee patient-centered care in a timely, efficient, and equitable manner. Informatics specialists with knowledge and skills in analyzing organizational culture, planning change within the organization, building and working in interprofessional teams, and leading information system development and implementation are key resources for the organization. In order for health care professionals and health care systems to embrace and meaningfully use informatics and other emerging technologies, a change in culture is critical.[19]

CONTEXT TO NURSING AND HEALTH CARE

Nurses are involved in informatics in terms of their own professional roles and responsibilities and with their interprofessional roles and responsibilities with other health care professionals within a health care institution. To best understand this, it is important to examine the evolution of health informatics and the domains of informatics and specific application in nursing.

Historical Perspective: The Evolution of Technology and Informatics in Health Care

One could argue that early ideas related to informatics date back more than 150 years (Figure 48-2). Various health information technologies have been available since the 1970s; the support for widespread use of information and communication technologies is a more recent occurrence. During the past decade, a convergence of driving forces has served as a major catalyst to move the health care informatics agenda forward and ensure that all health care professionals have the necessary "21st century knowledge and skills for practice in a complex, emerging technologically sophisticated, consumer-centric, global environment."[20,p58] Since 2000, the Institute of Medicine has consistently highlighted the use of health information technologies as one solution for ensuring safe and quality health care. Starting with *To Err Is Human: Building a Better Health System*,[21] using appropriate technologies has been one recommended solution to reduce errors and ensure patient safety. In *Crossing the Quality Chasm*,[22] there was general consensus that the current health care system was in need of

"In attempting to arrive at the truth, I have applied everywhere for information, but in scarcely an instance have I been able to obtain hospital records fit for any purposes of comparison. If they could be obtained they would enable us to decide many other questions besides the ones alluded to. They would show the subscribers how their money was being spent, what amount of good was really being done with it, or whether the money was not doing mischief rather than good."
Florence Nightingale (1863).

Longman, Green, Longman, Roberts and Green: Notes on Hospitals, 1863, London, p. 176

FIGURE 48-2 The First Nurse Informatician

reform. It is stated throughout the report that in order to achieve this reform, the health care system must make

effective use of information technologies to automate clinical information and make it readily accessible to patients and all members of the care team. An improved information infrastructure is needed to establish effective and timely communication among clinicians and between patients and clinicians.[22,p12]

This points not only to the need for the meaningful use of the EHR but also to the need to examine the use of communication tools and patient portals to foster communication between patients and clinicians, as well as the need to transform health professional education. The Institute of Medicine report titled *Best Care at Lower Cost: The Path to Continuously Learning Health Care in America*[8] continues to support an informatics infrastructure to ensure

the development of a learning health care system designed to generate and apply the best evidence for the collaborative health care choices of each patient and provider; to drive the process of discovery as a natural outgrowth of patient care; and to ensure innovation, quality, safety, and value in health care.[23,pix]

In 2009, the American Recovery and Reinvestment Act authorized the CMS to provide a reimbursement incentive for physician and hospital providers who are successful in becoming "meaningful users" of an EHR. As part of this act, the adoption of EHRs and other initiatives, such as meaningful use, was of paramount importance and served as the current catalyst for all hospitals, clinics, and providers to use EHRs.

According to the current draft of the Federal Health Information Technology Strategic Plan 2015–2020, the overall vision is that "health information is accessible when and where it is needed to improve and protect people's health and well-being."[24,p3] The mission is to "improve health, health care, and reduce costs through the use of information and technology."[24,p3]

The increased use of technology in society also is driving the integration of technology in health care. The Pew Research Center has noted three technology revolutions that have occurred during approximately the past 15 years: (1) greater access to broadband, which has increased access to the Internet and promoted its use in various facets of people's lives; (2) mobile connectivity and the concept of anytime/anyplace access; and (3) the presence of social media and social networks in daily life.[25] These three revolutions have impacted patients and their families, caregivers, and health care providers as increasingly more adults are using digital tools to not only access health information but also to manage their own health data and be an active participant in their health care.

Domains of Informatics

Health informatics is evolving as a discipline and its definition and standards are a work in progress. Although there is currently no universally accepted taxonomy for the major domains of informatics, for the purposes of this concept presentation, AMIA's three domains of informatics are used: clinical informatics, public health informatics, and translational bioinformatics.[7]

The domains overlap in various ways and are not exclusive to one another.[7] All domains integrate computer science and information science to manage and communicate data, information, and knowledge; however, they differ in the integration of the discipline-specific science and discipline-specific practice. The field of informatics has recently grown to reflect the substantive contribution of the various health disciplines to the generation and usage of health care data and related information, which has helped to differentiate the often confusing terminology. In the following discussion, each domain is defined and the major subtypes, if applicable, are described.

Clinical Informatics

Clinical informatics is the application of information and communication technologies to the delivery of health care services. Despite some variations, informatics, when used in health care delivery, is essentially the same regardless of the health professional group involved, whether dentists, pharmacists, physicians, nurses, or other health professionals. According to AMIA, clinical informatics has two subdomains: clinical health care informatics and clinical research informatics.

Clinical Health Care Informatics. Clinical health care informatics seeks to transform health care and enhance human health through a creative and innovative use of informatics. This transformation will be accomplished through a well-educated and properly trained informatics workforce, an enhanced performance of health care processes and systems, appropriate public policy, and a relevant research agenda. Clinical health care informatics includes the development of direct approaches to patients and their families and even to individuals who are not yet patients (consumers) who desire to seek the use of information and communications technology support to preserve and/or improve their health status.

A subset of clinical health care informatics is nursing informatics (NI). As defined by the ANA, NI is the specialty that integrates nursing science with multiple information and analytical sciences to identify, define, manage, and communicate data, information, knowledge, and wisdom in nursing practice.[13] NI supports consumers, patients, nurses, and other providers in their decision making in all roles and settings. The support is accomplished through the use of "information structures, information processes, and information technology."[13,p7]

Another subset of clinical health care informatics is consumer health informatics (CHI), which is defined by the AMIA as a form of health information technology geared toward delivering better health care decisions based on the consumer's perspective.[7] It is well recognized that consumer informatics stands at the crossroads of other disciplines, such as nursing informatics, public health, health promotion, health education, library science, and communication science, and is perhaps the most challenging and rapidly expanding field in health informatics. CHI is paving the way for health care in the age of connected health. CHI includes technologies focused on patients as the primary users of health information.[26]

Clinical Research Informatics. *Clinical research informatics* relates to informatics whose objective is to advance the biomedical/health sciences through the humane and ethical use of informatics. Included are issues relating to the use of information and knowledge as well as the sound and socially appropriate collection and maintenance of person-specific and/or de-identified patient data. EHRs will enhance the availability of clinical data for research and quality improvement initiatives.

Public Health Informatics

Public health informatics and its corollary population informatics are the application of information, computer science, and technology to public health science to improve the health of populations. Application of the principles and practices of public health informatics leads to the development of new tools and methodologies that enable the development and use of interoperable information systems for public health functions such as biosurveillance, outbreak response, and electronic laboratory reporting.

Translational Bioinformatics

AMIA refers to translational bioinformatics as the development of storage, analytic, and interpretive methods to optimize the transformation of increasingly voluminous biomedical and genomic data into proactive, predictive, preventive, and participatory health.[7] Translational bioinformatics is evolving with the support of the National Institutes of Health road map for medical research. The end product of translational bioinformatics is newly found knowledge from integrative efforts that can be disseminated to a variety of stakeholders, including biomedical scientists, clinicians, and patients.

Informatics in Nursing Practice

Nurses use various health information technology tools to support their clinical practice. EHRs are the most common tool and are more inclusive of the clinical data and information collected on a patient by numerous health care professionals to facilitate clinical decision making. Within EHRs, nurses also use nursing documentation systems to record the process and outcomes of their care. To facilitate the provision of care, evidence-based practice guidelines and alerts are incorporated to help nurses conduct their assessments, diagnose, and determine the nursing interventions to achieve optimal patient outcomes.

With the introduction of meaningful use criteria, EHRs are also becoming accessible to patients and their families as well as to caregivers and consumers. Patients, families, caregivers, and consumers are part of the interprofessional team and engage in health care decision making. The engagement of patients is not a new concept, but in recent years, health information technologies have made health information and patient records more accessible, thus giving patients the tools they need. Accessing social media sites, patient portals, and mobile health devices are all ways that engaged patients can participate in their health care.

The use of health information technologies across professionals, patients/consumers, and health care institutions is creating a connected health care delivery system. Connected health maximizes the use of technology-enabled tools to provide health care delivery beyond the walls of any one health institution.[27] The concept of connected health is integral to the notion of providing accessible health information for patients and families.

The transformation of health care is enabled by the future of health information technology and informatics. Widespread and meaningful use of fully functional EHR systems combined with a robust infrastructure for broad-based health information exchange has the potential to improve the quality, safety, and efficiency of health care for all Americans. As more organizations adopt EHRs, health professionals will have greater access to patient information, allowing faster and more accurate diagnoses and treatment. Patients will also have access to their own information and will have the choice to share it with family members securely over the Internet. This will allow better coordination of care for themselves and their loved ones. EHRs are becoming increasingly widespread across the health care system because of their efficiency in disseminating knowledge and promoting safe patient care. Health information technologies, network connectivity, and an informatics infrastructure provide the necessary strategies to transition to a continuously learning health system, one that aligns science and informatics, patient–clinician partnerships, incentives, and a culture of continuous improvement to produce the best care at lower cost.[8]

INTERRELATED CONCEPTS

Many interrelated concepts bear some relationship to health information technology and health informatics but do not necessarily share the same set of attributes. Related concepts identified here include data, information, knowledge, wisdom, trust, health, health care, meaningful use, bandwidth, and interoperability.

Interrelated concepts that are found in this book include Clinical Judgment, Leadership, Communication, Collaboration, Safety, Evidence, Care Coordination, and Health Care Quality, as well as Ethics, Health Policy, and Health Care Law (Figure 48-3). It is also important to note that the health and illness concepts in Section 2 of this book are interrelated concepts in that they provide the substance for the data, information, knowledge, and wisdom components that form the framework for meaningful use of health informatics.

CLINICAL EXEMPLARS

Box 48-2 displays some common exemplars of health IT and informatics that may be encountered in clinical practice. This list is not complete and is ever changing and expanding as new technology and new interfaces are developed and implemented in health care. Emerging new models of health care delivery will require informatics tools for improving quality and efficiency. Additional information for all exemplars presented can be found in multiple textbooks and websites related to health IT and informatics.

Featured Exemplars
Computerized Nursing Documentation

Computerized nursing documentation technology enables nurses to document all activities associated with the nursing process and serves as a repository for stored nursing data and information that can facilitate clinical decision making and interprofessional communication. Nurses can use an electronic documentation system to capture and store assessment data and to transform these data into

FIGURE 48-3 Technology and Informatics and Interrelated Concepts

---

BOX 48-2   EXEMPLARS OF TECHNOLOGY AND INFORMATICS

Clinical Informatics
- Bar code medication administration
- Clinical decision support systems
- Computerized acuity systems
- Computerized nursing documentation
- Computerized provider order entry (CPOE) systems
- Disease/patient registries
- Electronic health record (EHR) systems
- Electronic prescribing (eRx)
- Health information exchange (HIE)
- Telehealth tools
- Population health management tools

Consumer Health Informatics
- Personal health records (PHR)
- Patient portals
- Patient-generated health data tools (PatientsLikeMe)
- Social media tools for online support

- Health and wellness apps
- Chronic disease management apps
- Home and self-care monitoring devices
- Smart devices and sensors
- Public health informatics

Biosurveillance Tools
- Geographical information system tools
- Predictive modeling tools
- Disaster preparedness tools
- Immunization registries

Bioinformatics Tools
- Homology and similarity tools
- Protein function analysis tools
- Structural analysis tools
- Sequence analysis tools
- Data mining and data analytics tools

---

clinical information associated with diagnoses, nursing activities, and a plan of care to enable patients to reach desired outcomes. Electronic documentation systems facilitate effective, efficient, safe, and quality care to patients.

Bar Code Medication Administration

Bar code medication administration (BCMA) technology allows nurses to effectively and safely administer medications to patients. BCMA ensures that the right provider is giving the right patient the right medication in the right dose and right route at the right time for the right reason and documents the result of that administration. The BCMA system reduces errors and adverse drug effects.

Clinical Decision Support Systems

Clinical decision support systems (CDSSs) provide electronic tools that can provide the information and knowledge to assist the nurse in clinical decision making. CDSSs can include such tools as computerized alerts, reminders, clinical guideline protocols, condition-specific order sets, and diagnostic tools.

Electronic Health Record

EHR systems can decrease the fragmentation of care by improving care coordination. EHRs have the potential to integrate and organize patient health information and facilitate its instant distribution among all authorized providers involved in a patient's care.[28]

CASE STUDY

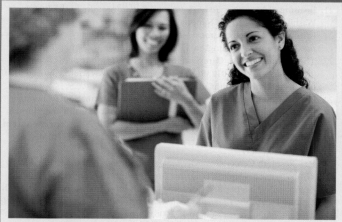

Source: Fuse/Thinkstock

Case Presentation

The Jayhawk Medical Center uses an electronic health record certified by the Office of the National Coordinator of Health Information Technology. To demonstrate nursing's contribution to patient care, the chief nursing officer supports the Council for Nursing Informatics and provides trained informatics nurses to help the Council achieve the goals of safe patient care and quality nursing data. Jayhawk Medical Center is a Magnet hospital and is actively engaged in a patient safety program, including National Database for Nursing Quality Indicators (NDNQI) quality metrics.

Cassandra Mendoza, MSN, RN, is one of the informatics nurse specialists. Her current informatics project is to design and implement a falls risk management protocol in the EHR that also collects data to submit to NDNQI. She first meets with the nursing staff to determine the evidence supporting falls risk management. Based on this evidence, they select a falls risk assessment tool and other data that need to be collected to document and manage the falls risk. They determine the levels of risk are none, moderate, and high risk, and they define order sets for each risk level. Next, Cassandra interviews and observes the staff to determine the workflow surrounding the assessment, documentation, and management of a falls risk.

With this information, she begins to design the screens for the assessment and order sets to facilitate accurate data entry and present the information in a way that all clinicians can understand and can use to make accurate clinical judgments about the care of the patient at the point of care. As she evaluates the evidence, she determines the data elements and their values (assessment questions and possible patient observation) and the appropriate data types (e.g., numeric, free text, and coded response list). For each question and coded response list, she matches each concept to a standardized language. Next, she ensures that the design reveals the nursing process and maps each component to the Reference Information Model of Health Level Seven. She adds a decision support rule that states, "When the falls risk assessment score indicates a risk, Falls Risk is added to the patient problem list and an order set for the indicated risk level is presented to the nurse for approval." Finally, she determines the staff members who may view and interact with the protocol to ensure confidentiality.

After Cassandra completes the implementation of the protocol, she meets with the nursing staff again to evaluate whether the protocol meets their needs and represents the evidence for falls risk management. After the final approvals for the protocol, she builds the screens in the EHR and implements a training program for the staff. Three months after implementation, Cassandra evaluates the protocol and its use by the staff. The number of falls had been reduced by 15%, all of the NDNQI falls metrics were collected electronically (saving money on data collection from charts), nurses were very satisfied with the decision support that saved them time by automatically adding the risk to the problem list and entering orders, and patient satisfaction increased by 10% based on free text comments about the staff's thoughtfulness in keeping patients safe.

Case Analysis

This case is an example of how an informatics nurse specialist works with staff nurses to design assessment and clinical decision support tools to improve quality and safety of patients at risk for falls. The informatics specialist collaborated with nursing staff to develop and implement an electronic fall assessment and prevention protocol that ultimately reduced fall incidence and increased patient and nurse satisfaction. Before designing the clinical tool, the informatics nurse involved the nursing staff to determine evidence to support level of risk and to examine workflow patterns to determine best fit for data collection within the EHR. These are key elements to increase usability of the tool. Also, note that the clinical decision support tool implementation included training and follow-up evaluation.

ACCESS EXEMPLAR LINKS IN YOUR GIDDENS EBOOK

REFERENCES

1. Merriam–Webster: *Technology* (n.d.) Retrieved from <http://mw1.merriam-webster.com/dictionary/technology>.
2. Buntin MB, Burke MF, Hoaglin MC, et al: The benefits of health information technology: A review of the recent literature shows predominantly positive results. *Health Aff (Millwood)* 30:464–471, 2011.
3. Chaudhry B, Wang J, Wu S, et al: Systematic review: Impact of health information technology on quality, efficiency, and costs of medical care. *Ann Intern Med* 144:744, 2006.
4. Shekelle PG, Jones SS, Rudin RS, Southern California Evidence-Based Practice Center, et al: *Health information technology: An updated systematic review with a focus on meaningful use functionalities*, Washington, DC, 2014, U.S. Department of Health and Human Services. Retrieved from <http://www.healthit.gov/sites/default/files/systematic_review_final_report_508_compliant.pdf>.
5. Saba VK: Nursing informatics: Yesterday, today, and tomorrow. *Int Nurs Rev* 48:177, 2001.
6. Proctor R: *Definition of health informatics. Personal communication to Virginia Van Horne, Content Manager, HSR Information Central, Bethesda MD*, 2009. Retrieved from <http://www.nlm.nih.gov/hsrinfo/informatics.html>.
7. American Medical Informatics Association: *The science of informatics*. Retrieved from <https://www.amia.org/about-amia/science-informatics>.
8. Institute of Medicine: *Best care at lower cost: The path to continuously learning health care in America*, Washington, DC, 2012, National Academies Press.
9. Thompson TG, Brailer DJ: *The decade of health information technology: Delivering consumer-centric and information-rich health care—Framework for strategic action*, Washington, DC, 2004, U.S. Department of Health and Human Services.
10. Lundberg CB, Warren JJ, Brokel J, et al: Selecting a standardized terminology for the electronic health record that reveals the impact of nursing practice on patient care. *Online J Nurs Informatics* 12(2): 2008.
11. Center for Medicare and Medicaid Services: *EHR incentive programs*, 2014. Retrieved from <http://www.cms.gov/Regulations-and-Guidance/Legislation/EHRIncentivePrograms/index.html?redirect=/ehrincentiveprograms>.

12. U.S. Department of Health and Human Services: *HIPAA regulations*, 2013. Retrieved from <https://www.federalregister.gov/articles/2013/01/25/2013-01073/modifications-to-the-hipaa-privacy-security-enforcement-and-breach-notification-rules-under-the>.

13. American Nurses Association: *Scope and standards of nursing informatics practice*, Washington, DC, 2015, American Nurses Publishing.

14. Gardner RM, Overhage M, Steen LB, et al: Core content for subspecialty of clinical informatics. *J Am Informatics Assoc (JAMIA)* 16:153, 2009.

15. Lorenzi N, Riley R: Managing change: An overview. *J Am Informatics Assoc (JAMIA)* 7(2):116–124, 2000.

16. McGonigle D, Mastrian K: *Nursing informatics and the foundation of knowledge*, Boston, 2009, Jones & Bartlett.

17. Shortliffe EH, Blois MS: The computer meets medicine and biology emergence as a discipline. In Shortliffe EH, Cimino JJ, editors: *Biomedical informatics: Computer applications in health care and biomedicine*, New York, 2006, Springer.

18. McCarthy M, Eastman D: *Change management strategies for an effective EMR implementation*, Chicago, 2010, Healthcare Information Management Systems Society.

19. Walker PH: Strategies for culture change. In Ball M, Douglas JV, Walker PH, editors: *Nursing informatics: Where caring and technology meet*, ed 4, New York, 2011, Springer.

20. Warren J, Connors H: Health information technology can and will transform nursing education. *Nurs Outlook* 55(1):58–60, 2007.

21. Institute of Medicine: *To err is human: Building a safer health system*, Washington, DC, 2000, National Academies Press.

22. Institute of Medicine: *Crossing the quality chasm: A new health system for the 21st century*, Washington, DC, 2001, National Academies Press.

23. The Learning Health Care System in America: *Institute of Medicine activity description*, 2012. Retrieved from <http://www.iom.edu/Activities/Quality/LearningHealthCare.aspx>.

24. Office of the National Coordinator for Health Information Technology (ONC), Office of the Secretary, U.S. Department of Health and Human Services: *Federal health IT strategic plan 2015–2020*, 2015. Retrieved from <http://www.healthit.gov/sites/default/files/federal-healthIT-strategic-plan-2014.pdf>.

25. Pew Research Center: *Three technology revolutions*, 2014. Retrieved from <http://www.pewinternet.org/three-technology-revolutions>.

26. Brennan PF, Greenes RA: Consumer health informatics. In Shortliffe EH, Cimino JJ, editors: *Biomedical informatics: Computer applications in health care and biomedicine*, New York, 2006, Springer.

27. Partners Healthcare: *Connected health*, (n.d.). Retrieved from <http://connectedhealth.partners.org>.

28. HealthIT: *Benefits of EHRs*, 2014. Retrieved from <http://www.healthit.gov/providers-professionals/improved-care-coordination>.

Evidence

Ingrid Hendrix

Evidence has become a ubiquitous term in health care and society as a whole. Public fascination with forensics and police and legal proceedings has proliferated in the media. Evidence uncovered at crime scenes or in autopsy rooms is vital to solving cases. Evidence can describe the course of events leading to a crime or a death and can solve the riddle of who committed the crime. An emphasis on evidence also permeates every aspect of health care. Evidence serves a similar function in health care as it does in the legal system. It provides proof of the usefulness of an intervention, the projected course of a disease, or the link between environmental insults and illness.

The phrase "evidence-based" is applied to every health discipline: evidence-based medicine, evidence-based nursing, evidence-based dentistry, and the more inclusive evidence-based practice or evidence-based health care. But what is evidence? This concept presentation examines evidence broadly and includes how the term is defined, describing the various forms of evidence and the way it is used in health care. Understanding approaches to recognize and classify evidence in clinical or educational situations aids in incorporating evidence in useful and meaningful ways.

DEFINITION

The concept of evidence is probably most closely associated with law and the sciences. In the legal system, evidence is used to establish guilt or innocence. In the sciences, evidence establishes expected benefit or harm. Evidence is defined as a testimony of facts tending to prove or disprove any conclusion, or something that furnishes proof. When used as a verb, evidence means to attest or prove. These definitions describe most aptly why evidence-based practice (EBP) is so fundamental to health care. Evidence supports or disputes the efficacy of a treatment, the use of a diagnostic tool, the transmission of a disease, or any number of scenarios relevant to health care. Similarly in the legal arena, evidence is a highly regarded and essential element in judging a situation. Evidence is "information, whether in the form of personal testimony, the language of documents, or the production of material objects, that is given in a legal investigation, to establish the fact or point in question."[1] Distilling this definition into its key elements, evidence is information given to establish fact. Synonyms for evidence include affirmation, attestation, confirmation, corroboration, data, documentation, information, substantiation, and testimony.

However, evidence is more than just data or documents. Aikenhead states that evidence, as opposed to data, is scrutinized by comparing it with other information and thus is more credible than raw data.[2] Examples of this definition of evidence in forensic and legal arenas can be witness testimony, phone records, toxicology reports, or DNA samples. In clinical practice and health research, evidence is usually exemplified by research studies. Clinical experience and expert opinion can be considered as evidence, but these forms of evidence are usually given less value because of their subjective nature.

Evidence-based nursing has been defined as "the conscientious, explicit, and judicious use of theory-derived, research-based information in making decisions about care delivery to individuals or groups of patients and in consideration of individual needs and preferences."[3,p152] Scott defines evidence-based nursing as "an ongoing process by which evidence, nursing theory, and the practitioners' clinical expertise are critically evaluated and considered, in conjunction with patient involvement, to provide delivery of optimum nursing care for the individual."[4,p1089] A commonality among these definitions is the use of evidence to guide practice while incorporating key elements of patient involvement and the expertise of nurses.

SCOPE

The scope of evidence can be thought of as a range from the discovery and generation of evidence on one end of the spectrum to the delivery of care at the bedside on the other end (Figure 49-1). Discovery of evidence is often referred to as "bench" research when discovery is on a molecular or cellular level. Moving bench evidence to studying the application in clinical practice is known as translational research. This is a bidirectional process because the focus of bench research is based on clinical problems observed, and advances in clinical practice are dependent on bench research. In health care, research can be done by an individual, but recently a greater emphasis and value have been placed on collaborative and interprofessional research, particularly with translational research efforts.

ATTRIBUTES AND CRITERIA

An attribute is a quality or characteristic that is associated with the concept that helps to clarify or confirm the concept. Several attributes

FIGURE 49-1 Scope of Evidence Scope extends from the discovery of evidence to the application of evidence into patient care through patient care standards.

BOX 49-1 Major and Minor Attributes of Evidence

Major Attributes	Minor Attributes
• Replicability	• Publicly available
• Reliability	• Understandable
• Validity	• Useable

BOX 49-2 U.S. Preventive Services Task Force Grading of Evidence

Grade A = Strongly Recommends
• There is high certainty that the net benefit is substantial.

Grade B = Recommends
• There is high certainty that the net benefit is moderate or there is moderate certainty that the net benefit is moderate to substantial.

Grade C = No Recommendations For or Against
• There may be considerations that support providing the intervention in an individual patient but not for the general population. There is at least moderate certainty that the net benefit is small.

Grade D = Recommends Against
• There is moderate or high certainty that the intervention has no net benefit or that the harms outweigh the benefits.

I Statement = Insufficient Evidence to Recommend For or Against
• The current evidence is insufficient to assess the balance of benefits and harms of the service. Evidence is lacking, of poor quality, or conflicting, and the balance of benefits and harms cannot be determined.

Source: From U.S. Preventive Services Task Force (http://www.uspreventiveservicestaskforce.org).

---

of evidence exist (Box 49-1). Major attributes of evidence include replicability, reliability, and validity:

• *Replicability*: Evidence is built on research findings. Findings can only be verified if they can be repeated. If other researchers are unable to achieve the same results using the same methodology as the original study, the evidence presented by that study is called into question.
• *Reliability*: Evidence must also be consistently and accurately measured.[2] Even clinical experience, as a form of evidence, demonstrates that the same treatment applied to similar patients over time leads to similar outcomes.
• *Validity*: For evidence to be valid, it must successfully measure what the study set out to measure. The definition of validity is producing the desired result, effective, sound.

Minor attributes of evidence include that it is publicly available, understandable, and usable.

Levels of Evidence

Unfortunately, not all evidence produced is of equal quality. Conclusions drawn from research are not necessarily valid just because they originate from a study. For this reason, levels of evidence have been created to help the busy practitioner determine the quality of a study. A hierarchy, based on how much trust can be placed in the results of a study design, has been developed. Unfortunately, there has been no standardization, and therefore different organizations have created their own versions. Initiatives such as GRADE (Grading of Recommendations, Assessment, Development, and Evaluation) are attempting to consistently measure the quality of research studies.[5] Basically, this system classifies studies as strong or weak based on the methodology of the study—such as sample size and blinding of the researchers and/or study subjects. For quantitative studies, numerous websites show detailed tables of what has become known as levels of evidence.[6,7] The design of qualitative studies makes them less well suited for categorization into these levels of evidence, but articles are available to help guide readers in evaluating these types of studies.[8,9]

Another level of evidence is applied to secondary literature, particularly practice guidelines. In this context, a grade or level is assigned to a recommendation to help a health care professional understand how well the recommendation is supported by the collective research. For example, the U.S. Preventive Services Task force has a grading of evidence A, B, C, D, and I (Box 49-2).

Evidence on the Internet

Levels of evidence are designed to be applied to original research studies—the primary literature. Because of the accessibility of information on the Internet, many health care professionals look to search engines such as Google to find the information that they need. This can be a risky practice. Anyone can post information on the Internet and create very authoritative-appearing websites, even if the information provided is false or misleading. Professional organizations have developed criteria to evaluate the credibility of online health information.[10] First, determine the author and sponsor of the information. This is not always easy to discern. Looking at the *About Us* or *Contact Us* page of a website can provide clues. However, as with research studies, information found online should limit bias as much as possible. For example, if the information about a particular drug is provided by the pharmaceutical company selling that product, it would be prudent to evaluate that information with such a bias in mind. Looking at a website's domain can help determine the source of the information—for example, *.edu* for educational institutions or *.gov* for a government website. In addition, determine who is providing the content of the website. Is it a health care professional, a concerned individual, or a government agency? Content on a website should be validated with evidence, such as references to research studies.

Otherwise, the information should be considered opinion. Currency is another important element of information found on the Web, especially in regard to health information. Organizations such as the Health on the Net Foundation (http://www.healthonnet.org) provide a seal of approval to websites adhering to their standards of quality. This seal provides a quick visual that the information on the site has met certain criteria.

THEORETICAL LINKS

Various models of evidence-based nursing (EBN) have been developed to help nurses understand how to incorporate evidence into practice on a routine basis. Some models address EBN from the standpoint of an individual, whereas others address it from an organizational viewpoint. Two such models that facilitate the use of evidence into practice are the Johns Hopkins nursing EBP model and guidelines and the Iowa model of EBP.

The Johns Hopkins Nursing EBP Model and Guidelines

This model provides a systematic method for applying evidence in the clinical, research, and educational settings.[11] Developed in collaboration with clinical and academic nurses, the Johns Hopkins model uses a mentored, stepwise approach to EBN. The model addresses three common barriers to implementing EBN—lack of knowledge, overwhelming amounts of information, and time constraints. Staff nurses are provided with educational opportunities and tools to facilitate gathering and evaluating evidence. The key elements of this model are individual mentoring and support from nursing leadership.

The Iowa Model of Evidence-Based Practice

The Iowa model takes a broader and more institutional approach to implementing EBP.[12] The flowchart of the model begins with either of two types of triggers—problem focused or knowledge focused. These triggers are initiated by events such as clinical problems, risk management or quality improvement data, organizational guidelines, or new evidence from the literature. What is unique about the Iowa model is the identification of triggers beyond a clinical practice question. Nurses can easily follow the steps of the flowchart to identify if there is a sufficient evidence base to guide a change in practice, to determine steps to take if there is insufficient evidence, and to establish outcomes to monitor after initiating a change. Another unique element of this model is consideration of the relevance of the question to the organization, which in turn guides the level of support that can be expected when piloting, adopting, and instituting the projected change and evaluating outcome data. The 2001 revision of the model provides even more feedback loops and detailed instructions for incorporating EBP.

CONTEXT TO NURSING AND HEALTH CARE

To provide safe, quality care, nurses must base their practice decisions on evidence. The context of evidence in nursing is nurses using the available evidence and producing new research evidence.

Origins of Evidence

Examining the origins and definitions of the phrase "evidence-based" is useful in determining the meaning of evidence within the context of health care. Although there has been a recent emphasis placed on the use of evidence in clinical practice, this is not a new phenomenon.

Examples of evidence-based medicine and evidence-based nursing can be found throughout history. One historical example is illustrated by the discovery of the link between an absence of hand washing and the transmission of infection. In the 1800s, Ignaz Semmelweis, a physician, was alarmed by the high rate of childbed (i.e., puerperal) fever in women delivered by physicians compared to those attended by midwives.[13] Semmelweis questioned the cause of this disparity, an essential element in uncovering the evidence to prove or disprove his theory. He observed that the women dying of this fever were being attended by physicians and students who had just finished working in the dissection lab. These physicians and medical students did not wash their hands after working on cadavers and so were spreading infections from the cadavers to the laboring women. The women who had a lower rate of puerperal fever were attended by midwives who did not attend the cadaver lab. Semmelweis did not purposely randomize the women but, rather, discovered the difference between the two groups through observation. Unfortunately, his discovery was met with some hostility; his colleagues were insulted by the suggestion that they were at fault.[13] Semmelweis was forced to move to another city, where he implemented hand-washing techniques and reduced the prevalence of puerperal fever significantly.[14] He questioned existing and entrenched practices, examined the variables involved, and then changed his practice based on the evidence he uncovered.

Florence Nightingale is well-known for her work in establishing the nursing profession and being instrumental in hospital reform. Her work and writings provide a classic example of the practice of EBN. She used observations and statistics as evidence to support her demand for improved hospital conditions to reduce infections and mortality.[15] Nightingale began evidence-based reporting during her work in the Crimean War, but she continued throughout her career to incorporate evidence in her lobbying for hospital design reform, patient record systems, nursing care, and patient outcomes.[16]

The more recent emphasis on using evidence to guide practice came from Dr. Archie Cochrane, a British epidemiologist who called on the medical profession to incorporate more evidence, in the form of randomized controlled trials, into the care of patients. He was disturbed that many health care professionals were not implementing information that could improve patient care and instead turned to colleagues for information or relied on historical methods of treatment. He also advocated for a regularly updated database of randomized controlled trials, which later developed into the *Cochrane Database of Systematic Reviews*.[17]

Types of Evidence

An expectation of the professional nurse is the incorporation of evidence into his or her practice. Evidence can present in many ways; thus it is important to recognize and understand the various types when encountered. Evidence created from research studies is presented in two major ways: through primary and secondary literature.

Primary Literature

Primary literature constitutes original research studies on which the secondary literature is created. Two broad types of primary literature represent research studies that are the building blocks of evidence: quantitative research and qualitative research.

Quantitative Research. Quantitative research has been defined as being "focused on the testing of a hypothesis through objective observation and validation."[18,p17] The types of studies that make up this category include randomized controlled studies, cohort studies, longitudinal studies, case–control studies, and case reports (Figure 49-2).

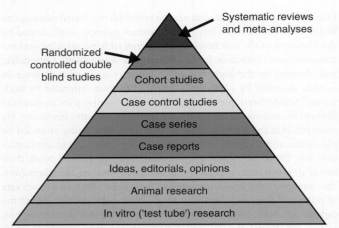

FIGURE 49-2 Types of Quantitative Studies Source: From SUNY Downstate Medical Centre: *Guide to research methods.* Retrieved from http://library.downstate.edu/EBM2/2100.htm.

Randomized controlled double-blind studies are considered the "gold standard" for quantitative research. The reason is that the methods used to conduct these types of studies introduce the least amount of bias. Patients are randomly assigned to the experimental or control group, and both researchers and subjects are "blind" to the intervention. Minimal bias in research studies allows the user of this information to have more confidence in the evidence created by that research. As Gugiu explains, "by 'credible evidence' we mean results for which the study design, conduct, and analysis has minimized or avoided biases that would otherwise raise doubt in their veracity beyond a reasonable doubt."[19,p234] Other study designs introduce more variables and thus the potential for increased bias. For example, case reports study only a few subjects, making it difficult to draw meaningful conclusions to other patients.

Qualitative Research. Qualitative research answers questions that cannot be answered using a quantitative study design. Qualitative research focuses on a person's experience and uses analysis of textual, or nonnumeric, data, such as interviews, surveys, or questionnaires. Morse argues that more attention needs to be paid and more funding needs to be given to qualitative research because these types of research studies answer questions essential to health care and are of particular interest to nurses.[20] Examples of qualitative study methods are ethnography, phenomenology, grounded theory, and case reports.

Mixed Design Research. Increasingly, mixed design studies are being conducted that feature both quantitative and qualitative approaches. Gilgun suggests that the two methodologies of qualitative and quantitative research complement each other and that the melding of the two provides a holistic approach to the research question.[21] As Gilgun notes, the quantitative study may prove the efficacy of a drug but not address patient compliance if the patient considers the side effects of the drug too harsh. The compliance issue can be addressed by examining the patient's response to treatment and barriers to compliance and therefore increase the usefulness of the treatment.[21]

Secondary Literature

Busy professionals tasked with providing evidence-based care are faced with an enormous body of literature to guide their practice. This information explosion in the health sciences has led to the development of several types of secondary literature designed to summarize findings from individual or multiple studies. Three categories of secondary literature are evidence summaries, systematic reviews and meta-analysis, and practice guidelines.

Evidence Summaries. Evidence summaries are categorized as secondary literature because they summarize original research studies. Summary publications have emerged in recent years to address the problem of the explosion of information and the timely incorporation of evidence into practice. Publications such as *Evidence-Based Nursing, WORLDviews on Evidence-Based Nursing,* and *ACP Journal Club* review individual studies and summarize the results for their readers.

Systematic Reviews and Meta-Analyses. Systematic reviews and meta-analyses have been referred to as synthesis of the evidence.[22] Systematic reviews include the available evidence on a topic in the form of randomized controlled trials that are summarized using a systematic methodology. Rather than conducting one very large study, the results of many studies can be evaluated and a conclusion can be drawn about the effectiveness of a particular treatment. Because creation of a systematic review is very labor-intensive—exhaustive searches of the literature and the complex methodology used to evaluate each study included in the review—relatively few of these types of publications are available. Their number is expanding with initiatives such as the Cochrane Collaboration, the Campbell Collaboration, and the Joanna Briggs Institute. As a result, the topics found in a systematic review tend to focus on areas of research that would be of the most interest to the greatest number of practitioners. Meta-analyses, similar to systematic reviews, summarize evidence from multiple studies. What differentiates a meta-analysis from a systematic review is that it combines the statistical results of numerous randomized controlled trials and analyzes that evidence.

Practice Guidelines. Practice guidelines are another type of summary publication. They are designed to summarize findings of the research and advise practitioners on the current standard of care. Ideally, guidelines result in a faster integration of new evidence into practice and address issues of cost and variation in practice. Guidelines are often developed by government agencies or societies, such as the U.S. Preventive Services Task Force, the American College of Obstetricians and Gynecologists, or the National Association of Pediatric Nurse Practitioners. They create guidelines by using evidence from the literature, research studies on the topic of the guideline, and expert opinion to craft the publications. These publications are then referred to as the standard of practice for a particular treatment. Unlike systematic reviews or meta-analyses, practice guidelines are less structured in their design. One source for guidelines is the National Guideline Clearinghouse (http://www.guideline.gov), a searchable database of available guidelines provided by the Agency for Healthcare Research and Quality (AHRQ).

Nurses as Researchers: Evidence Discovery

Many nurses are involved in research. Involvement may include leading a research study as a principal investigator, being a collaborating investigator on a study, or contributing to a study through data collection. Leading research studies requires a specific skill set that is acquired by completing graduate education at the doctoral level and by following research protocols outlined by an institutional oversight committee, such as an institutional review board. Most researchers are affiliated with an academic health sciences center, private organizations and foundations with dedicated research departments, or government agencies dedicated to research.

Nurses as Consumers of Evidence

All nurses must be skilled as consumers of evidence. Understanding research designs and learning to incorporate high-quality evidence into practice can make creating nursing research a less daunting endeavor. For nurses, being a consumer of the evidence generally assumes two forms: (1) practice policies and procedures and (2) finding solutions to practice problems.

Policies and Procedures

Policy and procedure manuals in health care agencies outline the practice standards for various care activities; nurses are expected to follow policies and procedures for the agency in which they practice. Policies and procedures should be regularly updated to reflect the current evidence and standards of practice and approved by a committee charged with this oversight. Nurses have a role in developing and maintaining policy and procedure guidelines by serving on such committees or volunteering to participate in updates. In this context, nurses must be skilled research consumers in order to make accurate and efficient recommendations for policy updates.

Finding Solutions to Practice Questions or Problems

There are many occasions when practicing nurses identify practice-related problems that require solutions. Nurses should use available evidence to systematically approach a question of patient care. The steps are outlined as follows:

1. Develop an answerable question.
2. Search the literature to uncover evidence to answer the question.
3. Evaluate the evidence found.
4. Apply the evidence to the practice situation.
5. Evaluate the outcome.

Step 1: Develop an Answerable Question. The first step in finding evidence is determining a question to ask. This may seem straightforward and obvious, but this step is often a stumbling block for many people. The reason is that most people start searching for information, or evidence, with only a vague idea of what they are seeking. It would be similar to searching for someone's house and knowing only that the person is located in the southeast part of town. One could spend hours or even days trying to find the exact location with such vague directions—and one would probably quit the search without success. To find the most direct route, one must start with a good map. A good map begins with the question, "Where do you want to go?" The best way to find evidence is to be clear about what information is needed. The question needs to be specific or answerable without being too vague or so specific that the probability of finding information about the topic would be unlikely. Entering a search query such as "breast cancer" or "diabetes" would lead to an overwhelming abundance of information. What particular aspect of breast cancer or diabetes is of interest: treatment, supportive services, or prevention strategies? Before searching for the evidence, define the question to be answered and map a strategy to get there.

There are two types of questions to consider: background and foreground questions. Background questions are those that provide foundational knowledge. An example of a background question is "What is scleroderma?" These types of questions can most easily be answered by a textbook, review article, or a reputable website. Foreground questions address issues of a more specific nature, such as "Is drug x more effective than drug y in treating scleroderma?" These questions are best answered by searching the primary literature, which is found in databases indexing research studies, such as PubMed

or the Cumulative Index to Nursing and Allied Health Literature (CINAHL).

One formula that can be helpful in designing an answerable foreground question is the PICO formula. The acronym stands for *popula*tion, *i*ntervention, *c*omparison, and *o*utcome. Using these elements clarifies the formulation of a question. The following is an example of a PICO question: "For inpatients (P), is turning every 2 hours (I) more effective than air mattresses (C) for preventing pressure ulcers (O)?" Another formula used to develop an answerable question is the PICOT formula. The difference here is the addition of the T, which represents time. This is the time frame in which the patient or population of interest is observed to determine if the outcome of interest is achieved. The following question is an illustration of the PICOT formula: In new mothers (P), do home visits by a nurse practitioner (I) versus no home visits (C) decrease the incidence of child abuse (O) in the first year postpartum (T)?

Step 2: Search the Literature. Once a question is developed, the next step is searching the literature. With a question mapped out, it is easier to determine which key words will be used in the search. Most databases accept quotes to search for phrases, such as "kangaroo care." Without quotes around the phrase, the search engine will look for the words "kangaroo" and "care" but not necessarily next to one another, which may lead to retrieval of unrelated studies. In addition, it is a good strategy to think of synonyms for any key words used. This saves time and frustration. For example, a search on the topic "AIDS" will result in articles discussing hearing aids or walking aids, for example, in addition to articles on the disease. Searching the phrase "acquired immunodeficiency syndrome" will retrieve only articles focused on the disease. If retrieval is too limited, remove a key word of less importance to the question. A large retrieval can benefit from limits such as language, age groups, or dates of publication.

It is virtually impossible to keep current with new findings and different approaches to patient care. On the topic of evidence-based nursing alone, the number of articles in the PubMed database has expanded from 1 in 1996 to 3870 in 2014. Bibliographic databases have been designed to help access and catalog the rapidly expanding body of literature. However, it is an imperfect system. There are many databases that cover different topic areas, and each has a different search engine, or interface, to learn. As a result, many clinicians resort to Google or Wikipedia because of the fast, user-friendly interfaces. However, there are drawbacks to using search engines such as Google. The amount of information retrieved is usually quite large. Using Google Scholar, a subset of Google, reduces somewhat the volume of information retrieved, but results are usually large. This can be beneficial for an initial search to discover how much is available on a topic. Mastrangelo et al. reported that Google Scholar has a higher recall than PubMed but that PubMed's retrieval is more precise.[23] Nourbakhsh et al. concluded that Google Scholar's retrieval reflects high-quality, relevant results compared to PubMed.[24]

Using databases specifically focused on health care research is more efficient, but it requires some training. Most searchers use only key words, but using the subject heading search feature of a database can significantly narrow a search and yield far more precise results. Consulting with a medical librarian or using tutorials provided by the database producer save valuable time in locating evidence to guide practice. Searching the literature is more an art than a science, and it requires creativity and perseverance. As with any skill, practice will increase satisfaction with the outcome.

Step 3: Evaluate the Evidence Found. Once information has been located as evidence for a change in practice, that information should be evaluated for its quality and applicability to a particular patient situation. The following questions are most commonly used to evaluate studies: Are the results of the study or systematic review valid? What are the results, and are they meaningful and reliable? Are the results clinically relevant to my patients? Many articles have been published in the nursing literature to help nurses assess the quality of the information found in research studies.[25-31] The American Medical Association has also published the book *Users' Guides to the Medical Literature*, which is a compilation of articles from *JAMA* covering topics on how to read and understand the information found in published studies. As stated previously, not all evidence is created equal, and nurses need to be critical consumers of the information they uncover. By reading the articles just referenced,[25-31] nurses can improve their skills in critically evaluating the literature.

Step 4: Apply the Evidence Found. If sufficient evidence is found to guide a change in practice, the next step of EBP is to apply that evidence to a particular patient situation. Although evidence provides proof of the validity of a course of action, it is not the sole reason for treatment decisions. A key element in any practice situation is the incorporation of patients' preferences for their health processes and outcomes: "Nurses play a pivotal role in empowering patients, engaging them in their care, and ensuring that they are fully activated to be personally accountable for their own health."[32,p110] An individual should be provided with the evidence and advice of a well-informed health care professional to support his or her decision to move forward with the care he or she desires. It is the responsibility of the health care professional to use the most appropriate and current evidence to guide practice and optimize care.

Step 5: Evaluate the Evidence. To complete the process, the nurse evaluates the outcome. Evaluation includes appraisal of the degree of success of the intervention and the patient's satisfaction with the outcome in addition to assessment by the nurse of the efficacy of the evidence. Outcomes, both successful and unsuccessful, provide a source of new evidence for others to use. Repeatedly following the steps of EBN will facilitate its use.

INTERRELATED CONCEPTS

Many concepts relate to and work in synergy with evidence; in fact, nearly everything in health care is impacted by evidence. In addition to guiding individual practice, evidence also impacts health care on a more global scale. Four concepts featured in this textbook have especially important interrelationships: Safety, Health Policy, Technology and Informatics, and Health Care Economics. Figure 49-3 illustrates the multidirectionality of evidence. The arrow pointing outward illustrates how evidence provides the foundation and evolution for these concepts. The arrow pointing toward evidence indicates that these concepts provide evidence to their efficacy; thus their connection to the evidence is not static. Outcomes inform future research to update previous evidence and thus a constant flow of evidence is maintained.

In 2003, the Institute of Medicine (IOM) released the report, *Keeping Patients Safe: Transforming the Work Environment of Nurses.*[33] The IOM used evidence from a variety of industries, other IOM reports, and expert testimony to develop policy recommendations related to nurse/patient ratios, work hours, and overtime—all factors that influence the delivery of safe patient care (Safety). A decade after the IOM report, the Robert Wood Johnson Foundation examined whether progress had been made on this important issue and concluded that efforts need to be increased.[34] Patient safety initiatives and the pursuit of quality health care are all built on the foundation of evidence.

Evidence provides a foundation for the creation of Health Policy. Benefits of new treatments and diagnostic tests are evaluated by examining the evidence proving their efficacy for policymakers to approve their use. Policies developed to guide practice are based on evidence found in the literature. Other factors such as modifying factors in specific settings, the degree of need (e.g., the prevalence of disease or risk facts or problems with delivery, financial or governance arrangements), values, costs, and the availability of resources also affect

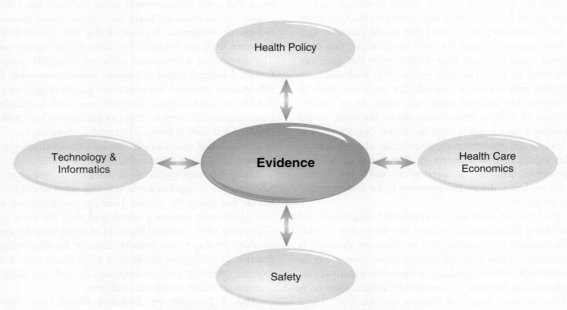

FIGURE 49-3 Evidence and Interrelated Concepts

guideline development.[35] Federal agencies and numerous global agencies, such as the World Health Organization, have developed initiatives to improve the uptake of scientific evidence into the development of health policy.[36,37]

Technology and Informatics is another concept related to evidence. Technology in the context of evidence allows for increased access to the literature through online databases, web content, electronic books, and online journal articles. Sophisticated search engines provide end users with increasingly intuitive interfaces that are faster and more powerful than computers of previous generations. Tablets and smartphones allow information to be accessed from anywhere the user is located. Evidence also influences technology in that new technology is not incorporated into practice until it has been tested for its validity and utility. The American Nurses Association defines nursing informatics as "the specialty that integrates nursing science, computer science, and information science to manage and communicate data, information, and knowledge in nursing practice."[38,p1] Informatics has been the driving force behind such innovations as the development of the electronic medical record (EMR).

Evidence plays a vital role in Health Care Economics through cost containment. Policymakers, governments, institutions, and the public are all demanding evidence to support health care resource decisions. One example of the relationship between economics and evidence is research showing that care provided by nurse practitioners has been shown to be more cost-effective in certain situations than that by physicians, a significant issue in an era of health care reform.[39,40]

BOX 49-3 EXEMPLARS OF EVIDENCE

Quantitative Research Studies
- Randomized controlled trial
- Cohort study
- Case–control study
- Case study
- Longitudinal study

Qualitative Research Studies
- Ethnography
- Phenomenology
- Grounded theory
- Case study

Practice Guidelines
- Standards of medical care in diabetes (American Diabetic Association)
- Lipid screening and cardiovascular health in childhood (American Academy of Pediatrics)
- Guideline for human papillomavirus (HPV) vaccine use to prevent cervical cancer (American Cancer Association)

Expert Opinion/Commentaries
Health Care Policies
- Healthy People 2020

CLINICAL EXEMPLARS

An exemplar is a specific example of a concept, and there are literally thousands of evidence exemplars. Although research studies, practice guidelines, and expert opinions are general categories of evidence exemplars, the studies or practice guidelines themselves are the exemplars. For example, in the category of practice guidelines alone, there are more than 7000 practice guidelines listed in the National Guidelines Clearinghouse. Box 49-3 presents common exemplars linked to this concept.

Featured Exemplars
Randomized Controlled Trial

Double-blinded randomized controlled trials are considered the gold standard for evidence related to therapies because these types of studies represent the least amount of design bias. Study subjects are randomly placed (randomized) into either a treatment or a control group of the study, so neither the subjects nor the researchers decide the subject placement, thus reducing the influence of preconceived ideas about the likely outcomes. Double-blinded studies are designed so that neither the researcher nor the subject knows which treatment is being given; thus they are both "blinded." By removing these sources of design bias, more confidence can be placed in the results of the study.

Longitudinal Study

Studies of a group of people over a specified period of time can be used to detect long-term health changes, such as the effects of exposure to particular environmental factors or lifestyle choices. Groups of people who are exposed and who are not exposed may be observed over time to determine if their health outcomes differ. The time frame can be as long as decades, as is in the case of the Framingham Heart Study, started in 1948, or the Nurses' Health Study, started in 1976.

Ethnography

Ethnographic studies are a type of qualitative research methodology. This type of study has historically been used by anthropologists to study cultural groups, such as indigenous peoples. In health care, the cultural groups can be patients in a particular unit or groups of nurses. These studies examine a particular cultural response to a variable such as a disease or a health behavior. Nurse researchers employ ethnography to understand their patients' environment and inform care.[41]

Practice Guidelines

Practice guidelines are recommendations for clinicians on the current best practices for treatment. These guidelines, created using the latest evidence available on a particular topic, are usually created by the consensus of experts. They can be developed by government agencies, nonprofit agencies, hospitals, or professional societies. Often, they are sponsored by government agencies to standardize the best treatment available and disseminate research findings as quickly as possible.

Expert Opinion

Opinion is at the opposite end of the spectrum of reliability from double-blind randomized controlled trials, due to the inherent bias. Individuals who are considered experts in their field by their peers produce information/evidence based on their experience. Although experience is an important and valid form of evidence, it needs to be considered in light of how it is produced. Examples of expert opinions are book chapters, review articles, and guidelines.

CASE STUDY

Source: Ablestock.com/
Thinkstock

Case Presentation

Mika Kimura, a registered nurse working in the neurosurgical intensive care unit (NSICU), observes that many of the patients under her care need to be transferred from their beds to wheelchairs. However, most of these patients have very little motor control and are unable to assist the nurses with transfers. As a result, she observes more absences among her coworkers attributable to back injuries. Mika realizes there is a need for change and is curious about how other similar units address this issue. She asks her coworkers who have worked in other units if they have seen a solution to this problem. No one reports a satisfactory solution.

Mika turns to the evidence from the published literature to determine if anyone has conducted a study to address this problem. The question she develops is, "In intensive care units, specifically neurosurgical ICUs, is there a method of transferring patients that does not cause injury to the nurse?" She starts her search in the PubMed database and types in the key words "neurosurgical icu," "patient transfers," and "nurses." This yields a few hits but nothing very useful. Thus she decides to broaden her search to include any ICU, and this time spells out "intensive care unit" and tries the key word of "lift*." By using an asterisk, Mika retrieves articles that use the word *lift* or

lifts or *lifting* or *lifted*. She omits the word "nurse" because she can still use the information if the article refers to other health care employees. She finds a few articles that she wants to examine in more depth, so she links to the full text of those articles and prints them. Later that evening, when it is quieter on the unit, she reads the articles. Mika learns that many hospitals have developed "no lift" policies and have also purchased moveable lift devices. One article discusses the cost-effectiveness of using a lift versus dealing with staff absences attributable to back injuries and workers' compensation claims. Mika then determines how many employees in her unit in the past year have missed work because of injuries caused by transfers. Armed with this information, she approaches the unit manager to request that the hospital purchase a lift that can be rolled from room to room. Based on the evidence that she provided to prove her point—both from the literature and from hospital injury reports—Mika's request is approved and a lift is purchased. Not only has she won the thanks of her coworkers but also she has saved the hospital substantial money in lost time from occupational injuries.

Case Analysis

Mika recognized a potentially dangerous work situation and followed the steps of practicing EBN to identify a solution. After formulating a question, she searched the literature for possible solutions, examined the evidence presented in the studies she found, evaluated the applicability to her situation, and pilot tested the change on her unit. After evaluating efficacy, she shared information and implemented the change with her coworkers. By incorporating evidence, she was able to get support from both her coworkers and her managers to make a change. The systematic steps she took and the evidence she presented gave her argument more credibility than just expressing her opinion.

ACCESS EXEMPLAR LINKS IN YOUR GIDDENS EBOOK

REFERENCES

1. OED Online: *Evidence*, 2014. Retrieved from <http://www.oed.com/view/Entry/65368?rskey=D3R4ku&result=1#eid>.
2. Aikenhead GS: Science-based occupations and the science curriculum: Concepts of evidence. *Sci Educ* 89:242–275, 2005.
3. Ingersoll G: Evidence-based nursing: What it is and what it isn't. *Nurs Outlook* 48:151–152, 2000.
4. Scott K, McSherry R: Evidence-based nursing: Clarifying the concepts for nurses in practice. *J Clin Nurs* 18:1085–1095, 2009.
5. Guyatt G, Oxman AD, Akl EA, et al: GRADE guidelines: 1. Introduction—GRADE evidence profiles and summary of findings tables. *J Clin Epidemiol* 64:383–394, 2011.
6. American Academy of Family Physicians: *Evidence-based medicine toolkit*, (n.d.). Retrieved from <www.aafp.org/journals/afp/authors/ebm-toolkit.html>.
7. Phillips B, Ball C, Sackett D, et al: *Oxford Centre for Evidence-Based Medicine—Levels of evidence*, 2009. Retrieved from <http://www.cebm.net/oxford-centre-evidence-based-medicine-levels-evidence-march-2009>.
8. Moon M, Wolf L, Zavotsky K, et al: Evaluating qualitative research studies for use in the clinical setting. *J Emerg Nurs* 39:508–510, 2013.
9. Pickler RH: Evaluating qualitative research studies. *J Pediatr Health Care* 21:195–197, 2007.
10. Medical Library Association: *Find and evaluate health information on the web*, (n.d.). Retrieved from <https://www.mlanet.org/resources/userguide.html>.
11. Dearholt S, Deborah D: *Johns Hopkins nursing evidence-based practice: Model and guidelines*, ed 2, Indianapolis, IN, 2012, Sigma Theta Tau International.
12. Titler MG, Kleiber C, Steelman VJ, et al: The Iowa model of evidence-based practice to promote quality care. *Crit Care Nurs Clin North Am* 13:497–509, 2001.
13. Lane HJ, Blum N, Fee E: Oliver Wendell Holmes (1809–1894) and Ignaz Philipp Semmelweis (1818–1865): Preventing the transmission of puerperal fever. *Am J Public Health* 100:1008–1009, 2010.
14. Loudin I: Ignaz Philip Semmelweis' studies of death in childbirth. *J R Soc Med* 106:461–463, 2013.
15. Aravind M, Hung KC: Evidence-based medicine and hospital reform: Tracing origins back to Florence Nightingale. *Plast Reconstr Surg* 125:403–409, 2010.
16. McDonald L: Florence Nightingale and the early origins of evidence-based nursing. *Evid Based Nurs* 4:68–69, 2001.
17. Shah HM, Chung KC: Archie Cochrane and his vision for evidence-based medicine. *Plast Reconstr Surg* 124:982–988, 2009.
18. Hamer S, Collinson G: *Achieving evidence-based practice: A handbook for practitioners*, ed 2, Edinburgh, UK, 2005, Baillière Tindall Elsevier.
19. Gugiu PC, Gugiu MR: A critical appraisal of standard guidelines for grading levels of evidence. *Eval Health Prof* 33:233–255, 2010.
20. Morse JM: Reconceptualizing qualitative evidence. *Qual Health Res* 16:415–422, 2006.
21. Gilgun JF: The four cornerstones of qualitative research. *Qual Health Res* 16:436–443, 2006.
22. Haynes RB: Of studies, summaries, synopses, and systems: The "5S" evolution of information services for evidence-based healthcare decisions. *Evid Based Med* 11:162–164, 2006.
23. Mastrangelo G, Fadda E, Rossi A, et al: Literature search on risk factors for sarcoma: PubMed and Google Scholar may be complementary sources. *BMC Res* 3:131–134, 2010.
24. Nourbakhsh E, Nugent R, Wang H, et al: Medical literature searches: A comparison of PubMed and Google Scholar. *Health Infor Libr J* 29:214–222, 2012.

25. Stillwell SB, Fineout-Overholt E, Melnyk BM, et al: Asking the clinical question: A key step in evidence-based practice. *Am J Nurs* 110:58–61, 2010.

26. Fineout-Overholt E, Melnyk BM, Stillwell SB, et al: Critical appraisal of the evidence: Part III. The process of synthesis—Seeing similarities and differences across the body of evidence, seventh article in a series. *Am J Nurs* 110:43–51, 2010.

27. Fineout-Overholt E, Melnyk BM, Stillwell SB, et al: Evidence-based practice step by step. Critical appraisal of the evidence: Part I. An introduction to gathering, evaluating, and recording the evidence, fifth in a series. *Am J Nurs* 110:47–52, 2010.

28. Fineout-Overholt E, Melnyk BM, Stillwell SB, et al: Evidence-based practice, step by step. Critical appraisal of the evidence: Part II. Digging deeper—Examining the "keeper" studies, sixth article in a series. *Am J Nurs* 110:41–48, 2010.

29. Stillwell SB, Fineout-Overholt E, Melnyk BM, et al: Evidence-based practice, step by step: Searching for the evidence. *Am J Nurs* 110:41–47, 2010.

30. Melnyk BM, Fineout-Overholt E, Stillwell SB, et al: Evidence-based practice: Step by step. The seven steps of evidence-based practice: Following this progressive, sequential approach will lead to improved health care and patient outcomes. *Am J Nurs* 110:51, 2010.

31. Melnyk BM, Fineout-Overholt E, Stillwell SB, et al: Evidence-based practice: Step by step. Igniting a spirit of inquiry: An essential foundation for evidence-based practice: How nurses can build the knowledge and skills they need to implement EBP. *Am J Nurs* 109:49–52, 2009.

32. Pelletier L, Stichler J: Ensuring patient and family engagement. *J Nurs Care Qual* 29:110–114, 2014.

33. Page A, editor: *Keeping patients safe: Transforming the work environment of nurses*, Washington, DC, 2004, National Academies Press.

34. Kurtzman E, Fauteux N: *Ten years after Keeping Patients Safe: Have nurses' work environments been transformed? Charting Nursing's Future*, 2014. Issue 22, Robert Wood Johnson Foundation. Retrieved from <http://www.rwjf.org/content/dam/farm/reports/issue_briefs/2014/rwjf411417>.

35. Oxman AD, Lavis JN, Lewin S, et al: SUPPORT tools for evidence-informed health policymaking (STP) 1: What is evidence-informed policymaking? *Health Res Policy Syst* 7(Suppl 1):S1, 2009.

36. World Health Organization: *Evidence-informed policy networks (EVIPNet)*, (n.d.). Retrieved from <http://global.evipnet.org>.

37. Global Health Group: *Evidence to policy initiative*, 2014. Retrieved from <http://globalhealthsciences.ucsf.edu/global-health-group/evidence-to-policy-initiative-e2pi/about-e2pi>.

38. American Nurses Association: *Nursing informatics: Scope and standards of practice*, ed 2, Washington, DC, 2014, American Nurses Publishing.

39. Bauer JC: Nurse practitioners as an underutilized resource for health reform: Evidence-based demonstrations of cost-effectiveness. *J Am Acad Nurse Pract* 22:228–231, 2010.

40. Kapu AN, Kleinpell R, Pilon B: Quality and financial impact of adding nurse practitioners to inpatient care teams. *JONA* 44:87–96, 2014.

41. Cruz EV, Higginbottom G: The use of focused ethnography in nursing research. *Nurse Res* 20:36–43, 2013.

Health Care Quality

P.J. Woods

Health care organizations have a duty to the communities they serve to maintain the quality and safety of care. Health care quality applies within the realm of health care delivery in any public or private setting. Whatever structures, systems, and processes an organization establishes, it must be able to show evidence that standards are upheld. Nurses are a crucial link in meeting the needs of patients and ensuring patient safety, patient-centered care, and communication as part of the health care team. This concept also includes patient preferences, access, cost, and quality as intertwined variables. In other words, the delivery of quality care is irrelevant if the patient cannot access care, the cost is prohibitive (either through insurance or self-pay), or the patient does not want it. Thus both the medical provider and the nurse who want to do the best for the patient may be at odds with the patient, society norms, and best practices. The purpose of this concept presentation is to help students gain a general understanding of quality in the delivery of health care.

DEFINITION

The term *quality* in health care has 19 definitions on a single quality dictionary website (http://dictionary.reference.com/browse/quality), and an Internet search turned up 2,680,000 results for defining quality. This includes definitions from the general meaning that it is merely an attribute of something (e.g., soft or hard) to more specific meanings associated with the degree of excellence or superiority (which, for the purpose of this concept analysis, applies more to how the term is used in health care evaluations).

The importance of quality dates back to Florence Nightingale when she assessed for quality by measuring patient outcomes.[1] Defining quality is difficult because the meaning of "quality" can vary based on context, expectations, and requirements. The expectations of patients, providers, and managers may be different. For example, according to Meade, quality care to the patient is determined by the patient's perception of whether he or she received extraordinary service.[2] This is the "wow" factor that makes the organization and the care, according to patients' perspectives, unique and unparalleled among competing facilities. An additional benefit to having superb overall quality according to patients' perspectives is that it leads to improved clinical outcomes.[3] Overall, these expectations of patients have come to be known as *patient-centered care*. This means that the patient and the patient's

family as he or she defines it are at the center of care, and the health care system seeks to empower them to be active participants and make shared decisions for all aspects of their care. This is particularly important for the nurse because the basis for patient-centered care is communication.[4]

The provider might consider quality as the effects of medical interventions and scientific knowledge resulting in successful and cost-effective recovery without complications. The nurse at the bedside might view quality as the delivery of safe, caring, and competent care, whereas the nurse manager might see quality as a ratio of volume of care in relation to the available resources or the score on a patient satisfaction survey. Regardless, the focus should be on providing patients excellent services via competent health care, comprehensive communication, interprofessional teamwork, and cultural sensitivity.[5]

Quality is also both tangible and intangible. The care delivered can be technically perfect, but if the patient does not improve, according to realistic expectations, or is very dissatisfied with the care, it is useless. Although quality can be a perception, a feeling, or an impression, it can also be something measured. Quality health care is competent and cost-effective. It meets the needs of the patient and utilizes the hospital's resources in a cost-effective way. It meets and/or exceeds an established standard. At times, it seems an impossible goal, but one for which we continually strive. For the purposes of this concept presentation, the Institute of Medicine's (IOM) definition of quality is used. The IOM defines quality of care as *the degree to which health services for individuals and populations increase the likelihood of desired health outcomes and are consistent with current professional knowledge.*[6]

SCOPE

Clearly articulating the scope of quality is challenging because of the abstract nature of this concept. However, as a starting point, it might be helpful to think about the scope of quality on a continuum ranging from consistently poor quality and poor patient outcomes to perfection—that is, always delivering error-free, high-quality care, resulting in optimal outcomes for every patient (Figure 50-1). Embedded within this continuum are multiple variables that collectively impact the overall quality of care.

FIGURE 50-1 Scope of Quality: A Continuum of Quality Consistency

The foundation of quality health care is based on the premise that those who want health care have access to it. Everyone should have access to quality health care, regardless of age, geography, or socioeconomic circumstance. The U.S. health care system is largely based on fee-for-service or insurance, creating a barrier to the poor and uninsured. In addition, because of large rural areas in the United States and health provider shortages, many individuals cannot access primary care or specialty care in their communities. Even in areas where providers are available, they may not accept new patients if they have a full complement of patients (referred to as a *full panel*). In addition, access is not just having access to a provider but also being able to navigate external and internal access demands. External demands include appointment requests, referrals, calls, walk-ins, or any other way patients can gain access to a provider. Internal demands include follow-up appointments that take the place of a new patient or a returning patient with a new problem.

Like all concepts, quality cannot be applied in isolation. From a broader perspective, quality is one element within the context of improving health care in the United States. The "Triple Aim" (developed by the Institute for Healthcare Improvement) focuses on improving the patient experience through quality care but also focuses on improvements in the health of our population and reducing cost.[6,7]

ATTRIBUTES AND CRITERIA

A fundamental attribute inherent in the concept of health care quality is that you cannot improve what you cannot or do not measure. For this reason the health care system uses measures to gauge progress and improve results. Measurement identifies gaps in performance and allows providers to gauge the quality of care delivered. Publicly reporting the results of measurement provides valuable information for patients choosing high-quality providers, purchasers and insurers shaping payment policies based on rewarding quality and efficiency, physicians making referral decisions, and patients recommending a specific health care system to their friends and family.[8]

It is difficult, if not impossible, to list or rank all of the many attributes associated with health care quality or to integrate them to identify a single measure that identifies quality. However, the IOM's *Crossing the Quality Chasm* identifies six characteristics or attributes for quality health care that are useful for this concept presentation: safe, effective, timely, patient-centered, efficient, and equitable (Box 50-1).[6]

BOX 50-1 Attributes of Health Care Quality

- Safe
- Effective
- Timely
- Patient-centered
- Efficient
- Equitable

Safe

All patients should expect care to be delivered correctly and without error. Unfortunately, tens of thousands of errors occur every day in the U.S. health system.[9] Safe health care delivery conforms to standards of practice and sound decision making. Health care professionals demonstrate appropriate knowledge of the health/illness status of the patients they are treating and practice within the appropriate scope of practice based on their licensure or certification. The outcome of a safe health care environment is the avoidance of injury in the delivery of care.[6]

Effective

Effective health care is care based on offering services that address the most important health care concerns to individuals and the most vulnerable population groups. Effective care involves integration of curative and preventative services and refraining from providing services to those who are not likely to benefit. In other words, effective care avoids underuse and overuse of health care services.[6]

Timely

Timeliness of care refers to reducing wait time for health care delivery services. This principle is particularly important to avoid harmful delays that can occur with certain medical conditions. In today's health care delivery system, there are many delays on many levels. Patients wait for parking, they wait in the clinic to get registered, they wait to be put in a room, and then they wait to be seen by the health care provider. If they need diagnostic testing, to fill a prescription, to see a physical therapist, or any other of a myriad of treatments, they will wait and wait again. Patients may have to wait for appointments, especially with specialists, for as long as 6–9 months. When health care is delivered in a timely manner, wait times and harmful delays for both the patient and the provider of care are reduced and care is offered before unnecessary complications occur.[6]

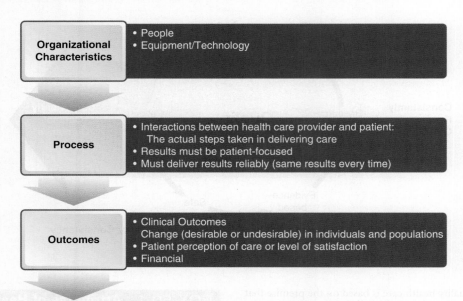

FIGURE 50-2 Donabedian Model of Structure–Process–Outcomes

Patient-Centered Care

Patient-centered care is responsive to individual patient preferences, needs, and values and ensures that these considerations guide all clinical decisions. It also means treating patients with respect and dignity, focusing on the patient, caring about the patient, and treating the patient the way you would like to be treated. Patient-centered care requires soliciting feedback from the patient and his or her family in every aspect of care.[6]

Efficient

Efficiency in health care delivery refers to efficient use of resources for care delivery, such as time, cost, supplies, and minimizing waste. Efficiency in care coordination is one example that increases the quality of the care experience and reduces redundancy and time wasted for patients and providers. Efficiency encourages best practices and prevention over a sick care model and strives to reduce reward based on volume in individual services.[6]

Equitable

Equitable care is providing care that does not vary in quality because of gender, ethnicity, geographic location, and socioeconomic status; it strives to serve the underserved and is delivered in a system that allows for exemptions.[5,9] When health care is equitable, all are afforded the same access, costs, and quality.[6]

THEORETICAL LINKS

Avedis Donabedian defined *quality* as values and goals present in the medical system and defined *outcomes* as a validator of the quality and effectiveness of medical care.[10] He stated that examining care processes instead of focusing on outcomes provided a more reliable indicator of the quality of medical care. Donabedian believed there was a framework that included all the various definitions and specifications, including how variations in care occur, or relate to one another, and the consequences they have on measuring, monitoring, and developing quality measurements in health care. This model is depicted in Figure 50-2.

The model identifies ways to define, categorize, and measure quality. This has become increasingly important in the era of managed care and cost containment. Most attempts at developing quality indicators have been based on the development of outcome measures. The framework in the Donabedian model is founded on quality using a three-part procedure—structure, process, and outcomes:

- *Structure* is defined as the attributes of settings in which care is delivered. These include the adequacy of facilities, equipment, supplies, staff training, provider knowledge and attitudes, and supervision. The context (structure) in which care is delivered affects processes and outcomes. For example, if the facility is lacking in amenities, wait times are too long, or the providers and staff are not adequately prepared, people will prefer to avoid the facility.
- Service *process* dimensions include the services offered; the technical quality of the services (i.e., the staff and providers perform the technical aspects of the task or job); the quality of interpersonal relations; and the adequacy of patient education, access, safety, and promotion of continuity of care (i.e., appropriate referral and follow-up).
- *Outcomes* are the impact of structure and process on the patient's satisfaction; perceptions of quality, knowledge, attitudes, and behavior; and health outcomes. For example, if a provider or facility is unavailable or if patients do not have accessibility, then the outcome will be a direct result of inadequate access.[11] The Donabedian model is the most common quality-of-care framework employed, and it has been universally accepted and used as the basis for much of the work addressing quality and outcome.[11,12]

CONTEXT TO NURSING AND HEALTH CARE

Delivering quality health care and monitoring its outcomes are inherent in all nursing practice environments, and all nurses are responsible for delivering safe, effective, and efficient care. Nurses are the front-line defense against actual and potential risks to patients; this requires an understanding of, and willingness to participate in, measures that promote and ensure the health and safety of patients. This includes being able to identify unsafe practices and respond appropriately to ensure a safe outcome for patients, clients, oneself, and others.

Quality is evaluated on the basis of process and outcomes. Process components include how health care is provided and how the system works. Outcome components include health status and the difference the process made. Improving health care quality is a shared responsibility among all health care professionals. Efforts to achieve quality through quality improvement, the adoption of quality improvement plans, and error reduction are expected in all health care organizations.

Error Reduction

According to IOM,[13] a medical error or adverse event is defined as the failure of a planned intervention or action to be completed as intended and includes a variation from the standard of care. This is referred to as an error of execution. Adverse events are caused by someone on the health care team or by a system failure rather than by the underlying disease or condition of the patient.[14] Another type of error is using the wrong plan to achieve an outcome, which is an error in diagnosis, planning, or delivery of care. As shown in Table 50-1, errors are classified as near-miss, adverse, or sentinel events.

Plsek and Greenhalgh define complex adaptive systems (CAS) as a collection of individuals who have freedom to act in ways that are not always predictable and who are interconnected so that small changes can affect other individuals in the CAS.[15] Our current health care system is a perfect example of a CAS. There are multiple relationships that are organized and evolving together to meet patient needs. These relationships are often nonlinear and dependent on individual behavior. Medical errors are rarely the result of personal negligence or criminal activity; rather, medical errors occur as a result of human fallibility compounded by poor system designs that allow for error. Error prevention management strategies include quality analysis tools such as

root cause analysis (RCA) and failure mode effective analysis (FMEA). These are used to analyze and report quality measures, including analyzing errors and near misses as well as preventing adverse events in the first place.

Regulatory Agencies

Multiple oversight bodies and regulatory agencies exist to ensure the safety of the public. These regulatory agencies license health care facilities for operation (e.g., specific state licensing regulations) and can fine organizations or restrict services and suspend operations if there is a failure to meet expected standards. For example, Medicare or Medicaid reimbursement can be withheld if the delivery of patient care does not meet national quality standards. The Centers for Medicare & Medicaid Services (CMS), The Joint Commission (TJC), and the Occupational Safety and Health Administration are the major agencies that regulate care provided in hospitals and in community-based settings. Other important regulatory agencies that ensure health care quality include the U.S. Food and Drug Administration, the U.S. Department of Justice, the Office of the Inspector General, and the U.S. Drug Enforcement Administration.

An example of the influence on quality from the regulatory agencies is the establishment of the National Patient Safety Goals (NPSGs) program by TJC to help accredited organizations address specific areas of concern with regard to patient safety.[16] The NPSG program (updated annually) covers nine health care delivery system areas, each of which has specific patient safety goals. For each of these goals, there are specific measures that the organization must attain.

Advisory Bodies

Advisory bodies have an important role in influencing standards for the delivery of quality health care. Although the focus of various advisory bodies varies, contributions to quality health care include efforts such as studies and recommendations regarding best practices for the improvement of health care, establishment of health care performance measures, provision of data on care and outcomes, and collaborative learning efforts.

One of the most influential advisory bodies is IOM, an independent, nonprofit organization that conducts studies and provides unbiased and authoritative advice to improve the nation's health.[14] Many of the studies that IOM undertakes begin as specific mandates from Congress, whereas others are requested by federal agencies and independent organizations. Examples of landmark studies that have directly influenced health care quality include *To Err Is Human: Building a Safer Health System*[17] and *Crossing the Quality Chasm: A New Health System for the 21st Century*.[18]

Some advisory bodies are specific to nursing. For example, an initiative of the National Center for Nursing Quality (NCNQ) originally developed the National Database of Nursing Quality Indicators (NDNQI), a research-based national comparative database on nursing care and its relationship to patient outcomes. NDNQI is the only national nursing database that collects and evaluates unit-specific nurse-sensitive indicators (such as patient falls, pressure ulcer rate, nursing hours per patient day, and nursing turnover rate, to name a few), and provides quarterly and annual reporting of structure, process, and outcome indicators to evaluate nursing care at the unit level.[19] Participating organizations receive unit-level comparative data reports to use for quality improvement purposes.

Quality Management Programs and Philosophies

Health care agencies deliver health care within the context of a quality plan or philosophy designed to continually improve the quality of care

TABLE 50-1 Classifications of Safety Events	
Type of Event	**Criteria**
Near-miss event: An error that could have caused harm to a patient, but did not, as a result of chance, prevention, or some intervention that mitigated the impact. The majority of adverse events are near-miss events.	• Mild variation in standard of care • Caused by human or system error • Does not reach the patient • Does not cause harm • Use FMEA to analyze causes
Adverse event: An error that results in moderate to severe harm to a patient. One of the most common adverse events involves medication administration.	• Moderate variation in standard of care • Caused by human or system error • Reaches the patient • Minimal or no harm • Use FMEA to analyze causes
Sentinel event: A serious error that results in patient death or a serious, undesirable outcome as a result of the error.[33]	• Severe variation in standard of care • Caused by human or system error • Reaches the patient • Death or major harm • Use RCA to analyze causes

FMEA, failure mode effective analysis; RCA, root cause analysis.

delivery and reduce the chance of causing harm to a patient. There are many quality management programs. Health care organizations adopt a program based on the type of care given, patients served, the mission and core values of the organization, and the perspective of organizational leadership. Regardless of the plan adopted, quality management plans should be comprehensive, incorporating all areas of the organization, including clinical areas, administrative and management practices, and facility operation. Common to all quality management plans is a focus on the patient with purposeful collection and analysis of data to improve outcomes and patient satisfaction. Quality measures are used to gauge how well a health care entity provides care to its patients. Measures are based on scientific evidence and can reflect guidelines, standards of care, or practice parameters. A quality measure converts medical information from patient records or patient satisfaction surveys into a rate or percentage that allows facilities to assess their performance.[20] Examples of quality management programs are total quality management (TQM), continuous quality improvement, Six Sigma, and Lean Six Sigma.

One example of a quality improvement process associated with the TQM approach is plan–do–study–act (PDSA).[21] The PDSA cycle includes developing a plan to test the change (plan), trying out the change (do), analyzing what happened from the change (study), and determining what was learned (act) (Figure 50-3). The team then refines the change based on what was learned, and then this cycle is repeated. The PDSA cycle is usually done on a small scale so the health care team can quickly determine what will provide the best results before they implement a change on a large scale.[21]

Integral elements of quality management systems are error prevention and management strategies. Health care organizations strive for an error-free environment. To develop and maintain the goal of zero errors, many organizations have adopted a *culture of safety*, defined as the shared commitment of management and employees to ensure the safety of the work environment. In a comprehensive literature review, the following seven subcultures were identified: leadership, teamwork, evidence-based, communication, learning, just, and patient-centered.[22]

A culture of safety acknowledges the inevitability of error and proactively seeks to identify latent threats.[23] The following are characteristics of such a culture:

- Acknowledgment of the high-risk, error-prone nature of an organization's activities
- A blame-free environment in which individuals are able to report errors or close calls without fear of reprimand or punishment
- An expectation of collaboration across ranks to seek solutions to vulnerabilities
- A willingness on the part of the organization to direct resources for addressing safety concerns

Health Information Technology

Health information technology (HIT) enables organizations to mine the data collected in the delivery of patient care and track performance against established benchmarks more quickly and economically than with manual systems. This speeds adjustments to improve outcomes, regardless of whether they are clinical nursing outcomes, workforce outcomes, patient and consumer outcomes, or organizational outcomes. The RAND Foundation estimates that widespread adoption of various HITs could save up to $77 billion annually.[24] HIT structural measures are intended to help providers assess the efficiency and standardization of current HIT systems and identify areas in which additional HIT tools can be used.[24] IOM emphasizes the importance of using HIT to accomplish the following:[6]

- Design care processes based on best practices
- Translate new clinical knowledge and skills into practice
- Support the work of multidisciplinary teams
- Enable the coordination of care across patient conditions, services, and settings
- Measure and improve performance

INTERRELATED CONCEPTS

This concept represents areas that relate to health care quality. Several concepts featured in this textbook have a relationship with this concept. Health Policy is used to provide overarching goals and set priorities for the allocation of valuable health resources. Health Care Economics is concerned with issues related to the scarcity of resources in the allocation of health and health care. Health Care Organizations and delivery systems provide the framework for the delivery of health care. The concept Safety examines how we prevent accidental injury or harm to patients, and Technology and Informatics provides tools to help deliver quality health care. These interrelationships are depicted in Figure 50-4.

CLINICAL EXEMPLARS

In the United States, nurses can expect to encounter health care quality in any setting and whenever they interact with a patient. Nurses will encounter regulations and standards that their health care organization must meet along with nurse-sensitive indicators for which they are personally responsible. A sample of exemplars, based on categories previously described, are listed in Box 50-2. It is beyond the scope of this text to describe all these in detail, but several are briefly presented next.

Featured Exemplars
The Joint Commission

The Joint Commission is a regulatory agency that has perhaps had the greatest influence on quality as the leader in developing the highest standards for quality and safety and evaluating organization

PLAN: Plan a change or test of how something works
DO: Carry out the plan
STUDY: Look at the results. What did you find out?
ACT: Decide what actions should be taken to improve

FIGURE 50-3 The Plan–Do–Study–Act Cycle of Quality Improvement (Source: From Topol EJ, Teirstein PS: *Textbook of Interventional Cardiology*, ed 6, Philadelphia, 2012, Elsevier.)

Health Policy

Technology & Informatics

Health Care Economics

Health Care Quality

Safety

Health Care Organizations

FIGURE 50-4 Health Care Quality and Interrelated Concepts

BOX 50-2 EXEMPLARS OF QUALITY

Regulatory Agencies
- Accreditation Association for Ambulatory Health Care (AAAHC)
- Accreditation Commission for Health Care (ACHC)
- Centers for Medicare & Medicaid Services (CMS)
- Community Health Accreditation Program (CHAP)
- Healthcare Facilities Accreditation Program (HFAP)
- Healthcare Quality Association on Accreditation (HQAA)
- National Committee for Quality Assurance (NCQA)
- Occupational Safety and Health Administration (OSHA)
- The Joint Commission (TJC)

Advisory Bodies
- American Nurses Association (ANA)
- Association for Healthcare Research and Quality (AHRQ)
- Institute of Medicine (IOM)
- Institute for Healthcare Improvement (IHI)
- Leapfrog Group
- National Center for Nursing Quality (NCNQ)
- National Quality Forum (NQF)

Quality Plans and Philosophies
- Baldrige
- Culture of safety
- ANCC Magnet designation
- Plan–do–study–act (PDSA)
- Six Sigma
- Synergy
- Total quality improvement (TQI)
- Total quality management (TQM)

Error Prevention Management
- Failure mode effective analysis (FMEA)
- Root cause analysis (RCA)
- Risk analysis

Health Information Technology
- Computerized physician order entry (CPOE)
- Electronic health records (EHRs)
- Medication administration systems

---

performance based on these standards.[25] TJC is also the only accrediting organization with the capability and experience to evaluate health care organizations across the continuum of care. TJC accreditation and certification is recognized nationwide as a symbol of quality that reflects an organization's commitment to meeting certain performance standards.[26] In order for a health care organization to participate in and receive payment from the Medicare and Medicaid programs, it must be certified as complying with TJC regulations.[16]

The National Quality Forum

As an advisory body, the National Quality Forum (NQF) has been instrumental in advancing efforts to improve quality through performance measurement and public reporting. NQF is a private, nonprofit organization with more than 375 members representing virtually every sector of the health care system. NQF has become the "gold standard"

for health care performance measures. Major health care purchasers rely on NQF-endorsed measures to ensure that the measures are scientifically sound and meaningful and to help standardize performance measures used across the industry. To date, NQF has endorsed more than 500 measures.[27]

The National Center for Nursing Quality

Created by the American Nurses Association, the NCNQ is a nursing-specific advisory body that addresses patient safety and quality in nursing care and nurses' work lives. The center advocates for nursing quality through quality measurement, novel research, and collaborative learning. Issues such as the nursing workforce shortages and impact on patient outcomes are dealt with through innovative initiatives, including the NDNQI and Safe Staffing Saves Lives.[19,28]

Root Cause Analysis

A root cause analysis (RCA) is an exemplar representing error prevention management and is used when a patient has been seriously harmed or has died as a result of a medical error. The RCA is a critical tool to identify the systems that failed during the course of a given patient's care. Each level of the adverse event is investigated in order to identify problems that affect the entire system. Dlugacz and colleagues identified a series of specific questions that dissect the causes of an event to uncover the fundamental flaws in the process, which is important in determining risk points.[29]

Failure Mode Effective Analysis

Failure mode effective analysis (FMEA) is designed to prevent the occurrence of errors or system failures. The first step is to define the critical problem and then identify potential failure modes, analyze causes of system failure, identify solutions to the problem, and evaluate the results.

Leapfrog Group

The Leapfrog Group, an employer-based coalition, works with medical experts throughout the United States to identify and propose solutions designed to reduce medical errors through the adoption of specific best

practices.[30] Leapfrog Group's "never events" policy (events that should never occur in health care) requires hospitals to do the following when a never event occurs:[31]

- Apologize to the patient and/or family affected.
- Report the event to designated agencies.
- Conduct a root cause analysis, consistent with instructions from the chosen reporting agency.
- Waive all costs directly related to the event.
- Make the organization's policy available to patients and payers upon request.

Computer Physician Order Entry

Computer physician order entry (CPOE) is a health information technology exemplar of quality. CPOE is an electronic prescribing system that intercepts errors when medications are ordered, before they reach the patient.[32] With CPOE, rates of serious errors can be reduced by nearly 90% because immediate information to physicians is provided (e.g., warning them about a potential adverse reaction with the patient's other drugs).[5,6] Although CPOE is focused on the physician, the role of the nurse remains critical in avoiding errors by adhering to the "five rights" of medication administration.

CASE STUDY

Source: monkeybusinessimages/iStock/Thinkstock

Case Presentation

While hospitalized on a cardiac step-down unit, a patient undergoing cardiac monitoring died when a lethal cardiac rhythm was missed by the hospital staff. Because of the severity of the outcome, an RCA was done. The RCA determined the central monitor screens for the cardiac units were at the nurses' stations, giving them primary responsibility for oversight. However, the nurses were so busy that the unit secretaries were eventually trained to watch the monitors because they sat at the desk where the monitors were located.

The unit secretaries were also very busy, making it almost impossible to keep a constant eye on the cardiac monitors, resulting in inconsistent monitoring, reporting, and follow-up related to monitor alarms. During the RCA, it was determined that the nurses did not intend the secretaries to be the only pair of eyes on the monitors and had every intention of being closely involved. Secretaries were instructed to notify a nurse of any monitor alarm, and it was the nurse's responsibility to respond. However, when the nurses assigned the responsibility to the secretaries, they became complacent in their primary responsibility to ensure someone observed, reported, and responded to any alarm. In the case of the death, the secretary had learned to silence the monitors once she had alerted the nurse because the noise was overwhelming.

The secretary reported, "I had seen the nurses do it all the time because they often complained that patients turning over could cause the alarms to go off." This statement was corroborated by the nursing staff, and they admitted that they often instructed the secretaries to "shut it off" based on their having just been in a patient's room several times for monitor alarms and the patient was fine.

On the day of the event, the monitor was alarming and the secretary told the nurse as usual, but on her way to the patient's room, the nurse was called to an emergency at the other end of the hall, preventing her from checking the patient immediately. The secretary silenced the alarm on two subsequent times after she had notified the nurse, believing it had been addressed. The patient had been in ventricular fibrillation and died before the nurse returned to the room.

During the investigation, it was discovered there had been five other incident reports filed for similar problems during the past 2 years, including two near-death cases. In a review of the other incident reports, it was documented that the solution to the early problems had been to train the secretaries as a backup because the nurses were often in the hallways or in patients' rooms. It was believed that having someone who was always near the monitors and who could watch them and report alarms to the nurses would solve the problem. It became clear, based on the recent death, that a more drastic solution was needed. After analyzing several proposed solutions, it was decided that having a centralized monitor room separate from the nursing station monitors and staffed with monitor techs was the best solution. In addition to the centralized monitor room, the ability to silence a monitor was removed from the central unit at the nurses' station, so the alarm could only be silenced by a nurse at the patient's bedside to ensure someone had seen the patient before silencing the alarm. Finally, in the event of a lethal alarm, the monitor room techs would call a code blue before phoning the nursing unit.

Case Analysis

This model case illustrated a system failure that did not meet the major attributes of health care quality of being safe, patient-centered, timely, effective, and efficient. This effort would be classified as a sentinel event because there was a severe variation in the standard of care caused by both human error and system error, resulting in death.

ACCESS EXEMPLAR LINKS IN YOUR GIDDENS EBOOK

REFERENCES

1. Montalvo I: The National Database of Nursing Quality Indicators (NDNQI). *OJIN* 12(3):Manuscript 2, 2007.

2. Meade C: *Alliance for health care research organizational change processes in high performing organizations: In-depth case studies with health care facilities*, 2003. Retrieved from <http://www.studergroup.com/content/ahc_research/associated_files/ahcr_study_final.pdf>.

3. Chilgren A: Managers and the new definition of quality. *J Healthc Manag* 53(4):221–229, 2008.

4. Needleman J, Hassmiller S: The role of nurses in improving hospital quality and efficiency: Real-world results. *Health Aff (Millwood)* 28(4):w625–w663, 2009.

5. Wharam JF, Sulmasy D: Improving the quality of health care. *JAMA* 310(2):215–217, 2009.

6. Institute of Medicine, Committee on Quality of Health Care in America: *Crossing the quality chasm: A new health system for the 21st century*, Washington, DC, 2001, National Academies Press.

7. Stiefel M, Nolan K: *A guide to measuring the triple aim: Population health, experience of care, and per capita cost*, IHI Innovation Series white paper, Cambridge, MA, 2012, Institute for Healthcare Improvement.

8. National Quality Forum: *Measuring performance*, (n.d.). Retrieved from <http://www.qualityforum.org>.

9. U.S. Department of Health and Human Services, Agency for Healthcare Research and Quality: *National healthcare quality report*, AHRQ Publication No. 10-0003, 2009.

10. Donabedian A: Quality assessment and monitoring: Retrospect and prospect. *Eval Health Prof* 6(3):63–75, 1983.

11. Donabedian A: *The methods and findings of quality assessment and monitoring: An illustrated analysis*, Ann Arbor, MI, 1985, Health Administration Press.

12. Donabedian A: The quality of care: How can it be assessed? *JAMA* 260(12):1743–1748, 1988.

13. Duke University Medical Center: *Patient safety–quality improvement: What is quality improvement?*, 2005. Retrieved from <http://patientsafetyed.duhs.duke.edu/module_a/module_summary.html>.

14. Institute of Medicine: *About the IOM*, 2010. Retrieved from <http://iom.nationalacademies.org>.

15. Plsek P, Greenhalgh T: The challenge of complexity in health care. *Br Med J* 323(7313):625–628, 2001.

16. The Joint Commission: *National patient safety goals*, 2015. Retrieved from <http://www.jointcommission.org/standards_information/npsgs.aspx>.

17. Institute of Medicine, Committee on Quality of Health Care in America: *To err is human: Building a safer health system*, Washington, DC, 2001, National Academies Press.

18. Institute of Medicine, Committee on Quality of Health Care in America: *Crossing the quality chasm: A new health system for the 21st century*, Washington, DC, 2001, National Academies Press.

19. *National Database Quality Indicators*, (n.d.). Retrieved from <http://nursingandndnqi.weebly.com/ndnqi-indicators.html>.

20. U.S. Department of Health and Human Services, Centers for Medicare and Medicaid Services: *Hospital quality initiative*, 2011. Retrieved from <https://www.cms.gov/HospitalQualityInits/20_Outcome Measures.asp>.

21. Taylor MJ, McNicholas C, Nicolay C, et al: Systematic review of the application of the plan–do–study–act method to improve quality in healthcare. *BMJ Qual Saf* bmjqs-2013, 2013.

22. Pizzi L, Goldfarb D, Nash D, et al: *Making health care safer: A critical analysis of patient safety practices*, Washington, DC, 2001, National Academies Press.

23. Institute for Healthcare Improvement: *Plan–do–study–act (PDSA) worksheet*, (n.d.). Retrieved from <http://www.ihi.org/IHI/Topics/Improvement/ImprovementMethods/Tools/Plan-Do-Study-Act%20%28PDSA%29%20Worksheet>.

24. RAND Foundation: *Health information technology: can HIT lower costs and improve quality?*, 2005. Retrieved from <http://www.rand.org/pubs/research_briefs/2005/RAND_RB9136.pdf>.

25. The Joint Commission: *About the Joint Commission*, 2015. Retrieved from <http://www.jointcommission.org/about_us/about_the_joint_commission_main.aspx>.

26. Brown A: *Deciphering TJC condition-level findings*, 2011. Retrieved from <http://www.compass-clinical.com/hospital-accreditation/2011/05/19/deciphering-tjc-condition-level-findings>.

27. National Quality Forum: *About the National Quality Forum*, 2015. Retrieved from <http://www.qualityforum.org/story/About_Us.aspx>.

28. American Nurses Association: *Nurse Staffing*, (n.d.). Retrieved from <http://www.nursingworld.org/MainMenuCategories/ThePracticeofProfessionalNursing/NurseStaffing>.

29. Dlugacz YD, Restifo A, Greenwood A: *The quality handbook for health care organizations*, San Francisco, CA, 2004, Jossey–Bass.

30. The LeapFrog Group: *Leaps in hospital quality, safety, and affordability*, 2015. Retrieved from <http://leapfroggroup.org>.

31. The LeapFrog Group: *Position statement on never events*, 2015. <http://www.leapfroggroup.org/for_hospitals/leapfrog_hospital_quality_and_safety_survey_copy/never_events>.

32. Berger RG, Kichack BA: Computerized physician order entry: Helpful or harmful? *Am Med Inform Assoc* 11(2):100–103, 2004.

33. Centers for Medicare & Medicaid Services: *Hospital quality initiatives*, 2013. Retrieved from <https://www.cms.gov/Medicare/Quality-Initiatives-Patient-Assessment-Instruments/HospitalQualityInits/index.html>.

Care Coordination

Janet Prvu Bettger and Nicole Moore

Care coordination is a central component of service delivery because of its role in attaining optimal patient outcomes and health care quality. It is recognized as essential for organizing care and information around patients' needs and preferences.[1] Although it is now a focal point of health care policy and research, care coordination was not as prominent before the turn of the century. Implementation of the advances in technology and renewed commitment to patient-centered and family-focused care have increased the visibility of this concept. Care coordination is now a top priority for health system redesign.[2] The Affordable Care Act included several key Medicare initiatives to improve quality and cost-effectiveness of health care by focusing on hospital discharge, home care, and chronic illness.[3] However, the concept in practice is still evolving and, in some settings, still emerging. Without the adoption of care coordination models, fragmented service delivery, cost inefficiencies, and poor health outcomes will continue. This concept presentation explores the defining characteristics, attributes, and theory supporting care coordination, highlighting clinical exemplars and other related concepts.

DEFINITION

A 2007 systematic review of care coordination published by the Agency for Healthcare Research and Quality (AHRQ) identified more than 40 definitions of care coordination and related terminology.[4] A universally accepted definition of care coordination does not yet exist. However, several professional organizations and consensus bodies have endorsed definitions to guide practice and measurement. The American Academy of Nurses Care Coordination Task Force called for the Centers for Medicare & Medicaid Services (CMS) to develop a clear definition of care coordination that is patient, family, and population centric; addresses services provided by qualified professionals based on risks and needs; and is easily used and understood by all stakeholders.[5]

Definitions of care coordination in the peer-reviewed literature vary by the population and care environments of focus. Several are provided here as examples. As a professional organization, the American Academy of Pediatrics made one of the earliest efforts to define this concept.[6] With a focus on children with special health care needs, care coordination was presented as a process connecting both services and resources and involving patients, providers, and families, with the goals of optimal health care and optimal patient outcomes.

The National Coalition on Care Coordination was formed in 2008 to promote better coordinated health and social services for older adults with multiple chronic conditions; the emphasis of its definition is on a "person-centered and assessment-based interdisciplinary approach" across settings and providers to coordinate medical and supportive services over time.[3] Discussions of care coordination for persons with mental illness suggest services also be coordinated across people and sites, functions, and activities.[7] For the purposes of directing measurement, the National Quality Forum endorsed a definition focused on patients' needs and preferences for health services over time but also explicitly acknowledged the role of information sharing across people, functions, and sites of care.[8]

Review of the definitions of care coordination developed thus far reveals several core components. The identification of these is important to be able to consider the types and attributes of care coordination and the theory that supports this concept in practice. Guided by the 2007 systematic review and the evolution of the concept to date, care coordination can be defined as *a set of activities purposefully organized by a team of personnel that includes the patient to facilitate the appropriate delivery of the necessary services and information to support optimal health and care across settings and over time.*

SCOPE

From the most abstract perspective, the scope of care coordination ranges from efficient, well-coordinated care across multiple health care entities and involving multiple health care professionals to poor coordination of care or, worse, a complete lack of care coordination (Figure 51-1). The goal for any health care system is to coordinate care well. Although the need for efficient coordination of care exists for all patients, it is especially important for the management of individuals with multiple and complex chronic conditions.

ATTRIBUTES AND CRITERIA

Analysis of this concept yielded a definition of care coordination that states a set of activities be purposefully organized by a team of personnel that includes the patient to facilitate the appropriate delivery of the necessary services and information to support optimal health and care across settings and over time. This definition facilitates the discussion of attributes into specific components as outlined in Table 51-1.[4,7,9–16]

FIGURE 51-1 Scope of Care Coordination

TABLE 51-1	Attributes and Description of Integrated Care Coordination Models
Attribute	**Description**
Interorganizational and interprofessional team that includes the patient	Existing care coordination structure, guidelines, and organizational links Team based and interprofessional Inclusive of patient and patient's support system Trusting interaction among team members Shared and appreciated understanding of roles Clinical integration and interdependence Central point of contact (a person, partnership of providers, agency, or organization) responsible for continuity of care and management of all other attributes (nursing identified as most common clinical discipline as designated care coordinator, followed by social workers and pharmacists)
Communication and information exchange	Information exchange across services and team members before and after each interaction Standardized communication template of a minimal set of care data elements accessible to all team members, particularly during transitions of care Electronic record system to allow team members timely access to plan of care and data at all points in time with efficient and effective integration of patient information, laboratory data, imaging results, referrals, medications, social and community services, and self-management support Built-in support for quality improvement and safety, evidence-based decision support tools, provider alerts, and patient reminders Comprehensive in-hospital planning, home-based visits, and telephone follow-up to ensure continuity over transitions in care
A proactive plan of care with goals	Created, documented, executed, and updated with every patient Comprehensive including community and nonclinical services with health care services that incorporate the patient's needs, preferences, and resources to achieve the patient's goals Developed and shared across providers and patient's support system Revised as needed Patients most likely to benefit identified Patient-centered and family-focused
Targeted set of purposeful activities	Individual's needs, preferences, and risks assessed Evidence-based standards of care and referrals followed Shared decision making Activities matched to goals Self-care skills and independence promoted Duplicated services and unnecessary cost avoided Health promotion activities included
Proactive follow-up	Systematic surveillance, evaluation, and monitoring of patient and process including follow-up assessments, tests, treatments, or services

Although evidence is mounting in favor of care coordination programs benefiting patients, the 2007 technical review for the AHRQ found evidence about key intervention components to still be lacking due to the existence of a vast number of care coordination models.[4,16] The Affordable Care Act has charged the CMS to develop policies for care coordination resulting in an ongoing CMS-funded initiative to develop a care coordination model across care settings for Medicaid/Medicare enrollees.[17] Intervention descriptions from randomized controlled trials and literature review converge on five key attributes of care coordination:

- Interorganizational and interprofessional team that includes the patient
- Communication and information exchange
- A proactive plan of care with goals
- A targeted set of purposeful activities
- Outcomes and proactive follow-up

THEORETICAL LINKS

The literature on organizational theory provides useful insights for addressing the interactions and relationships among organizations that are required for effective delivery of care coordination in complex situations. An exhaustive review of relevant theories is less important than understanding the applicability of organizational theory in supporting the concept of care coordination.

The AHRQ surmises that there are three main domains in current care coordination theories: specific patient care situation, coordination mechanisms, and outcomes of care.[4] An update to the AHRQ study by Van Houdt and colleagues further identified key concepts and their relationships within these domains.[16] Coordination begins with an assessment of the individual patient situation that includes needs and resources within the health care system, community, and home based on current standards of care.[16,18] Consideration of the patient's need for coordination by assessing health status, preferences, self-care knowledge, support system, culture, and personal resources helps to direct care.[16] Other external factors, such as national and local policy, economics, insurance coverage, and benefits, are not within individuals' control but can influence availability of assets.[19] For example, the coordination needs of a newly diagnosed diabetic with insurance coverage, excellent family support, and high income are very different from those of an individual with no insurance, no family, and no job.

The second domain involves coordination mechanisms that include goals, team dynamics, and exchange of information.[4,16] A team may consist of a nurse and patient alone or may include any number of specialists, social workers, ancillary medical staff, and liaisons for transitional care. Successful teams must have a trusting relationship that employs effective communication. In addition, processes to achieve these goals are most successful when communication among and between participants is frequent, timely, and accurate.[4,7]

The final domain involves patient, team, and organizational outcomes.[16,20] Consideration of outcomes is an ongoing process, and quality outcomes should be evidence-based, patient-centered, substantive, and interprofessional. The nurse should assess these aspects continually not only to improve patient outcomes but also to ensure quality, cost-effective care.[9,21]

CONTEXT TO NURSING AND HEALTH CARE

Target of Care Coordination Efforts

Care coordination is important for everyone. During the life course, everyone will have at least a temporary need for improved coordination and communication between providers, settings, or periods of time during an illness. Thus everyone is at risk for, at a minimum, an episodic illness with at least temporary needs for care coordination. However, the structure of health care in the United States today and the workforce supporting it does not allow for everyone to be supported by a fully integrated care coordination program or model of service delivery.

The general population needs to be stratified based on risk and need. To best support those in greatest need, care coordination may need to be reserved for those individuals particularly vulnerable to fragmented, uncoordinated care on a chronic basis and at highest risk of negative health outcomes. Currently, as evidence mounts and the translation, adoption, adaptation, and implementation of care coordination models is accepted throughout the country, the priority population will need to be those most vulnerable and frail. This may include a targeted focus on serving children with special health care needs, the frail elderly population, those in crisis situations or catastrophic events, and people at the end of life before other high-risk populations. People in the second tier of risk and need for care coordination are individuals with complex conditions or life situations elevating the likelihood of negative outcomes, including people with cognitive impairments, complex medical or mental health conditions, disabilities, low incomes, or unstable health insurance coverage. Unfortunately, it is only a matter of time before the latter high-risk group will also become vulnerable and in greater need, and the risk increases for people in the general population.

The paradigm shift in health care financing and delivery of holistic patient-centered, family-focused care is facing resistance; as a result, people in need are not benefiting from a structured model of care known to produce positive outcomes. It will take time and continued research to fully implement care coordination for everyone, at all levels of need and in all communities. Until then, holistic care coordination is best reserved for those most likely to benefit: vulnerable and frail children and adults.

Care Coordination Models

Several variations of care coordination models have emerged to improve care, promote health and independence, and reduce unnecessary service utilization. To understand and evaluate the different types, it is important to recognize that people—patients and consumers—live and have needs beyond the health care system. Health care services are just one component in our society of services supporting health. Care coordination for some people may also require the knowledge and organization of social services such as those in sectors of education, employment, and the community from housing to utilities, transportation, or insurance of all types. When considering a person's needs that may fall within these different arenas, the different care coordination models include social models, medically oriented models, and integrated models of both social and medical services.

Figure 51-2 illustrates the balance in an ideally functioning integrated model that is proactive, focuses on patient wellness using evidence-based methods, employs effective communication, and appoints appropriate use of resources.[1,22] Patient care is a continuum and incorporates both medical and community social resources across the lifespan. In the opposing, dysfunctional model, care is reactive and fragmented, which negatively impacts the patient. Resources are mismanaged, resulting in either unmet needs or redundancy. The patient is ill informed, lacks resources for wellness, and is not involved in decision making. Social, medical, and integrated models are described next,

FIGURE 51-2 Balance and Imbalance of Care Coordination Attributes

and whereas social and medically oriented models are distinctly separate from one another, integrated models incorporate aspects of both models and can be differentiated by the level of influence of each model.

Social Models

Care coordination models first emerged to manage home and community-based services and usually did not address medical care. For children and teens, the model would include school-based services. Adults also occasionally require these or other traditional vocational programs when returning to work. Elderly individuals or financially disadvantaged families may require utilities assistance programs or have other housing needs that range from finding a home to making the home arrangement safe and accessible. Food and meal services are organized at the community level from shelters to drop-in programs and home delivery, or they can be facilitated at the state level with vouchers and food stamps. State programs also support local organization and facilitation of transportation, insurance, and disability-related services. Health care needs are sometimes also addressed by a variety of community programs, particularly for people who have become disconnected from a regular source of care. However, the care provided in social models is usually to support activities of daily living rather than skilled care. Although services in a social model vary based on need, the models are organized to offer information, referral, screening and assessment, planning, authorization, and monitoring.[13]

Leadership and organizing responsibility for social models of care coordination can be at the local or state level. For example, Area Agencies on Aging are often designated as coordinators and administrators of care coordination programs that can then be standardized at some level across a state. County social service agencies also assume care coordination responsibilities and are often able to serve as a single entity for multiple funding sources, such as waiver services, block grants, state-funded services, and Medicaid. Having a single entity coordinate all relevant social services can reduce the likelihood of redundancy and duplication of efforts. Advances in technology and electronic social networking interfaces will continue to facilitate opportunities for partnership and referral to social services. Social models of care coordination

are an important part of promoting health and independence in the community.

Medically Oriented Models

Medical models coordinate medical services and were traditionally designed to be diagnosis specific. As health systems have evolved, so have medical models of care coordination. New models have emerged as payers and providers of health services are needed by individuals for coordination of multiple treatments and visits for multiple conditions. The infrastructure and attributes vary because of funding, financing, and availability of services. Financing medical models further challenges the ability to coordinate care across settings (e.g., hospital to skilled nursing facility to assisted living) as well as over time. Managed care has been the most stable vehicle to support coordination across settings and payers, particularly for individuals with complex conditions that increase the risk of hospitalization and adverse outcomes.

Provider initiatives for Medicare beneficiaries are most common in the literature on medical models of care coordination. There are several types, and most are limited models targeting a specific disease or patient population, a specific setting of care, or a prespecified amount of time. Examples of these include pharmacist-supported models focused on medication management and self-management programs designed to empower patients to actively manage their own health needs.[23,24] Models more common in practice and with a stronger evidence base include disease management programs that supplement primary care for ambulatory-based conditions such as heart failure or diabetes and case management models that collaborate with primary care to support patients in navigating available services.[25,26] Although each of these provider-driven medical models is supported with randomized controlled trials yielding positive patient and health service outcomes, providers and patients have come to realize the limitations of addressing only the medical needs of patients and their families.

Integrated Models

Models committed to the integration of health care, social support, and community clinical and nonclinical services are still evolving. They offer significant promise for supporting holistic, patient-centered, family-focused care, but building bridges between services and settings is fraught with barriers. In the United States, most challenges stem from having the different service types financed from different sources. Coordination is further complicated by the scope of authority for managing the different services and the level of involvement of each agency or organization. An example is the need to coordinate services across community programs supported philanthropically, social services supported with government financing, and medical services supported by a health system. It can also be difficult to determine the setting in which the coordination should reside and ultimately the relationship or nature of the partnership that should exist between agencies and service organizations. Fully integrated models need to be able to coordinate a full range of services across settings and over time; they should also be funded and financed by different entities and inclusive of service providers (both clinicians and nonclinical community leaders), patients, and their caregivers.

A well-documented example of a fully integrated model is the Program for All Inclusive Care for the Elderly (PACE).[27] The PACE program is provider based and integrates both acute and long-term health care and social services. Working in contract with Medicare and Medicaid, the program is designed to support people age 55 years or older who qualify for admission to a nursing home but prefer to continue residing in the community. Other integrated models have been tested, but translation to practice will take time because evidence is promising but limited. These include medical homes, outpatient

comprehensive geriatric assessment programs, and geriatric evaluation and management programs.[28]

INTERRELATED CONCEPTS

Care coordination is a generic term that is sometimes used interchangeably both with specific types, such as case or disease management, and with related concepts that share a subset of defining attributes. The most closely related concepts and the ways they distinctly differ from care coordination are discussed here and illustrated in Figure 51-3.

At the center of the care coordination is the patient. Patient factors affecting care coordination are shown at the top in Figure 51-3. These concepts influence care coordination at the individual level and are affected by both personal and interpersonal situations; they include **Functional Ability**, **Development**, ability for **Self-Management**, **Adherence** to treatment plan, **Family Dynamics**, and the influences of **Culture**. Concepts shown at the bottom of Figure 51-3 are those related to care coordination at a community and systems level. Delivery of care is influenced and associated with **Health Care Quality**, **Evidence**-based practice, **Technology and Informatics**, **Communication**, and **Collaboration**. Access to care is determined in part by **Health Policy**, **Health Care Law**, **Health Disparities**, and **Health Care Organizations**. Additional concepts at the systems level include **Health Promotion**, **Patient Education**, and **Safety**. Each concept is associated

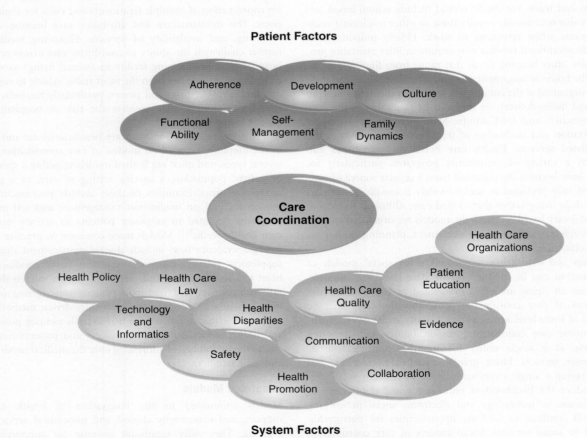

Patient Factors

Adherence · Development · Culture · Functional Ability · Self-Management · Family Dynamics

Care Coordination

Health Policy · Health Care Law · Technology and Informatics · Health Disparities · Safety · Health Promotion · Communication · Collaboration · Health Care Quality · Patient Education · Health Care Organizations · Evidence

System Factors

FIGURE 51-3 Care Coordination and Interrelated Concepts

BOX 51-1   EXEMPLARS OF CARE COORDINATION

Approaches to Care Coordination
- Case management
- Care management
- Discharge planning
- Integrated care
- Managed care
- Medical home
- Transitional care

Population Groups Most in Need of Care Coordination
- Children with special needs
- Disabled people
- Frail elderly
- High-risk pregnancy
- Preterm infant

Common Situations Requiring Care Coordination
- Catastrophic event
- Cancer care
- Cerebral vascular accident
- Chronic obstructive pulmonary disease
- Diabetes mellitus
- End-of-life care (hospice, palliative care)
- Heart failure
- Mental illness
- Myocardial infarction
- Substance use
- Traumatic brain injury

with care coordination at either the individual or the systems level and guides implementation and outcomes.

CLINICAL EXEMPLARS

The need for care coordination can be seen across the lifespan, ranging from simple plans involving just the patient and primary care provider to complex plans involving a team of specialized health care services in multiple locations. Box 51-1 presents a variety of exemplars associated with care coordination. The following featured exemplars provide insight on clinical conditions and situations associated with care coordination.

Featured Exemplars
High-Risk Pregnancy

Pregnant women who have a high-risk pregnancy are often stressed and often require more monitoring to promote the best possible outcome. Care coordination may include patient education, dietician or nutritionist referral, and coordination of specialty testing. A social work consult may be necessary for Women, Infants, and Children (WIC) and Medicaid program initiation.

Preterm Infants

Preterm infants typically have a myriad of needs. Depending on gestational age, preterm infants may be born with problems associated with breathing, feeding, temperature regulation, heart, brain, blood, and immunity. Care coordination may include specialty care, home health nursing or private duty nursing, family teaching, and social support.

Special Needs Children

Children with special needs "require interfacing among multiple care systems and individuals, including the following: medical, social, and behavioral professionals; the educational system; payers; medical equipment providers; home care agencies; advocacy groups; needed supportive therapies/services; and families."[9, e1451] Common conditions include autism, cerebral palsy, cystic fibrosis, Down syndrome, epilepsy, learning disabilities, intellectual disabilities, hearing loss, speech disabilities, and visual disabilities.

Frail Elderly

The frail and elderly spend the most health care dollars per capita. According to the Centers for Disease Control and Prevention, more than three-fourths of the geriatric population has at least one chronic disease, and half has two or more.[29] The frail and the elderly are vulnerable to negative outcomes following falls and serious illness, making this population ideal for care coordination to prevent such events.

Transitional Care

Preventing hospital readmissions through incentivized transitional care coordination is a targeted area for improvement across government initiatives and strategies, including the Affordable Care Act, the U.S. Department of Health and Human Services, and the CMS.[30] Effective communication of treatment plans and goals is essential for continuity of care. Kaiser Permanente Southern California recommends a standardized discharge summary, medication reconciliation, postdischarge hotline, postdischarge phone call within 72 hours, and timely primary care or specialist follow-up less than 7 days after discharge to reduce readmission rates.[31]

Mental illness

According to the National Alliance on Mental Illness, patients with mental illness are at increased risk of early death from treatable chronic diseases and substance use conditions; however, integrated care is lacking in the primary care setting.[32] Care coordination is beneficial for integrating behavioral health with medical care through screening, referral, and follow-up.

End of Life

End-of-life care espouses many aspects of care, including physical, psychosocial, spiritual, and cultural needs of both the patient and the family. Hospice and palliative care can take place in all health care settings, as well as in the home. Clinical guidelines of care established by the National Consensus Project for quality palliative care recommend care coordination as a key element to ensure quality communication between interdisciplinary team members and continuity of care during times of transition.[33]

CASE STUDY

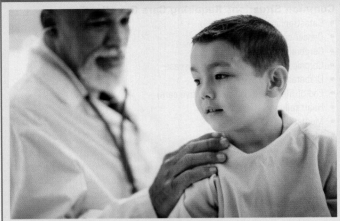

Source: Fuse/Thinkstock

Case Presentation

Shane is a 5-year-old boy who is having difficulty ascending the stairs to his family's second-story apartment. After diagnostic testing, Shane's family is informed that he has Duchene muscular dystrophy. Shane receives care from a medical home, and his team consists of a pediatrician, pediatric nurse practitioner, nurse, neurologist, physiologist, physical and occupational therapists, social worker, care coordinator, Shane, and Shane's family. The primary provider, in this case an advanced practice registered nurse (APRN), oversees the team, and the care coordinator facilitates organization. Mutually agreed upon goals include optimizing independence and attending school with his peers. The team communicates recommendations and changes in care through a patient care portal available to the medical home, inpatient, and outpatient services. This program also monitors prescriptions and provides prompts for the APRN when vaccinations and wellness activities are due.

During his initial evaluation, physical therapy makes recommendations for bracing. The social worker discusses when and how to file for social services programs such as Medicaid and disability. The social worker also contacts the local elementary school to make arrangements for bus transportation and accommodations so Shane can begin kindergarten in the fall. The care coordinator contacts the local chapter of the Muscular Dystrophy Association (MDA) for assistance with family and school support. The MDA also has supporters who assist the family's church to make the children's area accessible and help the family search for wheelchair-accessible housing within its school district. In addition, the care coordinator assists the APRN with compiling the documentation necessary for insurance approval of medications, durable medical equipment, and a physical and occupational therapy visit at the patient's home for family teaching. The care coordinator schedules a follow-up appointment in 3 months and will call Shane's mother in 3 weeks to determine if the current plan is meeting the needs of Shane and his family.

Summer camp and sports are important activities of childhood that can be facilitated through national and community programs for children with special needs. The MDA, Special Olympics, and other charitable organizations coordinate with the family and medical team to ensure safe and appropriate activities while complying with current medical treatment. When Shane enters high school, his care coordinator will work with the medical team, family, school counselor, and support group to help Shane develop a vocational plan for transitioning from school to higher education or the workforce, as well as a plan for independent living. Shane will also start transitioning from pediatric to adult care during this time; because both practices are located in his medical home, the same framework for care and electronic medical records are utilized, easing the transition and decreasing errors.

Case Analysis

This model case illustrates how Shane and his family's preferences and needs are recognized in a plan of care and met by a team of providers and services spanning health care and community-based programs supported by ongoing communication and follow-up. The case highlights the involvement of Shane's family and social network even before the disease progression necessitates.

This case presents an integrated care coordination model that spans across settings, from the medical home into the community. Although this appears to be an APN/social worker team model that addressed both social and medical needs, other clinical specialists were accessible and involved in this case to maximize wellness and respond to medical changes and hospital admissions. Community services were newly engaged to facilitate improved social and spiritual connectedness and ensure equal access to education and housing despite having a disability.

Communication is a key component of this case. Not only were the APRN and care coordinator in contact with one another and routinely in contact with the family but also an electronic health record was actively monitored for deviations from Shane's plan of care. Although not all attributes are fully presented in Shane's case, it is clear that this model of care delivery better suits his needs, particularly because he is at high risk for negative health outcomes as a child with special needs and chronic disease.

ACCESS EXEMPLAR LINKS IN YOUR GIDDENS EBOOK

REFERENCES

1. Camicia M, Chamberlain R, Finnie M, et al: The value of care coordination: A white paper of the American Nurses Association, *Nurs Outlook* 61(6):490–501, 2013.
2. Adams K, Greiner AC, Corrigan JM: *The first annual crossing the quality chasm summit: A focus on communities*, Washington, DC, 2004, National Academies Press.
3. National Coalition on Care Coordination: *Policy brief: Implementing care coordination in the Patient Protection and Affordable Care Act*, New York, 2011, New York Academy of Medicine.
4. McDonald, KM, Sundaram V, Bravata DM, et al: *Care coordination, Vol. 7: Closing the quality gap: A critical analysis of quality improvement strategies*, Technical Review No. 9, Rockville, MD, 2007, Agency for Healthcare Research and Quality.
5. Cipriano P: The imperative for patient-, family-, and population-centered interprofessional approaches to care coordination and transitional care: A policy brief by the American Academy of Nursing's Care Coordination Task Force, *Nurs Outlook* 60(5):330–333, 2012.
6. American Academy of Pediatrics, Committee on Children with Disabilities: Care coordination: Integrating health and related systems of care for children with special health care needs, *Pediatrics* 104(4):978–981, 1999.
7. Horvitz-Lennon M, Kilbourne AM, Pincus HA: From silos to bridges: Meeting the general health care needs of adults with severe mental illnesses, *Health Aff* 25(3):659–669, 2006.
8. National Quality Forum: *NQF-endorsed definition and framework for measuring care coordination*, Washington, DC, 2006, Author.
9. American Academy of Pediatrics: Patient- and family-centered care coordination: A framework for integrating care for children and youth across multiple systems, *Pediatrics* 133(5):e1451–e1460, 2014.
10. Antonelli RC, McAllister JW, Popp J: *Making care coordination a critical component of the pediatric health system: A multidisciplinary framework*, Publication No. 1277, New York, 2009, The Commonwealth Fund.
11. Bodenheimer T, Berry-Millett R: *Care management of patients with complex health care needs*, Research Synthesis Report No. 19, Princeton, NJ, 2009, Robert Wood Johnson Foundation.

12. Brown R: *The promise of care coordination: Models that decrease hospitalizations and improve outcomes for Medicare beneficiaries with chronic illnesses*, New York, 2009, National Coalition on Care Coordination.

13. Mollica RL, Gillespie J: *Care coordination for people with chronic conditions*, Baltimore, MD, 2003, Partnership for Solutions, Johns Hopkins University.

14. National Quality Forum: *Preferred practices and performance measures for measuring and reporting care coordination: A consensus report*, Washington, DC, 2010, Author.

15. Peikes D, Chen A, Schore J, et al: Effects of care coordination on hospitalization, quality of care, and health care expenditures among Medicare beneficiaries: 15 randomized trials, *JAMA* 301(6):603–618, 2009.

16. Van Houdt S, Heyrman J, Vanhaect K, et al: An in-depth analysis of theoretical frameworks for the study of care coordination, *Int J Integrated Care* 13:1–8, 2013.

17. U.S. Department of Health and Human Services and Centers for Medicare & Medicaid Services: *Medicare–Medicaid coordination office FY 2011 report to congress*, Baltimore, MD, 2011, Centers for Medicare & Medicaid Services.

18. Andersen RM: Revisiting the behavioral model and access to medical care: Does it matter? *J Health Social Behav* 36(1):1–10, 1995.

19. Wagner EH: Academia, chronic care, and the future of primary care, *J Gen Intern Med* 24(Suppl 4):636–638, 2010.

20. Institute of Medicine: *Crossing the quality chasm: A new health system for the 21st century*, Washington, DC, 2001, National Academies Press.

21. Perlin JB, Kolodner R, Roswell RH: The Veterans Health Administration: Quality, value, accountability, and information as transforming strategies for patient centered care, *Am J Managed Care* 5(4):10–24, 2005.

22. Coleman K, Austin BT, Brach C, et al: Evidence on the chronic care model in the new millennium, *Health Aff* 28(1):75–85, 2009.

23. Chisholm-Burns MA, Lee K, Spivey CA, et al: U.S. pharmacists' effect as team members on patient care: Systematic review and meta-analysis, *Med Care* 48(10):923–933, 2010.

24. Novak M, Costantini L, Schneider S, et al: Approaches to self-management in chronic illness, *Semin Dialysis* 26(2):188–194, 2013.

25. Chen A, Brown R, Archibald N, et al: *Best practices in coordinated care*, Princeton, NJ, 2000, Mathematica Policy Research.

26. Holtz-Eakin D: *An analysis of the literature on disease management programs*, Washington, DC, 2004, Congressional Budget Office.

27. Boult C, Wieland GD: Comprehensive primary care for older patients with multiple chronic conditions: "Nobody rushes you through," *JAMA* 304(17):1936–1943, 2010.

28. Boult C, Green AF, Boult LB, et al: Successful models of comprehensive care for older adults with chronic conditions: Evidence for the Institute of Medicine's "Retooling for an Aging America" report, *J Am Geriatr Soc* 57(12):2328–2337, 2009.

29. Centers for Disease Control and Prevention: *Healthy aging: Helping people to live long and productive lives and enjoy a good quality of life*, Atlanta, GA, 2011, Author.

30. Kocher RP, Adashi EY: Hospital readmission and the Affordable Care Act: Paying for coordinated quality care, *JAMA* 306(16):1794–1795, 2011.

31. Tuso P, Huynh DN, Garofalo L, et al: The readmission reduction program of Kaiser Permanente Southern California—Knowledge transfer and performance improvement, *Permanente J* 17(3):58–63, 2013.

32. National Alliance on Mental Illness: *Integration of mental health, addictions, and primary care, Policy brief*, Arlington, VA, 2011, Author. Retrieved from <http://www2.nami.org/Content/NavigationMenu/State_Advocacy/About_the_Issue/Integration_MH_And_Primary_Care_2011.pdf>.

33. National Consensus Project: *Clinical practice guidelines for quality palliative care*, ed 2, Pittsburgh, PA, 2009, Author.

Caregiving

Deborah Witt Sherman, Alexander Anzardo, Marieta Lima, and William Padron

One person caring for another represents life's greatest value.

—*Jim Rohn*

Love begins by taking care of the closest ones—the ones at home.

—*Mother Teresa*

An estimated 65.7 million Americans provide unpaid care for an adult or child with functional and/or cognitive limitations. These dedicated caregivers provide between 80% and 90% of the long-term care provided at home. Approximately 66% of caregivers are women, and 34% are men. Many caregivers of older people are also older adults themselves. Of those caring for someone older than age 65 years, the average age of the caregiver is 63 years; one-third of those receiving care are in fair to poor health, and one-third of caregivers provide care for two or more people.[1]

The need for family caregivers will escalate dramatically in the coming years because of the increase in our aging population and an overwhelmed formal health care system. People with chronic, debilitating diseases are being treated more effectively and they are living with rather than dying from these diseases. It is important for nurses to be aware of the role that caregivers play in health care delivery, the impact of this role on caregivers' lives, and supportive interventions that are needed to care for caregivers.

DEFINITION

Dentrea describes caregiving as providing unpaid support and assistance to family members or acquaintances who have physical, psychological, or developmental needs. Dentrea differentiates caregiving for a disabled child across his or her lifespan as different from routine child care, which is considered parenting.[2] Similarly, the National Alliance for Caregiving defines caregiver as "those who provide unpaid care to an adult or a child with special needs."[1,p2] The definition of caregiving offered by Hermanns and Mastel-Smith is as "a multidimensional concept that encompasses the action or process of helping those who are suffering."[3,p2] Furthermore, they explain that "caregiving is made up of actions one does on behalf of another individual who is unable to do those actions for himself or herself."[3,p5]

SCOPE

The scope of caregiving ranges from a temporary/limited caregiving role for an individual with an acute illness or condition to a long-term or permanent caregiving role (Figure 52-1). Examples of acute limiting conditions/illnesses include acute myocardial infarction, burns, influenza, pneumonia, and traumatic injuries. Chronic conditions/illnesses include dementia, including Alzheimer's disease; Parkinson's disease; cancer; diabetes mellitus; and stroke. Family caregiving is central to long-term care in the United States and the main source of assistance for the elderly and disabled. Family caregivers make enormous sacrifices to assist their loved ones and to care for them at home. Caregiving is known as the universal occupation that most of us take part in at some point in our lives.[4] It is estimated that 14% of family caregivers provide care for children with special needs younger than age 18 years, whereas 50% provide care for one's parent(s).[3]

Types of Caregivers

The caregiving role may be shared among family members so that it may be episodic. Caregivers are often categorized by their relationship to the person receiving care (care recipient). Although some caregivers may not have a familial relationship to the patient, the most common types of caregivers are spousal caregivers, adult children caregivers, grandparent caregivers, and parent caregivers.

Spousal Caregivers

Living with a chronically ill individual has an enormous impact on spousal caregivers; some studies have found that spouses experience greater levels of distress than those found in patients and they have a more pessimistic view of the patient's illness.[5] Spousal caregivers frequently find themselves having their own lifestyle interrupted and

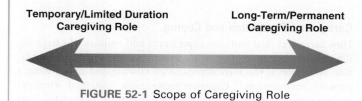

FIGURE 52-1 Scope of Caregiving Role

being emotionally affected themselves while serving as the primary caregiver for their spouse. They are commonly caring for their spouse with significant physical and/or cognitive disorders yet have their own significant health issues. With the increase in military war casualties, there is a new population of very seriously wounded service members who require extensive care and rehabilitation. Young spouses are now becoming caregivers for their husbands or wives with multiple physical injuries, including traumatic brain injuries. In addition to the physical injuries, the emotional "wounds" inflicted by war, combat stress, and the effects of the injuries are challenging for these young families. Spousal caregivers often have to face the reality that they have lost the husband or wife that they once knew.

Adult Children Caregivers

Adult children are often caregivers for their elderly parents. The increase in this phenomenon is due, in part, to medical and technological advances, which have extended life expectancy. In the United States, the population aged 65 years or older is expected to increase from 34 million in 2006 to 70 million by 2030.[1]

The impact of the caregiving role can be overwhelming for adult children caregivers who have to assume multiple roles and responsibilities while juggling employment and family responsibilities. They have to change their lives to meet the needs of their parent(s). Most adult children caregivers are in the "sandwich generation"—they must care for their children as well as their parents, either in their own home or in the home of their parents. Adult children caregivers also may experience forms of loss, including the following:

- Loss of their parent(s) as they knew him or her before the illness
- Loss of their jobs (or needing to cope with job changes)
- Change in their social networks

Adult children caregivers may be at higher risk of impaired health behaviors because their role as caregivers hinders their amount of time available for engaging in personal and preventative health behaviors.[6]

Grandparent Caregivers

Today, many grandparents are raising their grandchildren and providing care in a variety of ways. Approximately 5.8 million grandparents live with a grandchild. More than 6.5 million children throughout the United States live in households maintained by grandparents or other relatives. In approximately one-third of these homes, no parents are present.[7]

The most common reasons why grandparents become the primary caregivers are that their own children have died, have abandoned the grandchildren, have a mental illness or substance abuse problem, or are in prison. Other factors leading to grandparent-led households include child abuse and neglect. There has also been an increase in the number of pregnant teenagers unprepared for parenthood and an increase in unemployment and poverty, contributing to growing numbers of parents unable to care for their own children.[8] Grandparents are often overwhelmed in the role of caring for their grandchildren. This feeling of being overwhelmed may occur because they are

- raising their grandchildren on a fixed income and facing financial hardships;
- experiencing the effects associated with normal aging and/or the health problems that make caring for their grandchildren difficult;
- worrying about who will be the caregivers when they die or are physically unable to provide care; or
- raising children who may have mental, behavioral/emotional, or physical problems.[8]

In addition, a more subtle stressor occurs when grandparents become primary caregivers of children in that they lose the special relationship and unique role of being the grandparent. Grandparents may also be challenged with needing legal assistance and guardianship rights for their grandchildren in order to register them in school, apply for affordable housing, qualify for special community resources, and obtain medical care.

However, not all the demands of being a grandparent caregiver are negatives. Despite the challenging and stressful role grandparents endure to raise their grandchildren, aging caregivers frequently perceive caregiving as a rewarding experience.[8]

Parental Caregivers

Parental caregivers on average have been caregivers longer than those who have other relationships with their care recipient (9.5 vs. 3.8 years).[1] A primary role of parents is the provision of care for their children. However, parents become "caregivers" for their children when the children are at an age at which they would normally be expected to care for themselves. This can be due to a disability such as severe physical or cognitive limitations. It can also happen later in life from an accident (e.g., a spinal cord injury), a debilitating illness, or severe physical or emotional trauma experienced in military combat.

Stressors of parent caregivers of children will be unique to their situations. For parent caregivers of children with lifelong disabilities, stressors may include the fear of what will happen to their children when they outlive the parents. Parents of adult children who have experienced severe trauma or illness may suddenly be thrust into the parenting role again. Then these parents must decide how and when to relaunch their children into independence under a new context. Parental caregivers are in need of greater support at a community level, which can only be generated if health care practitioners and service providers have a better understanding of caregivers' experiences and perspectives.[9]

ATTRIBUTES AND CRITERIA

Concept attributes are identified characteristics that enhance a shared understanding and meaning to those discussing, observing, or experiencing the concept. In other words, attributes are the structural elements of a concept that are consistently described or observable. Antecedents describe experiences that lead to the concept, whereas consequences describe the human experience subsequent to the concept.[10]

The need for love, affection, empathy, compassion, and holistic care are identified as requisite emotions or antecedents to the concept of caregiving.[3] The attributes of the caregiver are specific to the person and are contextually based dependent on the caregiver/care recipient relationship and other relationships in the family. Caregivers have the following attributes or characteristics:

- Having the ability to care
- Adapting to a situation
- Being a good listener

- Showing affection
- Being responsible for someone other than self
- Being strong, protective, organized, patient, and understanding
- Serving as an advocate
- Assisting with activities of daily living
- Providing emotional and social support
- Managing and coordinating health care services[11]

THEORETICAL LINKS

Several theoretical frameworks have been suggested to assess the psychological burden or rewards, as well as other factors related to family caregiving. The stress process model identifies the positive and negative aspects of caregiving.[12] Caregiver stress is seen as the outcome of a multifactorial process that comprises caregiver resources, socioeconomic characteristics, and primary and secondary stressors to which a caregiver is exposed. Primary stressors are described as challenges directly related to the caregiving process, whereas secondary stressors are divided into two categories—the additional burden of roles and responsibilities external to caregiving and the psychological stress involving the depreciation of self-concept.[12]

Lazarus and Folkman proposed a theoretical model highlighting the concepts of stress, appraisal, and coping.[13,14] Stress is defined as a stimulus that can serve as a positive drive or a negative event. Stressors can be acute (sudden onset or time limited) or chronic. Prolonged caregiving is a chronic stressor. Psychological stress is a particular relationship between the person and the environment that is appraised by the person as taxing or exceeding his or her resources and endangering his or her well-being.[13,14]

The theory of caregiving dynamics describes the positive forces that make possible the change and growth of the caregiving relationship.[15] The model represents the relationship of caregiver and care recipient in the past, present, and future. The major concepts of the theoretical framework include commitment, expectation management, and role negotiation supported by the related concepts of self-care, new insight, and role support that maintains a caregiving relationship along the trajectory of an illness. Commitment refers to the caregiver intrinsic motivation to adapt and make changes to prioritize the care recipient's needs. Expectation management encompasses five dimensions: envisioning tomorrow, getting back to normal, taking one day at a time, gauging behavior, and reconciling treatment twists and turns. Role negotiation is defined as actions taken by the caregiver leading to patient recovery and independence.[15] The concepts presented in this theory serve as communication points with family caregivers, with the opportunity to explore their associated feelings and to discuss ways of promoting the caregiving experience.

CONTEXT TO NURSING AND HEALTH CARE

Caregiving involves daily demands that collectively become the experiences of the caregiver. Nurses can play an important role by maintaining an awareness of those experiences as well as connecting the caregiver with resources and providing supportive interventions for the caregiver.

Caregivers' Experience

As caregivers assume responsibilities for another person, they experience a tremendous amount of change in their lives. Caregiving involves unique experiences that may not be what most people expected during their lifetime. The realities of caregiving can be very rewarding and opportunities for positive changes or can produce a negative effect on the caregivers' physical and emotional health.

Caregivers' Perception and Coping

How caregivers deal with the experiences and realities of caregiving depends on their perception of the experience and their coping abilities. *Perception* is the mental process of viewing and interpreting a person's environment.[11] Caregiver experiences (potential stressors) are not stressful unless the individual *perceives* them as stressful. That is why what is stressful for one person may not be stressful for another. Important factors that may influence how caregivers perceive and react to the challenges of caregiving include their level of knowledge; their level of anticipatory loss and grief; and the availability of material, practical, and spiritual resources needed for self-care.[16]

Another factor that influences their perceptions and experience is their coping style and abilities. Coping can be either positive or negative. Positive coping includes activities such as exercising and spending time with friends and family. Negative coping may include substance abuse and denial.

Uncertainties and Inadequate Understanding

Caregivers often face uncertainties about the present and future along with an inadequate understanding of the disease. Caregivers simply do not know what is going to happen. For example, in the case of patients with dementia, patients' behaviors often change daily. There can be many fluctuations in the disease, especially early in its course. Sometimes the person can seem quite cognitively intact with no noticeable indication that anything is wrong. Then there may be other days when the person is combative and barely able to function. Many caregivers are unprepared to deal with variations in changes in cognitive status, and they become confused and hurt by the strange and/or difficult behaviors of the patient. Caregivers who do not understand a given diagnosis often can refuse to accept that certain symptoms are the result of a disease process.[9] This can result in caregivers feeling guilty, and they often express the idea that if they loved the person more and were more patient with him or her, then the individual would be less irritable or combative. Receiving a clear diagnosis and understanding the implications of a given disease process can provide caregivers with a sense of validation regarding their experience.[9]

Caregivers' Financial and Social Distress

Caregivers often experience negative financial consequences. The majority of family caregivers work full- or part-time. Nearly 60% of those caring for an adult older than age 50 years are working, with the majority working full-time.[17] They report late for work or leave early, need to take time off because of their caregiving responsibilities (e.g., to take their loved one to health care provider appointments), reduce their hours or take a less demanding job, decline a promotion, alter work-related travel, quit their job entirely, or take an early retirement. Grandparents find their retirement funds dwindle rapidly to cover the unexpected costs of raising their children's children. Many older adults do not have long-term care insurance, so the financial responsibilities of their care need to be paid for by the family. The caregiver may need to sell the family home to pay for health care or long-term care for the person with the disease, with their life savings quickly depleted.[18]

When caregiving responsibilities increase, caregivers may also become isolated as they sacrifice time with family and friends and give up their vacations, hobbies, social life, and sense of self. Giving up a professional career or work in general can have different consequences depending on the caregiver and his or her social support network. Evidence indicates that giving up work can in some cases increase the perceived burden and psychosocial and monetary distress.[9]

Changing Family Roles, Relationships, and Dynamics

When a person becomes very ill, his or her original roles and responsibilities in the family cannot be maintained and therefore need to be restructured. The family patriarch may no longer be able to fulfill that role; the family may struggle to find a new leader and existing roles are forced to change. For example, a woman who has never managed finances may now need to balance the checkbook. She may also need to learn how to do home and car repairs. Men, if in traditional roles, may have to learn how to cook and clean. Grandparents may also be unfamiliar with the roles of children being raised in today's world, which may be quite different from their past childrearing experiences. In addition, they may experience difficulty resolving legal issues and obtaining medical care for their grandchildren.

Many different situations exist with regard to how care is provided within a family. Some families share the responsibilities. Often, the primary care will fall to (or be designated to) one person with or without helpful (or often unhelpful) input from other family members.[11] These other family members may not be willing to be involved in the care, but their comments can be very stressful to the person who has become the primary caregiver. A common situation with spousal caregivers is that they find that their children do not help with the caregiving of their father or mother. Children may distance themselves because they cannot emotionally handle seeing their parent in a "sick" role. Parents may believe that their children are very busy with their own lives (career and children) and they cannot expect them to do anything. Spousal caregivers may believe it is their responsibility and they do not want to seem overbearing or demanding of their children.

Family members frequently do not communicate with each other about the needs of the patient or other important issues, such as the delegation of responsibilities and emotions related to the issues. This results in tension, which results in stress for the caregiver.[11] Ideally, one or several family members assume the central role of caregiver (usually a spouse or one of the care recipient's children) with the support and cooperation of the remaining members of the family. They share the burden of caregiving by providing emotional, financial, and spiritual support. They also relieve the primary caregiver for short periods of time in order to provide for respite and a recovering opportunity needed to focus and/or renew the primary caregiver's physical and emotional strength.[19]

The journey to achieve equilibrium after a drastic change that alters the family dynamics is a difficult one. Kim and Rose conceptualize this progression as family homeostasis. It involves processes and mechanisms that are based on knowledge of family dynamics, with an appraisal of those involved in the caregiving and receiving process, and the families' desire for stability or equilibrium.[19]

The burden of caregiving changes over time, requiring a constant adjustment of the family dynamics and also the relationship between the caregiver and health care providers.[20] An important issue among adult children is who will care for the mother or father. Even with the best of intentions, families can struggle. Preexisting patterns in the family, such as a history of disagreements or unresolved issues, influence how a family responds after a person is diagnosed with a disease and requires caregiving. If problems such as poor or bad relationships existed before the disease, they are probably going to worsen after the diagnosis of the disease.[21] Preexisting disagreements that are resolved during this process can help a family adjust to the new living situation and arrangements while improving communication and overall satisfaction.[21]

Influence of Culture on the Caregiving Experience

Culture permeates every aspect of the caregiving experience, from the initial demands placed on the caregiver to the final perception of the overall experience and the outcomes for the caregiver.[22] The culture in which the caregiver was socialized as a young person determines how caregiving duties are assumed, managed, and perceived. People from a culture that values individualism, competition, and independence may view the role of being a caregiver differently from people who come from collectivistic cultures in which interdependence and family take precedence over individual achievement. Although becoming a caregiver is an expectation in some cultures, caregivers in other cultures may feel captive in their role and perceive only the negative aspects of caregiving.[22]

A value shared in some cultures (e.g., Hispanic/Latino culture) is *familism*. This value refers to the central role of family in an individual's life and the individual's reliance on family as a priority. The Hispanic/Latino caregiver relies more heavily on unofficial sources of support, which include children, family members, and spouses.[23]

In addition, the support and resources that caregivers seek are largely determined by cultural values. The stressors in the caregiving experience are common to the vast majority of caregivers regardless of racial or ethnic background. However, how the caregiver perceives the situation and whether and when resources are mobilized to cope with the demands of caregiving are influenced by the cultural meaning given to the situation. The sense of duty and responsibility toward family members, especially parents, may determine whether a caregiver believes caregiving is an honor, a duty, an obligation, or a burden. The meaning attached to the caregiving experience is greatly influenced by cultural values.[24]

Outcomes of Caregiving

Caregiving can have both positive and negative consequences or outcomes. How caregivers perceive their caregiving experience may influence their abilities to focus on the positive aspects of caregiving, such as a sense of peace that they care for their family member. The caregiving experience has benefits and possible gains, but these outcomes have received little attention. The positive aspects associated with the caregiving experience may act as a buffer against overwhelming burden and traumatic grief.[25] Caregivers who have a positive approach to life are better able to cope with caregiving demands and are motivated to maintain their caregiving role.[26] A comprehensive review of quantitative studies reported post-traumatic growth of bereaved caregivers and a sense of existential meaning associated with the caregiver role, including a sense of pride, esteem, mastery, and accomplishment.[27,28] Using the stress process model, Haley and colleagues examined spousal caregiver depression and life satisfaction in the hospice setting and reported that caregivers found meaning and benefits of caregiving.[29] Concentrating on the positive aspects can "reframe" their role and help it seem more manageable and meaningful. It strengthens the bonds between caregiver and care recipient and elicits feelings of fulfillment at a personal level and satisfaction derived from the act of assisting others.[30]

In contrast, caregivers may become physically, emotionally, and financially overwhelmed with the responsibilities and demands of caring for a family member. Risk for negative, as well as positive, health events related to caregiving responsibilities is not homogeneous, and it varies depending on the activities involved and the coping abilities and resources available to caregivers.[30] Signs of caregiver stress include irritability, inability to concentrate, fatigue, and sleeplessness. Stress can progress to burnout and result in negligence and abuse of the family member by the caregiver. The combined action of multiple

BOX 52-1   Assessment of Family Caregivers

- What is your experience with being a caregiver?
- What are you doing to cope and how well are you coping?
- How well do you maintain your own nutrition, rest, and exercise?
- What is your level of social interaction versus social isolation?
- How much support do you get from outside sources (e.g., other family members, friends, church members)?
- How well are you taking care of your own health care needs (especially those with chronic illnesses of their own)?
- Are you aware of and do you use community and/or internet resources?
- Do you know about resources available for respite (someone caring for your loved one while you have time to yourself)?
- What kind of help or services do you think you need now and in the near future?

Source: Adapted from Lewis SL, Dirksen SR, Heitkemper MM, et al: *Medical-surgical nursing: assessment and management of clinical problems*, ed 9, St Louis, 2014, Mosby.

stressors, including monitoring and managing the patient's signs and symptoms, as well as emotional and spiritual needs can exhaust the caregiver's coping system and provoke a crisis for caregivers.[31] An understanding of the antecedents, attributes, and consequences of family caregiving are helpful when conducting a family caregiver assessment.

Nursing and Caregiver Support

Nursing care is framed within a holistic approach that includes the nurse, the patient, the caregiver, and the family as a whole.[32] When the nurse assesses a patient, he or she should include an assessment of the caregiver.

The nurse should listen attentively to the caregivers' stories. These stories provide clues as to what their lives are like and provide them the opportunity to share their perceptions, experiences, and coping as caregivers. Box 52-1 presents questions one may include when assessing a caregiver. The creation of a plan of care is developed in collaboration with members of the interprofessional team. The team includes, but is not limited to, the nurse; the medical doctor; physical, speech, and occupational therapists; the social worker; and a spiritual advisor or clergy. The plan of care attempts to identify the obvious and hidden needs or concerns of the caregiver and allows for the formulation of interventions that can reduce the impact of the caregiving process on the caregiver or family.[11]

Initially, caregivers may not identify with the term "caregiver." They may view themselves only as carrying out expected family responsibilities rather than as a caregiver. How does a nurse know when caregivers need help? The Alzheimer's Association has developed 10 signs of caregiver stress (Table 52-1). These are indicators that if the caregiver is not helped, he or she may develop serious health problems. Caregivers are frequently unaware that they have reached a breaking point. The first step in helping family caregivers is to identify persons as caregivers—either by health care professionals or by the caregiver him- or herself. Caregivers have been referred to as "hidden patients" because a common characteristic of caregivers is primarily having concern for their family member and often ignoring their own needs or being ignored by health care professionals.[33,34]

TABLE 52-1   Signs of Caregiver Stress

Sign	Description	What the Caregiver May Say
Denial	About the disease and its effect	"I know that Mom is going to get better."
Anger	At the person with the disease or others	"If he asks me that question one more time, I will scream."
Social withdrawal	From friends and family that once brought pleasure	"I don't care about getting together with the neighbors anymore."
Anxiety	About facing another day and what the future holds	"What happens when he needs more care than I can provide? What happens if I'm not here to provide his care?"
Depression	Begins to break the spirit and affects the ability to cope	"I don't care anymore."
Exhaustion	Makes it nearly impossible to complete necessary daily tasks	"I'm too tired to do anything."
Irritability	Leads to moodiness and triggers negative responses and reactions	"Leave me alone!!"
Sleeplessness	Caused by a never-ending list of concerns	"What if she wanders out of the house, falls, and hurts herself?"
Lack of concentration	Makes it difficult to perform familiar tasks	"I was so busy, I forgot we had an appointment."
Health problems	Begin to take their toll both mentally and physically	"I can't remember the last time that I felt good."

Source: Adapted from the Alzheimer's Association: Staying strong: Stress relief for a caregiver. Available at <http://www.alz.org/national/documents/aa_brochure_stressrelief.pdf>.

Identifying and Accessing Resources

Caregivers often need outside assistance and have difficulty asking for help because they do not want to be a burden on others; are afraid of being rejected if they ask for help; may be embarrassed or feel guilty for having a sick person in the family, especially when the disease has cognitive, memory, or behavior components; believe it is their duty to be the single provider of care; or do not have the financial resources to pay for assistance.

Many caregivers suffer in silence because they may not know *how* to ask for help or *where* to look for help, or they do not know that help is available for them. Nurses should encourage caregivers to seek and accept the support of family, friends, and community resources when needed. It is important for caregivers to understand that exhaustion and burnout are common consequences if they attempt to do everything themselves. Nurses can and should act as facilitators who can access and provide information about local, regional, and national sources of help and resources for caregivers and care receivers.[19]

In many cases of end-of-life caregiving, palliative care and hospice are options that are not mentioned or offered to the caregiver. The nurse can be in a unique position to provide information and support that can help reduce the burden of care and enhance the rewards of caregiving through the development of an individualized plan of care.[35]

Caring for the Caregiver

Another way nurses can assist caregivers is to help them to understand and cope with the stressors of caregiving. Nurses can communicate a sense of empathy to the caregiver by allowing discussion about the burdens and rewards of caregiving. According to McGuire and colleagues, there is not enough research focused on how caregiving affects the health and well-being of the caregiver. The authors state that there is need for research on post-traumatic stress disorder, differences between short- and long-term periods of caregiving burden, how caregivers react when they become receivers of care from health care professionals, and the effect of repeated episodes of caregiving responsibility.[35]

Nurses must monitor the caregiver for indications of declining health and emotional distress. A strategy to reduce stress is to help caregivers acknowledge feelings of stress and plan self-care activities.[36] Support groups provide self-help by sharing experiences and information, offering understanding and acceptance, and suggesting solutions to common problems and concerns. Encourage the caregiver to seek help from the formal social support system regarding matters such as respite care, housing, health care coverage, and finances. Respite care, which is planned temporary care for the patient, can allow the caregiver to regain a sense of equilibrium. Respite care includes adult day care, in-home care, and assisted living services. In addition, caregivers need to be encouraged to take care of themselves in all aspects of life.

Caregivers' quality of life is the cornerstone of effective caregiving interventions. Improved mental and physical health is essential in order for caregivers to continue to provide care. It is essential for health care providers to teach caregivers techniques to manage stressors and day-to-day challenges.[36] The care that nurses offer to family caregivers occurs on several levels:

- *Caring for the caregiver physically*: Nurses should reinforce the importance of eating a healthy diet at regular times, exercising to help relieve stress, and obtaining adequate sleep as essential. Lack of activity has been identified as one of the factors affecting caregivers' mood and propensity to depression.[37]
- *Caring for the caregiver emotionally*: Nurses can speak to caregivers about keeping a journal, which can help caregivers express feelings that may be difficult to express verbally. Humor is important, and its occasional use in some situations can provide distraction and relieve stress-filled situations. Humor can motivate caregivers and keep them focused on the importance of keeping a positive attitude.[9] Nurses should encourage caregivers to continue their social activities, interests, and hobbies to maintain a sense of balance in their own lives.
- *Caring for the caregiver socially*: Nurses can promote social support of caregivers. Physical contact with others provides emotional support and acknowledgment of the caregiver's own need for comfort and assurance. The main support sources for caregivers include friends, family, and health care professionals.[16]
- *Caring for the caregiver cognitively*: Nurses can encourage the caregiver to appraise his or her perception of situations and try to

maintain a positive perspective. Caregivers adapt to circumstances through a conscious procedure while dynamically making sense of the caregiving situation.[9]

- *Caring for the caregiver spiritually*: Nurses can nourish the spirits of family caregivers, help them to maintain a sense of awe about life, connect with the transcendent, and participate in spiritual or religious experiences that are important to the caregivers. Spiritual support from communities of faith can be a valuable resource for caregivers.[38]

INTERRELATED CONCEPTS

Many concepts presented in this textbook are related to the concept of caregiving and are presented in Figure 52-2.

Three concepts that are closely linked to caregiving are Family Dynamics, Culture, and Spirituality. Caregiving can trigger many changes in family structure and family roles. Culture influences a person's definition of family, the relationships among family members, and the perception of the caregiver's responsibilities or identity. Some caregivers report positive feelings such as increased self-esteem and a sense of purpose when cultural values and religiosity support positive family dynamics.[38]

Caregivers can be motivated to provide care for different reasons. Some caregivers report that their strong desire to provide care is due to a positive pre-illness/disability relationship with the care recipient and vice versa, and for others, caregiving is their main reason for living. Some may experience feelings of emptiness and lack of purpose the moment they do not have someone to care for.[9] Other reasons for Adherence to the caregiver role include feeling that their designated role is unavoidable, the need to keep a promise, or the lack of alternatives. These motives usually create a tense environment in which the caregiver may provide a minimum level of care, or there is a chance of neglect.[9] The caregiver may also feel unable to keep up with their own disease Self-Management.

Stress is the inability to cope with a perceived threat to one's mental, emotional, and spiritual well-being and can result in a series of physiological responses, including Fatigue.[39] The emotional and physical strain is caused by a person's response to pressure (stressors) in the environment. It leads to rapid changes throughout the body affecting almost every body system. Coping is the process through which a person manages the demands placed on the person–environment relationship and the emotions generated by a given situation and is influenced by a person's cognitive appraisal of an event. One's cognitive appraisal subsequently influences emotional arousal.[13,14]

Caregivers' Mood and Affect is influenced by their ability to cope with the experience. Mood swings can be expressive emotional responses to heightened tension and stress-related defensive mechanisms.[20] Caregivers may become overwhelmed and experience great Anxiety, which may result in Addictions of different kinds and may be a reflection of caregiver burnout, low self-esteem, or a history of psychosocial problems exacerbated by the act of caregiving.[40]

Establishing effective Communication between the caregiver, the care receiver, and the health care provider is essential in order to support the positive aspects of caregiving and minimize negative aspects.[20] Through an effective communication channel, all involved parties can be educated so that they can be aware of all of the complex intricacies of the caregiving process and understand the responsibilities associated with caregiving. Health Promotion is the expected result of an effective communication process and education.[20]

Deciding which is the right moment to request a Palliative Care consult in the case of patients with declining health status can make a major difference in the health care and treatment decisions going

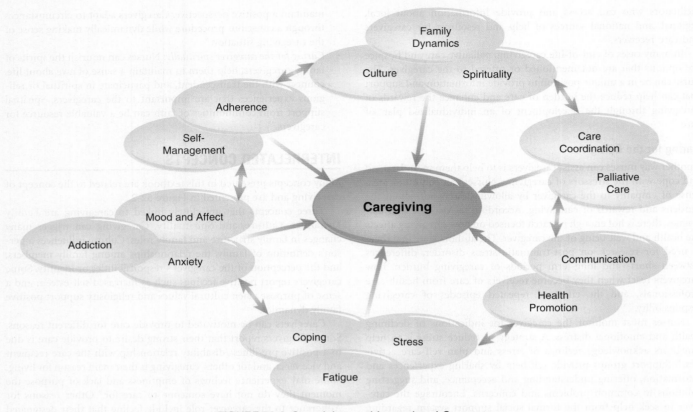

FIGURE 52-2 Caregiving and Interrelated Concepts

forward. Vigilant exploration of worrisome signs and symptoms and the analysis of functional and physical limitations can signal the need for the involvement of a palliative care specialist in order to coordinate the care that is appropriate on a case-by-case basis.[41] Care Coordination can be achieved when the needs of the patient and his or her family caregivers are discussed with other members of the interprofessional team. The results are positive outcomes for patients and their caregivers and efficient use of health care resources.[42]

CLINICAL EXEMPLARS

A wide variety of conditions and situations contribute to the need for an individual to require caregiving, and the variability in the level of care needed is influenced by multiple variables, including age and underlying health status. Although it is not possible to list all conditions or illnesses that require caregiving, Box 52-2 presents very common exemplars. It is beyond the scope of this textbook to describe all exemplars listed, but some of the most important are featured here.

Featured Exemplars
Impaired Physical Mobility
Many diseases and rehabilitative states involve some degree of immobility.[32] Examples include strokes, traumatic injuries, multiple sclerosis, Parkinson's disease, Huntington's disease, amyotrophic lateral sclerosis, and cerebral palsy.[43] With impaired mobility, individuals experience a decrease in muscle mass, strength, and function; their joints become stiffer and contracted; and their gait changes. The restrictions on movement affect the performance of activities of daily living (ADLs), and in some medical conditions or advanced medical conditions care recipients are totally dependent on caregivers.[32]

BOX 52-2 CAREGIVING EXEMPLARS

Short-Term Caregiving Needs
- Acute myocardial infarction
- Burn injury
- Influenza
- Pneumonia
- Recovery from surgery
- Sepsis
- Traumatic injury (nondisabling)

Long-Term Caregiving Needs
General Chronic Conditions
- Blindness
- Cancers
- Chronic kidney disease
- Chronic obstructive pulmonary disease
- Diabetes
- Heart failure

Impaired Cognitive Status
- Alzheimer's disease
- Dementia
- Huntington's disease
- Traumatic brain injury
- Stroke

Impaired Physical Mobility
- Amputation
- Amyotrophic lateral sclerosis
- Cerebral palsy
- Multiple sclerosis
- Parkinson's disease
- Stroke
- Spinal cord injury
- Traumatic brain injury

Mental Health Conditions
- Depression (severe)
- Post-traumatic stress disorder
- Schizophrenia
- Substance abuse

Impaired Cognitive Status

Changes in cognition can be highly stressful for caregivers. Individuals with moderate to severe changes in their level of cognition often require special care, which includes 24-hour-a-day supervision, special communication techniques, and management of their difficult behaviors.[32] They can become aggressive and unpredictable, and they will become totally dependent on their caregivers for assistance of ADLs, which include bathing, eating, transferring from bed to a chair or wheelchair, toileting, and other personal care.[44] Examples include traumatic brain injury, dementia, Alzheimer's disease, Parkinson's disease, and stroke.

Post-Traumatic Stress Disorder

Post-traumatic stress disorder (PTSD) occurs when individuals are exposed to traumatic events that engender extreme levels of fear for the safety of self and others. Although PTSD is treatable, it can become a chronic and disabling condition. In severe cases, PTSD leads to disability, and individuals may experience symptoms such as nightmares, hyperarousal, re-experience reminders of the trauma, flashbacks of the event, and increased startle reflexes. After a traumatic injury or experience, individuals must cope with psychological and physical factors, prolonged hospital stays, delayed recovery time, and treatment-related stressors. Frequently, the combination of physical and psychological factors can be disabling for the affected individual, and he or she becomes the responsibility of a caregiver.[45]

Impaired Respiratory Function

Impaired respiratory function can be the result of several diseases and conditions. Examples include chronic obstructive pulmonary disease, pneumonia, asthma, and cystic fibrosis.[32] Respiratory failure can be acute or chronic. In severe cases of lung disease, long-term care may be needed to provide continuous breathing support through mechanical ventilation. In the majority of these cases, individuals who require mechanical ventilation or continuous oxygen support to sustain their lives require the assistance of formal and informal caregivers.[32]

Substance Abuse

Substance abuse refers to the damaging and harmful use of psychoactive substances, including alcohol and illicit drugs.[46] The negative consequences of drug abuse are not only limited to the abuser; rather, they influence the families of the abuser particularly. Family members have an increased prevalence of experiencing domestic violence, stress, family cohesion problems, and, in the case of children, behavioral problems. In addition, close family members of drug-addicted individuals sometimes become the sole caregivers of abusers due to financial, legal, and physical restraints.[47]

CASE STUDY

Source: ands456/iStock/Thinkstock

Case Presentation

Maria, age 44 years, recently immigrated from the Caribbean to south Florida to live with her parents, grandmother, aunt, sister, and two teenage sons. Maria is a single mother and is struggling to find employment due to her language barrier. The family's main source of income is the Social Security benefits obtained from her parents, grandmother, and aunt. The Social Security pensions that the family receives are currently the minimum amount assigned by the federal government due to the limited employment histories of the retirees. Maria's father, Joseph, age 74 years, had stomach cancer 5 years ago and requires weekly injections of vitamin B12 and a specialized diet to maintain his nutritional health. Maria's 72-year-old mother, Luisa, suffers from depression and does not help around the house. Maria's grandmother recently turned 100 years old and requires moderate assistance with her activities of daily living. Approximately 1 month ago, Maria's 83-year-old Aunt Elsa (who has advanced Alzheimer's disease) suffered a subdural hematoma as a result of a fall. After 1 month in the trauma unit and the inpatient rehabilitation center, Aunt Elsa's Medicare benefits expired and she had to be relocated home because the family could not afford her care in a skilled inpatient facility. Elsa's health condition has deteriorated significantly since her accident. She now has a tracheotomy tube, requires permanent oxygen, tube feedings, and needs 24-hour care due to her bedbound status. Maria's sister Laura is 52 years old, unemployed, and undergoing chemotherapy for breast cancer. Laura has a 15-year-old daughter, whose father lives in another country and does not provide any financial support.

Three months after Maria arrived in the United States, her sister Laura passed away from breast cancer, leaving Maria in charge of the entire household, which now consists of three teenagers currently attending high school and three elderly individuals.

Six months after Maria's arrival from the Caribbean, she gained 30 pounds. She constantly complains that food has been the only pleasure in her life for the past 6 months. Maria now has become the sole caregiver of her entire family. She is always stressed, and she constantly complains to her sons and niece that she has no help and that she has become a slave as a punishment by God. Sometimes, she spends the entire day without speaking to anyone, and whenever she has a chance, she locks herself in her room to eat and watch TV.

Case Analysis

Maria is in a highly stressful situation as the family caregiver, and she is in a depressive state. In her current situation, she has limited coping abilities and resources. She needs to find support outside of her home. Maria needs assistance from a social worker, who can assist her with finding financial and medical resources to care for her elderly family members. Finding a senior day care center for her parents and grandmother would be beneficial to her. She could also make arrangements with a home health company to provide skilled nursing services for her aunt who requires 24-hour care. Maria may also benefit from joining an online caregiver support group. Maria is at risk for poor physical and emotional health due to the stresses of caregiving. Her culture may influence her perceptions about caregiving and the need to sacrifice her life for the well-being of her children, parents, and extended family. In multigenerational families, the role of caregiving often falls on the oldest daughter. A caregiver assessment is important in order to provide Maria much needed physical, emotional, and financial support. The well-being of her family is dependent on Maria's well-being. Palliative care addresses the patient and the family as the unit of care. Maria would benefit from a palliative care consult to support her in the caregiving role.

ACCESS EXEMPLAR LINKS IN YOUR GIDDENS EBOOK

REFERENCES

1. National Alliance for Caregiving: *Executive summary: Caregiving in the U.S.*, 2009. Retrieved from <http://www.caregiving.org/pdf/research/CaregivingUSAllAgesExecSum.pdf>.
2. Dentrea P: Caregiving. In *Blackwell encyclopedia of sociology*, 2007. Retrieved from <http://www.blackwellreference.com/public/tocnode?query=caregiving&widen=0&result_number=1&fields=content&from=search&type=std&id=g9781405124331_yr2012_chunk_g97814051243319_ss1-7>.
3. Hermanns M, Mastel-Smith B: Caregiving: A qualitative concept analysis. *Qualitative Rep* 17(75):1–18, 2012.
4. Family Caregiver Alliance: *Caregiving*, 2015. Retrieved from <https://caregiver.org/caregiving>.
5. Kuenzler A, Hodgkinson K, Zindel A, et al: Who cares, who bears, who benefits? Female spouses vicariously carry the burden after cancer diagnosis. *Psychol Health* 26(3):337–352, 2011.
6. Do EK, Cohen SA, Brown M: Socioeconomic and demographic factors modify the association between informal caregiving and health in the sandwich generation. *BMC J* 14:362, 2014.
7. Generations United: *Grandfacts: Data, interpretation, and implications for caregivers*, 2011. Retrieved from <http://www2.gu.org/OURWORK/Grandfamilies.aspx>.
8. Janicki MP, McCallion P, Grant L, et al: Grandparent caregivers I: Characteristics of the grandparents and the children with disabilities for whom they care. *J Gerontol Social Work* 33(3):35–55, 2008.
9. Williams KL, Morrison V, Robinson CA: Exploring caregiving experiences: Caregiver coping and making sense of illness. *Aging Mental Health* 18(5):600–609, 2014.
10. Bonis SA: Concept analysis: Method to enhance interdisciplinary conceptual understanding. *Adv Nurs Sci* 36(2):80–93, 2013.
11. Sherman DW, Cheon J: Family caregivers. In Matzo M, Sherman DW, editors: *Palliative care nursing: Quality care to the end of life*, ed 4, New York, 2014, Springer, pp 147–167.
12. Pearlin LI, Mullan JT, Semple SJ, et al: Caregiving and the stress process: An overview of concepts and their measures. *Gerontologist* 30:583–594, 1990.
13. Lazarus S, Folkman S: *Stress, appraisal, and coping*, New York, 1984, Springer.
14. Lazarus S, Folkman S: The relationship between coping and emotion: Implications for theory and research. *Social Sci Med* 26(3):309, 1988.
15. Williams LA: Whatever it takes: Informal caregiving dynamics in blood and marrow transplantation. *Oncol Nurs Forum* 34:379–387, 2007.
16. Epiphaniou E, Hamilton D, Bridger S, et al: Adjusting to the caregiving role: The importance of coping and support. *Int J Palliative Nurs* 18(11):541–545, 2012.
17. MetLife Mature Market Institute & National Alliance for Caregiving: *The MetLife caregiving cost study: Productivity losses to U.S. business*, 2006. Retrieved from <http://www.caregiving.org/data/Caregiver%20Cost%20Study.pdf>.
18. Kapp MB: For love, legacy, or pay: Legal and pecuniary aspects of family caregiving. *Care Manage J* 14(3):205–208, 2013.
19. Kim H, Rose KM: Concept analysis of family homeostasis. *J Adv Nurs* 70(11):2450–2468, 2014.
20. Rosser M, Walsh H: *Fundamentals of palliative care for student nurses*, Hoboken, NJ, 2014, Wiley-Blackwell.
21. Moore H, Gillespie A: The caregiving bind: Concealing the demands of informal care can undermine the caregiving identity. *Social Sci Med* 116:102–109, 2014.
22. U.S. Department of Health and Human Services, Office of Minority Health: *What is cultural competency?* 2015. Retrieved from <http://minorityhealth.hhs.gov/omh/browse.aspx?lvl=1&lvlid=6>.
23. Aranda M, Knight B: The influence of ethnicity and culture on the caregiver stress and coping process: A sociocultural review and analysis. *Gerontologist* 37(3):342–354, 1997.
24. Arevalo-Flechas LC: Factors influencing Latino/Hispanic caregivers' perception of the experience of caring for a relative with Alzheimer's disease, *Dissert Abstr Int*, DAI-B 69/06 (UMI 3311328), 2008.
25. Higginson IJ, Gao W: Caregiver assessment of patients with advanced cancer: Concordance with patients, effect of burden and positivity. *Health Qual Life Outcomes* 6:42–51, 2008.
26. Stajduhar KI, Martin WL, Barwich D, et al: Factors influencing family caregivers' ability to cope with providing end-of-life cancer care at home. *Cancer Nurs* 31(1):77–85, 2008.
27. Stajduhar K, Funk L, Toye C, et al: Part 1: Home-based family caregiving at the end of life: A comprehensive review of published quantitative research (1998–2008). *Palliative Med* 24(6):573–593, 2010.
28. Funk L, Stajduhar K, Toye C, et al: Part 2: Home-based family caregiving at the end of life: A comprehensive review of published qualitative research (1998–2008). *Palliative Med* 24(6):594–607, 2010.
29. Haley WE, LaMonde LA, Han B, et al: Predictors of depression and life satisfaction among spousal caregivers in hospice: Application of a stress process model. *J Palliative Med* 6(2):215–224, 2003.
30. Buyck J, Bonnaud S, Boumendil A, et al: Informal caregiving and self-reported mental and physical health: Results from the Gazel Cohort Study. *Am J Public Health* 101(10):1971–1979, 2011.
31. Li Q, Mak Y, Loke A: Spouses' experience of caregiving for cancer patients: A literature review. *Int Nurs Rev* 60(2):178–187, 2013.
32. Gulanick M, Myers J: *Nursing care plans: Diagnosis, interventions, and outcomes*, ed 8, St Louis, 2013, Mosby.
33. Saban K, Sherwood P, DeVon H, et al: Measures of psychological stress and physical health in family caregivers of stroke survivors: A literature review. *J Neurosci Nurs* 42(3):128–138, 2010.
34. Van Vliet D, de Vugt ME, Bakker C, et al: Impact of early onset dementia on caregivers: A review. *Int J Geriatr Psychiatry* 25(11):1091–1100, 2010.
35. McGuire D, Grant M, Park J: Palliative care and end of life: The caregiver. *Nurs Outlook* 60(6):351–356, 2012.
36. Lewis S, Miner-Williams D, Novian A, et al: A stress-busting program for family caregivers. *Rehabil Nurs* 34(4):151–159, 2009.
37. Mausbach B, Roepke S, Chattillion E, et al: Multiple mediators of the relations between caregiving stress and depressive symptoms. *Aging Mental Health* 16(1):27–38, 2012.
38. Hebert R, Weinstein E, Martire L, et al: Religion, spirituality and the well-being of informal caregivers: A review, critique, and research prospectus. *Aging Mental Health* 10(5):497–520, 2006.
39. Seaward BL: *Managing stress: Principles and strategies for health and well-being*, ed 7, Burlington, MA, 2011, Jones & Bartlett.
40. Lowder J, Buzney S, Buzo A: The caregiver balancing act: Giving too much or not enough. *Care Manage J* 6(3):159–165, 2005.
41. Leblanc TW, Currow DC, Abernethy AP: On Goldilocks, care coordination, and palliative care: Making it "just right." *Primary Care Respir J* 23(1):8–10, 2014.
42. Masso M, Owen A: Linkage, coordination and integration: Evidence from rural palliative care. *Aust J Rural Health* 17(5):263–267, 2009.
43. Arsenault L, Magafas M, Gulanick M: *Nursing diagnosis care plans*, ed 4, St Louis, MO, 2012, Mosby.
44. Family Caregiver Alliance: *Alzheimer's disease*, 2012. Retrieved from <https://caregiver.org>.
45. Mabey L, Servellen G: Treatment of post-traumatic stress disorder in patients with severe mental illness: A review. *Int J Mental Health Nurs* 23(1):42–50, 2014.
46. World Health Organization: Substance abuse. In *Health topic*, 2015. Retrieved from <https://www.who.int/topics/substance_abuse/en>.
47. American Psychological Association: *Family members of adults with substance abuse problems*, 2015. Retrieved from <http://www.apa.org/pi/about/publications/caregivers/practice-settings/intervention/substance-abuse.aspx>.

Palliative Care

Deborah Witt Sherman, Lucy Caicedo, Grethell Estrada,
Alissette Naveda, and Iliana Pena

The issues affecting the care of patients with serious, life-threatening, and chronic illness are expected to intensify during the next several decades, particularly given the aging population. It is predicted that by 2030, for the first time in history, people aged 65 years or older will outnumber the young.[1] Unlike a century ago, when most people died of infections, accidents, or other rapidly lethal diseases, the leading causes of death in the United States are now cardiovascular disease, cancer, cerebrovascular diseases, chronic obstructive lung disease, unintentional injuries, and dementia.[2] From a global perspective, it is estimated that 40 million people worldwide will need palliative care as a result of chronic, noninfectious diseases.[3]

Palliative care is becoming a part of mainstream health care in the United States. It is a highly structured and organized system of care intended to address the physical, emotional, social, cultural, and spiritual needs of patients and families experiencing serious, life-threatening, progressive or chronic illness.[4] Palliative care is offered across the lifespan, and across the illness trajectory from the diagnosis of serious disease to the bereavement period for families.[5] All nurses at every educational level must become generalists in palliative care, and some may choose to become educated and certified as specialists in palliative care.[6] Along with other members of the interdisciplinary team, palliative care practitioners combine their clinical judgment and expertise with the best level of evidence available through research and an understanding of patients' wishes and preferences, known as evidence-based care.[7]

DEFINITION

Palliative care is a holistic approach to care that focuses on the physical, emotional, social, cultural, and spiritual needs of both the patient and his or her family members across the illness trajectory.[4] The Worldwide Palliative Care Alliance supports the World Health Organization's definition of palliative care:

> *Palliative care is an approach that improves the quality of life of patients and their families facing the problem associated with life-threatening illness, through the prevention and relief of suffering by means of early identification and impeccable assessment and treatment of pain and other problems, physical, psychosocial, and spiritual.*[8]

The definition of palliative care recognizes not only the needs of patients and family members experiencing cancer but also its use and integration into the symptomatic management of chronic and end-stage organ diseases such as end-stage heart, lung, liver, or kidney disease, as well as neurodegenerative diseases or life-threatening infections such as HIV/AIDS.[3] Like hospice, palliative care was originally associated with end-of-life care or when curative treatments were no longer beneficial, effective, or desirable. However, in its current conceptualization, palliative care cures what illnesses can be cured, and it alleviates or relieves the symptoms of the disease or its associated treatment.[4] For example, it is unlikely that advanced ovarian cancer in a 94-year-old woman is curable or even treatable. However, a urinary tract infection causing delirium and pain to the woman may be cured with antibiotic therapy. With most advanced illness, patients become highly symptomatic, and palliative care needs intensify until the end of life.[8]

SCOPE

The changing demographics of populations, changing illness trajectories, advances in health care, and longer life expectancies have created a need for palliative care offered across the lifespan, from neonates to the frail elderly. Although palliative care was originally derived from the concept of hospice care, which focuses on the last 6 months of life, palliative care is offered across many health settings and the continuum of care from the time of diagnosis with a life-threatening illness until death and into the bereavement period for families.[9] Hospice now is recognized as a type of palliative care existing for patients at the end of life.

In the past, when cure of a disease was no longer considered possible and the prevalent medical thought was that "there is nothing more that we can do," the patient was offered "comfort," "supportive care," or "end-of-life" care. Remembering that not all patients want to enroll in "hospice" care or are eligible for the hospice Medicare benefit, a new type of care emerged termed "palliative" care. The term *palliative care* means to "cloak," "soothe," or "alleviate" the pain and suffering associated with serious, progressive, life-threatening or chronic illness.[10] Through the work of the National Consensus Project for Quality Palliative Care, which began in 2004, it was recognized that palliative and hospice care are part of a continuum of care, with palliative care beginning "upstream" at an earlier point in the illness trajectory. However, palliative care, like hospice care, can continue until the end of life in the care and support of patients and families.[4]

ATTRIBUTES AND CRITERIA

Palliative care is a comprehensive, holistic interprofessional approach to care of patients and families across the lifespan who have serious, life-threatening, progressive, or chronic illness or conditions.[11] Palliative care can transform the current disease-focused approach to a patient-centered philosophy, in which the needs of the patient and patient and family goals become essential to planning the patient's care.[12] Patient-centeredness broadens the focus of care and requires well-defined coordination across specialties and disciplines as well as access to palliative care physicians and nurses.[12] To promote, maintain, and even restore the patient's and family's quality of life, an interprofessional approach to care is of value. Optimal functioning of a team requires outstanding training, communication, and a description of the tasks and responsibilities of each team member.[13] Palliative care encompasses the following attributes: (1) total, active, and individualized care; (2) support for the family; (3) interdisciplinary team approach; and (4) effective communication.[14] Further attributes of palliative care include the following:

- Optimal assessment and management of physical and psychological symptoms (i.e., pain, dyspnea, nausea/vomiting, constipation, anxiety, agitation, and depression)
- Honoring the wishes and preferences of families and developing a comprehensive and individualized plan of care
- Assisting patients in identifying the goals of care and the completion of living wills or the appointment of a health care proxy
- Promoting communication among patient, families, and members of the interdisciplinary team
- Promoting continuity of care for transitions to home or other settings[6]

THEORETICAL LINKS

The conceptualization of palliative care, based on the National Consensus Project for Quality Palliative Care (NCP),[4] is broader than end-of-life care and stresses the need for palliative interventions earlier in the disease trajectory in conjunction with curative or disease-specific therapies. Palliative interventions can slow disease progression, maximize the benefits of treatment, and even prolong life. The NCP generated a clinical document that can be used as the theoretical framework for palliative care clinical practice, education, and research by setting the standard for palliative care across the lifespan and health care settings. The guidelines promote high-quality care; reduce variation in new and existing programs; encourage continuity of care across settings; and facilitate collaborative partnerships among palliative care programs, community hospices, and a wide range of other health care delivery settings.[4] Another goal of the guidelines is to promote recognition, stable reimbursement structures, and accreditation initiatives through projects such as the National Quality Forum (NQF).[15]

The NCP[4] and the NQF[15] work together to advance palliative care by formalizing the concept of palliative care and differentiating it from other types of care. The eight domains of the NCP guidelines can serve as a theoretical framework and are presented in Box 53-1. These domains have been cited in the growing body of literature regarding palliative care.[16] During the past few years, many organizations have implemented the clinical guidelines into practice and operationalized the domains to provide optimal palliative care.[4]

According to Fawcett, the use of a theoretical framework or conceptual model provides consistency in nursing by facilitating

---

BOX 53-1   National Consensus Project Guidelines

1. Structure and processes of care (i.e., offering holistic, comprehensive health care by an interprofessional team; education of generalists and specialists in palliative care; and patient–family focused care, including patient education)
2. Physical aspects of care (i.e., assessing and managing pain and other symptoms related to disease or its treatment)
3. Psychological and psychiatric aspects of care (i.e., assessing and managing anxiety, depression, and other common psychological symptoms or normal psychological reactions of patients/families to serious illness, and including the care of family caregivers associated with grief and bereavement)
4. Social aspects of care (i.e., conducting a family assessment, and facilitating patient/family meetings with members of the interdisciplinary team to provide information, discuss goals of care, offer support, and implement socially focused plans of care)
5. Spiritual, religious, and existential aspects of care (i.e., assessing spiritual needs of patients and families, religious practices or rituals, while providing spiritual and existential support)
6. Cultural aspects of care (i.e., conducting cultural assessments to determine locus of decision making and preferences of patient or family regarding the disclosure of information and truth-telling, language, and rituals)
7. Care of the imminently dying patient (i.e., recognizing and treating symptoms of the patient during the active dying phase while preparing family caregivers of the physical and psychological transitions that occur at the end of life; ascertaining and documenting patient/family wishes about site of death; and providing bereavement support to caregivers)
8. Ethical and legal aspects of care (i.e., determining and documenting patient/surrogate preferences for goals of care, treatment options, and setting of care; promoting advanced care planning; and signing of advance directives)

Source: Data from National Consensus Project for Quality Palliative Care: *Clinical practice guidelines for quality palliative care*, Pittsburgh, PA, 2013, Author.

---

communication and a mechanism that promotes a systematic approach to nursing practice, education, and research.[17] Mid-range theories also provide frameworks that can guide clinical care and research for patients with significant physical and psychological symptoms.[18] The theory of comfort is a humanistic, holistic theory that is based on human needs.[19] Comfort is defined in this model as the state of having addressed basic needs for ease, relief, and transcendence met in four contexts of experience: physical, psychospiritual, sociocultural, and environmental.[19] For example, physical comfort needs are physiological mechanisms that are disrupted; therefore, the palliative care team provides comfort measures directed at achieving homeostasis (e.g., fluid and electrolyte imbalance due to chemotherapy-induced nausea and vomiting). Palliative care practitioners pay close attention to the comfort needs of a patient by assessing pain and suffering and providing comfort measures.

CONTEXT TO NURSING AND HEALTH CARE

In 2011, more than 20.4 million people needed palliative care, 69% of whom were older than 60 years of age and 6% were children.[8] Millions of Americans are living with one or more chronic debilitating diseases, and 7 out of 10 Americans can expect to live with their diseases several years before dying.[12] When coupled with the advancing age of the 8 million baby boomers, who now qualify for Medicare, this will create a huge demand on health care resources and community-based services. These demands will force changes in patterns of care for patients living for several years with chronic illness and their complications before dying.[5] The early referral to palliative services can make a difference in the treatment approach, resulting in positive health care outcomes even in the face of serious illness or impending death. Nurses and primary care providers have an essential role in providing education to patients and family to facilitate their engagement in early palliative care when appropriate.[20]

Palliative Care as a Team-Based Approach

To promote quality of life, the comprehensive needs of patients and families are addressed by an interprofessional palliative care team. Interdisciplinary palliative care is characterized by a collaborative effort that includes information exchange and coordinated care planning; it actively places the patient and family at the center of team deliberations and maximizes the unique contributions of each member. Services commonly offered by the palliative care team are presented in Box 53-2. The central focus of the team is to engage and partner with patients and families to be able to provide effective and efficient care coordination.[6] The interdisciplinary team must have an appropriate number of dedicated and trained staff available for consultation and dedicated to provide quality palliative care.[13] It is also recommended that training must include cultural awareness and competence in order to deliver a culturally sensitive care.[21] The palliative care team often represents a variety of disciplines, including the following:

- *Nurses*—who assess and evaluate the ongoing needs of the patient and family, including physical, emotional, social, cultural, and spiritual well-being; advocate for the patient and family; and provide referrals to other health professionals when needed
- *Primary care practitioners*—who may be physicians or nurse practitioners and provide comprehensive and holistic assessment, diagnosis, management, or treatment of diseases and conditions or problems while working closely with nursing and other members of the interdisciplinary team.
- *Specialty services*—who may also be physicians or advanced practice nurses from diverse specialty services or who are specialists in palliative care providing consultation to the primary care team to offer

aggressive symptom management, related to illness treatments and comorbidities.
- *Social services*—who are social workers providing psychological care for the patient and family, helping to identify areas of need, such as communication, behavioral issues, educational, financial, guardianship, and other legal issues, including assistance with housing and access to community support and resources. In the event of death, social workers also provide support with the grief and bereavement process.[22]
- *Spiritual care*—who are members of the clergy, chaplains, and other spiritual advisors providing spiritual counseling and support for the patient and his or her family, as well as other members of the interdisciplinary team when they experience moral or ethical distress. Spiritual issues often are intertwined with other patient symptoms and can be masked by both physical and psychoemotional responses. Spiritual care goes beyond identification of the patient's or family's faith background to an understanding of the meaning and purpose in life, sense of hope, faith, love, trust, and forgiveness.[10] All health care providers can offer compassionate care that touches the human spirit of patients and families, whereas spiritual care providers have a deep understanding of human emotional and spiritual needs and issues.
- *Ancillary services*—who are other members of the health care team and support the care offered to patients and families. These roles include case managers, psychologists, psychiatrists, nutritionists, and nursing assistants; physical, speech, and occupational therapists; child life, art, and music therapists; pharmacists; bereavement counselors; family support specialists; and volunteers.[23]

All members of the interdisciplinary team contribute their expertise and knowledge in assisting patients and family members to establish goals of care and identify treatment wishes and preferences that facilitate patient/family choice and autonomy.[4,24]

National Strategic Direction for Palliative Care

The Institute of Medicine's 2014 report regarding the care of patients with serious and advanced illness recommended that the provision of palliative care should be covered by every health insurer.[25] Furthermore, standards of care should be evidence-based and continuously updated based on emergent research findings, and health care providers must achieve competence in palliative care. Thus, at least generalist-level palliative care competencies should be achieved by all nurses and other health care providers across all health care settings.[25]

The U.S. Department of Health and Human Services (USDHHS) commissioned a task force to recommend and produce a strategic framework to improve the health status of Americans living with concurrent multiple chronic conditions (MCCs).[1] The USDHHS aims to change the culture or produce a paradigm shift and implement new strategies that will provide a foundation to support and maintain optimal health and quality of life for patients with MCCs.[1] To achieve this vision, the following four overarching goals have been identified:

1. Provide better tools and information to health care and social service workers who deliver care to individuals with MCCs
2. Maximize the use of evidence-based, self-care management strategies and resources
3. Foster health care and public health system changes to improve health
4. Support research to fill knowledge gaps about individuals with MCCs[1]

Changing Models of Care

Changes in care models will require attention to the cost-effective management of chronic diseases and their associated symptoms.[1]

BOX 53-2 Common Palliative Care Services

- Access to community resources
- Advance directives
- Assessment
- Care coordination
- Counseling (patient and/or family)
- Family therapy
- Identification of goals for care
- Nutrition support
- Occupational therapy
- Pain management
- Patient/family teaching
- Patient safety
- Physical therapies
- Prevention of disease exacerbations
- Rehabilitation
- Respite services
- Speech therapy
- Symptom management

When palliative care is consulted at the time of diagnosis of a life-threatening condition or disease, quality of care is strengthened and quality of life is improved for patients and their families.[26]

The biomedical approach to chronic disease management typically has a curative rather than palliative care focus. Curative care is evidence-based and traditionally and historically practiced in routine health care, and it provides the familiar and expected approach to disease management.

The hospice care model was initially based on the cancer disease trajectory in which there are clear and obvious indications of decline based on the effects of metastatic disease and associated therapies. Patients who live with chronic disease states, such as congestive heart failure and chronic obstructive pulmonary disease (COPD), often experience disease exacerbations and remissions that ultimately have a poor prognosis. Patients who follow this disease trajectory often live for several years with their chronic disease and have varying fluctuations in their functional status. Each time these patients encounter an exacerbation of their disease and enter into the acute care setting, their disease becomes less responsive to curative or disease-specific measures. Furthermore, traditional curative treatments provided to patients with chronic and life-limiting conditions do not comprehensively address the countless patient and family needs throughout the trajectory of the disease. As such, the value of palliative care is the combination of curative, disease-specific, and comfort/supportive therapies offering quality care to the end of life.[20]

In addition to the care of adults, pediatric palliative care is focused on providing quality care to children with life-threatening, life-limiting chronic conditions by providing symptom management and emotional and spiritual support.[21] In the pediatric population, obtaining early referrals for palliative care can be a challenging process. Some nurses and practitioners in pediatrics do not feel comfortable communicating with parents regarding palliative care initial referral and services. Parents may still have the misconception that palliative care is their last resource and they feel guilty about "giving up" on the hope for a cure for their child. Therefore, it is important to improve communication with patients, families, and health care providers to increase their understanding of palliative care and its services. In pediatric and adult patient populations, collaboration between inpatient palliative care teams and community palliative services providers is essential for a successful transition from hospital to home.[21,23]

For individuals receiving palliative care across the lifespan, continuous evaluation of the care plan by members of the interdisciplinary team is necessary to ensure that it reflects "best practices" and "evidence-based" interventions while recognizing and addressing the individual needs of patients and families facing life-threatening illness across the illness–dying trajectory.

INTERRELATED CONCEPTS

Palliative care is a concept that is related to numerous concepts in this book. Using domains of the NCP as a framework, Figure 53-1

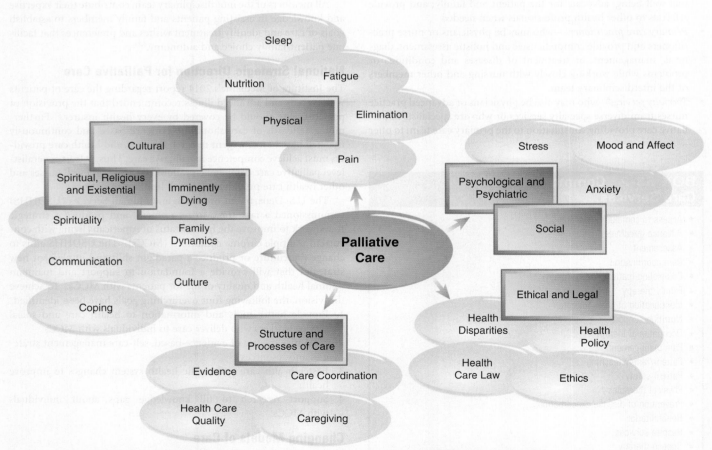

FIGURE 53-1 Palliative Care and Interrelated Concepts Using the National Consensus Project for Quality Palliative Care as a Framework

identifies the relationship between palliative care and other nursing concepts.

The structure and processes of care domain focuses on interdisciplinary team engagement and collaboration with patients and family members. Concepts such as Evidence, Health Care Quality, Caregiving, and Care Coordination are appropriately included in this domain. The use of evidence supports high-quality interventions in palliative care, resulting in improved quality of life.

The physical, psychological, psychiatric, and social domains focus on the assessment and treatment of the whole person. These domains integrate a variety of concepts, such as Fatigue, Sleep, Nutrition, Elimination, Pain, Mood and Affect, Anxiety, and Stress. These concepts present common symptoms and difficulties for patients in palliative care and require the best thinking of palliative care practitioners.

The cultural, spiritual, religious, existential, and imminently dying domains relate to the concepts Culture, Spirituality, Coping, Family Dynamics, and Communication. Again, the interdisciplinary team must be competent and able to deal with these issues along with any physical and psychological concerns of the patient and family.

The ethical and legal domains relate to the concepts of Ethics, Health Disparities, Health Care Law, and Health Policy because palliative care should be accessible to all individuals.

CLINICAL EXEMPLARS

There are multiple clinical examples of palliative care that are seen in diverse clinical settings. Box 53-3 identifies some of the most common exemplars in which palliative care is practiced. Some of the most important exemplars in which the patient and family would benefit from an either generalist level or specialist level of palliative care include cancers, end-stage organ diseases, neurode-

generative disorders, and infectious diseases such as HIV/AIDS. It is beyond the scope of this concept presentation to describe each exemplar in detail; however, breast cancer, leukemia, chronic obstructive lung disease, Alzheimer's disease, and stroke are presented as featured exemplars.

Featured Exemplars
Breast Cancer

Breast cancer is the most common cancer in women.[27] Depending on the stage of the disease, the patient needs support with the management of symptoms that may result from surgery, chemotherapy, and/or radiation. Palliative care also assists patients with psychosocial needs such as anxiety, depression, and possible concerns regarding changes associated with body image experienced by many breast cancer patients.[28]

Leukemia

Leukemia is a type of cancer that originates in the bone marrow and can present in an acute or chronic form, affecting children or adults. Often, children and their parents find it extremely difficult to accept the diagnosis of cancer given a young age. Members of the palliative care team spend considerable time talking to the young patient and teaching parents how to speak to their child about this serious illness, in addition to addressing their physical and emotional needs.[28]

Chronic Obstructive Pulmonary Disease

This disease actually refers to a group of lung diseases in which the airways and lungs become damaged, making it difficult for those affected to effectively breathe. The symptoms associated with the disease include shortness of breath, low oxygen in the blood, cough, pain, weight loss, and risk of lung infections. Patients may also experience depression, anxiety, insomnia, and social isolation due to the symptoms that accompany this disease. Reduction in symptoms is a key role of the palliative care team. Palliative care can also help by educating patients and their families regarding not only the pharmacologic management of COPD but also nonpharmacologic management such as use of fans, posture and positioning, respiratory hygiene, and relaxation techniques to lessen associated anxiety.[29]

Alzheimer's Disease

This disease is a type of dementia diagnosed primarily in older adults and in which patients suffer from progressive cognitive impairment, memory loss, and decreased level of functioning with all activities of daily living. Patients and families can benefit from palliative care by receiving symptom management, family support, and education regarding creation of a safe environment. The palliative care approach includes services such as cognitive retraining, physical therapy, and guidance to maintain a daily routine, which are all important to maintaining or protecting cognitive function.[30]

Stroke

Stroke occurs with a cerebral vascular accident in which there is ischemia to the brain. Stroke may happen suddenly, leaving patients and their families faced with life-altering challenges. Physically, patients may experience varying degrees of paralysis or weakness. Depending on the affected area of the brain, patients may also experience physical, emotional, behavioral, and motor sensory effects. Palliative care provides holistic care of the patient and family to help them cope with the residual effects of stroke while guiding them as to what to expect with regard to recovery and establishing a realistic plan of care.[30]

■■■ BOX 53-3   EXEMPLARS OF PALLIATIVE CARE

Adults
- Alzheimer's disease and other dementias
- Cancer
- Chronic obstructive pulmonary disease
- Chronic kidney disease
- Heart failure
- HIV/AIDS
- Liver failure
- Parkinson's disease
- Stroke
- Traumatic brain injury

Infants, Children, Adolescents
Chronic, Progressive, Degenerative, Malignant, Life-Threatening, or Life-Limiting Conditions
- Cerebral palsy
- Congenital malformations
- Chromosomal abnormalities
- Childhood cancers
- Cystic fibrosis
- Muscular dystrophies
- Severe traumatic brain injury
- Sickle cell disease

CASE STUDY

Source: Buccina Studios/
Photodisc/Thinkstock

Case Presentation

Patricia Thompson is a 46-year-old female who is married and has two adolescent children. Three years ago, she was diagnosed with stage II adenocarcinoma of the right lung, which was surgically removed. Mrs. Thompson has a long history of smoking. Although she quit smoking for a while following her lung cancer diagnosis, she started smoking again due to stress. Recently, she began having increased dyspnea, especially with exertion, and was diagnosed with COPD. A pulmonary function test suggested moderate staging of COPD (FEV_1 <70% predicted). Her laboratory analysis revealed normal values for her complete blood count and chemistries. However, she has had significant weight loss of 11 pounds during the past 6 months.

At this time, Mrs. Thompson complains of moderate to severe dyspnea, generalized weakness, insomnia, and depression. She states that her symptoms are very uncomfortable; that she is unable to work; and that she has become more homebound, engaging in limited family or church and community activities. These symptoms have impacted her activities of daily living, as well as her ability to care for her family. She needs to rest frequently, often sitting up in a chair even at night, which is upsetting to her husband. Mrs. Thompson's coping strategy is denial of the seriousness of her illness, which is of concern to her husband and children as they witness her significant physical and functional decline.

Following an appointment with the adult nurse practitioner in the oncology clinic, a comprehensive assessment indicates that Mrs. Thompson has not been taking her prescribed medications because of financial issues and her depressed mood. The nurse practitioner also learned that her husband decreased his hours of work to take care of his wife and the children. The nurse practitioner recognized the need for a referral to the ambulatory palliative care team and consulted with the social worker, dietitian, and spiritual advisor for additional assessment and supportive palliative care interventions. The nurse practitioner prescribed a pharmaceutical management regimen that included the following:

- Long-acting bronchodilator (maintenance medication) used for COPD and dyspnea
- Short-acting bronchodilator (rescue medication) for immediate dyspnea relief
- Short-term titrated systemic corticosteroid medication to improve breathing and also improve mood and appetite
- An antidepressant to be used at bedtime, which could also improve the patient's insomnia

After 1 month of coordinated palliative care, Mrs. Thompson has made positive improvement in her physical, emotional, social, and spiritual well-being. She has been provided education about the disease process and the importance of treatment adherence. She is now more willing to follow her plan of care, including a smoking cessation plan, which has improved her dyspnea and other symptoms. Mrs. Thompson has increased energy and has started to engage in the care of herself and her family. She has been able to sleep through the night and has gained seven pounds. The family has been actively involved in working with the social worker to access community support and resources. This interprofessional approach to care has allowed an effective management of the patient's symptoms, improvement of her and her family's quality of life, and the ability to gain and maintain a state of wellness despite illness.

Case Analysis

The case illustrates the effects of multiple chronic conditions on a person's life. Mrs. Thompson's symptoms, including insomnia, dyspnea, depression, and weakness, were preventing her from participating in activities of daily living and in regular community activities. Using an interprofessional and palliative care approach, the goals of reducing the symptoms associated with cancer and COPD and improving quality of life of a patient and family have been met.

ACCESS EXEMPLAR LINKS IN YOUR GIDDENS EBOOK

REFERENCES

1. U.S. Department of Health and Human Services: *Multiple chronic conditions—A strategic framework: Optimum health and quality of life for individuals with multiple chronic conditions*, Washington, DC, 2010, Author.
2. National Center for Health Statistics: *Health, United States, 2010: With special feature on death and dying*, Hyattsville, MD, 2011, Author.
3. Humphreys G: Push for palliative care stokes debate. *Bull World Health Organ* 91(12):902–903, 2013.
4. National Consensus Project for Quality Palliative Care: *Clinical practice guidelines for quality palliative care*, Pittsburgh, PA, 2013, Author.
5. Sherman DW, Bookbinder M, McHugh M: Palliative care: A response to the need for health care reform in America. In Matzo M, Sherman DW, editors: *Palliative care nursing: Quality care through the end of life*, ed 4, New York, 2014, Springer, pp 21–32.
6. Sherman DW, Matzo M, Metheny T: The interprofessional practice of palliative care nursing. In Matzo M, Sherman DW, editors: *Palliative care nursing: Quality care through the end of life*, ed 4, New York, 2014, Springer, pp 3–20.
7. Sherman DW, Evans S, Halstead L, et al: Palliative and hospice care. In *The Maryland comprehensive cancer control plan*, Baltimore, MD, 2011, Maryland Department of Health and Mental Hygiene.
8. Worldwide Palliative Care Alliance: *Global atlas of palliative care at the end of life*, 2014. Retrieved from <http://www.who.int/cancer/publications/palliative-care-atlas/en>.
9. Sherman DW, Free D: Nursing and palliative care. In Hank G, Cherny N, Christakis N, et al, editors: *Oxford textbook of palliative medicine*, ed 4, New York, 2014, Oxford University Press.
10. Sherman DW, Free D: Culture and spirituality as domains of palliative care. In Matzo M, Sherman DW, editors: *Palliative care nursing: Quality care through the end of life*, ed 4, New York, 2014, Springer, pp 91–128.
11. Teitelbaum HS, Travis LD, Heilig DL, et al: The epidemiology of hospice and palliative care. *Dis Mon* 59(9):309–324, 2013.
12. Grant M, Elk R, Ferrell B, et al: Current status of palliative care—Clinical implementation, education, and research. *CA Cancer J Clin* 59(5):327–335, 2009.
13. Vissers KC, Brand M, Jacobs J, et al: Palliative medicine update: A multidisciplinary approach. *Pain Pract* 13(7):576–588, 2013.
14. Meghani SH: A concept analysis of palliative care in the United States. *J Adv Nurs* 46(2):152–161, 2004.
15. National Quality Forum: *Palliative and end of life care consensus report*, 2014. Retrieved from <http://www.qualityforum.org>.
16. Reed SM: A unitary-caring conceptual model for advanced practice nursing in palliative care. *Holist Nurs Pract* 24(1):23–34, 2010.

17. Fawcett J: Criteria for evaluation of theory. *Nurs Sci Q* 18(2):131–135, 2005.

18. Peterson SJ, Bredow TS: *Middle range theories: Application to nursing research*, Philadelphia, 2009, Lippincott Williams & Wilkins.

19. Kolcaba KY: A taxonomic structure for the concept comfort. *Image J Nurs Sch* 23(4):237–240, 1991.

20. Wittenberg-Lyles E, Goldsmith J, Ragan S: The shift to early palliative care. *Clin J Oncol Nurs* 15(3):304–310, 2011.

21. Crozier F, Hancock LE: Pediatric palliative care: Beyond the end of life. *Pediatr Nurs* 38(4):198–227, 2012.

22. Paul S: Public health approaches to palliative care: The role of the hospice social worker working with children experiencing bereavement. *Br J Soc Work* 43(2):249–263, 2013.

23. American Academy of Pediatrics: Pediatric palliative care and hospice care commitments, guidelines, and recommendations. *Pediatrics* 132(5):966–972, 2013.

24. Hospice and Palliative Nurses Association: *HPNA position statement: Value of the professional nurse in palliative care*, 2013. Retrieved from <http://www.HPNA.org>.

25. Hinds PS, Meghani SH: The Institute of Medicine's 2014 Committee on Approaching Death report: Recommendations and implications for nursing. *J Hosp Palliat Nurs* 16(8):543–548, 2014.

26. Callaway C: Timing is everything: When to consult palliative care. *J Am Acad Nurse Pract* 24(11):633–639, 2012.

27. Centers for Disease Control and Prevention: *Breast cancer statistics*, 2014. Retrieved from <http://www.cdc.gov/cancer/breast/statistics>.

28. Guthrie A: Cancer. In Matzo M, Sherman DW, editors: *Palliative care nursing: Quality care through the end of life*, ed 4, New York, 2014, Springer, pp 269–294.

29. Brennan M: Chronic lung disease. In Matzo M, Sherman DW, editors: *Palliative care nursing: Quality care through the end of life*, ed 4, New York, 2014, Springer, pp 329–346.

30. Kovach K, Reynolds S: Neurological disorders. In Matzo M, Sherman DW, editors: *Palliative care nursing: Quality care through the end of life*, ed 4, New York, 2014, Springer, pp 347–372.

Health Disparities

Eun-Ok Im and Sangmi Kim

Health disparities refer to gaps in the quality of health and health care among population groups that often parallel differences in socioeconomic status, racial/ethnic background, and education level. Health disparities are prevalent throughout the world between countries and within countries. For example, when comparing the countries Malawi and Japan, there is a 36-year gap in life expectancy (47 years in Malawi compared to 83 years in Japan).[1] Within countries, health disparities occur by social status, family income, race/ethnicity, gender, disability, or sexual orientation.[1] Significant health disparities in the morbidity and mortality of the U.S. population exist. The Centers for Disease Control and Prevention reports health disparities and inequalities in various diseases; risk factors; environmental factors; social and behavioral determinants; and health care access by sex, race/ethnicity, income, education, disability status, and other social characteristics.[2] For example, premature death (before age 75 years) from stroke and coronary heart disease is higher in non-Hispanic African Americans compared to non-Hispanic whites.[2] As another example, the incidence of diabetes is highest among men, those aged older than 65 years, non-Hispanic African Americans, those of mixed race/ethnicity, and the disabled.[2]

Health disparities have long been a focus of nursing care; in fact, a number of nursing studies on health disparities in various populations have been conducted.[3,4] However, health disparities have rarely been explored as a major concept in nursing. When PubMed was searched with key words of "health disparity," "nursing," and "concept analysis," only 4 articles were retrieved, and only 1 of these was a concept analysis of health disparities.[5] Even when the search was expanded with the key words of "health disparity," "nursing," and "concept," only 14 articles were retrieved, and only 2 articles pertained to the concept of health disparity.[5,6] Here, the concept of health disparities is examined in the context of nursing.

DEFINITION

Various definitions of health disparities exist in the literature. For example, the National Institute of Health defined health disparities as "differences in the incidence, prevalence, mortality, and burden of diseases and other adverse health conditions that exist among specific population groups in the U.S."[6] The Institute of Medicine defined health disparities as "racial or ethnic differences in the quality of health care that are not due to access-related factors or clinical

needs, preferences, and appropriateness of intervention."[7] In *Healthy People 2020*, health disparities are defined as "differences that occur by gender, race or ethnicity, education or income, disability, living in rural localities, or sexual orientation."[8] The Health Resources and Services Administration provides a definition of health disparities as "population-specific differences in the presence of disease, health outcomes, or access to care."[9]

Common to these definitions is the notion of differences in health status between one or more population groups compared to a more advantaged group, and most mention social justice and equity as components. Since the mid-1990s when the term health disparities first came into use, it has generally been assumed to refer to health or health care differences between racial/ethnic groups, including differential access to screening and/or treatment options, or unequal availability of culturally or linguistically knowledgeable and sensitive health personnel.[10,11] However, equating health with health care draws attention primarily to diseases and health care services to alleviate the existing health inequality in the United States and could overlook the contribution of social determinants of health (e.g., race/ethnicity, socioeconomic status, or gender) to health disparities. Because the delivery of health care is a major source of health disparities, the term *health care disparities* is often used. Both terms and their distinctions are necessary to an understanding of the impact of health disparities in nursing practice. The term health care disparities is defined as

> *differences in the quality of care received by minorities and non-minorities who have equal access to care—that is, when these groups have similar health insurance and the same access to a doctor—and when there are no differences between these groups in their preferences and needs for treatment.[7]*

SCOPE

From the broadest and most simplistic perspective, the scope of health disparities is represented by unavoidable and avoidable disparities (Figure 54-1). In some cases, this categorization can be easily applied. For example, disparity in health outcomes by age may be unavoidable because aging as the biological process is not subject to intervention. However, in reality, this type of categorization does not represent the contextual factors that must be considered. For example, disparity in

FIGURE 54-1 Scope of Health Disparities

health outcomes due to unsafe living environments could be an avoidable cause of inequality. An avoidable disparity raises ethical questions of needless harm and justice. Indeed, many health disparities are avoidable, and continuous efforts are necessary to identify existing health disparities that are preventable.

ATTRIBUTES AND CRITERIA

Carter-Porkras and Baquet asserted that health disparity should be viewed by "a difference in environment, access to, utilization of, and quality of care, health status, or a particular health outcome that deserves scrutiny."[12,p427] These criteria could be used to identify health disparity. That is, if differences are observed in "environment, access to, utilization of, and quality of care, health status, or a particular health outcome,"[12] then we could say that a health disparity might exist.

Before determining existence of a health disparity, however, it is required to examine if the identified difference is inequality or inequity. Inequality does not necessarily mean being inequitable; health inequities indicate "differences in health, which are not only unnecessary and avoidable, but, in addition, are considered unfair and unjust."[13,p220] Thus, Whitehead's seven determinants of health disparities are useful as attributes for health disparity:[13]

1. Natural, biological variation
2. Health-damaging behavior that is freely chosen
3. The transient health advantage of one group over another when one group is first to adopt a health-promotion behavior
4. Health-damaging behavior in which the degree of choice of lifestyles is severely restricted
5. Exposure to unhealthy, stressful living and working conditions
6. Inadequate access to essential health services and other basic services
7. Natural selection, or health-related social mobility, involving the tendency for sick people to move down the social scale

The determinants of health disparity by Health Canada are also useful attributes to determine existing health disparity (although some overlap with Whitehead's determinants exists).[13,14] These include income and social status; social support networks; education; employment and working conditions; social environments; physical environments; personal health practices and coping skills; healthy child development; biology and genetic endowment; health services; gender; and culture.

THEORETICAL LINKS

There are several different theories associated with health disparities that are used in nursing, and each theory has strengths and limitations in explaining health disparities.[15] Three prominent theories used in nursing to explain health disparities are presented here.

The Social–Ecological Model

The social–ecological model aims to explain dynamic interrelations among various personal and environmental factors. This model

basically evolved from the ecological systems theory of child development by Bronfenbrenner, who proposed five socially organized subsystems related to human development: microsystem, mesosystem, exosystem, macrosystem, and chronosystem.[16,17] Each of these five systems interacts within the context of the person's life and provides diverse options and sources of growth. The interactions within and between systems are bidirectional and have impact from and toward the person. The mesosystem is beyond the dyad or two-party relation and links over two systems that a person lives.[16,17] Also, mesosystems link the structures of the person's microsystem. The macrosystem consists of cultural values, customs, and laws, and includes the overall patterns of ideology and organization that distinguish an individual society or social group.[16,17] The chronosystem includes time as a dimension as it relates to environmental contexts.[16,17] The chronosystem could be either external or internal. For instance, the timing of a family member's death could be an external chronosystem, and physiological changes due to aging could be an internal chronosystem.

The social–ecological model has been widely used in nursing research and practice related to health disparities because it provides an understanding of interrelationships of individuals and systems, and it can provide a perspective to identify health disparities at each system level and directions for interventions at each system level. For example, the social–ecological model allows nurses to identify cultural barriers in access to health care at the level of macrosystem and to develop an intervention to tackle the cultural barriers to reduce subsequent health disparities.

The Structural–Constructivist Model

The structural–constructivist model is based on an assumption of dual nature of human existence.[15] The model adopts a constructivist perspective that the reality of life is based on a mental representation constructed by combinations of socially shared understandings within a society. Simultaneously, the model adopts a structural perspective that people are constrained by the external structures in which they are embedded (e.g., social relations created by the shared and distributed expectations of others). Health disparities literature featuring this model asserts that the concept of race/ethnicity is socially or culturally constructed with the underlying logic that when we can control the ways in which race/ethnic groups differ, racial/ethnic disparities will disappear. This perspective/model strongly supports the idea of social and cultural construction of race/ethnicity that frequently results in health disparities observed in health care systems,[18,19] and it gives direction for nursing research and practice in understanding health disparities in both clinical and community settings.

The Cultural Competence Model

The cultural competence movement grew out of early efforts to bridge the divide between the largely biomedical, white, middle-class American culture perspectives of clinicians and the perspectives of patients (mainly immigrants) whose experience and language put them at a substantial cultural distance from American health care.[20]

BOX 54-1 Key Elements of Cultural Competence for Individual Interactions and Organizations

Interpersonal Interactions
- Explore and respect patient beliefs, values, meaning of illness, preferences, and needs
- Build rapport and trust
- Find common ground
- Awareness of one's own biases/assumptions
- Knowledgeable about different cultures
- Awareness of health disparities and discrimination affecting minority groups
- Use of interpreter services when needed

Organizations
- Diverse workforce reflecting the diversity of patient populations
- Health care facilities convenient and attentive to communities
- Language assistance available for patients with limited English proficiency
- Ongoing staff training regarding the delivery of culturally and linguistically appropriate services

Source: From Saha S, Beach MC, Cooper LA: Patient centeredness, cultural competence and healthcare quality. J Natl Med Assoc 100(11):1275–1285, 2008.

Cultural competence expanded in the late 1980s through the 1990s in three ways. First, the populations of interest expanded from primarily immigrants to essentially all racial/ethnic minority groups. Second, the conceptual boundary expanded beyond culture per se to such issues as prejudice, stereotyping, and the social determinants of health. Third, the scope expanded beyond the interpersonal domain (between patients and health care providers) to health systems and communities. Cultural competence in health care entails (1) understanding the importance of sociocultural influences on patients' health beliefs and behaviors, (2) considering how these factors interact at multiple levels of the health care delivery systems (organizational, structural, and clinical), and (3) devising interventions that take these issues into account to ensure the delivery of high-quality health care to diverse patient populations.[21]

Despite the existence of several different models of cultural competence, several key elements are shared at interpersonal and organizational levels (Box 54-1).[20] Interpersonal interactions focus on the ability of a provider to bridge cultural differences to build an effective relationship with a patient. Health care organizations focus on meeting the needs of diverse groups of patients. Nevertheless, the cultural competence model has been criticized due to its exclusive emphasis on health care providers to improve health disparities.[22]

CONTEXT TO NURSING AND HEALTH CARE

Health disparities seen in the context of nursing and health care largely represent health care disparities. These are seen in various nursing settings and/or situations and are roughly categorized as unavoidable and acceptable, unavoidable and unacceptable (unjust), avoidable and acceptable, and avoidable and unacceptable.

Unavoidable and Acceptable

The health disparities that are unavoidable and acceptable should not be a concern for nurses. For example, in an emergency room, nurses could observe health disparities in emergency visits by age; in general, older people make more emergency visits compared with younger people. In this situation, age becomes a determinant of the disparity, and aging is unavoidable and acceptable.

Unavoidable and Unacceptable

Health disparities that are unavoidable and unacceptable can also happen in health care settings and should be a concern for nurses. For example, the high prevalence of diabetes among Hispanic populations might be partially due to genetic factors so that such a disparity in the prevalence of diabetes could be unavoidable. However, health disparity due to differences in access to health care for diabetes treatment is unacceptable, which raises a concern for nurses.

Avoidable and Acceptable

Most health disparities that are avoidable are not viewed as acceptable, and these situations are rare in health care. However, there are unique or unusual circumstances in which avoidable health disparities could be viewed as acceptable. For example, a health disparity could exist among people involved and those not involved in a natural disaster. When a natural disaster occurs, unequal health outcomes among residents in the affected area may be acceptable even though the disaster and resultant health disparity could be avoidable.

Avoidable and Unacceptable

Health disparities that are avoidable and unacceptable unfortunately occur in health care settings, and these are the targets of interventions. For example, a disparity in cancer pain management exists between Asians and whites. This difference is attributable to Asian cultural values and attitudes related to cancer pain and pain medication distinguished from the cultural values of whites. The disparity is avoidable if Asian cancer patients are adequately educated and instructed on cancer pain management strategies, including pain medication and complementary and alternative medicine. Also, this disparity is unacceptable because this gives an unnecessary burden of pain to Asian cancer patients that could be easily managed by using existing strategies. Several avoidable and unacceptable disparities are worth further exploration from the perspective of health care disparities because they are frequently seen and experienced by nurses.

Lack of Health Insurance and High Health Care Costs

Health insurance is the most significant contributing factor to poor quality of care. Uninsured people are less likely to get adequate care for disease prevention (e.g., cancer screening, dental care, counseling about diet and exercise, and flu vaccination) and/or for disease management (e.g., diabetes care management), and they are more likely to visit the emergency department and be admitted to the hospital for ambulatory care-sensitive conditions.[23,24] Many racial/ethnic, low socioeconomic status (SES), and other minority groups lack adequate health insurance compared with their counterparts. For example, Hispanics and non-Hispanic African Americans have substantially higher uninsured rates compared to Asian/Pacific Islanders and non-Hispanic whites.[2] Also, minorities are disproportionately enrolled in lower cost health plans that place greater per-patient limits on health care expenditures and available services.[7]

Even with health insurance, the financial burden of health care is high and continuously increasing. High premiums and out-of-pocket payments can be a significant barrier to accessing needed medical treatment and preventive care.[23] From 2006 to 2011, the percentage of people younger than age 65 years whose family's health insurance premium and out-of-pocket expenses were more than 10%

of total family income was more than 3.5 times as high for poor individuals and low-income individuals and more than twice as high for middle-income individuals compared to that of high-income individuals.[23]

Language Barriers

Patients who face language and cultural barriers are less likely than others to have a usual source of medical care. They receive preventive services at reduced rates and have an increased risk of nonadherence to medication. Among patients with psychiatric conditions, those who encounter language barriers are more likely than others to receive a diagnosis of severe psychopathology.[25] Ad hoc interpreters, including family members, friends, untrained members of the support staff, and strangers found in waiting rooms or on the street, are commonly used in clinical encounters. However, the use of such unqualified interpreters results in increased medical errors, less effective patient–clinical provider communication, and poorer follow-up and adherence to clinical instructions, as well as possible conflicts with patient privacy rights.[25,26]

Lack of Transportation to Health Care Providers

The lack of access to affordable transportation could physically isolate people of color, households in rural areas, and people with disabilities from health care facilities. It also forces families to spend a large percentage of their budget on cars and other expensive options rather than actual health care costs. An increasing number of people are unable to reach health care providers and health care services because they reside in non-walkable areas with limited public transportation. Individuals of low SES, households in rural areas, and people with disabilities could face significant hurdles because many cannot drive and/or because public transportation is often unavailable, inaccessible, or unreliable.[27]

The poorest one-fifth of U.S. families spend approximately 42% of their income on transportation. This massive expenditure on transportation can wipe out their already limited budget for out-of-pocket medical expenses, nutritious foods, and healthy recreational activities. Because affordable housing is increasingly located far from main transportation lines and jobs, low-income people and people of color are more likely to have long commutes, which reduces their time for exercise, shopping for healthy foods, and additional earning opportunities.[27]

Provider–Patient Communication

Sociocultural differences between health care providers and patients often influence patient and provider communication. People from different backgrounds frequently have differences in their recognition of symptoms, thresholds for seeking care, comprehension of management strategies, expectations of care (e.g., preferences for or against diagnostic and therapeutic procedures), and adherence to preventive measures and medications.[28] Furthermore, patients with different sociocultural backgrounds from those of health care providers may not feel comfortable asking questions or disclosing personal health information. Due to the pressures of a fast-paced clinical setting, health care providers frequently experience difficulty determining what the patient does not understand and addressing this knowledge gap adequately. The printed health information materials that are frequently used in an effort to bridge the knowledge gap may be too complex or scientific for patients to understand.[29,30] Thus, when sociocultural differences between health care providers and patients are not appreciated or communicated effectively in clinical encounters, patient dissatisfaction, poor adherence, poorer health outcomes, and racial/ethnic disparities in health care easily happen.[28]

Biased Clinical Decision Making

Clinical decisions are shaped by the attributes of patients (e.g., age, sex, SES, race/ethnicity, language proficiency, religion, nationality, and insurance status), health care providers (e.g., specialty, level of training, clinical experience, age, sex, and race/ethnicity), and practice settings (e.g., location, organization of practice, form of compensation, performance expectations, and incentives).[28,31] Thus, health disparities, especially health care disparities, often result from health care providers' bias or prejudice against minorities, greater clinical uncertainty when interacting with minority patients, and beliefs or stereotypes about the health or health behaviors of minority patients. If a health care provider has difficulty accurately understanding his or her patient's symptom(s) or is less sure of his or her patient's signal, then the provider is likely to place greater weight on his or her prior beliefs, which may differ by the provider's age, gender, SES, and race/ethnicity, than on information gathered in a clinical encounter. This reliance on prior beliefs may result in discordance between health services and patient needs.[7]

Stereotyping often leads to biased clinical decision making. Stereotyping refers to the process by which people use social categories (e.g., gender or race/ethnicity) in acquiring, processing, and recalling information about others. Both implicit and explicit negative attitudes and stereotypes of health care providers significantly shape interactions with patients, influence how information is recalled, and guide expectations and inferences in systematic ways.[7] Stereotyping often occurs subconsciously, unlike prejudice or discrimination. If it is left unchecked, stereotyping has a detrimental clinical effect on certain groups deemed as less worthy of diagnostic or therapeutic procedures or resources.[28]

Biased clinical decision making also derives from the bias in health care, operationalized as discrimination on the basis of patient attributes. Patients with certain sociodemographic features have a propensity to be assessed, diagnosed, referred, and treated not only differently but also at a lower level of quality or to a lesser degree of adherence to established standards of care than different groups of people with comparable health problems.[31]

Prejudice, which refers to unjustified negative attitudes based on a person's group membership, is another source of biased clinical decision making. An example of prejudice related to race/ethnicity is the belief that African American patients are less intelligent, less educated, more likely to abuse drugs and alcohol, more likely to fail to comply with medical advice, and more likely to lack social support than white patients, regardless of an individual patient's actual income, education, and personality.[7]

Patient's Mistrust and Refusal

In response to historical factors of discrimination, segregation, and medical experimentation or to real/perceived mistreatment by health care providers, African American patients may convey mistrust, refuse treatment, or comply poorly with treatment. As a result, health care providers may become less engaged in the treatment process such that patients are less likely to be provided with more vigorous treatments and services.[7]

INTERRELATED CONCEPTS

Many concepts discussed in this book are interrelated to the concept of health disparities. Some of the most closely interrelated are presented in Figure 54-2 and described further. Health disparities is closely linked to Culture. Nursing scholars have suggested that marginalization due to cultural differences could decrease the

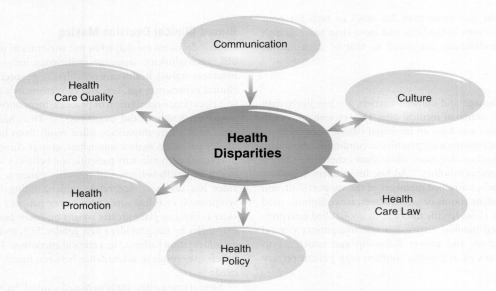

FIGURE 54-2 Health Disparities and Interrelated Concepts

opportunities to receive equitable health care, which subsequently leads to health disparities.[21,32] They also claim that marginalization due to cultural differences and subsequent disadvantages including financial, environmental, and linguistic barriers result in health disparities.[32–34] Furthermore, cultural differences frequently give rise to issues with Communication between health care providers and patients, and the miscommunication could cause health disparities.[33] Stereotypes, bias, or prejudice of health care providers can be activated or increased by miscommunication with patients, which can then lead to diminished Health Care Quality provided to the patients.[33]

The lack of Health Promotion in disadvantaged populations (e.g., physical inactivity of African American adolescents in poor urban areas) also results in health disparities.[2] The poor health outcomes or increased morbidity and mortality among ethnic minorities are frequently due to lack of health promotion activities and/or risky health behaviors in these populations.[2] Health Policy and Health Care Law powerfully influence health care utilization, particularly for vulnerable populations including minorities, people with low SES, and people with disabilities. The Affordable Care Act exemplifies the critical role of health policies and health care laws in addressing health disparities. The Affordable Care Act is expected to extend health insurance coverage to an additional 25 million people by 2019.[35]

CLINICAL EXEMPLARS

Unfortunately, there are many examples of health disparities. Although there are many types of health disparities, only the avoidable and unacceptable health disparities are presented in Box 54-2 because these are the ones that health care providers, including nurses, frequently encounter in clinical and community settings. Furthermore, these are the health disparities that health care providers need to target to intervene. A detailed discussion of each exemplar of health disparities is beyond the scope of this textbook; however, some of the most important exemplars across the age span are briefly described here.

Featured Exemplars
Unequal Receipt of Early and Adequate Prenatal Care

Early and adequate prenatal care is defined as the prenatal care initiated by week 28 of pregnancy and in which a woman has at least 80% of the expected number of prenatal visits.[23] Early and adequate prenatal

---

BOX 54-2 EXEMPLARS OF HEALTH DISPARITIES

- Breast cancer mortality
- Breast cancer screening
- Diabetes
- Early and adequate prenatal care
- Health care access
- Health insurance coverage
- Cardiovascular disease
- Immunizations
- Infant, fetal, and perinatal mortality
- Invasive cervical cancer
- Obesity
- Pain management
- Pap smear screening
- Pregnancy-related mortality rate
- Preterm birth rates
- Preventive care
- Prostate cancer mortality
- Quality of palliative care

---

care helps to promote healthy pregnancies through screening and management of risk factors and conditions and through education and counseling on healthy behaviors during and after pregnancy. Common barriers to getting prenatal care as early as desired (or at all) are limited resources, transportation issues, and not knowing that one is pregnant.[36]

Unequal Receipt of Recommended Immunizations

Immunization protects recipients from illness and protects others in the community who are not vaccinated. Beginning in 2007, the recommended vaccines that should be completed by the age of 19–35 months include diphtheria–tetanus–pertussis vaccine, polio vaccine, measles–mumps–rubella vaccine, *Haemophilus influenza* type B vaccine, hepatitis B vaccine, varicella vaccine, and pneumococcal conjugate vaccine.[23] However, the 2013 *National Healthcare Disparities Report* documented that African American children or children from poor, low-income, and middle-income households were less likely to receive all the recommended vaccinations compared with white children or children from high-income households in 2011.[23]

Unequal Pain Management

Judgments about pain are frequently influenced by the characteristics of patients (e.g., race/ethnicity), situations (e.g., medical evidence), and health care providers (e.g., experience).[37] In the face of such uncertainties, latent/implicit stereotypes may be activated, advantaging patients who fit positive stereotypes (e.g., pro-white) and disadvantaging patients who do not (e.g., African Americans).[37] For example, African Americans and Hispanics are seen as more likely to require scrutiny for potential drug abuse. Consequently, primary care providers are more likely to underestimate pain intensity in African Americans and Hispanics than in other sociodemographic groups.[37,38]

Unequal Breast Cancer Screening

Women without health insurance are much less likely to get a mammogram than women with health insurance. In the United States, breast cancer is the most common cancer in Asian American women, but these women have relatively lower rates of breast cancer screening than African American and white women.[39] Furthermore, disparities in breast cancer screening reportedly result from low income, lack of a local mammography center, lack of transportation to a mammography center, lack of a usual health care provider, lack of a recommendation from a health care provider to get mammography screening, lack of awareness of breast cancer risks and screening methods, and cultural and language differences.[40]

Unequal Palliative Care

Racial/ethnic minorities tend to receive lower quality palliative care across multiple domains, including satisfaction, communication, and pain management. Compared to whites, African Americans report less satisfaction with the quality of communication, including the extent to which health care providers listen and share information, with greater disparities in racially discordant patient–provider relationships. Moreover, racial/ethnic minorities are disadvantaged in terms of the access to hospice care. Minority older adults have lower rates of hospice use than their white counterparts across diagnoses, geographic areas, and settings of care.[41] Racial/ethnic differences in knowledge, cultural beliefs, and treatment preferences are regarded as barriers to the use of palliative care.[41]

CASE STUDY

Source: michaeljung/iStock/ Thinkstock

Case Presentation

Jones Antoinette, a 21-year-old pregnant African American woman, visited an obstetric clinic for prenatal care for the first time at 30 weeks of gestation. Her baseline vital signs were normal. She was assigned to a white nurse midwife for her prenatal care throughout the remaining pregnancy until her delivery.

The nurse midwife interviewed and assessed Jones' sociodemographic characteristics, past medical history, health behaviors, and psychological health status. Jones had a medical history of abnormal glucose tolerance and asthma, but she has not seen a health care provider to treat the asthma because she lacks health insurance. Prior to her pregnancy, she smoked five cigarettes a day, but she stopped smoking when she learned she was pregnant. She also said that she drank often during the weekends but has cut back. She complained of depressive feelings and sleep disturbances due to several life crises. She is at risk of losing her part-time job and has not had steady income for months. She has a car, but she often gets rides because she cannot afford gas. She wants to move from her current apartment because there is high crime activity in her apartment complex—even drug use in the hallways. Her asthma has become worse due to poor housing conditions. Furthermore, her boyfriend was recently arrested and has been asking her for money for legal help. Under these circumstances, she was not sure if it was right to carry this baby.

After the interview, the nurse midwife ordered a regular diabetes check, which should have been conducted at week 28 of gestation. The patient's history of abnormal glucose tolerance has a potential to put Jones and her fetus at high risk. The nurse midwife informed Jones of cystic fibrosis screening as well. This genetic test is not mandatory, but it is encouraged. Jones listened to the nurse midwife carefully and asked if it would be good for her baby. After getting information on the test, Jones wanted to be tested. The nurse midwife provided the test consent form and printed information on the screening test. Jones signed the consent form without reading the printed information. Before leaving, the nurse midwife asked if Jones had any questions or concerns, and Jones said "no." After meeting with the nurse midwife, Jones met a nurse coordinator who was responsible for scheduling of the next appointment and additional tests, case management, and patient education. When the nurse coordinator double-checked whether Jones really wanted cystic fibrosis screening, Jones said that she did not hear about the test from the nurse midwife.

Case Analysis

Health disparities in prenatal care by racial/ethnic group have been frequently reported in the literature, and African American women are less likely to have early and adequate prenatal care and more likely to have preterm births. Such health disparities are well reflected in this case. Jones has multiple risk factors that hindered early prenatal care in the first trimester, such as no income, poor housing conditions, lack of social support from her partner, and her reluctance to deliver a baby. Because she was unable to obtain an education, it is a challenge to find stable and well-paying employment. A poor employment situation can result in lack of health insurance, one of the major factors influencing health care disparities. She may live in an area far from the clinic, resulting in lack of access to health care. During the interaction with the nurse midwife, the information on cystic fibrosis screening was not appropriately communicated, which is also an influencing factor in health disparities, perhaps because the printed information was too technical for her to understand or too long. As a result, Jones signed the consent for the testing, not fully informed of its purpose, process, benefits, and harms.

Some of the risk factors could be addressed through interventions. For example, through collaboration with a social worker, the nurse midwife could help resolve Jones' financial issues by providing information on the resources that are available for prenatal care of low-income women and/or by referring Jones to the resources. Consequently, the health care team could ensure Jones' continuation of regular prenatal care until the delivery.

ACCESS EXEMPLAR LINKS IN YOUR GIDDENS EBOOK

REFERENCES

1. World Health Organization: *Fact file on health inequities*, (n.d.) Retrieved from <http://www.who.int/sdhconference/background/news/facts/en>.
2. Centers for Disease Control and Prevention: *CDC health disparities and inequalities report—United States 2013*, 2013. Retrieved from <http://www.cdc.gov/mmwr/pdf/other/su6203.pdf>.
3. Ancheta IB, Carlson JM, Battie CA, et al: One size does not fit all: Cardiovascular health disparities as a function of ethnicity in Asian-American women. *Appl Nurs Res* 28(2):99–105, 2015.
4. Cameron BL, Carmargo Plazas MDP, Salas AS, et al: Understanding inequalities in access to health care services for aboriginal people: A call for nursing action. *ANS Adv Nurs Sci* 37(3):E1–E16, 2014.
5. Fink AM: Toward a new definition of health disparity: A concept analysis. *J Transcult Nurs* 20(4):349–357, 2009.
6. National Institutes of Health: *National Institutes of Health strategic research plan and budget to reduce and ultimately eliminate health disparities*, 2000. Retrieved from <http://www.nimhd.nih.gov/documents/VolumeI_031003EDrev.pdf>.
7. Institute of Medicine: *Unequal treatment: Confronting racial and ethnic disparities in health care*, Washington, DC, 2002, National Academies Press.
8. U.S. Department of Health and Human Services: *Healthy People 2010: Understanding and improving health*, ed 2, Washington, DC, 2000, Author.
9. U.S. Health Resources and Services Administration: *Eliminating health disparities in the United States*, 2000. Retrieved from <https://archive.org/details/eliminatinghealt00usde>.
10. Adler NE, Stewart J: Health disparities across the lifespan: Meaning, methods, and mechanisms. *Ann N Y Acad Sci* 1186:5–23, 2010.
11. Braveman P: Health disparities and health equity: Concepts and measurement. *Annu Rev Public Health* 27:167–194, 2006.
12. Carter-Pokras O, Baquet C: What is a "health disparity"? *Public Health Rep* 117(5):426–434, 2002.
13. Whitehead M: The concepts and principles of equity and health. *Health Promot Int* 6(3):217–228, 1991.
14. Health Canada: *Toward a healthy future*, 1999. Retrieved from <http://publications.gc.ca/collections/Collection/H39-468-1999E.pdf>.
15. Dressler WW, Oths KS, Gravlee CC: Race and ethnicity in public health research: Models to explain health disparities. *Annu Rev Anthropol* 34:231–252, 2005.
16. Swick K: *Empowering parents, families, schools and communities during the early childhood years*, Champaign, IL, 2004, Stipes.
17. Roberts MC, Steele RG: *Handbook of pediatric psychology*, ed 4, New York, 2009, Guilford.
18. Gravlee CC: Emic ethnic classification in southeastern Puerto Rico: Cultural consensus and semantic structure. *Soc Forces* 83:949–970, 2005.
19. Gravlee CC, Dressler WW: Skin pigmentation, self-perceived color, and arterial blood pressure in Puerto Rico. *Am J Hum Biol* 17:195–206, 2005.
20. Saha S, Beach MC, Cooper LA: Patient centeredness, cultural competence and healthcare quality. *J Natl Med Assoc* 100(11):1275–1285, 2008.
21. Betancourt JR, Green AR, Carrillo JE, et al: Defining cultural competence: A practical framework for addressing racial/ethnic disparities in health and health care. *Public Health Rep* 118(4):293–302, 2003.
22. Meade MA, Mahmoudi E, Lee S-Y: The intersection of disability and healthcare disparities: A conceptual framework. *Disabil Rehabil* 37(7):632–641, 2015.
23. Agency for Healthcare Research and Quality: *National healthcare disparities report*, 2013. Retrieved from <http://www.ahrq.gov/research/findings/nhqrdr/nhdr13/2013nhdr.pdf>.
24. Kaiser Family Foundation: *Key facts about the uninsured population*, 2014. Retrieved from <http://files.kff.org/attachment/key-facts-about-the-uninsured-population-fact-sheet>.
25. Flores G: Language barriers to health care in the United States. *N Engl J Med* 355(3):229–231, 2006.
26. Regenstein M: *Language barriers in health care*, 2008. Retrieved from <http://www.rwjf.org/en/research-publications/find-rwjf-research/2008/09/language-barriers-in-health-care.html>.
27. The Leadership Conference Education Fund: *The road to health care parity: Transportation policy and access to health care*, 2011. Retrieved from <http://civilrightsdocs.info/pdf/docs/transportation/The-Road-to-Health-Care-Parity.pdf>.
28. Betancourt JR, Renfrew MR: Unequal treatment in the US: Lessons and recommendations for cancer care internationally. *J Pediatr Hematol Oncol* 33(Suppl 2):149–153, 2011.
29. Egbert N, Nanna KM: Health literacy: Challenges and strategies. *Online J Issues Nurs* 14(3):1–10, 2009.
30. Eiser AR, Ellis G: Cultural competence and the African American experience with health care: The case for specific content in cross-cultural education. *Acad Med* 82(2):176–183, 2007.
31. Alspach JG: Is there gender bias in critical care? *Crit Care Nurse* 32(6):8–14, 2012.
32. Meleis AI: Culturally competent scholarship: Substance and rigor. *ANS Adv Nurs Sci* 19(2):1–16, 1996.
33. Hall JM: Marginalization revisited: Critical, postmodern, and liberation perspectives. *ANS Adv Nurs Sci* 22(2):88–102, 1999.
34. Hall JM, Stevens PE, Meleis AI: Marginalization: A guiding concept for valuing diversity in nursing knowledge development. *ANS Adv Nurs Sci* 16(4):23–41, 1994.
35. Congressional Budget Office: *Effects of the Affordable Care Act on health insurance coverage—February 2013 baseline*, 2013. Retrieved from <http://www.cbo.gov/publication/43900>.
36. U.S. Department of Health and Human Services, Health Resources and Services Administration, Maternal and Child Health Bureau: *Child health USA 2013*, Rockville, MD, 2013, U.S. Department of Health and Human Services.
37. Tait RC, Chibnall JT: Racial/ethnic disparities in the assessment and treatment of pain: Psychosocial perspectives. *Am Psychol* 69(2):131–141, 2014.
38. Johnson TJ, Weaver MD, Borrero S, et al: Association of race and ethnicity with management of abdominal pain in the emergency department. *Pediatrics* 132(4):e851–e858, 2013.
39. American Cancer Society: *Breast cancer facts & figures*, 2012. Retrieved from <http://www.cancer.org/docroot/STT/STT_0.asp>.
40. Komen Susan G.: *Disparities in breast cancer screening*, 2014. Retrieved from <http://ww5.komen.org/BreastCancer/RacialEthnicIssuesinScreening.html>.
41. Johnson KS: Racial and ethnic disparities in palliative care. *J Palliat Med* 16(11):1329–1334, 2013.

Health Care Organizations

Teresa Keller

Health care organizations (HCOs) are complex and dynamic, a product of the interactions of mission and values, internal and external environments, and the motivations and actions of those who work in the organizations. The delivery of health care services in the United States is driven by the need to provide a broad spectrum of care in a variety of settings to diverse consumers. The delivery of these services requires a highly specialized, professional workforce financed by a mix of private and public funding and subject to oversight and regulation by many different public and private authorities. Whether they are rural clinics catering to migrant laborers, large teaching hospitals in urban environments, or integrated health systems providing a spectrum of services throughout the nation, HCOs face challenges that require them to adapt and innovate or face extinction.

The results are new service delivery arrangements, new kinds of health care workplaces, new types of service providers, and new treatments and services hardly imagined in prior times, all of which represent some innovation meant to serve a market, a population, or a social need. HCOs are social systems created by people and managed by people; therefore, the HCO is a socially created entity with no meaning outside of the collective actions and aspirations of the people involved. The significance of this perspective of the organization is that all people involved with an HCO, as members of a dynamic social system, are able to make creative and meaningful contributions to the success of the HCO. As members of the largest professional workforce, nurses can have a strong and positive influence on the HCO as it evolves and innovates.

DEFINITION

Organizations can be defined as a group of people who come together for a purpose[1] or as a collection of people brought together for a predetermined purpose in a defined environment.[2] Common to both of these definitions is that organizations are composed of people and have a purpose. Organizations could be further defined as having a socially determined structure provided by formal properties, such as rules, policies, and procedures, and by informal properties, such as customs, norms, and values.[1] A more robust definition for

organizations is that they are structured social arrangements that use systematic strategies to combine and coordinate a mix of resources (people and capital) to provide specific products or services. For the purposes of this concept presentation, the definition of HCO is *a purposefully designed, structured social system developed for the delivery of health care services by specialized workforces to defined communities, populations, or markets.*

SCOPE

There are so many different ways to organize an HCO that the result is a large variety of distinctive organizations in the U.S. health care sector, purposely designed to meet the need for health care services in a community or population or market.[3] There are HCOs specifically designed to deliver health care services, such as hospitals and clinics, and those that are designed for a health-related purpose but not to deliver services, such as pharmaceutical companies or manufacturers of medical equipment.

Obviously, a discussion of the concept of the HCO can be quickly complicated by all the different possible purposes and forms of organization. The variety of distinctive organizations with specific purposes defies simple classification. For the purpose of establishing a scope for this complex topic, only organizations that provide a range of health care services for health promotion, illness, and wellness care are considered. This encompasses a variety of organizations, including (but not limited to) hospitals, home health agencies, clinics or ambulatory care centers, nursing homes, and organizations that serve a particular market or population.

ATTRIBUTES AND CRITERIA

All organizations have defining attributes. Each has a purpose, a structure, and members who do the work of the organization. HCOs are no different from other kinds of organizations in this regard. As social systems, HCOs are situated within an environment from which resources are obtained and from which challenges are presented that require an organizational response. In daily operations, HCOs must be able to acquire resources, produce services, and change as necessary to sustain their existence within the challenging U.S. health care services sector.

Major Attributes

HCOs are distinguished from other types of organizations by their unique purpose, by their specialized workforce, and by a level of public trust that separates HCOs from other types of organizations.

Purpose

The purpose of HCOs is to help others by providing health care services. This distinguishes the HCO as distinct from other types of organizations involved in the business of health care. The primary purpose of companies that sell health insurance is to sell an insurance product. Schools for health professions have a primary educational purpose. The purpose of accreditation and public regulatory agencies is to support the work of the HCO, but these organizations do not directly deliver health care services. An HCO provides health care services to manage illness or promote health, whether those services are childhood immunizations, surgical interventions, diabetes education, family planning advice, or any of a wide variety of other health care services offered to individuals, families, and communities. This purpose remains the same—to provide health care services—regardless of profit status or ownership arrangements.

Specialized Health Care Workforce

HCOs are notable for the highly specialized workforce needed to deliver health care services. The work produced in an HCO is complex, variable, and, at times, urgent in nature. The margin for error is narrow with little tolerance for mistakes that can lead to life-threatening and costly consequences.[1] Health professionals who work in HCOs undergo extensive education and experiential learning. The knowledge and skills that these specialized workers bring to the HCO are necessary for the effective delivery of services in an ambiguous, challenging work environment. The compelling need for this specialized workforce increases the costs for HCOs, but it also benefits the organization in terms of maintaining standards and ensuring quality services. An additional benefit is that the strong professional ideals of these workers promote and strengthen the service values that support the purpose of the HCO.

Furthermore, the work of managing the health of humans is not easily divided because people present with health problems that affect the whole person, their families, and perhaps the entire community. The need to treat a person, rather than a disease or problem, is central to the work of health care professionals. This creates an interdependence among these workers that is another notable characteristic of HCOs.[1] Although labor might be divided among numerous specialized personnel, the need to address the person or patient as a whole means that each of these professionals is dependent on the knowledge and skills of others. An interprofessional approach to the treatment of human health problems not only is a distinguishing feature of the HCO but also serves to increase the complexity of the organization.

Although the HCO is uniquely defined by its specialized workforce of health care professionals, a discussion of the health care workforce is not complete without reference to the numerous other personnel essential to the effective functioning of the HCO. For example, the human resource department of any large HCO provides critical services necessary for the daily operations of the HCO because most health care professionals expect to receive a salary and benefits. Dietary and housekeeping personnel provide important services within the HCO that support the work of health care professionals, as do the administrators responsible for ensuring adequate supplies and equipment. Because the HCO is a specialized organization with unique functions, all of these workers could be considered a part of the specialized health care workforce.

Public Trust

The historical development of HCOs demonstrates a long record of service to others. Early organizations were created by religious orders or by social service groups to provide services to society's most vulnerable members—the ill and infirm. The work of these early organizations gained the confidence of the public that their altruistic purpose was to serve others by providing care and comfort, regardless of personal circumstances. These laudable efforts helped to establish a social contract between the public and HCOs, one from which HCOs have benefitted in both financial terms and public regard.

Currently, the level of public trust in HCOs has eroded with the growth of managed care, national corporate chains of for-profit HCOs, and allegations of fraud and abuse by health care providers.[4] However, people still turn to their physicians and nurses for help and advice, and they still seek the services offered by HCOs for health concerns. This indicates that the social contract is still intact, if a little worn. As such, HCOs are still distinguished by their relatively positive image of institutions designed to provide valuable and needed services to others. As mentioned previously, all organizations must generate income to remain viable, so the for-profit/not-for-profit status of the HCO is less important than managing the tensions created by financial issues versus the need to preserve altruistic values. HCOs that provide quality health care services and are good corporate citizens will be able to maintain their positive image and their part of the social contract, regardless of their profit status.

Minor Attributes

The minor attributes of HCOs differ from major attributes in terms of HCOs' relationship to other kinds of organizations. The major attributes of HCOs discussed in the preceding section are identified with health care and the health care services sector. The minor attributes of HCOs are those that define them as forms of purposeful organizations and are features they share in common with other types of organizations.

Structure

Structure is the collective of formal rules and policies that govern organizational practices and that promote the effective management of materials and resources. Structure also creates the various roles and associated responsibilities that are required for organizational function. Different organizational roles carry varying levels of authority for decision making relative to the assigned responsibilities of those roles. Organizational rules, policies, and authority are necessary for the integration of diverse functions and activities across the organization into a coordinated system capable of supporting the purpose of the organization. However, too much structure can be stifling, causing the HCO to be so encumbered by rules and regulations that meaningful action is hampered. An organization needs sufficient structure to support important processes and operations; otherwise, it will disintegrate into anarchy. A balance needs to be maintained that provides the structure necessary for sustaining the HCO while not producing unnecessary constraints.[5]

The requirement for supportive structures that minimize constraints is especially important for HCOs because of the type of personnel working within these organizations. As noted previously, the workforce of HCOs is composed of a large number of health care professionals. These professionals possess valuable knowledge and skills that are critical to the delivery of health care services. These professionals also have a strong allegiance to a set of professional values. Most health care professionals possess a state-licensed authority to manage their own practice and are responsible for the outcomes of their work.

For an HCO, this means management authority and control is relatively weak in relation to professional authority because decision making related to practice is not subject to control by those outside the profession.[1] This requires additional lines of authority to be established within the HCO; for example, nurses are accountable to nursing officers, and physicians are accountable to medical executives. This is true for most of the institutional arrangements that create authority within an HCO. Professional control of licensed practice is the basis for the interdependency between health professionals in the HCO, but it can also fuel the typical conflicts and "turf wars" seen in an HCO.

The result of these divided lines of authority is that management control by those outside of the profession is limited to those work activities that lie outside the professional's scope of practice. For example, nurses can expect that their professional practice will be directed and evaluated by other nurses and that they will be accountable for maintaining the standards of the profession. However, they can also expect that they will need to meet the requirements established by non-nursing administrators for other expected work behaviors, such as the use of vacation time or maintaining appropriate licensure.

Organizational Environments

Organizations possess an internal environment, but they also interact with an external environment. The internal environment of the HCO consists of an integrated web of factors such as organizational culture (where *culture* is defined as a set of values, beliefs, and practices), systems such as information systems or the human resources management system, and structural elements such as role responsibilities, rules, and practices. All of these factors affect the decisions and responses of the HCO to demands and challenges encountered during daily operations.[6]

The external organizational environment consists of those external forces, conditions, or events that affect the organization, such as economic trends or new laws and government regulations.[3] Examples of external environmental forces are a widespread economic recession and government funding changes that affect HCOs. These kinds of forces in the external environment provide resources and/or feedback as inputs to the organization and are major factors that drive organizational change.

There is an ongoing interplay between the internal and external environments of the HCO, where organizational decisions and operations are affected by perceived forces from the external environment. Organizations integrated into their environments will also change those environments in some ways, adding to the complexity of the relationship. For example, a national economic recession can prompt workers to expand their work hours, either by increasing the hours they work or by seeking additional employment. This holds true for nurses. If experienced professional nurses are working more hours or seeking additional employment, the effect on the HCO could be human resources changes that mean fewer new and inexperienced nurses are hired. The decline in demand for new nurses has the potential to affect the admission decisions of nursing schools or the funding

decisions made by government organizations that support nursing education. As these resources are curtailed, there are fewer new nurses prepared and, subsequently, fewer new nurses for the HCO to hire to replace nurses who leave or retire.

Before the 20th century and the rise of organized health care delivery, the health care industry was unregulated, health care workers were less knowledgeable, and health care markets were small and relatively simple.[7] Currently, multiple interacting forces in the health care environment have profound effects on HCOs, especially because they increase uncertainty and create instability. While HCOs evolve to meet the challenges presented by their environments, they are still expected to maintain the service orientation that is fundamental to their purpose. An example of the internal pressures created by external environmental demands is tying government reimbursements to HCOs for meeting evidence-based standards of quality care and for ensuring optimal patient safety. Meeting quality and safety standards is highly desirable, but it is also costly in terms of training personnel, providing additional staffing, and building work processes that support quality care and patient safety. This creates tensions within the HCO while workers seek to meet expectations for safe and effective care with limited additional resources.

HCO policies created to meet environmental challenges might conflict with professional values or with legal guidelines, requiring actions to negotiate and resolve the conflict. New technologies might need to be adopted that require a shift of resources from one part of the organization to another. The need to change (rapidly in some cases) in response to environmental effects means that HCOs are complex and their work environments are notably ambiguous.

THEORETICAL LINKS

The industrial revolution led to the development of large organizations. As these organizations grew, they became the vehicle through which many different kinds of human activities are organized and coordinated. This prompted social scientists to study the phenomenon of purposive, organized systems and to create theories to explain these systems. A complete description of the organizational theories of the past 100 years is beyond the scope of this concept presentation. Instead, an overview of the major directions in theory development related to organizations is useful to understanding the HCO concept.

Bureaucracy

Early conceptualizations of organizations were that they were closed systems and were a rational, machine-like collection of components to be coordinated and controlled through authoritative management. Max Weber, German sociologist and economist, developed the first theoretical model of bureaucracy in the early 20th century. Weber described the principles of organization that created efficiency in work design and were thought to be the most effective way to organize work. He also described the distribution of authority in bureaucracies, noting that authority grounded in position and divided into hierarchies was preferable to authority derived from personal characteristics. Weber viewed the bureaucracy as the organizational design most likely to create the stability needed to sustain an organization.[8]

Bureaucratic design was common to the large organizations that developed during the industrial revolution because the manufacturing and distribution of goods required a rational system of centralized control to effectively acquire resources and efficiently convert them to a finished product.[9] Bureaucratic organizations were made of functional parts, or divisions, all welded together through management control made possible by hierarchical authority. These organizations were believed to be capable of achieving a high degree of coordinated precision in production, leading to the common metaphor of a "well-oiled machine."

The drawback to this model of rational efficiency is that it takes little account of the organization as a social system within an environment. Bureaucratic theory mainly focuses on authority and control to achieve efficient production within a closed system. The human dimension of the organization is not well-defined outside of the role of management. Other organizational theorists of that time attempted to describe and explain the social dynamics of organizations, but the main theoretical approach taken was mechanical and emphasized the role of management in attaining maximal productivity from workers through planning and control.[8] The effects of environmental factors on the production and efficiency of an organization were also not considered by these early theorists. The bureaucratic organization was a self-contained, closed system.

Systems Theory

The view of organizations as social systems had an early beginning with the human relations school of organizational theorists. This group focused their study on the needs and desires of people who work in the organization. From this field of study grew an understanding that the organization has social components that interact and that these components are affected by factors from the outside environment.[9] These social components (people, relationships, and roles) interact with environment, technology, and organizational structure in an integrated manner to create a unified, dynamic system.[2,10] This open systems perspective paved the way for interesting new theories that not only intrigue organizational theorists but also provide for new ways to organize and new ways to empower the people who work in these systems (Figure 55-1).

Complex Adaptive Systems

Current organizational theory describes the organization as having biological characteristics that allow the organization to react and

change when stimulated. This understanding of the organization defines a new way of viewing organizations as organic and lifelike entities that are open to the environment and capable of transforming themselves in light of perceived opportunities and threats. Organizations can "read" and interpret the environment,[5] and they can adjust and adapt through the coordinated action of their interdependent parts. The changes that occur within an organization in response to environmental stimuli are necessary for sustaining the organization, just as metabolic processes within the human body change to allow the body to adapt to environmental challenges. In the case of the HCO, the need for change and adaptation requires that all organizational members be engaged and motivated to meet the organization's goals. Viewing the organization as a living social system recognizes the creative energy of the people who innovate to produce desirable products and services in uncertain, changing environments. Understanding the HCO as a complex, adaptive system is probably the most realistic of the organizational theories developed to date because it is able to account for the complexity created by interrelated and interdependent social systems responding to internal and external stimuli.

CONTEXT TO NURSING AND HEALTH CARE

In the context of health care, HCOs can be broadly classified by their mission, financial structure, and ownership.

Mission

The purpose of an HCO is determined by the organization's mission, vision, and values.[2] Mission statements issued by HCOs describe each organization's purpose based on a vision of what the HCO is meant to achieve. Mission statements also describe the values that drive the work of the organization, such as quality and excellence. Even if the HCO is a for-profit, privately owned corporation that pays dividends to shareholders, the mission statement will reflect values commonly associated with helping others, such as service and professionalism. Because mission statements reflect strategic vision, they focus and drive the work of the HCO toward organizational goals. Mission statements that reflect values that primarily benefit shareholders, such as seeking higher profits, would drive the work of the HCO in a direction that may conflict with the goal of helping others with their health care needs. Mission statements that prominently feature service ideals and values and that promote assistance and support to others serve to sustain the primary purpose of the HCO.

Financial Structure

Another way to classify HCOs is by their financial purpose as either for-profit or not-for-profit entities. The difference between the not-for-profit and the for-profit HCO is not the profits generated but, rather, how the profits are distributed. For-profit HCOs are designed to generate profits for shareholders while also providing health care services. Not-for-profit HCOs also generate profits, but these are used for organizational purposes, such as building additional facilities, providing improved services, or acquiring new equipment.

In reality, this distinction between for-profit and not-for-profit HCOs is less clear because all HCOs must pay attention to financial viability. The need to generate revenues to meet expenses is important to all organizations, whether for-profit or not-for-profit, because the failure to cover expenses creates risks to the continued existence of HCOs. Unprofitable HCOs that collect less revenue than what is required to meet expenses—even if they are publicly supported—will eventually have to close or be reorganized.

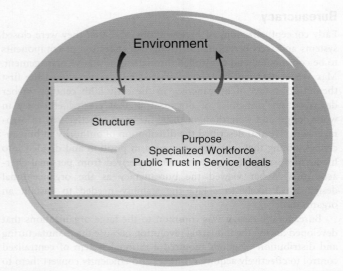

FIGURE 55-1 Health Care Organizations: Open Systems Model

Ownership

Health care organizations, in addition to their mission and financing, can also be classified as publicly or privately owned.[2,3] Publicly owned HCOs are commonly seen as community organizations that are supported by government funding. The typical example of this type of ownership is the tax-supported county or state hospital that provides generalized health care services or specific health services, such as behavioral and mental health. State and local public health departments could also be considered publicly owned HCOs. Investor-owned corporations are considered privately owned, but private ownership could also include HCOs owned by religious or social organizations. Privately owned HCOs are not generally supported by public funding.

The defining characteristics of mission, finance, and ownership noted previously can be combined to create a myriad of HCOs designed to meet the challenges of the health care environment. The variety seen in HCOs can be illustrated using hospice as an example. Hospice services provide specialty care to a specific population—the terminally ill and their families. As an HCO, the hospice might be for-profit and privately owned (by investors) and any profits generated by services are returned to the investors in the form of dividends, or the hospice might be nonprofit and privately owned by a religious organization and any profits realized are returned to the HCO to improve the quality of services and infrastructure or to sustain other services offered by the organization. Both of these types of hospice provide the same unique service and play a distinct role in the health care community, although they vary by ownership and by profit status. Furthermore, a hospice could be a part of an integrated, national network of HCOs delivering a full spectrum of coordinated health care services. Regardless of the structure and institutional arrangement, as an HCO, the hospice must be ready to manage costs and maintain services while evolving as the health services environment changes.

Regardless of the mission, financing, or ownership, nurses can be found in almost any kind of HCO, in which they are responsible for ensuring the safe and effective delivery of care. The nursing profession in the United States is the largest health professional group. Nurses are working throughout the health services sector and in all HCOs because their knowledge and skills are integral to the delivery of health care services.[11]

However, nursing contributions to successful HCOs go beyond providing bedside, patient-focused care to include active management and administration of patient care and patient units, conducting research and collaborating with other professionals to coordinate and deliver safe and effective patient care. Nurses work as case managers, infection control specialists, managers of information technology, human resources specialists, and quality/risk managers. Nurses are also directors and executives, advanced practice providers, and administrative specialists in HCOs and HCO networks. Furthermore, professional nurses affect the environments of HCOs by creating partnerships with other institutions, educating future nurses in universities and community colleges, and working with public policy decision makers to create policies that enhance health services environments. It is likely that professional nurses will be associated in some way with HCOs for most, if not all, of their professional nursing careers.

INTERRELATED CONCEPTS

Other organizational concepts featured in this textbook are important to understanding the HCO as a dynamic social system (Figure 55-2).

Contemporary **Leadership** is required for HCOs—a leadership that creates inspiration, is able to sustain motivation to achieve results, and that values the contributions of all members. Leaders have to be able to "read" the environment and interpret the trends or changes for others. They must be able to lead others through turbulent and uncertain environments and must be able to adapt to change as readily as their followers.[5,12]

Timely, current, and accurate **Communicaton** is an essential component of safe and effective care delivery. Delayed, diminished, or compromised communication not only hampers the organization's activities and productivity but also can lead to serious deficiencies in patient care. Ineffective communication is linked to many instances of catastrophic errors in patient care,[13] such as wrong-site surgery or unexpected patient death.

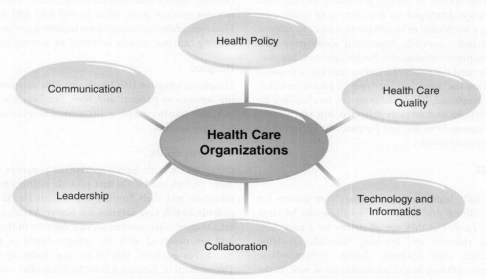

FIGURE 55-2 Health Care Organizations and Interrelated Concepts

Collaboration can be defined as partnerships developed for the purpose of achieving optimal patient care outcomes.[14] It is essential that nurses be able to collaborate with other members of the HCO, the patient, and the patient's family to deliver quality health care that is safe and effective. The ability to collaborate also creates the conditions necessary for effective mentoring of new nurses and for professional control of practice.

Technology and Informatics is essential to the HCO for ensuring the delivery of safe patient care, and the collection and meaningful use of patient care information provides the basis for much of the evidence used in health care decision making. The era of the electronic health record has arrived and is proving to be a disruptive innovation that will fundamentally change how health care is delivered. Clinical informatics provides data and statistics about health care services and the outcomes of these services.[15] Coupled with new government payment systems, these outcomes will drive the products and services provided by HCOs.

In 2001, the Institute of Medicine issued a clarion call for an increased focus on Health Care Quality. Since then, many HCOs and health care leaders (including nurses) have worked to identify gaps in care that lead to patient care errors and to propose solutions to address the conditions that lead to these errors. Many of these proposals are aimed at correcting the problems in organizational design and function that promote an error-prone environment in HCOs. For instance, the strategies developed for improving communications in handoffs are meant to promote greater patient safety during transfers between units.[16]

Health Policy is a major force driving change in HCOs. Obvious pressures are changes to HCO revenue related to the increased focus on reimbursements for quality outcomes or on changes to health insurance markets that result in greater access to health care. Less obvious are the pressures that arise from other policy decisions. To illustrate, consider the impact of decisions by a state board of nursing on the nursing workforce. Suppose a board of nursing moves to require a bachelor's degree as a condition of professional licensure. A decision such as this will greatly affect the staffing patterns and pay scales of nurses hired by an HCO.

CLINICAL EXEMPLARS

Examples of HCOs are numerous. As defined previously, an HCO can be any type of organization developed for the delivery of health care services and employing a workforce of health professionals to achieve this mission. These include hospitals, clinics and ambulatory care centers, nursing homes, public/community health agencies, hospice, and HCOs developed to meet the needs of a unique market or population (Box 55-1). These are the more familiar types of HCOs in which nurses are likely to be employed. These facilities can be classified by ownership, financial purpose, and services delivered, but when combined with their organizational mission and purpose, the variety to be found among HCOs expands greatly.

Featured Exemplars
Hospitals

Hospitals have traditionally been viewed as tertiary care centers for the treatment of acute illness and disability. Hospitals can be large or small and urban or rural, but they are all driven by a particular mission. For example, research and teaching hospitals are large HCOs usually associated with academic health centers whose mission includes the education of health professionals as well as the delivery of health care services. Community hospitals offer general

---

BOX 55-1   EXEMPLARS OF HEALTH CARE ORGANIZATIONS

Hospitals
- Teaching/academic medical centers
- Community hospitals (rural and urban)
- Specialized care (rehabilitation)

Nursing homes

Clinics and ambulatory care facilities
- Federally qualified health centers
- Nurse-managed centers
- Retail walk-in clinics (urgent care)
- Same-day surgery centers

Hospice

Specialty HCOs
- U.S. Department of Defense military HCO
- U.S. Department of Veterans Affairs
- Indian Health Services

---

medical and surgical services to a surrounding community, but most will not have a research or teaching mission.[3] Hospitals can also specialize in the care of a particular health condition, a market, or a population.

Clinics and Ambulatory Care Centers

Clinics and ambulatory care centers are generally viewed as HCOs with a mission to deliver services in an outpatient setting. For example, federally qualified health centers offer primary care services such as well-child examinations, immunizations, and the diagnosis and management of chronic conditions such as diabetes. Another example of a clinic is a nurse-managed center offering a range of primary care services for adults, children, and families. Clinic facilities and ambulatory care centers are not usually equipped to provide prolonged acute care, so patients requiring these types of services are referred to a hospital for treatment.

Nursing Homes

Nursing homes and assisted living facilities offer long-term, skilled nursing services most often to the frail and ill elderly population. However, adults with conditions requiring prolonged periods of skilled nursing care may also be admitted to nursing homes.

Hospice

Hospice is a type of HCO with a specific mission—to provide end-of-life services to patients and their families. The intent is to provide palliative care to patients with terminal illnesses and to provide support for their families.

Specialty HCOs

Other HCOs with highly specialized purposes include U.S. Department of Defense HCOs that provide health care services to military members and their families and Indian Health Services HCOs that provide health care services for Native American populations. These HCOs most often confine service delivery to the specified population and are designed with the unique needs of these populations in mind. For example, the HCOs that make up the network of U.S. Department of Veteran Affairs facilities offer services only to military veterans.

CASE STUDY

Source: Steve Hix/Fuse/Thinkstock

Case Presentation

A form of HCO that offers nurses the opportunity to fully realize their professional role is the Magnet organization. Magnet organizations are those HCOs, primarily hospitals, that have adopted organizational practices that promote excellence in nursing practice. The HCO that adopts Magnet principles is committing to an organizational design and structure that empowers nursing staff to achieve higher levels of performance through engagement and participation. The Magnet designation is only obtained after a process of learning and self-evaluation followed by changes to the organization's structure.[17] These design changes provide a decentralized authority structure created to support participative management and professional autonomy for nurses.[18,19] Nurses working in Magnet facilities are expected to be active participants in organizational processes, to govern themselves, to collaborate with other professional colleagues, and to be both responsible and accountable for the outcomes of nursing care.

Magnet designation is an empowerment model that captures the main features of the complex adaptive system. Adopting Magnet principles meant to attract and retain excellent nurses is, fundamentally, recognition that professional nursing is a valuable and scarce resource essential to the effective function of the HCO. Nurses are not simply workers in the system but are instead a critical component of the organization making substantial contributions to the success of the HCO. To achieve this recognition, an HCO must be able to demonstrate the full integration of professional nursing into its operations through authority structures that move decision making, power, and control of practice to nurses throughout the organization. This is usually accomplished through the creation of governance councils in which all nursing staff are able to voice their concerns with care issues and then make decisions that will affect how care is delivered in that facility. Professional decision making is no longer the exclusive domain of the nursing executive and directors. Instead, there is a flattening of hierarchical relationships related to authority and control over practice, with more of the responsibilities for care outcomes being assumed by nursing staff.

The HCO must also demonstrate that appropriate processes are in place that allow for the development of innovative care strategies and that nurses can implement and review the results of their innovation efforts. Quality management in Magnet organizations is robust, and nurses are fully involved in creative activities that encourage continuous quality improvement and the achievement of excellence in nursing care. These facilities promote the continuing professional development of their nurses by supporting education and career-ladder programs.[19]

Case Analysis

This case exemplifies the concept of HCOs' major and minor attributes of purpose, public trust, structure, and organizational environment. Although Magnet designation is specific to nursing, the adoption of a Magnet design by an HCO has spillover benefits for the entire organization. Because the HCO is an integrated system and professional nursing is the largest workforce in most of these organizations, an active and engaged nursing workforce positively influences other members and other components of the HCO. Empowered nurses act as transformative agents in the Magnet structure, leading efforts to improve the quality of care and inspiring others in the organization to join in the effort to create better systems and improved HCO outcomes. In summary, the HCO with Magnet designation benefits from increased collaboration, self-determination, and participation by nurses because this increases the capacity of the organization to adapt to uncertainty and change.

ACCESS EXEMPLAR LINKS IN YOUR GIDDENS EBOOK

REFERENCES

1. Shortell S, Kaluzny A: Organization theory and health services management. In Shortell S, Kaluzny A, editors: *Health care management: Organization design and behavior*, ed 5, Clifton Park, NY, 2006, Delmar, pp 5–41.
2. Mancini M: Healthcare organizations. In Yoder-Wise P, editor: *Leading and managing in nursing*, ed 5, St Louis, 2010, Elsevier, pp 116–136.
3. Longest B, Darr K: *Managing health services organizations and systems*, ed 6, Baltimore, 2014, Health Professions Press.
4. Zazzali J: Trust: An implicit force in health care organization theory. In Mick S, Wyttenbach M, editors: *Advances in health care organization theory*, San Francisco, 2003, Jossey-Bass.
5. Porter-O'Grady T, Malloch K: *Quantum leadership: Advancing innovation, transforming health care*, ed 3, Sudbury, MA, 2011, Jones & Bartlett.
6. Ledlow G, Coppola N: *Leadership for health professionals: Theory, skills, and applications*, Sudbury, MA, 2010, Jones & Bartlett.
7. Scott K, Mesnick J: Creating the conditions for breakthrough clinical performance. *Nurse Leader* 8(4):48–52, 2010.
8. Olden P, Diana M: Classical theories of organization. In Johnson J, editor: *Health organizations: Theory, behavior and development*, Sudbury, MA, 2009, Jones & Bartlett, pp 29–46.
9. Diana M, Olden P: Modern theories of organization. In Johnson J, editor: *Health organizations: Theory, behavior and development*, Sudbury, MA, 2009, Jones & Bartlett, pp 47–62.
10. Cummings T, Worley C: *Organization development & change*, Mason, OH, 2009, South-Western Cengage Learning.
11. Buerhaus P, Staiger D, Auerbach D: *The future of the nursing workforce in the United States: Data, trends and implications*, Sudbury, MA, 2009, Jones & Bartlett.
12. *Institute of Medicine*: *The future of nursing: Leading change, advancing health*, Washington, DC, 2010, National Academies Press.
13. Altmiller G: Interprofessional teamwork and collaboration. In Kelly P, Vottero B, Christie-McAuliffe C, editors: *Introduction to quality and safety education for nurses: Core competencies*, New York, 2014, Springer, pp 131–160.
14. Liesveld J: Collaboration. In Giddens J, editor: *Concepts for nursing practice*, St Louis, 2013, Elsevier, pp 425–433.

15. Connors H, Warren J, Popkess-Vawter S: Technology and informatics. In Giddens J, editor: *Concepts for nursing practice*, St Louis, 2013, Elsevier, pp 443–451.

16. Havily C, Anderson A, Currier A: Overview of patient safety and quality of care. In Kelly P, Vottero B, Christie-McAuliffe C, editors: *Introduction to quality and safety education for nurses: Core competencies*, New York, 2014, Springer, pp 1–37.

17. Sportsman S: Care delivery strategies. In Yoder-Wise P, editor: *Leading and managing in nursing*, ed 6, St Louis, 2015, Elsevier, pp 249–271.

18. Folse V: Managing quality and risk. In Yoder-Wise P, editor: *Leading and managing in nursing*, ed 6, St Louis, 2015, Elsevier, pp 361–381.

19. *American Nurses Credentialing Center: Magnet Recognition Program*, 2015. Retrieved from <http://nursecredentialing.org/Magnet.aspx>.

Health Care Economics

Teresa Keller

The future of the health care system is one of the most important issues facing the United States. This system is funded by a patchwork of public and private insurance programs and philanthropies, in contrast to many other nations in which the central government manages financing of the delivery of health care for the majority of its residents. Most people in the United States finance their health care through some form of insurance, but not a single form. The health care market is complicated and involves insurance companies, employers, and regulators. This loose system of health insurance coverage impacts individuals' and family's interactions with the health care delivery system, particularly in terms of the type of care and the providers that can be seen along with the out-of-pocket costs. Even with the major overhaul of the health care insurance market by the Patient Protection and Affordable Care Act of 2010 (PPACA), gaps in coverage still exist and there are still issues with access to quality, affordable care for all. Determination of those who qualify for access to health care markets, the amount of care received, and how to pay for it are moral and practical challenges to our society.

A foundational element in this discussion is the concept of health care finance, including the economic principles that influence the insurance markets. Economics, as a discipline, can provide insight into the issues of the distribution of health care because the fundamental problem of resource scarcity requires making choices in the health care market. Health care resources are limited, creating a situation in which scarcity propels the costs associated with health care delivery and the financial arrangements made to meet these costs. Health care economics is concerned with both efficiency (getting the most out of a fixed amount of resources) and distribution (determining who receives resources and who will be denied). Sellers of medical goods and services (physicians, nurses, pharmacists, hospitals, and clinics) are motivated by economic interests as well as patient needs.[1]

DEFINITION

Health care economics focuses on how people deal with scarcity and finite resources. For the purpose of this concept presentation, health care economics is defined as *a behavioral science that begins with two propositions about human behavior. First, human behavior is purposeful or goal directed, implying that persons act to promote their own interests. Second, human desires and demands are unlimited, especially for something such as health care.* However, resources are limited and cannot meet unlimited demands. Thus the basic problem addressed by health care economics and finance is how to allocate limited resources among unlimited demands and how to pay for these resources.[2] The term *health care finance* refers to the arrangements made to pay for these goods and services.

SCOPE

Health care economics represents the availability (or scarcity) of health care resources and financing, or payment mechanisms, to pay for these resources. Whether or not there is payment influences utilization of resources, regardless of the availability and distribution of health care. Therefore, health care economics and finance are twin sides of the same coin and are appropriately considered together. The delivery and financing of health care is highly influenced by government and public and private organizations because they define and control payment for health care services. Economic behavior in the health care marketplace is highly sensitive to the actions of all participants, leading to ongoing changes in health care goods and services and their costs.

ATTRIBUTES AND CRITERIA

The characteristics commonly associated with the concept of health care economics are price and cost, supply and demand, cost-effectiveness, efficiency, and value. In a health care market, financing is driven by economic principles and the effect these principles have on market participants (Box 56-1).

Price and Cost

The United States spends more money on health care than any other nation. By 2017, it is estimated that $13,000 per person will be spent on health care, according to the annual projection by the Centers for Medicare & Medicaid Services (CMS). Annual health care spending in the United States is estimated to surpass $4.2 trillion in 2018, representing 19% of the gross domestic product by 2018.[3] Payment mechanisms are needed to cover these costs. Approximately 60% of Americans have employer-provided health care insurance (including military health care), and 9% self-pay for their health insurance.[4] However, for many employees, growth in health care insurance premiums displaces wage increases. For other employees, increasing insurance premium costs mean their employers struggle to offer coverage at all. Older Americans (>65 years of age) are eligible for the government insurance programs, Medicare and Medicaid. Rising costs associated with these

FIGURE 56-1 Relationship among Attributes of Health Care Economics

government programs are paid for by taxpayers, include the insured participants, through taxes.

Supply and Demand

The relation between supply and demand is an economic model of how prices are determined in a market. In a competitive market such as the United States, the unit price for a particular good will vary until it settles at a point where the current price will equal the quantity supplied by producers. This results in an economic equilibrium of price and quantity. The two important concepts to understand are the laws of supply and demand. For supply, this means that when the selling price of an item rises, more people will produce the item because they can make a profit. The law of demand states that when the price of an item is reduced, the demand for it increases. This means there is a balance. As a price increases, demand decreases, and vice versa. Generally, supply reflects demand because individuals would not continue to develop a product or supply a service for which demand has declined, nor would they buy something when the price is too high.[5] Regardless of where the market is in terms of supply and demand, long-term sustainability of health care entities depends on delivering care that is cost-effective, efficient, and has value.

Cost-Effectiveness

Health economics aims to find the best way to satisfy the increasing demand for health care given the limited resources. The resources used to provide care services are scarce, and decisions about the services to be provided and who will receive these services usually have resource and cost implications. The overall aim of economic evaluation is to aid decision makers to make efficient and equitable decisions about the allocation of resources by comparing the cost-effectiveness and benefits of health care interventions.[6] Cost-effectiveness analyses of health care interventions have become one of the focal points in the decision-making process in health care. The introduction of any health technology, whether it is a new drug or a new medical device, is often associated with an increase in health care costs and can limit the funding available for other interventions. Using health economics and measuring the cost-effectiveness helps policymakers, health care providers, and insurance companies determine whether the new intervention is cost-effective in comparison to other options.[7]

Efficiency

Efficiency in the delivery of health care can be thought of as avoiding waste (including waste of equipment, supplies, and people) or as using health care resources to get the best value for the money. The definition of efficiency used by economists was formulated by the Italian economist Vilfredo Pareto. Achieving a Pareto efficiency would be a balanced allocation of resources where no one can be made better off without making someone else worse off.[5]

Today, health care system financial resources in the United States are less frequently controlled by physicians and nurses and more often by administrators, financial managers, third-party payers, and politicians. These people view reduced illness and death as a reasonable goal, but they also seek objective evidence that this goal is achieved with fiscal efficiency (i.e., by the least expenditure of increasingly scarce financial resources).[8] Economic analysis is based on the fundamental notion of efficient use of available resources. Two basic points are that economics is about resource allocation and efficiency in resource use (getting the most from available resources).[2]

Value

Cost-effective and efficient delivery of health care is needed to achieve value and thus is a critical attribute of economics in health care. The best way to drive system progress is rigorous, disciplined measurement and improvement of value. However, value in health care remains largely unmeasured and misunderstood.[9] Achieving high value for patients must become the overarching goal of health care delivery, with value defined as the health outcomes achieved per dollar spent. This goal is important for patients and unites the interests of all who interface with the system. If value improves, patients, payers, providers, and suppliers all benefit, and the economic sustainability of the health care system increases. Because value depends on results, not inputs, value in health care is measured by the outcomes achieved, not the volume of services delivered, and shifting focus from volume to value is a central challenge. Nor is value measured by the process of care used; process measurement and improvement are important tactics, but in economics they are not substitutes for measuring outcomes and costs.[10] The interrelationship among the attributes of cost-effectiveness, efficiency, and value is shown in Figure 56-1.

The interrelationship of how these attributes build on one another is represented as a bull's-eye because the "target" for the concept of health care economics is to have cost-effective care; thus it is in the center of the bull's-eye. Close to the center of the bull's-eye is efficiency in delivery of care. Even if the care is cost-effective, inefficiency wastes resources and the system becomes unsustainable. At the outer rim of the bull's-eye is value. If a fire at the target hits value, there will be contributing economic benefits to the health care delivery system, but without the others, value alone cannot sustain the system. For example, if a patient were to spend a full hour with a primary care provider during a routine visit that normally would be a 20-minute visit, the patient would likely perceive value. However, the time involved is not efficient, cost-effective, or sustainable. Alternatively, if no value is perceived by the patient, the system is still not sustainable.

THEORETICAL LINKS

An important theoretical link to the concepts of health care economics is *risk*. Risk is the uncertainty and unpredictability of a loss—for example, the loss of a home due to fire. Typical health care risks are generally related to the debilitating effects of serious health conditions and their effect on an individual's or family's quality of life. For example, if the health of one of the income earners in a household deteriorates, there is likely to be a loss of income to sustain the family. Health insurance mediates this risk by transferring the risk to an insurance company in a contractual arrangement between the insured and the company. In the case of a loss, the insurance company compensates the insured for their loss.[11]

CONTEXT TO NURSING AND HEALTH CARE

Nursing is the largest segment of the nation's health care workforce. With more than 3 million members who often provide the largest bulk of patient care, nurses can play a vital role in helping realize the objectives set forth in the 2010 Affordable Care Act—legislation that represents the broadest health care overhaul since the 1965 creation of the Medicare and Medicaid programs. Working together with government, businesses, health care organizations, professional associations, and the insurance industry, nurses can play a vital role in ensuring that health care is equitable and accessible to all and leads to improved health outcomes.

Health care economics affects all professional nurse practice environments as well as the individual nurse and his or her family. Nurses delivering patient care in an organization may be unaware of the many issues of economics and finance that they encounter on a daily basis. Health care organizations of all types usually have a finance office that manages income and payments so health care personnel can provide patient care. Nurses will often encounter the economic and finance issues that directly affect their patients at discharge, such as insufficient resources to pay out-of-pocket costs or to purchase medications. In such cases, the nurse should work with the interdisciplinary team, including the patient, to problem solve these issues. Nurses will experience almost daily a constant concern for achieving efficiencies in practice, reducing unnecessary waste, and working together to reduce the costs of care. In addition, as health care consumers themselves, nurses will have to make choices and trade-offs about the resources they use to keep themselves and their families healthy.

Patient Protection and Affordable Care Act (Public Law 11-148)

One of the major impacts on health care economics in recent years has been the PPACA. This legislation has elicited much debate among policy experts and the public. No one knows exactly how this new complex law will evolve. The objective evaluation of its effectiveness is extremely important.[12]

The American College of Physicians wants legislation to advance key priorities on coverage, workforce, payment, and delivery system reform. The goal of the PPACA is to help provide affordable health insurance coverage to most Americans and to improve access to primary care. What remains to be seen is to what extent the PPACA will ensure affordable coverage and sufficient numbers of primary care physicians.[13]

The PPACA is expected to cover an estimated 32 million uninsured Americans.[14] Without the PPACA, the Census Bureau estimates the number of uninsured persons would reach to more than 60 million or one out of five U.S. residents.[15] The Congressional Budget Office (CBO) estimates that 95% of legal U.S. residents will be covered under the legislation, including the aforementioned 32 million who otherwise would have been uninsured.[16] Despite the challenges that initially existed when the enrollment process began, the number of previously uninsured individuals enrolled reached nearly 17 million people by May 2015.[17]

According to the Kaiser Foundation,[18] the following are some of the law's major provisions:

- The requirement that most U.S. citizens and legal residents have health insurance by 2014
- The creation of state-based exchanges through which individuals can purchase coverage, with subsidies available to lower income individuals
- A major expansion of the Medicaid program for the nation's poorest individuals
- The requirement for employers to cover their employees or pay penalties, with exceptions for employers with few employees
- New regulations on health plans in the private market requiring them to cover all individuals, regardless of health status
- Establishment of a national, voluntary insurance program for purchasing community living assistance services
- Increases in payments for primary care services
- Greater support for prevention, wellness, and public health activities

Pay for Performance

Current health policy initiatives to reduce market distortions are directed at both supply and demand. Pay for performance is designed to enhance the communication and coordination of care among patients, providers, and clinicians (including nurses) by offering additional reimbursement to clinicians and hospitals for the provision of health care services considered appropriate and of high quality. This will ensure that patients receive important care that may not have been prioritized before the program's existence. More than half of commercial health maintenance organizations (HMOs) use pay for performance, and recent legislation requires the CMS to adopt this approach for Medicare.[19]

There is much debate about whether pay for performance should be at the individual provider level, for a provider group, or at an organizational level. An example of this is the use of generic drugs. Unless contraindicated for a particular patient, a provider who prescribes a generic drug is saving the health care system money; thus the provider should be rewarded. One of the struggles with pay for performance is how to develop performance reporting on both cost and quality measures and then to use the same performance data to calculate financial rewards. Many current pay-for-performance programs offer rewards for high relative performance (being among the top 10% of physicians) rather than absolute performance. Rewarding only the top providers creates competition and can stretch a small bonus pool. On the other hand, competition may limit collaboration and sharing of best practices and may create or sustain quality gaps between high- and low-performing providers.[20]

Nurses are indirectly part of pay for performance with new Medicare reimbursement guidelines. Currently, Medicare will not cover the cost of preventable hospital-acquired conditions, mistakes, and infections that can occur during a patient's hospitalization. For example, if a patient admitted to a hospital develops a pressure ulcer during his or her hospital stay, Medicare will not pay for the extended admission related to acquiring the pressure ulcer. Other nurse-sensitive indicators included in Medicare's new ruling are falls from bed, catheter-associated urinary tract infections, blood incompatibility mistakes, and vascular catheter-associated infections. This is placing an additional financial burden on hospitals because nurses need the time to assess all of these indicators on an ongoing basis and hospitals must code for infections and other conditions as "present on admission" so they are not liable for a reduction in their payment. Therefore, staff nurses have the ability to contribute to the organization's efforts to achieve pay-for-performance standards, including education, documentation, team collaboration, and patterns of care.[21]

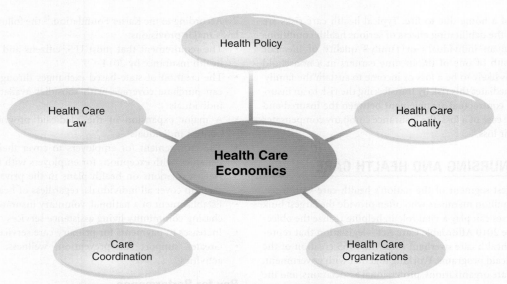

FIGURE 56-2 Health Care Economics and Interrelated Concepts

INTERRELATED CONCEPTS

This concept represents areas that relate to health care economics. Several concepts featured in this textbook have a relationship with this concept. Health Policy is used to provide overarching goals and to set priorities and values for the allocation of health resources. Health Care Quality is concerned with issues related to ensuring standards of care and outcomes are achieved in the delivery of health care. Health Care Organizations provide the framework for the delivery of health care. Care Coordination involves the marshaling of personnel and other resources needed to carry out all required patient care activities. Health Care Law affects health care economics because it governs the insurance industry and is illustrated in the application of health care funding and reform. These interrelationships are depicted in Figure 56-2.

CLINICAL EXEMPLARS

The ability to deliver patient care is affected by a wide variety of categories involved in health care economics. These include the factors that constitute our health care markets, such as the distribution of health care that results in health disparities and the principles of free market and supply and demand, and the influence these have on creating health care that is efficient, cost-effective, and has value. In addition, health care financing, which includes government-sponsored care, managed care, and private insurance, is the driving force behind health care economics. Payment mechanisms dictate the use of care, and this influences the availability and scarcity of resources. These exemplars are shown in Box 56-2 and further described next.

Featured Exemplars
Medicaid

Medicaid is the nation's major public health insurance program for low-income Americans. Enacted in 1965, Medicaid has improved access to health care for low-income individuals, financed innovations in health care delivery, and functioned as the nation's primary source of long-term care financing. Medicaid is now one of the centerpieces of expanding coverage in the national health reform bill.[22] By 2019, the program is expected to cover nearly one in five Americans. Medicaid is funded by state and federal government sources such as legislative appropriations, intergovernmental transfers, certified public

---

expenditures, permissible taxes, and provider donations. Medicaid eligibility is determined by income and need.

State Children's Health Insurance Program

The State Children's Health Insurance Program (SCHIP) was enacted in 1997 to provide coverage to uninsured low-income children who did not qualify for Medicaid. Like Medicaid, SCHIP is jointly funded by state and federal governments and eligibility is determined by income and need. Payments are only distributed to qualified hospitals and health care facilities and home health agencies, and they cannot exceed a reasonable estimate of the amount Medicare would pay for the same services.[23]

Medicare

Medicare provides health care coverage for all people ages 65 years or older, people who are permanently disabled, and individuals with end-stage renal disease. It is a federal health insurance program that individuals or their spouses have paid into through employment or self-employment taxes.[24] Medicare includes hospital insurance (Part A), supplemental medical insurance (Part B), Medicare Advantage plans (Part C), and outpatient prescription drug coverage (Part D). Part A includes hospital coverage, and Part B includes outpatient coverage and is optional—the recipient must contribute a premium each month to preserve coverage. Patients with Part A may opt to add Part B, which covers 80% of the fees for outpatient services.[25]

Accountable Care Organizations

The 2010 PPACA provided for the creation of accountable care organizations (ACOs). ACOs are organizations of health care providers that are accountable for the quality, cost, and overall care of Medicare patients, for whom they provide the bulk of primary care services.[26] ACOs must have defined processes for promoting evidence-based medicine and reporting data to evaluate the quality, cost, and coordination of care. ACOs that meet specified quality standards will receive a share of the savings if Medicare's cost for the care of their assigned patients is below a certain benchmark.[27] Critical to the achievement of these ACOs is regulation by the Centers for Medicare & Medicaid Services and the Federal Trade Commission. One of the most important judgments these agencies will make includes assurances that ACOs foster, not hinder, competition in health care markets.[28]

Managed Care Organizations

In managed care, health care providers and insurance companies assume a part of the financial responsibility for health care. Patients pay a monthly premium for health care insurance. Patients choose from several different plans under the managed care system, including preferred provider organizations (PPOs) and HMOs. Patients receive health care from a list of providers who participate in the PPO or HMO.[29] Current trends show insurance companies have multiple health care plans that they manage for different employers. Health care services covered by the plans are determined by the employer. Insurance payment varies according to geographic region and depends greatly on the type and plan of coverage. This may often leave the patient with unpaid medical expenses or the need to obtain prior authorization before seeking treatment or medication.[29]

Private or Indemnity Health Insurance

Private health insurance may be purchased on a group basis (e.g., by a firm to cover its employees) or purchased by individual consumers. Most Americans with private health insurance receive it through an employer-sponsored program. Nearly 60% of Americans are covered through an employer, whereas approximately 9% purchase health insurance directly.[15] The PPACA has expanded access to Medicaid and to private insurance markets for individuals and families who were previously unable to obtain insurance benefits. An example of private indemnity health insurance that can be purchased either by an employer for its employees or by an individual is that provided by the Blue Cross Blue Shield Association.[30]

CASE STUDY

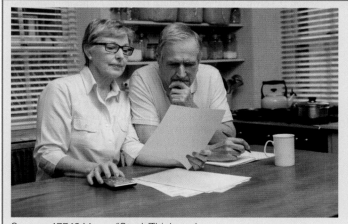

Source: 4774344sean/iStock/Thinkstock

Case Presentation

Raymond Wiley operates a small business in a rural area. In his community, there is a 10-bed hospital that has a 2-bed intensive care unit (ICU). A large hospital with comprehensive services is located in a nearby city 100 miles away.

Mr. Wiley became ill with a fever and cough. Because his regular physician was out of town, he went to the local hospital, where he was diagnosed with pneumonia and admitted. Mr. Wiley received supportive care, but after 3 full days with no apparent improvement, the admitting physician transferred him to the city hospital for a referral with a pulmonologist.

Mr. and Mrs. Wiley wanted to drive to the city hospital in their private vehicle, as opposed to having Mr. Wiley transported by ambulance. Their rationale was based on the fact that Mrs. Wiley could drive, Mr. Wiley was stable, and their insurance did not cover ambulance transport unless it was a medical emergency. Up to this point, Mr. Wiley had only received supportive care; his IV had been capped, and he was taking oral antibiotics. The Wileys' request to drive themselves was refused, and Mr. Wiley was transported by ambulance; they were charged $1300 for the transport.

Once Mr. Wiley arrived at the city hospital, it took 2 days for the pulmonologist to see him because the admitting unit mixed up his name with another patient. A computed tomography scan was completed, which revealed he had a large mass and pleural effusion. Mr. Wiley was then seen by a thoracic surgeon, who scheduled him for a thoracotomy the next day— a Sunday. This required assembling an on-call surgical team at the higher weekend rate.

Following surgery, Mr. Wiley was in the ICU. He experienced several postoperative complications precipitated by the initial delay in correct diagnosis and treatment. On postop day 11, an order was written to transfer Mr. Wiley out of the ICU to the medical unit, but because of a shortage of nursing staff on the medical unit, he remained in the ICU for 2 additional days before being transferred to a medical unit and discharged home later that day.

Mrs. Wiley spent 10 months disputing many of the charges because her husband's care had been delayed by the medical team, causing his complications and extensive hospitalization. The Wileys believed that they should not be charged and held responsible for the 3 days in the rural hospital, the "emergency" transport, the 2 days in the city hospital before Mr. Wiley was seen by the specialist, and the 2 additional days spent in the ICU because the hospital was short staffed. The insurance company and hospital finally agreed on how much the insurance company would pay of the $136,000 worth of services billed. The hospital wrote off $60,000, and the Wileys paid $5000 in co-payments.

Case Analysis

Mr. Wiley's care was not cost-effective because there were many delays that were costly both from a systems standpoint and from the exacerbations to the seriousness of his illness. The hospital eventually was forced to write off nearly half of the billed charges, which will eventually result in higher charges across the system to compensate for these and other losses. Mr. Wiley's story highlights how a lack of communication resulting in a lack of effectiveness in timely treatment continues to haunt health care, affecting the quality of patient care and outcomes as well as patient costs. Value was not attained because Mr. Wiley's care was delayed in both the rural and the tertiary care hospitals.

ACCESS EXEMPLAR LINKS IN YOUR GIDDENS EBOOK

REFERENCES

1. Wells DA, Ross JS, Detsky AS: What is different about the market for health care? *JAMA* 298(23):2785–2787, 2007.
2. Solomon S, McGowan J, Jr: Applying economic principles to health care. *Emerg Infect Dis* 7(2):282–295, 2001.
3. Pulcini JA, Hart MA: Financing health care in the United States. In Mason DJ, Leavitt JL, Chaffee MW, editors: *Policy and politics in nursing and health care*, St Louis, 2007, Saunders.
4. *Centers for Medicare & Medicaid Services: Office of the Actuary, National Health Statistics Group: Projected data from NHE projections, 2009–2018.* Retrieved from <http://www.cms.hhs.gov/NationalHealthExpendData>.
5. Besanko D, Braeutigan DS: *Microeconomics*, ed 2, Hoboken, NJ, 2005, Wiley.
6. Ratcliffe J, Laver K, Couzner L, et al: Not just about costs: The role of health economics in facilitating decision making in aged care. *Age Ageing* 39(4):426–429, 2010.
7. Giang N: *The role of health economics*, 2009. Retrieved from <http://www.brighthub.com/health/technology/articles/6763.aspx>.
8. McGowan J, Jr: Cost and benefit in perioperative antimicrobial prophylaxis—Methods for economic analysis. *Rev Infect Dis* 13(Suppl 10):S879–S889, 1991.
9. Porter M: What is value in health care? *N Engl J Med* 363:2477–2481, 2010.
10. Porter M, Teisberg E: *Finding health care: Creating value-based competition on results*, Boston, 2006, Harvard Business School Press.
11. Rejda G, McNamara M: *Principles of risk management and insurance*. New York, 2015, Pearson.
12. *Affordable Care Act: HR 3590*, 2010. Retrieved from <http://www.ncsl.org/documents/health/HlthWrkfrceProvHR3590>.
13. Doherty RB: The certitudes and uncertainties of health care reform. *Ann Intern Med* 152(10):679–682, 2010.
14. Dubay L, Holahan J, Cook A: The uninsured and the affordability of health insurance coverage. *Health Aff* 26(1):22–30, 2007.
15. *U.S. Census Bureau: Health insurance: Current population survey, annual social and economic supplement*, 2009. Retrieved from <http://www.census.gov/hhes/www/hlthins/hlthins.html>.
16. *Congressional Budget Office: Preliminary estimate of the direct spending and revenue effects of an amendment in the nature of a substitute to H.R. 4872, the Reconciliation Act of 2010.* Retrieved from <https://www.cbo.gov/ftpdocs/113xx/doc11355/hr4872.pdf>.
17. Reinberg S: *Almost 17 million gained coverage under Obamacare. Medicine. net*, 2015. Retrieved from <http://www.medicinenet.com/script/main/art.asp?articlekey=188359>.
18. *Kaiser Foundation: Health policy education: health reform*, 2010. Retrieved from <http://www.kaiseredu.org/Topics/Health-and-Government.aspx>.
19. Rosenthal M, Dudley R: Pay-for-performance: Will the latest payment trend improve care? *JAMA* 297(7):740–744, 2007.
20. Belshe K: But pay for performance is unlikely to be a panacea: California's role in ensuring that the potential of health reform becomes reality. *JAMA* 298(23):2785–2787, 2007.
21. Bedrock J, Mion L: Pay for performance in hospitals: Implications for nurses and nursing. *Qual Manage Health Care* 17(2):102–111, 2008.
22. *Centers for Medicare & Medicaid Services: Community services and long term supports*, 2010. Retrieved from <http://www.medicaid.gov/medicaid-chip-program-information/by-topics/long-term-services-and-supports/long-term-services-and-supports.html>.
23. *Medicaid.gov: Children's Health Insurance Program*, n.d. Retrieved from <http://www.medicaid.gov/chip/chip-program-information.html>.
24. *U.S. Department of Health and Human Services, Centers for Medicare & Medicaid Services: Hospital-acquired conditions and present on admission indicator reporting provision*, 2009. Retrieved from <http://www.cms.gov/Outreach-and-Education/Medicare-Learning-Network-MLN/MLNProducts/Downloads/wPOAFactSheet.pdf>.
25. Pulcini JA, Hart MA: Financing health care in the United States. In Mason D, Leavitt J, Chaffee M, editors: *Policy and politics in nursing and health care*, St Louis, 2007, Saunders.
26. McClellan M, McKethan A, Lewis J, et al: A national strategy to put accountable care into practice. *Health Aff* 29:982–990, 2010.
27. Thomas L, Greaney JD: Accountable care organizations—The fork in the road. *N Engl J Med* 364:e1, 2011.
28. Sinaiko A, Rosenthal M: Patients' role in accountable care organizations. *N Engl J Med* 363:2583–2585, 2010.
29. Kreitzer MJ: Successes and struggles in complementary health care. In Mason DJ, Leavitt JK, Chaffee MW, editors: *Policy and politics in nursing and health care*, ed 5, St Louis, 2007, Saunders.
30. *Blue Cross and Blue Shield: About the Blue Cross Blue Shield Corporation*, 2011. Retrieved from <http://www.bcbs.com/about-the-association>.

Health Policy

Nancy Ridenour and Teresa Keller

Health policy is a legitimate government interest because the desire for good health is common to all. Ill health can disrupt an individual's ability to participate in personal and civic activities and can also have a major impact on family members and communities. Widespread ill health threatens entire communities and even larger social systems, potentially disrupting the delicate web of social obligations and activities that are the supporting infrastructure of modern life. The creation of public policies that address health concerns has become an accepted responsibility for governments and a means for ensuring some level of security from the personal and public consequences of ill health.

In the United States, decisions about health policy are made at many levels of government and by a variety of political institutions.[1,2] Health policy is determined through laws, regulatory actions, judicial decisions, and the administrative actions of government agencies.[3] Health policy decision making in the United States is also affected by the numerous cultural and social trends that arise from technological change, shifting demographics, economic pressures, and consumer demands.[4] The results are health policies that support a decentralized health services sector in which there is no single source of decision-making power. The health care policies created within this dynamic environment are meant to address policy goals through a political process of negotiation and compromise, subjected to public review and comment, and, ultimately, acceptable to the widest possible majority of interested parties. However, the outcome of widespread, decentralized health policy decision making can also be that the policies are fragmented, complex, contradictory, and even unconstitutional.

This slow and sometimes cumbersome process reflects the realities of the health care environment in the United States. A mix of private and public systems, the health care environment is constantly changing and constantly creating new opportunities for innovations that are both a part of and in response to the political and cultural values of Americans. It is also this type of health policy environment that provides opportunities for nurses to intervene in the interests of their patients, families, and vulnerable populations as well as for the interests of the nursing profession. To effectively participate and advocate in the health policy decision-making process, nurses should have a clear understanding of the concept of health policy, including its definition, major characteristics, and ways it is differentiated from related concepts.

DEFINITION

A clear definition of health policy needs to account for the variety of ways that health policy is determined and controlled in the public sector. Initially, health policy can be defined as a form of public policy, differentiating it from other kinds of decision making. A classic and basic definition of public policy is what governments decide to do or not to do.[5] Public policy can also be defined as the choices made by a society or social entities that relate to public goals and priorities as well as the choices made for allocating resources to those goals and priorities.[6] Health policy would therefore be the result of choices and resource allocation decisions made to support health-related goals and priorities. Public policy is further defined as "authoritative guidelines that direct human behavior toward specific goals,"[7] so health policy is also authorized and directed toward health goals. Longest and Darr define health policy as public policies pertaining to health that are the result of an authoritative, public decision-making process.[3] A realistic definition of the concept health policy is *goal-directed decision making about health that is the result of an authorized, public decision-making process*. Health policy is further defined as *those actions, nonactions, directions, and/or guidance related to health that are decided by governments or other authorized entities*.

Examples of this definition of health policy include decisions related to federal subsidies for the education of health professionals, state regulations that cover insurance benefits, and court decisions that overturn these same state regulations based on constitutional arguments. This definition also includes a variety of other health policies related to Medicare reimbursements to nurse practitioners, state-mandated immunizations for schoolchildren, and the decisions of a state or federal court that establish the rights of families to make health care decisions for their children or for elderly parents. This definition also provides for government *inaction*, as is the case when a legislative committee defers a decision on a health-related matter or when a proposed health program is not adopted by a government agency because of resource restraints. All of these examples demonstrate the public, goal-oriented, and authoritative nature of health policy decision making. They are also examples of the divided nature of health policy decision making in the United States.

SCOPE

Health policy as a concept can first be differentiated by locating it within the realm of public decision making by political authority including executive order, legislation, judicial process, or regulatory rule-making agencies. Health policy determined through a presidential executive order or by legislation is easily recognizable as the legitimate responsibility of elected leadership. Health policy that is the result of regulatory actions or results from the administrative decisions of government agencies is not as easily identified. However, the decisions made in these other policy arenas may have significant impact on the distribution and quality of health care services.

The scope of health policy is wide and as varied as the numerous entities responsible for decisions, funding, enactment, and oversight as well as the many populations and individuals who are affected by these decisions. Health policy decisions can have both macro-level (Medicare program funding) and micro-level effects (co-payments for episodes of care) and can be made on the basis of economics, social justice, political trends, and/or changing social values. Health policy can also be the source of much political conflict because it has the potential to affect a large number of people, depending on the health policy goal.

Because health policy, as defined previously, is the result of authoritative, public decision making, a simple way to categorize it is to use the major types of political institutions established in the United States for politically determined decisions. These major government institutions decide, implement, and regulate policies, including health policy, and are legally authorized to do so by constitutional arrangements. Each of these authorities uses a public process for decision making. The major public authorities operating at the federal, state, and local levels are (1) state and national legislatures, (2) state and national as well as local courts and judiciary, (3) the executive branches of federal and state governments, and (4) regulatory agencies.[3,7]

Legislatures

The U.S. Congress and state legislatures are deliberative bodies that establish laws to serve some policy goal. Along with the authority to create laws, legislatures are also tasked with determining the appropriate funding for a legislative act and for providing oversight for policies that are administered by government agencies. Health policy that results from law is legally binding as long as it is consistent with the authorizing constitutional framework.[3] The multiple perspectives embodied by the independently elected representatives to legislatures ensure the consideration of a diversity of different values in the political process.[2]

Courts and Judiciary

Health policy is the result of the political integration of values and interests. The enactment of new health laws can result in the establishment of new rights related to health programs or benefits. At the same time, it might be necessary to ensure preservation of previously established rights. Court systems play an important role in the development of health policy because the federal and state courts are often the staging ground for determining rights in health policy disputes through judicial review. Judiciary review can be addressed to widely varying concerns, including challenging unreasonable government action, supporting the establishment of newly created rights through legislation, and ensuring protections provided by health care law.[8]

Executive Branch

The executive branch of federal and state governments is responsible for the execution of laws passed by legislatures. Government executives, such as state governors and the U.S. President, oversee a vast apparatus of agencies and personnel tasked with the implementation of laws. The chief executive plays a major leadership role in health policy because of the legitimate powers of the office. Chief executives develop and implement institutional budgets, control the vast resources of the executive branch, and are usually able to use veto authority to influence policy changes. The office is also a clearly identified leadership position that provides the chief executive with a stage from which to influence the direction of health policy goals and decision making.

Regulatory Agencies

Regulatory agencies either can be a part of the executive branch or may be independent or semi-independent organizations. These agencies are established by legislatures to implement and enforce laws through a rule-making process.[3] The rules developed by these agencies are made through public administrative processes and have the force of law. Health care is a highly regulated industry, so many health policies are established through administrative rule making by regulatory agencies. Decisions related to nursing licensure by state boards of nursing are an example of administrative rule making.

ATTRIBUTES AND CRITERIA

Health policies relate to a health concern or issue and are meant to address a public policy goal. Health policies result from a public decision-making process that directs the action or inaction of governments. The following are the *major attributes* of health policy:
1. Decisions are made by authorized government institutions such as legislatures or courts or by government-authorized entities.
2. The decision-making process is subject to public review and public input.
3. Health policies address a public policy goal.

Minor attributes of health policy include the following:
1. Health policies are subject to ongoing review by governing institutions and by the public.
2. Health policy goals change according to changes in political and social values, trends, and attitudes.

THEORETICAL LINKS

The attributes described previously provide one means for understanding the concept of health policy. The concept can be further understood by developing an understanding of the process by which health policy is made. Anderson provides a simple framework for understanding how health policy is created through sequential stages of activities.[9] In the first step or stage, *agenda setting*, a health-related issue is identified, usually as a problem. Nurses can be especially effective in this stage by helping to frame the issue. Framing the issue means creating a particular perspective for the issue—for example, that assisted suicide is ethically justified because patients have a right to make their own health care decisions.

Once defined and framed, an issue is refined through a political process that involves negotiation and debate as well as the mobilization of support from interested politicians and interest groups. The next stage is *policy formulation*, in which different policy interventions are proposed and considered. *Policy adoption* is the next stage; during this stage, a proposed intervention is selected. Selection is followed by *policy implementation* (carrying out the proposed intervention), and the process ends with *policy evaluation* or determining if the policy achieved the desired policy goals (Figure 57-1).

FIGURE 57-1 The Policy Process

This simple process model does not fully describe the complexities of health policy, but it does provide a structure for building conceptual understanding. As defined previously, health policies result from political processes. A basic understanding of health policy is impossible without consideration of key political concepts that affect policy development and implementation in the United States. These concepts are basic to the operations of constitutionally grounded governments in the United States and are necessary for ensuring health policies that account for the myriad of perspectives present in a multicultural, democratic society. These include the dynamics of intergovernmental relationships, the social expectations created by a system of participative governance, and the effect of dominant cultural values on political processes.

Intergovernmental Relationships

The United States consists of 50 sovereign states and a federal government, united by a mutually agreed upon constitution. The U.S. Constitution provides for a division of power between the federal government and the states that seeks to balance one against the other. The result is divided and limited government powers that create the need for political collaboration through systems of intergovernmental relations. The concept of *federalism* explains the dynamics of these intergovernmental relationships. Since 1965, federal funding for health policy initiatives has increased significantly. Policy initiatives requiring collaborative federal–state relations may result in state governments ceding some of their decision-making authority in return for federal funding. The reverse can also be true: The federal government may devolve more decision-making responsibility for health policy to state governments. This results in a complex mix of collaborative strategies supported by a web of shared responsibilities between state and federal governments.[10] The effect on health policy can be profound, leading to ongoing policy changes as authority and discretionary power shift.

Participative Governance

State and federal constitutions also provide for governments to operate through *consent of the governed*. Government power, especially in the United States, is limited to that allowed by the governed, U.S. citizens. Representatives of the governed are elected through a public voting process to conduct the business of government and to be accountable to voters for their decisions. Citizens are also expected to attend to the actions of government and participate in the political process. Paying attention and participating include a range of activities, from the simple act of voting in elections to more active political participation such as lobbying or running for office. Participative governance is fundamental to American democratic institutions because government powers are limited and subject to the will of the governed. It is a necessary check on government power that promotes the interests and values of the citizenry rather than a few elected officials. Health policies created by governments but that do not engender support from the governed do not enjoy much prolonged success.

Values

The dynamic relationship between the levels of government and sustained participative governance provide for the negotiation of diverse values through the political process. All health policy in the United States should be viewed as a product of negotiated values. Fairness and efficiency are the two competing values that are at the heart of most public policy decisions.[11] These values are decision drivers and the source of much health policy conflict because decision makers must be accountable for prudent use of public funding while also considering the needs of different constituencies. The values of fairness and efficiency are subject to interpretation and highly influenced by time, social trends, cultural expectations, economic priorities, and political situations. To ensure fairness in health policy might mean that legal rights are preserved, whether an individual right or communal rights established by law. Fairness might be interpreted as equitable distribution of health resources or as improved access to those resources. Establishing a fair policy might mean a trade-off with efficiency. Less efficient health policies may be more impartial, but they are also more costly. The additional costs must be balanced against the benefits to be derived from the policy. American democratic institutions are uniquely crafted to provide the mechanisms for negotiating values through open, clearly identified political processes.

Dynamic Tension

Federalism, participative governance, and the need to negotiate values produce a dynamic tension between competing health policy interests at the intersection of access, cost, and quality (Figure 57-2). Providing access to care for uninsured Americans, for example, will require increased government expenditures and increases the need for tax revenue. Depending on state and national policy goals, increasing access to health care for the uninsured would bring into play the forces of federalism, politics, and economic interests from both public and private sectors. Current national concerns with the quality of health care are another major focus of U.S. health policy since the publication of two Institute of Medicine (IOM) reports that emphasized the morbidity and mortality caused by medical errors.[12,13] In an effort to address the issue of quality care while also managing costs, the federal government has issued new Medicare and Medicaid guidelines that provide incentives for quality outcomes while reducing reimbursements to providers for poor quality outcomes. Improving access to quality care while decreasing overall costs also creates tensions among a variety of interested parties, including state and federal governments, regulatory agencies, legislatures, professional provider organizations, and advocacy groups.

FIGURE 57-2 The Dynamic Tension among Cost, Quality, and Access

CONTEXT TO NURSING AND HEALTH CARE

Health Care Delivery

Health policy, as defined previously, is the result of authoritative, public decision making and is negotiated through a political process. The potential is always present that some interests will be disadvantaged compared to other interests as a result of the competition of ideas and values that is the American political process. Because health policies, especially at the national level, have the potential to affect large portions of the public, an awareness of social policy, institutional policy, and markets is central to understanding health policy.

Social Policy

Social policy, in its broadest sense, relates to decisions that promote the welfare of the public.[6] Social policy can be directed at a wide variety of social concerns and issues in which the primary policy goal is not necessarily health but the policy still has an impact on health. For example, government policies related to a social policy goal that addresses obesity may result in legislation or regulation that governs the sale of high-fat/high-sugar content foods available in public schools. A state or federal law might govern WIC (women, infants, and children) payments for healthy foods at farmers' markets. A linked health policy goal would be directed at ensuring Medicare/Medicaid payments for exercise and weight loss programs.

Institutional Policy

Social policies are also not always public policies that result from political decision making. Institutional policies govern the workplace.[6] Nurses are often familiar with the policy and procedure manual of their unit or clinic or home health agency. An organization might have specific institutional policies developed for their workforce that relate to the prevention of obesity, such as providing exercise facilities onsite. Nurses also work with institutional policies that govern nursing practice, such as professional job descriptions. Social policies can take the form of organizational position statements established by professional organizations and advocacy groups. For example, the Student Nurses Association might adopt a resolution supporting exercise classes for student nurses.

Markets

The U.S. health care system is situated within an economic system that emphasizes capitalism and markets. In capitalism, markets function to ensure efficient distribution of resources to those goods and services that are the most desirable among many options. A major assumption of market systems is that the exchange of goods and services takes place among knowledgeable participants in a transparent and equitable process. This ideal is not always present in the sophisticated and expensive U.S. health care markets. Most Americans are dependent on the expertise of health care professionals to help them manage serious health problems. If they also lack adequate health insurance, they might have limited access to necessary health services if they cannot afford to pay for their care on their own.

Market ideals in these circumstances break down as the pursuit of efficient resource allocation results in resources being directed away from important social needs. An example is overallocating health care resources to relatively lucrative health markets such as cardiovascular care in the hospital but limiting resources for childhood immunizations. This creates a need for government interventions to direct resources to goods and services that serve some public interest, provide for equity in market transactions, or subsidize care for vulnerable or neglected populations. In the complex U.S. health care system, the marriage of governments and markets is inevitable as policy goals shift between the twin values of efficiency and equity.[14]

Professional Nursing Practice

Within the framework of professional nursing practice, policy can be understood within the context of nursing practice regulation and the role of the professional nurse through engagement and advocacy.

Scope and Standards of Professional Nursing Practice

The licensing and regulation of health professionals, including nurses, are the responsibility of state governments. States create laws that establish professional practice acts meant to regulate health professionals. A state regulatory agency and a politically appointed board of nursing are tasked with the implementation and administration of nurse practice acts, including issuing licenses to individuals to legally practice nursing. Some state regulatory boards are specifically created for nursing and some boards are tasked with regulation of several health care professions, but all of these regulatory boards establish the scope of legally licensed practice and minimum standards for professional performance under that license. Regulatory boards have authority delegated by the state legislature to make rules, and these rules have the force of law. Professional practice errors that violate the provisions of the practice act are subject to disciplinary action by boards and are adjudicated by the regulatory agency through established disciplinary procedures. Boards have the authority to revoke licenses for unsafe practice as defined by the practice act, including actions or behaviors by the nurse that lie outside of the scope and standards of practice established by the license.

Negligence and Malpractice

Related to professional licensing are health policies that govern professional negligence, or malpractice. Professional negligence occurs when the actions of the nurse are judged as substandard to what is expected in "reasonable and prudent" standard of practice and that result in harm to others. Whether a nurse is in violation of these standards is dependent on the minimum standards for practice set by the relevant state board of nursing, by practice standards published by professional societies, and by standards established through similar cases decided in state courts.

Engagement and Advocacy

Nurses have a profound influence on health policy by becoming engaged in the political process and through their actions in everyday practice. Lipsky introduced the concept of "street-level bureaucracy" to define the impact of frontline workers on public policy.[15] He demonstrated that these frontline workers, such as police officers and social workers, have great influence in implementing policy at the "street level," or where the policy meets its intended beneficiaries. Street-level decision making works to ensure that *policy intent* becomes the *policy as experienced*. Nurses work very closely with the patients and families who are the intended recipients and beneficiaries of health policies; therefore nurses are "street-level" workers who have the potential to greatly impact the implementation of policy at the bedside as well as in the community. Nurses deal with policy issues daily while ensuring the confidentiality of patient information, allocating health care resources through staffing assignments, or teaching patients about their health care rights—these actions all have a health policy impact for patients and their families that can be traced back to an authorized decision-making process. In addition, the clinical expertise of nurses can be used to influence policy at local, state, national, and international levels. Nurses are always engaged in health policy at many different levels, whether as frontline workers or as policy advocates in the regulatory, legislative, judicial, and executive arenas.

Health policies and the economic consequences of these policies are everyday realities for most working nurses, regardless of their specialties or their workplace. Access to care is a national health policy issue that is driven, in part, by economics. Americans with health insurance are able to access available health care resources with relative ease. Uninsured Americans either do not seek care or they obtain care through federal- and state-sponsored clinical facilities or in the nation's emergency departments. The lack of secured access to primary care or to needed tertiary care results in a chaotic and costly health care system in which financial incentives drive health behavior and health outcomes. Nurses encounter a variety of patient care dilemmas caused by economic factors in daily practice. These situations can be the source of frustration and moral distress for many professional nurses, although they can also be the motivation for nurses to engage in the political processes that produce health policies.

Nurses are in a unique and pivotal position to impact the cost/quality/access equation through advocacy. The IOM report developed in collaboration with the Robert Wood Johnson Foundation provides a road map for nurses to become active in health policy at the local, state, and national levels.[16] This report calls on all health professionals, regulatory bodies, and policymakers to improve health care by removing scope of practice barriers and increasing educa-

tion, leadership, and standardized workforce data collection and analysis (Box 57-1).

Advocacy is providing support to others and rallying that support to a cause. Nursing interest groups might unite for the purpose of advancing national health policy reform that ensures greater access to health care for all Americans. In another example, nurses can advocate for nurse-managed centers to be eligible for Federally Qualified Health Clinic (FQHC) status. Nurse practitioners working in an FQHC are eligible to receive a higher rate of reimbursement. Nurse-managed centers have a long history of providing primary health care to underserved patients. By advocating for FQHC status, nurses can support increased access to quality care at an affordable cost.

INTERRELATED CONCEPTS

Health policy is not an autonomous concept. Several additional concepts discussed in this book are closely related to health policy (Figure 57-3). Data and research are used to generate support and

---

BOX 57-1   Eight Recommendations from *the Future of Nursing* Report

1. Remove scope-of-practice barriers.
2. Expand opportunities for nurses to lead and diffuse collaborative improvement efforts.
3. Implement nurse residency programs.
4. Increase proportion of nurses with BSN degree to 80% by 2020.
5. Double the number of nurses with a doctorate by 2020.
6. Ensure that nurses engage in lifelong learning.
7. Prepare and enable nurses to lead change to advance health.
8. Build an infrastructure to collect and analyze health care workforce data.

Source: Reprinted with permission from Institute of Medicine: *The future of nursing: Leading change, advancing health,* 2011 by the National Academy of Sciences, Courtesy of the National Adademies Press, Washington, DC.

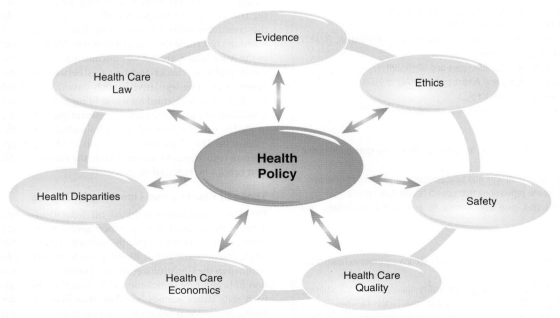

FIGURE 57-3 Health Policy and Interrelated Concepts

interest for a specific health policy agenda. This use of Evidence supports advocacy. Distribution of scarce resources and policy development to enhance the greater good while minimizing harm require use of ethical decision making. Negotiation of diverse values in the context of balancing the competing values of fairness (Ethics) and efficiency (Health Care Economics) epitomizes the challenge of designing and implementing successful health policy, particularly addressing Health Disparities. The tension described previously among cost, quality, and access highlights these competing values. Nurses are in a unique position to combine their advocacy role of ensuring patient Safety and Health Care Quality with the ethics and health economics values of fairness, access, and cost efficiency. In some contexts, it may be difficult to distinguish health policy from Health Care Law. Health professionals often respond to the laws and regulations that have been promulgated as a result of health policies.

CLINICAL EXEMPLARS

In the United States, nurses can expect to encounter a wide variety of health policies that have a direct impact on their work. A sample of some of the more visible and relevant health policies that shape the environment of nursing is listed in Box 57-2. Although it is beyond the scope of this book to describe each exemplar in detail, a few are featured here with a brief description.

BOX 57-2   EXEMPLARS OF HEALTH CARE POLICY

Federal
- Americans with Disabilities Act of 1990
- Emergency Medical Treatment and Labor Act of 1986
- Health Information Technology for Economic and Clinical Health Act of 2009 (electronic health records)
- Health Insurance Portability and Accountability Act of 1996
- Patient Protection and Affordable Care Act of 2010
- Patient Safety and Quality Improvement Act of 2005
- Patient Self-Determination Act of 1998
- Promoting Health/Preventing Disease: Objectives for the Nation, *Healthy People 1990, 2000, 2010, 2020*
- Social Security Act of 1965 (Medicare and Medicaid)
- The Mental Health Parity and Addiction Equity Act of 2008
- U.S. Preventive Services Task Force
- Mandated Health Coverage and Medicaid Expansion 2012[25]

State
- Scope of practice and licensing for nurses as defined by state professional practice acts
- State public health programs and policies related to infectious diseases
- State public health regulations that govern health care facilities
- State statutes and case law related to professional negligence and malpractice

Local
- City and county fire codes that govern safe occupancy limits in health care facilities
- City and county ordinances that govern facility maintenance, signs, utilities, parking, and/or traffic around hospitals and other health facilities
- City and county tax districts for publicly supported facilities

---

Featured Exemplars
Patient Self-Determination Act

The Patient Self-Determination Act (PDSA) requires health care facilities such as hospitals and nursing homes to provide patients with information related to their preferences for end-of-life care. For example, some patients will choose to accept all life-saving measures should their condition deteriorate while hospitalized. Under PDSA, the facility should inform the patients of their right to make their own decisions about their end-of-life care and the facility's policies respecting those decisions. A statement by the patient that informs the family, the provider, and the facility of the patient's wishes is known as an *advance directive* and is covered by the guidelines of this law.[17]

Emergency Medical Treatment and Labor Act of 1986

This act, commonly referred to as EMTLA, was enacted to prevent the denial of emergency services to patients chiefly because they are uninsured and unable to pay for their care. Common practice before this law was to transfer patients to "safety-net" hospitals, usually tax-supported public hospitals. EMTLA was meant to stop private hospital facilities from "patient dumping" to public hospitals at taxpayer expense.[18]

Health Information Technology for Economic and Clinical Health Act of 2009

The Health Information Technology for Economic and Clinical Health Act of 2009 (HITECH) amends the Public Health Service Act to establish a nationwide health information technology infrastructure, including the development of health IT standards, interoperability and certification, reports on quality, and reimbursement incentives to improve health care quality. A section of the act also addresses privacy and security concerns associated with the electronic transmission of health information through several provisions that strengthen the civil and criminal enforcement of the HIPAA rules.[19,20]

2012 Supreme Court Ruling on Mandated Health Coverage and Expansion of Medicaid

The Supreme Court has final authority for determining if the laws of Congress are acceptable by interpreting the Constitution in relation to the law. In the case *Independent Business v. Sebelius*, the court upheld the constitutionality of mandating health coverage (the *individual mandate*) but ruled that the expansion of Medicaid eligibility outlined in the Affordable Care Act was unconstitutional. This is an example of the interplay of checks and balances between the three branches of government. The legislative branch passed the Affordable Care Act. The judicial branch ruled on a case brought before the Supreme Court upholding one part of the law as constitutional and ruling another part of the law unconstitutional. The administrative branch under the auspices of the U.S. Department of Health and Human Services (USHHS) rewrote regulations to accommodate the ruling that Medicaid expansion cannot be required of states.[21]

Scope of Practice and Licensing for Nurses

The U.S. Constitution is based on federalism—sharing of powers between the national, state, and local governments. The federal government is granted powers explicitly outlined in the Constitution. The 10th Amendment of the Bill of Rights provides that states have powers not outlined in the Constitution and not prohibited by the states.[22] Regulation of health care professionals is one of the powers granted to states. Each state issues licenses based on state licensure rules and regulates health professional behavior based on state laws and regulations. For nurses, state licensure is usually regulated through a *nurse practice act*.

CASE STUDY

Source: shironosov/iStock/Thinkstock

Case Presentation

The confidentiality of medical information became an *agenda* item for Congress when electronic data systems became widely adopted throughout the United States. The increased use of computers in health care had created the capacity for critical health care information to be efficiently shared among health care providers and among insurance companies. Advocates for patient confidentiality and information privacy argued that the ease of information sharing through electronic transmission of records would result in personal health information becoming available to a wide variety of interested parties. Access to this information could result in a variety of actions, including denial of coverage through employer-sponsored plans to individuals or family members with chronic or debilitating conditions. Other unfavorable outcomes from the unrestricted sharing of private health information could also result, such as the sale of mailing lists of individuals with particular medical conditions to companies with a commercial interest in obtaining those lists.

The intent of the Health Insurance Portability and Accountability Act (HIPAA) of 1996 was to limit the ability of employers to deny health insurance coverage to their employees based on preexisting medical conditions. In the *formulation* of a policy response, the intervention chosen by Congress was to limit access to health care information to only those parties with a legitimate role in the financing and delivery of services, specifically health care providers, insurance companies, and third-party contractors.[23] Through HIPAA, Congress directed the USDHHS to *implement* the policy by developing privacy rules that protect electronically transmitted health information. These rules cover any entity that must have access to this information for legitimate purposes and provide guidelines for determining access to and disclosure of protected health information. Criminal and financial penalties are provided for proven HIPAA violations, including federal prison sentences for perpetrators and fines of up to $250,000. Investigations and prosecutions of HIPAA violations are the responsibility of the U.S. Department of Justice.[23]

One of the federal agencies tasked with public review and reporting for federal policies is the U.S. Government Accounting Office (GAO). The GAO has published different reviews of HIPAA at the request of government officials throughout the years since passage of the statute, and these reports are publicly available on the GAO website. A recent review documents the ongoing issues of implementation of this widespread policy that governs the electronic transmission of health care information.[24] HIPAA provides broad guidelines for the protection of patient information that must be interpreted for implementation. Covered entities targeted by the statute are expected to develop HIPAA-compliant policies that govern the treatment of protected health information in their organizations and during transactions with contracted third parties. The GAO report notes that there is still much guidance to be issued by USDHHS to assist these entities in complying with HIPAA guidelines. This guidance will be created through USDHHS rule-making authority and will be publicly available for comment and feedback by affected organizations and the general public during the rule-making process.

Case Analysis

This case demonstrates some of the major components of the health policy concept. HIPAA is the result of public concerns about the privacy of health care data. The electronic transmission of data potentially involves disparate entities, persons, and companies, across a variety of states. This called for a federal response because the federal government is responsible for regulating interstate commerce. However, insurance—including health insurance—is regulated at the state level as a part of state responsibilities. This federal law, meant to address the confidentiality of health data as they are transmitted electronically throughout the country, is the result of a public process of information exchange and negotiation among different levels of government and a variety of interested parties. The rules and regulations created by federal agencies tasked with implementing this law are under continuous review as is expected with the dynamic political processes that exist in the United States.

ACCESS EXEMPLAR LINKS IN YOUR GIDDENS EBOOK

REFERENCES

1. Cummings T, Worley C: *Organization development & change*, Mason, OH, 2009, South-Western Cengage Learning.
2. Peterson M: Congress. In Morone J, Elke D, editors: *Health politics and policy*, ed 5, Clifton Park, NY, 2014, Delmar, pp 30–55.
3. Longest B, Darr K: *Managing health services organizations and systems*, ed 5, Baltimore, 2010, Health Professions Press.
4. Shortell S, Kaluzny A: Organization theory and health services management. In Shortell S, Kaluzny A, editors: *Health care management: Organization design and behavior*, ed 5, Clifton Park, NY, 2006, Delmar, pp 5–41.
5. Dye T: *Understanding public policy*, ed 7, Englewood Cliffs, NJ, 1992, Prentice Hall.
6. Mason D, Leavitt J, Chaffee M: Policy and politics: A framework for action. In Mason D, Leavitt J, Chaffee M, editors: *Policy and politics in nursing and health care*, ed 6, St Louis, 2013, Saunders, pp 1–16.
7. Hanley B, Falk N: Policy development and analysis: Understanding the process. In Mason D, Leavitt J, Chaffee M, editors: *Policy and politics in nursing and health care*, ed 6, St Louis, 2013, Saunders, pp 75–93.
8. Betts V, Keepnews D, Gentry J: Nursing and the courts. In Mason D, Leavitt J, Chaffee M, editors: *Policy and politics in nursing and health care*, ed 6, St Louis, 2013, Saunders, pp 825–834.
9. Anderson JE: *Public policymaking: An introduction*, ed 7, Boston, 2010, Wadsworth Cengage.
10. Thompson F, Cantor J: Federalism. In Morone J, Elke D, editors: *Health politics and policy*, ed 5, Clifton Park, NY, 2014, Delmar, pp 94–115.
11. Stone D: Values in health policy: Understanding fairness and efficiency. In Morone J, Elke D, editors: *Health politics and policy*, ed 5, Clifton Park, NY, 2014, Delmar, pp 2–13.
12. Institute of Medicine: *To err is human: Building a safer health system*, Washington, DC, 2000, National Academies Press.
13. Institute of Medicine: *Crossing the quality chasm: A new health system for the 21st century*, Washington, DC, 2001, National Academies Press.
14. Rice T: Markets and politics. In Morone J, Elke D, editors: *Health politics and policy*, ed 5, Clifton Park, NY, 2014, Delmar, pp 14–25.

15. Lipsky M: *Street-level bureaucracy: Dilemmas of the individual in public services*, New York, 1980, Russell Sage Foundation.

16. Institute of Medicine: *The future of nursing: Leading change, advancing health*, Washington, DC, 2010, National Academies Press.

17. American Bar Association: *Health care advanced directives*, 2015. Retrieved from <http://www.americanbar.org/groups/public_education/resources/law_issues_for_consumers/patient_self_determination_act.html>.

18. Rosenblum S, Cartwright-Smith L, Hirsch J, et al: Case studies at Denver Health: "Patient dumping" in the emergency department despite EMTALA, the law that banned it. *Health Aff* 31(8):1749–1756, 2012.

19. U.S. Department of Health and Human Services: *HITECH act enforcement interim final rule*, 2009. Retrieved from <http://www.hhs.gov/ocr/privacy/hipaa/administrative/enforcementrule/hitechenforcementifr.html>.

20. HealthIT.gov: *Health IT legislation and regulation*, 2015. Retrieved from <http://www.healthit.gov/policy-researchers-implementers/health-it-legislation>.

21. Courts US: *About the Supreme Court*, (n.d.). Retrieved from <http://www.uscourts.gov/educational-resources/get-informed/supreme-court/about-supreme-court.aspx>.

22. The White House: *State & local government*, (n.d.). Retrieved from <http://www.whitehouse.gov/our-government/state-and-local-government>; see also <http://bensguide.gpo.gov/9-12/government/federalism2.html>.

23. Flores J, Dodier A: HIPAA: Past, present and future implications for nurses. *OJIN Online J Issues Nurs* 10(2):Manuscript 4, 2005.

24. Harman L: HIPAA: A few years later. *OJIN Online J Issues Nurs* 10(2):Manuscript 2, 2005.

25. Rosenblum S, Westmorland T: The Supreme Court's surprising decision on the Medicaid expansion: How will the federal government and states proceed? *Health Aff* 31(8):1663–1672, 2012.

Health Care Law

Nikki Austin

Ours is a government of liberty, by, through and under the law. No man is above it, and no man is below it.

—Theodore Roosevelt

Health care and the systems in which health care is delivered are constantly evolving, highly regulated, and increasingly complex for all disciplines, including nursing. The underlying reasons for this complexity can be understood through the lens of health care law. The rule of law has a profound impact on health care in the United States. Thus, health care law is a fundamental concept for all health care professionals. Nurses must be aware of health care law as it applies to health care in general and specifically the impact and consequences of these laws on nursing practice.

DEFINITION

In a civilized society, laws are enacted for purposes of regulating behavior and guiding conduct. A law is a rule or a set of principles enacted by a government or government agency that details how an individual or group must behave in a given circumstance. A law may be *prescriptive*—it defines something that must be done—or *proscriptive*—it prohibits something from being done. As a concept, health care law represents both prescriptive and proscriptive principles covering a wide spectrum of topics. Just as the health care industry is composed of a vast network of people, places, and things, health care law is likewise broad in its definition and scope. There are many ways to define and examine health care law. For the purposes of this concept presentation, health care law is defined as *the collection of laws that have a direct impact on the delivery of health care or on the relationships among those in the business of health care or between the providers and recipients of health care.*

SCOPE

Health care law is a complex concept representing a wide spectrum of both creation and application of laws. The executive, legislative, and judicial branches of federal and state governments hold the authority for the creation of law. The process for creating law is through legislation, litigation, or through regulatory activities by government agencies. These processes are not linear; rather, they represent an interwoven process that fosters a continuing evolution in health care law (Figure 58-1). For example, laws may begin by a legislature identifying

an issue and drafting a law to address the issue. Authority may be given to an existing federal agency to draft rules that support compliance with the policy goals of the initial law. If a situation arises that does not completely fit within the law as drafted by the legislature or an individual affected by the law believes that the law is unconstitutional or in conflict with other laws, a legal challenge in court may be presented. Sometimes the judicial ruling will stand alone as a law, and sometimes the legislature will revise the law to be consistent with the court's ruling. Or perhaps the legal challenge preceded the legislation and the legislature may or may not decide to make a formal declaration of law.

Sources of Law

Health care law is derived from primary and secondary sources of law, including constitutional law, statutory law, administrative law, tort law, common law, contract law, and criminal law (Figure 58-2).

Constitutional Law

The powers of the federal government are specifically defined in Article I Section 8 of the U.S. Constitution. The powers specifically given to the federal government do not have a direct relationship to health care, so a link to the Constitution (e.g., due process or equal protection) creates the necessary authority to draft federal health care laws. For example, the due process clause of the Fourteenth Amendment was the constitutional legal principle under which the Supreme Court decided the landmark 1973 case of *Roe v. Wade*,[1] which forbid states from criminalizing or otherwise banning first-trimester abortions and recognized a constitutional right to privacy inclusive of a woman's right to terminate her pregnancy, and the 1990 case of *Cruzan v. Missouri*,[2] which clarified a competent patient's right to refuse treatment. State constitutional authority bears a more direct relationship to health care than the federal powers and influences areas such as public health and public safety.

Statutory (Legislative) Law

Statutory law is an important source of health care law. Statutes are laws enacted by a legislative body. Many laws at both the federal and the state level have been enacted with the intent to directly impact the business or relationships of health care. Some laws have evolved with time. Other laws may not have been enacted with the intent to directly affect health care, but they may have an effect on the business of health care nonetheless. Each of the 50 states has independent legislative bodies, so the laws that are enacted by the states may vary in title, but the underlying authority to legislate for the general health and welfare of the people is the same.

FIGURE 58-1 Scope of Health Care Law

Administrative Law and Regulation

In general, administrative agencies protect a public interest and act as agents for the executive branches of the federal and state government. Many government agencies have the power to make laws in the form of rules and regulations to promote public health. Examples of administrative agencies that have a significant effect on health care law are the U.S. Department of Health and Human Services (USDHHS) and state licensing boards. Federal and state regulations aim to address several health care system objectives, such as protecting the public's health by preventing and controlling communicable disease and protecting the public against bioterrorism; promote quality of health care services; reduce health care costs and promote access to care; and protect consumers in the market for health insurance and other types of coverage.[3]

Tort Law

The most common basis for liability of nurses, physicians, and other health care providers is rooted in tort law. A civil tort refers to an action or omission that results in harm to a person. Tort law has been responsible for shaping and defining many health care quality and safety standards. The tort must cause an injury that the law believes entitles the injured party to compensation. Tort law includes unintentional and intentional conduct. An unintentional tort, such as negligence, is based on the concept of fault, meaning that liability (fault) attaches to an incorrect act or mistaken omission that caused harm even if the act or omission was unintentional. An intentional tort is based on the perspective that the wrongdoer acted intentionally to harm the patient or violate the patient's rights and should be held responsible. Examples of intentional torts include assault and battery, false imprisonment, invasion of privacy, defamation, intentional infliction of emotional distress, abuse of process, and malicious prosecution.

Common Law

The role of the judge or the judicial branch of government is to interpret the law, but often their interpretation of the law leads to law itself. This type of law is referred to as common law (or case law) whereby

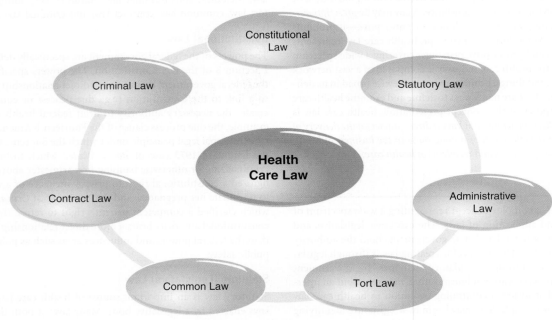

FIGURE 58-2 Sources of Law

statutory laws, applicable regulations, and legal precedents are analyzed in the context of the situation under review. A decision is made based on this analysis. Sometimes the decision is limited to the exact facts of a case or limited to a specific state or area of the country, and sometimes the decision impacts the country as a whole. Sometimes one area of the country may not have addressed a question that another area of the country has already answered in the courts, and it may adopt the ruling of another area without going through the process of litigating the question in the courts.

Contract Law

Contract law has also shaped and influenced health care law. To some degree, routine conditions of admission and consent forms represent a contract between the patient and the health care facility or the health care provider. Principles of contract are also used to define the work agreements of those who provide services of health care, such as an employment contract between a nurse and a health care organization.

Criminal Law

Criminal penalties have increasingly influenced health care laws, with felonies associated with Medicare or insurance reimbursement fraud, misrepresentation of qualifications, or even purposeful breaches of protected health information becoming more commonplace.[4] There are specific situations in which the act of negligence is so reckless or done with such purposeful disregard that the act may be considered criminal. Criminal liability considers the nature of the action, not necessarily the resultant harm, and can attach even when there is no resulting injury or harm. Health care professionals have been found guilty of criminal neglect or abuse when they have shown extreme indifference to the needs of their patients, such as restraining patients and then ignoring their cries for help or needs for repositioning, toileting, or other care. In Arizona, a physician was found guilty of manslaughter for refusing to return to attend to a patient after she developed complications from an elective procedure.[5]

ATTRIBUTES AND CRITERIA

There are many accreditation requirements, social expectations, and customs that can influence and have an effect on the delivery of health care decision making and organizational behavior. However, these are not the same as health care laws. For example, health care standards such as The Joint Commission accreditation standards can influence health care law, but these standards are not laws. Health care law can be distinguished and differentiated from accreditation requirements, social expectations, and customs by considering major and minor attributes presented in Box 58-1.

CONTEXT TO NURSING AND HEALTH CARE

Many state and federal laws have been enacted that impact health care and thus also affect nurses. This section discusses some of the most important laws that impact the professional practice of nurses and health care.

Federal Statutory Laws Impacting Health Care

Throughout the years, a number of federal laws have had sweeping effects on the delivery of health care. The Social Security Act of 1965[6] and 1983 amendment,[7] the Patient Self-Determination Act of 1981,[8] the Health Insurance Portability and Accountability Act,[4] the Patient Protection and Affordable Care Act,[9] and the Controlled Substance Act are several such laws. Implementation of these laws requires significant effort in the development of policy and in monitoring to ensure compliance.

BOX 58-1   Attributes of Health Care Law

Major Attributes
- Created by a government body with appropriate authority, such as a legislature, agency, or judiciary
- Usually has enforceable sanctions (e.g., fines or imprisonment)
- Publicly available and accessible by any individual or group
- Consistent with national and state constitutions
- Can be modified, changed, or upheld through authoritative action

Minor Attributes
- May contain incentives
- May be self-limited, expiring after some time period
- May vary in scope (some are wide and sweeping, but some are small and narrowly focused)
- May be established to promote a policy goal

Administration and Regulation
Federal Regulation

The USDHHS is the federal government's principal agency for the administration and regulation of federal laws associated with health care. It is also charged with providing essential human services, especially for those who are least able to help themselves.[10] The Secretary of USDHHS is a member of the President's Cabinet. There are 11 divisions within USDHHS, including the Centers for Disease Control and Prevention, the U.S. Food and Drug Administration, the National Institutes of Health, the Agency for Healthcare Research and Quality, and the Centers for Medicare & Medicaid Services (CMS). CMS has been given broad authority to draft the Medicaid and Medicare Conditions of Participation for Hospitals (CoPs), which are safety and health standards that define quality and patient safety expectations for health care organizations participating in Medicaid and Medicare programs. For example, when CMS became concerned about patients dying while in restraints or in seclusion, it enacted a regulation that delineates specific rules regarding the use of restraints and seclusion in participating hospitals. This regulation also requires hospitals to report any deaths that occur during or are reasonably assumed to have resulted from restraint or seclusion.[11] The CoPs regulations are now a part of the restraint policy for any hospital that expects to receive Medicare and Medicaid funding.

Licensing and Scope of Practice

The area of health care law that has an immediate and direct impact on nurses and health care providers is state licensing laws. Licensure grants permission to a person to perform professional services and/or activities of an occupation based upon the person's demonstrated qualifications and competency to perform such activities, which are illegal if performed without a license.[12] Licensure laws are commonly referred to as practice acts. Practice acts create regulatory bodies, such as a state board of nursing, that are responsible for several functions, including creating and enforcing rules consistent with the state practice act, investigating and deciding cases involving violations of the state practice act, and licensure. In addition to establishing the educational, examination, and competence requirements necessary to obtain a license in a particular health-related discipline, practice acts and regulatory agencies also establish and enforce the context and scope of licensure within which regulated professionals must comply in order to retain their status as licensees in good standing. The scope of practice for professional nursing is the range of permissible activity as defined by the law; in essence, it defines what nurses can and, sometimes more important, what nurses cannot do.[13]

Because the scope of nursing practice is defined by state legislation, there is great variation from state to state both in specificity and in the range of activities that are legally authorized. Many state legislatures have enacted very specific scope of practice statements, whereas others have drafted very vague and broad scope of practice statements and have left the task of describing the specific activities to the state board of nursing. Some state scope of practice statements are very restrictive, whereas others allow a much broader range of activities. It is important that a nurse become very familiar with the practice act and the scope of practice as defined by the legislature or the state board of nursing in the state in which he or she intends to practice. Although there is general consistency for the scope of practice for the professional registered nurse, there is significant variability for the scope of practice of licensed practical or vocational nurses and even more variability for the scope of practice for advanced practice registered nurses (APRNs).[13]

In *The Future of Nursing: Leading Change, Advancing Health*, the Institute of Medicine identified the variability of scope of practice for APRNs as one of the barriers to transforming practice and meeting the health care needs of the 21st century.[14] Because of the restrictive nature of the scope of practice statements of many states, all APRNs are not able to practice to the full extent of their education and training. However, there is evidence that when nurses play an integral role in the delivery of primary care, there are improvements in quality, access to care, patient satisfaction, and value. Allowing nurses to practice to the full extent of their education and training would likely benefit patients and the health care system as a whole.

Licensure is an important privilege that should not be taken lightly due to the enormous responsibility borne by licensees and certificate holders. When a health care professional demonstrates that he or she is in violation of the practice act by virtue of mental or physical incompetence, substance abuse or impairment, criminal violations, practice deficiencies, or a variety of other concerns established in the practice acts, the state board exercises its power to discipline the licensee to a degree consistent with the board's assessment of the severity of the problem and potential risk to the public. Disciplinary actions can range from censure and penalties to progressively more undesirable consequences, such as probation, suspension, and revocation or denial of licensure. Boards are required to report disciplinary actions to the Healthcare Integrity and Protection Data Bank and the National Practitioner Data Bank, two federal companion data banks established for public protection. Unlicensed practice is a criminal violation and, if a person is convicted, may result in fines and/or imprisonment in most states.[15]

Licensing of Health Care Institutions

In addition to licensing individual practice, states also have the authority to license and regulate health care institutions. Licensure requirements vary in terms of building size, structure, safety requirements, staffing requirements, duties of the administrators, and types of services that can be offered. These requirements can become entangled with municipal (city) building and fire codes as well as federal laws such as CMS regulations that outline requirements that hospitals must meet in order to participate in Medicare and Medicaid services.

Negligence

Tort is the area of law under which cases of negligence are argued. Negligence is the failure to use reasonably prudent care in the same or similar circumstances. Also referred to as malpractice, negligence is the most common tort holding nurses, physicians, and other health care providers liable to patients for damages. For tort liability to attach to negligent conduct, the individual actor must have done more than simply act in a negligent manner. There are four elements that must be satisfied to establish liability: duty, breach, injury, and causation.

Duty

All persons owe a duty to exercise ordinary care to avoid harming another person, place, or thing. When negligence is alleged by a patient, however, the evidence must establish that the nurse or health care provider owed a professional duty to the person harmed beyond the duty to exercise ordinary care. This higher standard and professional duty arises from a special relationship between health care providers and patients. In relation to health care law, the physician–patient relationship or nurse–patient relationship is traditionally viewed as a special relationship that gives rise to a professional duty of care. Nurses owe a professional duty of reasonable care to all of their assigned patients.

The evidence must also establish the standard of care, which refers to an approved behavior or conduct established by the profession. The standard of care for nurses is the degree of care that would be exercised by a "reasonably prudent nurse" acting under the same or similar circumstances. From a legal standpoint, the nurse in a rural setting might be held accountable to a different standard of care than the nurse in an urban, tertiary care setting. Likewise, a nurse is held accountable to a different standard of care than other health professionals (e.g., a physician), and nurses with different areas of expertise or specialty practice are held accountable to the standard of care applicable to that specialty.

The practice of nursing often involves the exercise of professional judgment as well as the application of advanced clinical and scientific knowledge. Because it may be confusing for a jury of laypersons to determine how a nurse violated the standard of care, the standard of care is a critical element that must be established by common sense, expert testimony, evidence-based standards, and/or other published standards, such as accreditation or licensing regulation standards. Several states have laws that require expert witnesses to have the same or a similar clinical background as that of the defendant. In Arizona, for example, the law requires that an expert witness in a medical malpractice action be licensed as a health professional in the state of Arizona and have devoted a majority of professional time to active clinical practice of the same health profession as the defendant in the same specialty if the defendant claims to be a specialist.[16] Several state courts have held that nurses may be used as experts to establish the standard of care for nurses instead of physicians, who historically testified as expert witnesses on the standard of nursing care.

Breach of Duty

The second element that must be satisfied to establish liability is breach of duty. Health care providers breach their duty to patients when they fall below the standard of care or deviate from the standard in a manner that causes injury. It is important to remember that not all deviations from the standard of care will result in negligent tort liability. For example, it is below the standard of care for a nursing professional to administer the wrong dose of medication to a patient. If the medication error does not result in harm or injury to the patient, the nurse will not face tort liability for his or her actions but may face termination from employment or licensure discipline depending on the circumstances.

Causation

Causation is the link between breach and injury. Would the injury have not occurred "but for" the defendant's actions? Causation answers this question and establishes that the breach of duty legally caused injury to the patient. The breach of duty or violation of standard of care must be the direct or proximate cause of the harm that the patient experienced; in other words, if the breach had not occurred, no harm would have come to the patient. In many instances, causation can be difficult to prove in negligence cases.

Injury or Harm

The final element to be satisfied in a negligence action is proof of injury or harm. The resultant harm may be physical or a combination of physical, mental, emotional, or financial harm. In other words, in some states, a patient cannot recover from emotional harm alone without an accompanying physical disability. After injury is established by a preponderance of the evidence, there is often considerable disagreement among the parties to the lawsuit about the monetary value to be placed on the injury.

Employer/Employee Liability

Professional liability can attach to an employer for the negligent acts of its employee. This is known as vicarious liability, and it arises from the common law doctrine of *respondeat superior,* a Latin term that means "let the master answer." Under vicarious liability, an employer can be liable for the acts of its employee if the employee was acting as the agent of the employer and the actions that resulted in injury occurred within the scope of employment. Thus, an employer would not be liable for injury that happened while the employee was not at work or injury that resulted from activities that were outside of the employee's scope of practice.

Laws That Empower Patient Decision Making
Consent for Treatment

Although consent laws have been largely shaped by the common law, many states have enacted laws that designate who can consent or make decisions for an incapacitated patient if the patient has not already designated someone. The concept of consent arises from the ethical principle of autonomy and the fundamentally accepted tenet that patients have a right to be involved in decisions about their health care. It is also a protective response to the tort of battery, which is the purposeful, unwelcome, harmful touching of another. Performing a procedure without patient consent could constitute battery even if the procedure was done competently and the outcome was good.

To obtain a valid consent, the provider who will be performing the procedure must provide the patient with a description of the procedure, an explanation of the risks and benefits of the procedure, and a discussion of any alternatives to the proposed procedure. Consent by the patient must be voluntarily given, and the person who consents must have the capacity to consent. Capacity can be determined by the health care provider and may be affected by drugs or the current/underlying medical condition. In short, the provider must be sure that the patient understands the information provided and the consent is voluntarily given. If the patient is unable to give consent directly, he or she may designate a person who can give consent on his or her behalf. If such a person is not designated by the patient, most states provide a statutory solution, a law that lists "statutory surrogates"—individuals who, based on their relationship to the patient, would be given priority to consent on the patient's behalf.

Advance Directives

All states have laws that provide guidelines for the execution and enforcement of health care directives. These directives include living wills, medical power of attorney for health care decisions, and prehospital do not resuscitate orders. These directives identify how a patient wishes to be treated in the event of certain medical conditions and also identify who the patient wants to make decisions on his or her behalf in the event that the patient is unable do so. These laws encourage compliance with the patient's directive by giving health care providers who act in reliance on these documents immunity from civil or criminal liability, and some states impose criminal liability if a patient's advance directives are not followed.

Death with Dignity Laws

National discussion regarding whether mentally competent but terminally ill patients should have the right to hasten their death has been a topic of health care law since Jack Kevorkian championed the issue in the early 1990s. In the midst of the so-called "right to die" or "assisted suicide" movement, Oregon enacted the nation's first Death with Dignity Act in 1997.[17] Washington passed a similar initiative in 2008,[18] the Montana Supreme Court ruled in favor of physician-assisted death by lethal medication dose in 2009,[19] and Vermont passed the state's Patient Choice and Controls at End of Life Act in 2013.[20] These laws allow physicians to write a prescription for a lethal dose of medication that a mentally competent but terminally ill patient can use to end his or her life if the patient has less than 6 months to live. Each state's law contains various safeguards and protocols to be followed by the prescribing physician. For instance, Oregon's Death with Dignity Act requires, in part, that the patient make two oral requests at least 15 days apart to the physician followed by a written request signed in the presence of two witnesses, one of whom cannot be a relative of the patient. It also requires two physicians to confirm the patient's diagnosis and prognosis and assess the patient's competency and mental health. In the landmark case of *Gonzales v. Oregon*, the U.S. Supreme Court upheld Oregon's Death with Dignity Act and ruled that the federal government's Controlled Substances Act did not bestow upon the Attorney General of the United States the authority to ban physicians from prescribing lethal doses of controlled substances for use in physician-assisted suicide under state law permitting the procedure.[21]

INTERRELATED CONCEPTS

Three concepts are closely interrelated to health care law: health policy, ethics, and health care economics, as shown in Figure 58-3. At its most basic level, a law is a set of rules that is designed to help meet a specific policy or goal. Analogizing to the nursing process, Health Policy is the goal or expected outcome, and health care laws are the interventions that are intended to affect the expected outcome. Ethics are the framework or boundaries in which many of those policies and laws are made. In other words, adherence to an ethical principle may drive a desire to adopt a policy and create laws that promote the policy.

Another concept that is closely interrelated is Health Care Economics. As previously described, many laws have a financial incentive to compel compliance with the law. There are organizations and departments within health care organizations whose job it is to ensure compliance with many health care laws and regulations. Within a health care organization or hospital, this task may be the responsibility of the compliance officer or compliance department. The compliance officer monitors the organization's activities so that the organization can continue to receive payments from the government and is not subject to any fines.

CLINICAL EXEMPLARS

There are a multitude of exemplars of health care law; the most common and important of these are presented in Box 58-2. Some

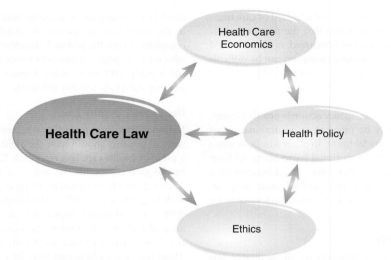

FIGURE 58-3 Health Care Law and Interrelated Concepts

exemplars are listed in more than one category; this illustrates the intertwined nature of the source of laws. Some of these are featured here.

Featured Exemplars
Social Security Act of 1965 (Medicaid and Medicare)
The Social Security Act of 1965 created a trust fund for the establishment of Medicaid and Medicare, a form of health insurance for those who do not have medical insurance through employment (retired individuals and the unemployed).[6] Reimbursement under the Medicare program has undergone many changes since it was initially enacted, and the federal government can decide what rules the health care organizations must follow to be eligible for reimbursement. One of the most significant changes was the adoption of payment based on diagnosis-related groups in 1983,[7] which was also eventually adopted by insurance companies as a means to compensate health care organizations for the care of those patients.

Emergency Medical Treatment and Active Labor Act of 1986
The Emergency Medical Treatment and Active Labor Act (EMTALA) was a provision of the Consolidated Omnibus Budget Reconciliation Act (COBRA) of 1986.[22] The policy underlying EMTALA is that hospitals that have emergency departments have a duty to care for those requiring emergency medical services irrespective of patients' ability to pay. Any Medicare-participating hospital that offers emergency services must provide an appropriate medical screening exam to any person who presents for treatment of an emergency medical condition and must stabilize any emergency medical condition before transfer to another facility.[23,24] At the patient's request, or if the hospital is unable to stabilize the patient's condition, the hospital can arrange for transfer to appropriate level of care.

Patient Self-Determination Act of 1991
The Patient Self-Determination Act was enacted to promote discourse about end-of-life medical treatment and to ensure that patients received appropriate education about their right to decide future care in the event of incapacitation. A health care organization (not individual physicians) that participates in Medicare is required to (1) provide patients, upon admission, information regarding advance directives (medical power of attorney and living will) and advise

---

■■■ BOX 58-2 EXEMPLARS OF HEALTH CARE LAW

Federal Statutory Laws
- Social Security Act of 1965
- Social Security Amendment of 1983
- Emergency Medical Treatment and Active Labor Act of 1986 (EMTALA)
- Patient Self-Determination Act of 1991
- Health Insurance Portability and Accountability Act of 1996 (HIPAA)
- Patient Protection and Affordable Care Act of 2010
- Americans with Disabilities Act of 1990 (ADA)

State Statutory Laws
- Licensing boards/practice acts
- Immunizations
- Public health and safety—disease surveillance, sanitation
- Consent/statutory surrogates
- Advance directives
- Death with dignity or aid-in-dying
- Good Samaritan acts
- CMS Conditions of Participation for Hospitals
- Practice acts
- Scope of practice

Torts
- Negligence/malpractice
- Standard of care
- Breach of duty
- Abandonment

Criminal Liability
- Insurance fraud
- Active euthanasia
- Sexual assault

---

patients of their right to participate in medical decision making; and (2) document in the medical record whether or not a patient has completed an advance directive.[8] The Patient Self-Determination Act prohibits a Medicare-participating health care organization from discrimination against patients based on the presence or absence of an advance directive.[8]

Health Insurance Portability and Accountability Act of 1996

The Health Insurance Portability and Accountability Act (HIPAA) of 1996 was enacted to provide individuals with preexisting medical conditions access to health insurance specifically if they changed or lost their job. The other element of HIPAA was to prevent health care fraud and abuse and medical liability reform. The act also included a provision (known as the Privacy Rule) for health information privacy requirements for individually identifiable health information. The Privacy Rule protects the confidentiality of health information relating to the provision or payment of health care for a past, present, or future physical or mental health condition but does permit the "minimum necessary" use and disclosure of protected health information without patient authorization for purposes of treatment, payment, and health care operations.[25]

Health Information Technology for Economic and Clinical Health Act

The Health Information Technology for Economic and Clinical Health (HITECH) Act was enacted as part of the American Recovery and Reinvestment Act of 2009. HITECH broadened the scope of HIPAA's Privacy Rule and provided for more enforcement of noncompliance by establishing increased levels of culpability and raising penalty amounts for compliance violations.[26] In addition, HITECH includes specific requirements for notifying individuals when their protected health information has been breached or improperly used or disclosed without authorization.[26]

Patient Protection and Affordable Care Act of 2010

The Patient Protection and Affordable Care Act includes provisions to enable Americans with preexisting conditions to more easily afford insurance, the creation of health insurance exchanges to make insurance coverage more accessible and affordable for some individuals and small businesses, and the elimination of insurance co-pays for preventive care.[9] The law also requires that every American have minimum essential health insurance.[9] This controversial provision of the law (whether or not it is constitutional for the government to compel individuals to purchase insurance) was upheld by the U.S. Supreme Court.[27]

CASE STUDY

Source: Wavebreakmedia Ltd/Wavebreak Media/Thinkstock

Case Presentation

On July 4, 2006, Julie Thao, RN, an experienced nurse with years of obstetrical expertise, worked an extended shift that ended at midnight, and she returned to duty at 7 a.m. on July 5. Shortly before noon on July 5, Thao made a lethal medication error while assigned as the primary nurse for a teenage patient admitted to the birthing unit at St. Mary's Hospital for induction of labor.[28]

On July 5, Thao spent almost an hour with the patient on admission explaining the birthing process and answering questions, with much of her focus on alleviating the patient's anxiety. During that time, Thao failed to place an identification wristband on the patient's wrist, in violation of hospital policy. Because the patient tested positive for group B *Streptococcus*, the physician ordered an antibiotic to be administered intravenously (IV) at 11:00 a.m. Anticipating that the patient would need an epidural during labor, Thao gathered epidural medications (bupivacaine and fentanyl) without a physician's order, took these to the patient's room, and placed them on the counter where the antibiotic was ready and waiting to be administered. At 11:30 a.m., Thao picked up the IV bag that she believed contained the antibiotic and began the infusion intravenously. However, Thao actually administered the IV bag containing the unordered epidural medication (which is supposed to be administered into the spine).

Almost immediately, the patient appeared to be seizing, and Thao stopped the infusion. Despite efforts to resuscitate the patient, Thao's error resulted in the death of the patient, whose baby was saved by an emergency C-section at 12:20 p.m. Thao was terminated from her position at St. Mary's Hospital, and the patient's family filed a civil lawsuit against the hospital.

The Wisconsin Board of Nursing suspended Thao's license for 9 months, followed by a 2-year practice limitation with terms and conditions including a requirement to make educational presentations to nurses or nursing students on the topic of preventing medication errors.

A subsequent criminal complaint charged Thao with patient abuse and neglect causing great bodily harm, a felony that carried a penalty of imprisonment and a significant monetary fine.[29] Thao's alleged criminal conduct was characterized as "(1) failing to obtain a doctor's order before introducing medication into the patient's room, (2) not looking at the medication prior to administration, (3) failing to adhere to the 5 'rights' of medication administration, and (4) failing to scan the barcodes on the medication as required."[29,p28] Thao eventually received probation after pleading no contest to two criminal misdemeanors counts related to the unlawful dispensing and possession of the epidural medication.[30]

Case Analysis

Historically, physicians and nurses have rarely faced criminal charges for providing negligent care to a patient.[31] Accountability for negligent conduct has generally been confined to the established health law domains of malpractice lawsuits based on tort law and state licensing board disciplinary actions. The reports of criminal medical negligence charges brought against both physicians and nurses represent a chilling trifecta of punishment involving the convergence of three sources of health care law: criminal law, tort law, and administrative law.

Negligent torts are based on unintentional breaches of the standard of care owed to a patient resulting in injury. It is difficult to know when a nurse has crossed the threshold from committing civil negligence to committing criminal negligence. Criminal negligence is based on a criminally culpable state of mind in addition to a flagrant deviation from the standard of care resulting in injury particularly significant harm or death. The lapse in standard of care need not be intentional for criminal prosecution.

ACCESS EXEMPLAR LINKS IN YOUR GIDDENS EBOOK

REFERENCES

1. *Roe v. Wade*, 410 US 113, 1973.
2. *Cruzan v. Missouri*, 497 US 261, 1990.
3. Harris DM: *Contemporary issues in health care law and ethics*, ed 2, Chicago, 2003, Health Administration Press and Association of University Programs in Health Administration.
4. *Health Insurance Portability and Accountability Act*, 42 U.S.C. § 1320(d)(6), 1996.
5. Sowers C: Doctor guilty in abortion death: Jurors convict Biskind, assistant, *The Arizona Republic*, A1, A4, February 21, 2001.
6. *Social Security Act of 1965*, Pub. L. No. 89-97, 79 Stat 285, 1965.
7. *Social Security Amendments of 1983*, Pub. L. No. 98-21, 97 Stat. 65, 1983.
8. *Patient Self-Determination Act*, 42 U.S.C. § 1395cc(f), 1991.
9. *Patient Protection and Affordable Care Act*, Pub. L. No. 111-148, 124 Stat.119, 2010, as amended by the Health Care and Education Reconciliation Act of 2010, Pub. L. No. 111-152, 124 Stat. 1029, 2010.
10. *U.S. Department of Health and Human Services: About HHS*, (n.d.). Retrieved from <http://www.hhs.gov/about>.
11. *Conditions of Participation for Hospitals, Standard: Restraint or Seclusion*, 42 CFR § 482.13 (e-g), 2006.
12. Trandel-Korenchuk DM, Trandel-Korenchuk KM: *Nursing & the law*, Gaithersburg, MD, 1997, Aspen.
13. Safriet BJ: *Federal options for maximizing the value of advanced practice nurses in providing quality, cost-effective health care*, paper commissioned by the Committee on the RWJF Initiative on the Future of Nursing, Institute of Medicine (Appendix H), 2010.
14. *Institute of Medicine: The future of nursing: Leading change, advancing health*, Washington, DC, 2011, National Academies Press.
15. *Goldfarb v. Va. State Bar*, 421 U.S. 773, 792, 1975.
16. *A.R.S. § 12-2604(A)*.
17. *Oregon Death with Dignity Act*, Ore Rev Stat §§ 127.800–127.897:800–995, 1994.
18. *Washington Death with Dignity Act*, Rev C Wash 70:245, 2008.
19. *Baxter v. Montana*, 2009 MT 449, 2009.
20. *Vermont Patient Choice and Control at End of Life Act*, 2013 Vt. Acts & Resolves 292, 296 (codified at Vt. Stat. Ann. Tit. 18, ch 133 (Supp. 2013)).
21. *Gonzales v. Oregon*, 546 U.S. 243, 2006.
22. *Consolidated Omnibus Budget Reconciliation Act of 1986*, Pub. L. No. 99-272,100 Stat 82, 1986.
23. *Consolidated Omnibus Budget Reconciliation Act*, 29 U.S.C. § 1161–1168, 1986.
24. *Emergency Medical Treatment and Active Labor Act*, 42 U.S.C. § 1395dd, 1986.
25. *U.S. Department of Health and Human Services, Office for Civil Rights: Summary of HIPAA privacy rule*, Washington, DC, 2003, Author.
26. *Health Information Technology for Economic and Clinical Health Act*, 42 U.S.C. § 17921, 2009.
27. *National Federation of Independent Business v. Sebelius*, 567 U.S., 2012, 132 S.Ct 2566.
28. *In the matter of the disciplinary proceedings against Julie Thao, R.N., State of Wisconsin Board of Nursing, December 14, 2006, Final Decision and Order LS0612145NUR*.
29. Collins S: Criminalization of negligence in nursing: A new trend? *Fla Nurse* 28, 2007.
30. *Wisconsin Court System: Circuit court access*, (n.d.). Retrieved from <http://wcca.wicourts.gov>.
31. Filkins J: With no evil intent: The criminal prosecution of physicians for medical negligence. *J Legal Med* 22:467–499, 2001.

INDEX

Page numbers followed by "*f*" indicate figures, "*t*" indicate tables, and "*b*" indicate boxes.